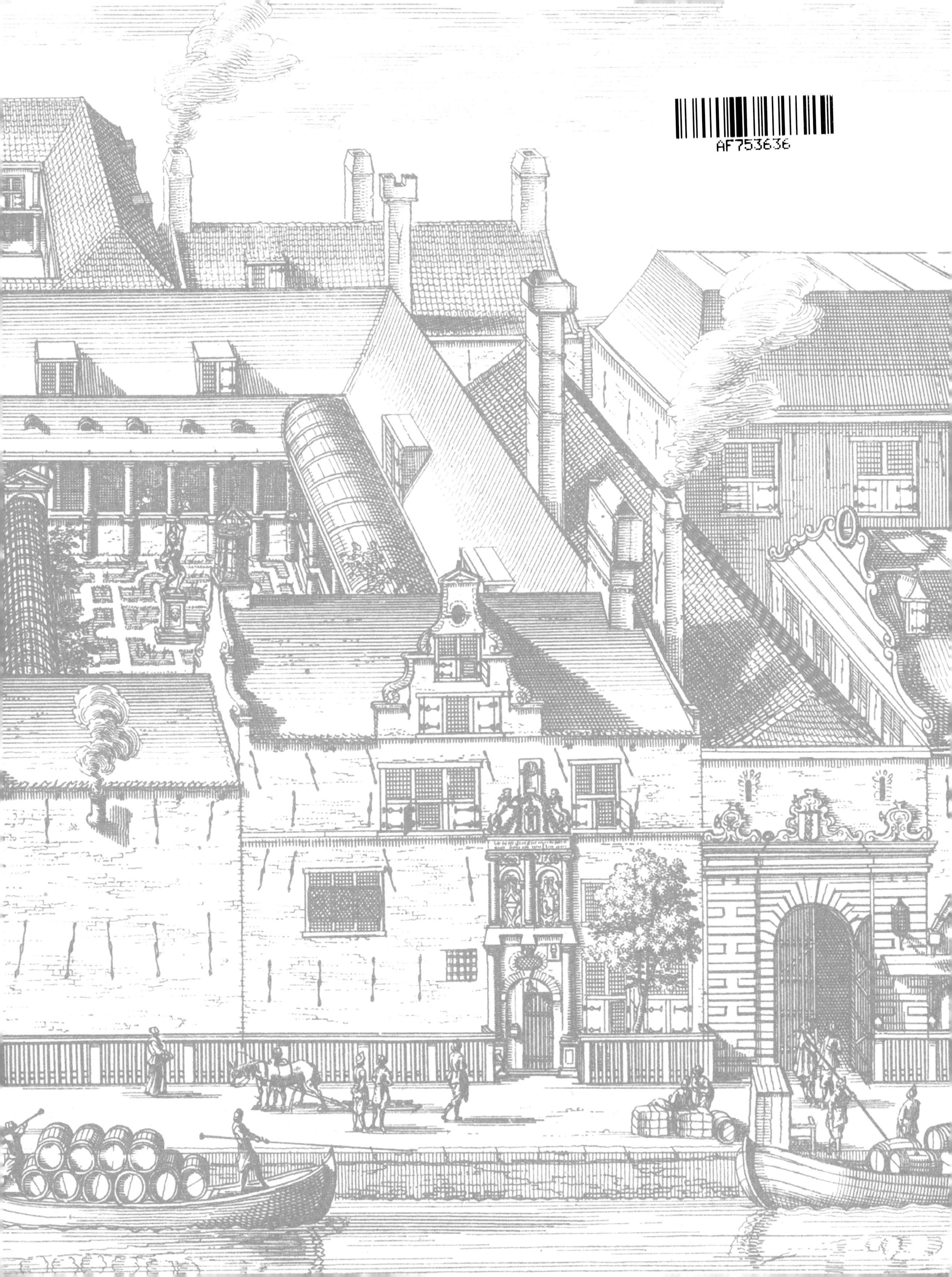

Health care architecture in the Netherlands

Front cover:
Ed. Cuypers, extension Jozefziekenhuis, Heerlen, 1920–1923 (photo a/d Amstel Architecten)
Architectenbureau Koen van Velsen, Groot Klimmendaal rehabilitation centre, Arnhem, 2009 (photo Rob 't Hart)

Back cover:
B. Poyet, design for the Hôtel-Dieu, Paris, 1785 (Bibliothèque nationale de France, Paris)
Van Tijen en Maaskant, Huis in de Duinen, Zandvoort, 1952–1955 (photo Jan Versnel/MAI)

Health care architecture in the Netherlands

Noor Mens / Cor Wagenaar

NAi Publishers

Contents

Preface

This book offers a survey of health care architecture in the Netherlands. It is more than a collection of best practices; it deals with hospitals, psychiatric institutions and housing and health care provisions for the elderly that are characteristic of developments in health care. These buildings tell a story, and health care plays an important role in that story. Nevertheless, the protagonist is architecture. Architecture is particularly significant in health care – it reflects developments in care, the ensemble of buildings can be read as a documentary journal of medico-technological innovations, changing insights in psychiatry, and socio-cultural opinions on the position of old people. Much more important is the fact that architecture is directly connected with the raison d'être of these buildings. There is no type of building in which the relation between function, structure and design is revealed so clearly as in health care architecture, and nowhere is the relation between buildings and the physical and mental wellbeing of the people for whom they are designed so intense. This is true not only of the patients and the elderly in need of care, but also of the staff – the doctors, psychiatrists and psychologists, nurses and technical staff without whom these buildings cannot function. This book is in the first place a plea for the (re)discovery of this quality of architecture, a quality that coincides with the essence of architecture.

What is the particular significance of architecture in health care? Here everything boils down to the way in which the patients and the elderly in need of care experience their stay. That experience has many facets. In the first place there is the effect of the treatment. A decisive factor in psychiatric institutions and hospitals is eventually whether the therapy is successful or not. That depends partly on the way in which the architecture supports or frustrates the therapy and everything connected with it. Whether housing for the elderly fulfils its function depends on how it promotes the wellbeing of the residents. It is increasingly recognised (again) that the way in which patients and the elderly are approached has an influence on their wellbeing. Architecture proves to have a direct influence on the experience of the users, and this influence extends to medical and psychological effects. Stress is the key concept to describe the negative effects of the wrong design decisions, and the negative effect of stress on health and healing has been proven. So these factors, which were regarded as 'soft' until recently, really do have 'hard' consequences, and they are directly connected with the core function of these buildings. The great merit of Evidence Based Design is that it has convincingly demonstrated that at least some of these consequences can be identified and measured: the view from the patient's room, single or shared rooms, routing, social support, privacy, et cetera.

Architecture, however, covers a wider area than Evidence Based Design, even apart from the way in which it accommodates processes – which are determined above all by the theme of the internal logistical organisation that dominates all else. Architecture also makes statements about the relation between staff and patient that go further than the necessary professional interaction – must the patient come to the specialist's own consultation or treatment room, or should the specialist renounce having a domain of his own in which he used to be lord and master? Can an outpatient unit also be conceived as a normal form of the provision of services and designed accordingly? Does it help psychiatric patients who are accommodated on remote terrains in the countryside if housing for normal residents is added? There is a long tradition of designs with a critical edge, and examples of that can be found in health care too, some of which have found their way into this book. Every kind of architecture – and health care architecture is no exception – transcends its function and forms a part of a long and dynamic evolution of this time-hallowed discipline as the designer of culture. Here it touches on the position of the design, the way it marks the evolution of the type, the relation with other types of building (especially housing, hotels and offices, but also airports, shopping centres, conference buildings); its social ambitions are at stake, and so is the relation with other design disciplines (art, design, fashion).

This publication throws light on the role that architecture has been able to play in the development of health care buildings. The survey covers the whole spectrum and aims at a dual renaissance: in the first place the rediscovery of the exceptionally direct impact of architecture on the care processes and thereby on how they are run and, in connection with that, on the real estate value (which, paradoxically enough, proves to increase with the generic character of the majority of the buildings); and secondly the direct effects of design on the wellbeing of the patients and staff. This book is thus above all a plea for the importance of architecture in health care. Now that hospitals, psychiatric institutions and nursing homes have been made responsible for their own real estate and have to raise funds for that purpose on the capital market, it is important to underline that investing in architecture pays off. The extra that is spent on quality is recuperated in savings in running expenses. Sustainable high-quality materials give the users that feeling that they matter and last so much longer that it is here in particular that the rule applies: cheap is expensive. Oversizing is still the best strategy to ensure flexibility. It saves the expense of renovation in the long term but immediately guarantees a spacious ambience. By taking into account not only the psychological but also the medical consequences of the design, a design makes a direct contribution to what will always remain the core function of health care buildings: the promotion of the welfare of the patients, residents and staff. In the last resort they are the benchmarks, these buildings are in the first place for them, not for the institutions that run them. The contours are slowly emerging of a trend that recognises the public character of health care architecture and no longer isolates the buildings from the social and physical context of the city, but integrates them in it. They are, when all is said and done, public amenities that directly benefit urban life.

This publication continues the tradition set by three previous monographs that were published in Dutch on the initiative of the University Medical Centre Groningen, *The Architecture of Hospitals*, and the series of activities organised under the umbrella of 'Architecture in Health'.[1] The book brings this work up to date and at the same time forms the crown and coping stone of this project – but hopefully also the stimulus for a follow-up. The fundamental role of architecture presented in this book deserves the opportunity to develop to the full – not in the service of architecture, but above all in the service of health care.

Frans C.A. Jaspers, MSc. M.D.
Member of the Executive Board University Medical Centre Groningen, Chairman Thomassen à Thuessink Foundation, Groningen

Introduction

This book contains a wide selection of Dutch health care buildings. Something special goes on in all of these buildings that is not experienced so intensely in any other building: the treatment and care of physical and mental disorders. Sometimes they are life-threatening, sometimes they only affect the quality of life, but they are always experienced as exceptional. Patients are confronted first with themselves, and afterwards with the people who take care of them. The most frequent and intensive contact is with the nursing staff. Interaction with doctors and specialists is less frequent and long-term, but all the more intensive and crucial. Health care buildings are designed to create the right environment for the medical processes that take place there. The examples collected in this publication illustrate the important role that architecture can play in this respect.

Every building has to comply with the purpose for which it is designed. All the same, the structure and physical appearance of a building are not always determined by its function. It is only since the last quarter of the eighteenth century that function has played a major part in the history of architecture, when principals and designers started to think about use in a rational way. In the case of hospitals and psychiatric institutions, this change was connected with the emergence of new insights into the treatment and accommodation of people with physical or mental disorders. The relation with tradition and convention was severed. This was also when the practice of relating all buildings, irrespective of their function, to the four architectural prime models – churches, palaces, town halls and merchants' houses – was dropped. The hospital, for instance, was often somewhere between a church and a merchant's home.

This double emancipation – from the shackles of tradition regarding use, and from the architectural practice of following a limited number of models – led to particularly specific types of building. The more exactly a building was tailored to its function, the more specific it was, the better it would be. The evolution of health care architecture is almost entirely determined by insights into its functioning. This often resulted in one-dimensional buildings: perfectly able to accommodate a particular vision, but completely outdated as soon as new insights appeared. A corollary of the classic functional approach is the need to keep adapting or replacing buildings. Hospitals, nursing homes and psychiatric institutions only appear in their original guise for a brief period. This is followed by the process of renovation, extension or demolition.

The functionalist approach was to predominate until the end of the twentieth century, when a new emancipatory movement appeared with the aim of freeing the building as much as possible from its functionalist shackles. The direct relation between function and building typology was called into question. Analysis of the actual use showed that only a small part of what goes on in hospitals, for instance, is really different from what goes on in other types of building: the hospital ward approximates the hotel, the offices with or without consultation rooms are not so different from the back and front office of regular office buildings. There was doubt about the need to cluster highly diverse medical functions, often bearing hardly any relation to one another, in large complexes. Moreover, smaller, more generic buildings seem to represent a higher value on the real estate market. The next stage in the evolution of health care buildings consists of a fundamental reappraisal of the relation between function and building. It presents the designers with challenges in which crucial episodes from the evolution prove to have lost none of their topicality. The question of the added value of architecture is fundamental. Thinking on this score oscillates between two extremes.

On the one hand, there is the experience of the space: the ambiance, the succession of rooms and encounters determined by the logistical organisation, the colour, the material, and the rural or urban setting outside the building. Architecture is manifested here as the art of manipulating spatial effects. The recipient and judge in this case is the patient. Apart from the effectiveness of this strategy, which at first was explicitly regarded as an essential component of the therapy offered in hospitals, this approach does justice at any rate to the fact that the patient's experiences form the ultimate criterion anyway. On the other hand, the architecture either facilitates or frustrates the medical and technological processes. Are the different flows of traffic separated from one another, or is it all a big confusion? What about the internal logistics? Such factors have a direct effect on how health care buildings are run, and thus on the expenses. In practice the opinions of the medical and technical staff, the programmers and managers are determinant here. In the ideal situation, the two approaches are mutually complementary rather than exclusive.

Inspired by other types of building, the contours of a new care landscape are coming into view. A number of recurrent pairs of concepts define a wide range of options: generic or specific? Central, large-scale and general, or decentralised, small-scale and specialised? Integrated in the urban context or isolated at the junctions of the infrastructure? Separate focused factories or networks of organisationally connected but physically separate branches? What is a suitable course of treatment in one case may be fatal in another – the interaction between designer and principal is still decisive. But the side that places the commissions is in flux too: health institutions are merging with similar ones or with organisations that offer complementary services; private parties are appearing, insurance companies are trying to increase their influence on the providers of care. It is in this dynamic world in which all the borders seem to be growing blurred that new opportunities for architecture arise. This leads to contradictory trends: while in Europe health care architecture is opening up to non-specialists, a trend can be discerned in the United States towards the certification of agencies specialised in health care who try to provide a scientific basis for their design methods (Evidence-Based Design).

The eight chapters of this book present health care architecture in the Netherlands. The structure is chronological and thematic – hence the first chapter is devoted to the origins of the separate building types. As a rule, each chapter devotes separate sections to the three main types (hospitals, psychiatric institutions and accommodation and care for the elderly in particular). Although the focus is on health care architecture in the Netherlands, considerable attention is paid to developments elsewhere too, at least when those developments have influenced Dutch ones. Each chapter is accompanied by an essay that goes into specific themes in more depth, and a selection of projects.

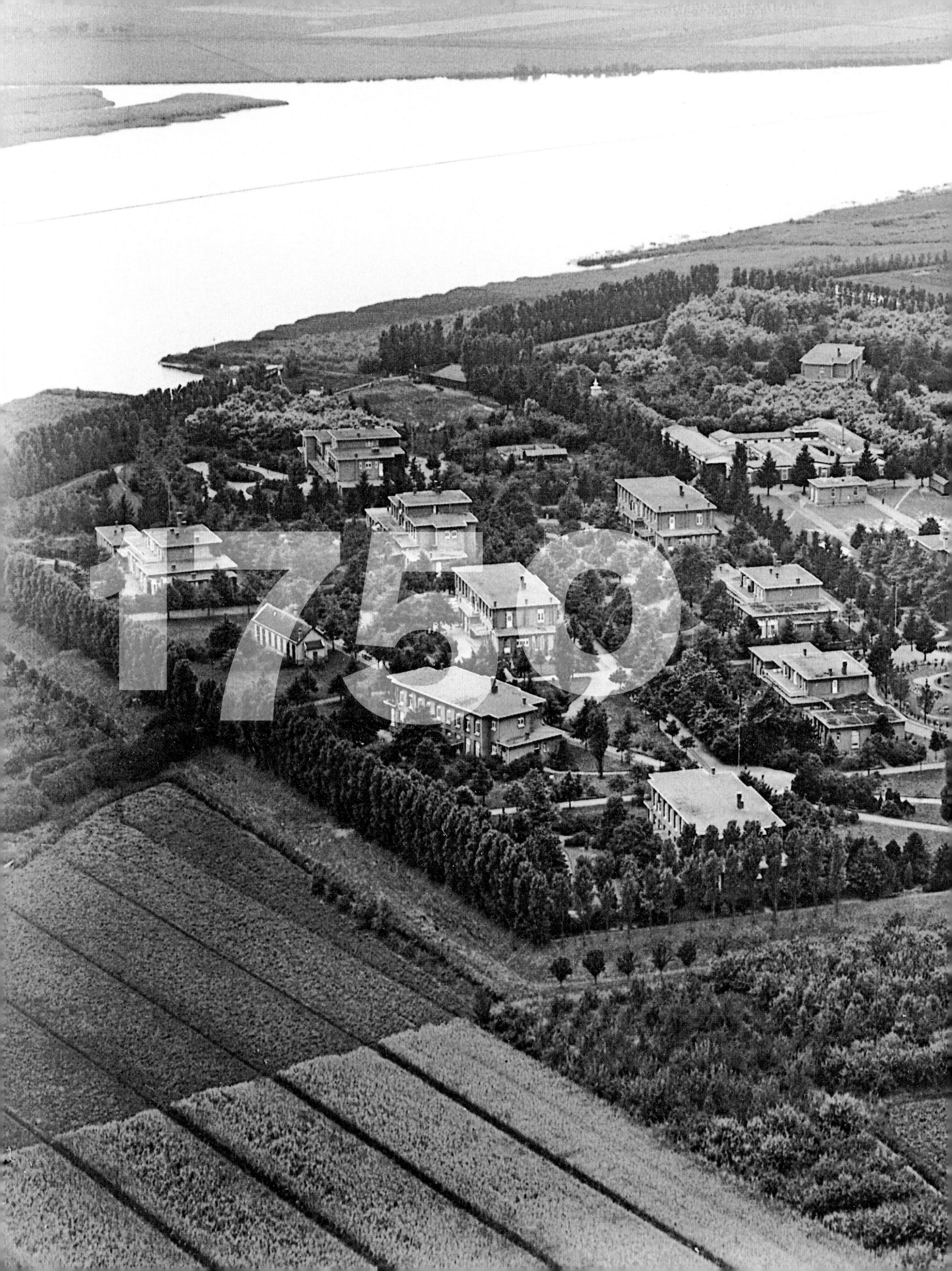
1750

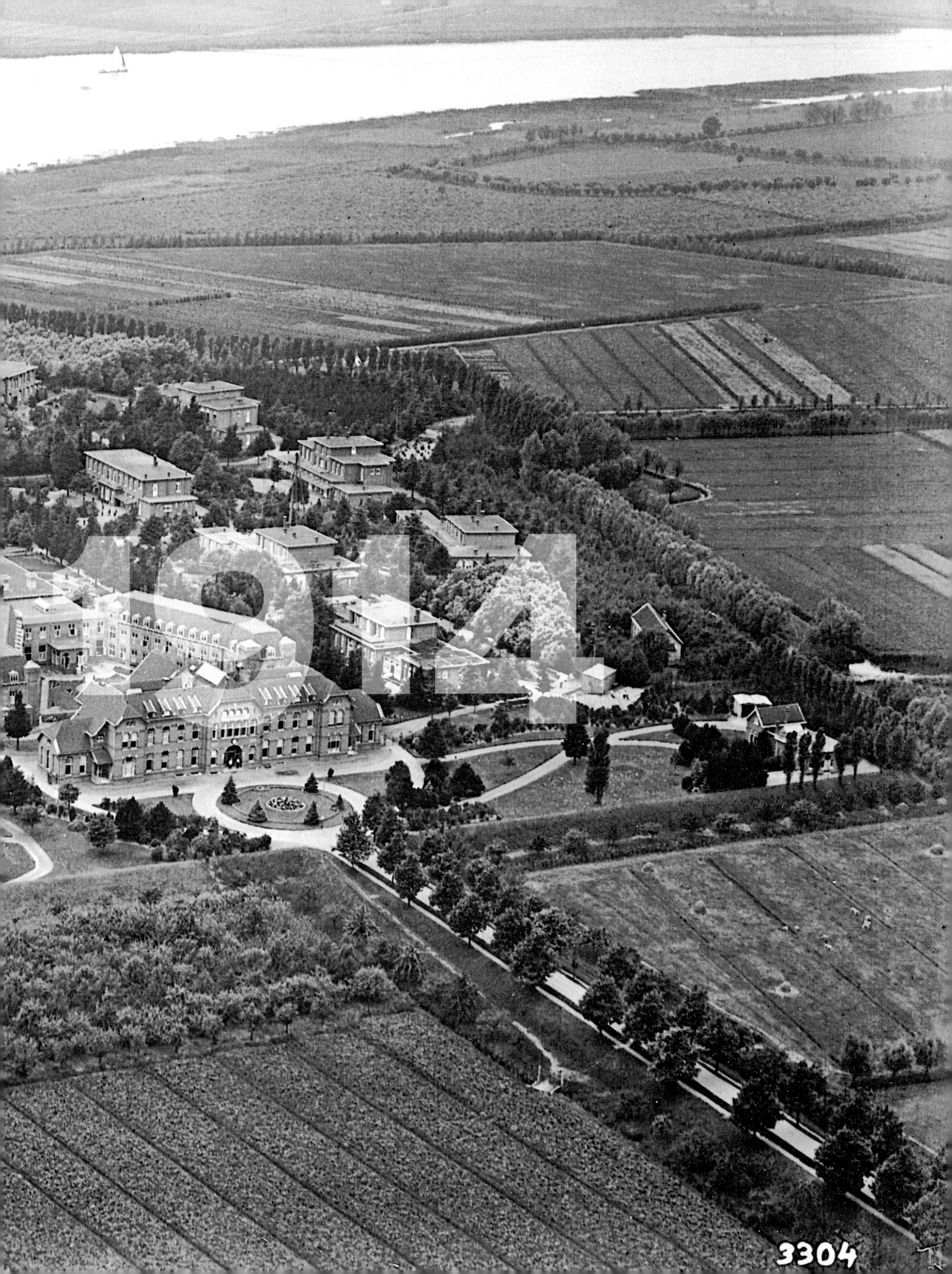
1914
3304

The origin of health care buildings

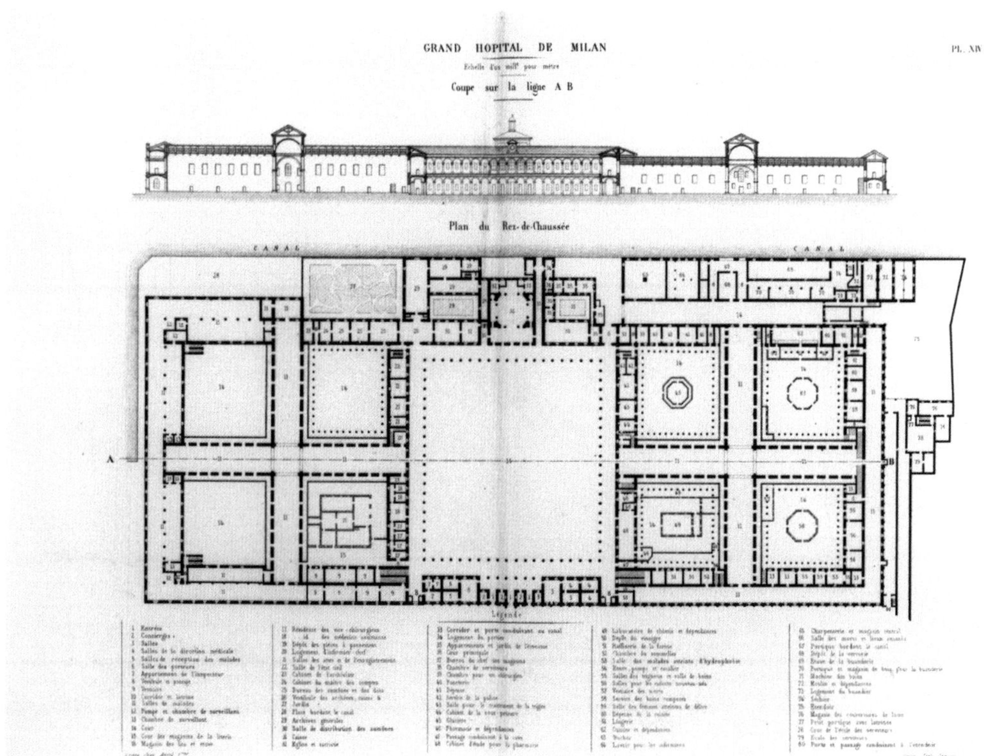

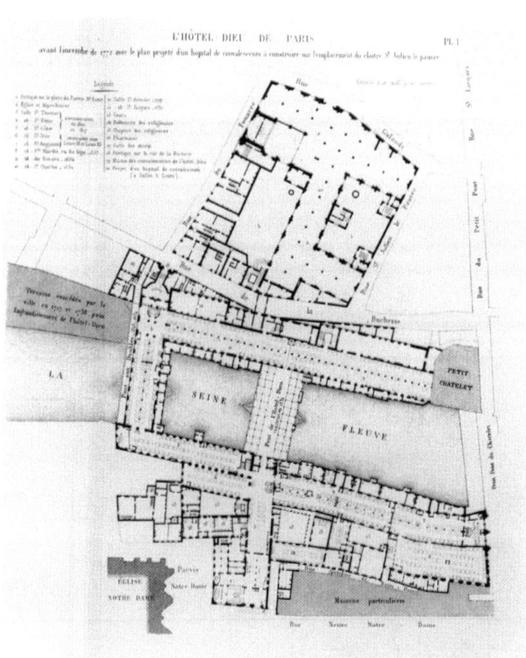

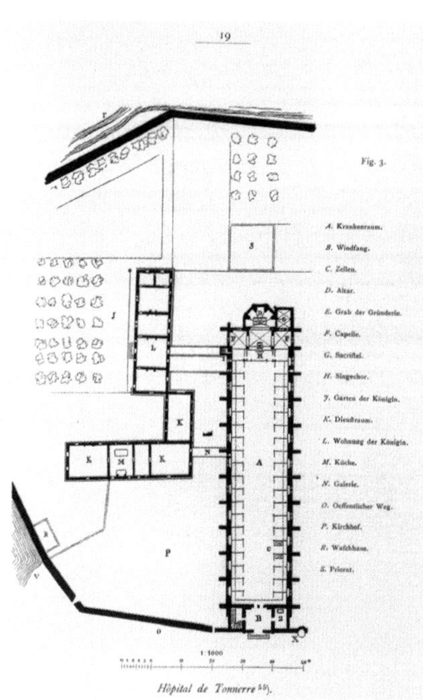

Hospitals as healing machines: the influence of the Enlightenment

The confrontation with health problems or the consequences of accidents affect people at the core of their lives. It is hardly surprising that this experience was traditionally connected with religious notions of the origin and meaning of life, nor that the first buildings for the sick were of a religious nature or were often erected in close proximity to religious buildings. It is no coincidence that the Hôtel-Dieu occupies a significant place in the evolution of the hospital. The link between religion and health had already been made in antiquity, when temples arose where the sick could gather to work on their healing. In the course of the eighteenth century the Enlightenment philosophers laid a scientific foundation for the organisation of the social order. They opposed everything that was not rational, especially belief and superstition. They went much further than their predecessors from the sixteenth and seventeenth centuries had done: they connected their insights with radical social consequences and explicitly addressed the general public. This cleared the way for the hospital and psychiatric clinic as institutions where the promotion of physical and mental health was practised on a scientific basis. This is where the roots of modern health architecture lie – modern in the sense of breaking away from tradition and aiming at a scientifically founded basis for dealing with ill health and discomfort.

The Enlightenment ideals also had major consequences for the architecture and design of cities, landscapes and buildings: the human habitat was supposed to reflect the universal laws of nature. The ultimate ideal was to bring the city closer to nature and to 'civilise' the countryside. The landscape park with Neo-Classical villas is a perfect illustration of these views (it is not fortuitous that Neo-Classicism was welcomed as the most appropriate style: in going back to classical antiquity, it was taken to be the most suitable to refer to the universal laws of nature). This combination resulted in splendid complexes, especially in psychiatry. The main focus of these developments was in France, as well as in Great Britain and Germany.

On the basis of the scientific study of methods derived from nature, the radical Enlightenment regarded interventions in physical and mental health not just as a possibility but even as an obligation – illnesses were taken to be a consequence of the growing separation of people from nature. The concept of a gap between civilised humankind and untrammelled nature is still a recurrent theme today, and it is still connected with the claim that the limited arsenal of therapeutic activities must be supplemented by interventions in the environment. Initially far more weight was attached to the latter. This view too goes back to the Enlightenment. The environment in general, and the built environment in particular, can be designed and this is where architecture comes into the picture. Although the Enlightenment was accompanied by a Scientific Revolution, its consequences in health care were at first not manifested in new therapies, but in proposals to make the environment healthier (to bring it closer to nature). Hospitals and psychiatric institutions were in the vanguard. The hospital even developed to become the first building to be designed by scientific insights into its function, in this case its contribution to the healing of the sick. The credit for having introduced thinking in typologies is thus due to the history of architecture. It was not until the middle of the nineteenth century that these concepts were embodied in stone. The splendid Hôpital Charenton that opened in Paris in 1838 is the first example.

This chapter describes the roots of modern health architecture. These storms bypassed care for the elderly, and it was not until the middle of the nineteenth century that the architectural consequences made headway in the Netherlands, but from then on the pace speeded up. Within a few decades the foundation was laid for a fully equipped institutional health care system. It was repeatedly modified in the twentieth century. Now, at the beginning of the twenty-first century, it is once again confronted with far-reaching changes.

p. 10
***G.J. de Jongh*, Maasoord mental asylum, Poortugaal, 1907**

p. 12
***Filarete*, Ospedale Maggiore, Milan, 1456**

Hôtel-Dieu, Paris, mid-eighteenth century (before the fire)

Hôtel-Dieu, Tonnerre, 1293

p.13
***Sir Christopher Wren*, Royal Naval Hospital, Greenwich, 1694**

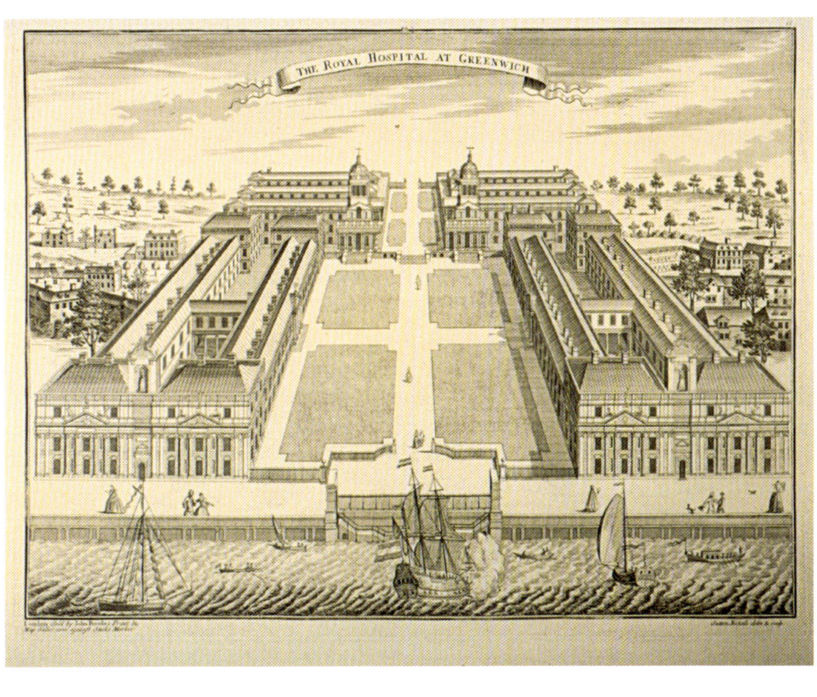

Hospitals

There were already special health care facilities in antiquity. The Greeks had *asclepeia*: complexes consisting of various buildings with the most important, the temple, in the centre. In the course of the first centuries AD health care was absorbed by Christianity. The first Council of Nicaea in 325 AD laid down that every town must have a place for the sick and the poor. The *xenodochia* were precursors of the institution of the Hôtel-Dieu, which was entrusted to the bishops at the Council of Aix-la-Chapelle in 816.[1] The best-known is that of Paris, while the most interesting in terms of its architecture is that of Beaune (1443-1451). Together with the convent hospitals, such as those in Tonnerre (1293) and Angers (1153), they were among the foundations of charitable, religious care for the sick in the Middle Ages. Usually, their architecture emulates that of churches.

The rise of the cities in the thirteenth century, first in Italy and Flanders, later elsewhere, encouraged the development of non-religious forms of care for the sick. Among the most famous city hospitals is the Ospedale Maggiore that was founded in Milan in 1456 and replaced a number of smaller institutions. This impressive complex was designed by Antonio Averulino, better known as Filarete. Although it was no more specifically designed for its function than the religious hospitals, the Ospedale Maggiore is regarded as a novelty: it was the first hospital to be structured in accordance with the geometric design principles of the Renaissance.

In the eighteenth century church and city were joined by the state as advocate and stimulus behind the building of hospitals. After the identification of the people as one of the most important foundations of its prosperity and (military) power, the state focused in the first instance on the construction of military hospitals. They took the latest scientific insights into account and were way ahead of their time in technical terms.[2] In England, the Royal Hospital Chelsea was founded in London in 1682 and the Royal Naval Hospital in Greenwich in 1694, both designed by the architect and physician Sir Christopher Wren. In dividing the wings of the Naval Hospital into separate hospital wards connected with one another on two sides, Wren anticipated the pavilion system. Alexander Rovehead went a step further. His Royal Naval Hospital at Stonehouse near Plymouth, built between 1756 and 1764, was striking for the fact that he split the wings into separate pavilions and left the courtyard open on the side facing the sea.

The non-military hospital was also increasingly deployed as an instrument in health policy. Unlike the military hospital, its civilian counterpart was to accommodate the poor. That made the hospital what it was to continue to be for years: a poor relief institution. Dozens were built within a few decades, particularly in the German-speaking countries. That was where the corridor hospital emerged. Usually they were relatively small institutions that, although specially designed to cater for the ailing poor, did not essentially differ in their structure from other representative buildings. The first corridor hospital, the Inselspital, was designed by the architect F. Beer between 1718 and 1724 in Bern, Switzerland. The wards were situated on either side of a long corridor. The introduction of open spaces gave the hospital, which had forty-five beds, a luminous air.[3]

The Bern hospital was followed by the Charité in Berlin. The Charité, founded in 1727 after the Parisian model and with two hundred beds, was considerably larger than the hospital in Bern and had a virtually square shape. The

p.14
***Sir Christopher Wren*, Royal Hospital Chelsea, London, 1682**

***A. Rovehead*, Royal Naval Hospital, Stonehouse near Plymouth, 1764**

p. 15
***J. Gerl*, Allgemeines Krankenhaus, Vienna, 1784**

Charité, Berlin, 1727

***F. Beer*, Inselspital, Bern, 1724**

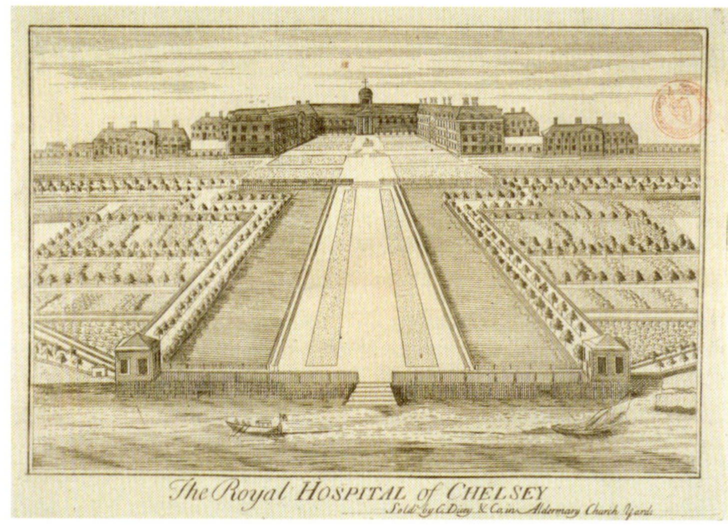

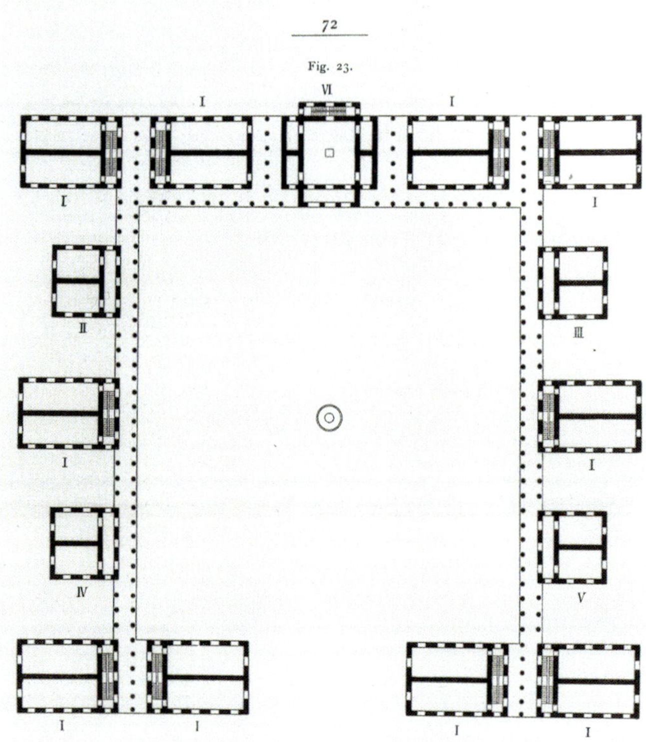

I. Krankengebäude.
II. Gebäude für Blatternkranke.
III. Küche und Speifefaal.
IV. Magazin für den Oekonomen.
V. Magazin für Lebensmittel.
VI. Capelle.

Royal naval hofpital zu Plymouth [181]).
Arch.: *Rovehead.*

Sein Grundrifs hat Hufeifenform; doch find die Flügel in ganzer Länge durch Höfe und zweimal quer durch Bogengänge unterbrochen. Die Säle haben nur 2 Reihen Betten, und es ftofsen nur je 2 an ihrer Querfeite zufammen. An jedem Ende eines folchen Doppelfaales liegen Treppe und Nebenräume. Jenfeits diefer folgt die Halle, welche das Compartiment von dem nächften trennt [188]).

71. Frankreich. In Frankreich wurde 1751 die *École Royale militaire* gegründet. Sie hat ihre

[188]) Der Plan findet fich in: HOWARD, J. Nachrichten von den vorzüglichften Kranken- und Pefthäufern in Europa. Aus dem Englifchen mit Zufätzen des deutfchen Herausgebers, welche befonders die Krankenhäufer angehen. Leipzig 1791. Pl. 4.

corridor ran around an open courtyard, the wards were designed for ten to twelve beds and were situated on the outside. The only medical staff in charge were three physicians; a separate surgical department was made available to them in 1730.[4] The most famous example of this type of hospital was the Allgemeines Krankenhaus in Vienna, which dates from 1686. The principles of this hospital were formulated by the imperial court physician, J. von Quarin, assisted by the architect J. Gerl. They opted to renovate an existing sanatorium, which was fitted out to accommodate two thousand ill citizens.[5]

Ventilation machines: radiators and pavilions

The Allgemeines Krankenhaus was one of the first hospitals to have special provisions for the artificial supply of fresh air and the extraction of stale air that had probably become contagious through contact with the patients being nursed. The conviction that illness was the result of harmful vapours, called *miasma*, went back to the second century. Statistical analysis and medical cartography – two important scientific innovations of this period – demonstrated the connection between the emergence, frequency and seriousness of illnesses and the physical qualities of the different districts of the city. This also provided the logic of combating diseases by manipulating the environment in which people lived. Architectural and urban interventions were to prevent the formation of *miasma*. The beneficial effects of fresh air were regarded as the best remedy, which explains why the first hospitals were designed as ventilation machines.

This concept was developed after the fire in the Hôtel-Dieu in Paris in 1772. The appalling conditions in this hospital had been a cause for complaints for a long time. The mortality rate was enormous: roughly 1 to 4.5 between 1721 and 1773. The corresponding ratios for the same period were roughly 1 to 13 in the Hôtel-Dieu in Lyon and about 1 to 11 in the Ospedale di S. Spirito in Rome.[6] The fire triggered a genuine protest movement that, on the eve of the French Revolution, was not free from political motives. If there was one field where the state system could be shown to be inadequate, it was in the treatment of poor and ill citizens.

In 1784 the French Academy of Sciences was asked to form a commission consisting exclusively of scientists. In the following year the state architect and draughtsman of the commission, B. Poyet, and C.Ph. Coquéau presented a radial plan for a colossal hospital. They published it in their *Mémoire sur la nécessité de transférer et reconstruire l'Hôtel-Dieu de Paris* (1785). The plan, that had the structure of a large ventilator, had sixteen wings and a total capacity of 5,184 beds. Another radial plan had already been presented a few years earlier, in 1774, by A. Petit. In his project the six radials functioned as a kind of wind tunnel; he projected a round building in the middle from which a cone-shaped ventilation shaft emerged (its shape was derived from the glass furnace illustrated in the *Encyclopédie*).[7]

The prototype of the rival concept – separate pavilions – was published in 1787. The physician J.B. Leroy presented himself as the designer; it was not until 1814 that it was

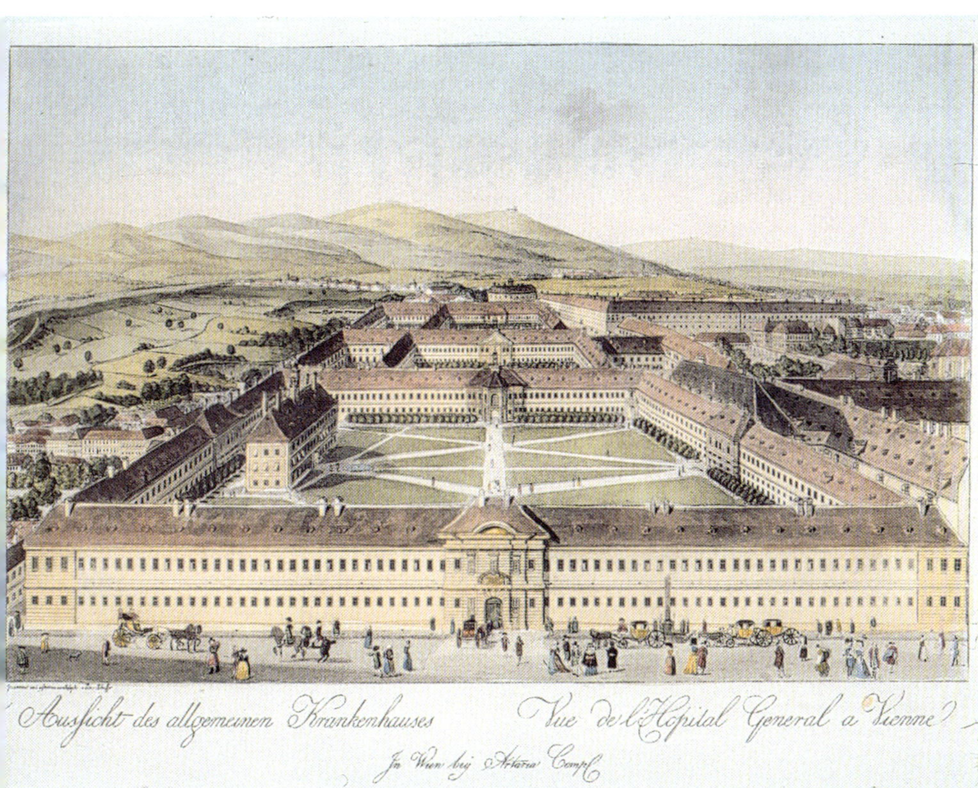

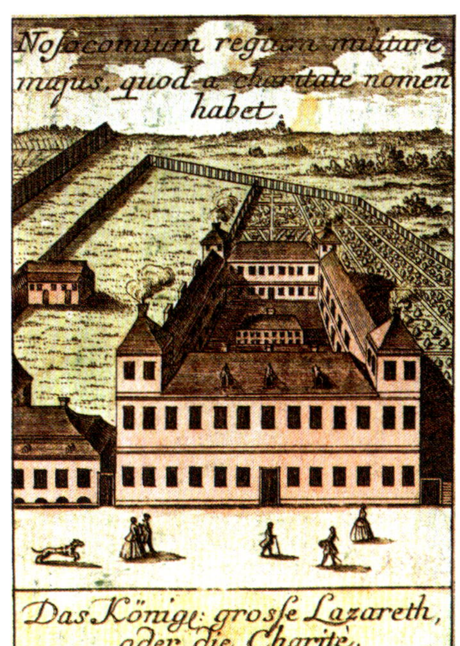

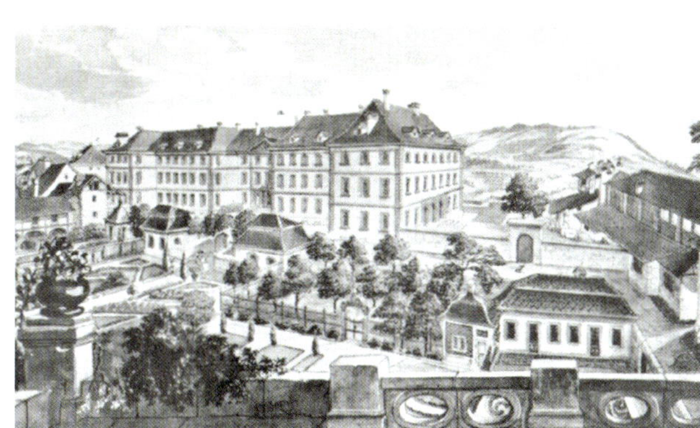

discovered that not he but the architect C.F. Viel had been responsible for the drawings. The 1787 report is one of the first explicit references to a building as a machine, what Leroy called 'une machine à traiter les malades'.[8] His report referred to the arrangement of hospitals like tents in an army camp or, in a more friendly tone, like the pavilions in the garden of Château Marly (1679) by J.H. Mansart. The pavilions were given roofs in the shape of mine shafts to guarantee optimal ventilation.[9] The commission eventually preferred the pavilion type to the radial model. Still, the first hospital of this kind – the Hôpital Lariboisière (1839-1854) by M.P. Gauthier – was not built for a further forty years. Gauthier followed the recommendations of the commission down to the last detail. This is hardly surprising since he had been instructed to take them into account in his design.[10] Lariboisière was acclaimed as a great success, although with six hundred beds it was only half the size of Poyet's sketch design.

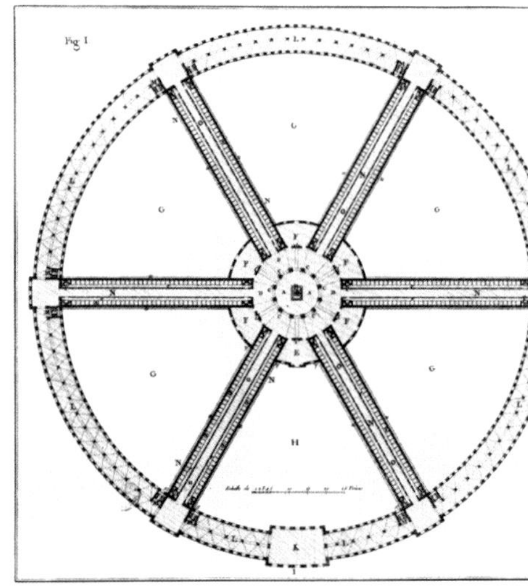

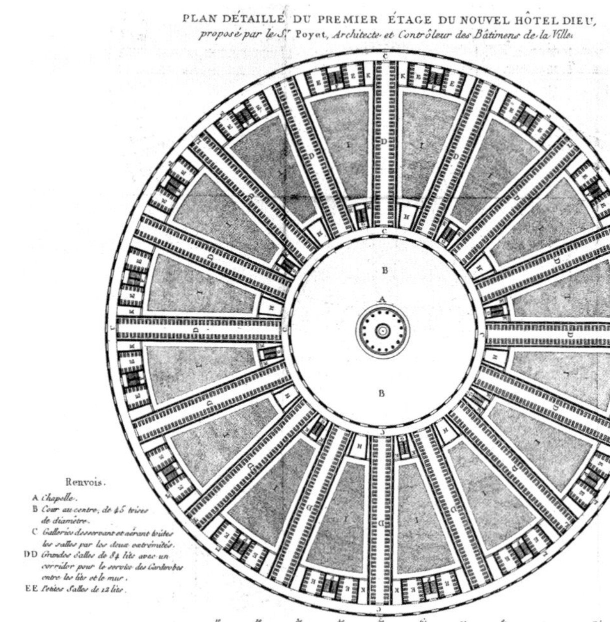

Lariboisière proved that the pavilion system was the model of the future. Once again, however, the breakthrough came from a military quarter. During the Crimean War (1854-1856), hospitals consisting of separate barracks were set up near the field of battle, a solution that was passionately propagated in the succeeding years by F. Nightingale, who proved to be an admirer of Lariboisière. She described the advantages of this type in her well-known *Notes on hospitals* (1859). In England her efforts resulted in D. Galton's Royal Herbert Military Hospital in Woolwich, which was built between 1859 and 1864, H. Currey's St. Thomas Hospital in London (1866-1871) and other buildings. Probably the most perfect pavilion hospital, however, was built in Paris, where a new Hôtel-Dieu opened its doors more than a century after the fatal fire of 1772. It was designed by E. Gilbert, who – not by chance – had previously made his name with the building of a psychiatric clinic (Charenton, definitive design 1838) and a prison (Mazas, built between 1840 and 1850).[11] The place of the new hospital was determined by G.E. Haussmann: on the northern side of the square in front of Notre-Dame, between the square and the main artery of the Seine. Napoleon III took a personal interest in the architecture: it was at his insistence that Gilbert's Neo-Gothic design was replaced by Neo-Renaissance façades.[12]

Hospitals in the Netherlands in the nineteenth century

The developments abroad had little influence in the Netherlands before the middle of the nineteenth century. The corridor system was still the favourite long after it had been rejected in France and Great Britain as outdated. This type proved to be amenable to important innovations in the hands of skilled designers, but these were mainly in the field of building construction. Typical is the building of the Coolsingelziekenhuis in Rotterdam (1855) designed by W.N. Rose. The Coolsingelziekenhuis was fairly literally inspired by Diakonissen Anstalt Bethanian designed by T.A. Stein that had been built in Berlin between 1845 and 1847. The Coolsingelziekenhuis was famous for a long time outside the Netherlands too: 'The visitors book that has survived from that period', M.J. van Lieburg, author of a monumental study of this hospital, remarked, 'contains the signatures, often with passionate laudations, of the most famous physicians and architects of the time.'[13] This fame was entirely due to the technical facilities, which were extremely modern at the time. The hospital had a sophisticated ventilation system and its own water purification installation. The potential of the steam engine, *the* invention of the nineteenth century, was

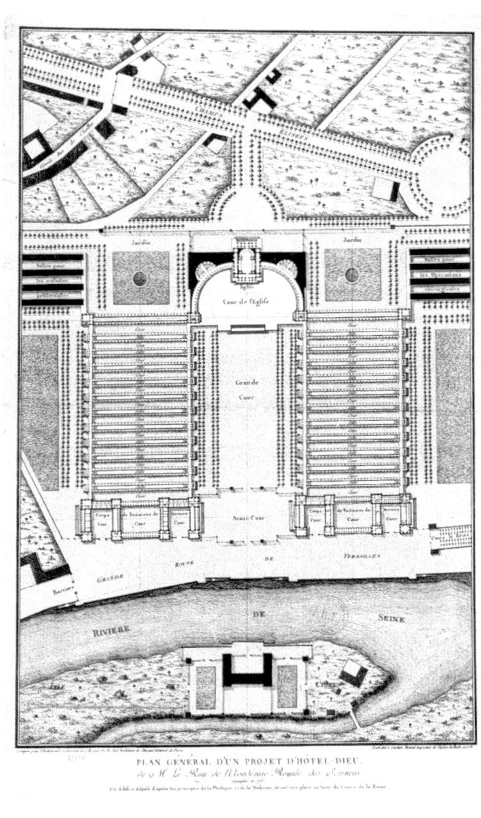

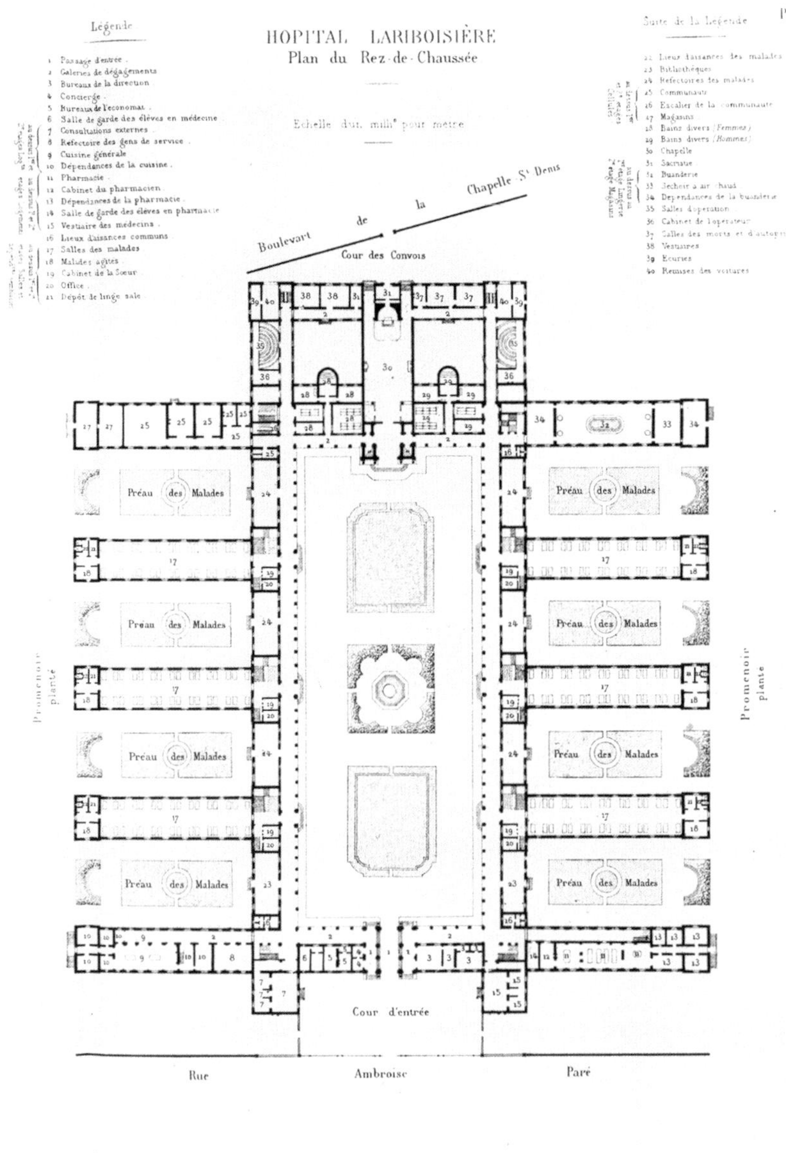

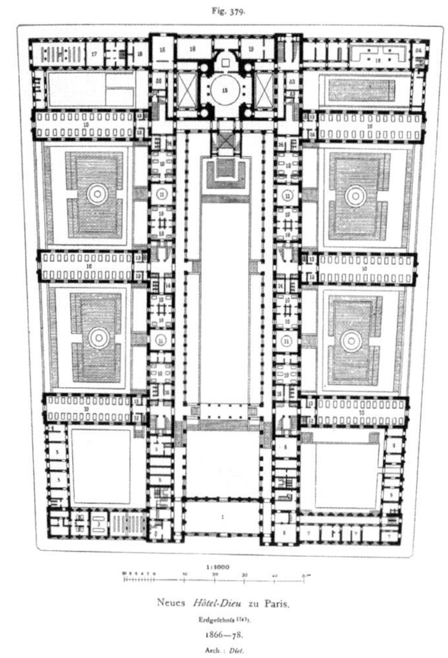

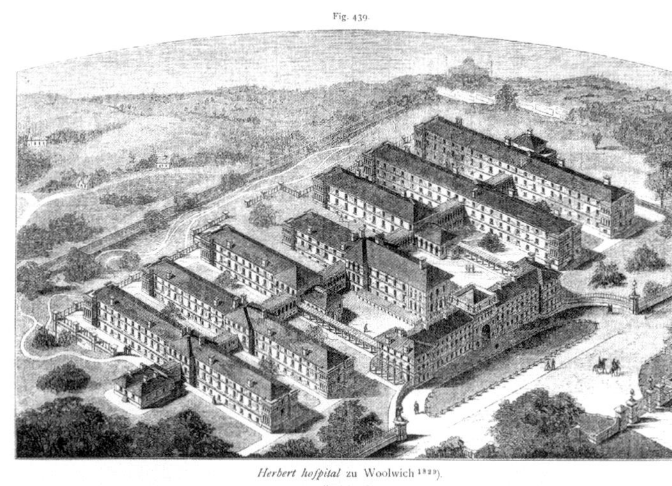

p. 16

***A. Petit*, design for the Hôtel-Dieu, Paris, 1774**

***B. Poyet*, design for the Hôtel-Dieu, Paris, 1785**

***J.B. Leroy, C.F. Viel*, design for the Hôtel-Dieu, Paris, 1773**

p. 17 | <

***M.P. Gauthier*, Hôpital Lariboisière, Paris, 1839-1854**

***H. Currey*, St. Thomas Hospital, London, 1866-1871**

***W.N. Rose*, Coolsingel-ziekenhuis, Rotterdam, 1855**

p. 17 | >

***E. Gilbert*, Hôtel-Dieu, Paris, 1866-1878**

***D. Galton*, Royal Herbert Military Hospital, Woolwich, 1859-1864**

Coolsingelziekenhuis. Transition to the pavilion model.

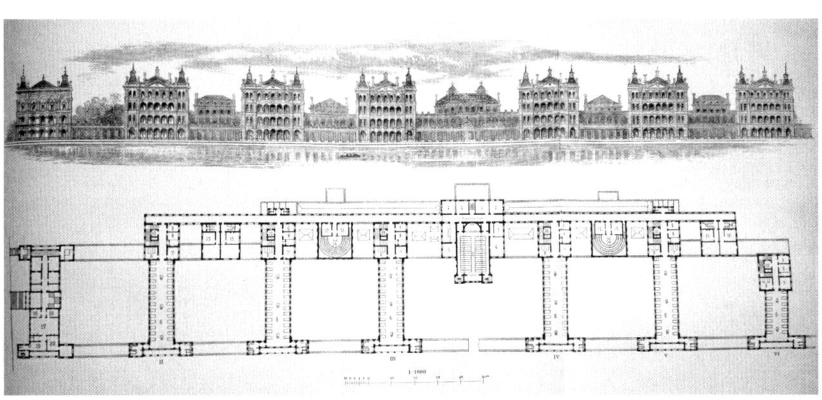

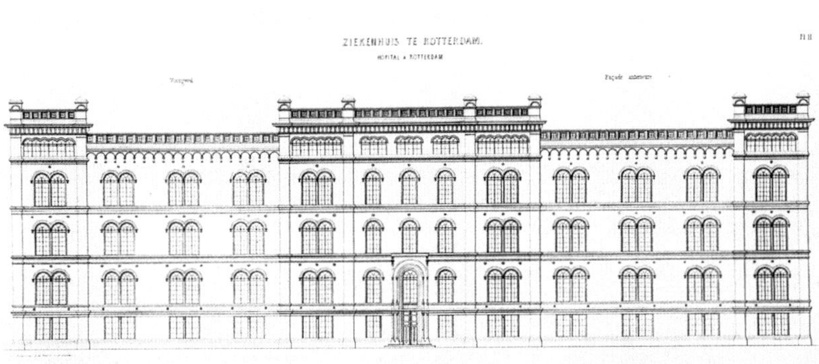

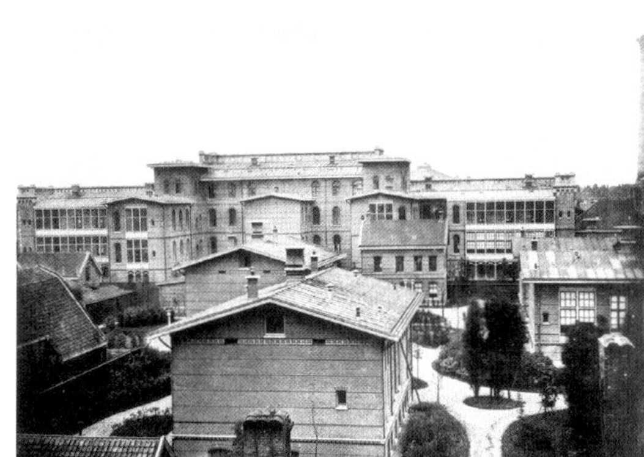

p. 18 | <
***T.A. Stein*, Diakonissen Anstalt Bethanien, Berlin, 1845-1847**

***J.A. van der Kloes*, municipal hospital Dordrecht, 1878**

***A.C. Bleys*, Onze Lieve Vrouwe Gasthuis, Amsterdam, 1894**

p. 18 | >
***H. Leguyt*, Wilhelmina Gasthuis, Amsterdam, 1891**

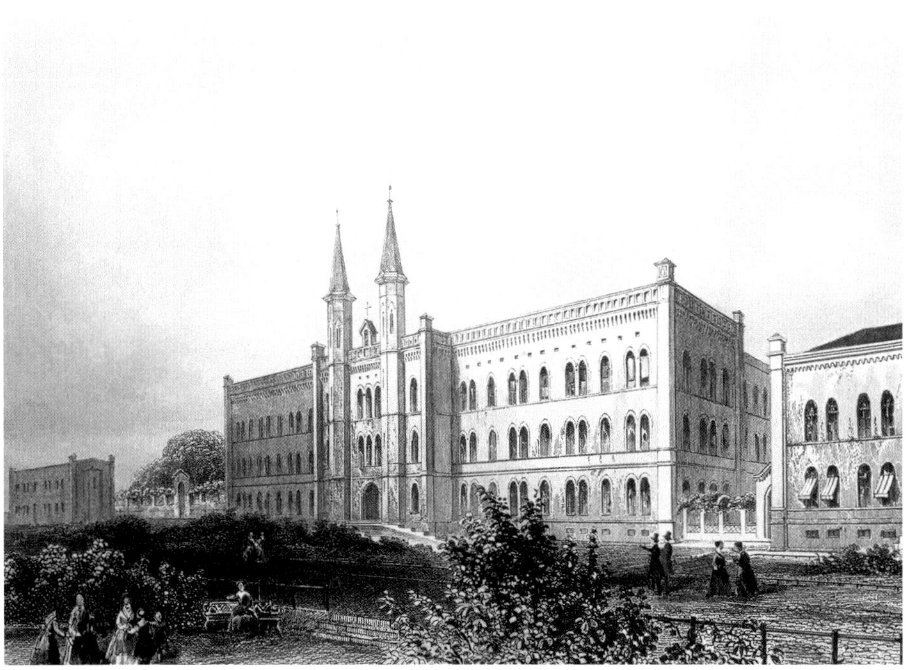

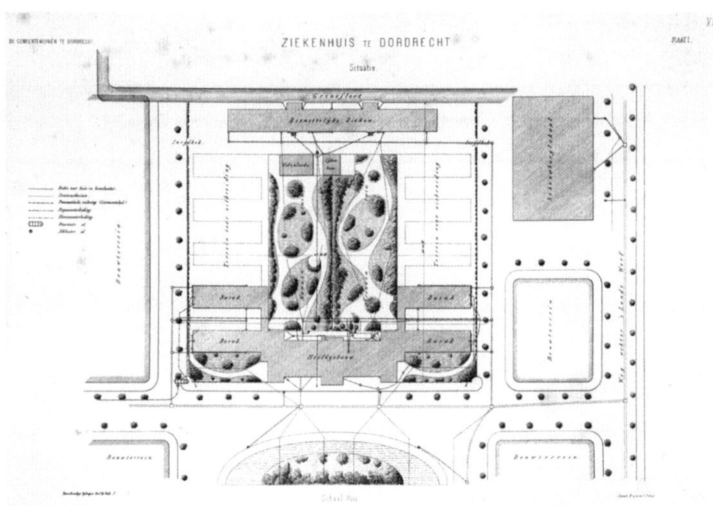

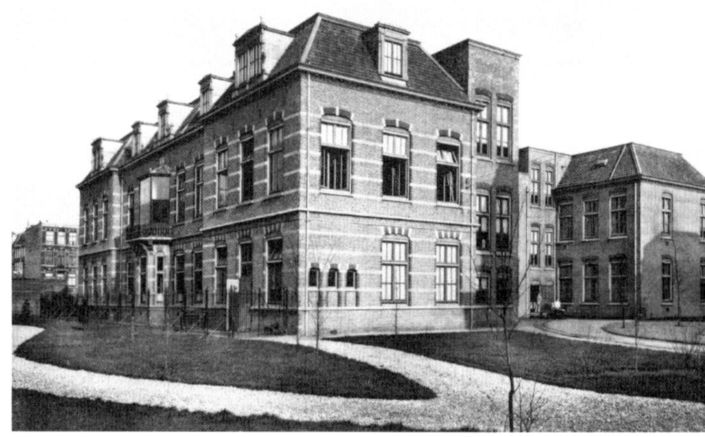

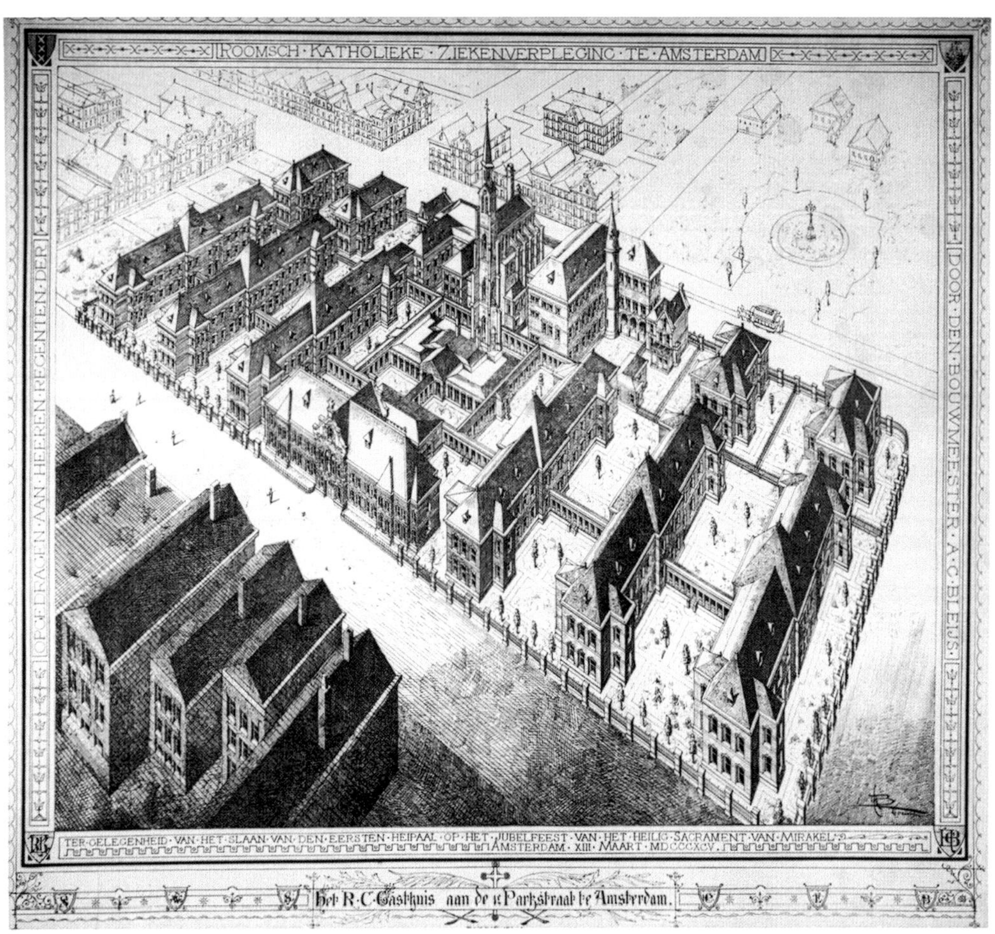

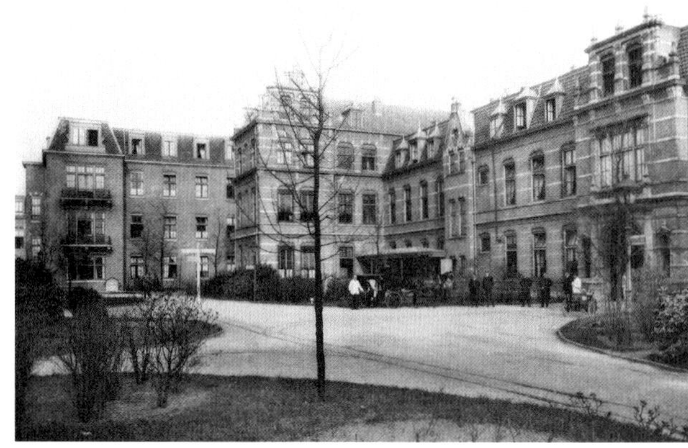

exploited to the full. Yet in spite of being so ahead of its time with regard to its architecture and in particular the technical installations, the corridor system on which it was constructed was behind the times. A pavilion system was adopted for later extensions.[14]

The first nineteenth-century Dutch hospital to be regarded as exemplary abroad for its design was built in Dordrecht in 1878. The architect J.A. van der Kloes first made a design for a corridor hospital.[15] It was above all the possibility of later extension already envisaged in the later pavilion design that was viewed so positively.[16] The Wilhelmina Gasthuis in Amsterdam (1889) designed by the architect H. Leguyt was also built as a pavilion hospital. Julius Petrus Bilmeijer and Joseph van Riel, who completed the Stuyvenberghospitaal in Antwerp in 1885, constructed a similar pavilion hospital in Maastricht between 1887 and 1891. After almost half a century of debate the Amsterdam council eventually also adopted this type for the Onze Lieve Vrouwe Gasthuis, designed by A.C. Bleys in 1894.[17] The 392-bed hospital had an administrative building, a financial building, three pavilions and four barracks. The pavilions (for men, women and neurasthenics) were symmetrical and had a wing on either side of the entrance.

As had been the case in the earlier corridor buildings, the pavilion hospitals comprised sections for men and women and for infectious illnesses. However, the importance of the pavilions was soon to change. Medical science took rapid strides ahead at the end of the nineteenth century. The various specialisations such as gynaecology, obstetrics and ophthalmology were accommodated in separate pavilions. This approach was particularly applied in practice to the building of university hospitals, such as the design by J. van Nieukerken for the Algemeen Provinciaal-, Stads- en Academisch Ziekenhuis in Groningen.[18] To prevent pavilion hospitals from spreading out over vast terrains, intermediate types were developed in between the corridor and the pavilion types. In many cases the pavilions were connected by corridors, as in the Onze Lieve Vrouwe Gasthuis in Amsterdam.

The psychiatric hospital

The roots of the psychiatric hospital partly coincide with those of the modern hospital: the identification of mental illnesses as complaints which could be treated with the help of recent scientific insights. There was no large-scale public agitation like that which followed the fire in the Hôtel-Dieu. At first it was mainly British models that were emulated. William Tuke, a coffee and tea merchant and a Quaker, had developed the concept of moral treatment at the end of the eighteenth century. He applied this philosophy in his Retreat, an attractive country house for some thirty patients. The most extreme forms of physical coercion were abolished, and the patients were given work to do and received education. Their living conditions were improved and the result was that at least some of the patients in the Retreat showed signs of recovery.

The method attracted wide attention thanks to a publication by his grandson Samuel Tuke. Ph. Pinel applied a similar method in the two Parisian institutions with which he was successively associated, the Hôpital Bicêtre from 1793, and the Salpêtrière from 1795. He too abandoned coercive methods where possible. Although Pinel also campaigned to adapt the buildings to the new philosophy, the big breakthrough did not come until 1838, when work on the Hôpital Charenton began. The location on the outskirts of Paris on a hill overlooking the Marne was idyllic, the architecture by E. Gilbert was strictly Neo-Classical, and the result was the marriage between nature and culture that had been propagated as an ideal since the Enlightenment.

Psychiatric institutions in the Netherlands

While the introduction of new forms of nursing and new institutions adapted to them was taking place abroad, the old 'madhouses', many of which had been set up in the Middle Ages, were still used for years in the Netherlands. Reinier van Arkel in 's-Hertogenbosch is the oldest of these, dating from 1442. It was followed by the Willem Arntsz Huis in Utrecht in 1461. The founders of these asylums were well-to-do citizens who, motivated by the Christian duty of charity, left a legacy in their will. Until late in the eighteenth century no attempt was made to heal the patients in these asylums; they were simply kept there. The 'mad' were often chained like animals and locked up naked in dark closets, usually because their deviant behaviour made them a threat to law and order in the city. Its function as a place of confinement was reflected in the structure of the asylum, which usually consisted of a number of cells (few at first) grouped around a square courtyard.

The number of such institutions gradually grew in the following centuries. There were a total of fourteen initiatives to set up specific institutions or special departments of an existing hospital for the mentally ill between 1550 and 1650.[19] The decision to construct an asylum in Amsterdam was taken in 1562; the Simpelhuis in Middelburg was opened in 1611; and the St. Caeciliagasthuis in Leiden, which was exclusively for the mentally ill, was inaugurated in 1635.

On 11 April 1818 King Willem I issued a Royal Decree calling for improvement of the care for the mentally ill in asylums. This 'philanthropic decree' provided first of all for a wide-ranging inquiry into the state of affairs at the time. The conclusion was that all the existing asylums should be closed down and replaced by five or six state asylums, each catering for between five and six hundred patients. In 1825 Reinhart Scherenberg, an official at the Home Office, published his *Ontwerp ter Oprigting van een Gesticht tot Verzekerde Bewaring, Verzorging en Genezing van Krankzinnigen* (Design for the Creation of an Asylum for the Safe Keeping, Nursing and Healing of the Insane), which was intended as a prototype. It envisaged a semicircular building that would accommodate six hundred patients. This was certainly an interesting plan, and so was the plan by the Ghent physician and architect J. Guislain, who published his findings in 1826 under the title *Traité sur l'aliénation mentale et sur les Hospices des Aliénés* (Treatise on Insanity and on the Hospitals for the Insane).

However, the intention of replacing the existing buildings by new ones proved to be overambitious, so it was decided to thoroughly renovate the old ones. The insights of. J.L.C. Schroeder van der Kolk (1797-1862), who was appointed Professor of Physiology and Anatomy at the University of Utrecht in 1827, played a decisive role. He became director of the Willem Arntsz Huis in the same year, which was apparently what prompted a speech entitled 'Rapport bij wijze van algemeen overzicht of voorslag tot verbetering van het Krankzinnigenhuis' (Report in the form of a general survey or proposal for the improvement of the mental asylum). Based on the latest insights, this report contains a number of guidelines for the architecture of the building. The rooms must have high ceilings and admit plenty of light and fresh air. The floors in the cells should be fairly sloping and there should be openings in the walls so that they could easily be swilled with water. Each room should have a WC, and the chair and table should be fixed to the floor. If the cells adjoined a public street or garden, they must be separated from it by a corridor to prevent passers-by from staring at the patients.

The Willem Arntsz Huis became a model institution. It was followed by the renovation of the old city asylums in other cities, in accordance with the example that Schroeder van der Kolk had set in Utrecht. Architecturally the results may not have been interesting, but thanks to them the intentions of the Law on the Insane could be put into practice everywhere within a few decades.

Meerenberg

In the province of North Holland, it proved impossible to modernise the sole general asylum, which was located in Haarlem. The only other approved institution, the home for poor Jews in Amsterdam, was too denominational to be able to accommodate non-Jewish patients as well. This provoked the building of an entirely new institution that was to be the

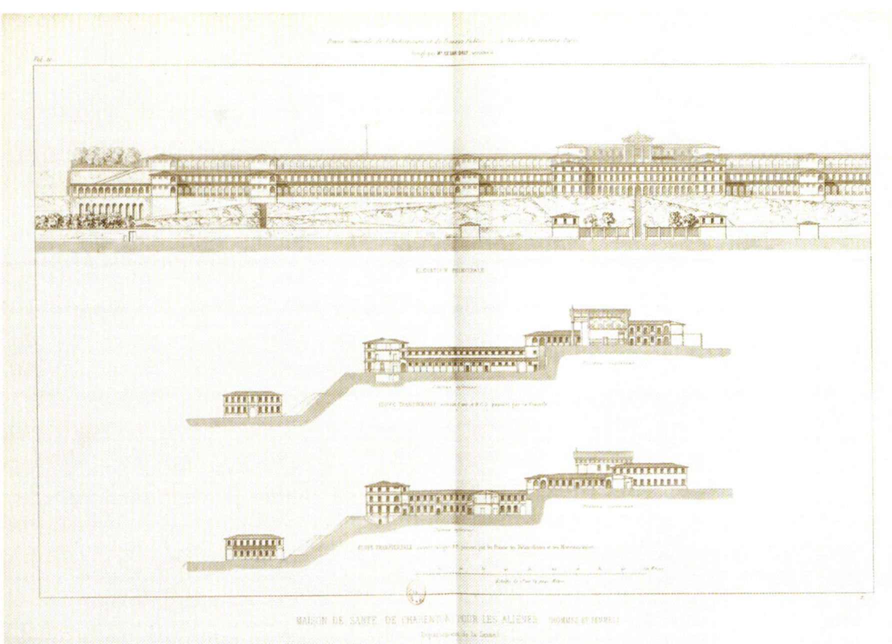

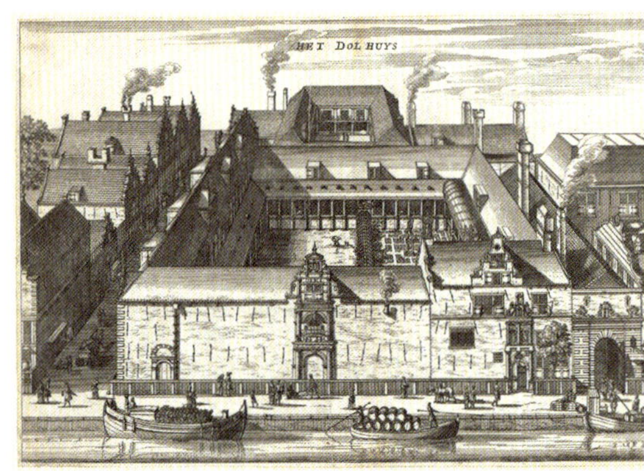

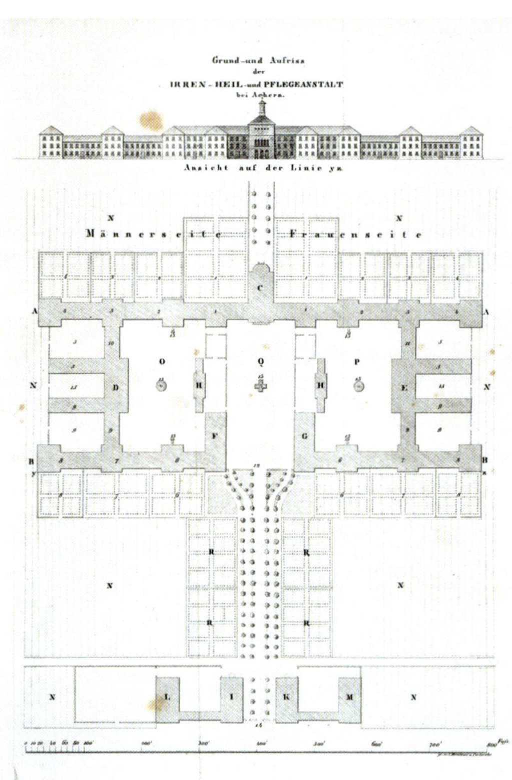

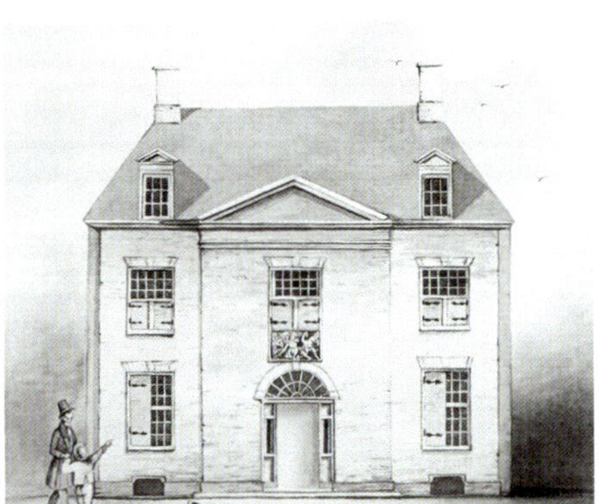

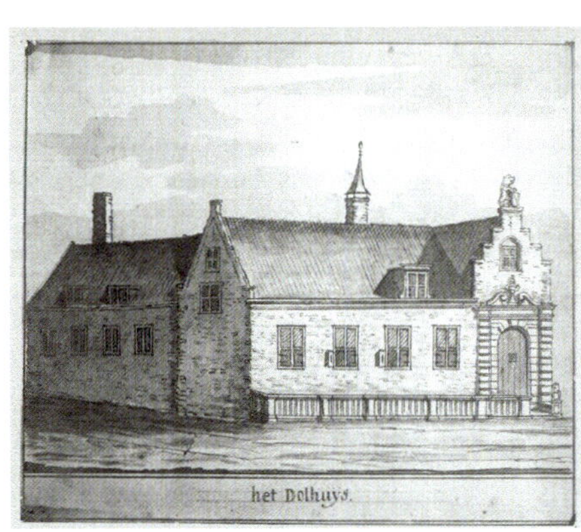

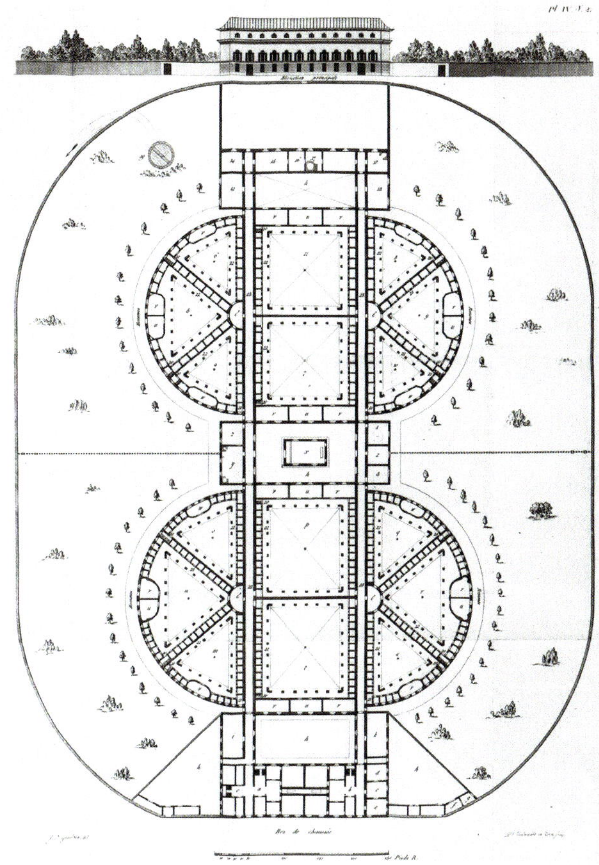

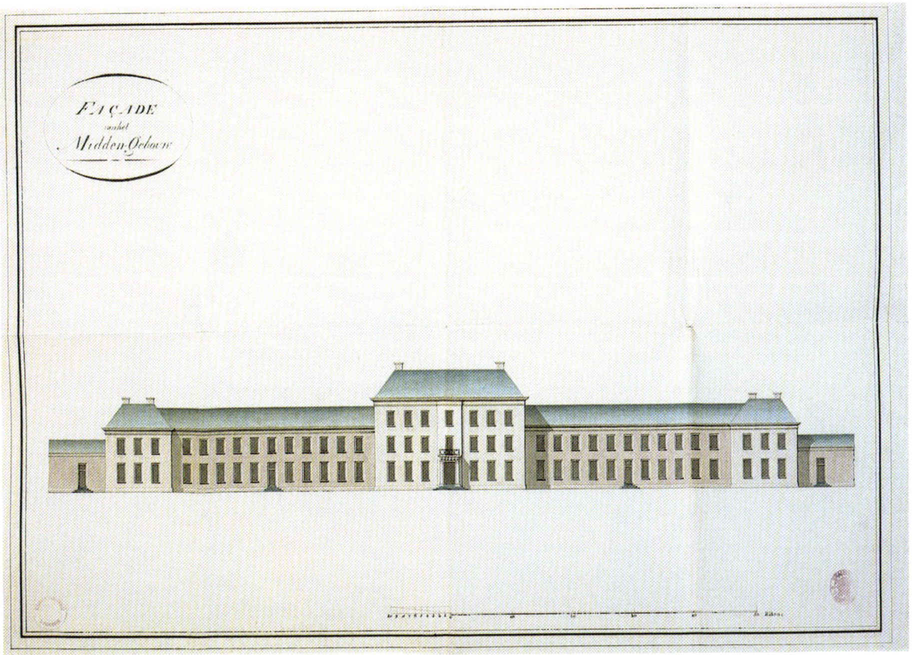

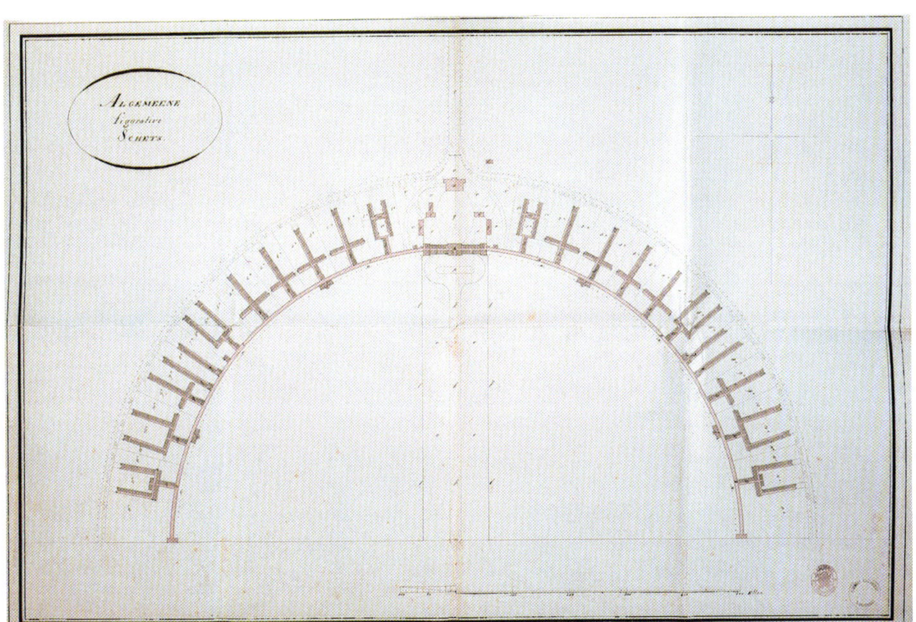

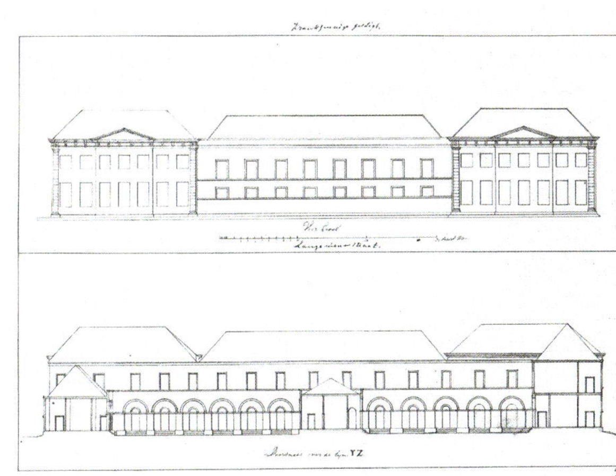

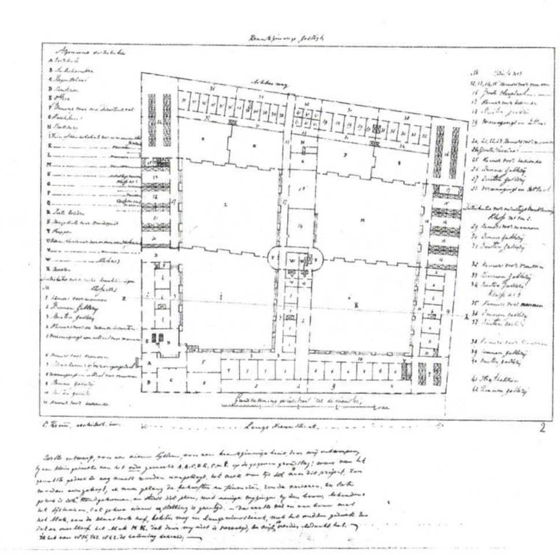

p. 20 | <

***E. Gilbert*, Hôpital Charenton, Paris, 1838**

Zinnelooshuis, 's-Hertogenbosch (Reinier van Arkel), 1442

Het Dolhuys, Utrecht (Willem Arntsz Huis), 1461

p. 20 | >

Kloveniersburgwal asylum, Amsterdam, 1562

Irren-, Heil- und Pflegeanstalt Illenau, Achern (Baden), 1838

p.21 | <

***R. Scherenberg*, 'Design for the Creation of an Asylum for the Safe Keeping, Nursing and Healing of the Insane', 1825-1826 (elevation main building and ground plan)**

p. 21 | >

***J. Guislain*, plan for an institute for 300 mental patients, 1826**

***C. Kramm*, design for the renovation of the Willem Arntsz Huis, Utrecht, 1836-1842 (front elevation and section and ground plan)**

showpiece of Dutch psychiatric institutions for years: Meerenberg in Santpoort. In June 1849 the first patient was admitted to this beautifully located institution on the edge of the dune landscape. At the time it was the only mental asylum to be situated in the countryside. Its idyllic setting and Neo-Classical architecture seem to have been inspired by Hôpital Charenton, but the direct model was Illenau near Baden. Meerenberg was designed by J.D. Zocher Jr (1791-1870), who was extremely successful as a garden and landscape architect and designer of Neo-Classical buildings. Thanks to a two-year period of study in Paris between 1809 and 1811, he was fully informed about the developments in France.

Zocher's design for Meerenberg was of a large symmetrical building. The square ground plan is divided into a side for men and another for women, with the cells arranged around courtyards. The rooms at Meerenberg were connected by wide corridors, hence the type is sometimes referred to as the square-corridor system. Meerenberg was divided into three classes, which were strictly separated from one another, and four departments per sex for calm and continent patients, less calm ones, very wild ones, and the incontinent. Elements of Neo-Classical architecture were combined and repeated, following the basic principles of sobriety and symmetry.

In 1852 the local authority gave permission for the asylum to be expanded to take a further two hundred patients. The architect A. van der Linden was commissioned to enlarge the asylum. Regular work, physical movement, hygiene, relaxation and the rural setting were supposed to stimulate the physical, moral and intellectual capacity of the patients. They were taught self-control and self-respect by work therapy and a strict daily schedule. In order to apply the new treatment the staff had to keep a close eye on the patients all the time, both day and night. That called for good material facilities such as generous living rooms and bedrooms for both patients and staff and work areas inside the building. The surrounding grounds could also be used for this purpose.[20] Two new side wings were added to the main building: a wing for female patients in 1853, and another for male patients three years later. The wings were connected by a corridor placed at right angles to the existing central corridor. Following the British model, each wing on the ground floor had a section for unruly patients with many single rooms and a few cells. The alterations to the building had considerably modified the original design, but in the end the physicians B.H. Everts and R.R. van Leeuwen had managed to create an institution where the new methods of moral treatment and non-restraint could be applied. Not only was this new in the Netherlands; it was considered to be extremely innovative all over the European continent.

The benefits of nature

The building of institutions in the countryside caught on in the Netherlands too in the middle of the nineteenth century. The pavilion system was preferred for these new buildings. Its great attractiveness lay in the possibility of an optimal embedding in the rural setting, the physical separation of the different categories and classes of patients, and a large degree of transparency within each pavilion.

In 1884 the Vereeniging tot Christelijke Verzorging van Krankzinnigen en Zenuwlijders in Nederland (Association for the Protestant Care of the Insane and Neurasthenics in the Netherlands) created a textbook example of a rural institution in the eastern part of the country: Veldwijk in Ermelo. The architect was E.G. Wentink. He and a few others involved in the initiative visited Währendorf near Hannover, Friedrichsberg near Hamburg, a clinic in Zehlendorf near Berlin, the Alt Scherbitz – which was regarded as extremely progressive – near Leipzig, the Protestant institution in Kaiserswerth near Düsseldorf, and an asylum in Düren. They concluded that the 'special' institutions were preferable to the regular public ones, at least 'as far as the warmth of tone and loving care' were concerned.[21] None of the clinics they visited could be copied in the Netherlands without some modification, because they were too grand, too big and far too expensive. All the same, the compilers of the report were definitively won over in favour of the pavilion system.

For many years Veldwijk functioned as a model asylum. It set a trend. Work on a new rural asylum just outside Deventer, Brinkgreven, was based on the pavilion model and commenced in 1892. The design was by J.A. Mulock Houwer, the Deventer town architect, while the park was laid out by L.A. Springer. The terrain was surrounded by extensive heath and woods, which offered plenty of opportunities for work therapy. Intensive work therapy was used in Brinkgreven right from the start.[22] The association that had set up Veldwijk established a total of five mental institutions before 1914. After the completion of Veldwijk and a further institution, Bloemendaal, in Loosduinen, in 1892 the association purchased the land for Dennenoord in Zuidlaren (Drenthe) close to the border of the province of Groningen. The advantages of the pavilion system were used there too, as Dennenoord was built in various stages. In the first stage four pavilions were built to accommodate a total of 110 third-class patients, an administrative building, a home for the director-physician, and a few other buildings. Building operations commenced in April 1895. Three years later Dennenoord had 193 patients, and by 1902 their number had risen to some five hundred.

Catholic institutions were built in Venray and Noordwijkerhout. The Brothers and Sisters of Love, two Belgian religious orders that played an important role in psychiatric reform, created two psychiatric institutions in Venray. Sint Servatius, designed by H. van der Plas, was opened in 1907. Sint Anna, specially designed for female patients, followed in 1907. The plan was made by Jozef César Haché (who was to reuse it several times in Belgium, where he built three virtually identical institutions). The Venray asylums soon became overcrowded. In order to offer a facility for their Catholic brethren who lived further to the north, the Brothers of Love bought thirty five hectares of land in the dunes in Noordwijkerhout. The Amsterdam architect P.J. Bekkers based his design on the ground plan that had been used in Venray.

The fully-fledged rural institution

One of the advantages of the pavilion type was that one could start on a small scale and slowly expand afterwards. Around the turn of the century, however, a drastic increase in scale took place. Meerenberg had already been enlarged with a second rectangular block, Meerenberg II, in 1887 to reach a total capacity of around thirteen hundred places. The decision to build the Duin en Bosch institution in the dunes near Castricum was taken in 1902. The architect was F.W.M. Poggenbeek, who designed six large pavilions, three for male and three for female patients, with a total capacity of 620.

The first building of a new institution in Den Dolder in the province of Utrecht, the Willem Arntsz Hoeve, was completed in 1907. It was primarily intended to offer care for

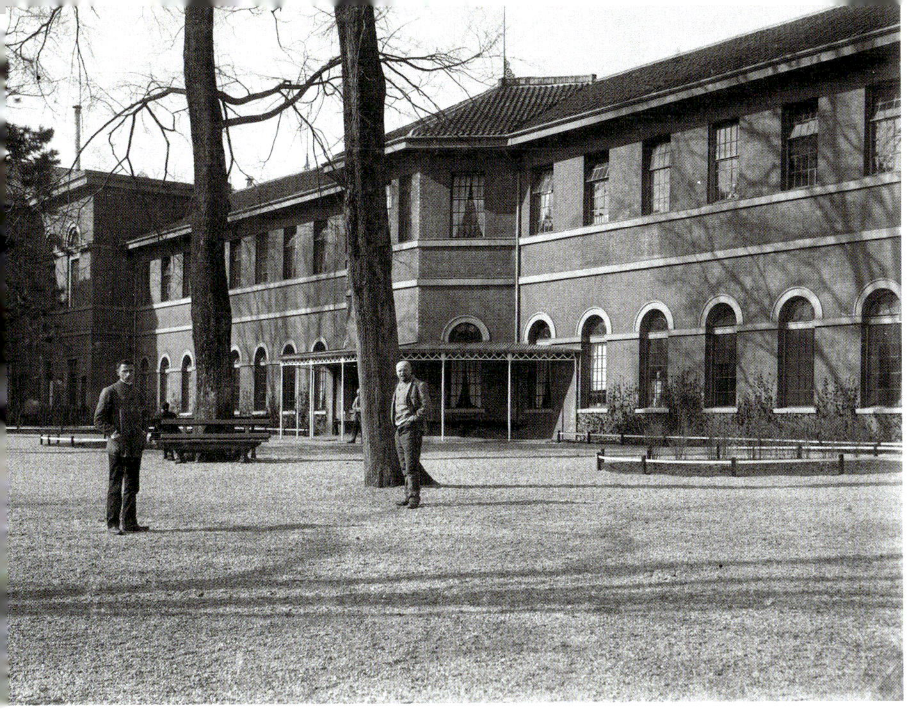

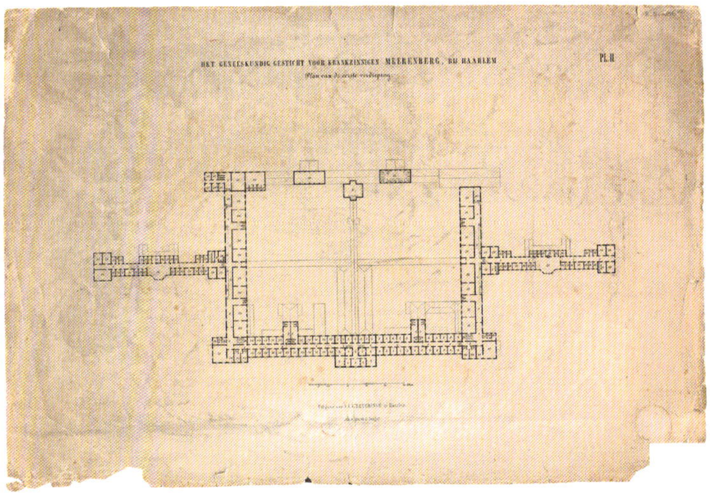

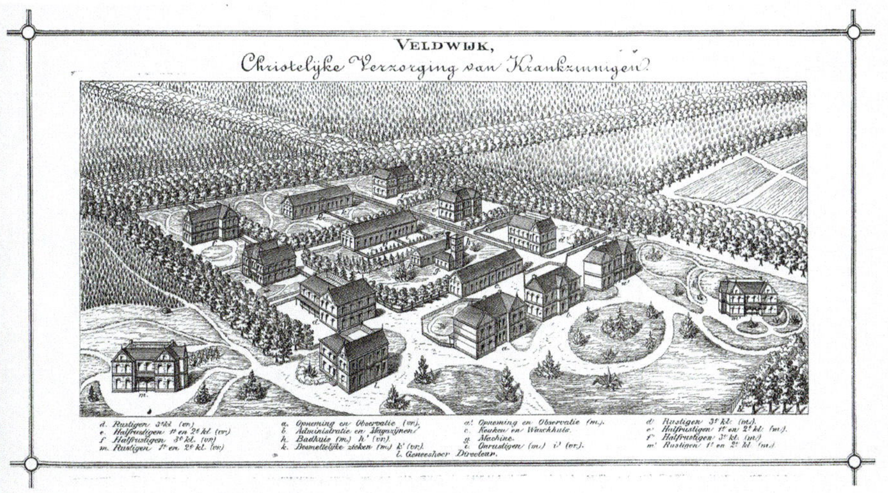

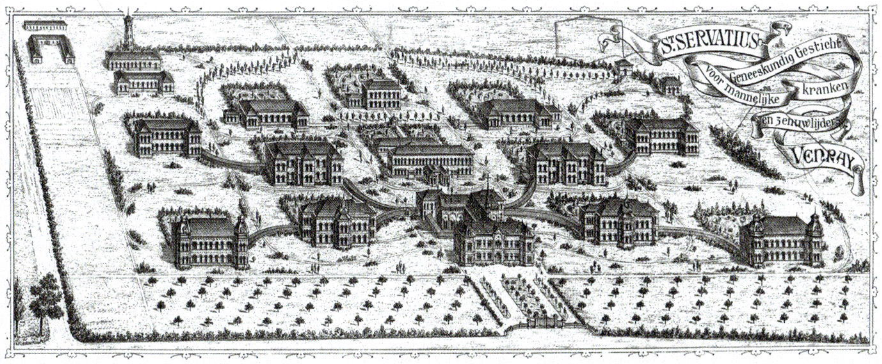

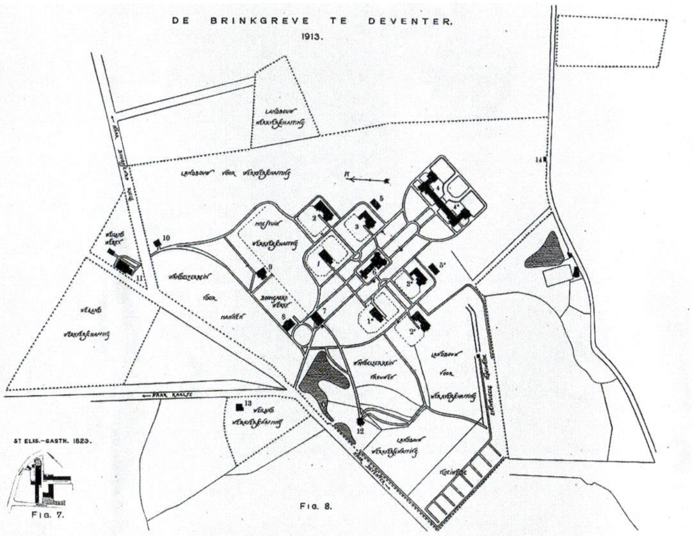

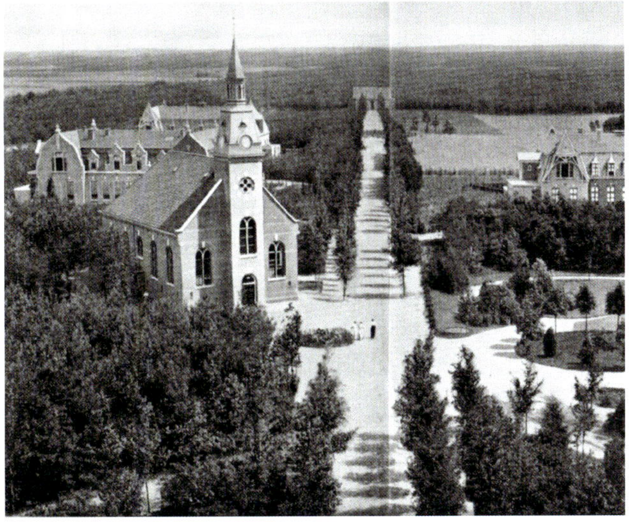

p. 23 | <
Meerenberg, Santpoort, with an expansion by A. van der Linden, 1853-1856

E.G. Wentink, design for Veldwijk, Ermelo, 1884

***H. van der Plas*, Sint Servatius, medical asylum for insane and neurasthenic male patients, Venray, 1907**

p. 23 | >
***A. van der Linden*, extension of Meerenberg, Santpoort, 1853-1856**

***J.A. Mulock Hower*, Brinkgreven, Deventer, situation 1913**

***K. Hoekzema*, Dennenoord, Zuidlaren, 1895**

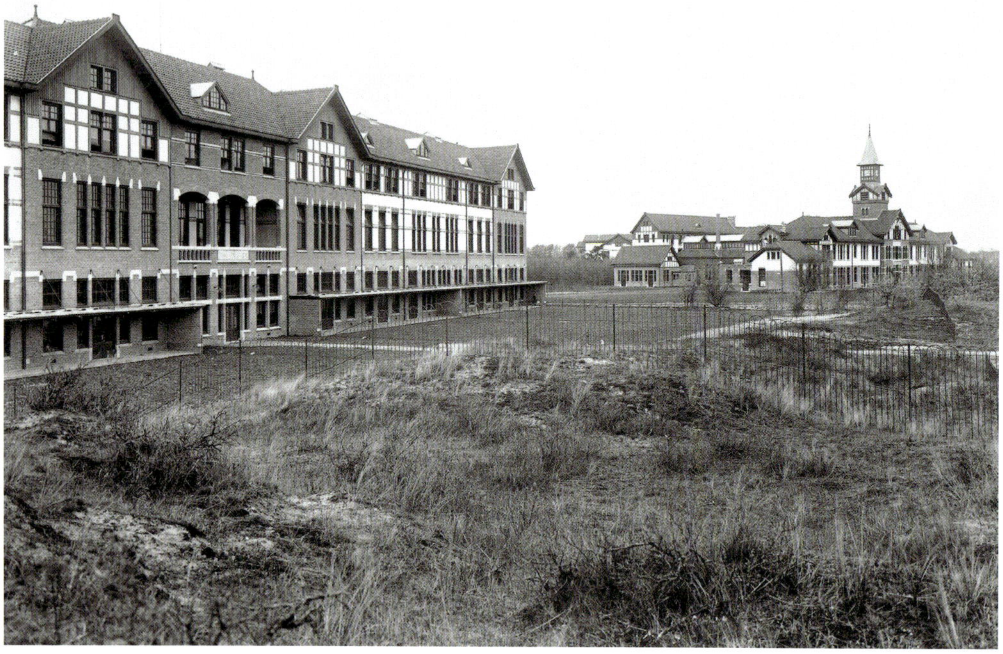

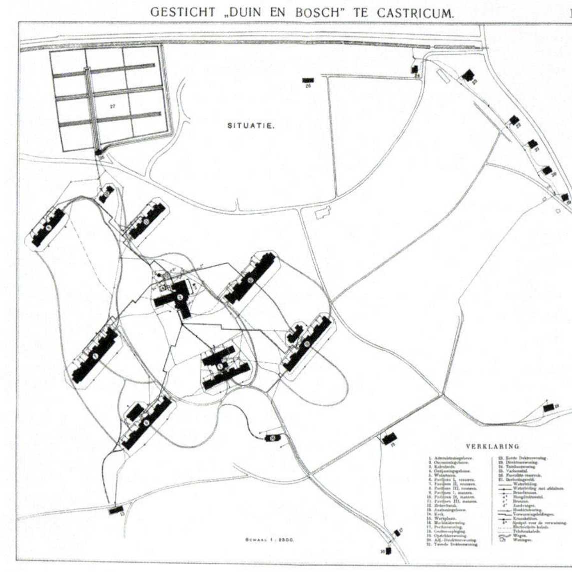

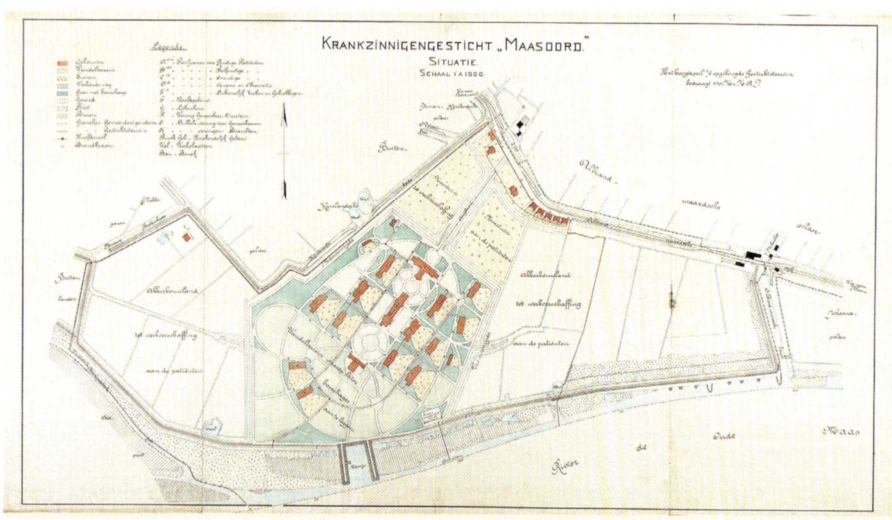

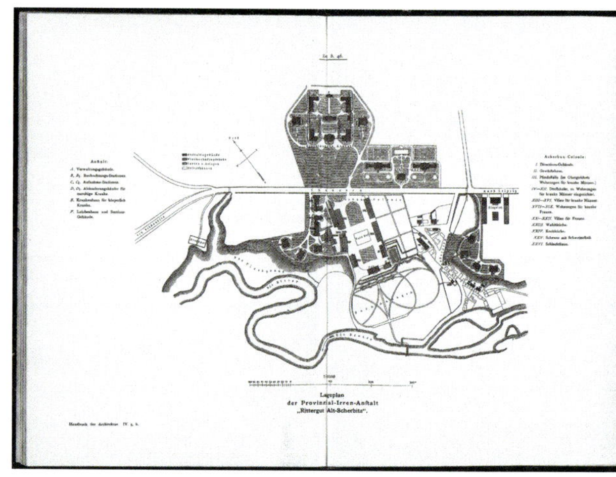

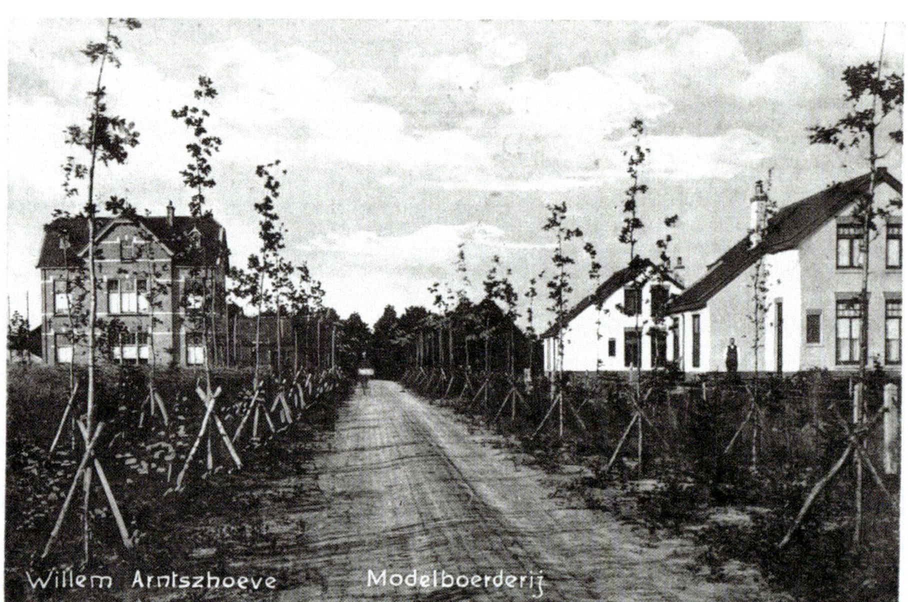

p. 24 | <
***F.W.M. Poggenbeek*, Duin en Bosch, Castricum, 1909**

***G.J. de Jongh*, Maasoord mental asylum, Poortugaal, 1907**

***G. van Heerde and H. Masselink*, Willem Arntsz Hoeve, model farm, Den Dolder, 1907**

p. 24 | >
***F.W.M. Poggenbeek*, Duin en Bosch, Castricum, 1909**

Alt Scherbitz asylum, Halle, 1876

p.25
***Jozef César Haché*, Sint Anna, Venray, 1908**

rural patients in a family-like setting. The architects G. van Heerde and H. Masselink first designed a farm for six patients and two nurses. F.W.M. Poggenbeek went on to design the core of the complex, which was built between 1909 and 1912. The institution measured at the time 207 hectares, surrounded by woods. Arranged on a central axis were a management building, a utilities building with the central kitchen, and sleeping quarters for the staff. Between these buildings was the auditorium, a communal area for the patients. Ten spacious pavilions, arranged in rough symmetry, flanked the central axis.

When the Rotterdam city council decided to build a municipal mental asylum for some six hundred patients in December 1902, it was already clear that there was no land available for it within the city boundary. A site near the Oude Maas below the village of Poortugaal was the solution. G.J. de Jongh, director of the city's urban planning board, and W. Vos, the future director-physician, put together the list of requirements. Simplicity was one of the most important demands to keep the cost within limits. De Jongh and Vos visited a number of institutions in the Netherlands and Germany, including Alt Scherbitz near Halle. Two years after the decision to create a new asylum had been taken, they presented an extensive report to the council. Assuming between forty and fifty patients per pavilion, between fifteen and twenty pavilions would be needed.

The sanatorium

In the second half of the nineteenth century a new category of the mentally ill was identified who differed from the category of the insane in that they did not usually pose a threat to society and were highly aware of their specific problem.[23] This group of patients had probably always existed, but now they were classified as a separate group: neurasthenics.[24] Their identification is usually attributed to the American physician George Beard, who launched the term neurasthenia for this type of disturbance in 1869.[25] He located the cause of the emergence of this group in the discrepancy between the increasing tempo of social change and the slow evolution of the human species. Civilisation therefore represented a threat to mental health. Although this view implies a reformulation of the classical Enlightenment idea, Beard did not refer to it. As neurasthenic disorders were most common among the well-to-do (the most civilised classes), this distinguished the group socially from the poor and insane.[26] This made them an exceptionally lucrative target group for the numerous small private clinics that sprang up everywhere in the last quarter of the nineteenth century. The regular asylums, however, could not join in the gold rush. The Law on the Insane of 1841 stipulated that only the insane could be treated in an asylum.

There was little scientific justification for such a strict

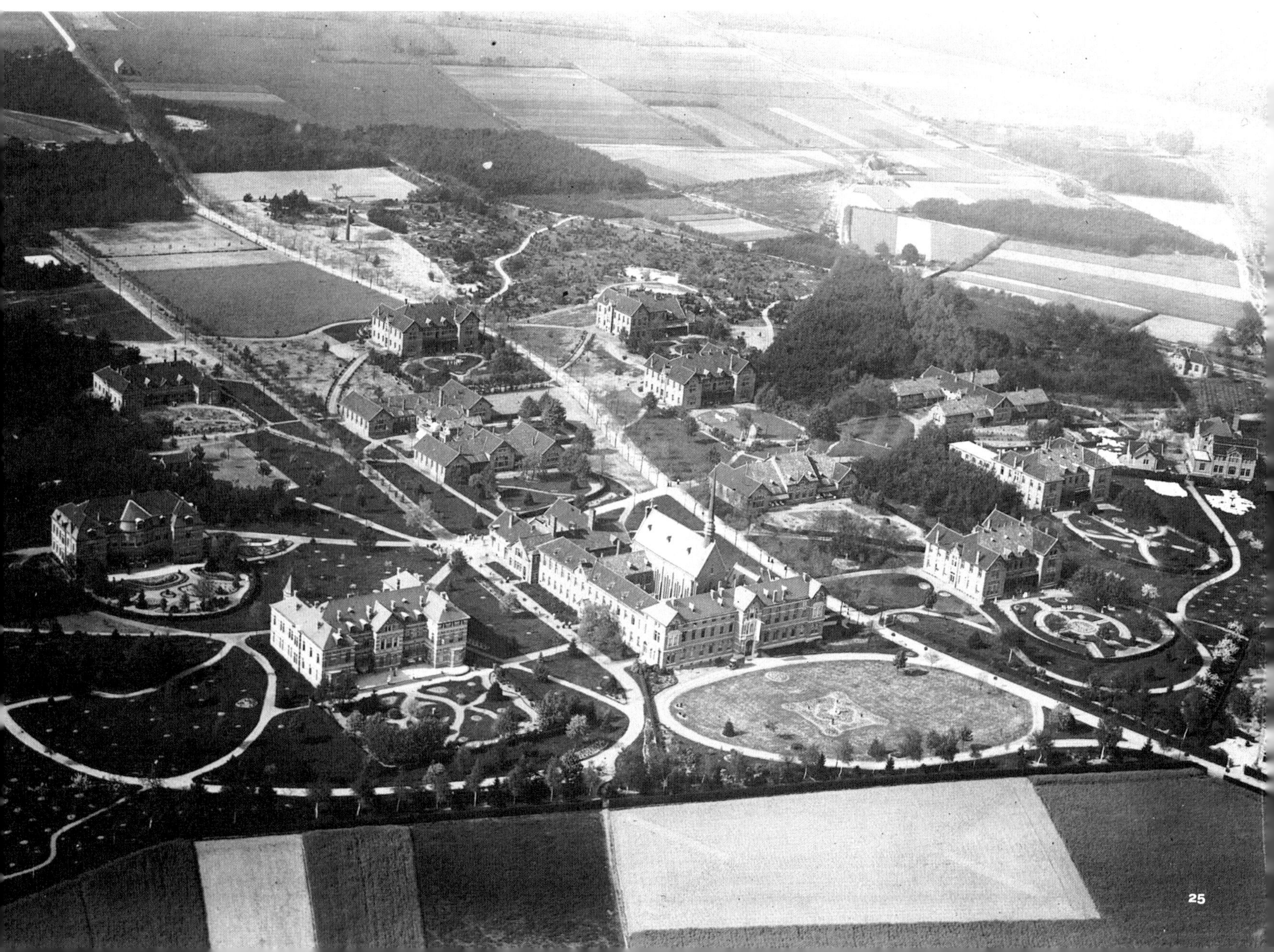

distinction, however. After all, both categories of patients were mentally ill, and at least some of them were potentially amenable to treatment. That was behind the introduction of an amendment to the law in 1904 to create 'designated departments'.[27] Regular asylums were now allowed to create special facilities for neurasthenics. In principle these departments were nothing but regular hospitals for a specific type of patient. The need to draw the distinction with the traditional mental asylum can be seen in the conventional name of the designated departments, that were often referred to as sanatoria. (The term is ambiguous: for example, the centres created later to provide tuberculosis patients with fresh air were usually called sanatoria too.) More than the hospital, the sanatorium evoked associations with the relatively luxurious health centres where the patients were treated in a healthy natural setting. The target group was initially similar: the more well-to-do neurasthenics who were able to bear the expense of a stay in a sanatorium. The first asylum to put the possibility opened up by the amendment into practice was Huize Padua in Boekel (Brabant) in 1916. This example was followed on a large scale. After the success of Veldwijk and the various subsidiary asylums, it was decided in 1900 to set up a smaller association besides the Vereeniging tot Christelijke Verzorging van Krankzinnigen en Zenuwlijders in Nederland to campaign for the foundation of one or more sanatoria. In October 1900 a commission including E.G. Wentink, the house architect of the Reformed Church, travelled to Switzerland and Germany in search of suitable models for a new sanatorium. They visited a large number of institutions. Each of these had its own specific character, though they all also had much in common. They were always accommodated in luxurious villas. Wentink concluded that clinics for neurasthenics would have to be located in idyllic surroundings with woods, gardens, meadows and agricultural land close at hand, because the landscape was not just for country strolls but also for work on the land. A dairy farm on the site was advisable where possible. A location near the city was recommended. Not only did that facilitate communications for all kinds of practical necessities, but it also made church attendance easier and offered the patients an opportunity for entertainment.

A clinic should start off with two large pavilions, one for first-class and second-class patients, the other for third-class patients. The design must offer opportunities for expansion that would not mar the beauty of the complex. Sanatoria for neurasthenics imposed high demands on the architectural appearance. 'The building looks agreeable, not sombre, and the style should be smart. The sight of it should arouse the thought: "I would like to be treated here". The entrance should be welcoming. (...) The rooms receive plenty of light and have as many balconies as possible. A large, spacious verandah should cover the south side, or the south-east or south-west side of the building depending on its orientation.'[28] The Protestant sanatorium in Zeist opened in 1903. Wentink's luxurious architecture set the tone; the influence of his study trip can be seen in the chalet style that was regularly applied in villas and country homes at the time. The sanatorium was clearly not designed as an institution for poor patients; it targeted the wealthier classes and offered accommodation of the most appropriate kind.

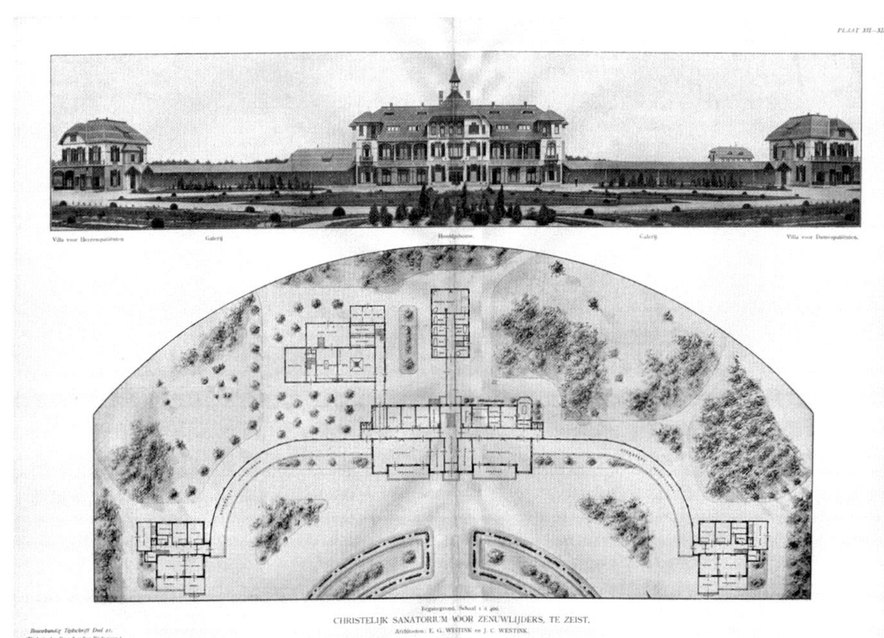

Housing and care for the elderly

Growing old is not an illness, but it can involve some handicaps. Of course, elderly people with physical or mental complaints are eligible for treatment in hospitals or psychiatric institutions. The origin of what has come to be called care for the elderly lies therefore not in the building of care institutions, but in the creation of housing specially intended for that target group. Housing was to be the foundation of care for the elderly down to the 1990s. Types of housing with integrated care go back to the 1940s; the nature and intensity of this care determined a number of building types (apartment buildings for the elderly, old people's home, nursing home, self-sufficient housing). Afterwards a distinction was implemented between housing and care which, paradoxically enough, has led to the present situation in which only care institutions count as care for the elderly. But we are getting ahead of the story – this is the place to trace the origin of care for the elderly, which can be done without much difficulty back to the Middle Ages. From the thirteenth century clusters of almshouses (*hofjes*) were created in many cities. These formed small communities for the elderly away from the bustle of city life. They were often founded thanks to the legacies of wealthy citizens. The construction of these almshouses expanded dramatically in the seventeenth and eighteenth centuries, and many Dutch cities have examples that, after thorough renovation and modernisation, still retain their original function today, such as the Hofje van Bakenes from 1395 in Haarlem, the Pepergasthuis (1405) in Groningen, that was designated as housing for the elderly in 1594, the Hofje van Nieuwkoop built in The Hague between 1658 and 1661 after a design by Pieter Post, and the Deutzenhofje (1692) in Amsterdam. The most characteristic feature of the *hofje* was not the type of house, which did not differ fundamentally from other houses of the time, but the urban setting: closed complexes of small, independent houses grouped around an open space that was usually arranged as a flower garden, often with a church or chapel. The architectural qualities are often evident. Most of them achieved the status of a protected monument long ago. The urban setting of the *hofje* anticipates the later old people's home, while the architecture of the houses anticipates the design of small homes specifically for fit old people. The small scale and urban setting are what still make this model attractive today.[29]

Many of the elderly had a much less fortunate lot. They had to fall back on charity. Care of the elderly was contracted out by the poor boards, but this was fairly expensive, which is why they decided to set up homes for the elderly themselves in the sixteenth century. In the second half of the eighteenth century workhouses were set up in many places. One was established in the Roetersstraat in Amsterdam in 1782; its name was changed to Armenhuis (Poorhouse) in 1875, and to municipal home for the elderly in 1933.

Between 1681 and 1683 the Deaconate of the Dutch Reformed Church in Amsterdam set up a home for elderly women, to which elderly men were also admitted after 1719. The location on the bank of the River Amstel was in use as a home for the elderly for more than three centuries; for many centuries it was the largest of its kind in the Netherlands. In 1843 the St. Ignatiusgesticht (Huize Goirke) was built in Tilburg (Brabant). It was intended for elderly men who needed care. They were tended by the Sisters of Love, who lived in the same complex. The building had a square ground

p.26
***E.G. Wentink & J.C. Wentink*, Christelijk Sanatorium voor Zenuwlijders, Zeist, 1903**

p.27
Hofje van Bakenes, Haarlem, 1395

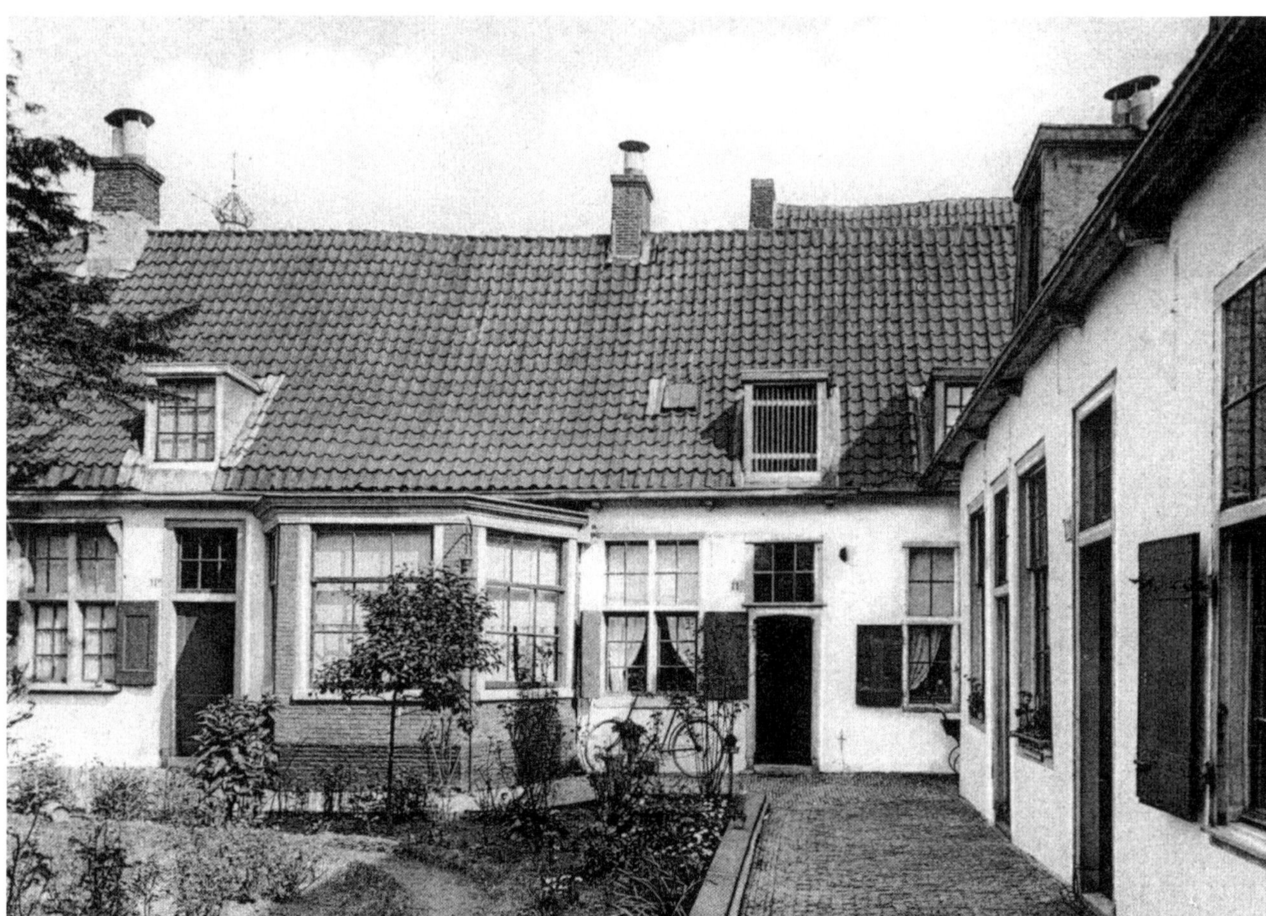

plan with two floors and a saddle roof. Two wings were added at the front in 1855.

While the elderly with sufficient means had little cause for concern, the vast majority of the poor and elderly had to fall back on the cheapest and worst housing available until late in the twentieth century. Even then they were sometimes only able to pay thanks to religious or private charity. Those with a little more money at their disposal could pay a one-off sum to obtain board and lodging in a *proveniershuis*. A new type of housing for the elderly was created in the 1920s that concentrated a relatively large number of apartments specially designed for the elderly in a complex that also included communal facilities. This type (known as *pensiontehuis*, *tehuis voor ouden van dagen* or *rusthuis*) was thus a forerunner of the later old people's home that was so popular in the 1950s. It is an example of what would later be referred to as an institutional form of housing.

p. 28
Deaconate home for elderly women, Amsterdam, 1681

Refectory in the municipal home for the elderly, Amsterdam (the former Nieuwe Werkhuis from 1782)

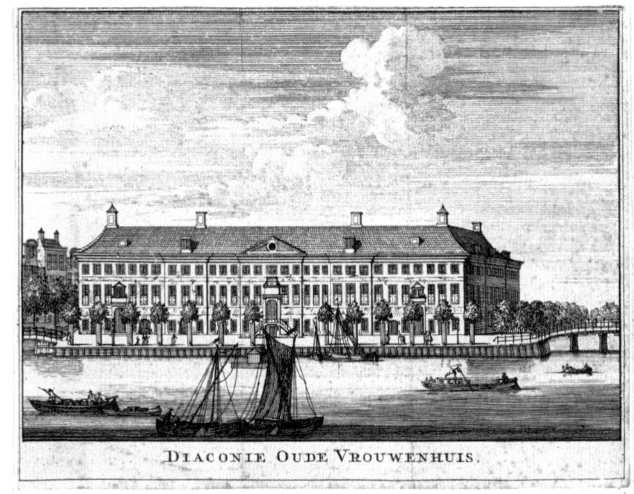

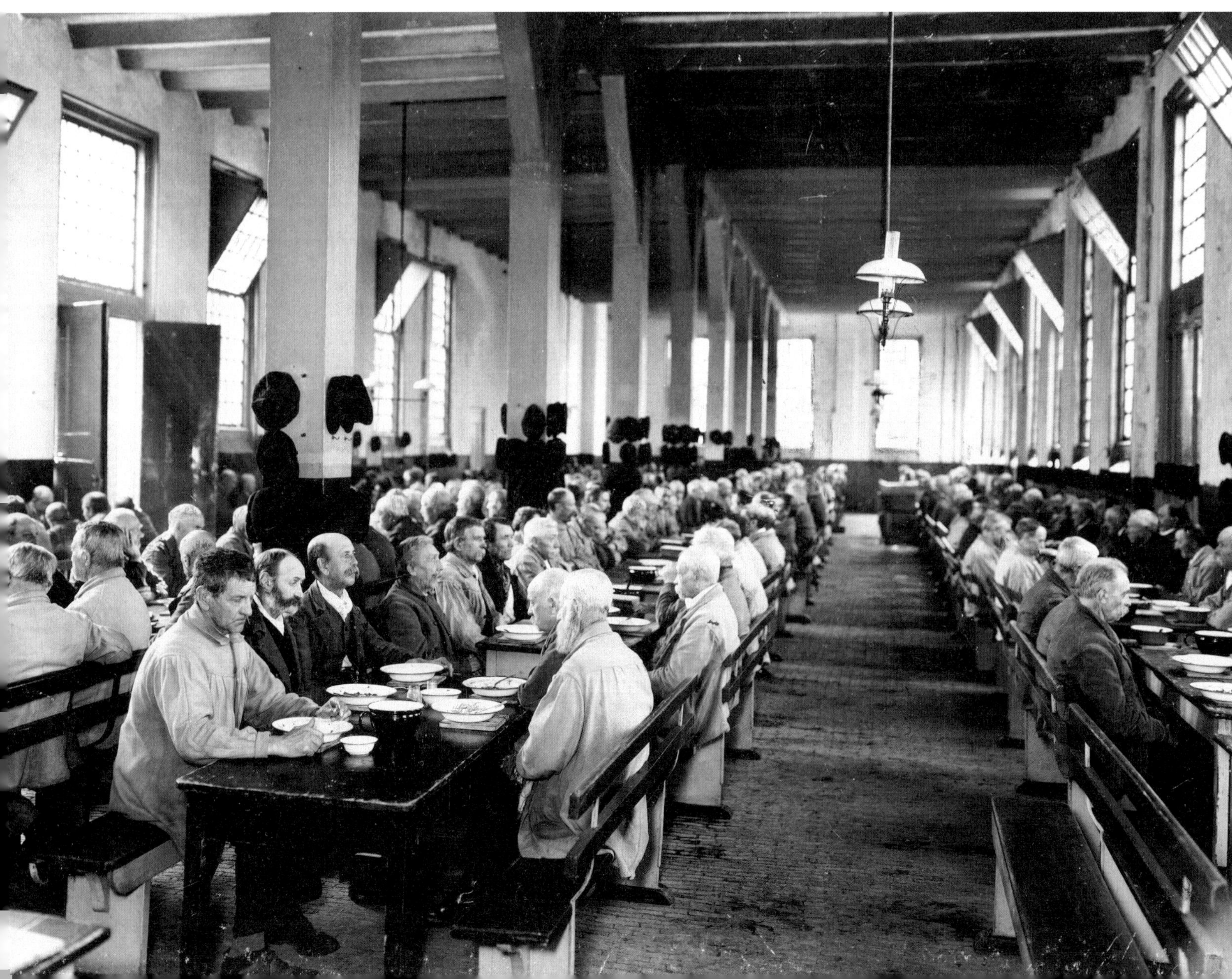

p. 29 | <
***Pieter Post*, Hofje van Nieuwkoop, The Hague, 1661**

Nieuwe Werkhuis, Amsterdam, 1782

p. 29 | >
Deutzenhofje, Amsterdam, 1692

Proveniershuis, Rotterdam, 1690

Huize Goirke, Tilburg, 1843

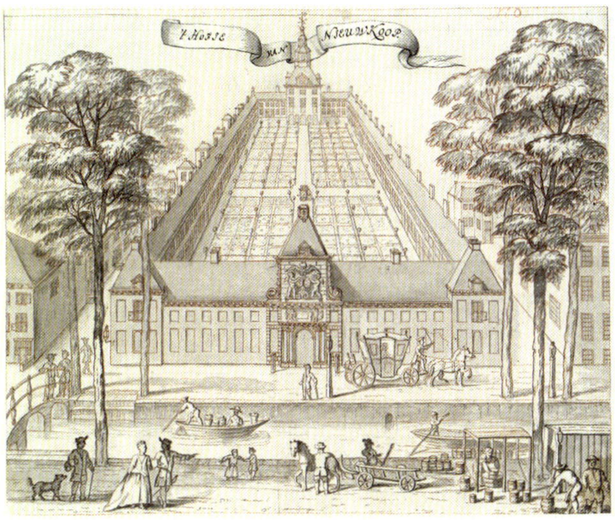

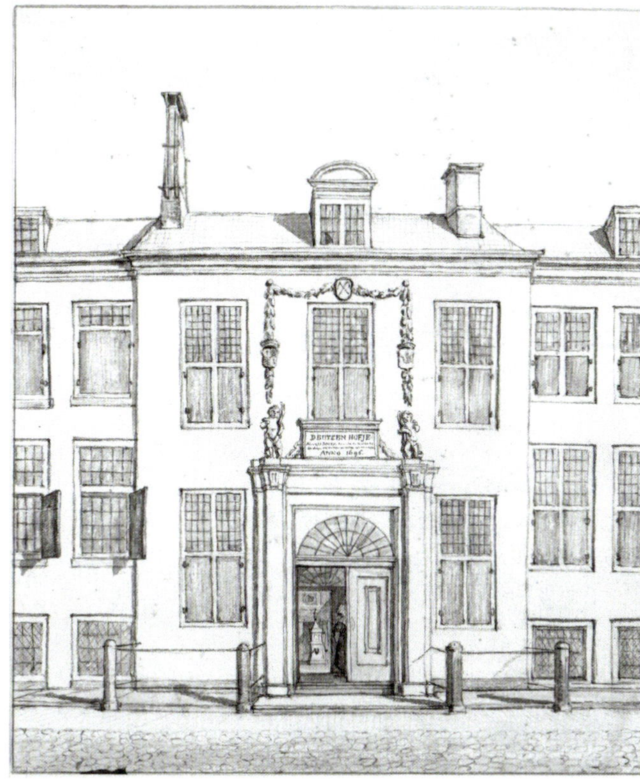

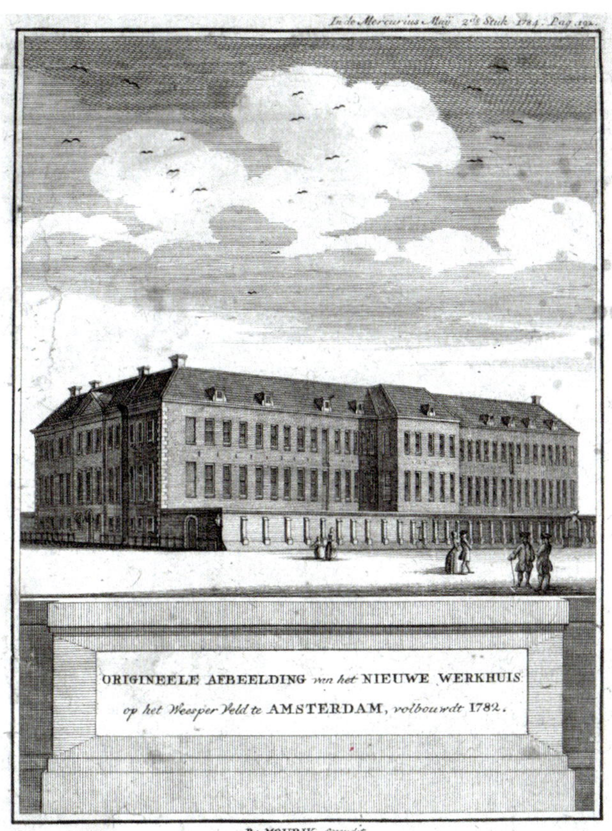

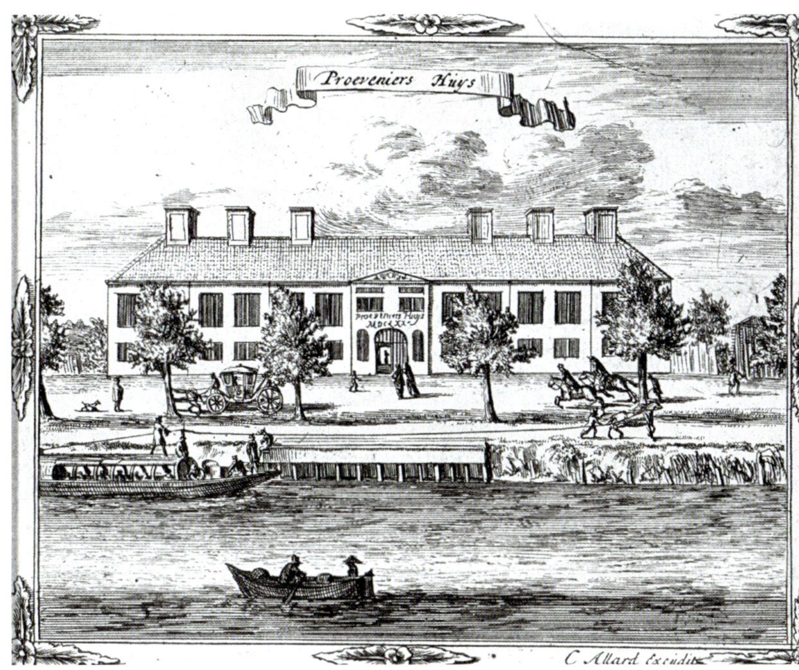

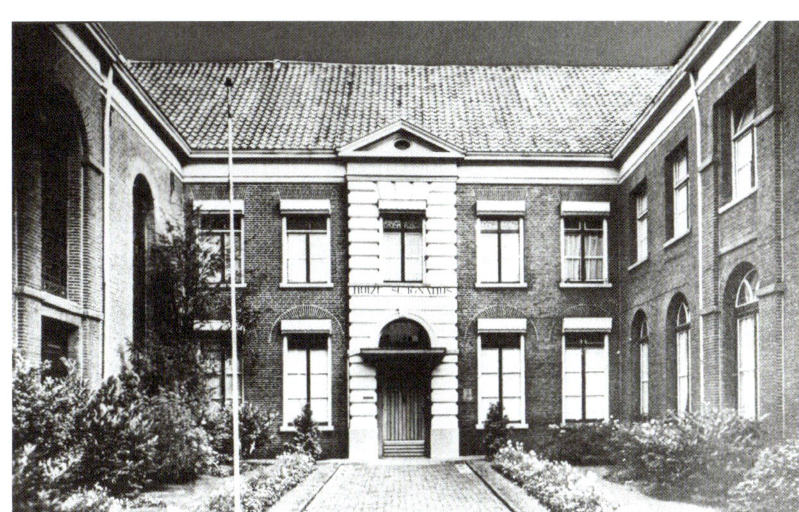

Carré

J.D. Zocher Jr.

Meerenberg
Santpoort
1844-1849

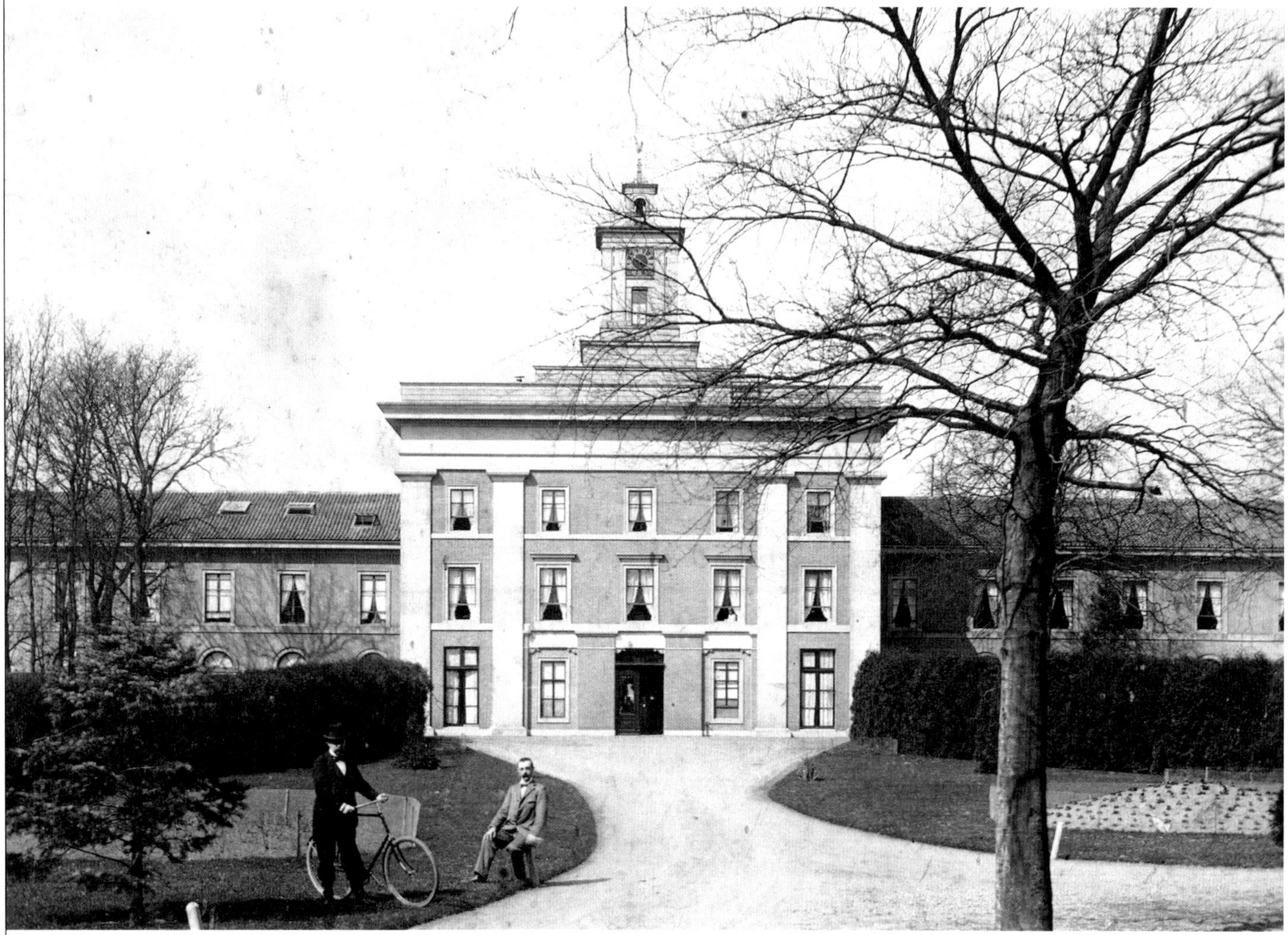

In 1843 the provincial administration of North Holland purchased the Meer en Berg estate in the dunes in Santpoort to build a provincial mental asylum. Surrounded by high dunes and a variegated park landscape, Meerenberg was the first asylum to be situated in a rural setting. The 300-patient asylum was designed by the well-known Haarlem architect and garden architect J.D. Zocher Jr. He applied the square-corridor system. The complex consists of four wings that enclose a courtyard. A long central corridor separates the men's ward from the women's. The central volume that stands out from the façade houses the director's office, the trustees' room, accommodation for physicians and non-medical staff, the archive, the kitchens, the depot and the pharmacy. On either side of the central volume are the wings for the first-class and second-class patients. The corner pavilions and the wings behind them are for third-class patients. The isolation cells for the third class are at the rear. The therapeutic bath installations, ranging from jets of water and showers to less vigorous forms of therapy, are placed at strategic points where the units of the different classes border on one another.

The wings are connected with one another by long, wide corridors which the patients can use for walks when the weather is bad. The gardens, where the patients of the first and second class can take a stroll, are situated in front of the asylum, where there are also verandahs. The designated walking areas for the third class are indoors. All employees live in the main building; the nurses have rooms of their own near the patients. The medical superintendent is accommodated in the renovated coach-house of the former estate.

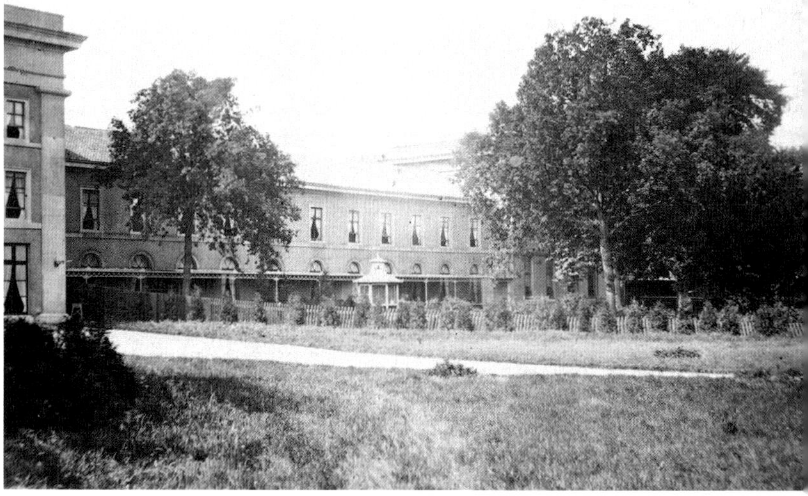

bottom
Ground floor and first floor

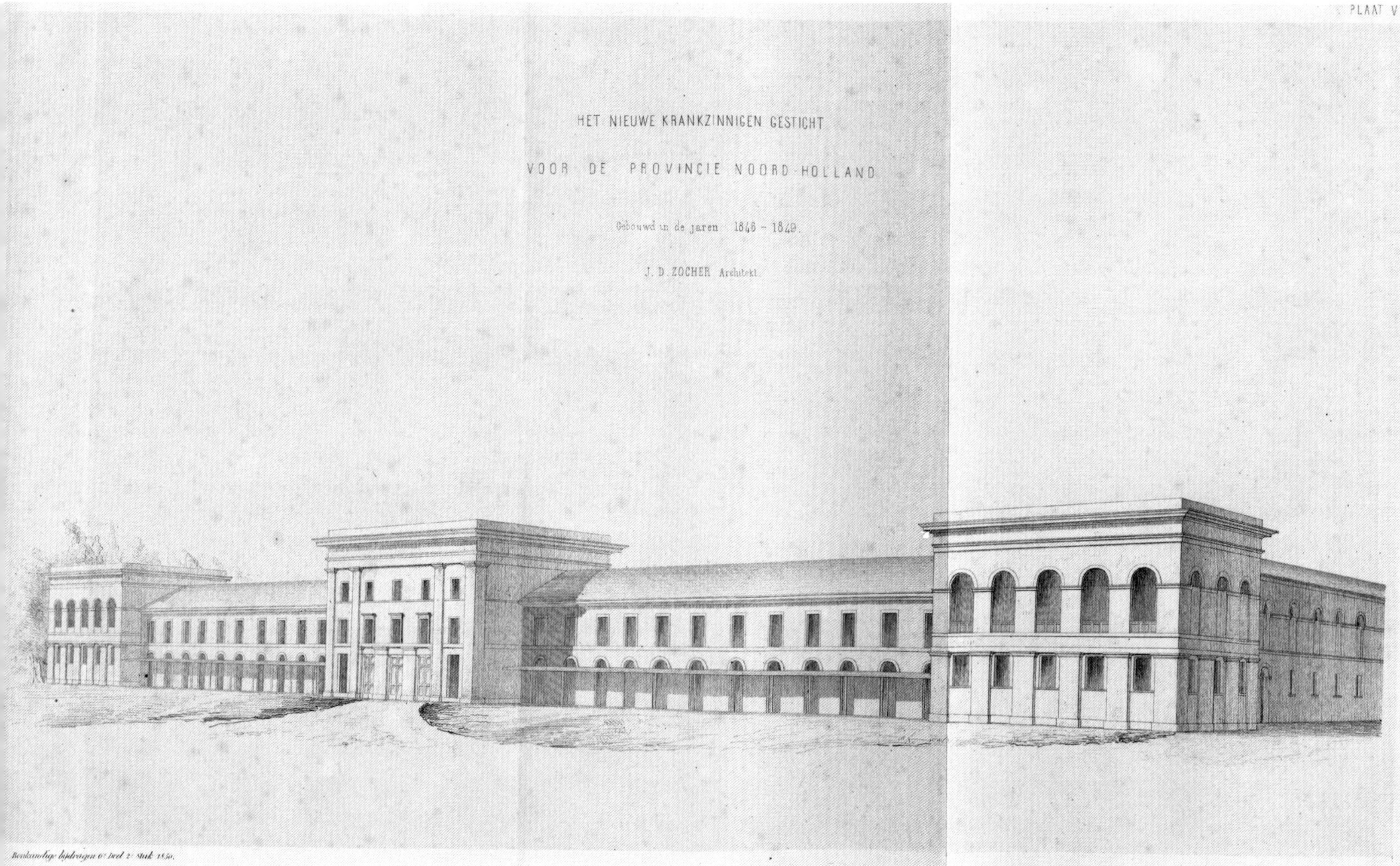

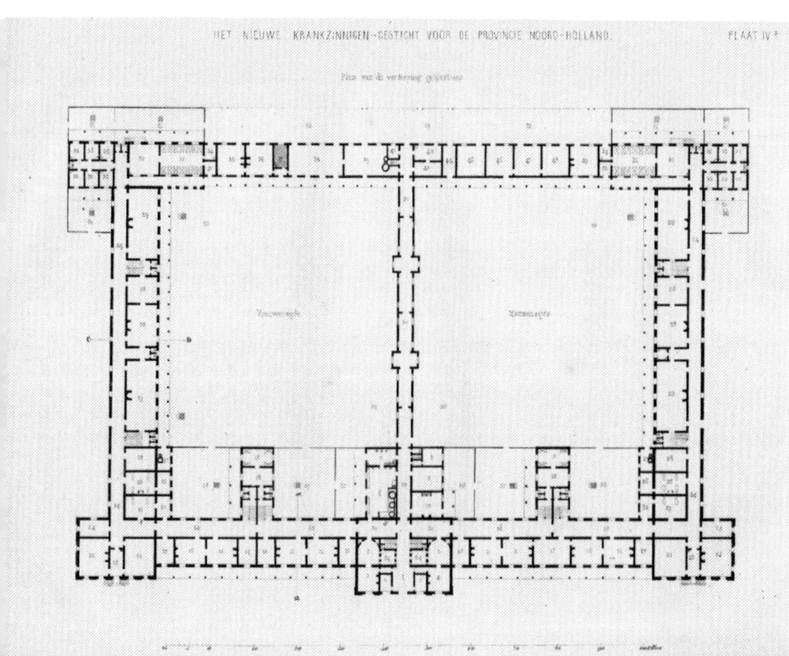

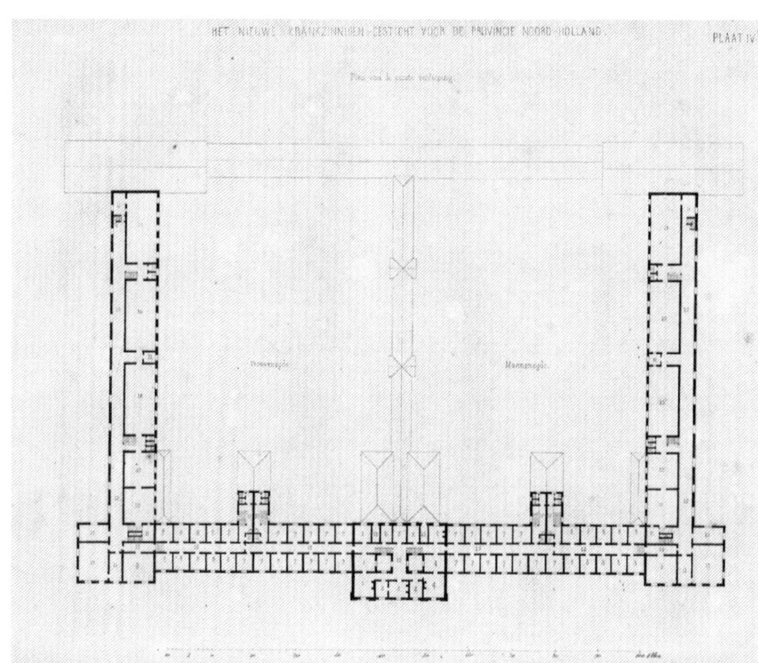

Pavilions

E.G. Wentink

Veldwijk
Ermelo
1884

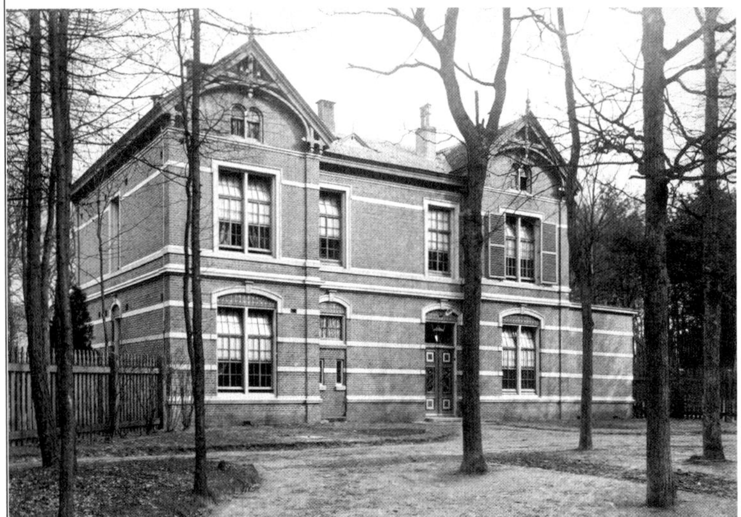

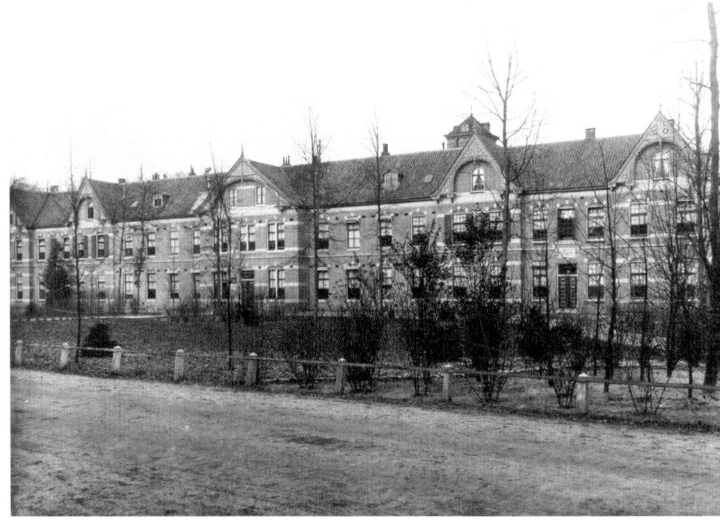

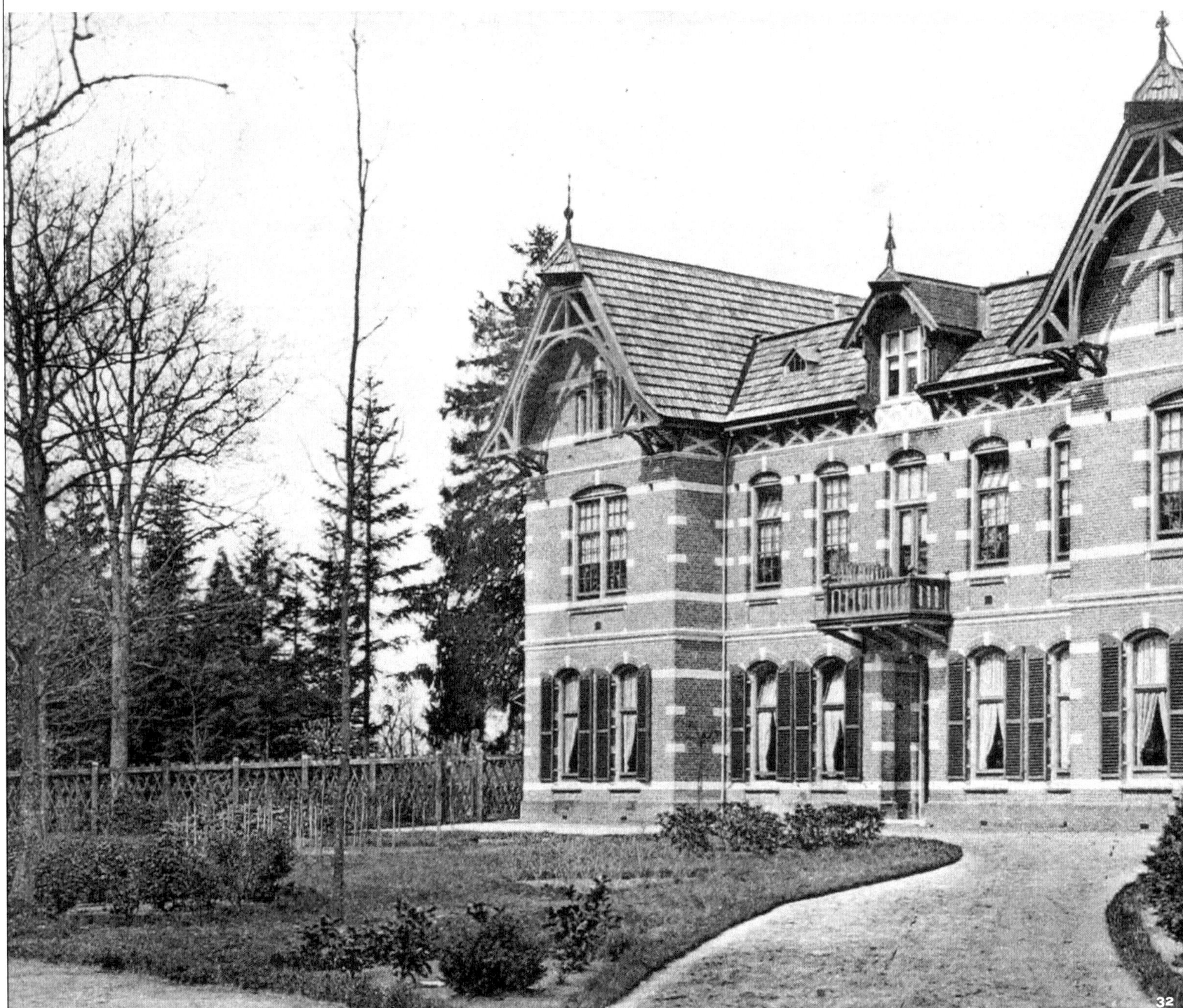

p. 32 | <
Heesteroord, pavilion for semi-quiet patients, first and second class

p. 32 | >
Main building

Sparrenheuvel, pavilion for women, first and second class

p. 33
Situation

The Association for the Protestant Care of the Insane and Neurasthenics in the Netherlands of the Dutch Reformed Church commissioned the architect E.G. Wentink to design its first mental asylum. Inspired by German models, Wentink applied the pavilion system to the Veldwijk asylum. This was entirely new to mental institutions in the Netherlands. Each pavilion is supervised by a male and a female superintendent who form a kind of family with the patients. The association believed that the cosiness of the family had a positive influence on the healing process. That was quite in accordance with Christian morality.

Wentink's design is fairly symmetrical. An axis divides the site into two. The west side is for female patients, the east side for male ones. The main building that houses the administration and the storage rooms is in the middle of the axis. On either side of the main building are the pavilions where the patients are first brought for observation. Along the axis behind the main building are the kitchen with the laundry, the chapel, a cell building for restless patients, and the building for patients with contagious diseases. The pavilions for first-class and second-class quiet patients are close to the main building, but are placed somewhat out of line with the other pavilions. Behind the observation pavilions are the pavilions for the third-class quiet patients and the semi-quiet patients from all three classes. Apart from the pavilions for first-class and second-class quiet patients, all of the pavilions have an enclosed garden of their own. The first-class and second-class quiet patients have full use of the asylum grounds.

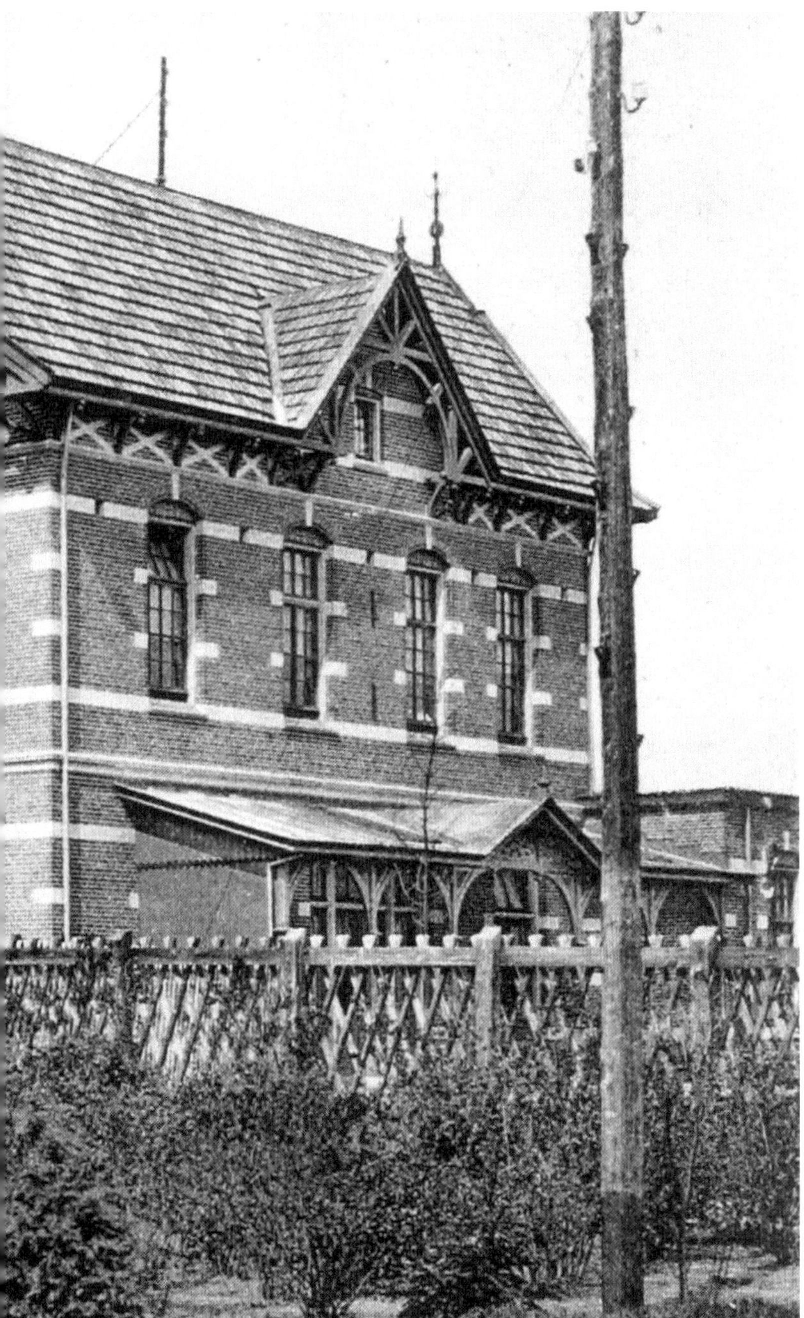

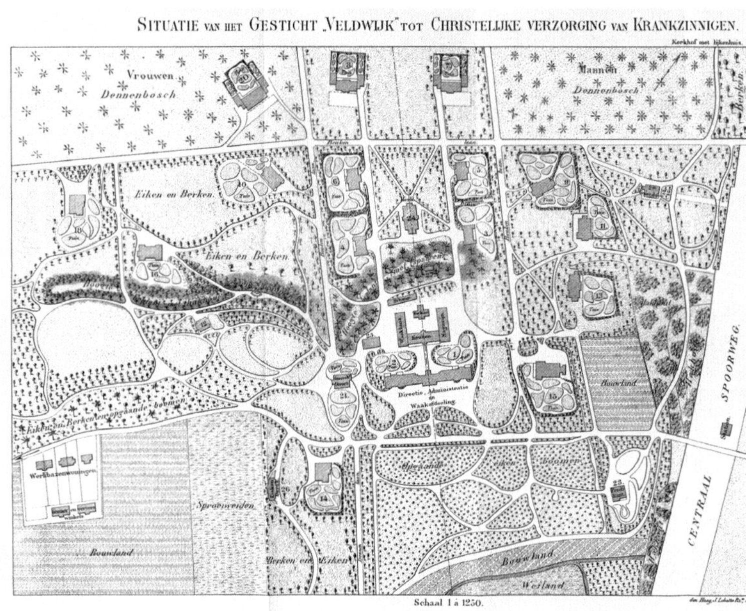

J.J. van Nieukerken

Algemeen Provinciaal-, Stads- en Academisch Ziekenhuis
Groningen
1903

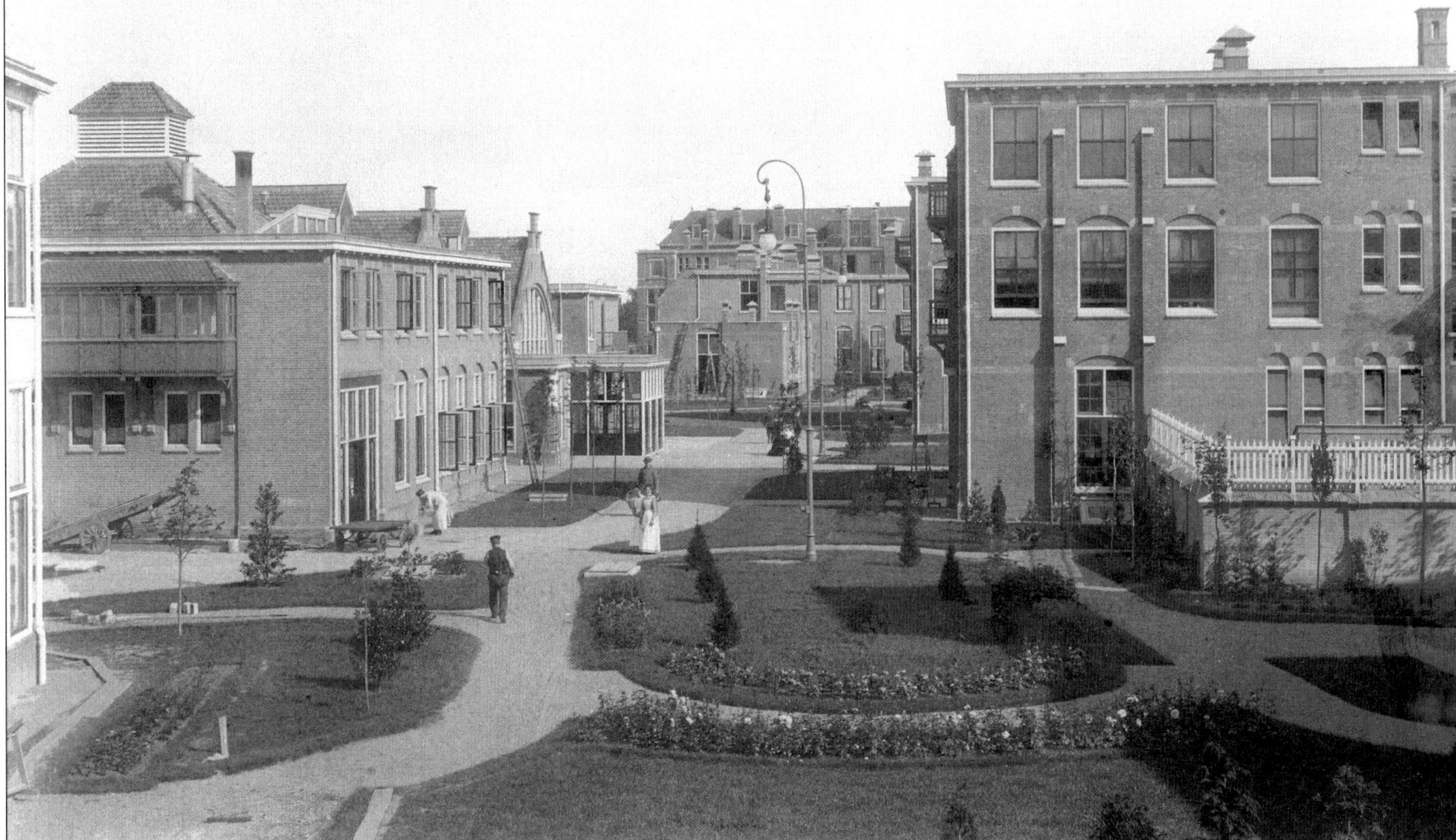

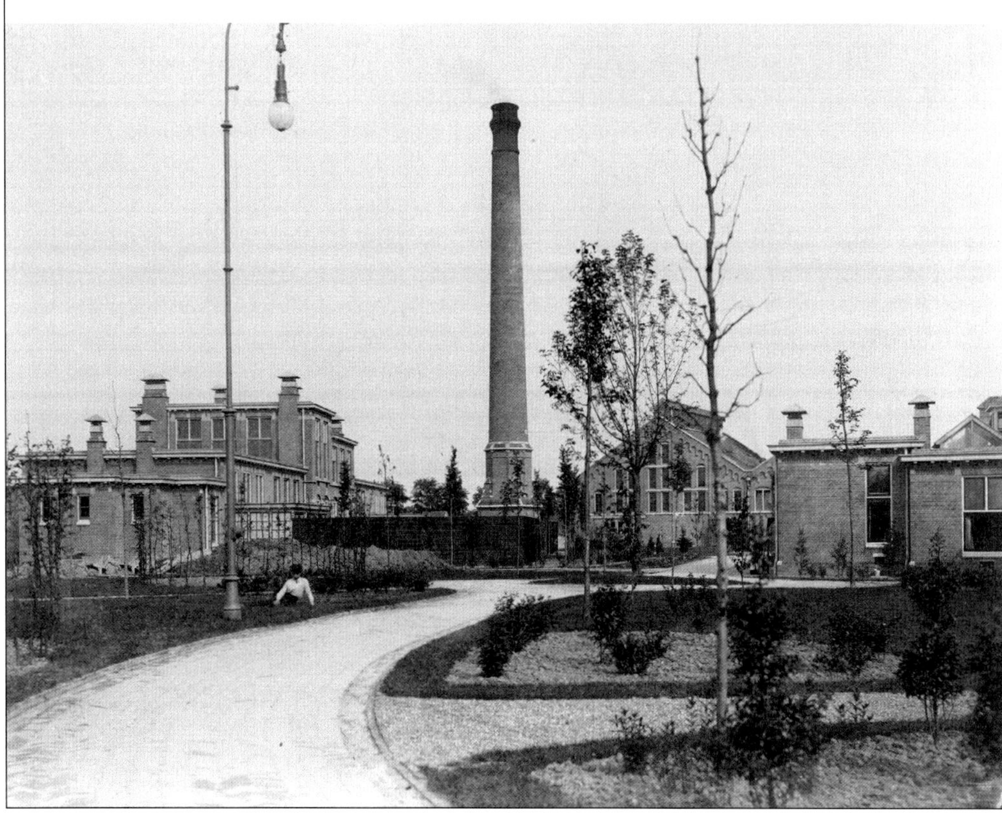

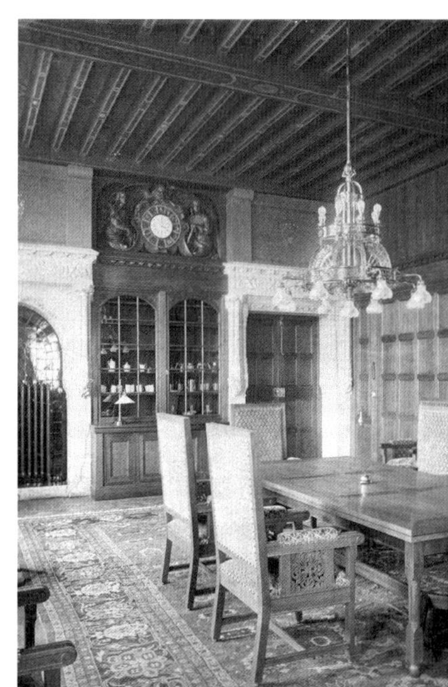

J.J. van Nieukerken built a new complex on the former fortifications to the east of the inner city. It functioned as a general hospital for the city and environs as well as a university teaching hospital. Van Nieukerken distributed the programme among three clusters. The medical cluster contained buildings for internal medicine as well as rooms for the psychiatric unit and barracks for contagious diseases. The surgical cluster also contained rooms for paediatric illnesses and a pavilion for syphilis patients. The third cluster targeted gynaecological complaints. The complex was completed by an administration building and a boiler house. The historicising style is typical of the late nineteenth and early twentieth centuries, but although the architect harks back to the past, his design can immediately be recognised as characteristic of the period in which it was built. The construction and the mechanically manufactured brick are contemporary, and the solution to the logistical challenges that the architect faced was only possible thanks to modern methods of construction. In the meantime the disadvantages of the pavilion system had been revealed. They were mitigated in this design by a well-conceived internal traffic structure in underground tunnels. Each cluster had laboratories, outpatient rooms, medical investigation rooms and teaching and observation rooms where the students could train in medical science.

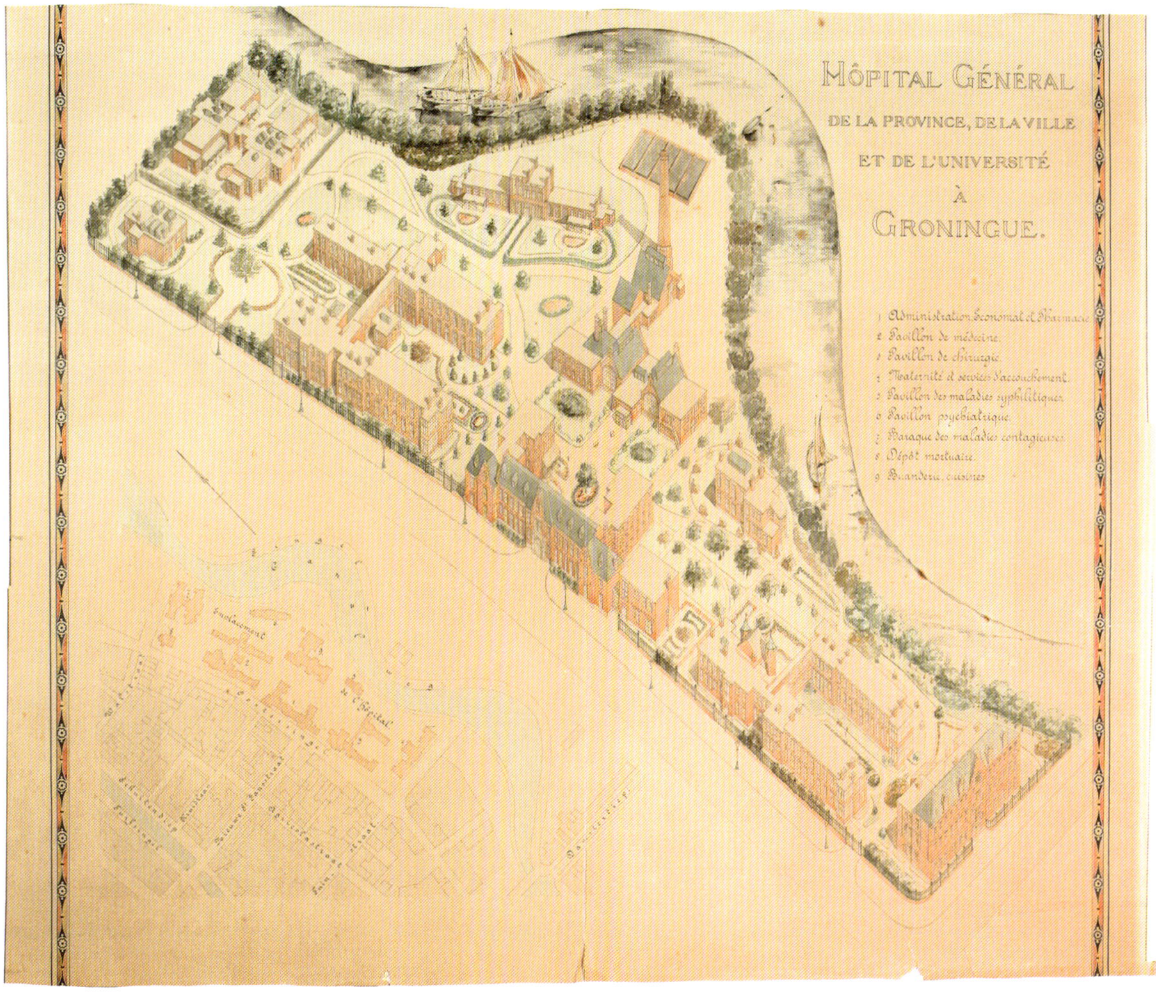

p. 34
View from the north, with at the left the kitchen, on the background the women's clinic and at the right the administration building

View from the northwest, with the psychiatric department at the left, the boiler house in the centre and the kitchen at the right

Board room

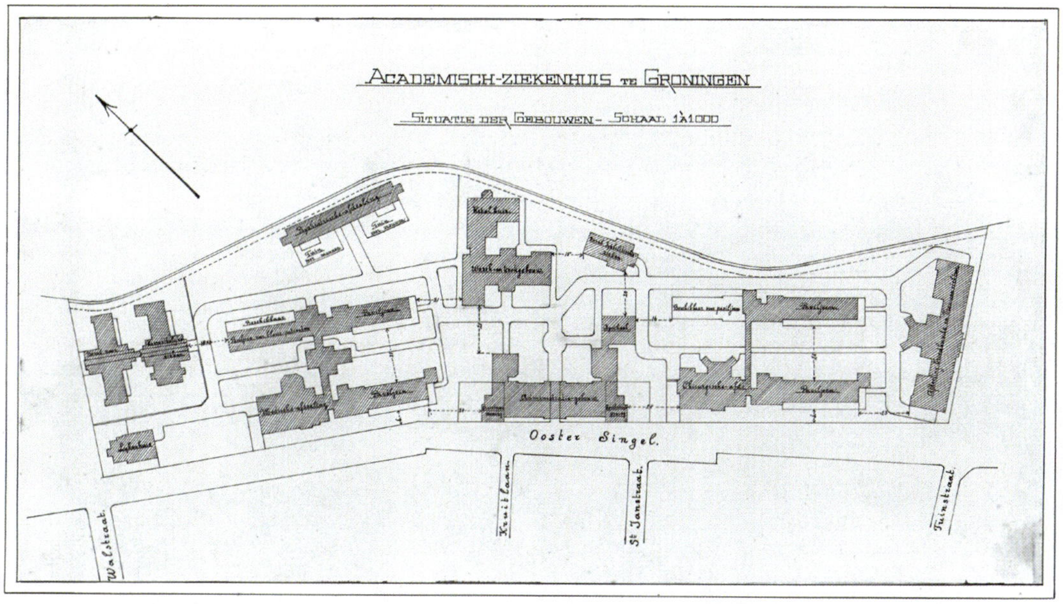

Chalet

F.W.M. Poggenbeek

Willem Arntsz Hoeve
Den Dolder
1909-1912

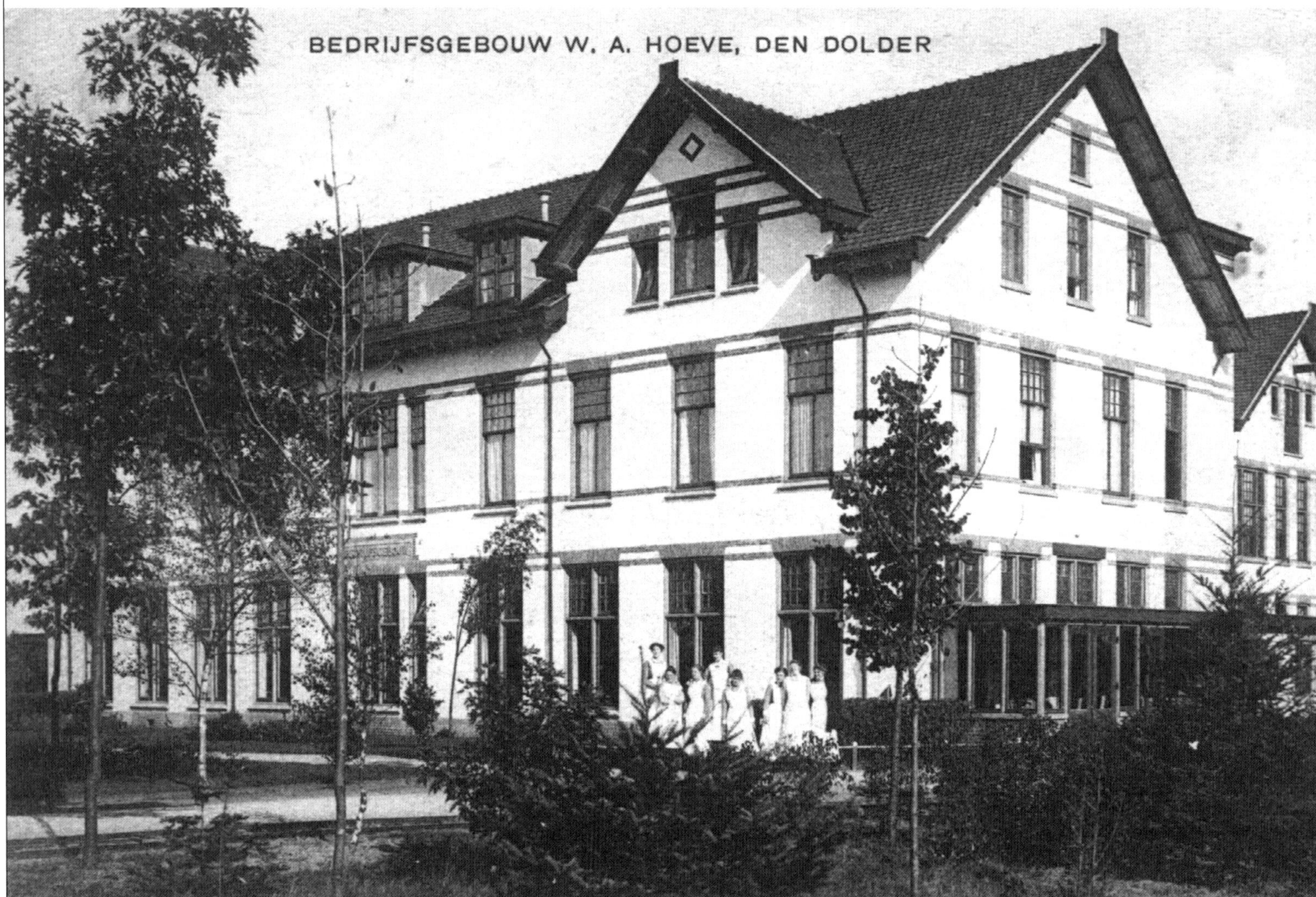

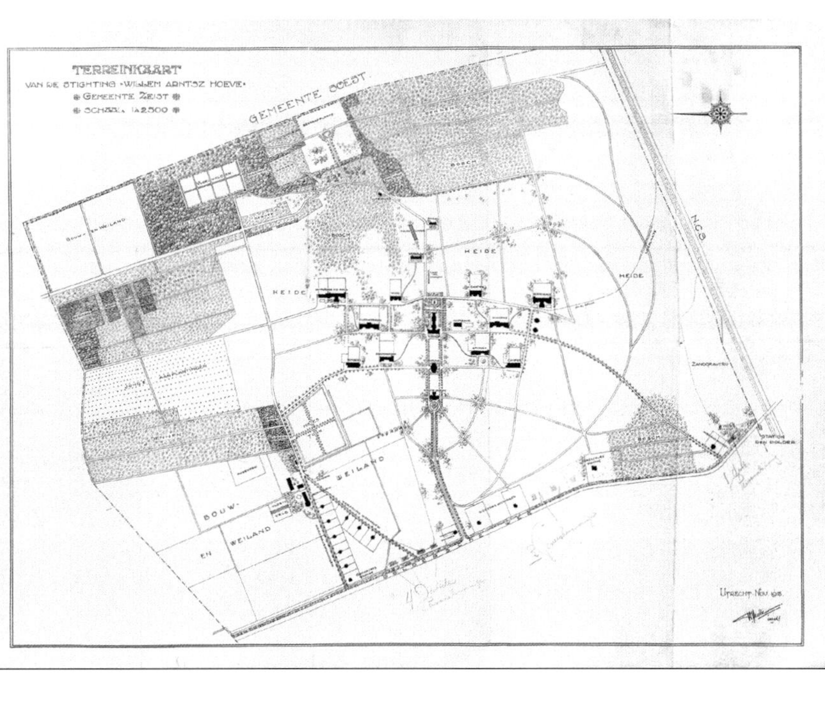

p. 36
Utilities building

p. 37
Pavilion for ill and weak patients, third class

Auditorium

Management building

Van Leeuwenhoek pavilion, for ill and weak male patients, third class

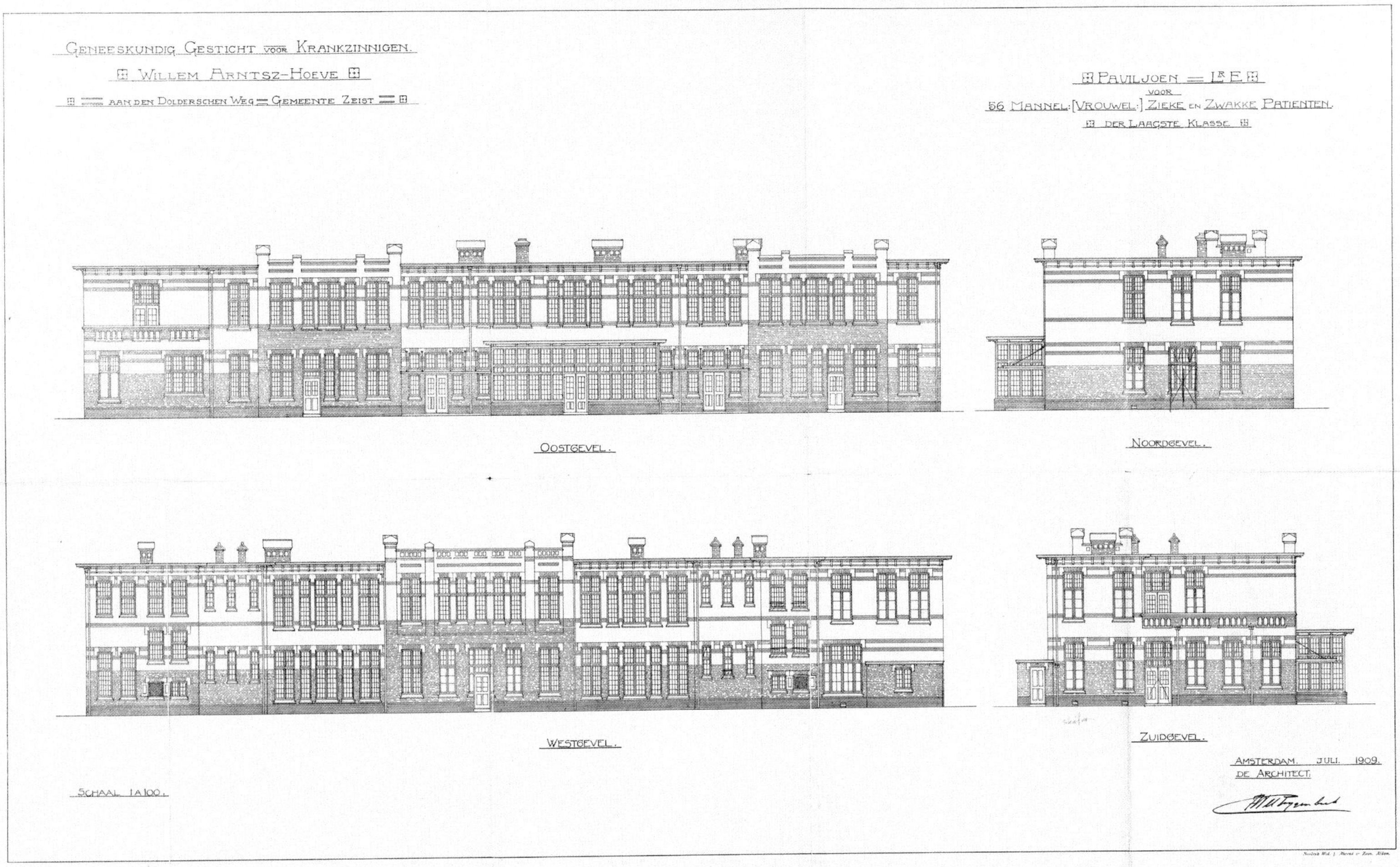

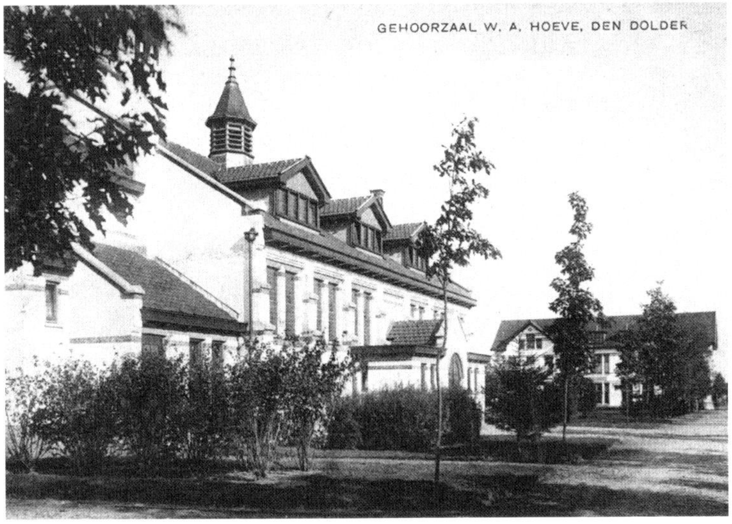

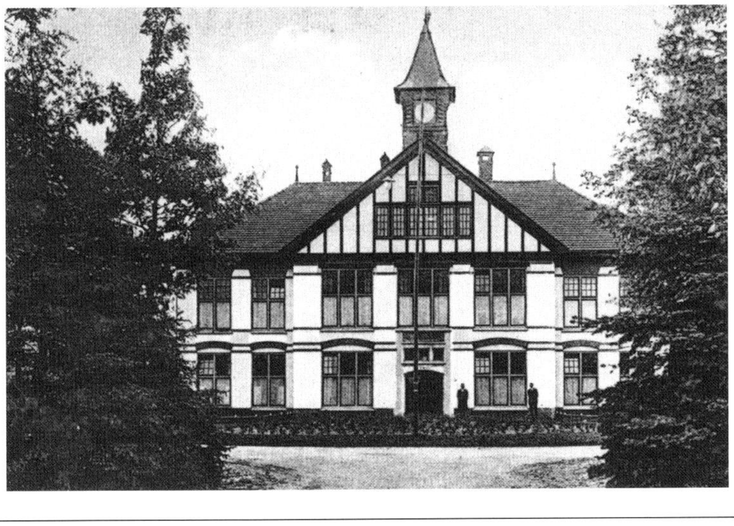

The Willem Arntsz Huis in the historic city centre of Utrecht is one of the many examples of psychiatric hospitals in the Netherlands to found a 'rural asylum' towards the end of the nineteenth and the beginning of the twentieth century. Part of the treatment in the Willem Arntsz Hoeve involved working on the farm and in the workshops, a form of work therapy. The annex expanded to become a large-scale complex that would have been inconceivable in or near the city. The whole complex was set up in accordance with the pavilion system.

In 1906 the Willem Arntsz Huis in Utrecht commissioned the architects G. van Heerde and H. Masselink to build a farm that was intended primarily to nurse rural patients in a family-like situation. The core of the complex, designed by F.W.M. Poggenbeek, was built between 1909 and 1912. The buildings are in the chalet style that was particularly common for villas. The outside walls are plastered and decorated with brick safety arches above the window-frames and doors and horizontal strips above and below the windows. The 207-hectare site is surrounded by woods. Arranged on a central axis are a management building, a utilities building with the central kitchen, and sleeping quarters for the staff. Between these buildings is the auditorium, a place where the patients could relax and where musical and stage performances were given. Ten spacious pavilions, arranged in rough symmetry, flank the central axis.

The pavilions on one side were for men, those on the other side for women. A distinction was made between three classes of patient. The pavilions for the first class were closest to the management building, while the third-class pavilions were further away.

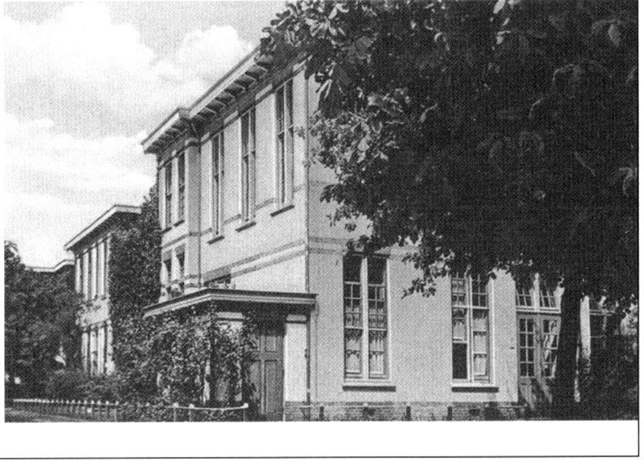

Representation

W. Kromhout

De Engelenbergstichting
Kampen
1911-1916

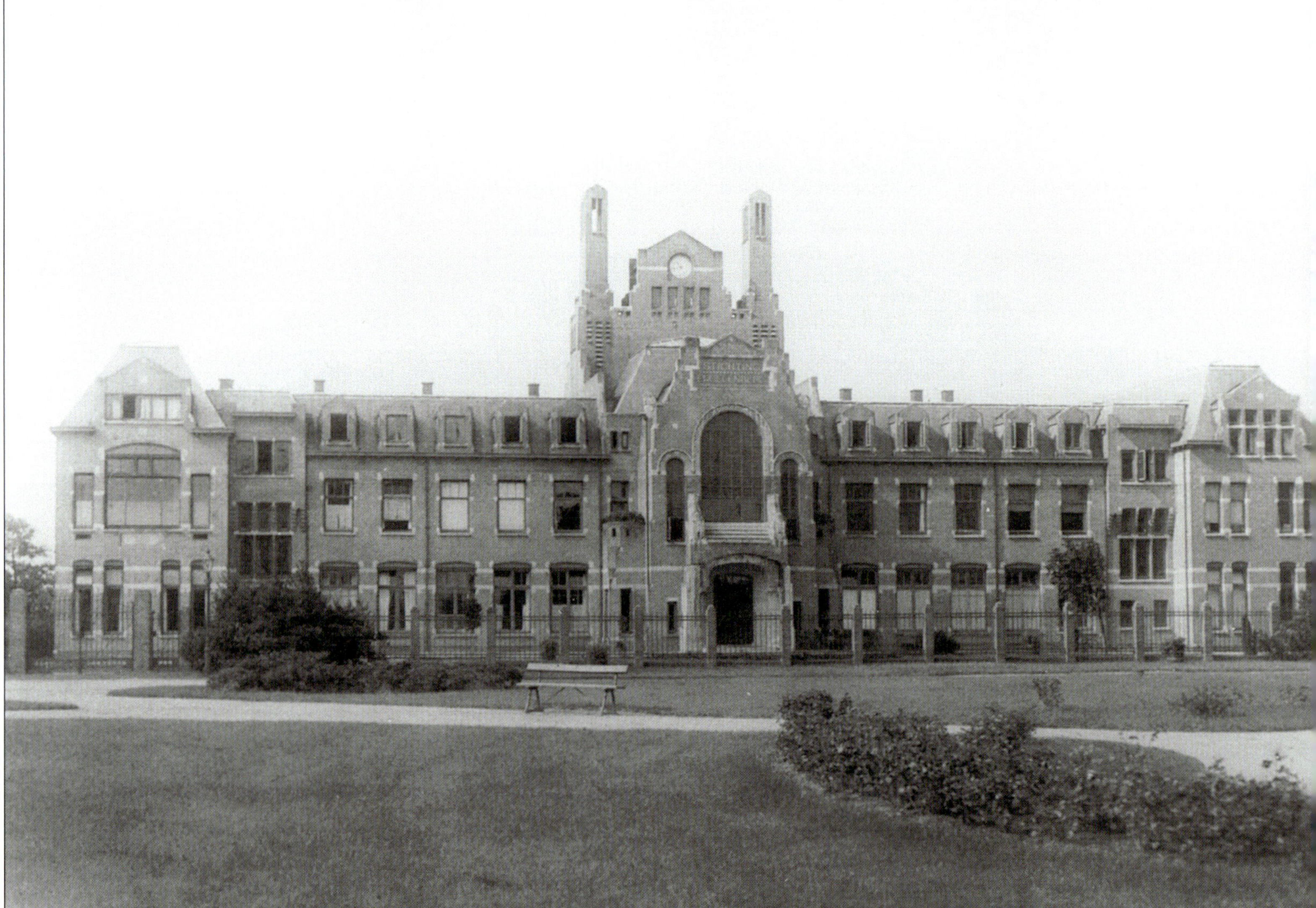

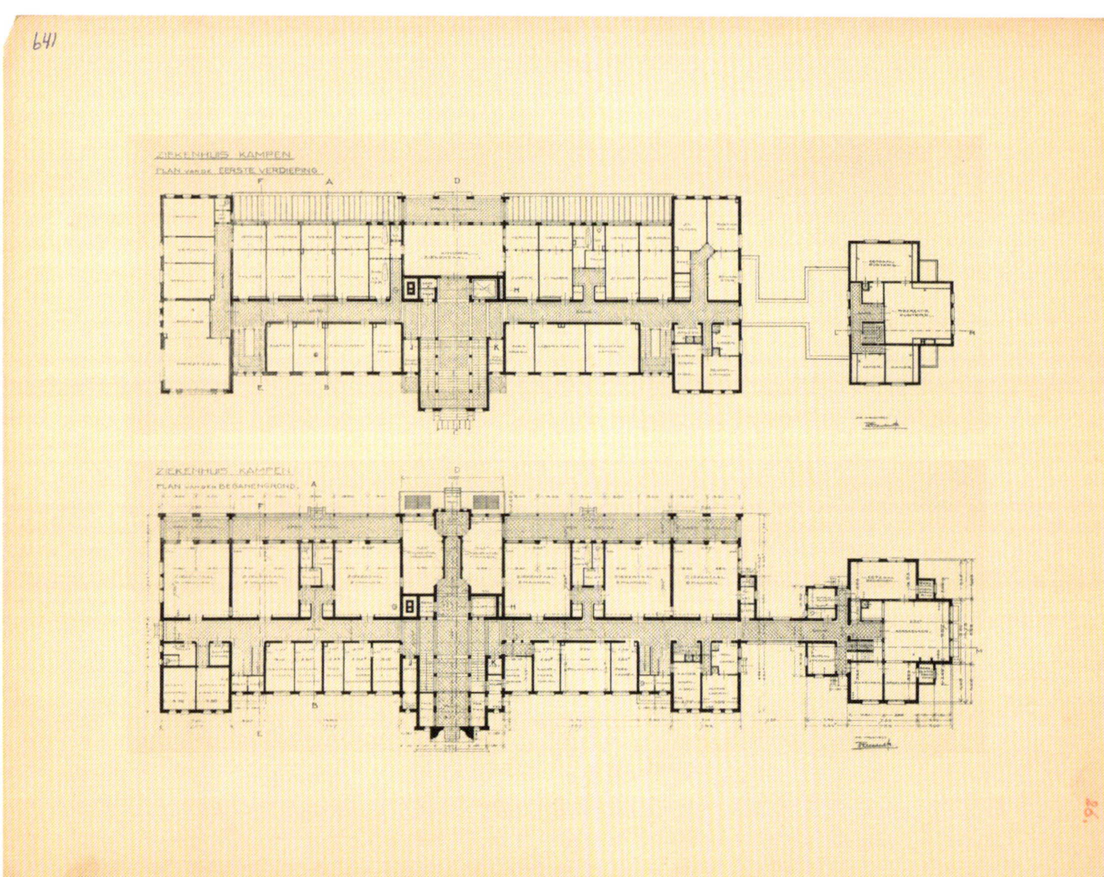

De Engelenbergstichting is a relatively small hospital. The design was by W. Kromhout, who was considered one of the big three Dutch architects – together with K.P.C. de Bazel and H.P. Berlage – at the beginning of the twentieth century. The building had 72 beds (eight or nine per ward), a few rooms for well-to-do patients, and a children's ward. The structure was symmetrical with a prominent central section. The remarkably tall chimneys heightened the architectural effect. This was where the ventilation ducts from the wards emerged. The demand for constant fresh air necessitated special solutions of this kind, which had been unnecessary in the old pavilion system. The architecture is typical of the attempt of the big three to break with the historicising styles that flourished in the nineteenth century and were only gradually yielding ground under pressure of modern views. With this hospital, Kromhout demonstrated that the contemporary design style could produce public buildings with a pronounced representative character.

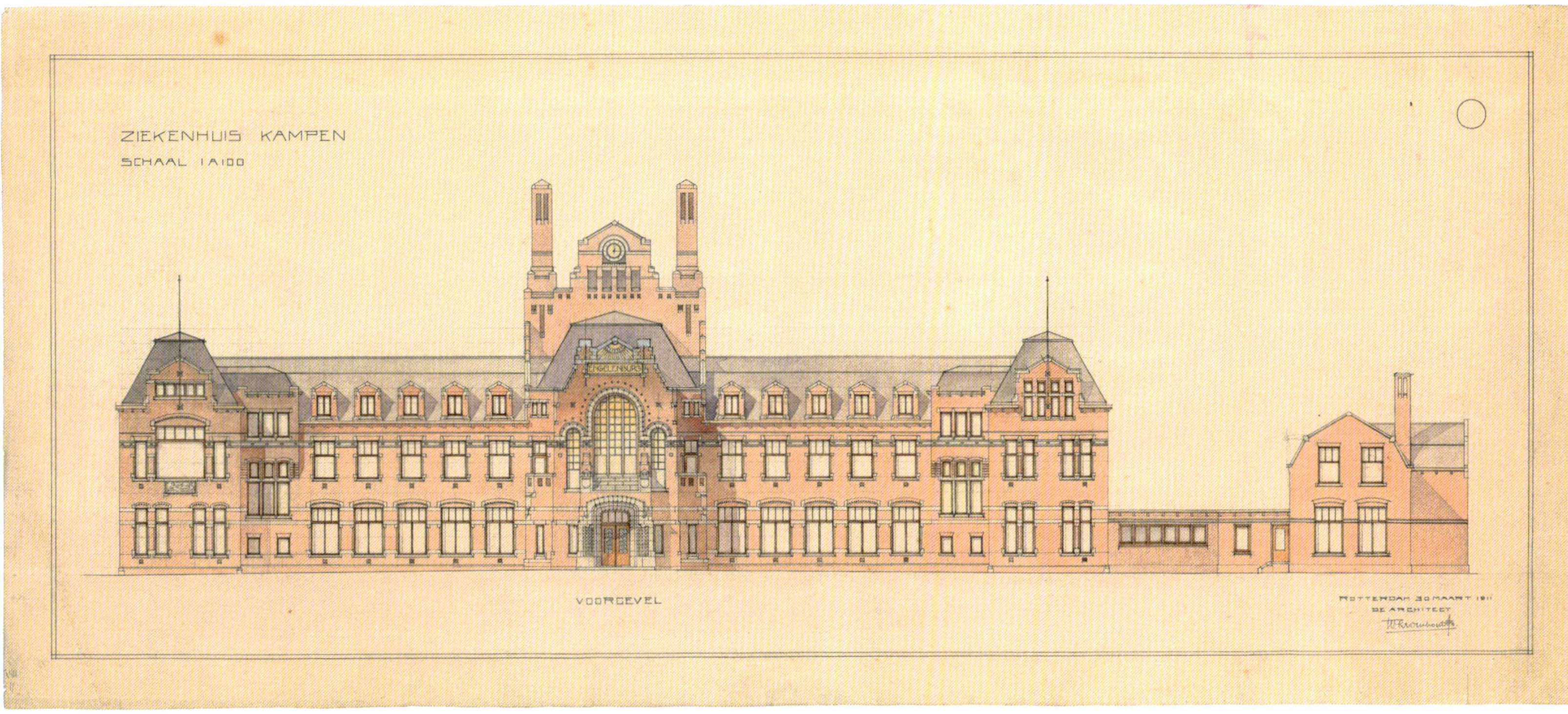

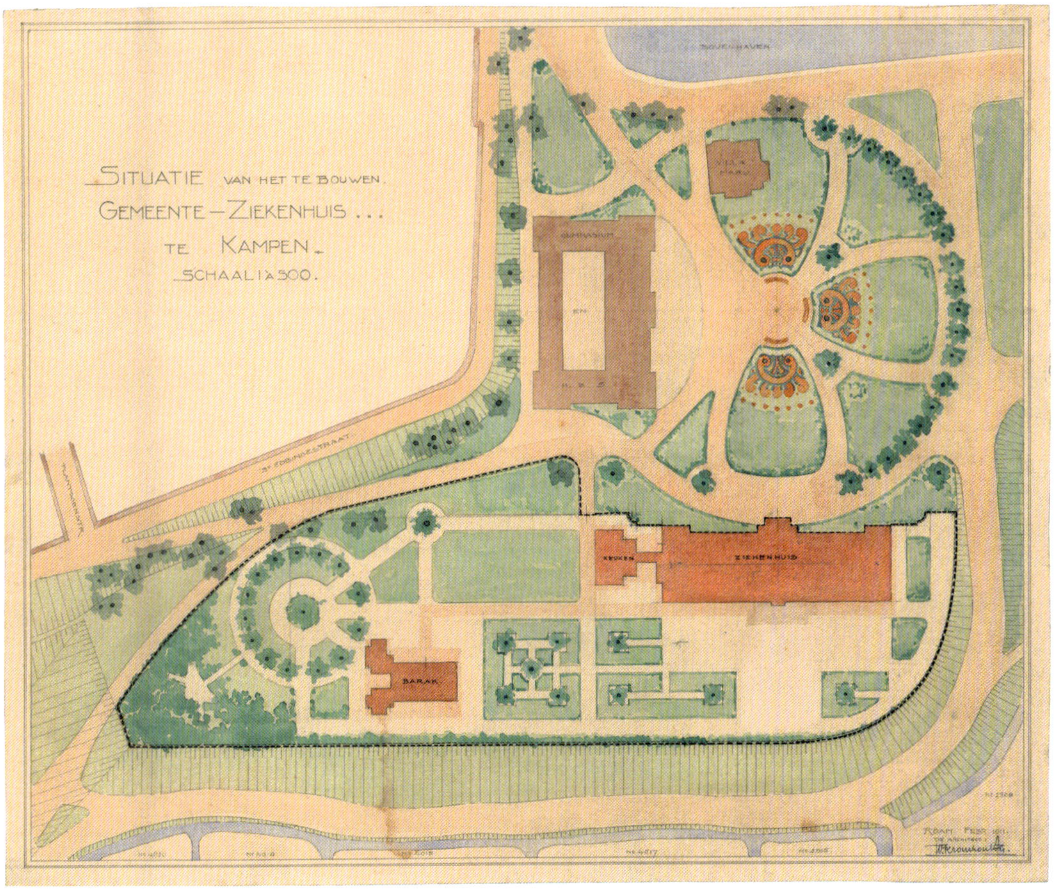

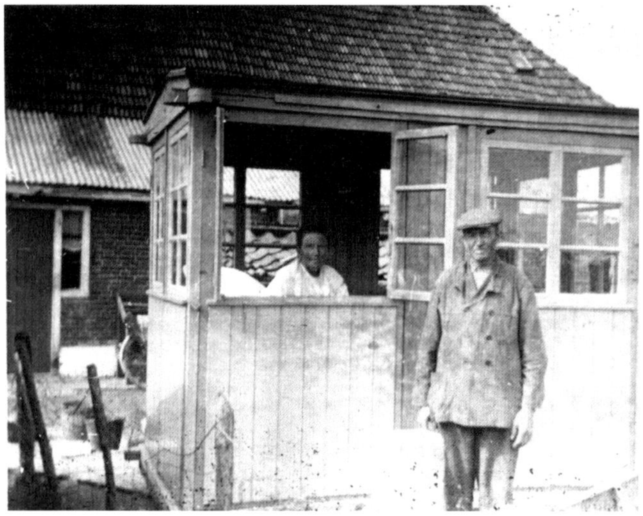

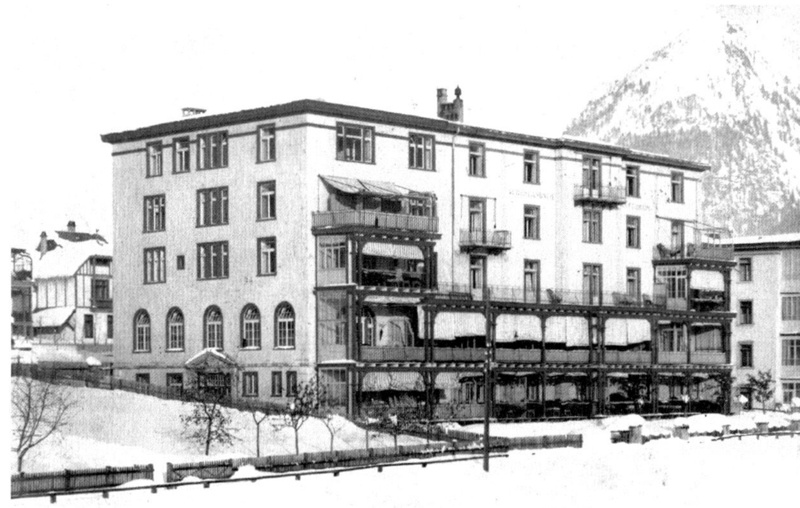

Sanatoria for tuberculosis patients

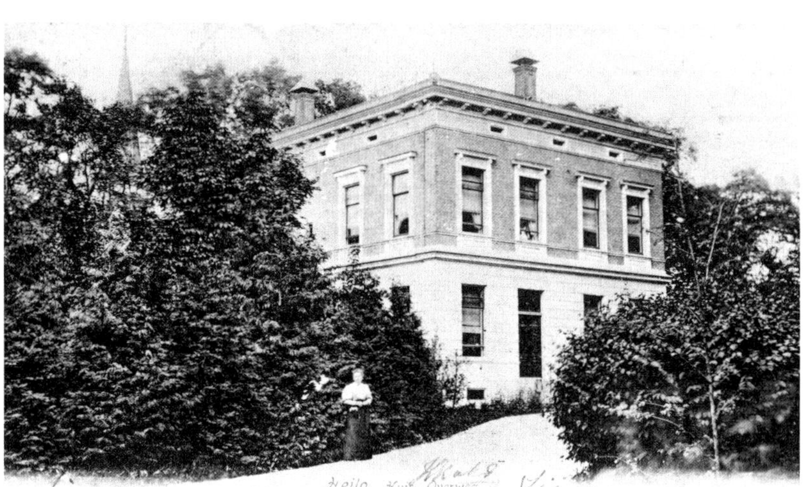

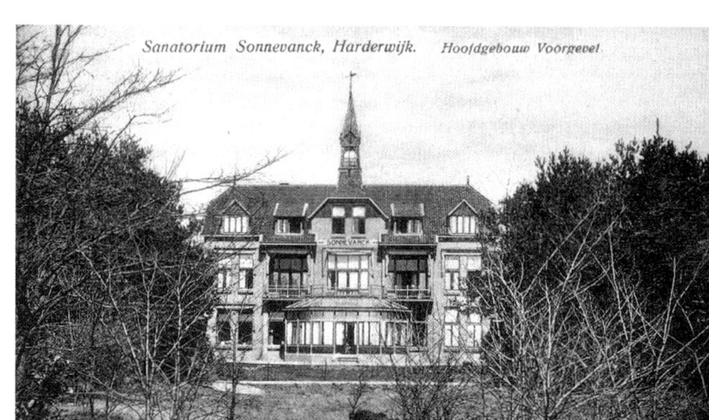

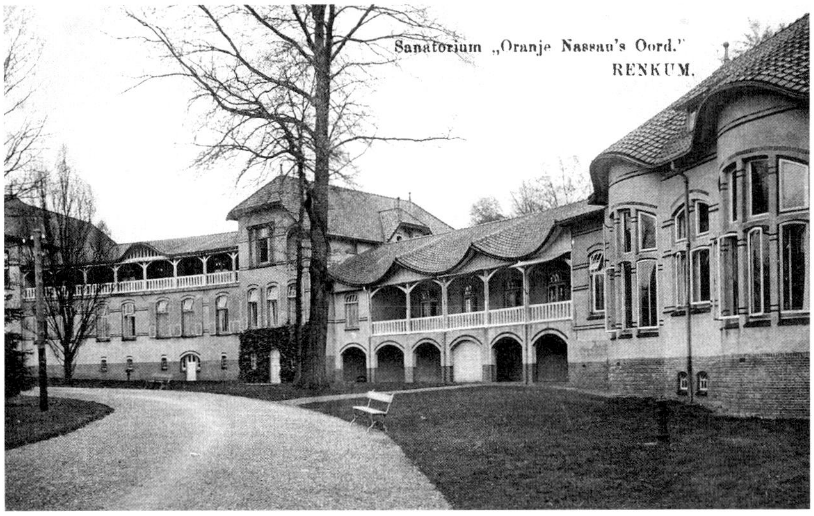

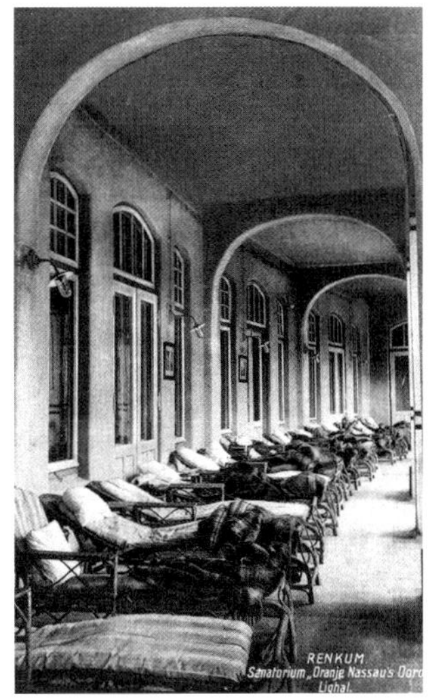

Top
Pavilion for home nursing

M.A. van Nieukerken, Dutch sanatorium, Davos, 1907

R. Kuipers, Oranje Nassau's Oord, Renkum. Main building and lounge.

Bottom
Huis Overweg, Heiloo, 1898

H.J. Tiemens Jr, Sanatorium Sonnevanck, Harderwijk, 1910. Main building.

J.J. van Nieukerken, Sanatorium Beekbergen, Beekbergen, 1910

Ed. Cuypers, Sanatorium Dekkerswald, Groesbeek, 1913. The garden with the main building and a swivelling lounge.

The word sanatorium literally means a building that makes people healthy. It has been used for a variety of institutions since the last quarter of the nineteenth century. In psychiatry it referred to buildings for patients who voluntarily requested treatment, which was different from the situation in the psychiatric institutions. The pendant of this was the tuberculosis sanatorium. Tuberculosis (TB) was a frequent complaint until late in the twentieth century. Although it is highly contagious, at first no one new exactly how it is transmitted. There were no medicines for it. The only remedy was to spend time in a climate with plenty of clean and fresh air. The fact that tuberculosis was much more common in the cities than in the countryside led the English physician George Bodington to propose this remedy first. The aim of the TB sanatorium is to offer this climate inside a building. This type thus harks back to the origin of the hospital, which began its remarkable evolution at the end of the eighteen century as a ventilation machine. The building of a respectable number of TB sanatoria began towards the end of the nineteenth century, and by 1950 the Netherlands had fifty-nine with a total capacity of nine thousand beds. There was thus only room for a fraction of the patients. Small, partly open pavilions were made available for individual patients for whom the sanatorium was not an option.

The ideal, however, was to spend time in the mountains – nowhere was the air purer than there. The basis for a successful method of treatment was laid by the German physician Hermann Brehmer. He had himself become infected by tuberculosis during his student years and gone to the Himalayas on the advice of his doctor. After returning home a cured man, he changed his course of study in order to be able to devote himself to the illness. As a physician he opened a sanatorium for the treatment of tuberculosis patients in Görbersdorf (then in Germany, now in Poland) in 1854. The most important element in the treatment that he recommended was spending time in the open air. Though situated in a low-lying mountainous region, the observance of strict schedules could yield results comparable with those from a stay in the higher regions. His sanatorium was situated in the middle of a large park and consisted of pavilions, grottos, and a dense network of paths with a total of 360 benches beside them. His assistant Peter Dettweiler continued Brehmer's work and opened the Falkenstein sanatorium in 1876. He placed more emphasis on rest in the treatment. His patients spent the day in lounges reclining on *chaises longues*. This phenomenon was widely copied in the Netherlands. Many sanatoria were built from the end of the nineteenth century on. It is noteworthy that the sanatorium movement got under way at the same time as the discovery of the tuberculosis bacillus by Robert Koch in 1882. The cause of the disease was now known, but it was years before an effective medicine was found.

The first Dutch sanatorium was built outside the country in the Swiss mountains near Davos in 1897. The Association for the Promotion of the Interests of Needy Dutch Pulmonary Patients, which was founded in the same year, collected money to enable impecunious TB patients to travel to Davos too. A new building near the villa that had initially been used was completed for the sanatorium between 1905 and 1907. The architect was M.A. van Nieukerken, who also spent some time there, as well as writing a booklet on TB sanatoria.[1] This booklet included recommendations on suitable grounds for a sanatorium. Dry sandy soil, preferably on a high location and near pine forests, was preferred. The air in the surroundings must be clean; dust, dirt, water and smoke were taboo. The building should be sheltered from northwesterly and

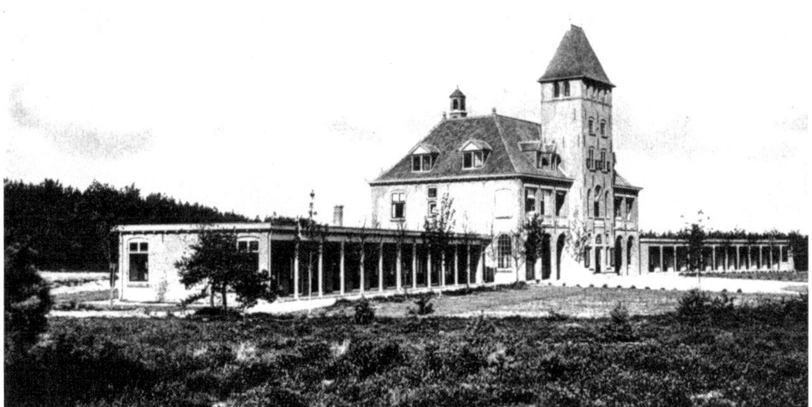

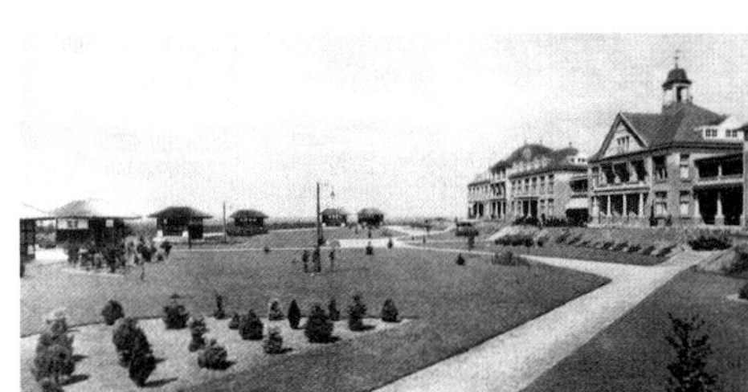

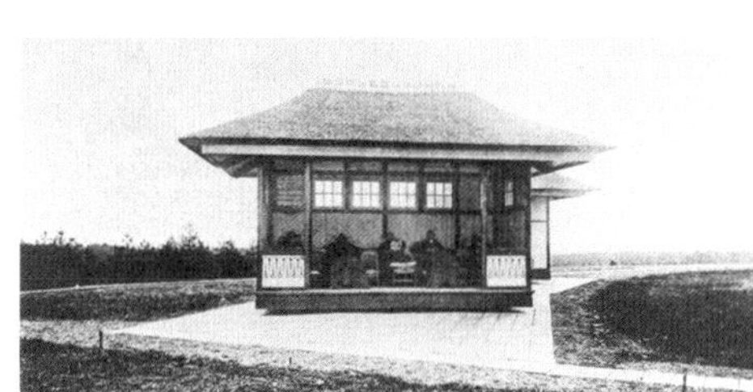

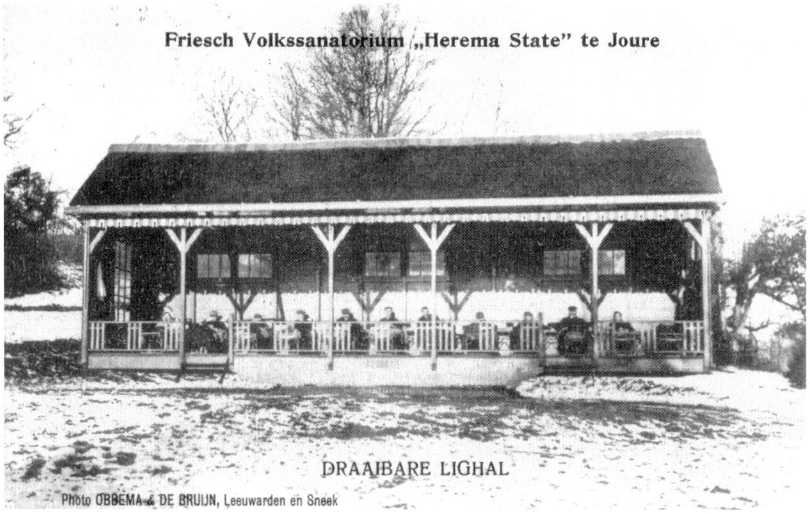

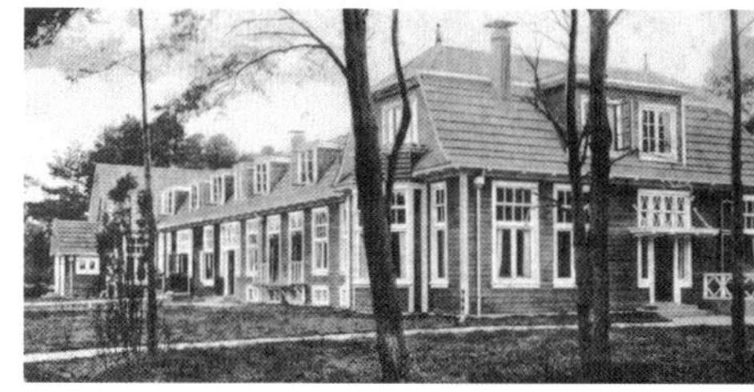

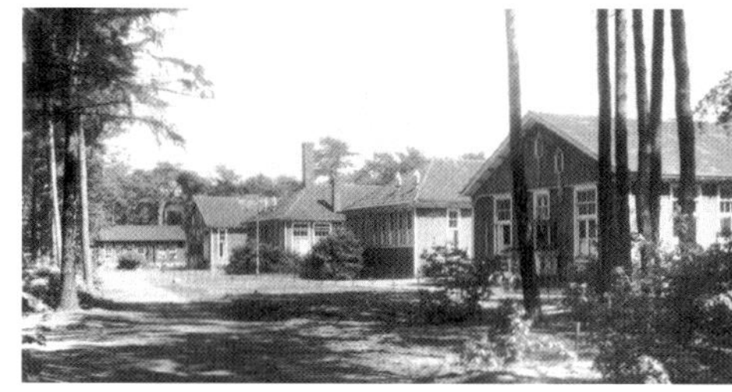

northeasterly winds, while sunlight should be admitted unimpeded on the south side. The main component of the sanatoria was the lounge. It was ideal if this could be turned towards the light, but Van Nieukerken considered this less necessary if the sanatorium was given broad verandahs.[2]

Long stays in Switzerland were expensive, which is why sanatoria were built in the Netherlands as well. The first was Huis Overweg in Heiloo in 1898, followed by Oranje Nassau's Oord near Renkum in 1899. The location on the south bank of a hill was regarded as particularly favourable, while tall trees provided shelter from the northeasterly wind.

The Association for Protestant Assistance to Tuberculosis Patients was set up in 1905, and with it the system of denominational compartmentalisation entered the world of the TB sanatoria. The association opened Sanatorium Sonnevanck in Harderwijk in 1908, with one pavilion for men and one for women. The main building, designed by H.J. Tiemens Jr, was completed two years later. This building contained not only the administration, laboratories, X-ray unit and so on, but also small rooms for one or two persons, each with its own lounge facing south, and larger rooms for eight to ten persons. Smaller pavilions, each with its swivelling lounge for reclining patients, were situated a little way from the main building. A large pavilion was added to the complex in 1925.

Sanatorium Beekbergen, situated in the village of the same name, was opened in 1910. It was designed by J.J. van Nieukerken. It is a symmetrical, fairly robust building with a somewhat higher Neo-Romanesque tower in the middle. It has a gently curving lounge for reclining patients on either side.

Naturally, there was also a demand for an institution for the treatment of Catholic pulmonary patients. Sanatorium Dekkerswald in Groesbeek was established for this purpose. A competition was organised and the design by Ed. Cuypers was selected from the fourteen entries. The plan has the shape of a half moon. After obtaining the commission, Cuypers went abroad on a study tour. He came to the conclusion that a T shape was more suitable than the half moon. He had already used the T shape himself before for the Hoog-Laren sanatorium in Laren, North Holland. He had encountered the same structure in the St. Gallisches Lungensanatorium near Wallenstadt in Switzerland and in the English King Edward VII Sanatorium in Midhurst. His submission to the competition was revised and approved in 1912. The opening took place at the end of 1913. The pavilions on either side of the main building are connected with it by wide corridors on the first and second floors. Above them is the sun terrace area. The medical service is accommodated in the central building. The patients' rooms for one or two patients are situated on the south side of the two pavilions on the ground floor; rooms for larger groups of patients are situated on the first and second floor.

The Friesch Volkssanatorium voor Onvermogende Beginnende Borstlijders (Friesian Sanatorium for Needy Incipient Pulmonary Patients) was established in the Herema State in Joure between 1910 and 1922. The nursing fee was low and affordable for the poor, whose ranks included many of the victims of the disease. In 1922 the sanatorium moved to a new complex in Appelscha. Sanatorium Berg en Bosch (1919-1920) was a small village of wooden buildings in the woods near Apeldoorn. Its small wooden cabins made it look more like a campsite than a sanatorium. It was intended as a temporary measure, and was closed down and replaced by a new sanatorium in Bilthoven in 1933.

The Protestant Association for the Establishment and Maintenance of Sanatoria for Tuberculosis Patients was

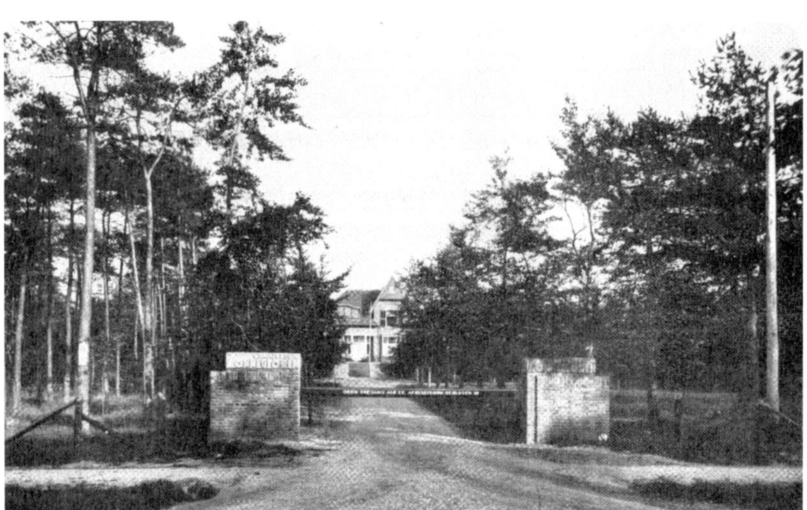

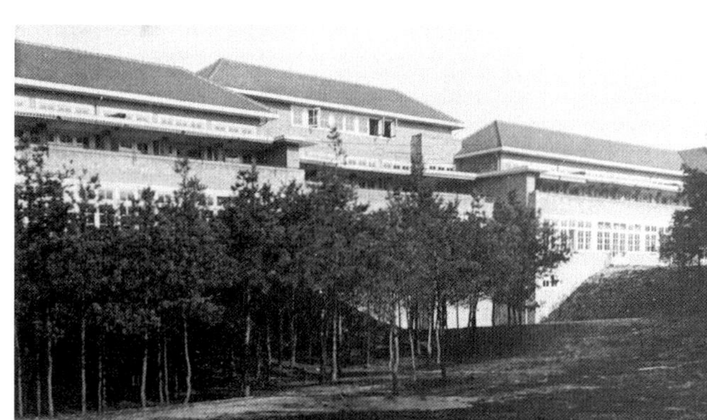

Top
Swivelling lounge, Friesch Volks-sanatorium, Joure

Friesch Volkssanatorium, Appelscha, 1922. Service building and pavilion for male patients.

B.J. Koldeweij and C.M. van Moorsel Pzn., Sanatorium Berg en Bosch, Bilthoven, 1933. Pavilion for male patients and lounge

Bottom
H.F. Mertens, Sanatorium Zonnegloren, Soest, 1927. Entrance with homes for nurses and sanatorium complex

A. Aalto, Paimio sanatorium, Finland, 1932

C.H. de Bever and C.M. van Moorsel Pzn., De Klokkenberg sanatorium, Breda, 1953

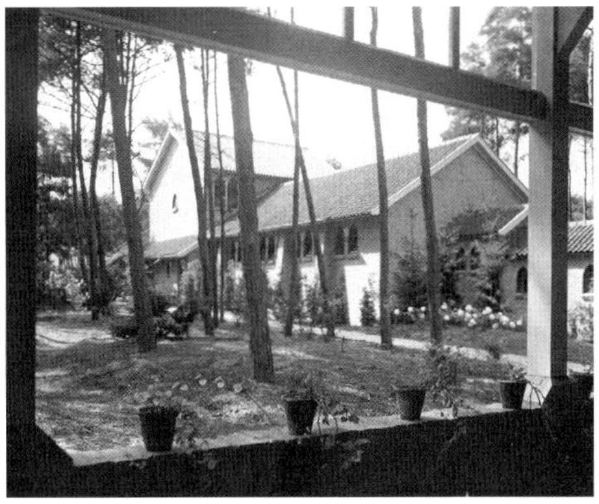

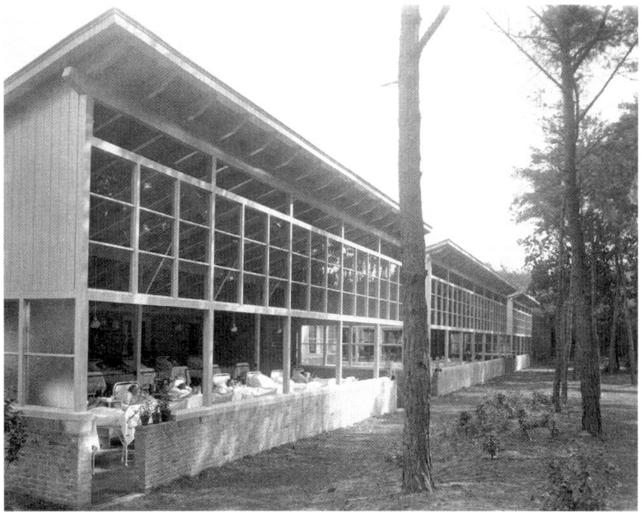

founded in 1921. The brochure extolling this institution of the Dutch Reformed Church naturally praised the endeavour to build Dutch Reformed sanatoria for members of its own persuasion.[3] The association purchased the Tjemara estate near Soestduinen, located in the woods and easy to reach by train. H.F. Mertens gave Zonnegloren the character of a chalet.

Many sanatoria were built in Europe in the 1920s and 1930s in accordance with the Modernist principles of the New Building movement. Light, air, sun, openness and hygiene determined their form to a large extent. Among the most famous are the sanatorium in Paimio, Finland, by Alvar Aalto, and the Zonnestraal sanatorium in Hilversum by J. Duiker. While Aalto's sanatorium that opened in 1936 is a high-rise building whose most striking feature was the stacking of open balconies, Duiker preferred a low-rise building. The initiative was taken by the Amsterdam union of diamond cutters, who also raised the funds. The official opening was on 15 October 1931. With its vast surfaces of glass and the fresh, white façades, Zonnestraal, which was intended for patients who were recovering, was immediately acclaimed as a textbook model of International Modernism. The main building forms the centre and contains the communal areas; the therapy consisted mainly of residence in one of the four pavilions arranged to form a letter V on either side of it and consisting of rooms with balconies. The use of a lot of glass guaranteed an unimpeded view of the wooded surroundings.

The Sanatorium Berg en Bosch, built in the 1930s to replace the Apeldoorn facility, was implemented in accordance with plans by the architects B.J. Koldeweij and C.M. van Moorsel Pzn. The complex consists of a symmetrical main building with which the patient units are connected. The lounges are situated at the ends of them.

In the 1940s medical science managed to bring TB under control. Success was achieved in France in 1921 with inoculation according to the Calmette-Guérin method, but it was not until more than twenty years later that Selman Waksman managed to take a big step forwards with his bactericidal antibiotic streptomycin; when Norwegian researchers discovered that side-effects like deafness could be counteracted by the simultaneous administration of para-amino salicylic acid, humanity seemed to have been rid of the 'white plague' once and for all. However, these discoveries also heralded the end of one of the most striking types of health care architecture. Not many sanatoria were built after 1950. In the meantime most of them have been demolished or given a new function. One of the last complexes to be built was De Klokkenberg in Breda (1953) designed by C.H. de Bever and C.M. van Moorsel Pzn. It was built for 550 patients, but it soon proved difficult to fill all the beds.

Since the 1990s, the bacillus discovered by Koch a century before and that, as scientists have discovered, has caused havoc for thousands of years has resurfaced. What is particularly worrying is that it seems to have become immune to medicine. Whether or not that will trigger a renaissance of the sanatorium, however, remains to be seen...

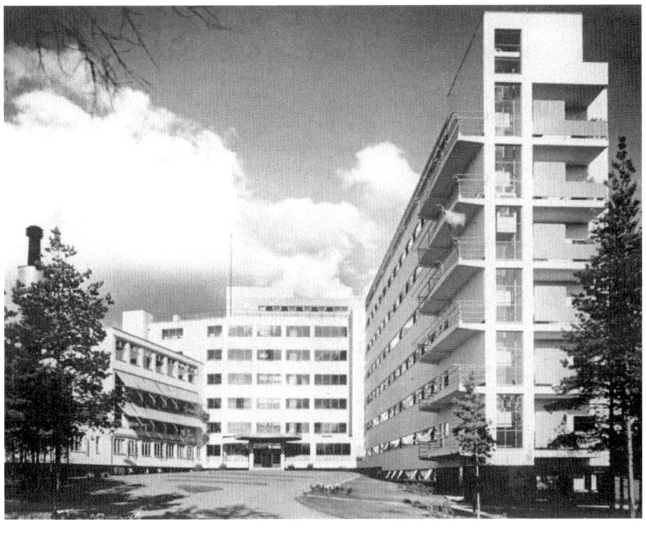

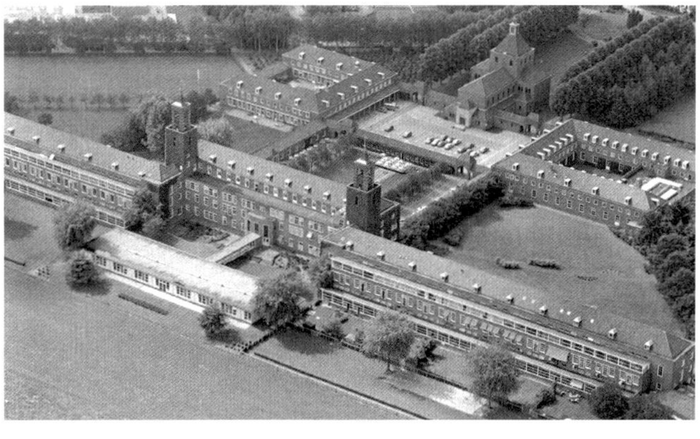

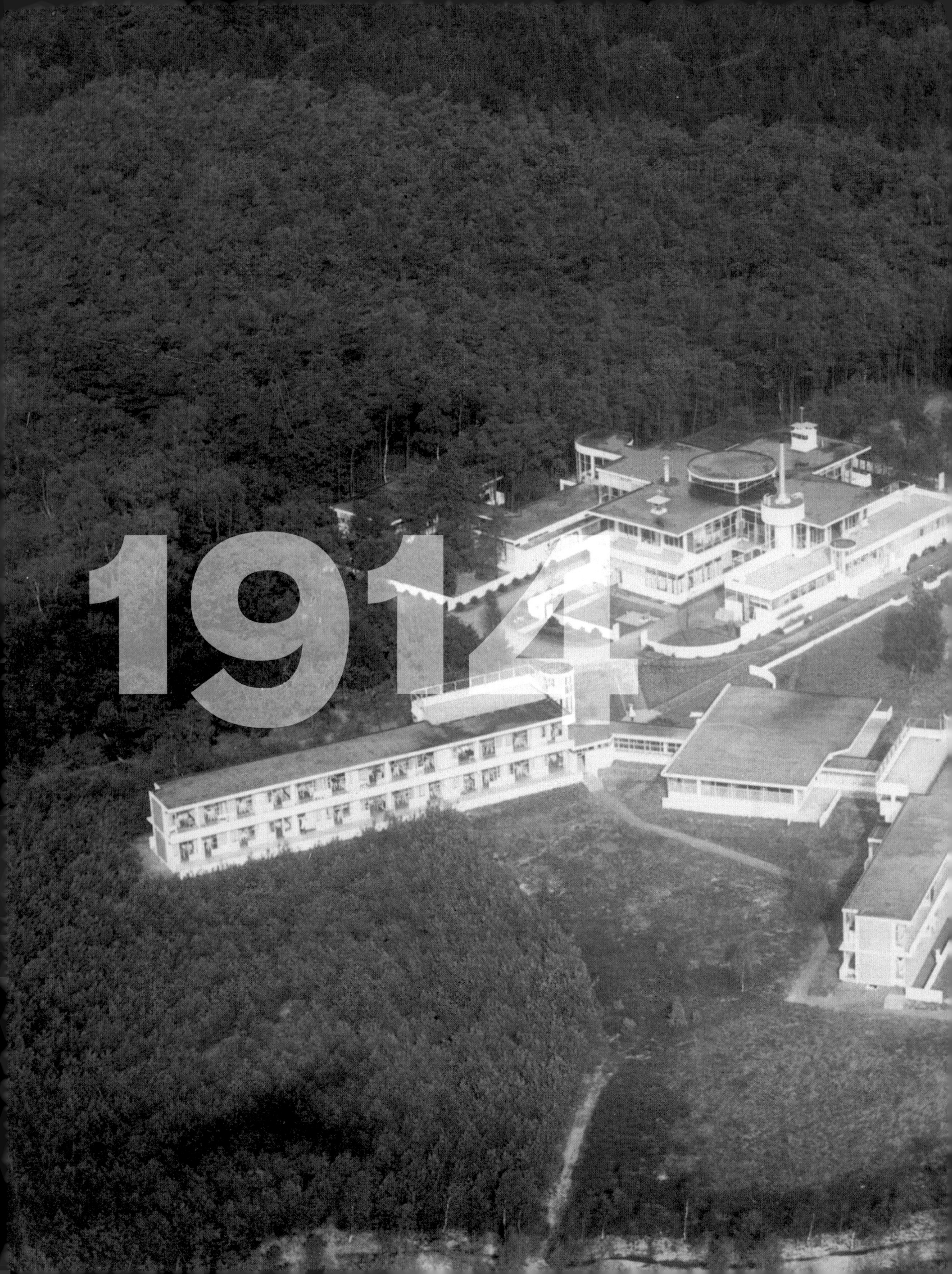
1914

1940

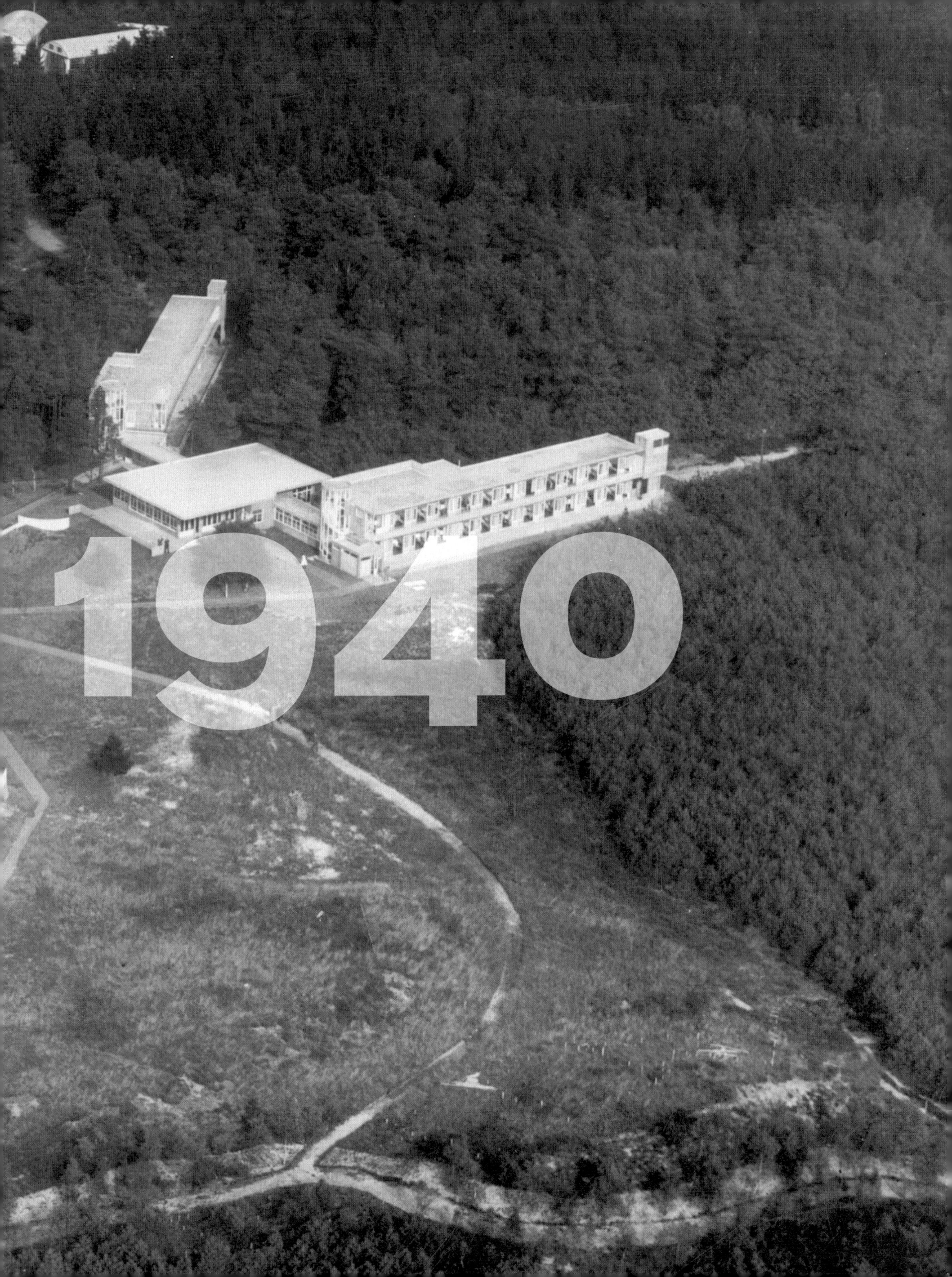

Light, air and space

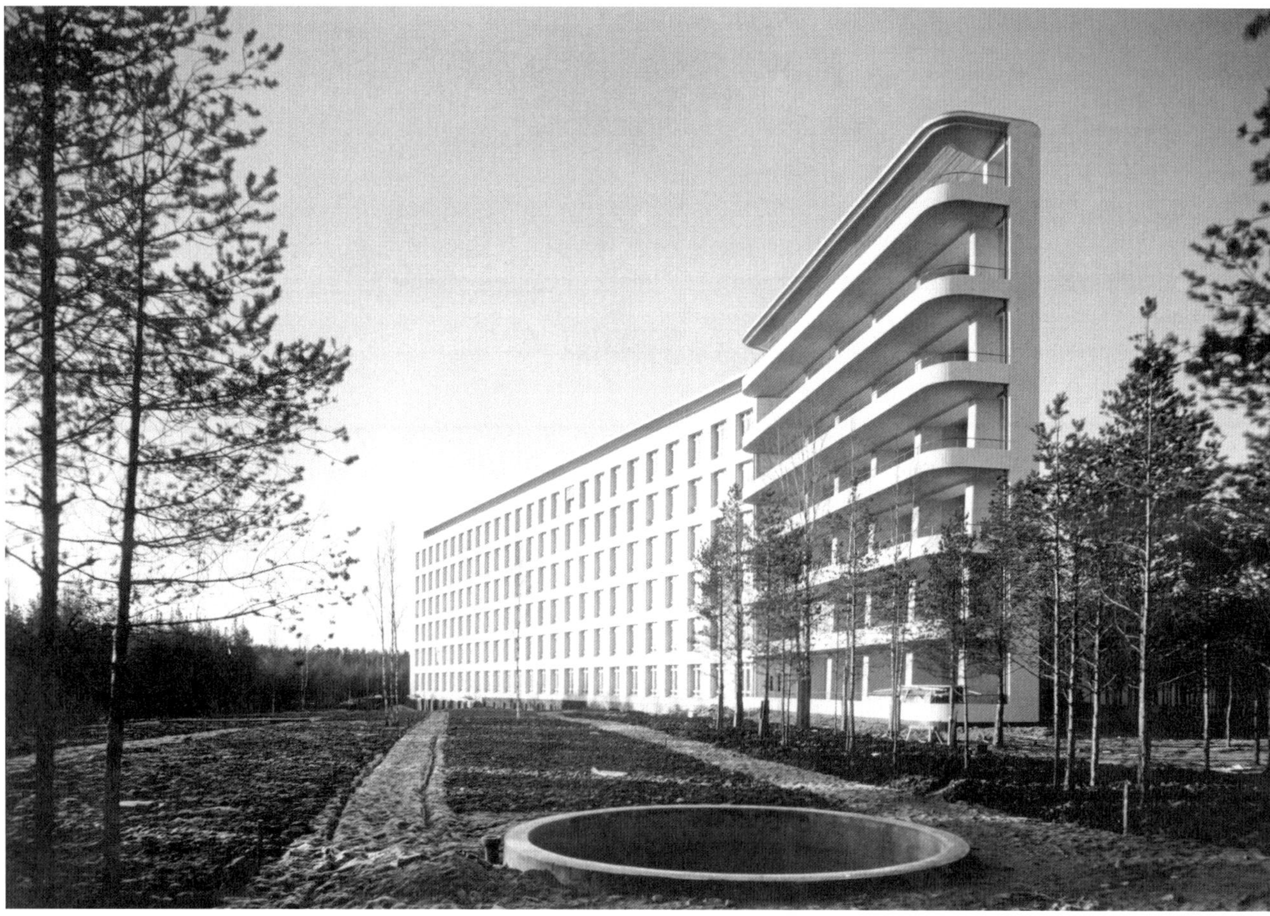

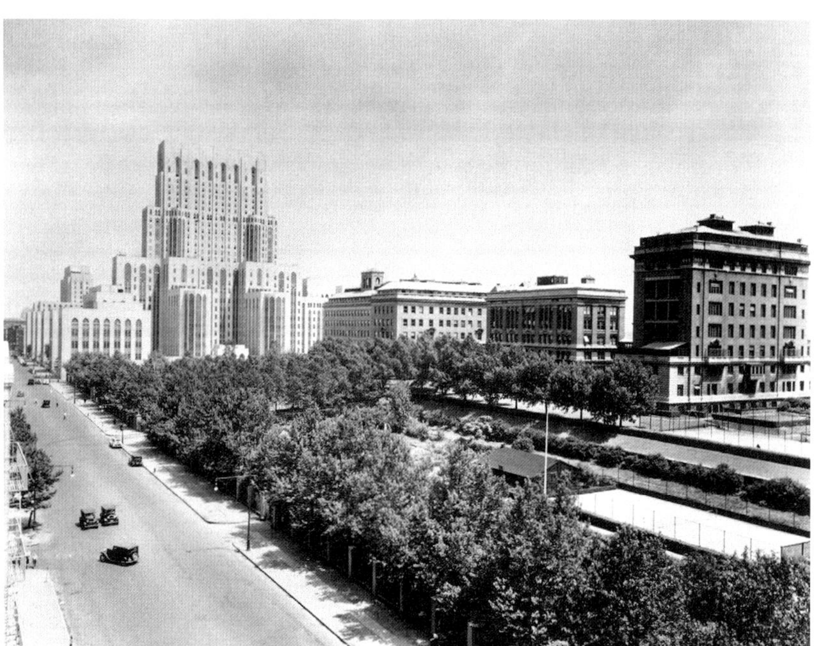

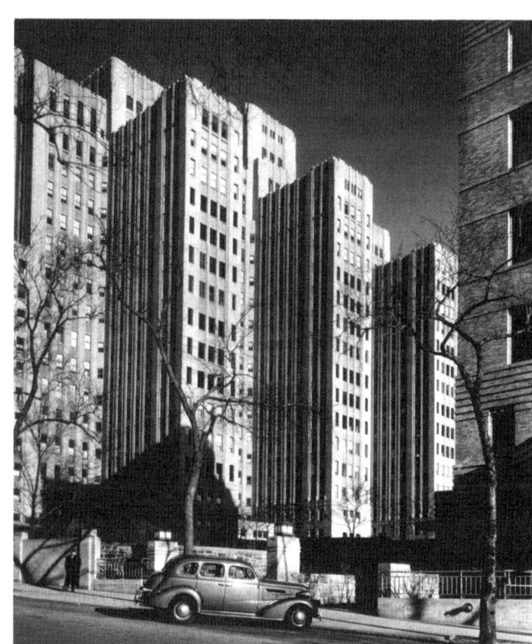

Temples of medical technology and active therapy

Slowly but surely, the principles that had led to the emergence of the modern hospital and modern psychiatric clinic towards the end of the eighteenth century were losing ground by the beginning of the twentieth. Clean air and rural surroundings were still considered important, but belief in the infectious properties of miasma disappeared once it was discovered that it was not the polluted air itself, but the bacteria it contained, that were contagious. Moreover, only a small proportion of those bacteria turned out to be disseminated by the air. The discovery of bacteria made the design of hospitals as ventilation machines redundant. The frontline of medical thought shifted to the laboratories, where a search was going on for ways of rendering bacteria harmless.

In the same period, medical technology took over the hospital. The first device to make a lightning appearance everywhere was the X-ray machine, followed soon afterwards by other wonders of technology. The triumph of medical technology turned the hospital from a poorhouse to a top clinical institution. This put it out of reach of the traditional clientèle of paupers. More compact forms were sought again in hospital architecture, and the new status of the building was reflected in an often pronouncedly representative look. Progress was made in the world of psychiatry too, where it led not to the abandonment of the extensive pavilion complexes but to a greater differentiation, partly due to the introduction of new therapies. Active therapy in particular led to the addition of rooms specially equipped for this purpose. Progress was also made in housing and care for the elderly, where the contours of new types of buildings came into view.

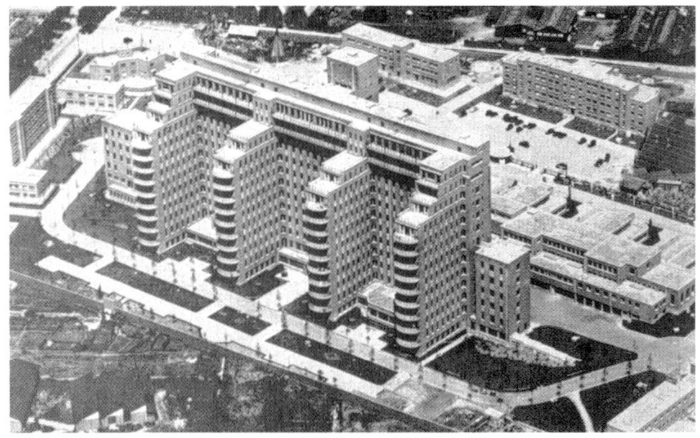

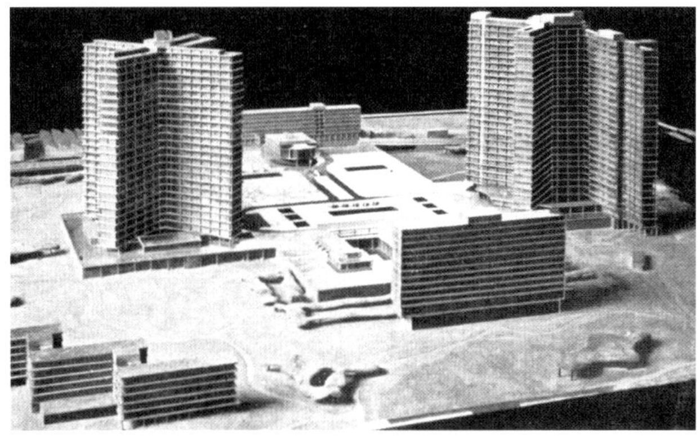

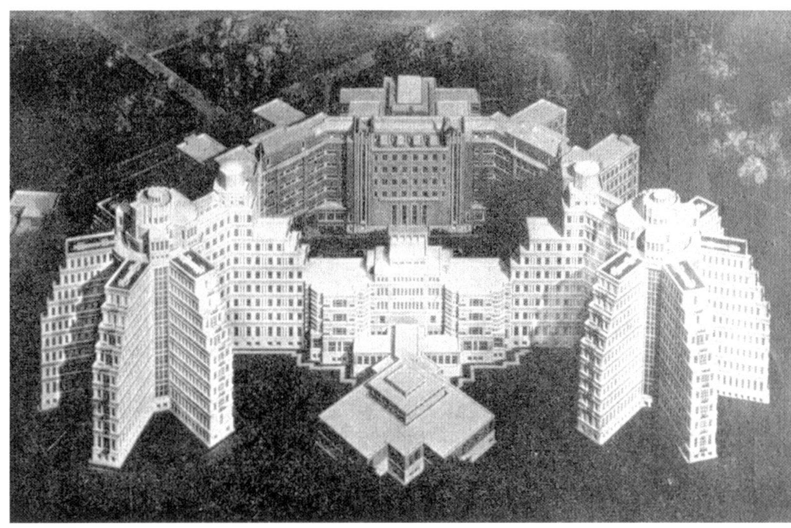

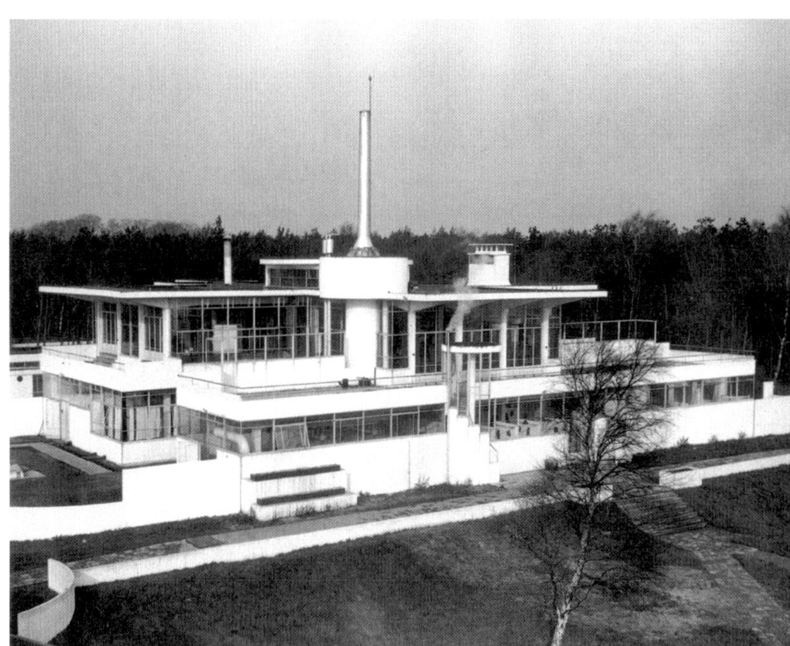

p. 44
***J. Duiker & B. Bijvoet*, Zonnestraal sanatorium, Hilversum, 1928**

p. 46
***A. Aalto*, Paimio sanatorium, Finland, 1932**

***Coolidge Shepley Bulfinch and Abbott*, Cornell Medical Center, New York, 1933**

***J. Gamble Rogers*, Medical Center (Presbyterian Hospital), New York, 1930**

p. 47
***L. Plousey, U. Cassan and J. Walter*, Hôpital Beaujon, Clichy-la-Garenne, 1935**

***P. Nelson*, design for the Cité hospitalière, Lille, 1933**

***J. Walter*, Cité hospitalière, Lille, 1953**

***J. Duiker & B. Bijvoet*, Zonnestraal sanatorium, Hilversum, 1928**

Hospitals

The popularity of the dominant pavilion typology gradually began to wane in the 1920s and 1930s. It was replaced by a more concentrated type of architecture that reflected a great confidence in technology. Fresh air, light and space remained important, but instead of providing these qualities by inserting pavilions in a park-like setting, emphasis shifted to the design of compact buildings. It is striking that the architectural movement for which light and space are key concepts – Modernism – barely gained a foothold in hospital architecture. At the core of Modernism were purity and sobriety and the designation of function as the essence of design in architecture and urban planning. Functionalism, it was believed, would be eminently capable of doing justice to what were regarded as positive developments of the day: technology, social factors (the rise of the lower class as a socio-economic force), science (nature brought under control), hygiene and the modern Zeitgeist: speed, mobility and simultaneity, characteristics that were first aesthetically deployed in modern art.

Prewar Modernism presented itself as an alternative movement that was opposed to the status quo in architecture, urban planning, art, culture and politics. It is this oppositional character that explains why functionalism failed to take root in hospital architecture, even though the philosophy behind it seemed to be exactly the right one for this type of assignment. There are a couple famous examples of Modernist sanatoria (Jan Duiker's well-known Zonnestraal sanatorium near Hilversum, 1925-1927 and Alvar Aalto's Paimio sanatorium in Finland, 1929-1933), but they were exceptions.

Tower blocks or pavilions?

In the twentieth century it became increasingly clear that the pavilion system and its variants were expensive and inefficient. Walking distances were too large and the grounds became built up. Besides, after the discovery of bacteria and antibiotics, there was no longer any need to resort to the pavilion typology. People grew increasingly aware that the demands that a hospital had to meet were changing. That process took place first in the United States, where the high-rise hospital appeared on the scene. High-rise building was an answer to the uncontrollability of the pavilion hospitals, which kept on expanding to eventually form complete districts, and to the high price of land in the US cities. Partly thanks to advances in building technology, it became possible to make more compact buildings and high-rise architecture seemed to offer a far more economical solution. Important high-rise hospitals are the Medical Center (Presbyterian Hospital), New York (1926-1930) by James Gamble Rogers, and the Cornell Medical Center in New York (1933) designed by Coolidge Shepley Bulfinch and Abbott.

There were hardly any high-rise hospitals in Europe before the Second World War. France was the only country to experiment with tower-block hospitals. It is noteworthy that the lead was taken by US architects who came to Europe during the First World War in the wake of the US army. Paul Nelson's project for a gigantic health centre in Lille attracted particular attention.[1] It combined a medical faculty, an out-patient clinic, a hospital, a nursing home and block of apartments for the elderly. The enormous complex, which was inspired by the Columbia University Presbyterian Hospital, was praised as a 'health city', but Nelson's plan was never implemented. A US-inspired French engineer, J. Walter, also specialised in hospital design, made his name with the design for the high-rise Hôpital Beaujon in Clichy. This was very different from Nelson's hospital city: Walter's design was characterised by a rigorous separation of the internal traffic flows, which yielded logistical advantages and subdivided the colossal building into small units.

Projects on this scale were exceptional. Usually other methods were found to avoid the disadvantages of the pavilion typology. To economise and to achieve a more efficient solution, the Swedish architects H. Cederström and B. Lindgren introduced a concept in which the nursing unit was central. Whatever demands might be made on a hospital in the future, they were convinced that at any rate it would always have to have nursing facilities. They proposed accommodating patients in nursing units consisting of twenty-five to thirty-five beds in rooms with one, two, four or

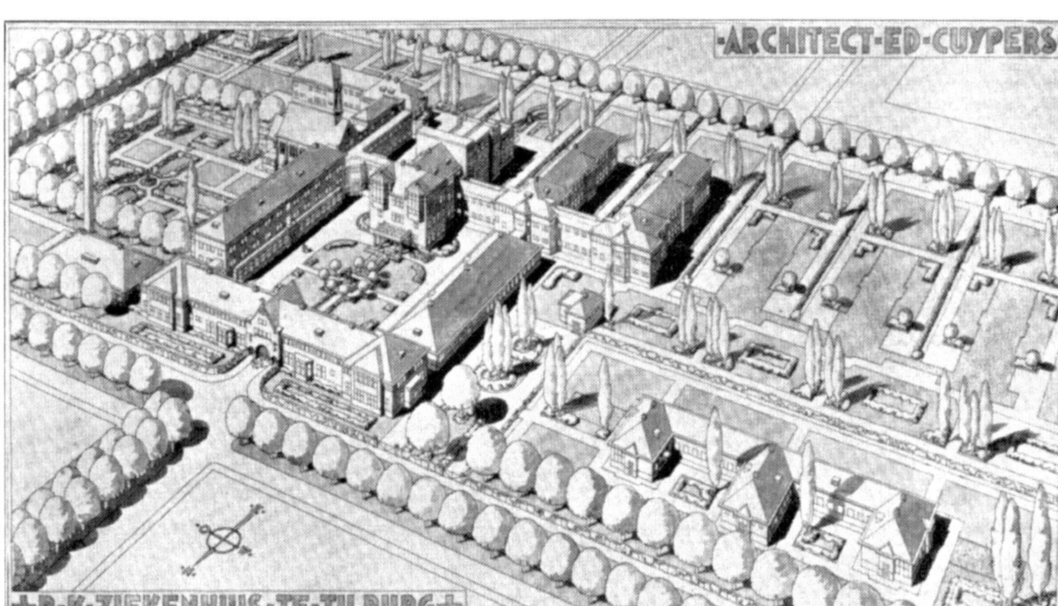

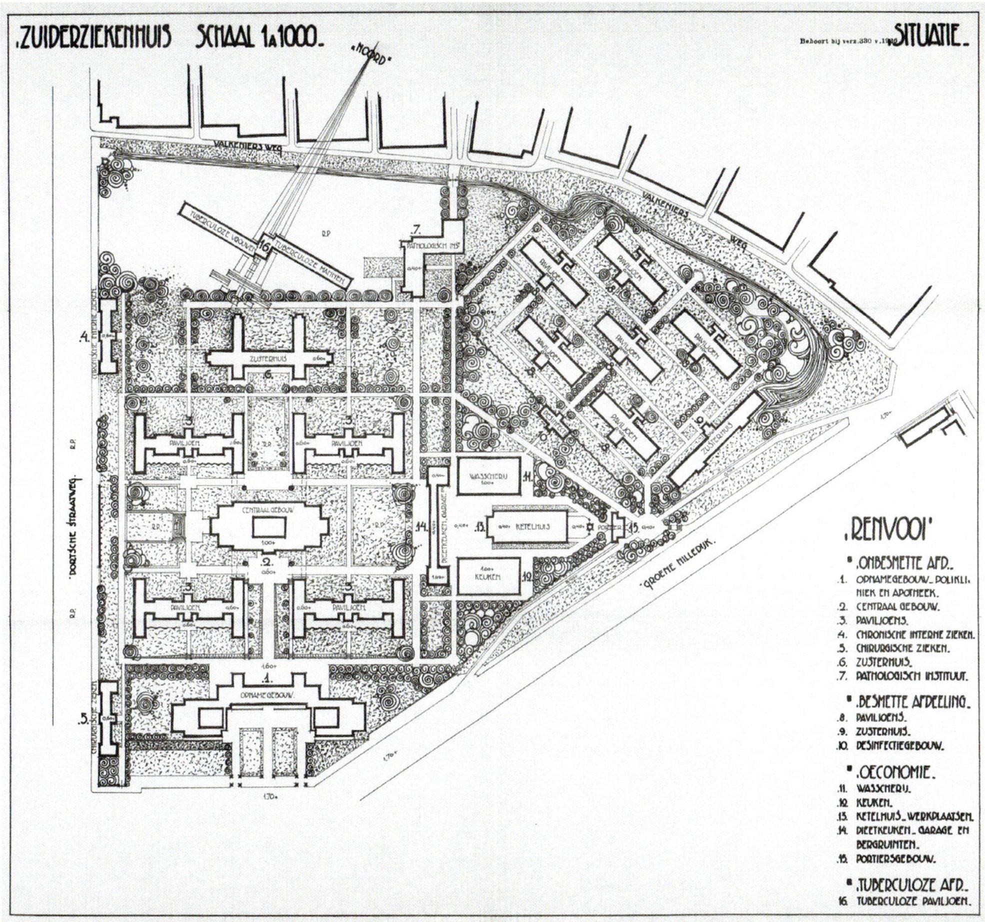

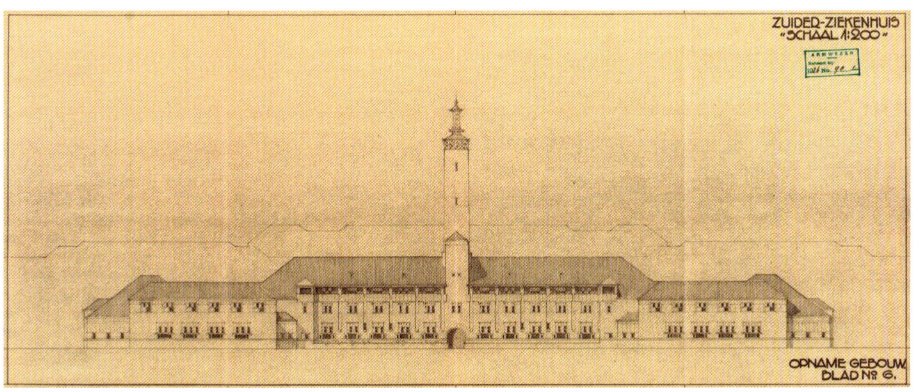

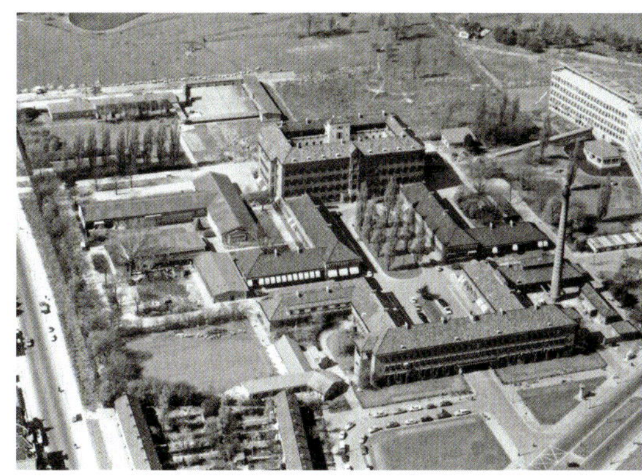

p. 48
***Ed. Cuypers*, Sint Elisabeth Ziekenhuis, Tilburg, 1926**

p. 49
***W.G. Witteveen*, design for a hospital on the left bank of the river Maas (Zuiderziekenhuis), Rotterdam, 1926**

***W.G. Witteveen*, design for the main building**

***A. van der Steur*, Zuiderziekenhuis, Rotterdam, 1939**

***Ed. Cuypers*, Sint Canisius Ziekenhuis, Nijmegen, 1922–1926**

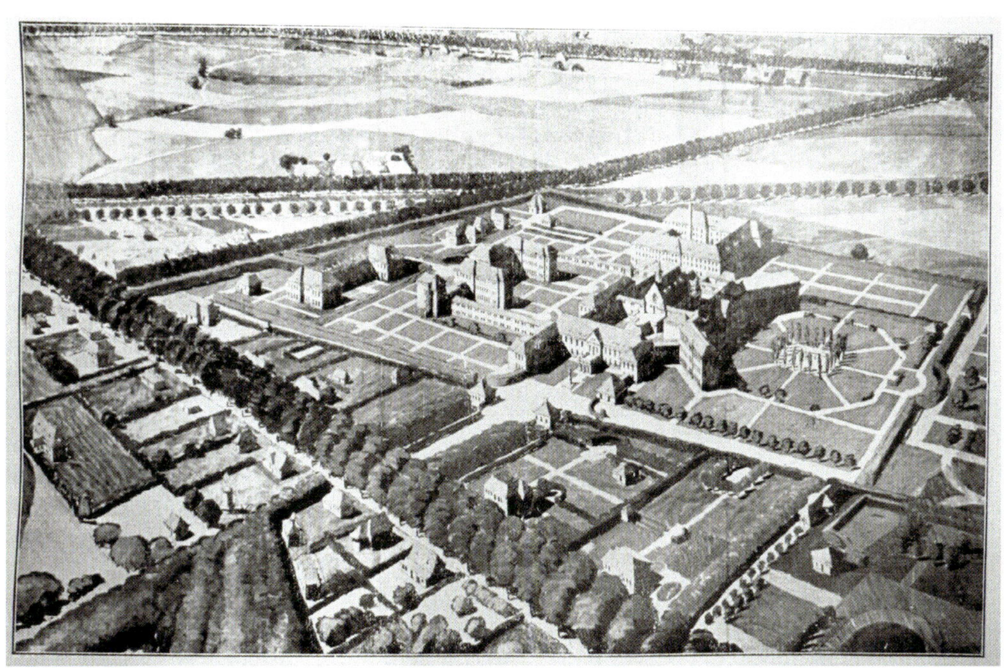

six beds. The nursing unit could be repeated several times; the total number of nursing units would form the nursing ward. There would also be a department for medical treatment with operating theatres, examination and treatment rooms, laboratories and technical facilities. The architects predicted that this was the part where most of the changes would take place.[2] Cederström and Lindgren thereby redefined the hospital: by separating the treatment areas from the nursing areas, the wards became an autonomous component of the modern hospital. Separating the nursing wards enabled various types.

In spite of the major objections to the pavilion system, hospitals of this type were still being built in the Netherlands in the 1920s. It is symptomatic of what had by then become a generally accepted conviction that the system was outdated that these projects often met with protest. Some of these buildings marked the completion of hospitals whose construction was already under way when it was stopped by the First World War; others were the implementation of designs that had remained at the planning stage because of the war. The medical superintendent of the Leids Academisch ziekenhuis, J.W. Wicherink, concluded that 'initially the choice of a pavilion system seemed entirely justified, but if today, in 1923, the building operations were still to be begun – assuming that there were any plans to build at all – then the design of a pavilion-style hospital would be out of the question'.[3] Having to walk from one pavilion to another was supposed to involve an enormous waste of time for the nurses; in the US it had been estimated that a waste of three hours a day was not unusual. Pavilion hospitals had become fossils from a previous era. The future was high-rise, only compact tower blocks could reduce the enormous waste of time that was inevitable in pavilion hospitals. The Hôpital Beaujon near Paris demonstrated that high-rise building was possible in Europe too. Various factors were in its favour: high land prices, limited plot size, and reduction of walking distances.[4] A tower-block hospital for the left bank of the river Maas in Rotterdam was given serious consideration for a while, but although high-rise was by now an accepted idea, it was not applied in the Netherlands before the Second World War.

Hybrid forms

The vast majority of hospitals that were built in the Netherlands before 1940 were designed in a hybrid form of pavilion and corridor system to combine the advantages of both types. The term *corridor-pavilion type* was used if a main corridor provided direct access to smaller rooms and areas and if the large pavilion rooms were also linked by a passage to the main corridor. The *pavilion-corridor type*, on the other hand, consisted of a number of pavilions connected with one another by corridors; these corridors in turn might be flanked by smaller areas and corridor rooms. The various hybrid forms and their development can be best traced in the impressive series of hospitals by Ed. Cuypers, who designed no less than eight in the last ten years of his life and was involved in the construction of the most important Roman Catholic hospitals. It is known that when Cuypers embarked on a project, he – often accompanied by his principals – went on study trips abroad. These included visits to the Städtisches Krankenhaus Lindenburg in Cologne (pavilion type) and the Städtisches Krankenhaus in Düsseldorf (concentrated system).[5]

From 1920 Cuypers was responsible for a series of extensions to the Sint Jozef Ziekenhuis in Heerlen that anticipate the later comb structure (referred to as herringbone system at the time). Cuypers elaborated two plans for the Sint Canisius Ziekenhuis in Nijmegen (1903, 1922-1926): one in what he called the full pavilion system and the other in a partial corridor system. The architect himself preferred the pavilion system because of 'the strict separation of functions and the specific character of each building', but for economic reasons his principals chose the more concentrated plans . The strong predilection for the pavilion system is particularly evident in the Sint Elisabeth Ziekenhuis in Tilburg (1926).[6]

A system combining the advantages of the pavilion and the corridor typologies was also adopted for the hospital for the left bank in Rotterdam. Studies had convinced W.G. Witteveen, head of the Rotterdam Urban Planning Department and responsible for the design of public buildings, that all the important institutions for the treatment of patients should be centralised in a modern hospital. A large area of the terrain was occupied by a symmetrically designed hospital for acute cases (the so-called germ-free department). At the front end of the central axis was an admission building and in the middle the central building that accommodated all of the examination and treatment rooms. Two pavilions flanked the central axis, each with a capacity of two hundred patients. The pavilions were connected with each other and with the central building by means of underground corridors. At the end of the central axis was a home for nurses. The plan envisaged a department for infectious diseases that would be entirely separate from this hospital. It would consist of eighteen separate pavilions, a tuberculosis department, and the economy department with a kitchen, laundry and boiler house. Besides large wards, the plan also envisaged rooms with up to six beds. (The only hospital with exclusively one-person rooms is that of the Ford plant in Detroit – apparently even a structure of this kind was briefly considered for Rotterdam.) The various buildings were designed in a style reminiscent of Frank Lloyd Wright.

The plan was further elaborated in 1929 by a team headed by A. van der Steur, who had been appointed head of the Buildings Department in that year. Building was already under way (the rough structure of the central part and of the administration building and the foundations of the economy building had been completed) when the plan was considerably simplified in 1931. This was necessitated by the poor financial state of the local authority. Van der Steur adjusted the plan so that it would be suitable in the first instance for four-hundred patients and could later be expanded to a hospital with 1,400 beds in accordance with the original plan.[7] The choice of a 'more individual nursing', prompted by the improvement in the conditions of the working class, is noteworthy. The large wards were cancelled and only rooms with three or four beds were built.[8] When the hospital was finally opened in 1939, it was a relatively small complex with no more than 250 beds.

The psychiatric hospital

By the last quarter of the nineteenth century, the fulfilment of the ideals of the late eighteenth century – the careful design of buildings to contribute to the healing of the mentally ill – seemed further away than ever. The major improvements of the first psychiatric revolution had been largely cancelled out by then by the explosive growth in the number of patients in care. The building of more and more new institutions could not prevent a situation of overpopulation almost everywhere. The disappointing results of the treatment gave the asylums the stigma of a prison for the chronically deranged poor. There was a sore need for improvement, but above all a lot of new buildings were required. The pavilion typology was preferred, above all because it could easily accommodate changes in therapeutic methods.

Active therapy

Unlike the situation in regular hospitals, in psychiatry technology plays a subordinate role. As a consequence, psychiatric institutions are less sensitive to the speed of technological innovation that obliges hospitals to adapt, expand and renovate all the time. The lack of centralised, heavy medical facilities rendered the pavilion type, in which the various departments are far away from one another, less disadvantageous, which is why this type was maintained. Differentiation between the pavilions increased. That was a result of the development of new therapeutic insights. A new period of reforms broke out at the end of the 1920s when work therapy and relaxation became increasingly important. The difference from the work therapy that had already been in use for some time (and which often resembled forced labour) lay in the fact that more attention was paid to activities that matched the capacities and needs of the patient.

The centre of active psychiatry was Germany, where the major innovations in psychiatry took place during this period. The latest trends in active therapy were introduced into the Netherlands by W.M. van der Scheer in the Provinciaal Ziekenhuis Santpoort. After a visit to H. Simon in Gütersloh, Van der Scheer became so enthusiastic that he dedicated several articles and a book to the subject: *Nieuwere inzichten in de behandeling van geesteszieken. Arbeidstherapie, actievere therapie volgens dr. H. Simon. De verpleging van onrustige krankzinnigen in geheel nieuwe banen* (Newer insights into the treatment of the mentally ill. Work therapy, more active therapy according to Dr H. Simon. The nursing of restless mental patients in entirely new directions). In terms of the distinction between neurology and psychiatry that was made at the time, enhanced active therapy was a technique of psychiatry. Its novelty lay in '... the explicit highlighting of the exceptional importance that environmental, *external* factors can have on the insane too, in a more accurate appraisal of the interaction between the outside world and the individual, even though a part of the potential has already been destroyed by illness'.[9]

The technique is based on the premise that patients are social beings who suffer from a disturbed relation with society and are in need of re-education. Van der Scheer's conviction that architecture plays a great role here is striking: 'In the first place, this can be done by making the communal dayrooms as cosy as possible. Paint the verandahs and rooms with cosy, warm or fresh bright colours; patients too feel more at home in such a setting; ensure the necessary variation. Pay attention to the furniture

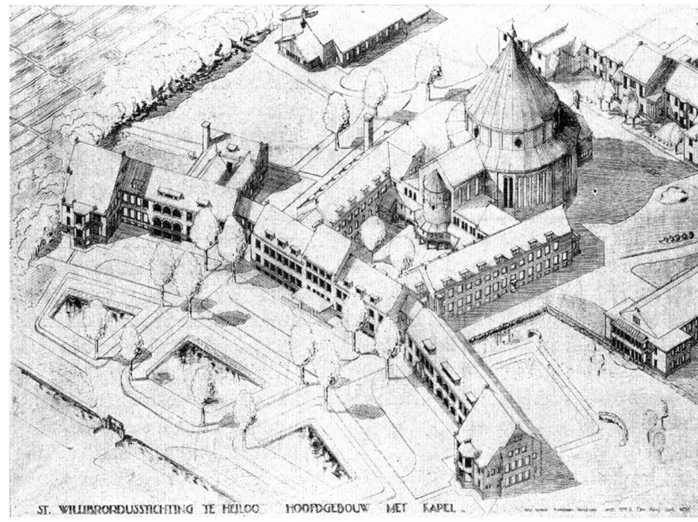

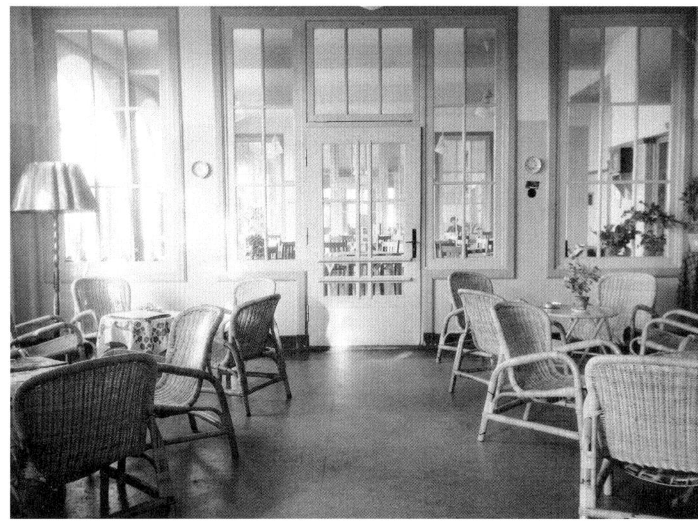

p. 51
***H.J.W. Thunissen & J.H. Hendricks*, main building Sint Willibrordusstichting, Heiloo, 1928**

Interior Sint Willibrordus-stichting, Heiloo

***J.G. & P.K. Mensink*, Licht en Kracht, Assen, 1936**

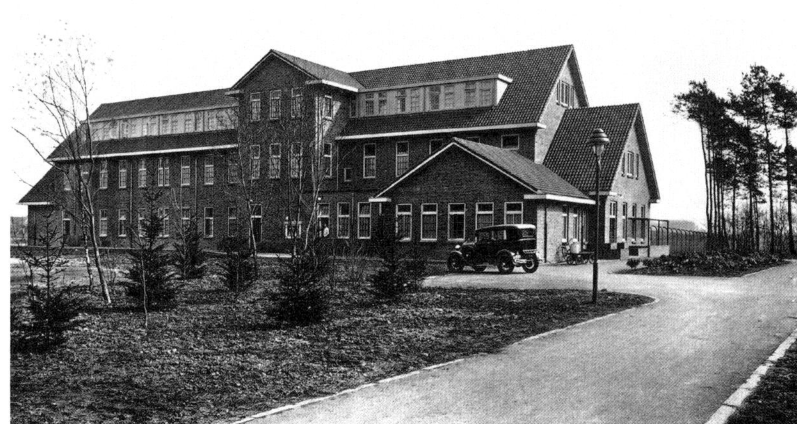

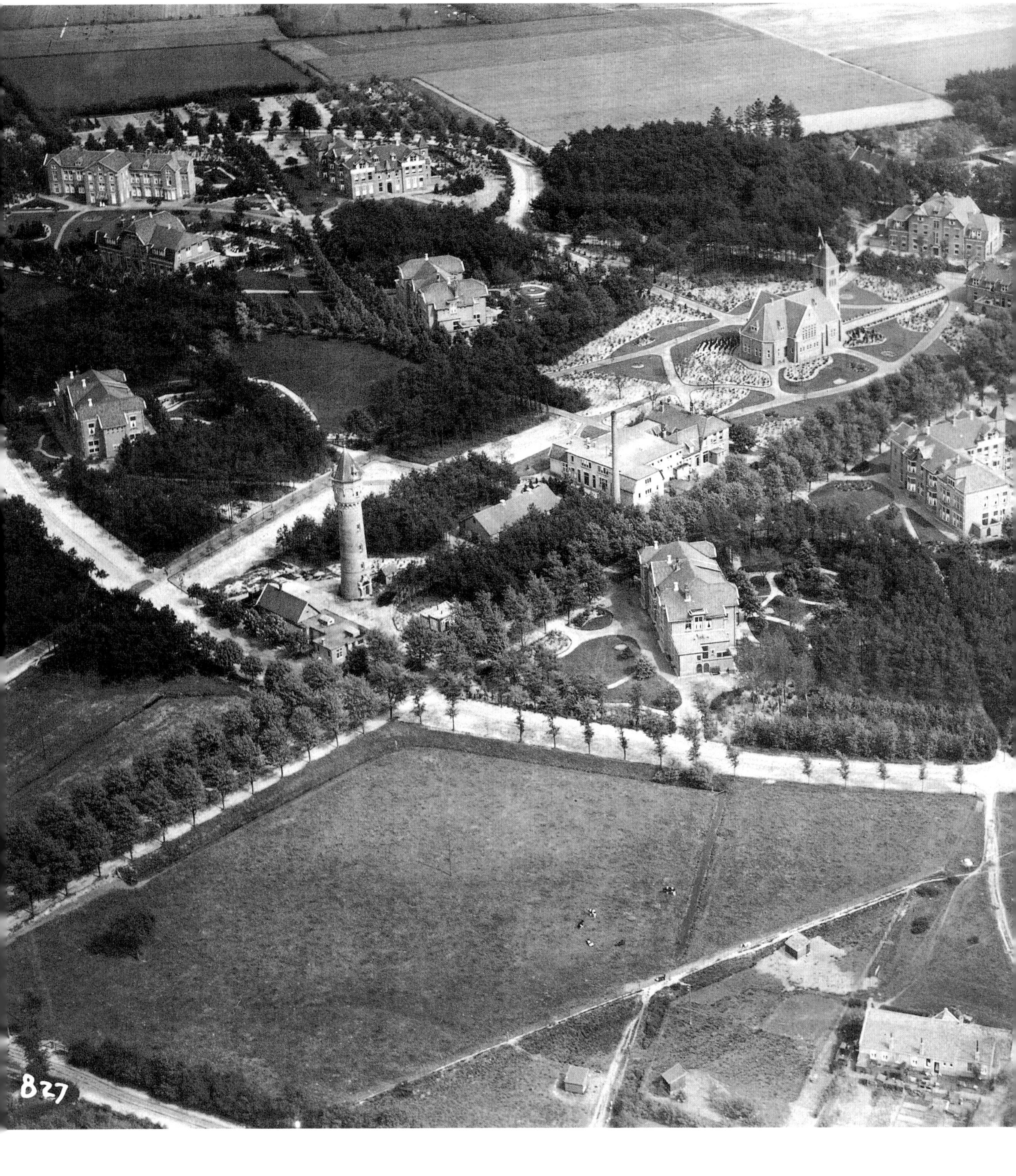
827

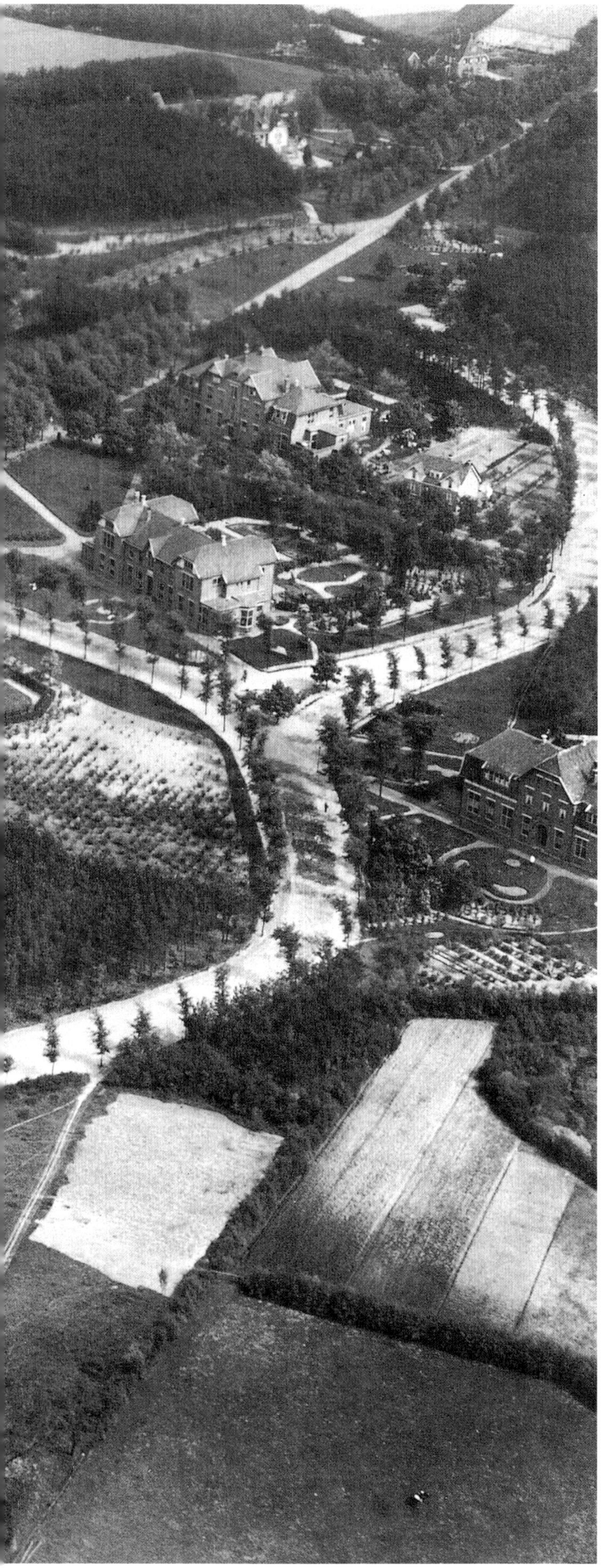

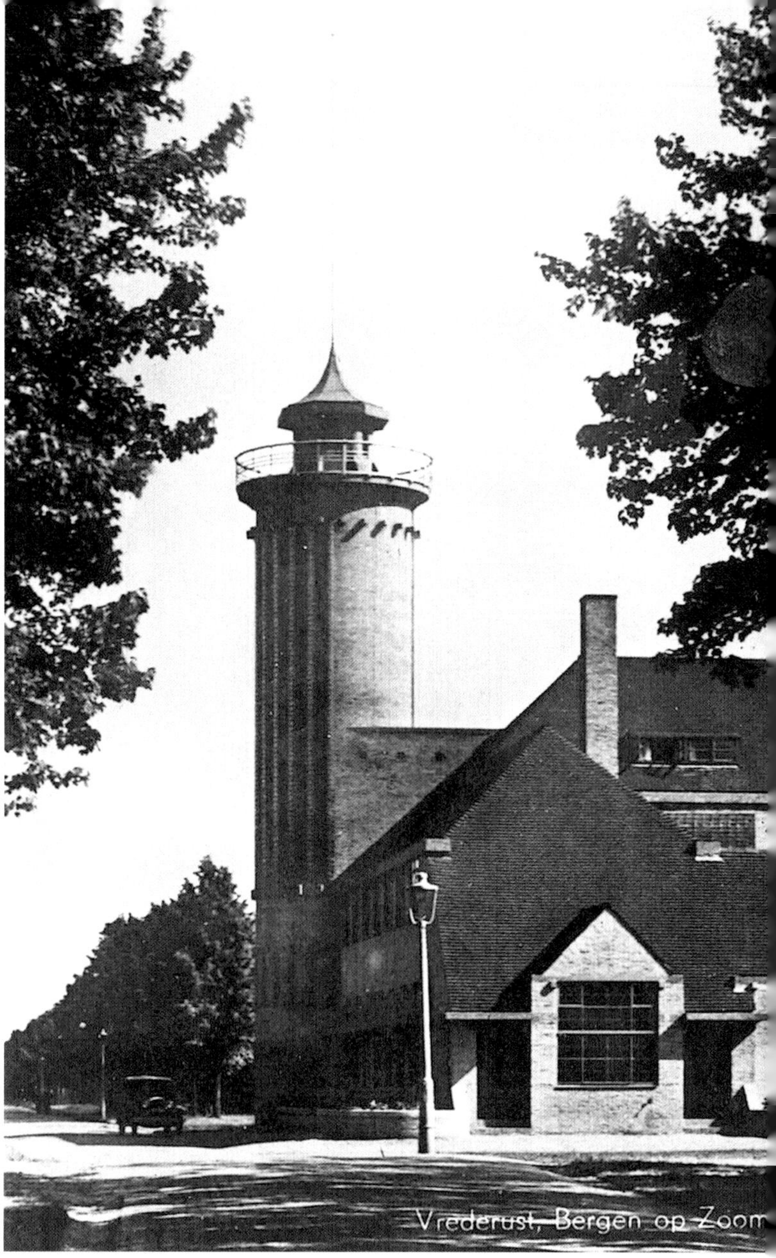

p. 52
***E. Knevel*, Vrederust psychiatric hospital, Halsteren, 1912**

p. 53
***B.T. Boeyinga*, Vrederust, main building, Halsteren, 1931**

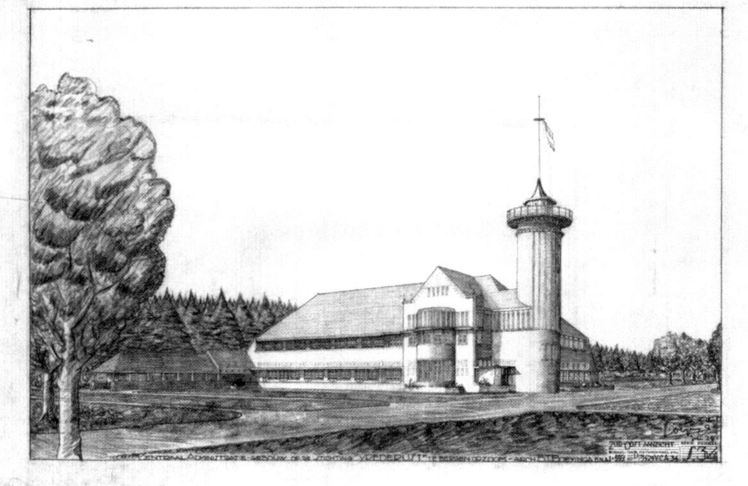

and create a tasteful whole; hang paintings and engravings on the wall, put flowers on the window-sill, introduce a hanging plant here and there; create a cosy corner with a rug and a standard lamp. A great deal can already be achieved with extremely simple means, with simple cretonne, with a simple type of wood, with simple linoleum. The care lavished on it, the love with which you prepare an agreeable spot for your patients, will be echoed in their mental life.'[10]

A wave of building construction

Many new psychiatric institutions were built and many others enlarged in the first half of the twentieth century. An example is Zon en Schild, which was built in Amersfoort in various stages between 1931 and 1938. It consists of an administration building linked with and flanked by an admission pavilion, two pavilions for paying patients, two pavilions for restless patients, and a church. The design was by Gebroeders Mensink from Apeldoorn and Van Hoogevest from Amersfoort. Licht en Kracht near Assen also consisted of pavilions on either side of a central axis on which the administration building, kitchen and depot were situated. The buildings had a modern look and met the demands for light, fresh air and space.

One of the most remarkable new institutions was the Sint Willibrordusstichting in Heiloo (1929), designed by the architects H. Thunissen and J. Hendricks from The Hague. It was an initiative of the Brothers of Our Lady of Lourdes. The choice of location was made under pressure from the state because of the lack of a Catholic institution above the North Sea Canal. The most striking part of the complex is the Mariakoepel, a circular church in the centre of the building. The monastery was also situated here until 1994. J.A.J. Barnhoorn, medical superintendent of the institution, drew attention to the fluid transition between treatment and nursing in psychiatry and delivered a plea for 'airy, cheerful, cosy rooms' and 'aesthetically sound furniture designs'.[11] Some of these pieces of furniture were designed by I. Falkenberg-Liefrinck, a fervent supporter of the Modernist movement in architecture and closely involved with the periodical *De 8 en Opbouw*, the flagship of Dutch Modernism. The opening of the Glorieux sanatorium followed in 1933.

Thunissen & Hendricks were also involved in the building of the Ursulakliniek in Wassenaar, which they designed with G.J. Simons. The latter had designed the St. Jacobuskliniek on the same site in 1926, which now set the tone for the architecture of its sister clinic. Vrederust in Halsteren (North Brabant) is interesting for its Expressionist design. It was founded by the Vereniging tot Christelijke Verzorging van Krankzinnigen in Zeeland (Association for the Protestant Care of the Insane in Zeeland). The first stage of Vrederust was carried out between 1908 and 1912 by E. Knevel. He broke with convention in grouping the pavilions not more or less symmetrically on either side of a central axis, but scattered beside idyllic winding lanes. This open-ended arrangement proved to be a good basis for the expansion by B.T. Boeyinga in the 1930s. He was a representative of the Amsterdam School who managed to achieve a remarkable symbiosis with the existing complex.

If new buildings were out of the question, part of the increased demand was catered for by expanding existing complexes. A successful example is the expansion of the Willem Arntsz Hoeve by H.F. Mertens between 1928 and 1940. Four generously designed pavilions were the result: Winkler for 136 restless women, Lorentz for 78 restless men, Van 't Hoff for 82 bedridden men, and Eykman for 54

p. 54

***H.F. Mertens*, Willem Arntsz Hoeve, Den Dolder, pavilion for 136 restless women, 1927**

***H.F. Mertens*, Willem Arntsz Hoeve, Den Dolder, homes for nurses, 1931**

***H.F. Mertens*, site map Willem Arntsz Hoeve, Den Dolder, 1928; the existing buildings, the extension in progress and the planned extension are indicated.**

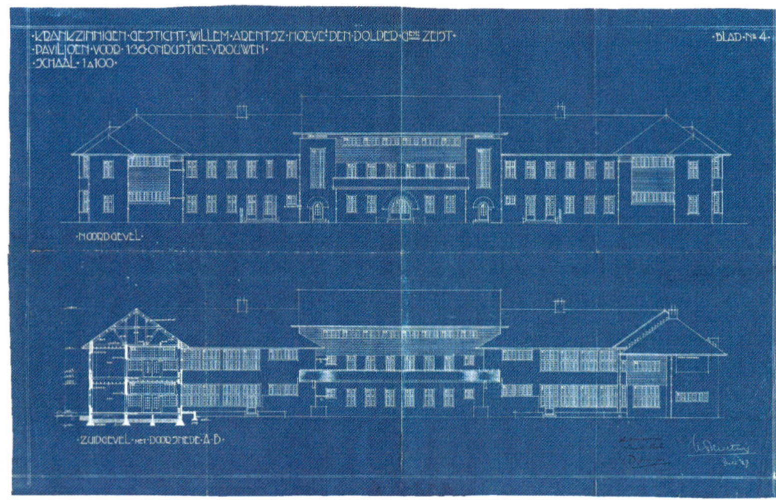

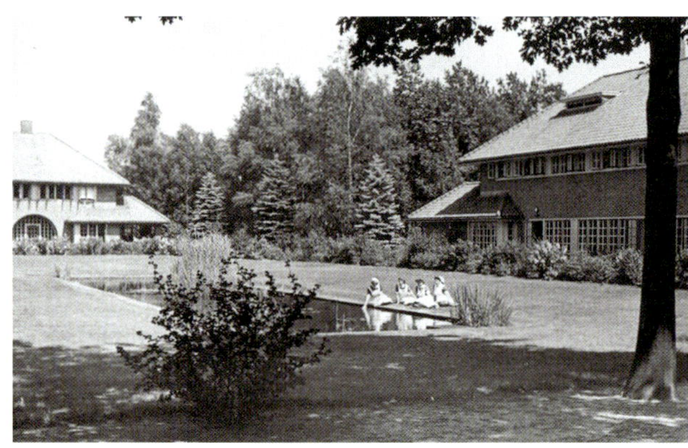

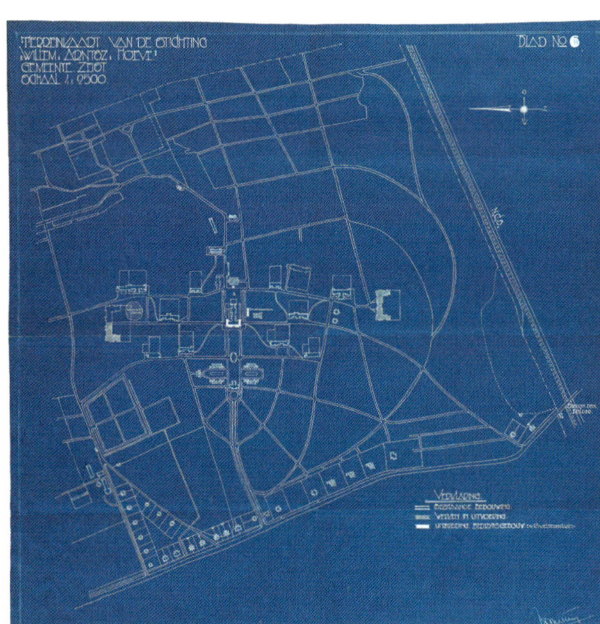

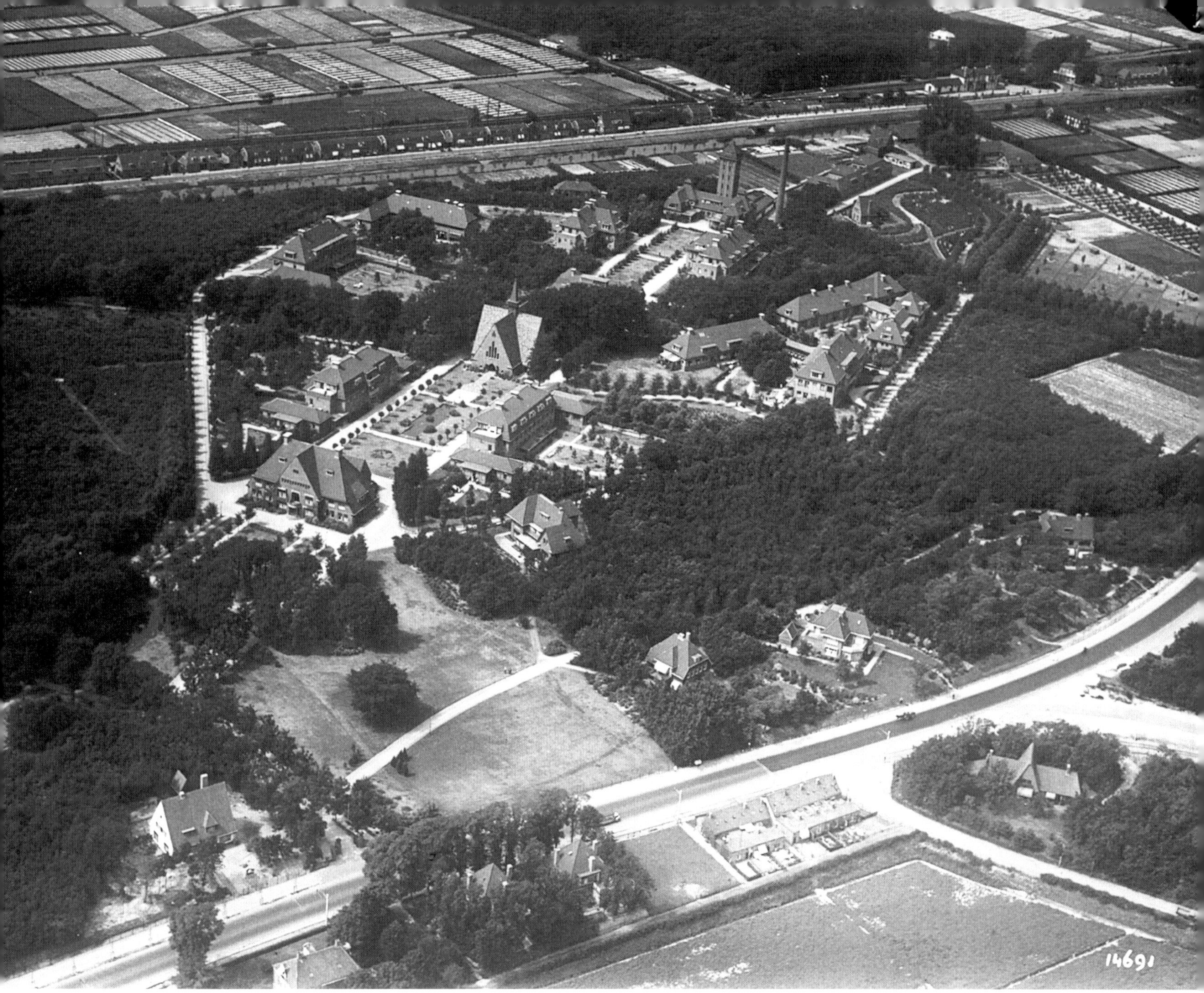

p. 55

Vogelenzang psychiatric hospital, Bennebroek

***A.T. Kraan*, Vogelenzang, administration building, Bennebroek, 1927**

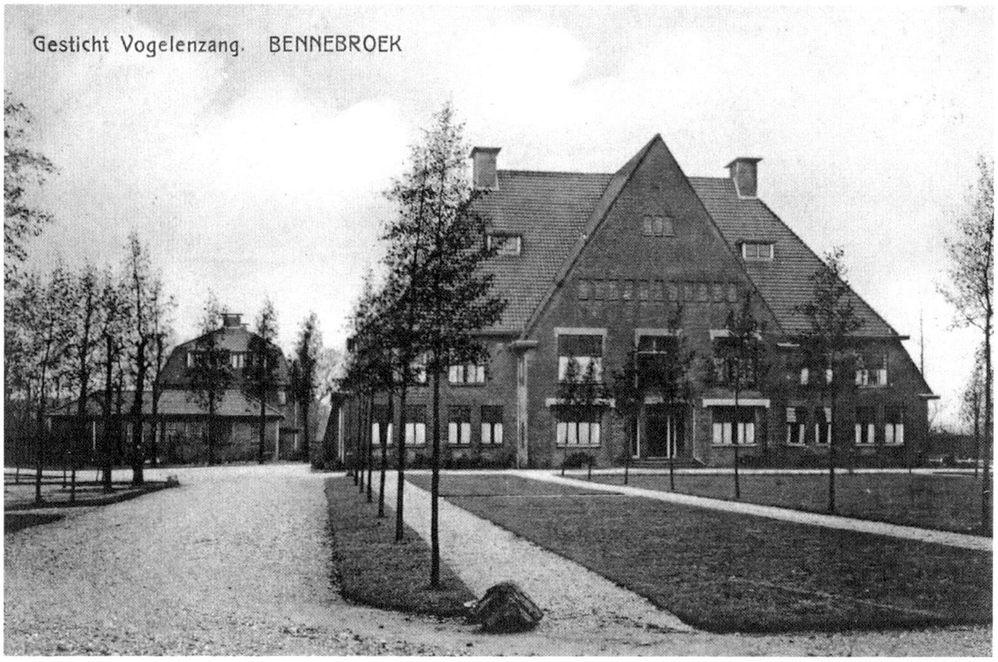

bedridden women. Characteristic of these pavilions are the use of reddish-brown brickwork, the overhanging roofs, and the high continuous window strips. Between 1928 and 1931 Mertens also designed a symmetrical complex of six houses for nurses projected on either side of two ponds, and a house for the female managerial staff. The complex intersected by the pavilion system of Poggenbeek was given the name Vijverhof because it was situated near the ponds (*vijvers*). Each of the six twin houses for nurses could accommodate twice ten nurses. Each nurse had a bedroom of her own, and each twin house had two pairs of living rooms, each for five nurses. The trainee nurses, as the annual report for 1929 stated, 'young and inexperienced as they are when they enter service and drawn from often a very simple circle, can (...) learn here, in a setting that satisfies certain demands of well-being and culture, to deal with one another in friendship and harmony and with a relatively large measure of freedom by comparison with the conditions in an ordinary, large communal home for nurses'.[12]

Sanatoria

The psychiatric sanatorium, which initially targeted primarily the more well-to-do patients, represents the major innovation in psychiatry in the 1920s and 1930s. The sanatorium was also a breakthrough in architectural terms, not so much for the logistical organisation and the way in which specific functions were organised as for the attempt to build relatively luxurious buildings that represented the new status of psychiatry. Numerous sanatoria sprang up within a couple of decades, often as separate complexes far from the existing asylums, but sometimes connected to them, though strictly separated from the other departments. Some of them were built as independent institutions, such as the open department of Vogelenzang in 1929, initiated by the Vereeniging tot Christelijke Verzorging van Krankzinnigen en Zenuwlijders in Nederland (Association for the Protestant Care of the Insane and Neurasthenics in the Netherlands), which had in the meantime changed its name to Vereniging tot Christelijke Verzorging van Geestes- en Zenuwzieken (Association for the Protestant Care of Mental and Neural Disorders).[13]

The building plan for Vogelenzang envisaged an administration building situated on the conventional asylum axis, a central kitchen, workshops, and a total of six pavilions: two for observation, two for restless men and women, and two for calm men and women. Posthumus Meyjes & Van der Linden built the Koningsheide sanatorium, for a mere sixteen female and fifteen male patients, in Arnhem. It comprised a main building with two wings. An attempt was made to create a friendly, domestic atmosphere: 'Since the nature of the patients makes them exceptionally sensitive to their surroundings, the aim has

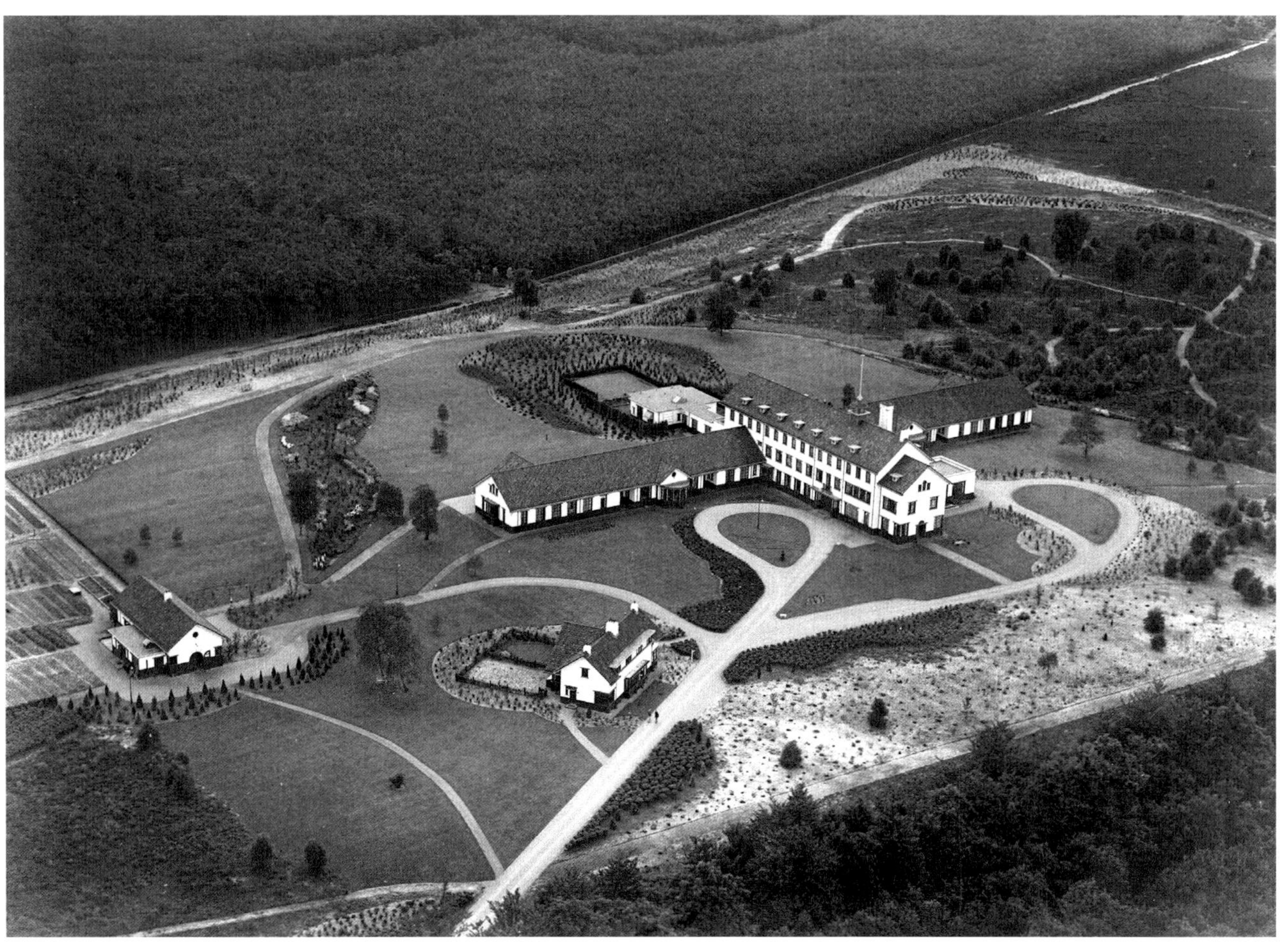

p. 56
***Posthumus Meyjes & Van der Linden*, Koningsheide sanatorium, Arnhem, 1936**

p. 57
***E.J. Rothuizen*, De Hooge Riet sanatorium, Ermelo, 1935**

p. 57 | <
***J.G. & P.K. Mensink*, Port Natal sanatorium, Assen, 1935**

***Gebroeders Mensink & Van Hoogevest*, Hebron sanatorium, Amersfoort, 1931**

p. 57 | >
***E.J. Rothuizen*, De Hooge Riet sanatorium, Ermelo, 1933-1935**

***E.J. Rothuizen (Architecten en Ingenieurs-bureau 'Buvani')*, Nederveluwe sanatorium, Wolfheze, 1933-1935**

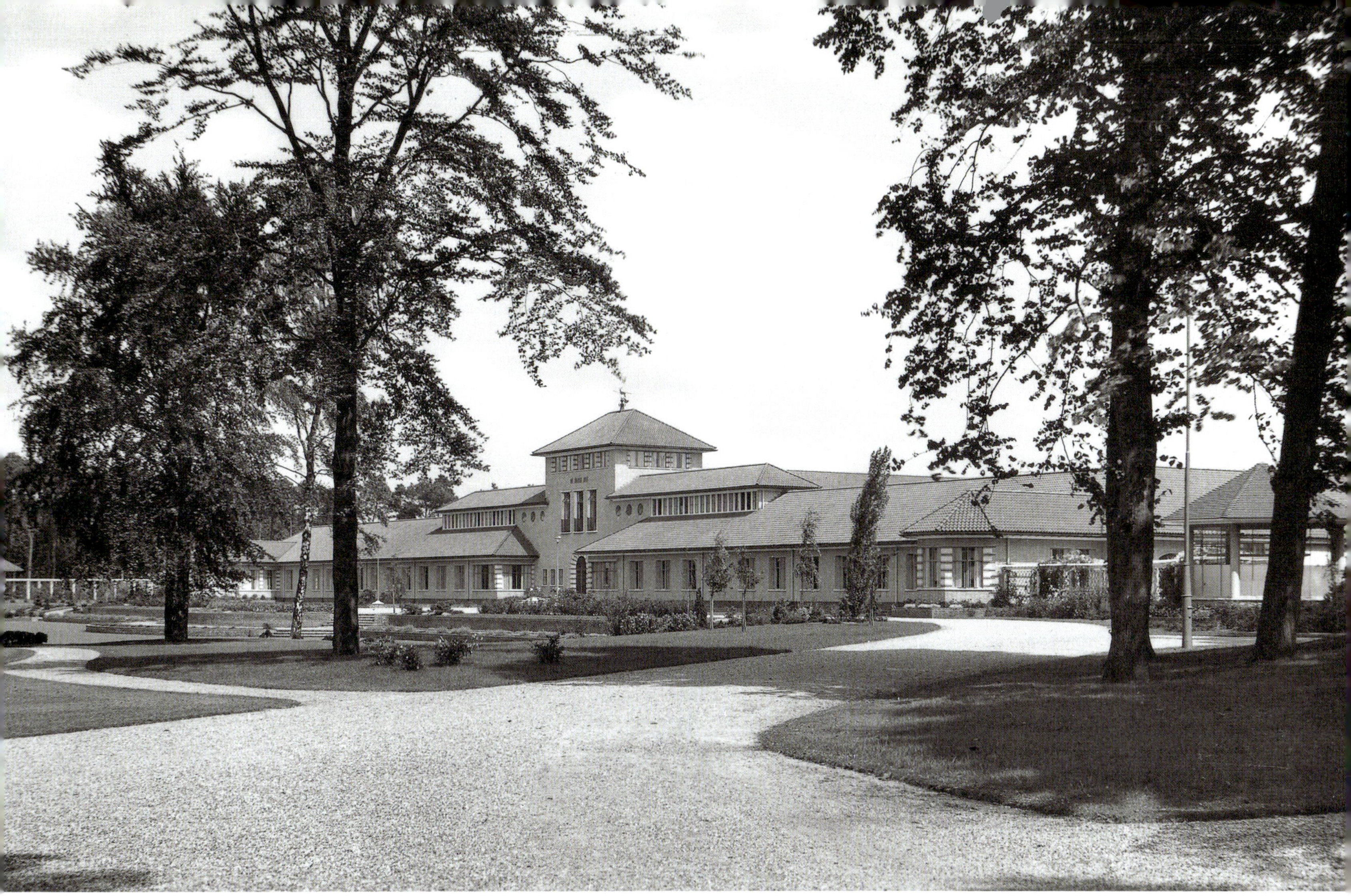

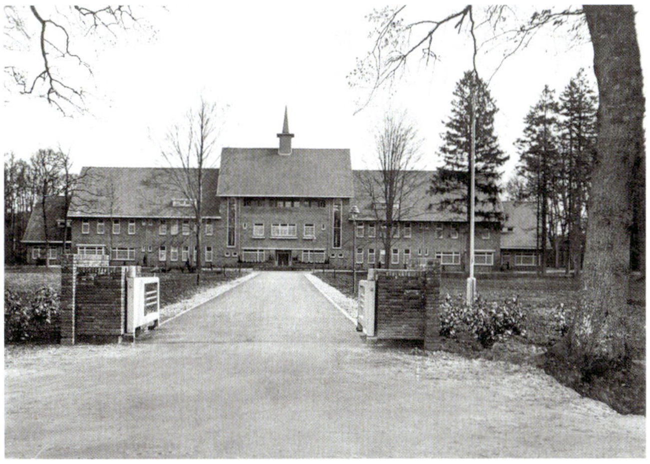

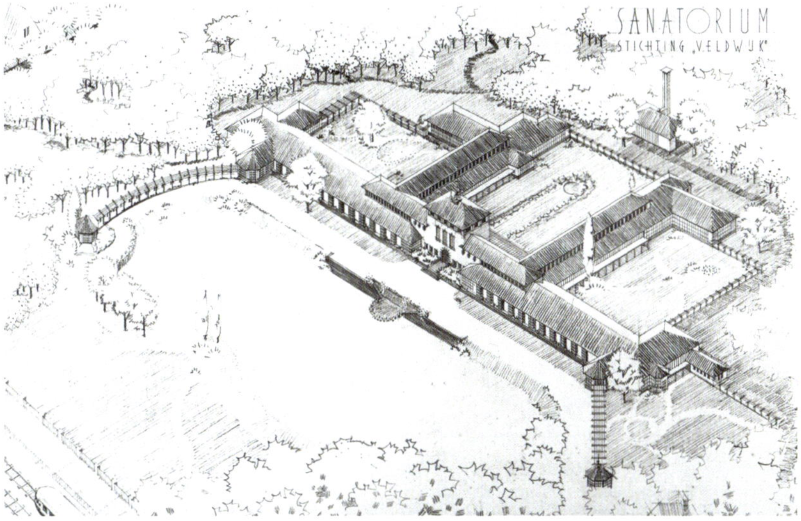
SANATORIUM
STICHTING „VELDWIJK"

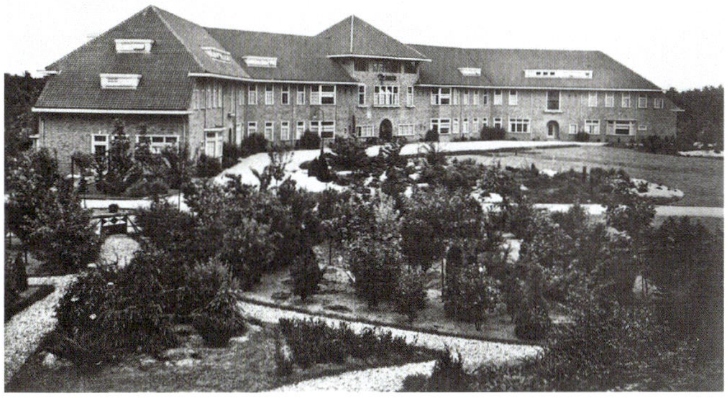

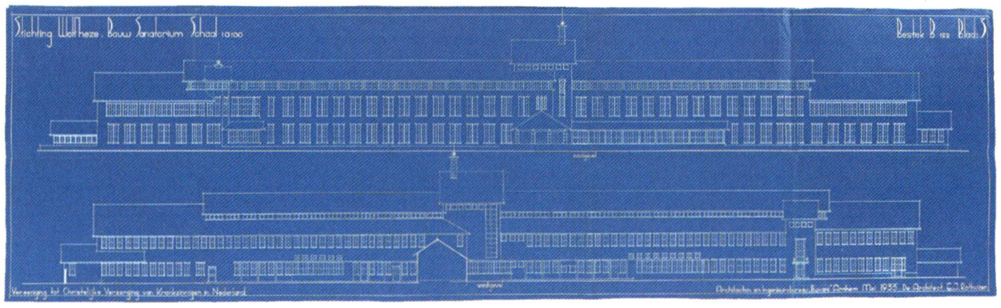
Stichting Wolfheze. Bouw Sanatorium
Vereeniging tot Christelijke Verzorging van Krankzinnigen in Nederland

been above all to give the building a friendly and domestic character totally lacking the depressing atmosphere of an asylum. On the outside the plinth is painted in a dull black and the walls above it are in a broken white silica. The roof, that is covered with dull black glazed tiles, hangs far beyond the walls to reinforce the rural character.'[14]

Such independent sanatoria, however, were rare. Most of them were built as annexes to existing asylums. Zon en Schild, the asylum built for the Dutch Reformed Church in Amersfoort in 1931, founded in turn the Hebron sanatorium some distance away. Hebron had two buildings with joint departments that were differentiated by class. After the completion of Licht en Kracht in Assen around 1935, the Port Natal sanatorium was created, which was physically separated from the asylum by the railway line to Zwolle. Work on building Hulp en Heil, the third complex commissioned by the Dutch Reformed Church, commenced in Leidschendam during the war. It was designed by the Mensink brothers. With its main building, various pavilions and a few service buildings, Hulp en Heil was more sober in design than the two earlier complexes of the Association.

The Association for the Protestant Care of Mental and Neural Disorders added a number of specially built pavilions to the existing asylums: Ockenburg to Bloemendaal (1930), Nederveluwe to Wolfheze (1935), the Noordersanatorium to Dennenoord (1935), and De Hooge Riet to Veldwijk (1939). The Noordersanatorium was opened in Zuidlaren in 1935. It is one of the most unusual buildings in the history of Dutch psychiatry and was described at the opening as a 'permanent monument' and a 'symphony of stone, glass and steel'.[15] It marks a climax in the oeuvre of the architect E. Reitsma. The effect of the architecture is reinforced by the carefully conceived garden design by J. Vroom, who developed around the middle of the twentieth century to become a specialist in the design of asylum gardens. Sanatoria like this mark a turning-point in psychiatry. What had proved impossible in the preceding decades was achieved between the two World Wars, when the asylums managed to shake off their negative aura and to replace it with the much more positive image of the modern hospital.

Housing and care for the elderly

Although the heyday of care for the elderly only began after the Second World War, it was anticipated by innovations in the 1920s and 1930s. The precursor of what was later to be known as the self-sufficient home for the elderly – homes that were specifically designed for that category without any care facilities – can already be found in the expansion plans of the larger cities in particular. Attempts to break away from the poorhouses for the elderly led in the same years to several competitions. Under the influence of religious compartmentalisation, the number of institutions that were later to be classified as a *pensiontehuis* – the concentration of a fairly large number of apartments for the elderly in a complex that also included communal facilities – increased slowly but surely. Although a systematic approach to housing and care for the elderly was still lacking , it cannot be said that housing for the elderly was entirely neglected.

Urban expansion and homes for the elderly

The awareness that at least a percentage of the elderly needed homes geared to their specific needs led designers to think about the architectural and urban planning requirements that they would have to meet. That led to proposals for small homes, usually with one storey, which were sometimes built in rows. These were integrated in the expansion plans of the larger cities. An example of this is the urban development plan that B.T. Boeyinga drew up for the Nieuwendam district; J. Boterenbrood designed the eighteen homes for the elderly that were included in that plan.[16] Some homes for the elderly were built by municipal housing departments, others by housing corporations, but in both cases usually within the provisions of the Housing Law. In 1927 the director of the Amsterdam Municipal Housing Department, A. Keppler, decided to build homes for the elderly in North Amsterdam: 230 were built between 1927 and 1931, most of them as part of garden villages.[17]

The homes for the elderly that were commissioned in South Amsterdam by the Remonstrant Brotherhood are stacked and there is no clear demarcation from the surrounding buildings. The two small blocks with a total of forty-two housing units for singles and couples were designed by the architect Th.J. Lammers and completed in 1937. The intention of the Remonstrants was to provide the residents with a self-sufficient housing unit with the advantages of a communal home. A concierge who lived on the premises was responsible for the central facilities.[18]

Attempts were made in Rotterdam to tackle the incorporation of homes for the elderly in a systematic way. Willem van Tijen, who achieved a reputation in the 1930s as a protagonist of modern principles in housing, designed a large complex of standardised housing units for the left bank of the River Maas, some of them designated for the elderly, within the framework of W.G. Witteveen's expansion plan. If this complex had been built it would have been a milestone in the history of modern prewar housing. It was an initiative of the N.V. Volkswoningbouw Rotterdam – a housing corporation that Van Tijen had helped to set up in 1929 – and envisaged four-hundred working-class homes and one-hundred middle-class ones. The challenge was to take increase of scale to such lengths that they would be profitable without the need for grants.[19] By working on a large scale, the N.V. Volkswoningbouw hoped 'to be able to benefit from the application of modern methods of labour and organisation and had confidence that by degrees they

p. 59 | <
***Th.J. Lammers*, home for the elderly, Amsterdam, 1937**

***A.J. Kropholler*, Mariënhof, Vught, 1939**

p. 59 | >
***J. Boterenbrood*, homes for the elderly, Amsterdam-Nieuwendam, 1931**

***J. Duiker & B. Bijvoet*, Karenhuizen, Alkmaar, 1919**

***J. Duiker & B. Bijvoet*, Karenhuizen, Alkmaar, 1919**

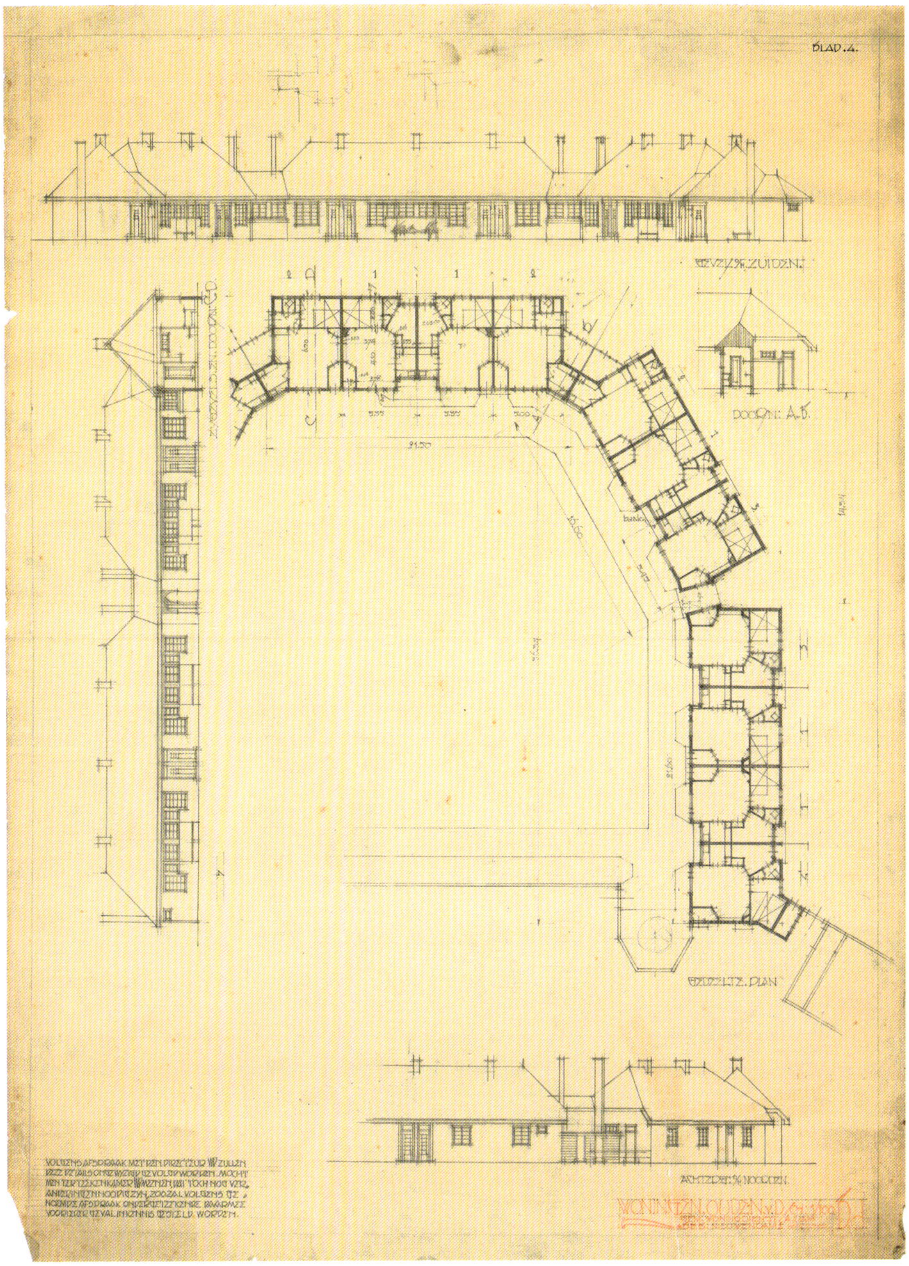

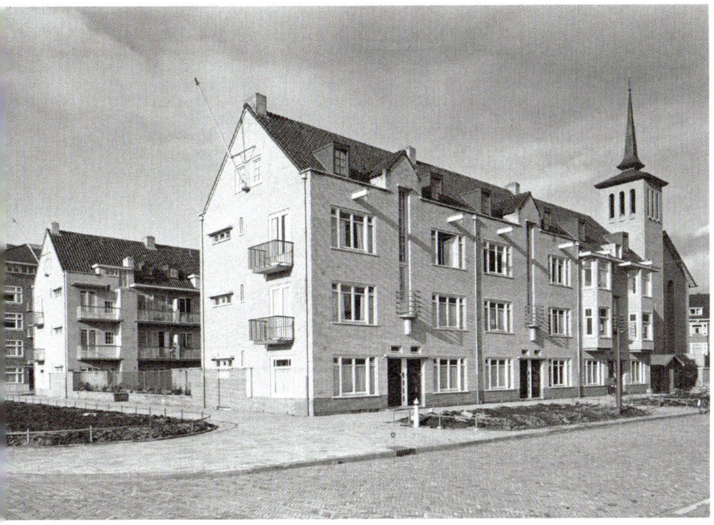

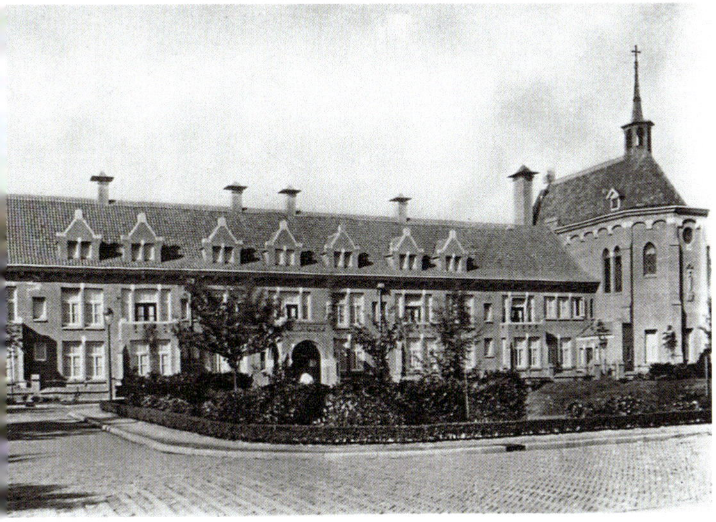

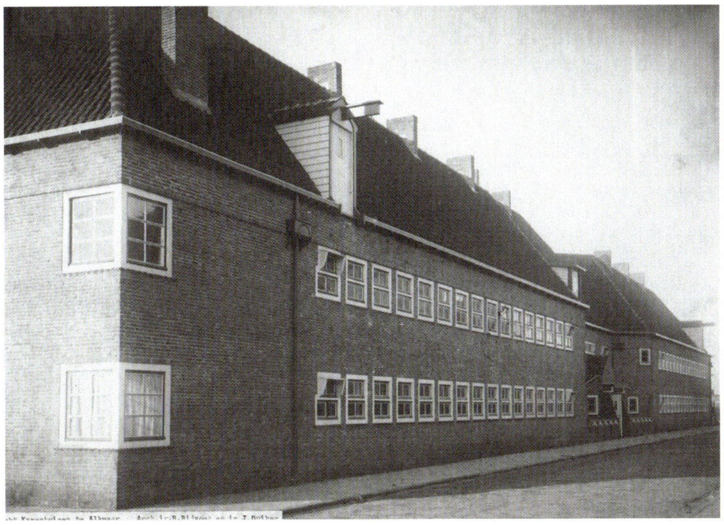

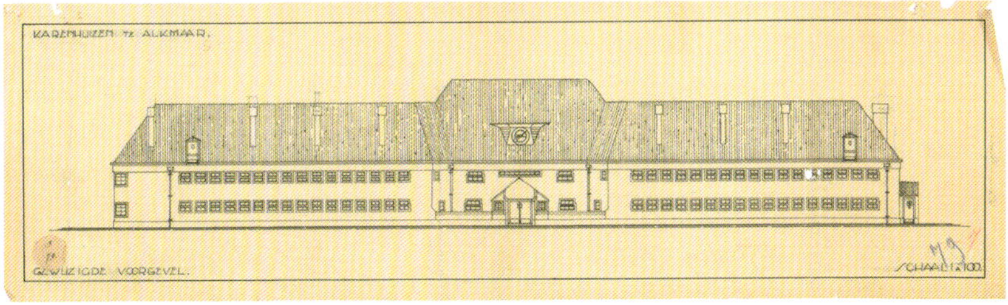

would be able to achieve appreciable savings, which will benefit the occupants first of all in the form of comfortable homes and low rents'.[20]

What did this pioneering design look like? It consisted of five long building blocks with a north-south orientation. The living rooms extended from the front to the back wall in accordance with the principle of what would later be known as the crosswall or through living room (*doorzonwoning*). Shops and garages sheltered the complex from the busy traffic on the northern side. The southern side was much quieter and therefore highly suitable for flats for the elderly. 'The open ends of the blocks and the strips of greenery that divide up each long block confer on the whole that openness on the one hand, that intimate contact between communal and individual vegetation on the other, that combine to form the characteristics of a good garden village.'[21] By charging a part of the rent to the ordinary working-class homes, these homes for the elderly could be kept very inexpensive. That the plan was not implemented was because there were delays in expropriating land in South Rotterdam, so that the local authority was unable to make the sites available here. The housing corporation decided to look for land elsewhere in the city, but the economic crisis threw a spanner in the works.

Predecessors of the old people's home

For most people, old age was synonymous with poverty until the 1940s, and this was reflected in their often appalling living conditions. If they were no longer able to live at home, there were poorhouses for the elderly, but these left a lot to be desired. The improvement of this situation was one of the reasons for the Vereeniging voor Volkshuisvesting 'Alkmaar' ('Alkmaar' Association for Housing) to organise an open competition for Karenhuizen, an old people's home. An important requirement was the generous admission of light and air. This meant that the corridor had to be placed on the northern side. The outside walls 'must give a harmonious expression of the organs behind them and of the function of the building'.[22] So the building was to have truth and character, two criteria that stem directly from the tradition of nineteenth-century architectural theory.[23] It must be able to accommodate as many old people as possible to meet the economic criteria. The names of the winning submissions are typical: Motto Sun II (first prize), Motto Sun I (second prize), Motto Old (third prize), Motto Pipe and Puss (fourth prize), Motto *Hofje* (fifth prize). The architects of Motto II Sun were Bernard Bijvoet and Jan Duiker. The jury wrote about their entry: 'The design is as a whole very good and has an attractive and intimate character. It satisfies the economic demands very satisfactorily (35 two-room and 11 one-room units) so that if implemented, this plan need not expect any objections from this quarter. The architecture is highly characteristic, except for the roof moulding, which is weak; the treatment of a few details is somewhat superficial.'[24] The design was implemented and was completed in 1919. It has a central volume that protrudes from the symmetrical façade, with one U-shaped wing on each side.

Karenhuizen is an early example of a complex that anticipates the later old people's home, but there were more. It is not fortuitous that the first attempts to build rest homes and old people's homes on any substantial scale date from the 1920s and 1930s and were completely dominated by the religious compartmentalisation. The most active were the Catholics, who erected many complexes that combined individual and communal facilities (*pensiontehuizen*) for both poor and more well-to-do old people, especially in the southern provinces of Brabant and Limburg. The Catholic complexes bear traces of the cluster of almshouses (*hofje*) typology, but the convent seems to have been a more important source of inspiration. Examples are the complexes designed by the Catholic architect A.J. Kropholler, such as Mariënhof in Vught commissioned by the Sisters of St Francis, built between 1939 and 1941 for affluent women, and Pension Mariëngaarde in Tilburg for more or less well-off elderly women, which opened its doors in 1935. Although its architecture may not be representative of Catholic taste in every respect, its aversion to experiments with modern materials and to an abstract modern idiom certainly was. Catholic institutional homes from these years seldom display any daring experiments and the accumulation of larger numbers of identical units was avoided or camouflaged. Traditional craftsmanship plays a large role, and it can clearly be seen that these complexes had to satisfy certain representative demands.

The Protestants focused on the poorer segment: the ambition of catering for the whole socio-economic spectrum was even rejected as late as the 1950s for being 'clerical'.[25] As a result, Protestant care for the elderly before 1945 was closely related to the traditional care for the poor, which does not mean that there were no attractive examples

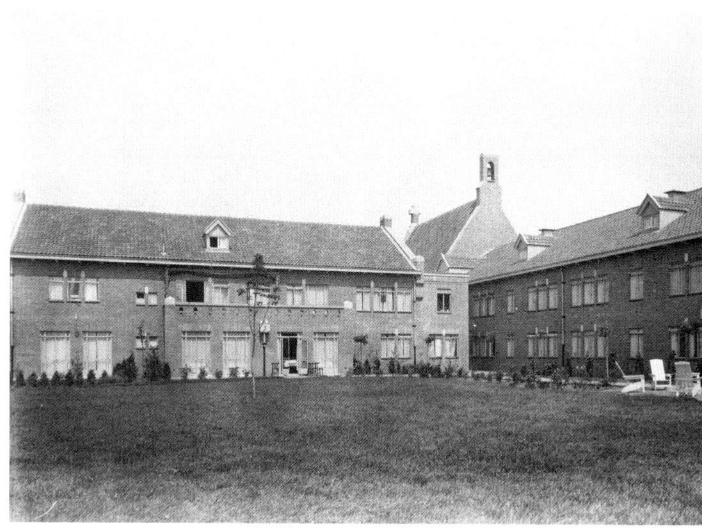

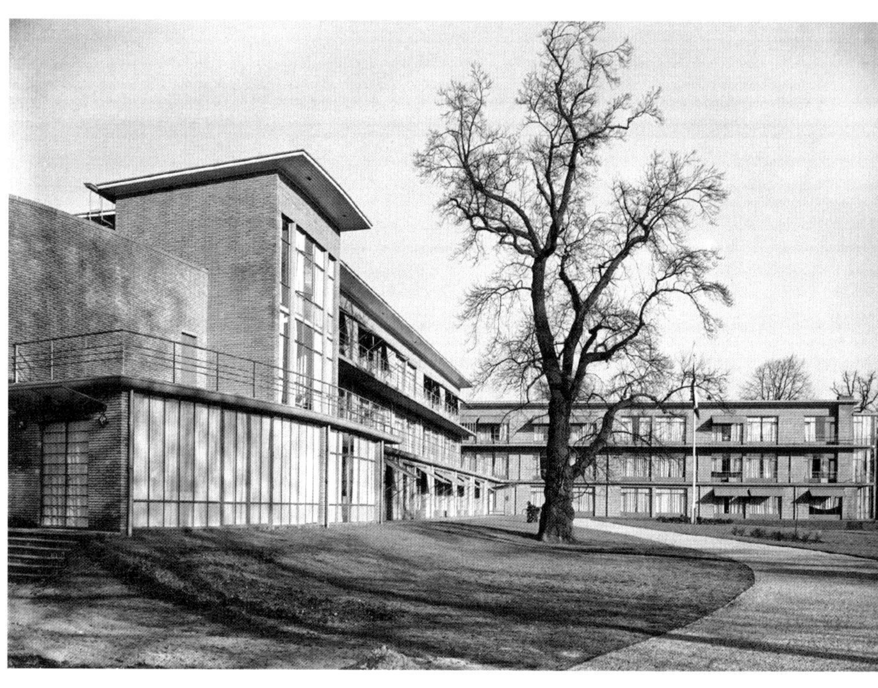

among the institutional homes that were implemented at the time. The Vereeniging van Hervormde Diaconieën in de Classis Edam (Association of Reformed Deaconates in the Edam Presbytery) commissioned Wieger Bruin to design a rest home for the elderly, De Rusthoeve, in Purmerend. It was partly intended for the elderly who could not afford the expense themselves (*bestedelingen*), and in this case also for more well-to-do old people.[26] Whereas this design followed traditional parameters, the rest home in Driebergen by J.B. van Loghem reflects the modern ideals of its architect.

The functionalist J.H. Groenewegen praised the building in *De 8 en Opbouw*, the fortnightly organ of the functionalists. He wrote that it had nothing in common with the conventional sombre, villa-like buildings with rooms on the north and communal areas that were oppressive in spite of their height of often four metres: 'How different from this type of rest home is the new rest home in Driebergen illustrated here. You notice it the moment you enter the building: here there is none of the oppressive feeling of being shut up, those who seek rest here do not feel that they are treated as patients. The long horizontal windows afford an unobstructed view of the beautiful pines, the frisky squirrels; in a room like that, you can actually be said to be resting in nature.'[27] Huize Avondzon in Velp, designed by the architect J.J. Hornstra, is an example of an old people's home that incorporated functionalist features in a more traditional design.

However modest the efforts were in the field of housing for the elderly, it is not that it was an unknown phenomenon before 1945. Several main types of specific housing for the elderly had already been developed, namely the combination of communal facilities with individual rooms (*pensiontehuis*) and the old people's home (*bejaardenwoning*). Their number was limited, however, and the number of old people who could make use of them was very small. A striking absentee is the later nursing home. It was not entirely unknown; in 1929 the Vereniging Het Zonnehuis established one of the first nursing homes in an old villa in Beekbergen (Gelderland). It offered a home not only to the elderly and infirm but also to younger people with a chronic illness. The Rotterdam architects Lockhorst and Overeynder extended the villa in 1937. Their extension was designed in a style typical of the 1930s with an emphasis on the horizontal dimension and gently sloping overhanging saddle or hip roofs and masonry.

p. 60
***A.J. Kropholler*, Pension Mariëngaarde, Tilburg, 1935**

***J.J. Hornstra*, Huize Avondzon, Velp, 1938**

p. 61
***Lockhorst & Overeijnder*, extension nursing home Het Zonnehuis, Beekbergen, 1937**

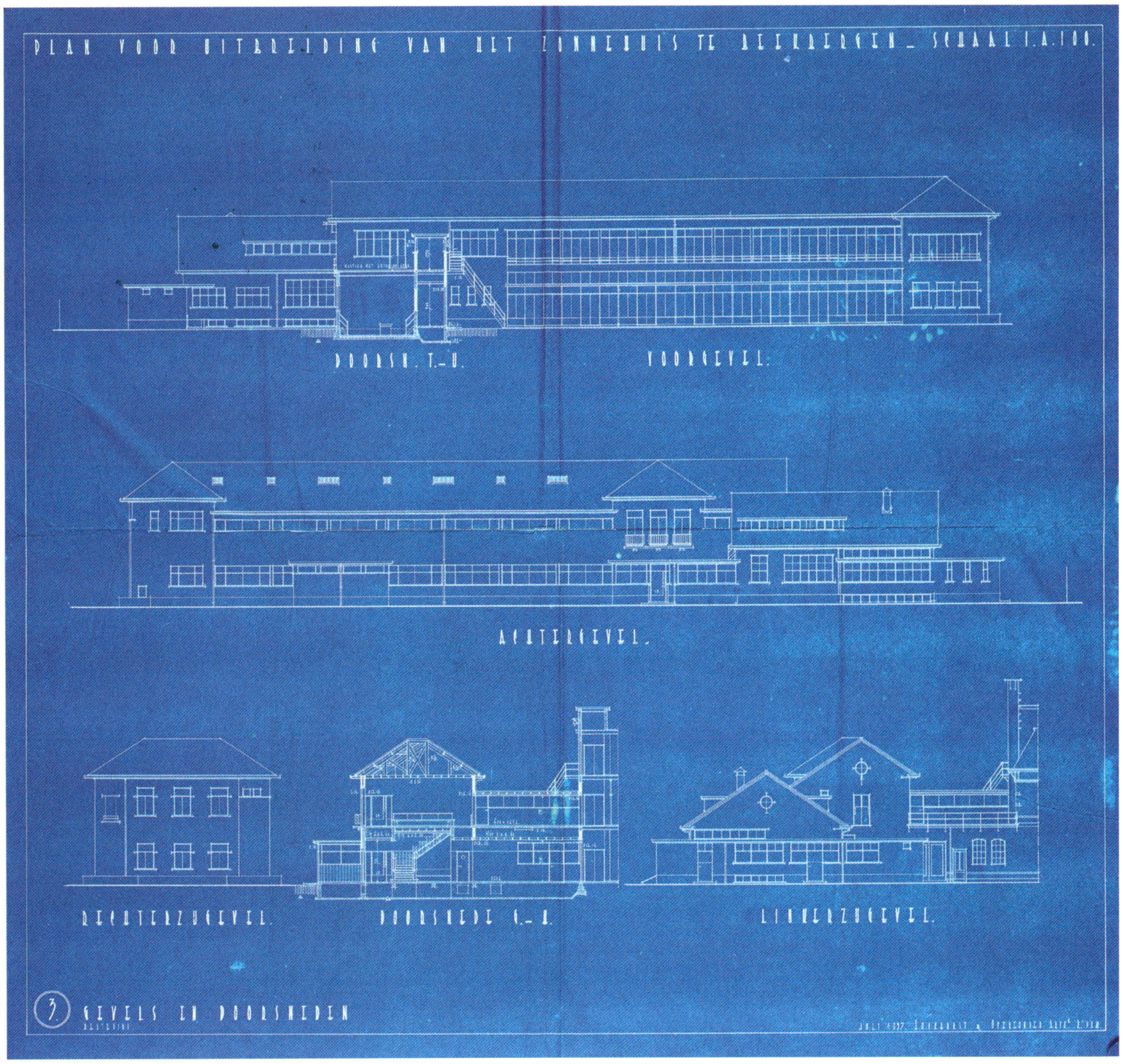

Connecting corridor

Ed. Cuypers

Extension Sint Jozefziekenhuis
Heerlen
1920-1923

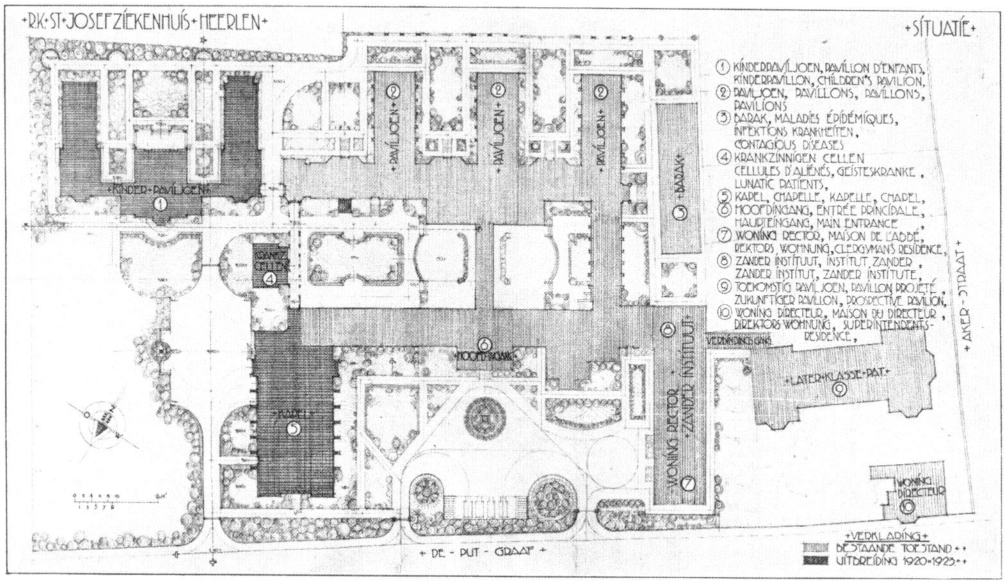

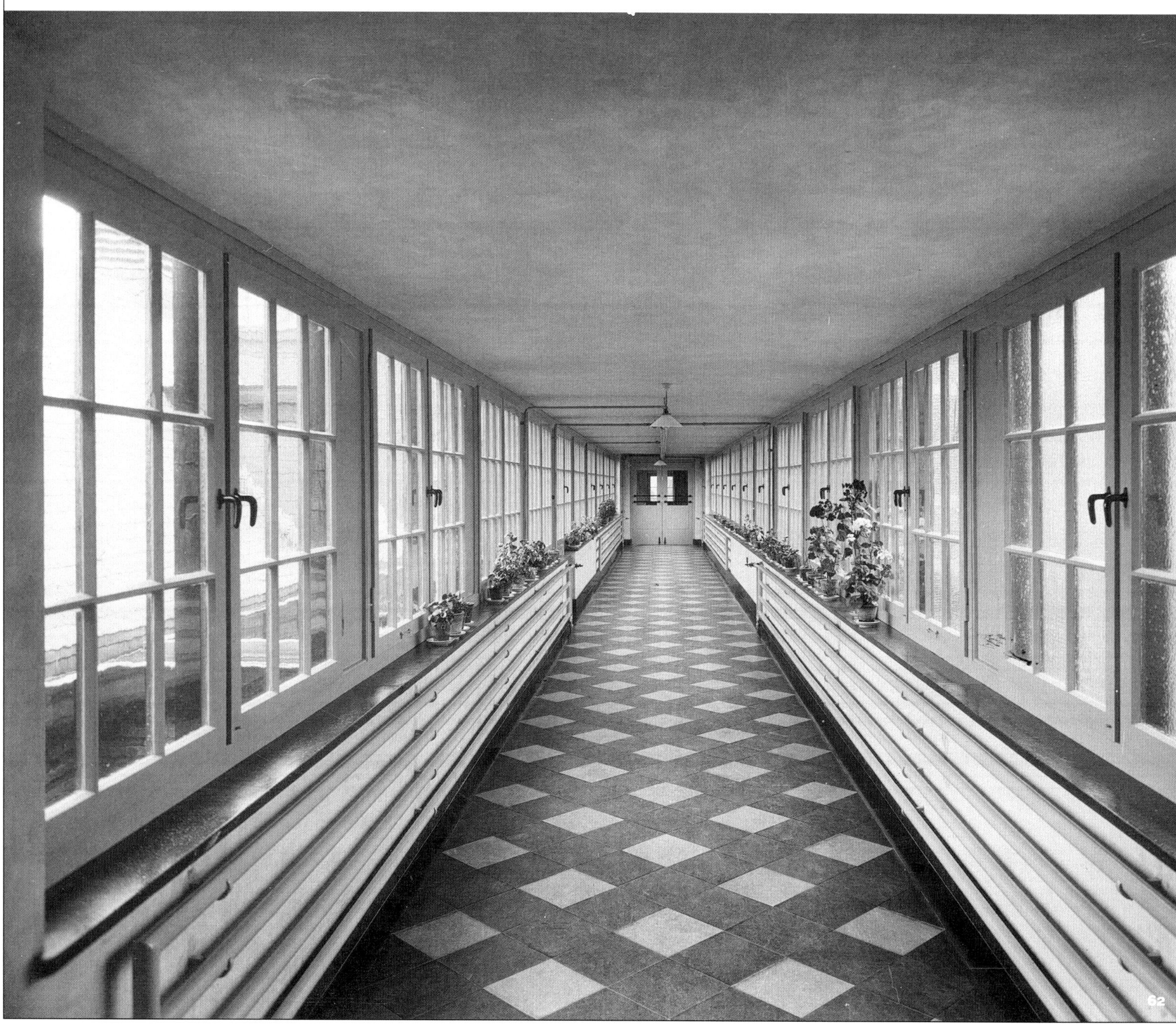

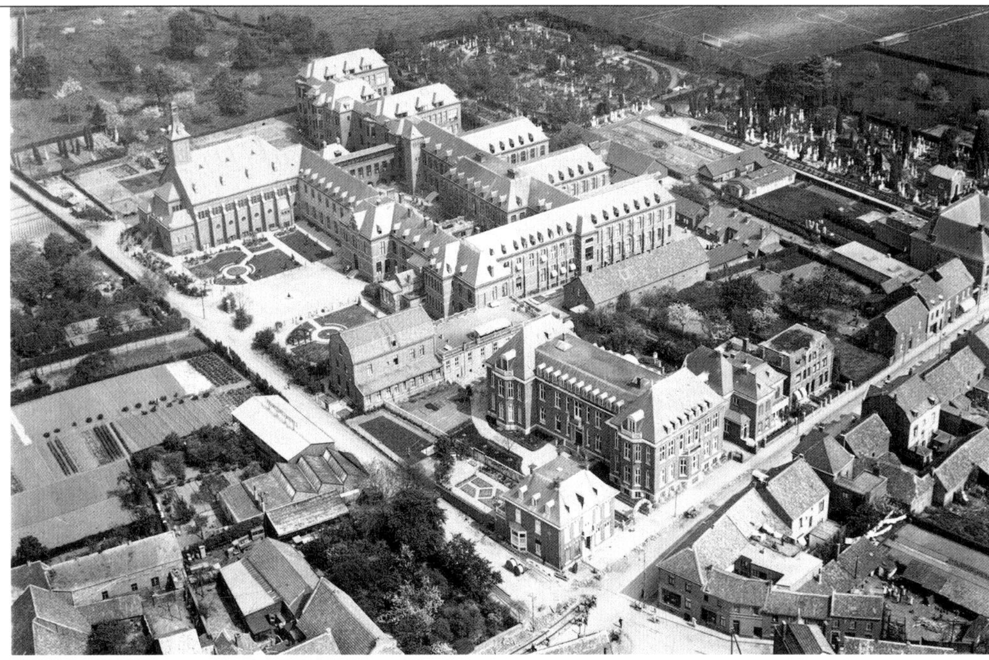

The Sint Jozefziekenhuis opened in 1904 and was extended several times afterwards. As the population of Heerlen grew rapidly because of the mining industry, a new extension was required by 1920. At that moment the hospital had 360 beds, whereas a capacity of 450 was called for. Ed. Cuypers was commissioned to draw up a design for an extension of the hospital with a pavilion for women and children, a church, living quarters for the staff, bedrooms for the nurses, a unit for mental patients, a mortuary, a laundry, connecting corridors, and a garage.

The hospital was conceived on a spacious scale from the first extension according to the corridor-pavilion system, a hybrid form that combined the advantages of both corridor and pavilion types. In this case the different pavilions are connected with one another by roofed corridors.

The extension of the hospital coincided with the implementation of several technical installations, including central heating and ventilation, hot and cold water, electric lighting, telephone, a lift, sanitary fittings, and drains. There is a lift to every floor large enough to carry an ambulance.

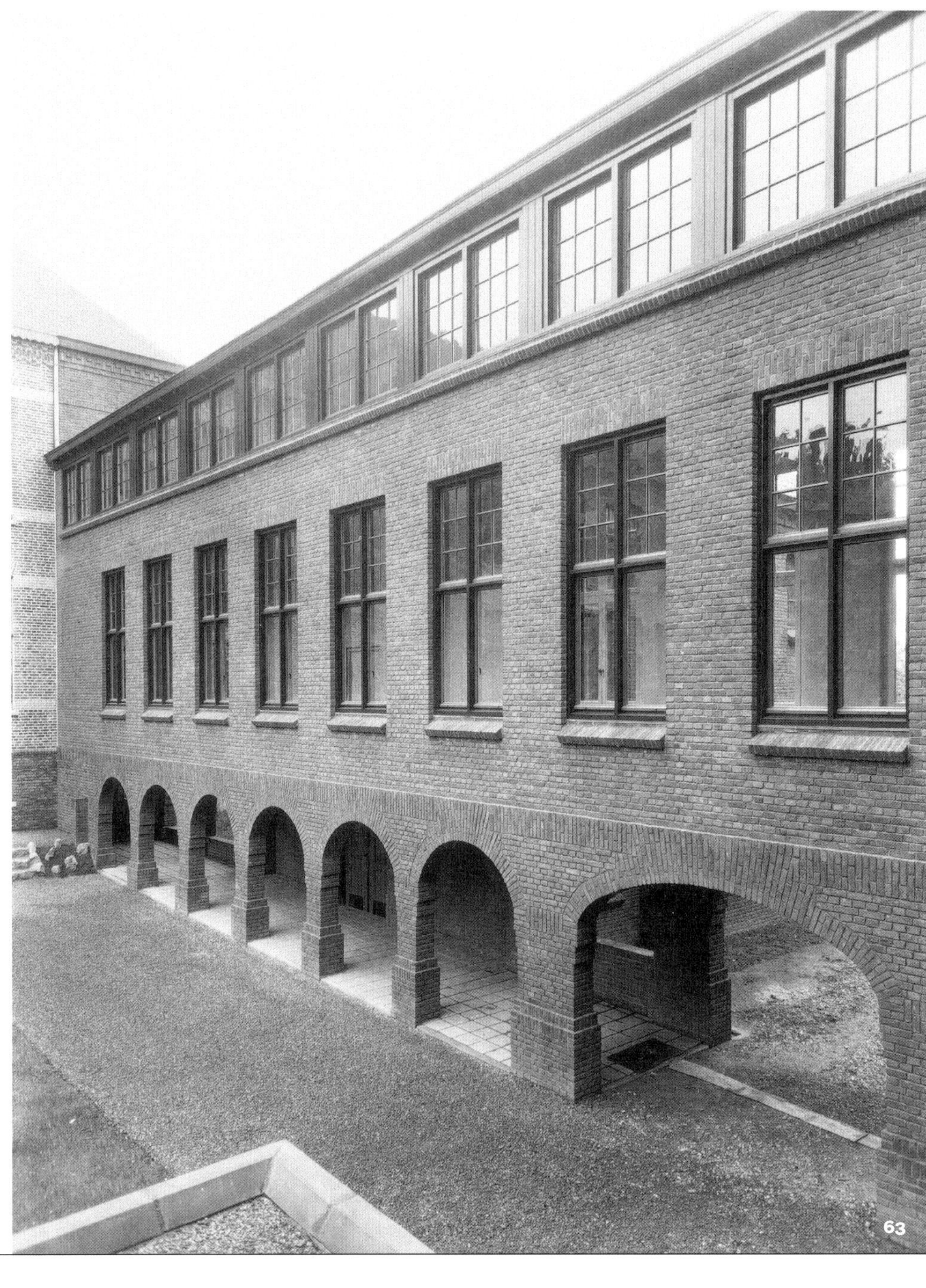

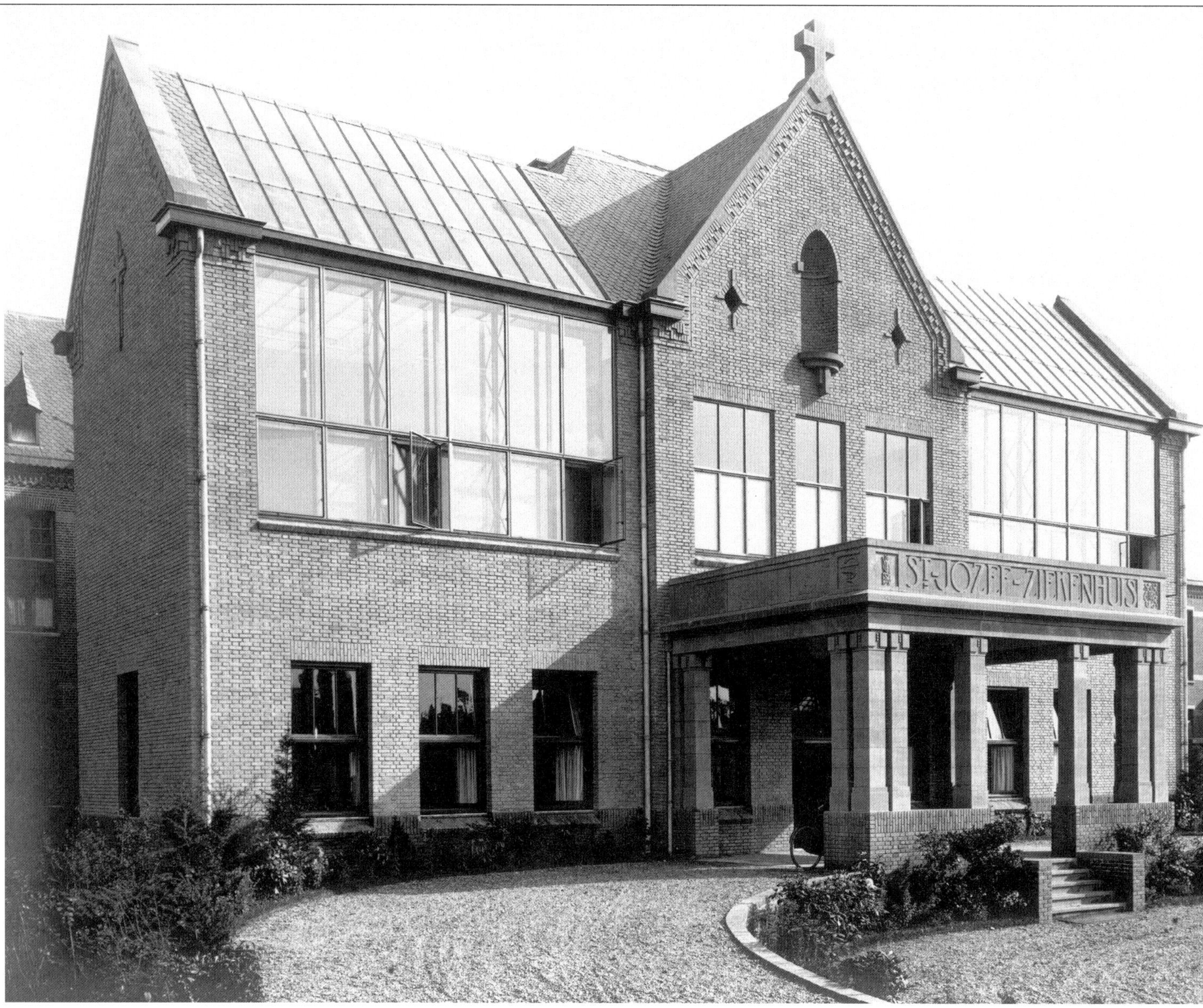
ST-JOZEF-ZIEKENHUIS

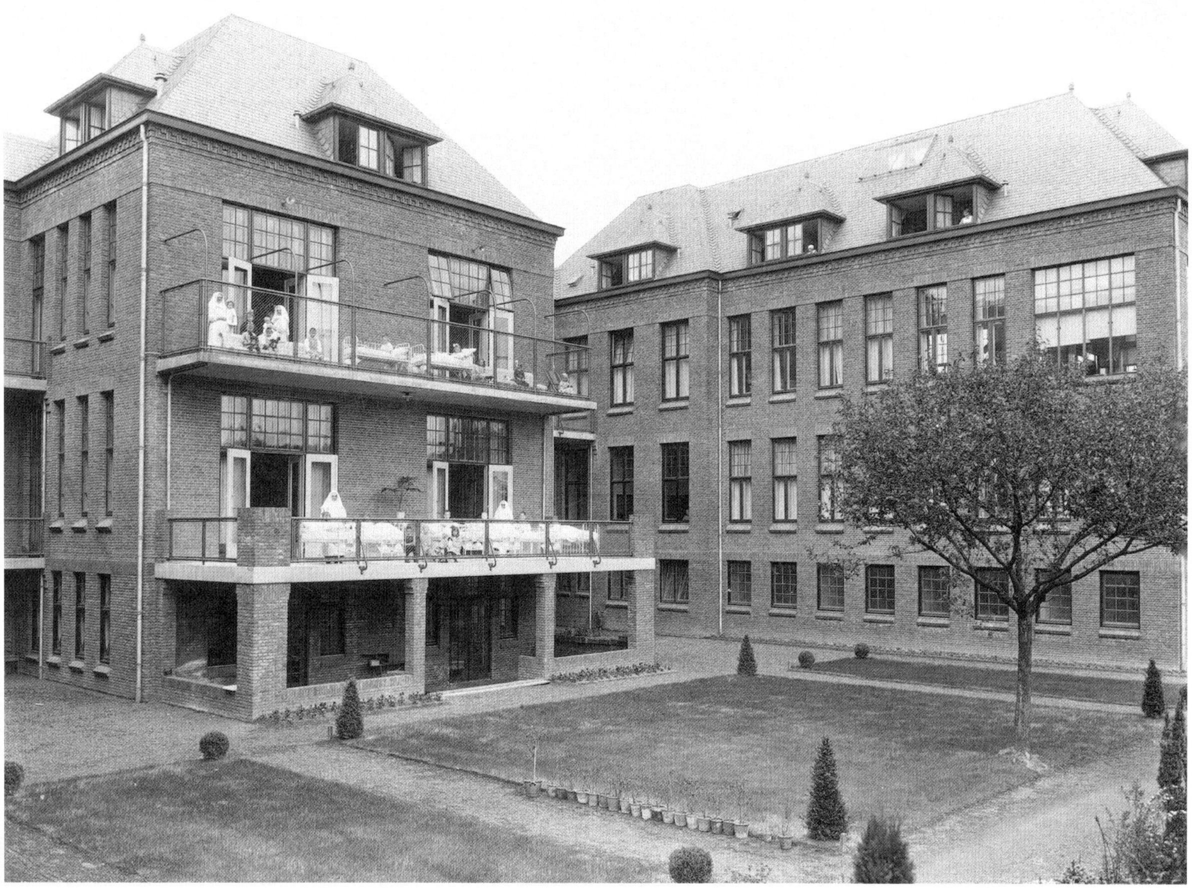

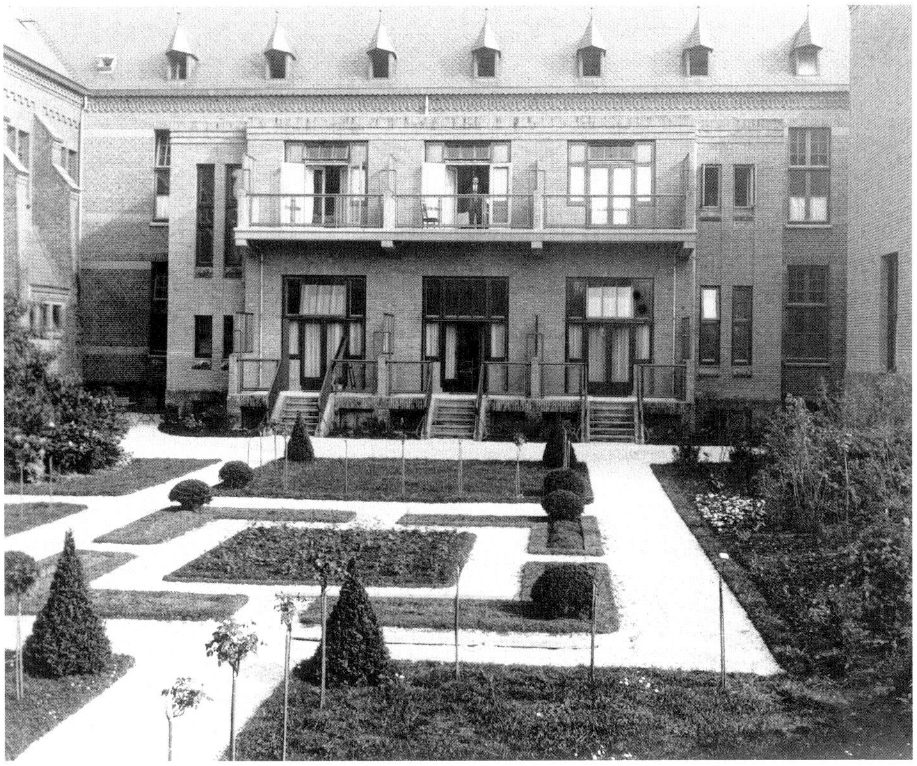

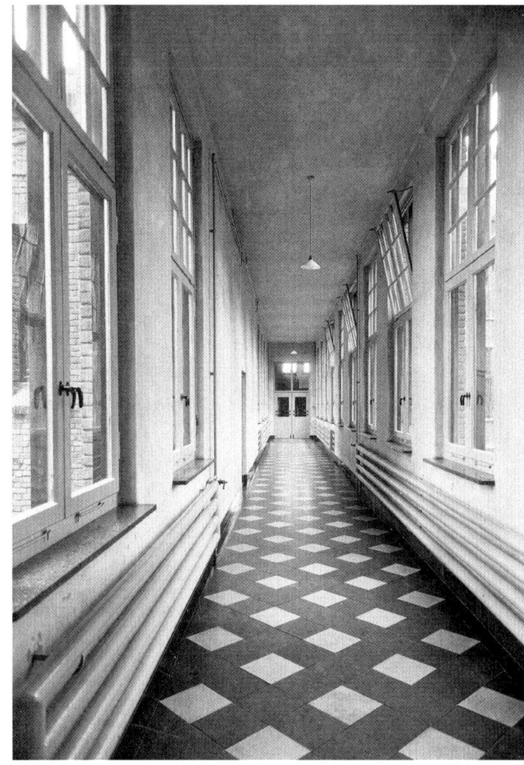

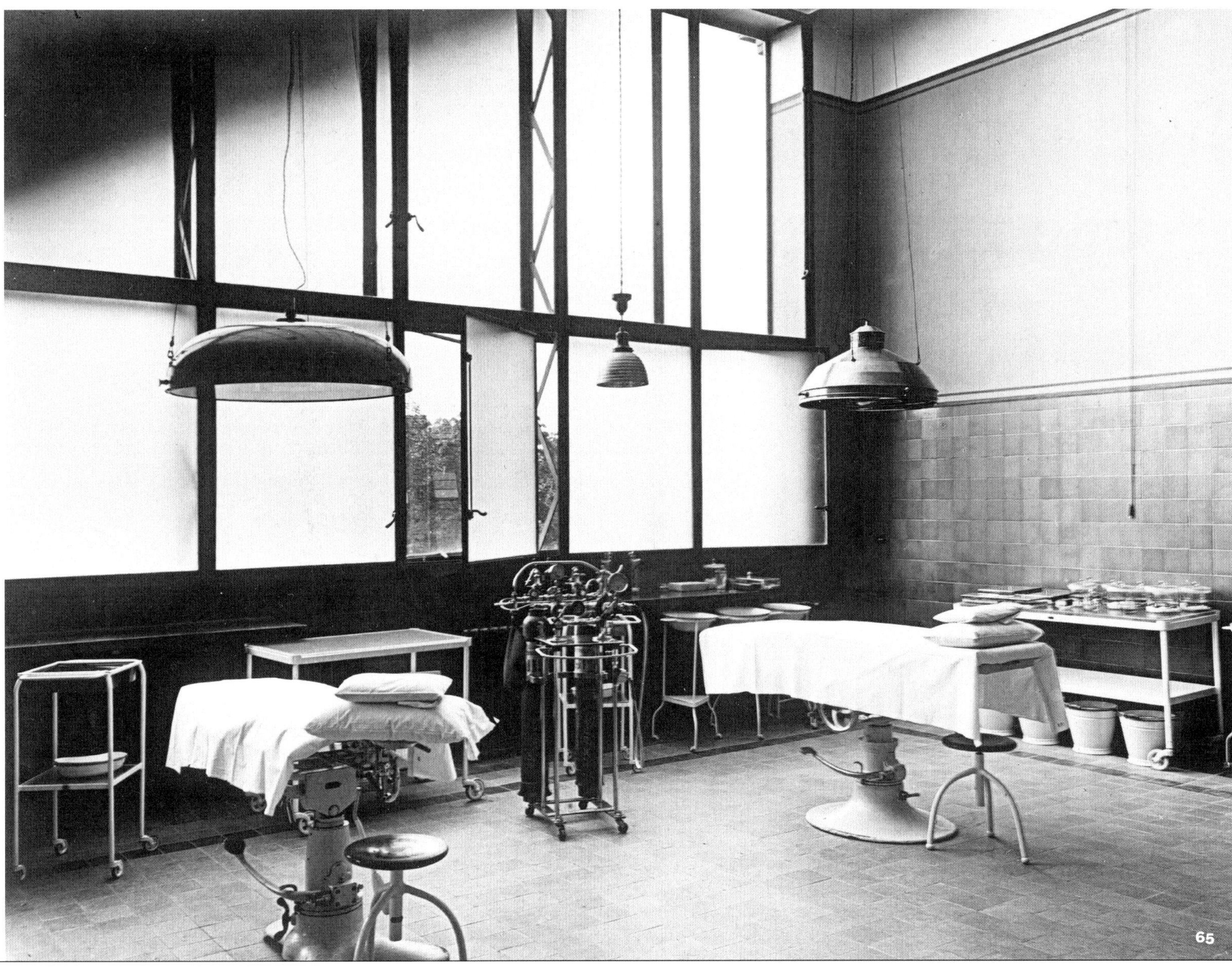

Shelter

Gebroeders Mensink &
Van Hoogevest

Zon en Schild
Amersfoort
1928-1940

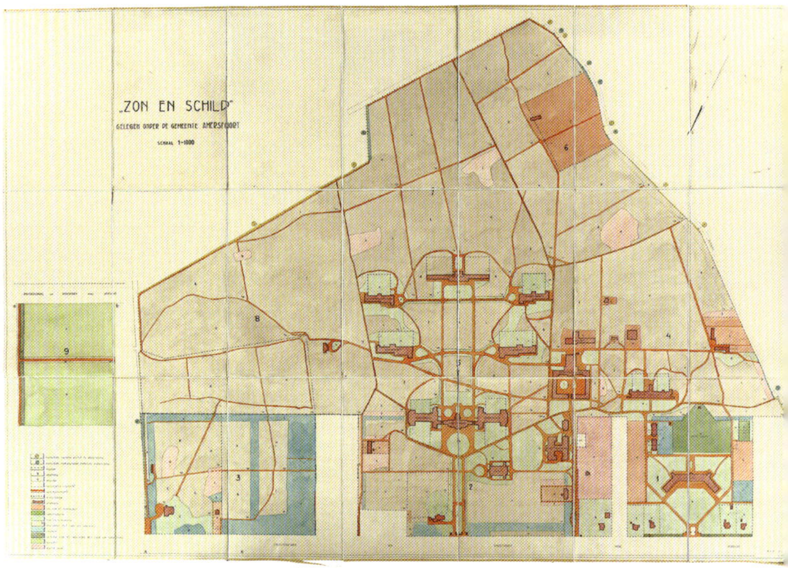

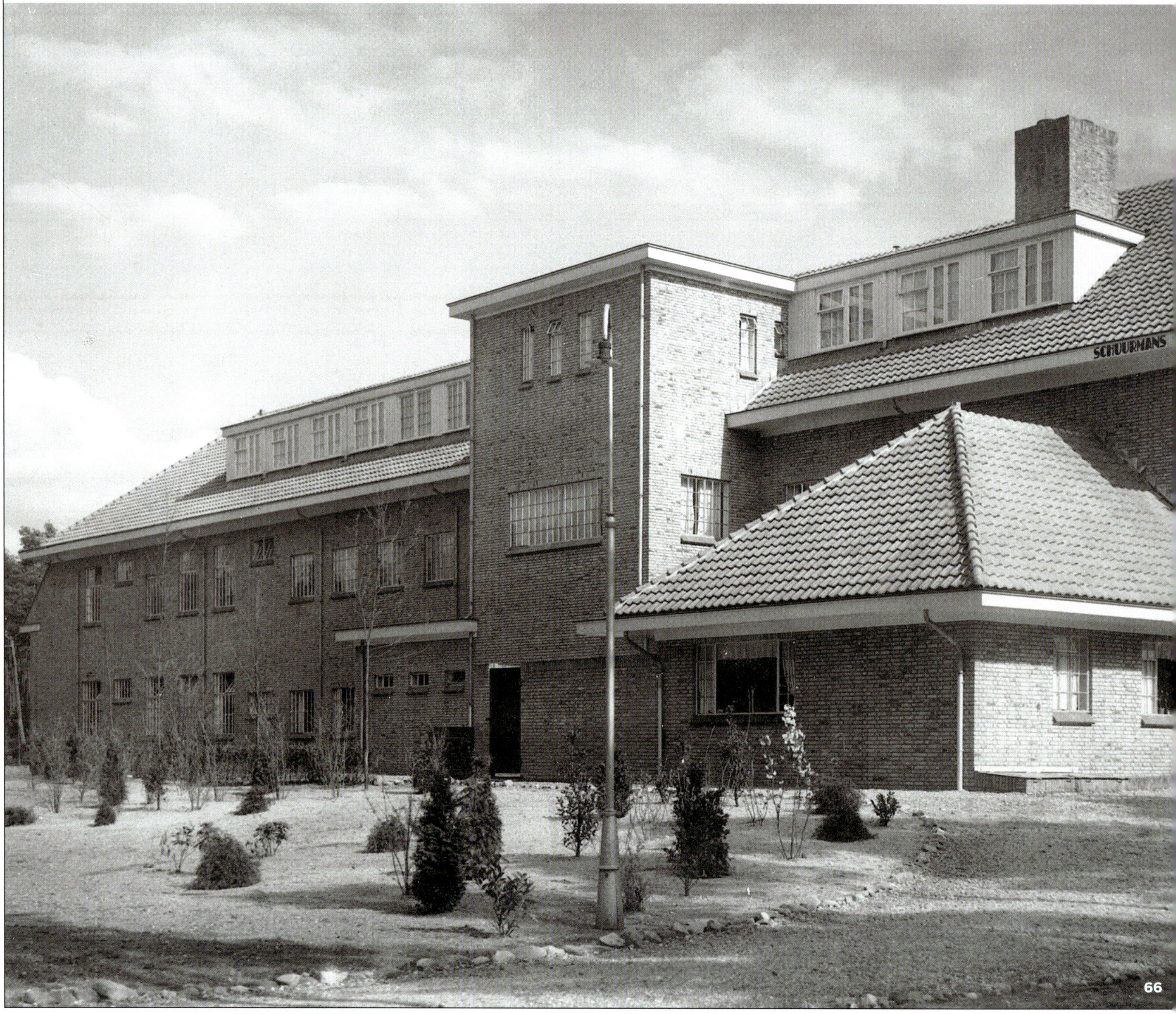

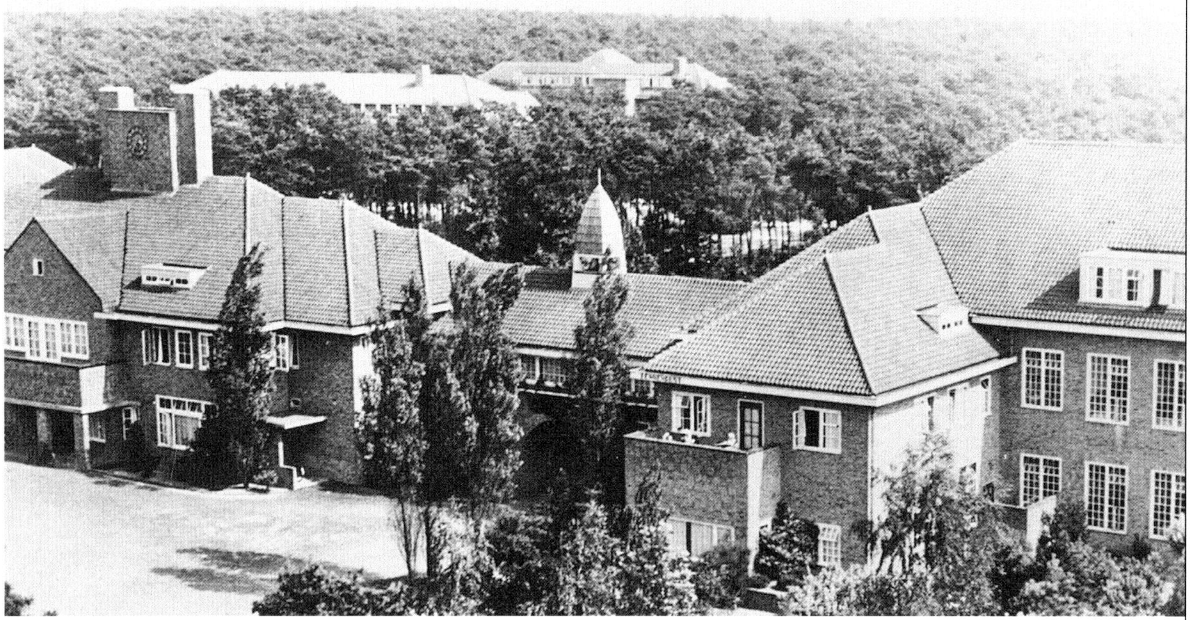

The Association of Dutch Reformed Foundations for Neural and Mental Illness set up the Zon en Schild institution in Amersfoort in the period between the two World Wars. The name is taken from *Psalm* 84:11: 'For the Lord God is a sun and shield'. The complex provides shelter for its residents amidst fellow sufferers of the same faith. It can accommodate approximately 600 patients. As was still common during this period, Zon en Schild was designed in accordance with the pavilion system and was implemented in several building stages. The complex has a predominantly symmetrical structure, with the most important buildings arranged on either side of a central axis. The main building, completed in 1931 and flanked by a wing on each side, occupies the position in the middle. Female patients are accommodated in the east wing and in pavilions, male patients in the west wing. South of the main building are two pavilions on both sides to accommodate patients. The calm patients are housed in the wings of the main building, those with the most restless behaviour in the pavilions at the rear. The 'semi-restless' patients are accommodated in the intervening pavilions. The complex also includes a church, a recreational building, a kitchen building, a therapy building, a laboratory, greenhouses, a gardener's house and a mortuary. The Hebron sanatorium with a pavilion for those who could afford to pay more was implemented in 1932. The director's villa is situated beside the main entrance, and there are several houses for the doctors beside the Utrechtseweg. In 1940 a pavilion was built for tuberculosis patients at the southern end of the main axis of the terrain.

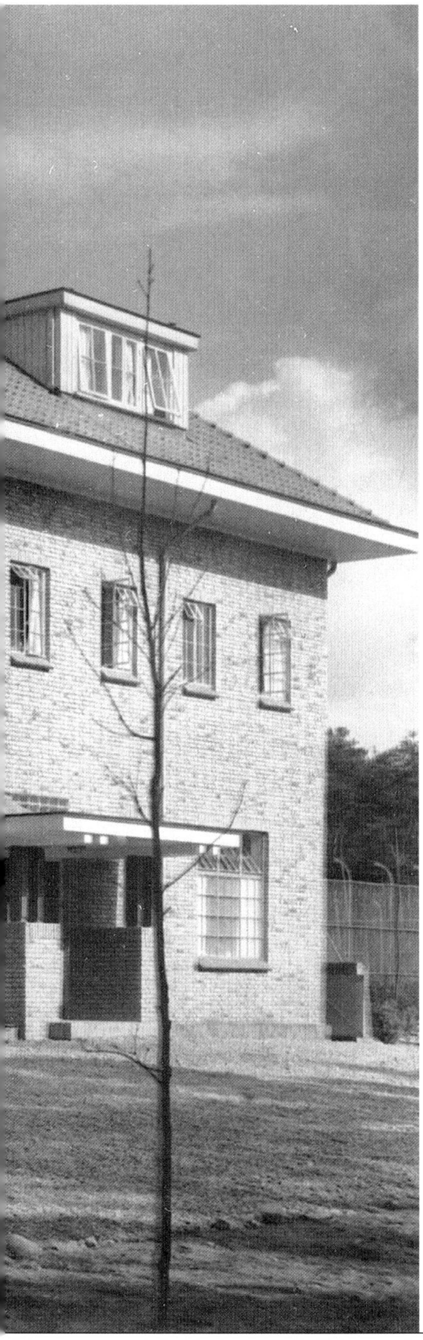

p. 66
Schuurmans Stekhoven pavilion

p. 67
Overview with on the foreground the main building and Dennenrust pavilion

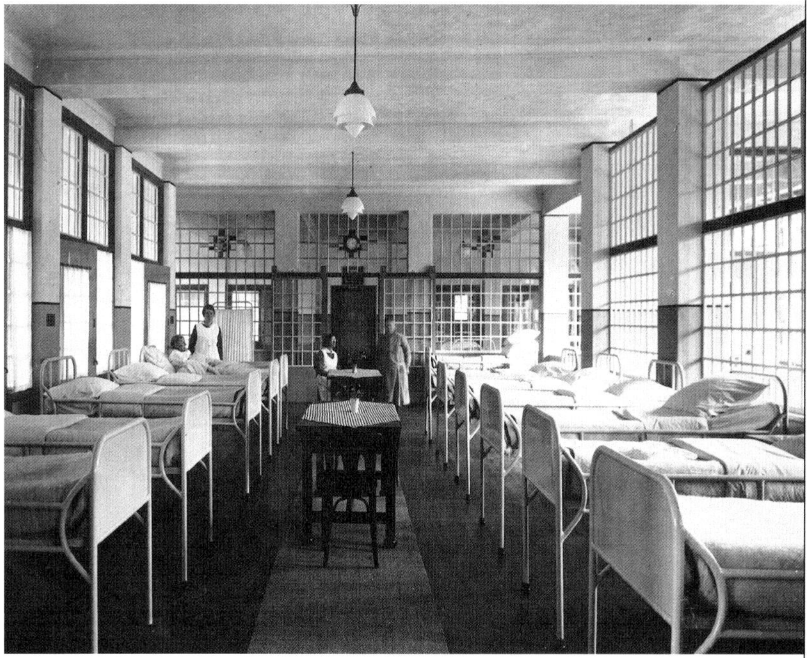

Villa

J.B. van Loghem

Rusthuis De Blauwvoet
Driebergen
1930

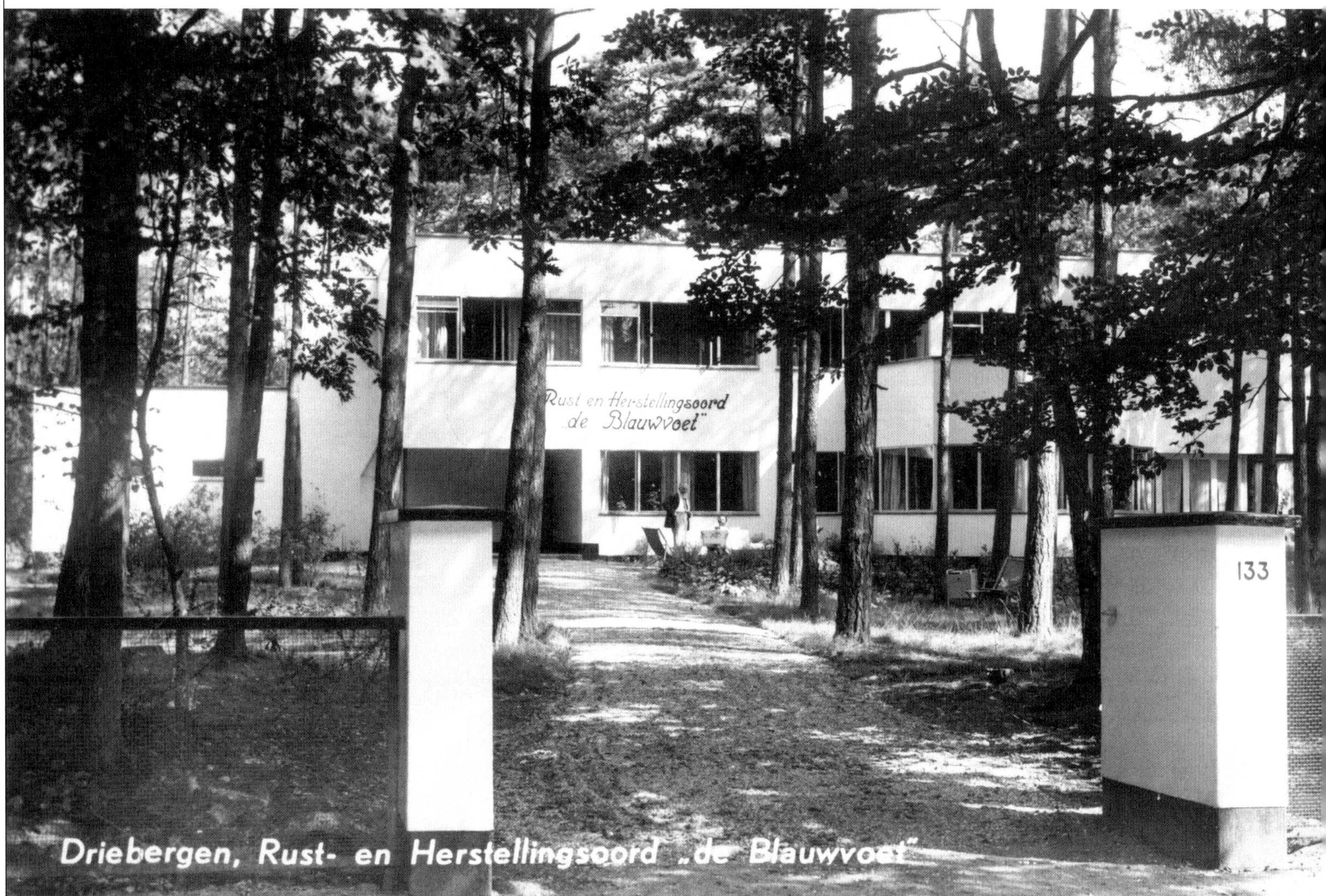

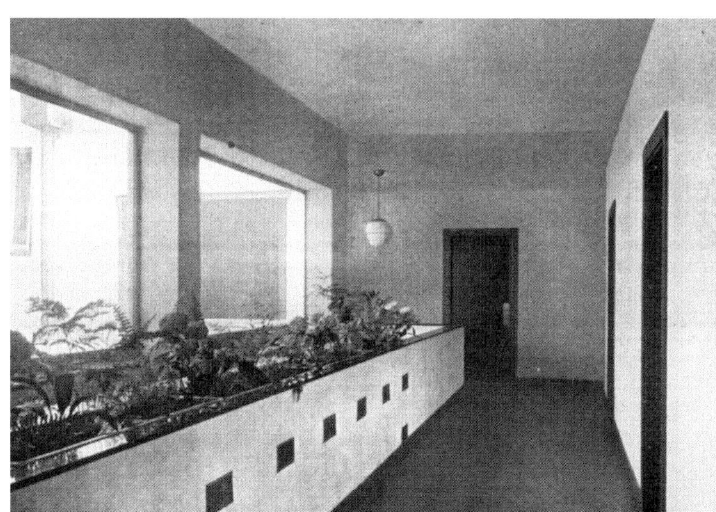

This rest home in Driebergen designed by J.B. van Loghem is inspired by the ideas of Functionalism. It was commissioned by the physician and psychiatrist Pieter Bierens de Haan. De Blauwvoet, a rest and convalescent home, accommodated a small number of (mild) neurasthenics on a non-permanent basis. Most of them were old people. The detached villa is situated in the woods in the middle of a large 5500 m² terrain. It has three storeys: a basement, ground floor and first floor. The lounges and dining rooms face south and west, with the bedrooms for the patients above them. The medical superintendent's quarters are in a separate wing. The east wing accommodates the kitchen and service areas on the ground floor and the bedrooms for the staff on the first floor. There are several roofed porches for the patients. The villa has horizontal strips of windows and is plastered white.

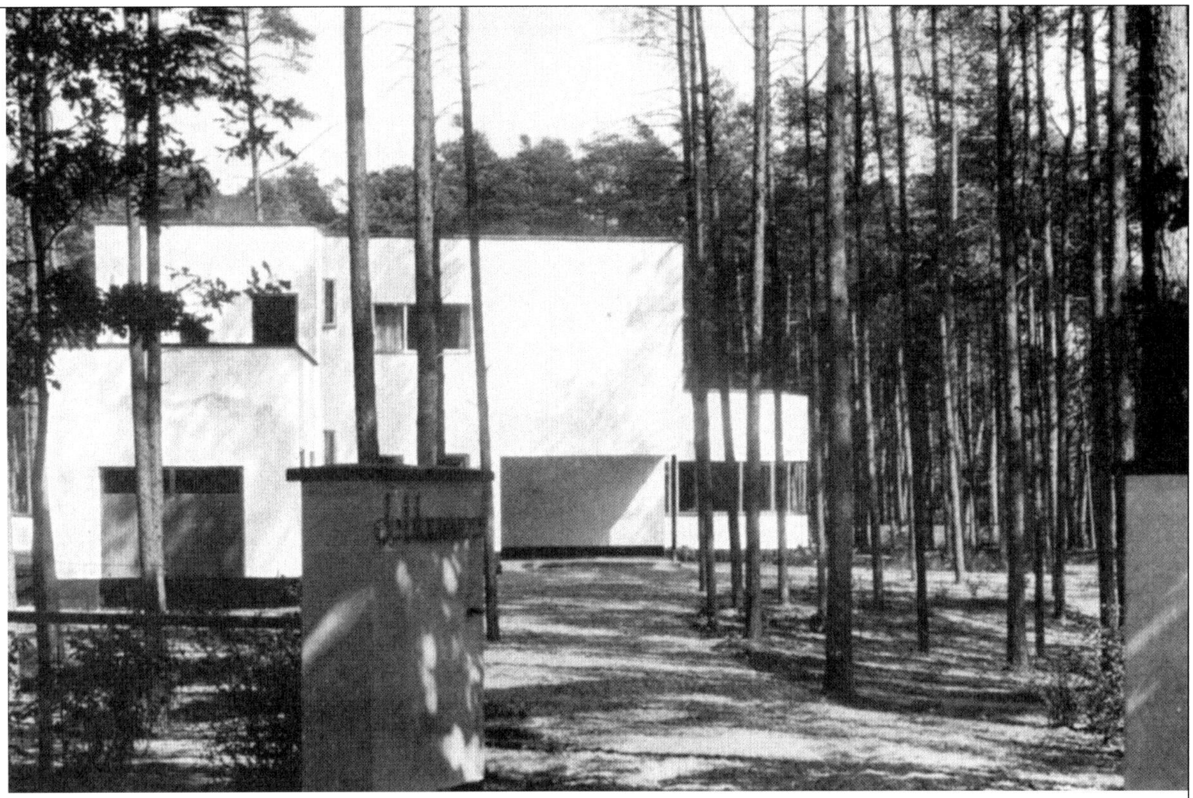

Ground floor and first floor
1 *bedroom*
2 *servant room*
3 *storage room*
4 *bathroom*
5 *garage*
6 *kitchen*
7 *dining room*
8 *living room*
9 *wardrobe*

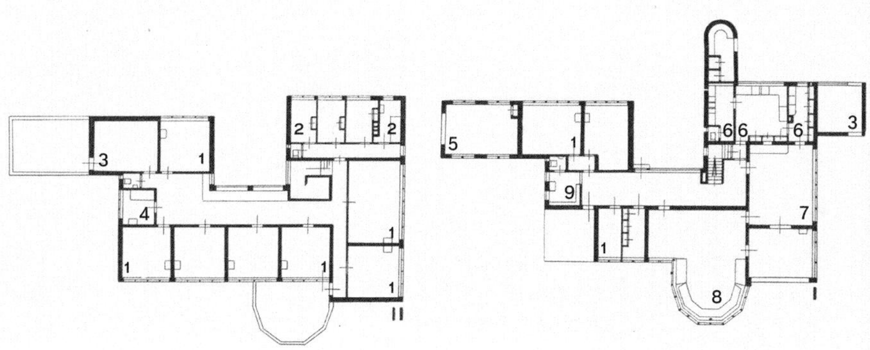

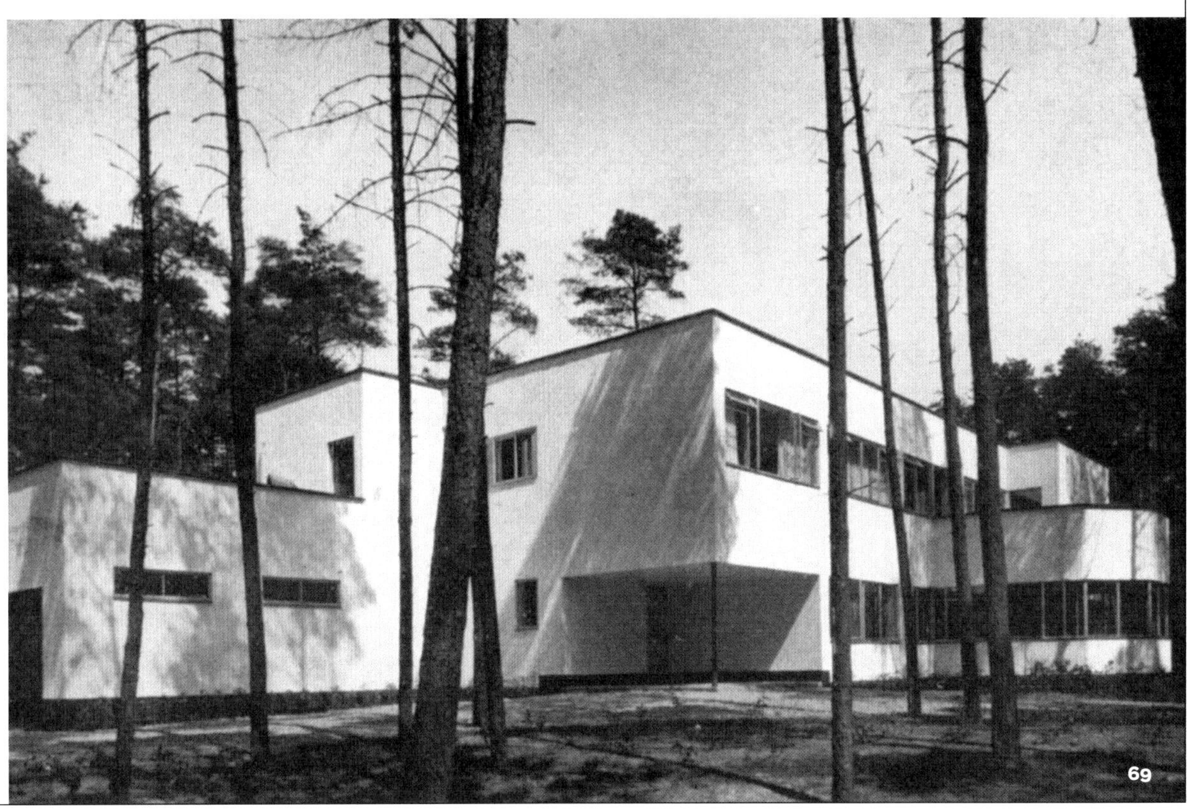

Cantilever

J.G. Wiebenga with
J. van der Linden

Extension Sophiaziekenhuis
Zwolle
1935

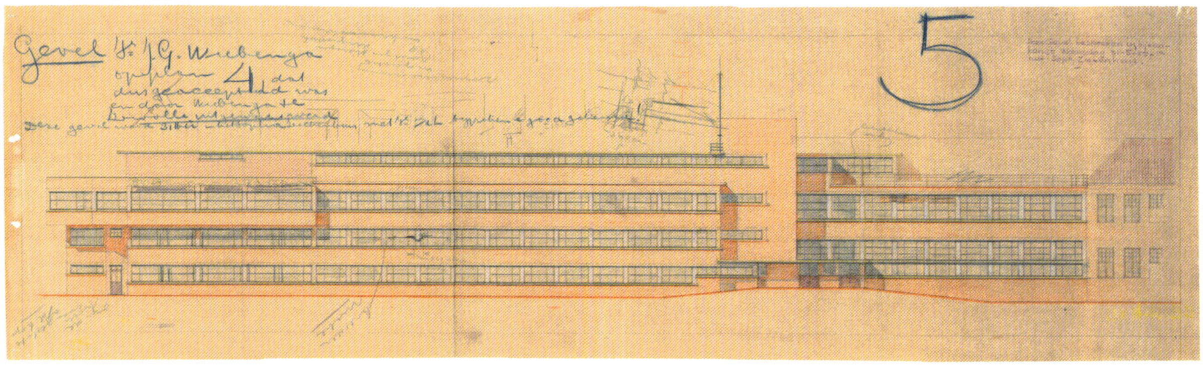

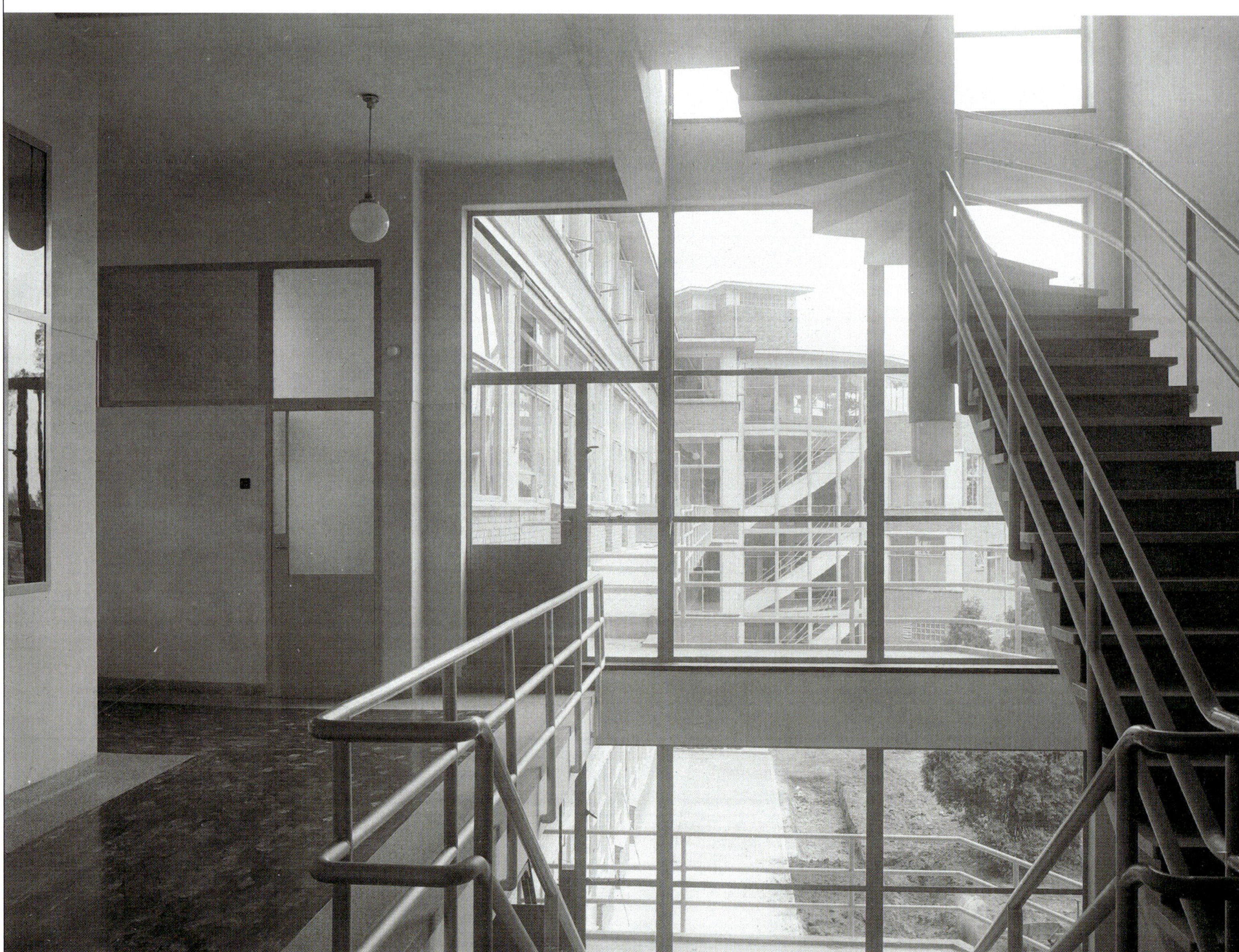

Wiebenga's plan for an extension of the Sophiaziekenhuis in Zwolle was intended to create order in the chaos that characterised the existing complex after numerous additions and modifications. The design was the result of the sketches that J. van der Linden, who had experience in building hospitals, put down on paper as a reaction to Wiebenga's earlier proposal. It filled the corner of the hospital grounds with a symmetrical narrow building containing the operating theatres, X-ray unit, a laboratory and teaching rooms for the nurses. Characteristic are the bold cantilevers, which show how Wiebenga managed to exploit the potential of reinforced concrete to the full.

An elongated wing, interrupted by the lift tower, extended from this narrow building to a previous extension of the old premises dating from 1883. The plan envisaged a similar wing on the other side to create an enclosed garden, but the latter wing never materialised. The main entrance is next to the lift tower and also has a cantilever canopy that juts out far from the wall. Most of the concrete has been left in view and plastered white on the outside. The use of yellow brick gives the building a light, fresh appearance.

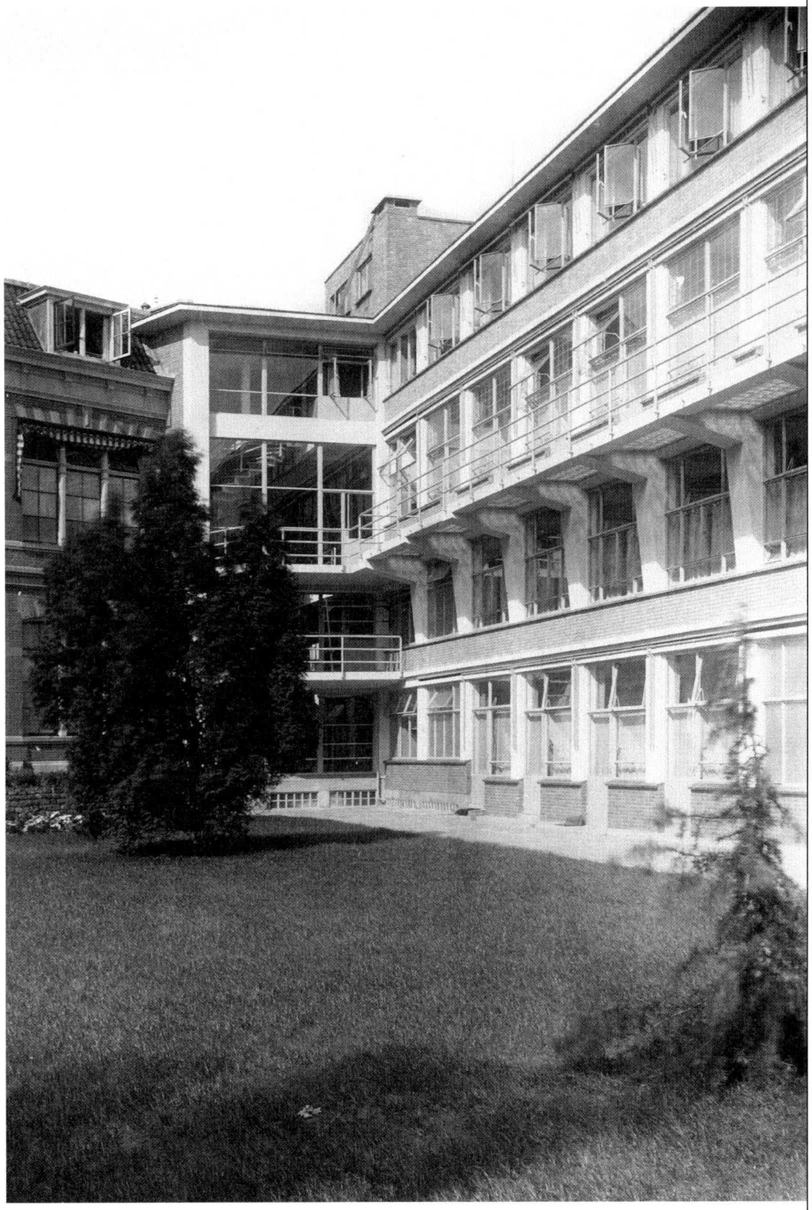

Situation with the existing buildings and the extension
1 *main building*
2 *kitchen*
3 *nurses' dormitory*
4 *wing*
5 *barrack contagious diseases*
6 *department for disinfection*
7 *mortuary*
8 *utilities building*
9 *extension by Wiebenga*

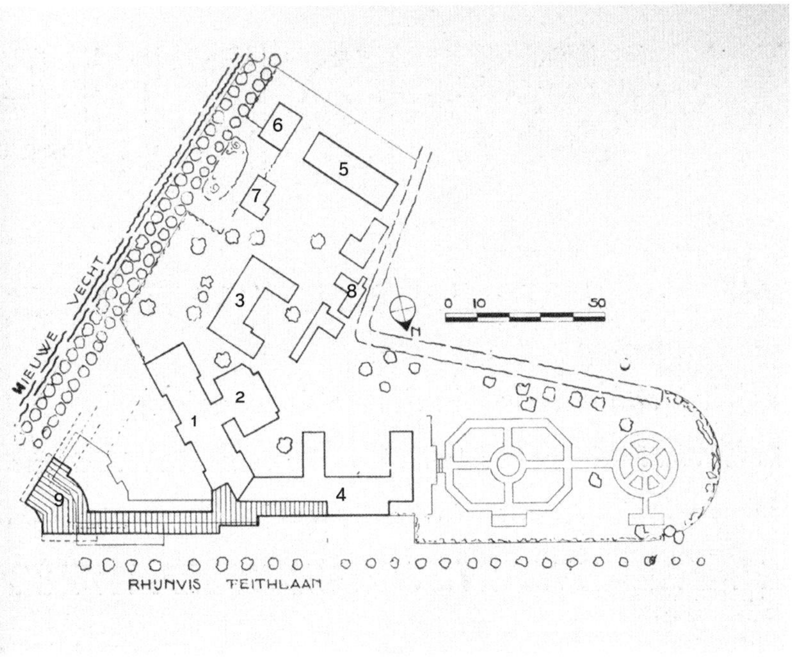

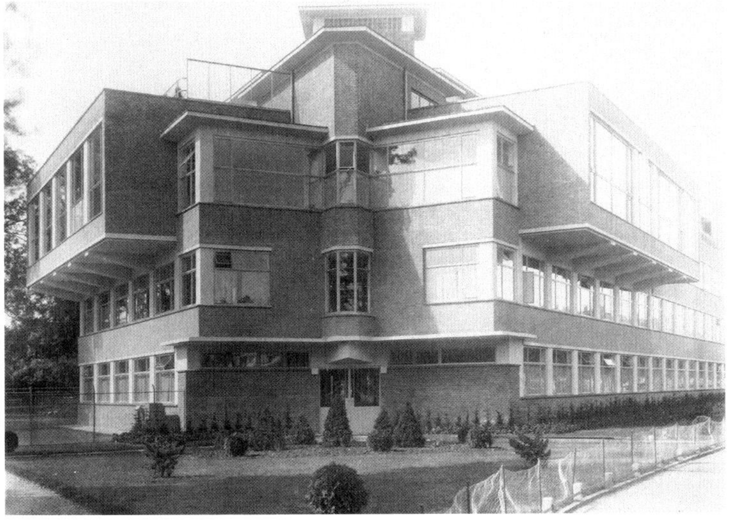

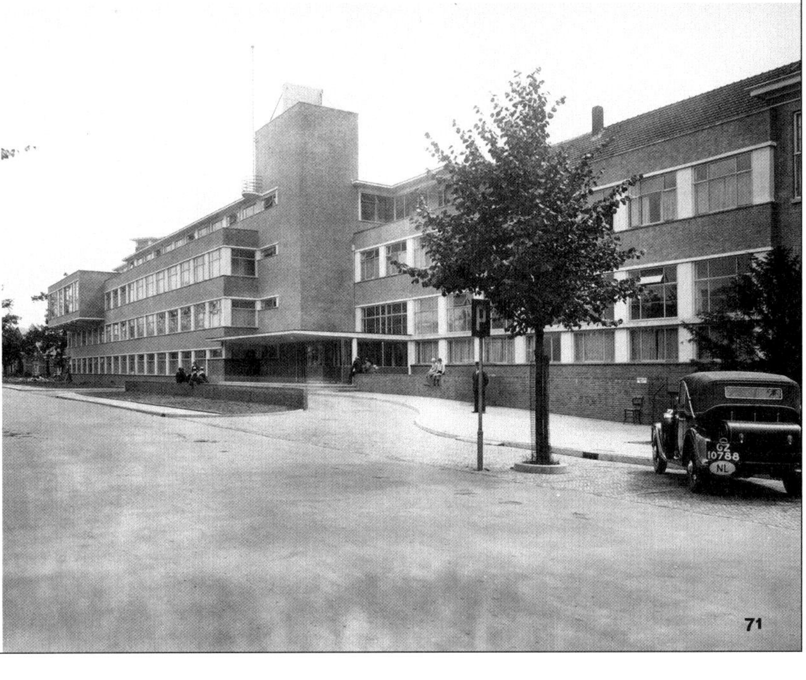

Expression

E. Reitsma

Noordersanatorium
Zuidlaren
1935

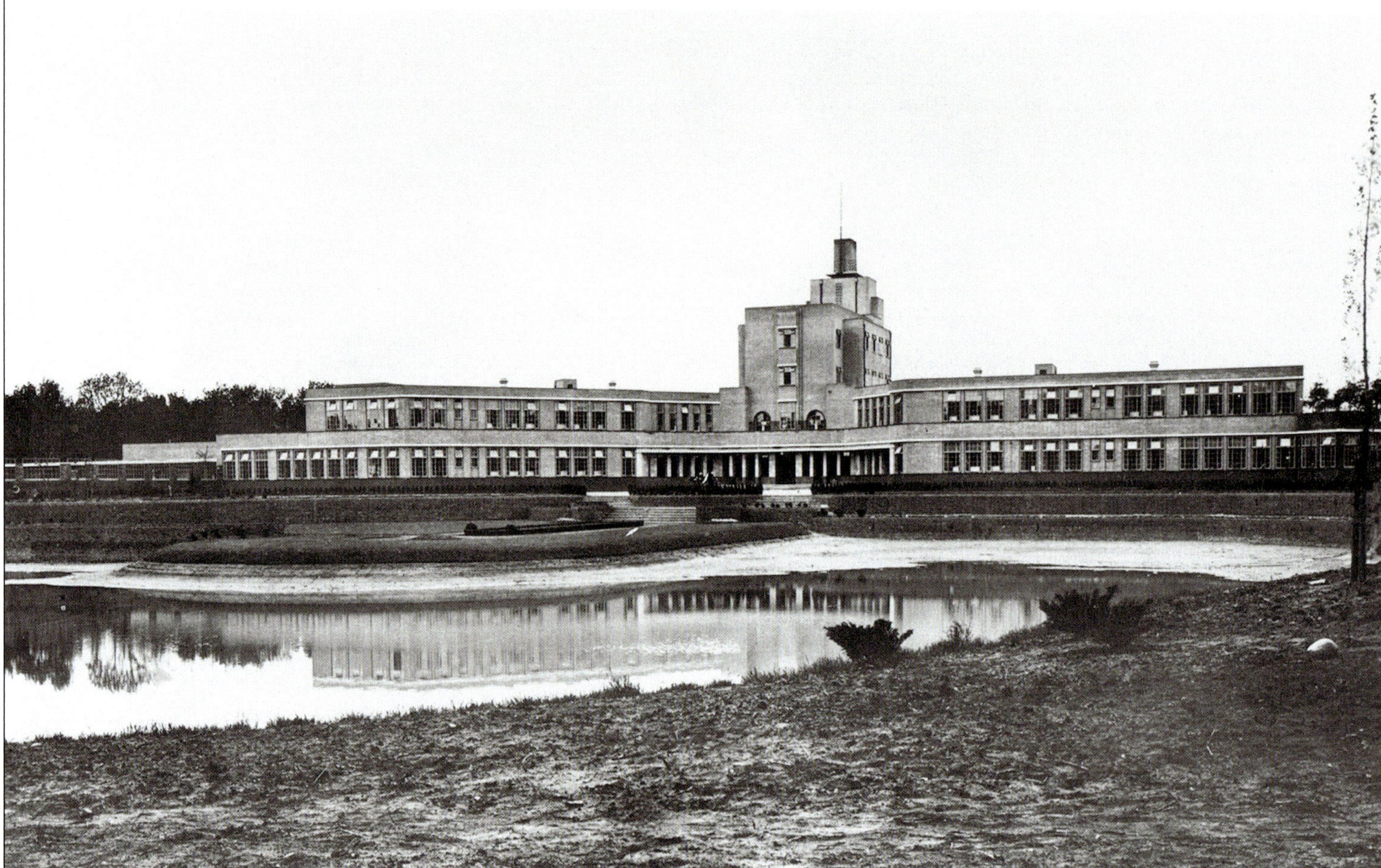

The main volume of the sanatorium consists of a robust tower block with three floors and a central staircase beside the north side of the tower. Four wings fan out from the tower. Entirely in accordance with the latest insights, in which the admission of sunlight is an important principle, the patients' rooms receive the maximal sunlight through their orientation towards the south, south-east and south-west. The areas for facilities and the isolation cells are located on the less favourably orientated sides of the wings. Each wing accommodates a different category of patients. The two eastern wings are for female patients, the two western wings for male patients. The calm patients are accommodated in the two front wings with a second floor. The two rear wings have only one storey and are reserved for the restless patients.

The day rooms are on the ground floor of the two front wings, while the bedrooms are on the first floor. The two rear wings consist mainly of rooms for bed nursing and single rooms. Each wing has its garden with a sunny terrace so that the bedridden patients too can enjoy the garden in the summer.

The tower contains the central functions, such as the administration and the medical service. On the ground floor next to the hall luxuriously clad with Italian marble are the administrator's office, the room of the medical superintendent, the treatment rooms, the examination rooms and a laboratory. The rooms of the nursing staff are distributed over three floors next to the corridors that run around the tall light well. The light well in the hall extends to the glass roofing so that daylight can be diffused evenly through the hall.

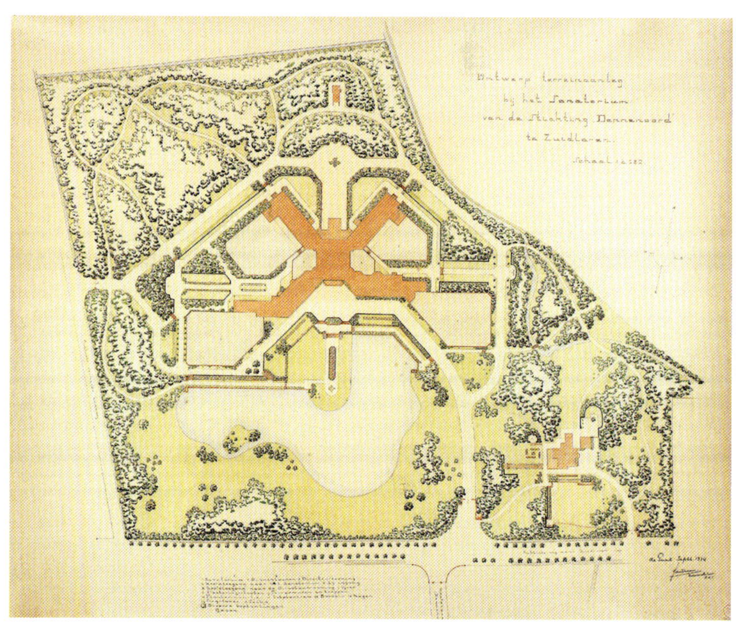

J. Vroom, garden design

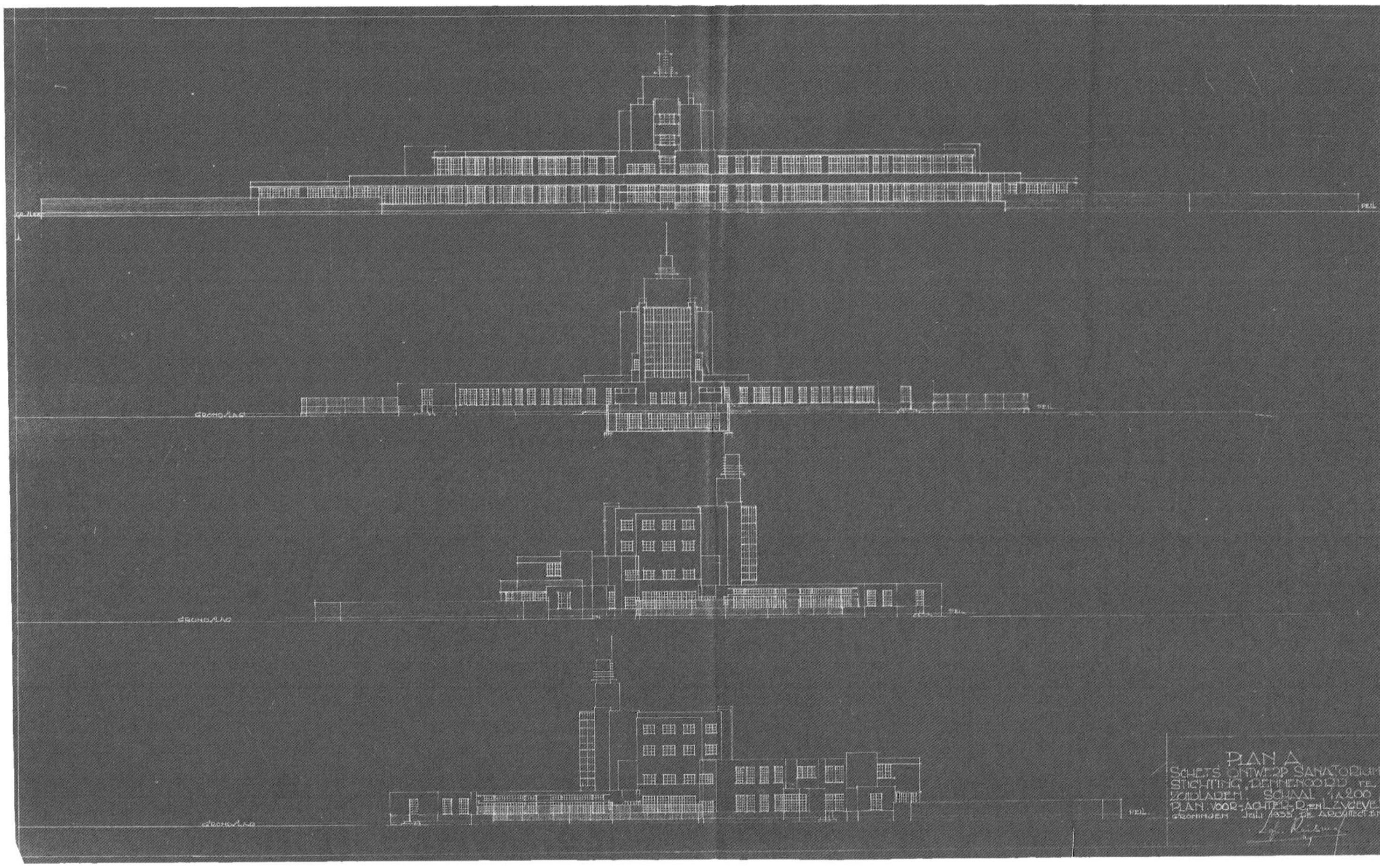
PEIL
PLAN A
SCHETS ONTWERP SANATORIUM
SCHAAL 1 à 200

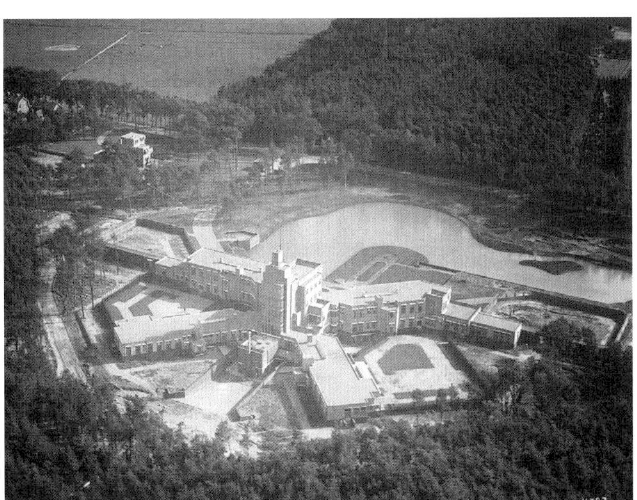

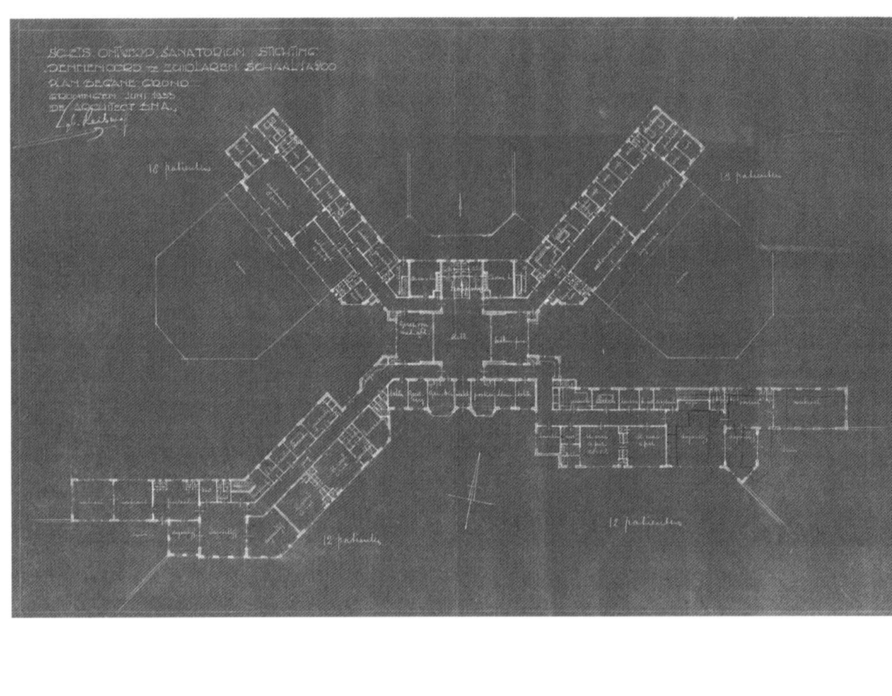
PLAN BEGANE GROND
18 patienten
12 patienten

Brick

Wieger Bruin

De Rusthoeve
Purmerend
1933-1936

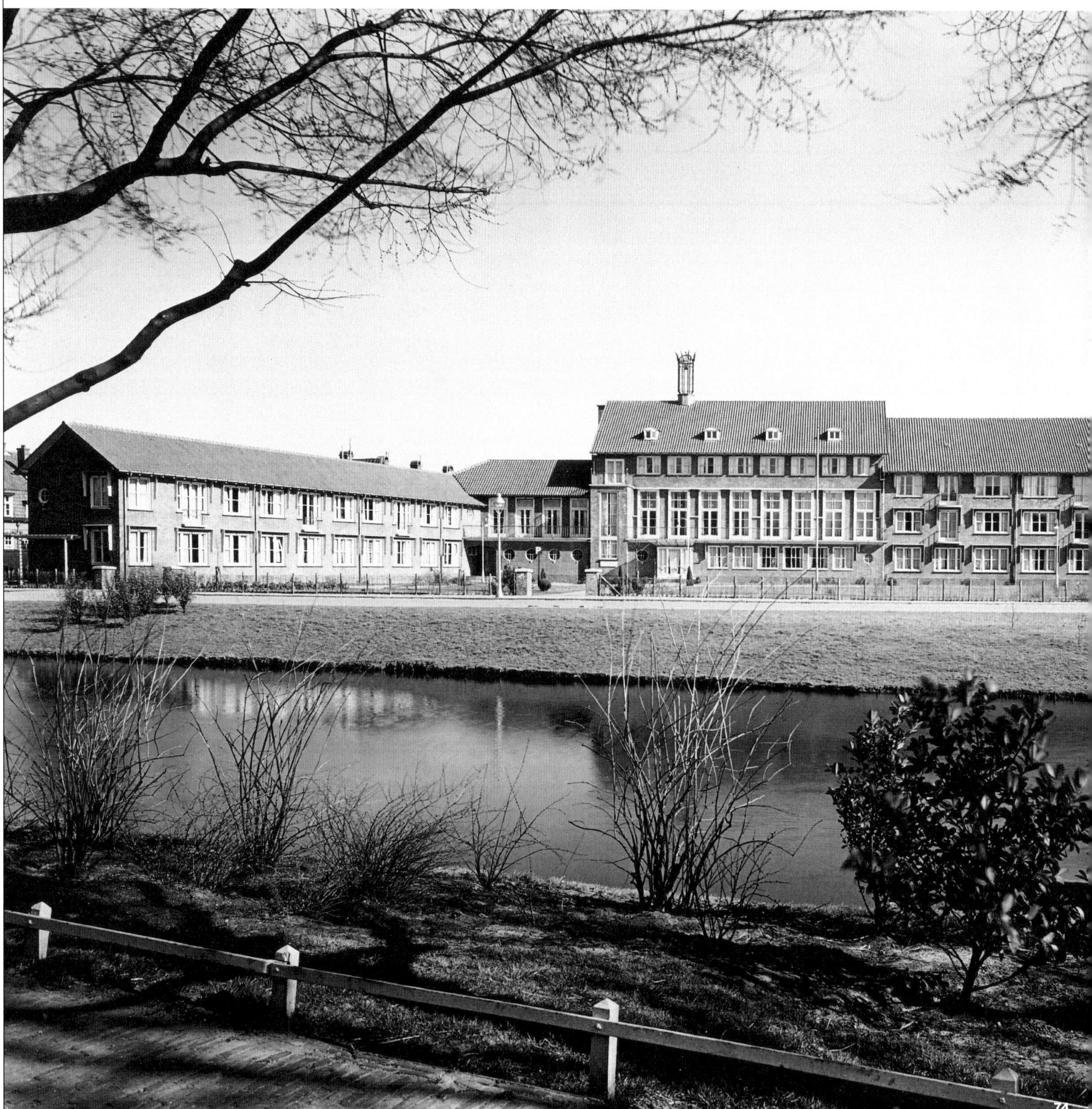

De Rusthoeve was an initiative of the Association of Reformed Deaconates in the classis Edam. The aim was to create a home free of any suggestion of an asylum. De Rusthoeve provided not only accommodation for eight invalid and infirm patients as well as 26 old people who were unable to pay their way, but also 86 residential units for more well-to-do elderly residents. The brick complex united the different categories of residents in their own wings. The residents who paid more had bed-sitters on either side of a central corridor in a volume running from north to south. At right angles to this were a short, low wing with several two-room apartments facing south. The communal facilities were located in the raised central section, which formed the link between the apartments for the better off and the diaconal wing for the less well off residents, whose bed-sitters also faced south. The invalid and infirm patients were accommodated in a low wing opposite that was also connected to the central section. The building was partly implemented as a steel construction. Every room had an unimpeded view of the garden. That gave it a measure of luxury, which is characteristic of this complex.

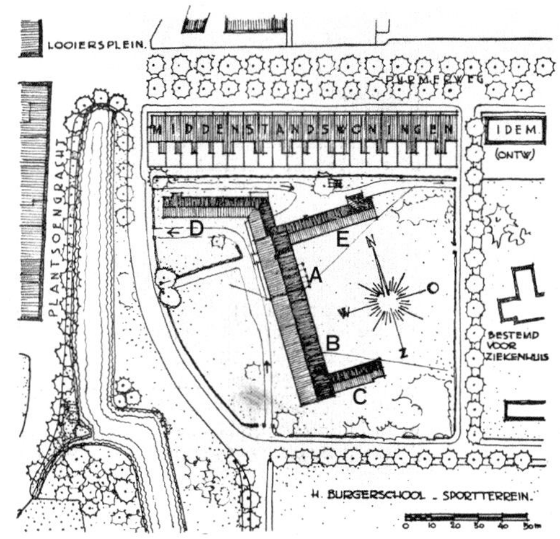

Situation
A *central section with the communal facilities*
B *main wing with apartments for the better off*
C *side wing with two-room apartments facing south*
D *wing for less well off residents*
E *wing for the invalid and diseased patients*

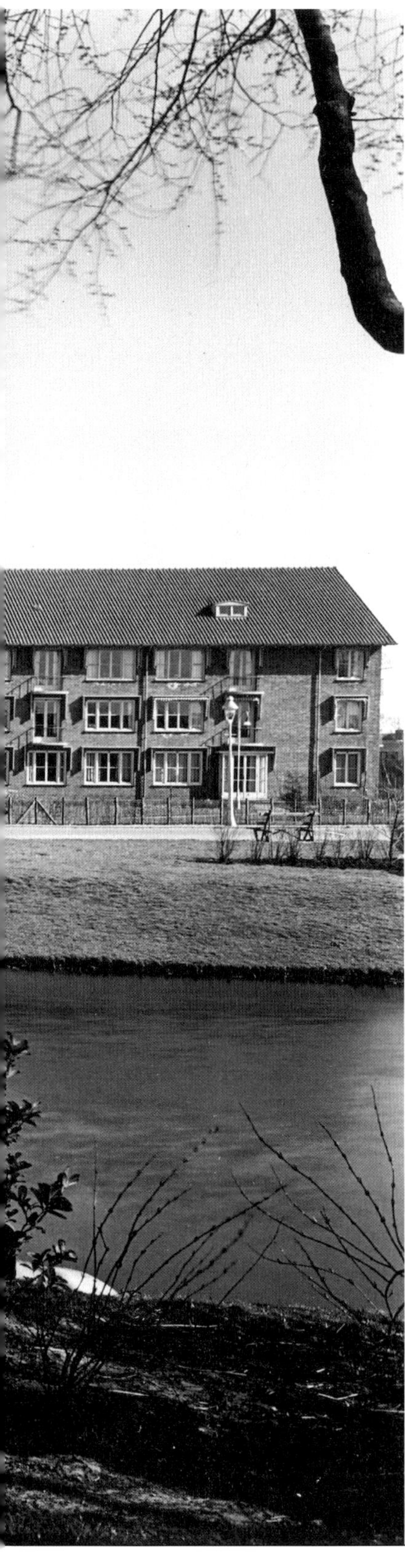

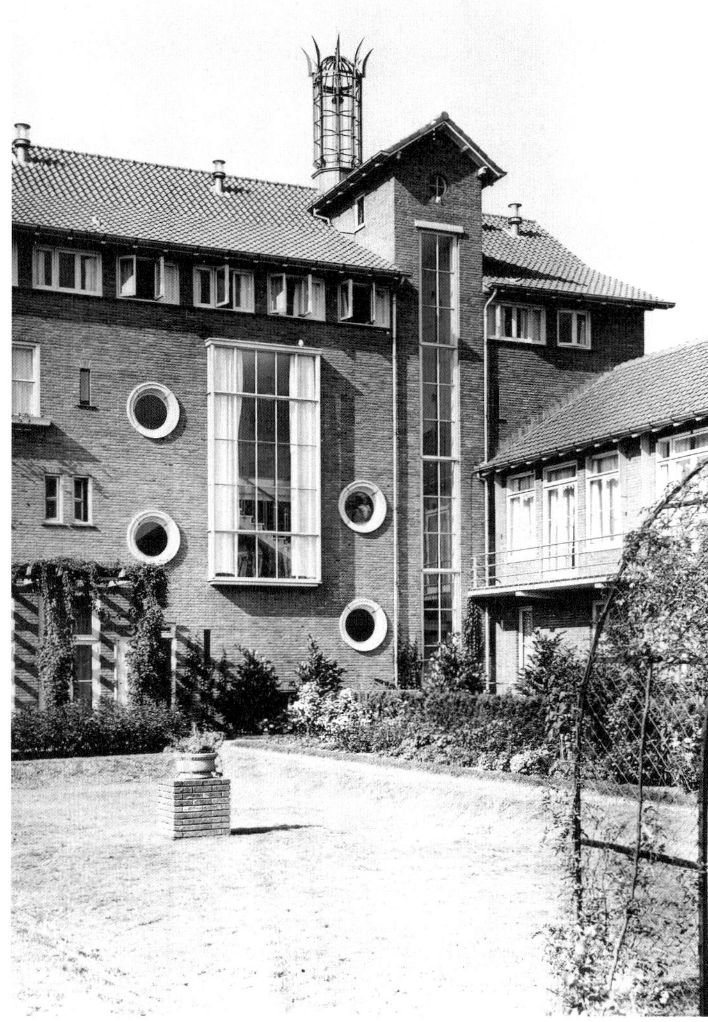

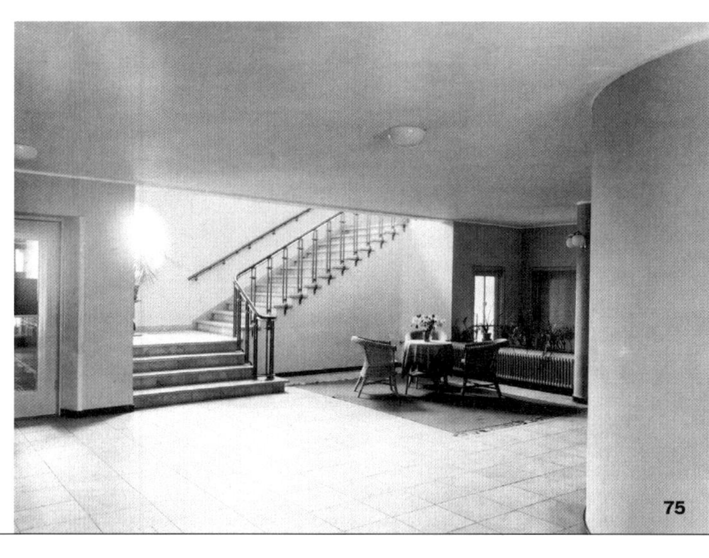

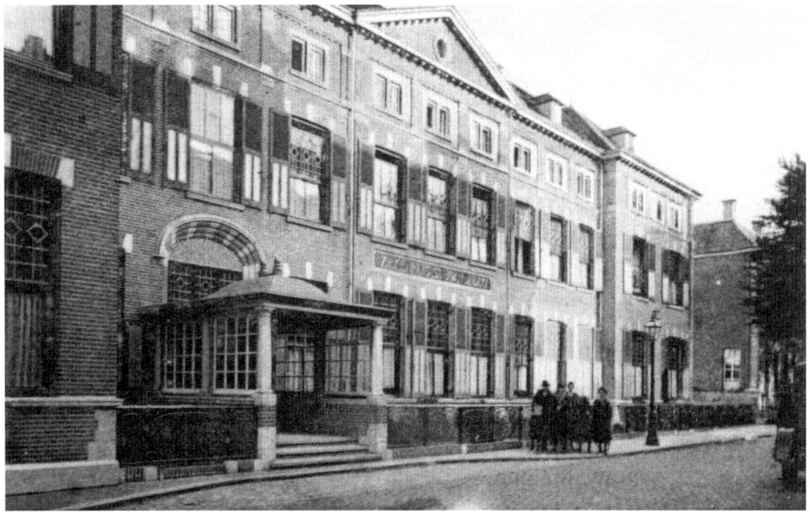

Utility and aesthetics

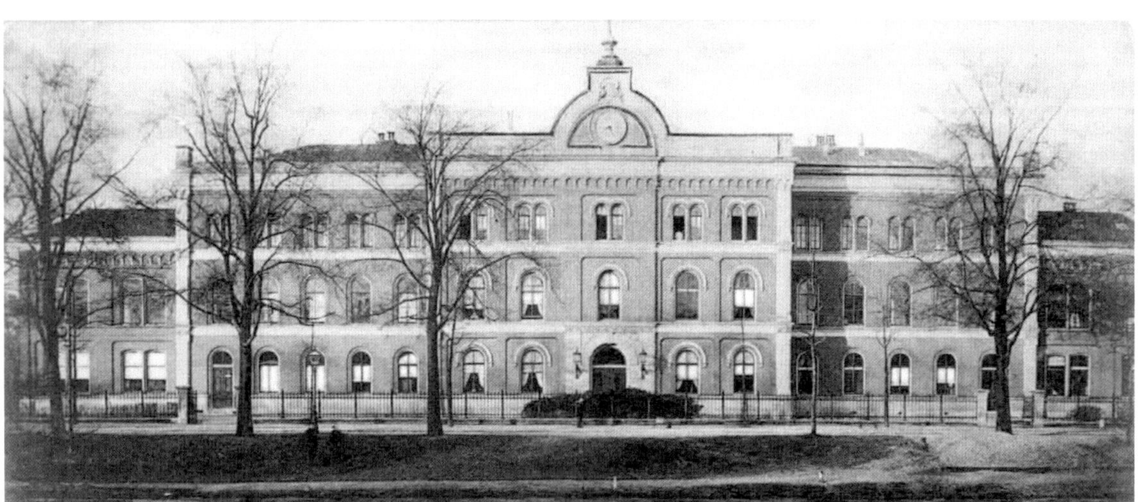

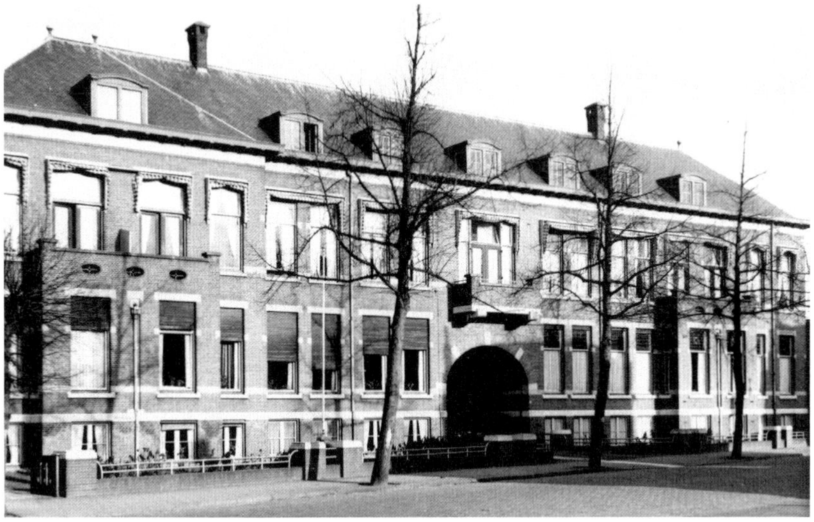

Top
Hospitals as monuments of bourgeois architecture: Ziekenhuis St. Joan de Deo in 's-Hertogenbosch and the Sint Jozefgesticht hospital in Oosterhout.

Bottom
Municipal hospital, Utrecht

Bronovo Ziekenhuis, The Hague

J.G. Wiebenga, Sophiaziekenhuis, Zwolle, 1935

It seems only natural for buildings to be determined by their function. All the same, a stage in the evolution of architecture and urban development can be pinpointed that is regarded as the origin of the view that, before designing a building, every facet of its functioning should be analysed in an almost scientific way. That conviction first took hold in the last quarter of the eighteenth century, first in France and first in hospital design. The idea gained ground that a hospital was first and foremost a utility. The designers drew their inspiration for the revolutionary late eighteenth-century types from mining engineers and winter garden designers – specialists in air conditioning. They learnt that this was the crucial element from the medical experts. What about the architect? His position was only saved by the fact that hospitals and psychiatric institutions were representative public buildings. They were monuments of progress that anchored the emergence of well organised networks of services in the city. Until late in the nineteenth century, health care buildings were uncontroversial monuments of bourgeois architecture.

When industrialisation and urbanisation disrupted bourgeois society and the traditional city, the distinction between functional and artistic once again led to a crisis in architecture. The crucial question of the identity of the profession was back at the centre of attention. What is architecture? If the hospital was the first functional type of building, it was by no means the only one. Since the industrial revolution the number of buildings with a technical function exploded: factories, railways, mines, docks – new challenges sprang up everywhere. Mass housing, offices, banks, and factory administration buildings were new architectural assignments that differed from the traditional ones through their function. The concentration of factory workers in the industrial cities, a new phenomenon that was manifested in its fullest form mainly outside the Netherlands, heralded the emergence of new social conditions. Architecture was in danger of being left behind and losing contact with everyday reality.

The more the gap between society and architecture grew, the louder was the call to bridge it. One possibility was an attempt to target assignments that had not previously been considered to belong to the natural preserve of architects and that by now had come to form a part of the field of operations of engineers and constructors. Once architects appropriated the field formerly left to the engineers, the question arose of what their specific contribution was. What distinguished an architect from an engineer? What did assignments of this kind have to gain from the artistic expertise that was traditionally sought among architects? The old dilemma reared its head again: is architecture the packaging of the programme, or also its logistical and functional organisation? Specifically in terms of the hospital, this boiled down to the question: if it increasingly becomes a building determined by medical processes, who possesses the most expertise – the medical expert or the architect? J. Hudnut, dean of the famous Graduate School of Design of Harvard, hit the nail on the head: 'No art is more widely misunderstood than the art of architecture, and no building illustrates the misunderstanding more clearly than the hospital. The hospital has become so completely a product of the technologies of medicine and of manufacture, so precisely adapted to the uses of sciences, as to become in effect a scientific instrument not essentially different from the X-ray machine or the operating-table which it encloses. It is hard for people to imagine any relationship between such a building and that great tradition whose flowers are the Parthenon and the Cathedral of Chartres. It is hard to think of a hospital as a work of art.'[1]

In the Netherlands, reflection on hospital

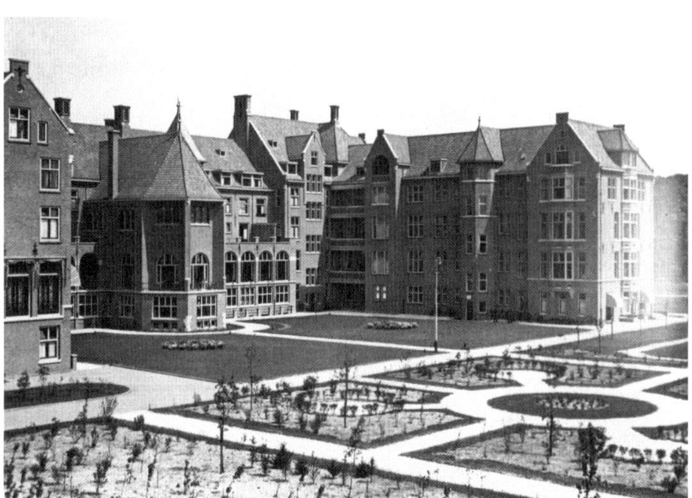

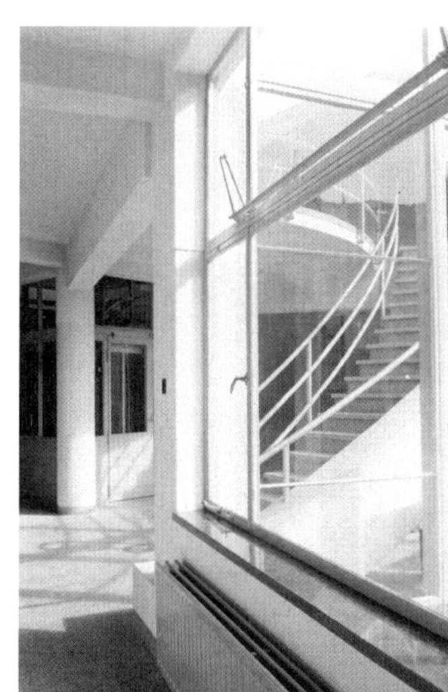

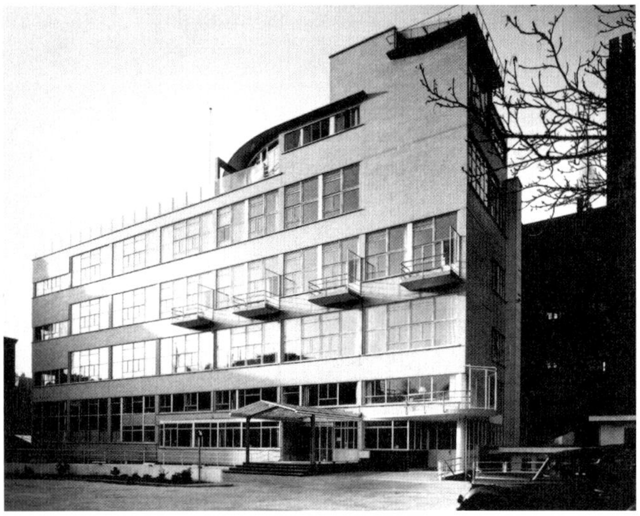

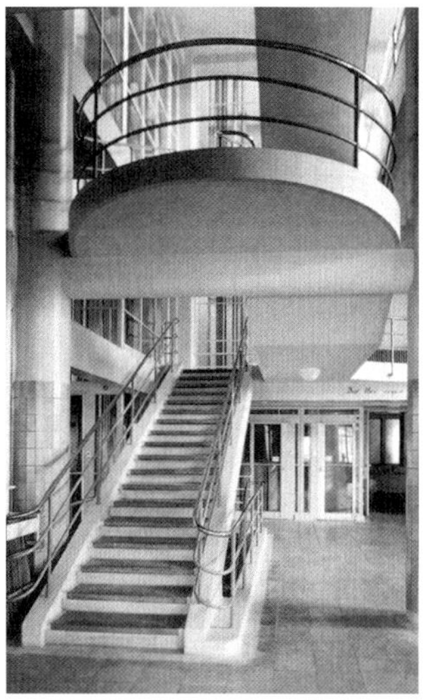

architecture was for a long time the exclusive preserve of the medical experts. They had clear ideas about the task of the architect and the role that they should be able to play in the design process. Wortman put it as follows: 'The key to the question of architecture (...) is the grouping of all the elements to form a whole. The architect is not free in the implementation of that task; he must follow the wishes presented to him from the medical side.'[2] Moreover, the architect was expected 'to give the whole an external form that is pleasing to the eye without making use of expensive decoration on the façade or roof.' In practice it was even not uncommon for a medical expert to design the ground plan before it was passed on to the architect for further elaboration. How different the situation was in the United States, where a standard work on hospitals, *Hospital Management*, with contributions not only from medical experts and (economic) managers but also from architects and constructional engineers, had appeared as early as 1911. There was no such multidisciplinary network of hospital experts in the Netherlands, and the first Dutch manual in the field was not published until 1939.[3]

This time-hallowed controversy between the principal and the designer went to the heart of the matter: was architecture just packaging, fashion and expression, or did the expertise of the profession reach much further? This dilemma was closely connected with the status of the hospital as a building. The emergence of the Modernist movement in the late 1920s threw new light on this distinction between an aesthetic and a utilitarian assignment by pronouncing it redundant: the aesthetic and the utilitarian were declared complementary concepts. It is not surprising that precisely the hospital was at stake several times in the polemic between the advocates of Modernism and their more conservative colleagues. J.B. van Loghem, considered one of the founders of Modernism, was crushing in his verdict on the classic, still representative hospital architecture. He had nothing positive to say about the Bronovo Ziekenhuis in The Hague; it was '(...) in its pitiful fragmentation a witness to such impotence that it is better to pass over it in silence'.[4] When J.G. Wiebenga was commissioned to extend the Sophia-ziekenhuis in Zwolle, the board had so little confidence in him that it appointed a second architect; Van Loghem cast scorn on this procedure, which had reduced the whole to a 'uniform mediocrity'.[5] One of the best examples of functionalist hospital architecture in the Netherlands was the extension of the Diaconessenhuis in Rotterdam by J.A. Brinkman and J.H. van den Broek. All the same, Van Loghem raised objections here too. He considered the board room and the chapel too sober, while the main staircase was too spectacular, too much of a 'film object'.[6] Architecture was supposed to contribute to the creation of a new sense of life in which light, air and sun were the key concepts. As a healing and health machine, the hospital seemed pre-eminently suitable for that. For the time being, however, hospital architecture was virtually a closed door for the architects who embraced Modernism. Their most important contribution to health care remained mainly confined to a few well-known sanatoria, including J. Duiker's Zonnestraal in Hilversum (1926-1931).

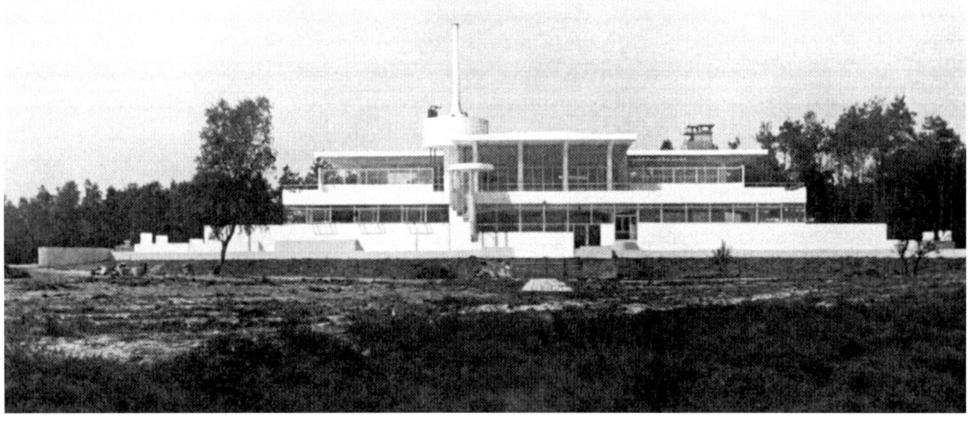

Top
Architectenbureau Brinkman en Van den Broek, extension Diaconessenhuis, Rotterdam, 1938

Bottom
J. Duiker and B. Bijvoet, sanatorium Zonnestraal, Hilversum, 1928

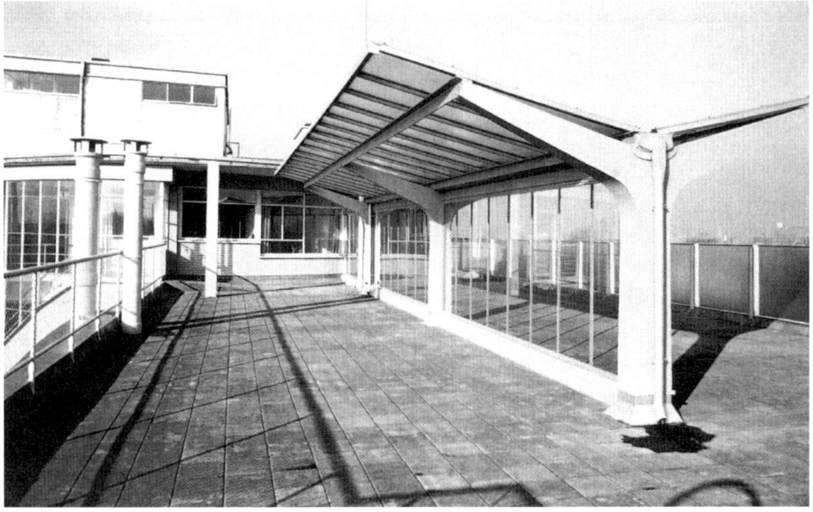
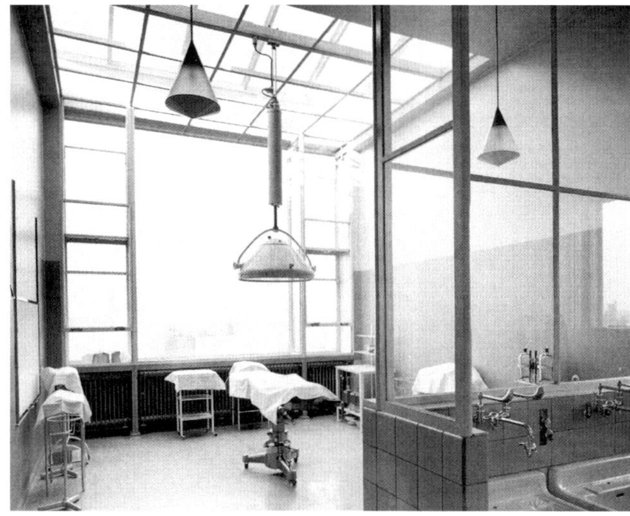
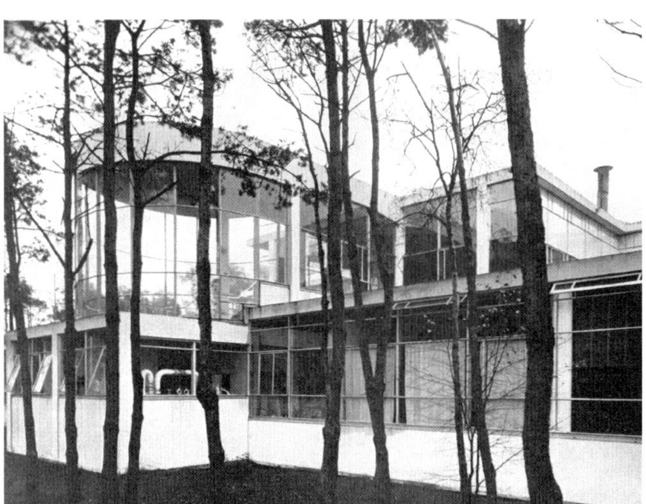
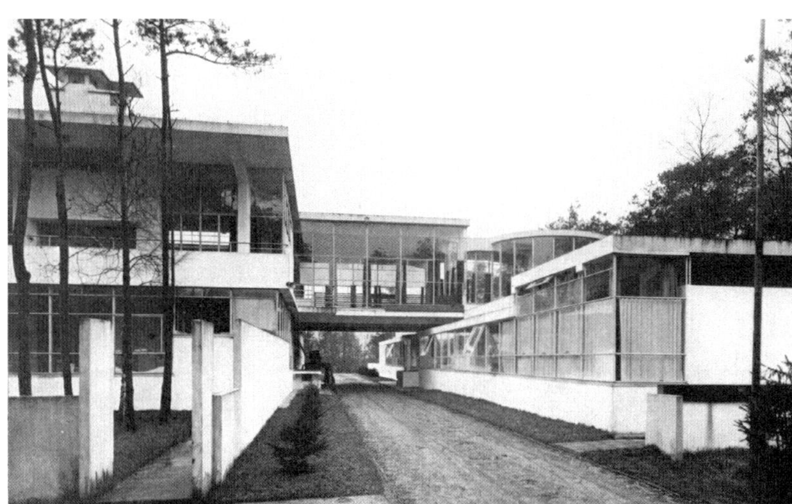

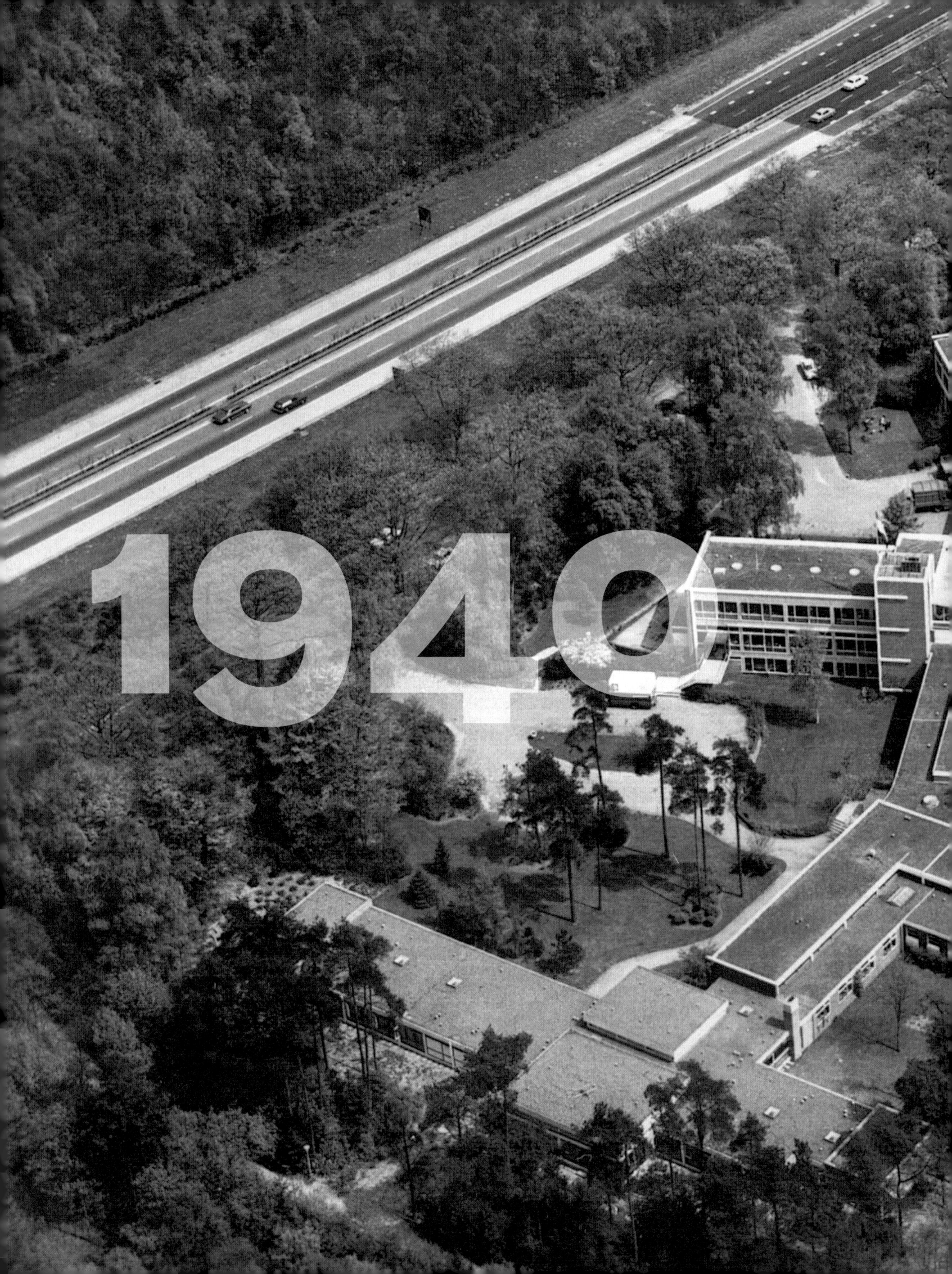
1940

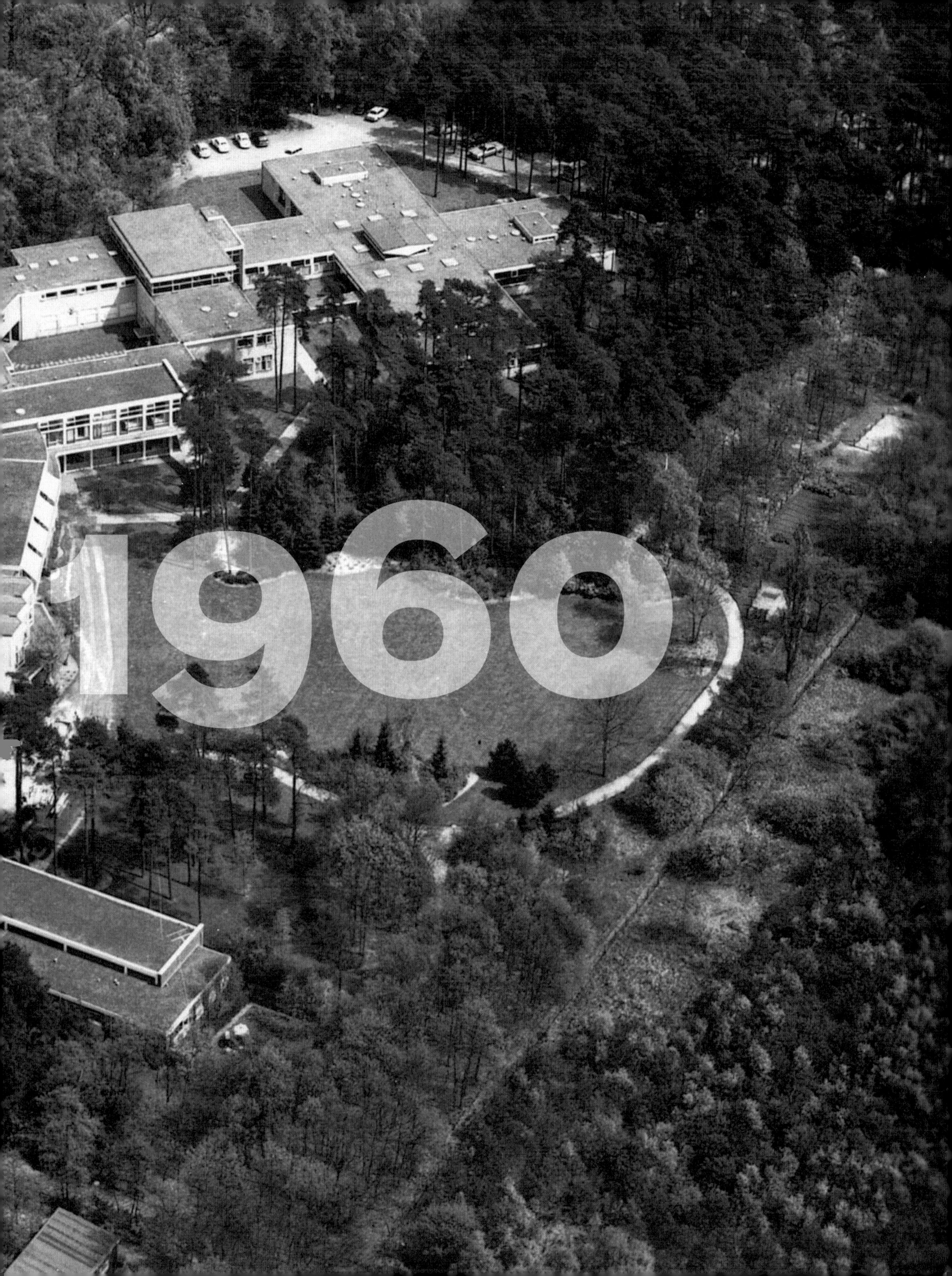
1960

The Reconstruction

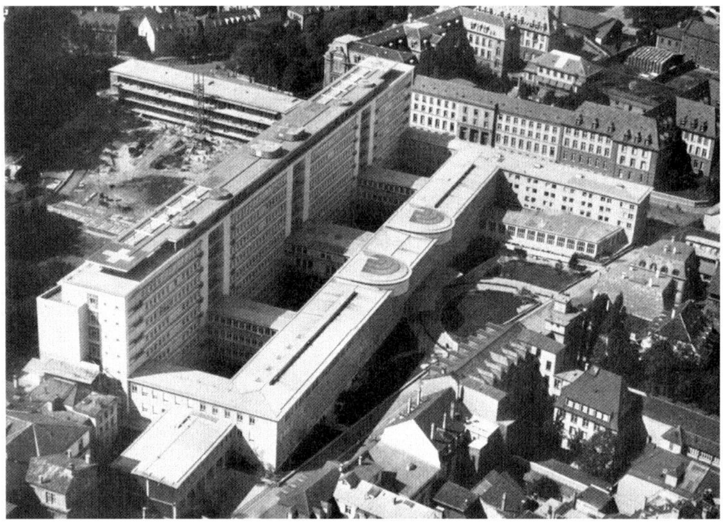

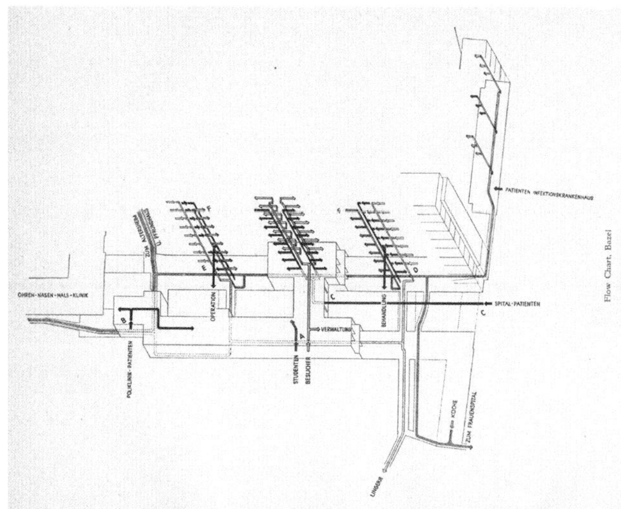

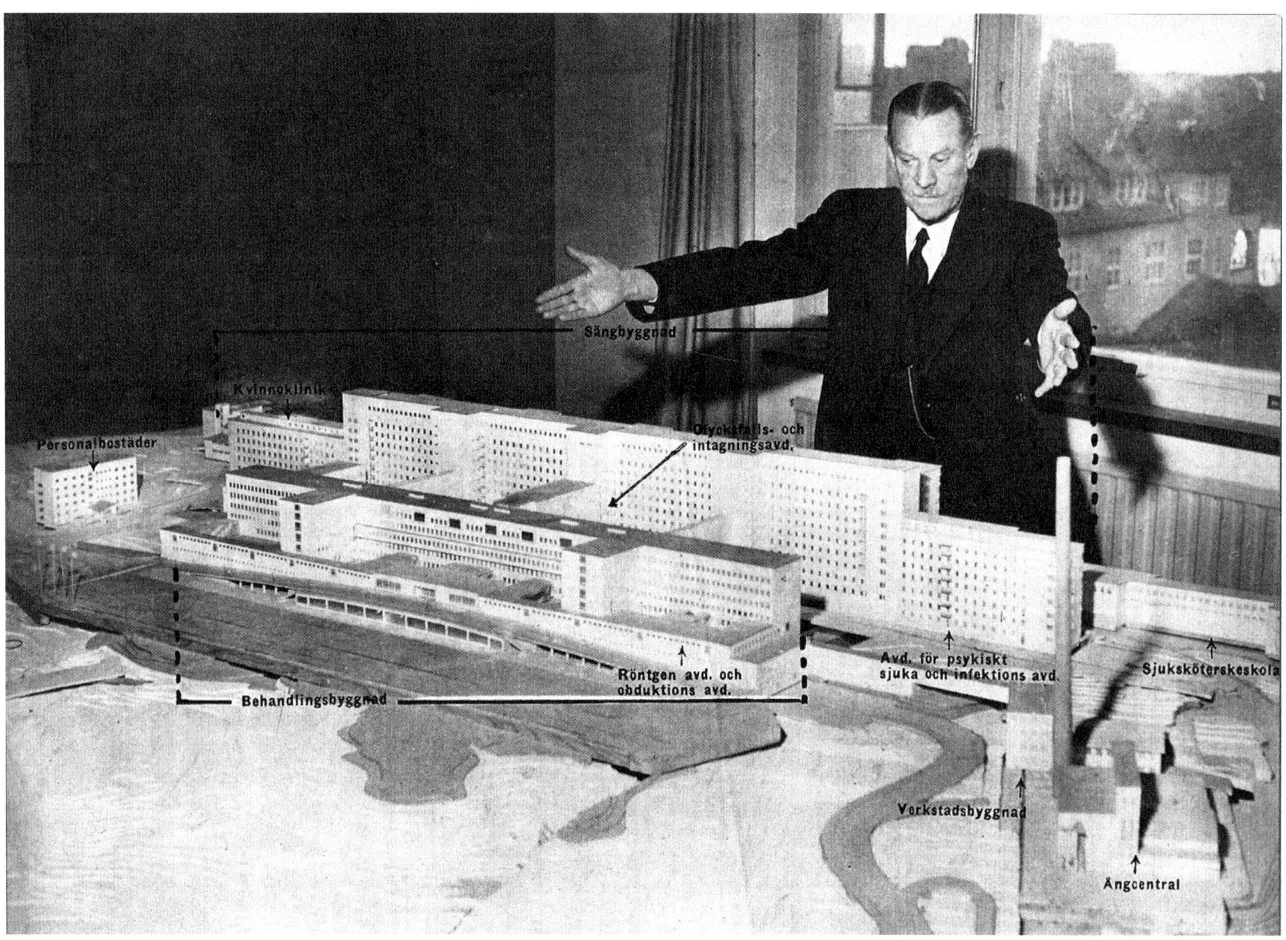

Postwar Netherlands

The government took the initiative for a fundamental modernisation of Dutch society between 1945 and 1970. Industrialisation, the increase of scale and mechanisation of agriculture, the reintroduction of social housing (which now determined by far the largest part of building production and thereby became the driving wheel of the economy), the introduction of a wide-ranging system of social security – this all marked a radical break with society as it had been before 1940. It is only in the last few decades that systematic research has been conducted on just how far-reaching this process was. Standard works like *1950. Welvaart in zwart-wit* (1950: Prosperity and Welfare) show the eagerness with which the remains of the past were cleared up.[1] Social deprivation, now regarded as one of the deeper causes of the Second World War, the mass destruction and the Holocaust must be avoided at all costs. Health care must be available for all social classes. As soon as the elderly had been identified as a particularly vulnerable group, a campaign was unleashed on an unprecedented scale to change that situation. All of a sudden, care for the elderly became one of the spearheads of an attempt to achieve a virtually complete social reconstruction.

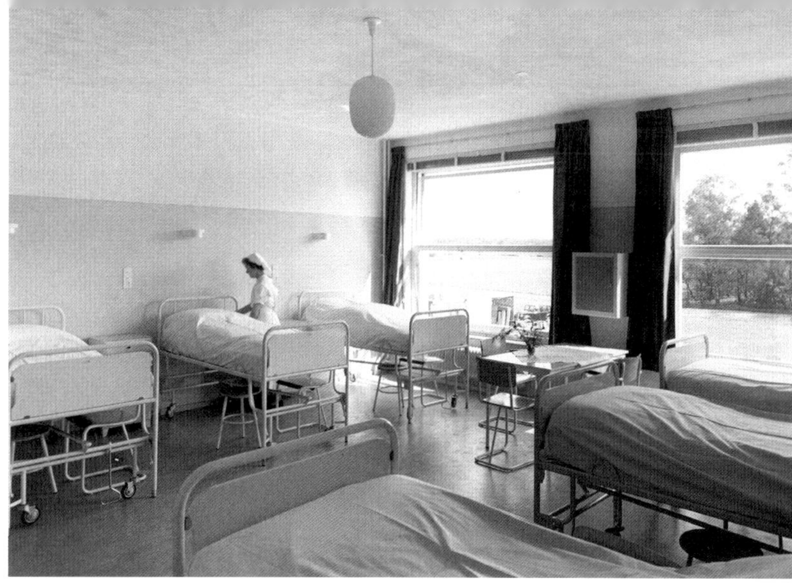

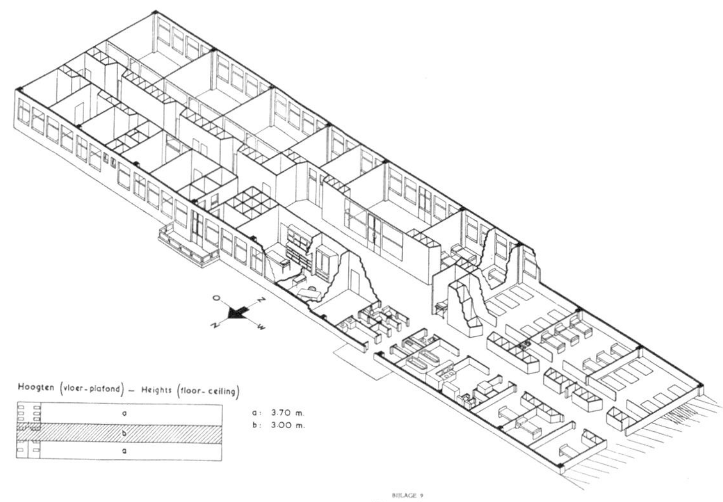

p. 80
***L.H.P. Waterman*, Sinai Centrum, Amersfoort, 1960**

p. 82
***E. & P. Vischer, Hermann Baur & Bräuning, Leu, Dürig*, Bürgerspital, Basel, 1946. At the right the flow chart.**

***H. Cederström*, Södersjukhuset, Stockholm, 1944**

p. 83
Room with six beds in Streekziekenhuis Bennekom

***P.C. Cleyndert*, standard nursing unit**

***J.P. Kloos*, Prinses Irene Ziekenhuis, Almelo, 1960**

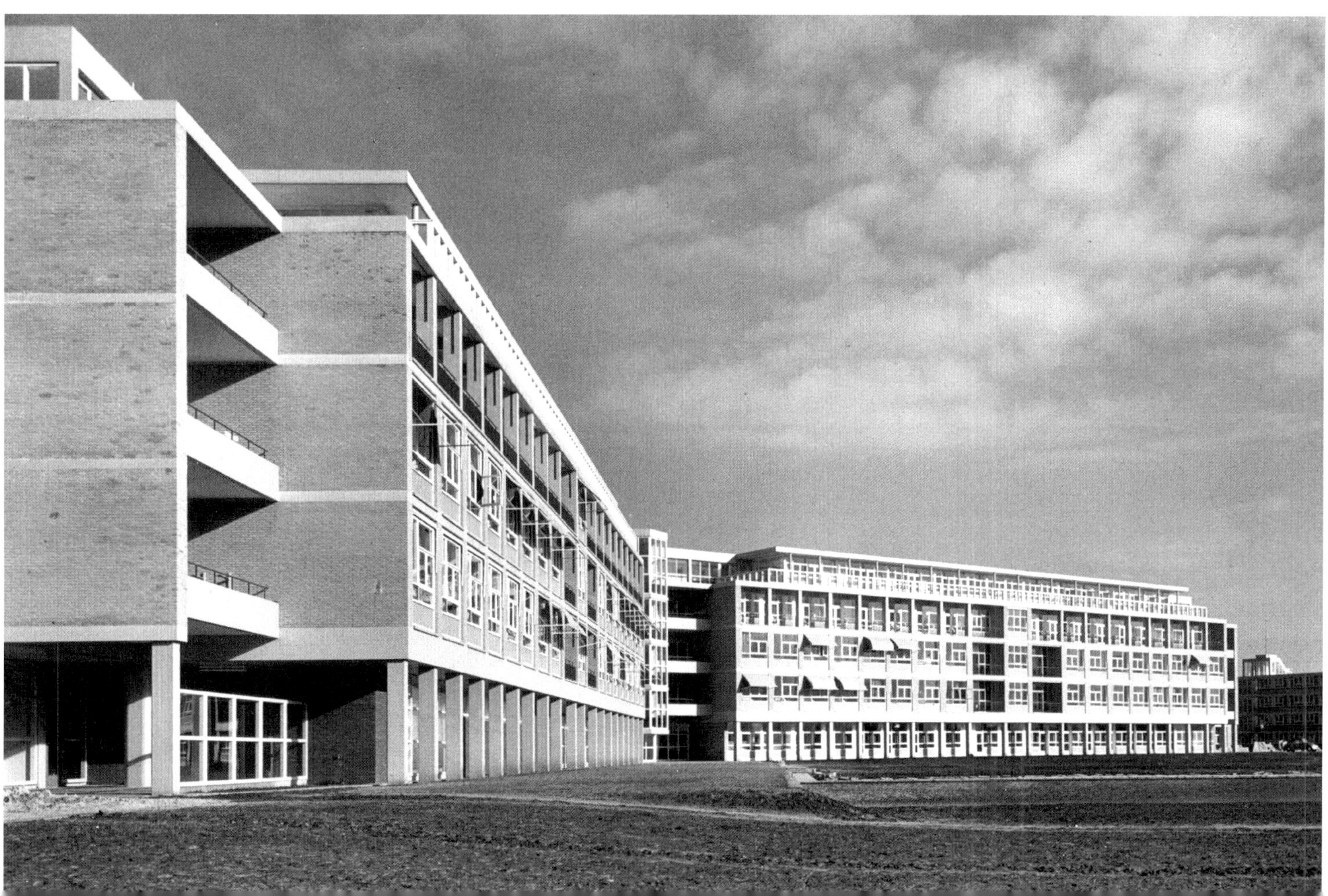

Hospitals

Once hospitals had grown to become the scientific and technological frontline of the medical system, there was a danger that the care they offered would be beyond the financial reach of the lowest classes, who had originally formed their major target group. This development was diametrically opposed to the ideals of the welfare state. The integration of the health insurance policies introduced by the occupying forces in the Dutch social security system was intended to bridge the financial gap, while the construction of new hospitals was to meet the predicted shortage of capacity. The building of hospitals had ground to a halt during the Second World War, not only in the Netherlands but practically all over Europe. They could all start afresh after the liberation. That created new opportunities that were gratefully welcomed. The desire for renewal that characterised other fields was also displayed in architecture, particularly so in the case of hospital architecture. The idea that architecture should play a crucial role in the construction of a new, socially minded society was also accepted in the Netherlands by almost all designers, no matter to which movement they subscribed. One of the attractive facets of the hospital of the future was that it was a communal amenity that was open to all. Was not hospital design a pre-eminently social task? That seemed to call for a different approach from what had been common practice before the war, when most hospitals were still designed as representative monuments.

Inspiration from Sweden and Switzerland

In so far as one can speak of a tradition in Dutch hospital architecture in the 1920s and 1930s, it came to a halt with the occupation; no attempts were made to resume the thread after the liberation. A few hospitals were completed in accordance with plans that had been drawn up before the war, but a new direction was deliberately sought for the new buildings. What were the sources of inspiration? In the search for new insights into hospital architecture, a number of hospitals abroad were the first to be considered, although there were not many of them. Only two hospitals had been completed during the war that met the latest demands and acquired a sort of exemplary function: the Södersjukhuset in Stockholm designed by H. Cederström, the 'inventor' of the nursing unit in the 1930s, and the Bürgerspital in Basel designed by the architect H. Baur.

The Södersjukhuset consisted of an eight-floor complex of nursing wards, and a parallel building for treatment with operating theatres, an X-ray unit and laboratories. One reason not to opt for the pavilion system was the consideration that it would isolate the specialists too much, while the organisation of the modern hospital called for their intensive cooperation. The two 330-metre blocks were linked by transversal corridors. The nursing units consisted of sixteen beds, divided into four-bed, two-bed and isolation rooms. Two such nursing units, which combined to form an L-shape, formed a station. There were waiting rooms and dayrooms at the point where they met.

Switzerland had already been discovered as an important source of inspiration before the war broke out; the Bürgerspital in Basel confirmed this reputation.[2] The team of architects E. and P. Vischer, Hermann Baur and Bräuning, Leu, Dürig and started work on the design in 1937. The first stage of this university hospital was completed in 1945. The nursing wards, that could accommodate a thousand patients, consisted of sixteen-bed nursing units, which were in turn divided into two six-bed and two two-bed rooms. There was a clear distinction between the nursing area, on the one hand, and the treatment, research, laboratory, administration and university areas on the other. This separation 'affords the patients the necessary rest and enables the medical and laboratory staff to work without interruption'.[3] Five bridges served to connect the two buildings.

The Building Centre

Inspiration from abroad was the first element in the modernisation of hospitals in the Netherlands, while Dutch research was the second. The Building Centre (*Bouwcentrum*) played a remarkable role in this research. Preparations for this institute were made by the Government Commission during the war and it was officially established in 1945 to modernise the building industry, which was outdated compared with other technical branches of industry, and to equip it for its new task as the driving force of the economy.[4] It seemed only natural to coordinate that activity and to bring it under the aegis of the Building Centre. A centre especially for hospital buildings, the Dutch Hospital Foundation, was to be incorporated in the Building Centre to form a link between the government, industry and the international hospital world.[5]

A part of the preparations was the setting up of a Hospital Commission in 1949 that comprised representatives of the Building Centre, the Dutch Hospital Foundation, the Dutch Organisation for Applied Scientific Research (TNO), the rational building foundation Ratiobouw, architects and hospital superintendents. Various members of this commission were selected and united in the Hospital Architecture Study Group to intensively tackle the question of hospital documentation. The chairman of the commission and the study group was W.K. van Oppen from the Special Buildings Department of the Ministry of Reconstruction and Housing. Van Oppen had previously headed a government study commission which had tried to develop a method for analysing the existing hospitals. The study group included experts in the field of hospital architecture such as P.C. Cleyndert and the architects H. Hoekstra, J.A. van der Laan, and A. Viergever.

The Hospital Building Centre, a joint initiative of the Building Centre, the Dutch Hospital Foundation, the Association of Catholic Hospitals and the Royal Institute of Dutch Architects (BNA), was officially opened on 28 February 1950 by the Minister of Social Affairs, A.M. Joekes. Its main task was to make standardised sheets (*normaalbladen* or *documentatiebladen*) to serve as comparative material for the appraisal of new projects. The standardisation of a particular feature, such as the nursing unit, was to standardise the function, the dimensions, and the physical implementation; only the latter was entirely seen as the task of the architect. It is obvious that the work of the Hospital Building Centre was entirely inspired by that of the Hospital Facilities Section and the Swiss Association of Hospital Establishments (VESKA).[6]

The activities of the study group included the study of the nursing units, the hospital kitchens and the outpatient units. The first standardisation sheets completed by the study commission of the Hospital Building Centre were those for the nursing unit, which were published in 1951 in *Het Ziekenhuiswezen*. It comprised a 34-bed nursing unit and was accompanied by ground plans of all the rooms involved.[7]

Although the role of the Building Centre was certainly important, there were other players in the field too. The

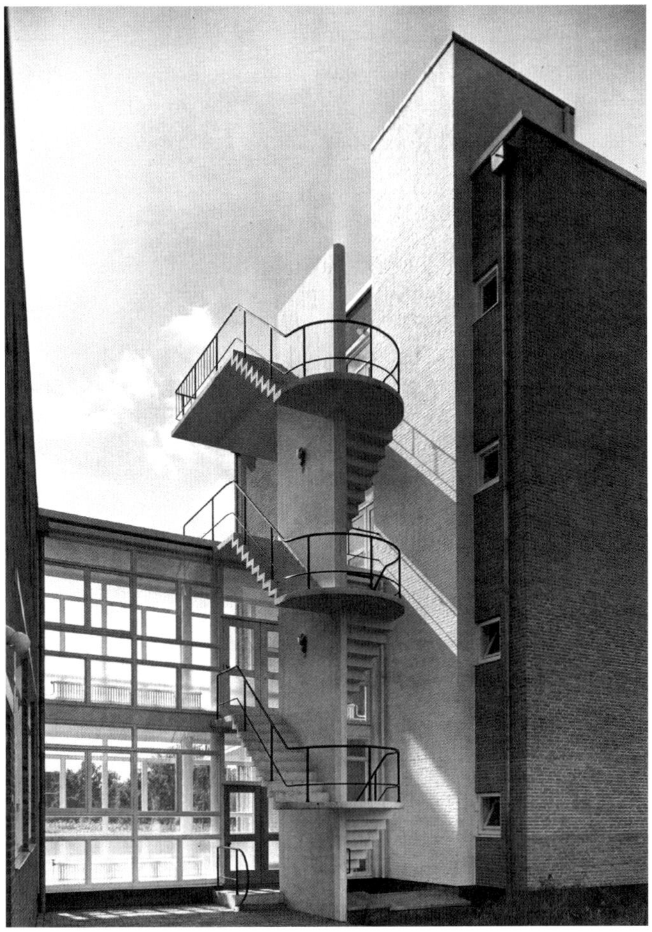

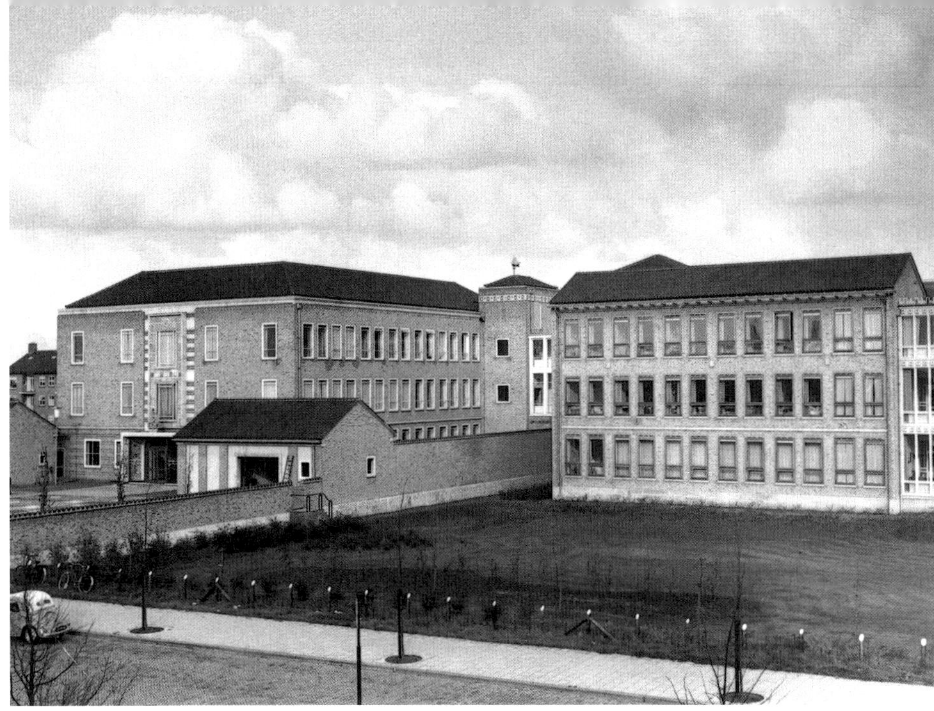

p. 85 | >
***Van der Laan Hermans Van der Eerden*, Sint Jozefziekenhuis Deventer, 1956**

p. 85 | <
***K.L. Sijmons*, Streekziekenhuis Bennekom, 1957**

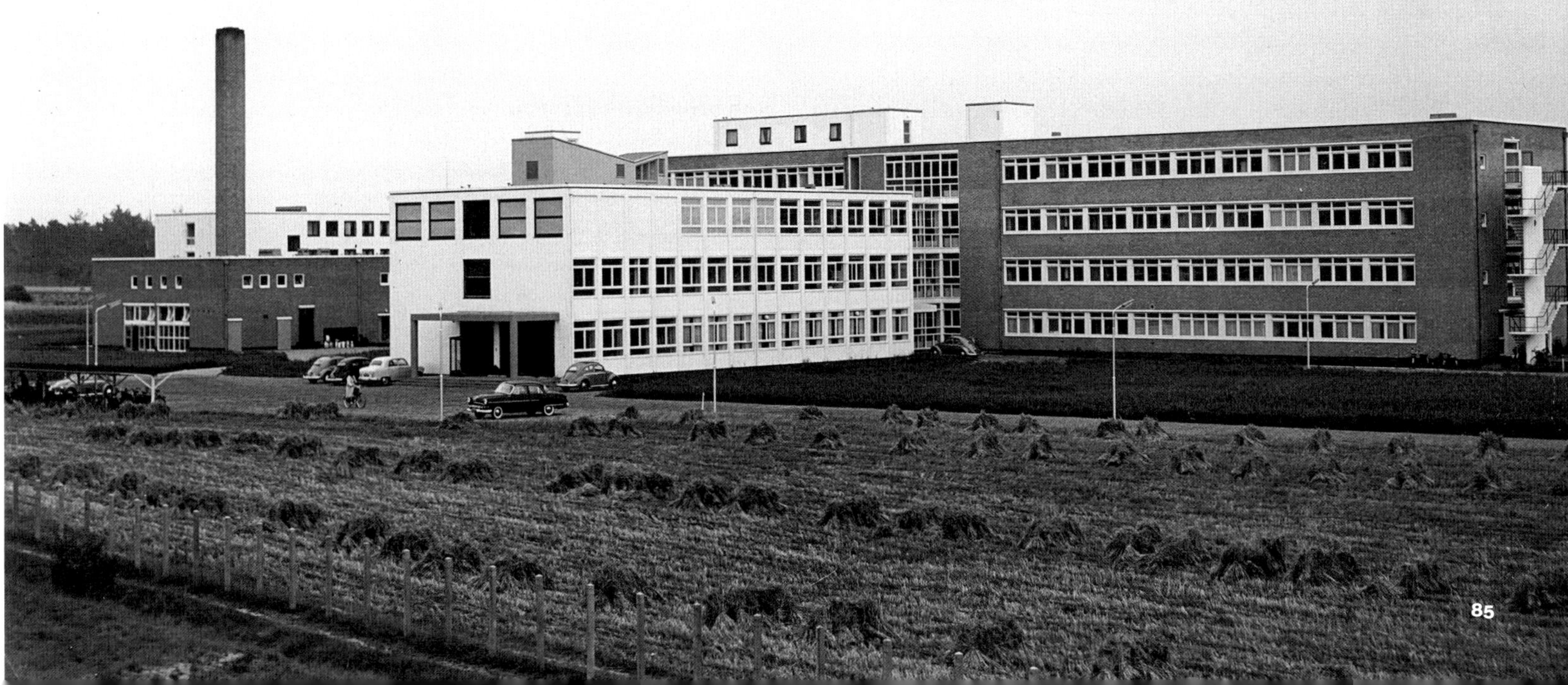

Hospital Institute came into action and the influence of the Hospital Commission, which advised on the usefulness and necessity of new projects and also took an interest in the design aspects, gradually increased. But focusing entirely on the architecture itself, it is above all the standardisation sheets of the Building Centre that illustrate the emergence of Synthetic Modernism.

Synthetic Modernism

A crucial aspect of the models from abroad was the way in which attention to function determined their structure and visual impact. Although functionalism had failed to gain control of hospital care before the Second World War, that situation now changed. The problem was that hospitals consist of units with very different functions and are thus not amenable to a uniform design, which would deny the differences in use. Synthetic Modernism accepted the need for justice to be done to the different units.[8] So what does a hospital comprise?

Nursing wards

The nursing units, identified by Cederström in the 1930s as the point of anchorage of the hospital building because it was the one where the least changes occurred, were the basic modules of the hospital wards and were seen as the most important components of the hospital. Everyone was agreed that large wards were a thing of the past. A modern nursing unit consisted of rooms with one, two, four or six beds as well as many secondary rooms (dayrooms, isolation room, kitchen, washing-up room, bathroom, toilet and storage area). The nursing unit's character was largely derived from the fact that a ward sister was in charge. A nursing unit in the Netherlands therefore had between twenty-four and thirty-six beds. As far as the size of the nursing unit was concerned, a distinction was made between the graded unit (first class, second class, and sometimes an intermediate class) and the general one. The large wards of thirty to forty beds that had been very common in the prewar period were no longer to be found.

To encourage the process of standardisation, Cleyndert – a physician – designed a standard type. His ideas were derived from personal experiences, trips abroad and study of the literature. Two 25-bed units were combined to form a double nursing unit. This solution was first applied in the Prinses Irene Ziekenhuis in Almelo, where Cleyndert worked in close collaboration with the architect J.P. Kloos. To reduce walking distances to a minimum, intensively used subsidiary areas such as washing-up rooms, kitchen and bathroom were placed in the middle. Facilities such as an examination room, a room for the ward sister, a dayroom and a storage facility could be shared. The bedrooms had a maximum of six beds; Cleyndert did not consider the four-bed rooms that had been applied in the Södersjukhuset in Stockholm to be economical. A nursing unit consisted of three six-bed, two two-bed and three one-bed rooms. The six-bed rooms were to be provided with a partial glass partition to create a sort of vestibule with washbasins and cupboards.[9] Cleyndert adopted the 'Prussian regulations' for the surface area per bed: 7.5 m^2 of floor space and a total volume of 25 m^3 per bed.[10]

The standard nursing units devised by the study commission of the Hospital Building Centre could be combined in different ways to form a ward. During lectures in Delft, J.H. van den Broek demonstrated the elongated system, the Y-system, the cross or star system, the comb system, and the triangular chevron system.[11] One of the most remarkable solutions was tried out in Rotterdam. Viergever introduced the double corridor system for the nursing units in his Dijkzigtziekenhuis. It had been developed in the United States by the hospital consultant Ch. Neergard, who experimented with it in the Saint Luke Hospital in Bethlehem (1946). The motto that he put into practice here, 'to save nurses steps', became a household motto in hospital architecture.[12] By projecting bedrooms on two sides, it became possible to reduce the length of the ward. As a result, the conventional view that bedrooms should have a southern orientation was abandoned.

Outpatient unit

Although the nursing ward was still the determinant component of the hospital, it had to yield ground to the outpatient clinic. Initially intended only for poor patients in need of medical assistance, its field of operations widened later – a development whose end is not yet in sight.[13] It was soon realised that these developments would lead the outpatient clinic to become a more integrated part of the hospital in terms of administration, organisation and architecture.[14]

Treatment units

The 'healing machines' were no longer the wards but the treatment units, which with their priceless medical equipment formed the core of the modern hospital. The most important elements in the treatment units were the operating theatres. According to the latest insights, they no longer required daylight, which meant the end of the large windows facing north that had been such a characteristic feature of the prewar hospitals. They were abandoned with regret. The most important requirements of the operating unit were that it should be easily accessible from the surgical unit and that it should form a closed entity so that it would not be disturbed by other units. Working with radioactive materials also imposed specific requirements on the X-ray unit. The increasing number of laboratories usually operated as auxiliary services for the treatment unit. The position of the kitchen was a point for discussion.

The view that a large central kitchen was the ideal solution enjoyed the largest support, but decentralised kitchens had been applied in the famous Södersjukhuset, which were stocked from a central kitchen for preparation. Although this system had its natural advantages, the central kitchen model was applied almost everywhere in the Netherlands.[15]

For a long time the nurses' home, though not an integral part of the hospital proper, was an essential appendage to it. The nurses lived there in immediate proximity to their work. This form of housing was believed to offer several advantages. It was practical, as well as enabling the hospital management to train the nurses in the right setting. Another essential appendage to the hospital proper in all denominational institutions was the chapel. Many Catholic hospitals also had a convent where the congregation of nurses lived. An example is the Sint Jozefziekenhuis in Deventer (1956) designed by J.A. van der Laan. The chapel and convent often offered an escape from the sobriety that was an inevitable part of the treatment and nursing units.

Finally there were the administrative units, which grew increasingly in importance as a clear-cut, standardised processing of patient data became the norm. It called for the creation of bulky card index systems.

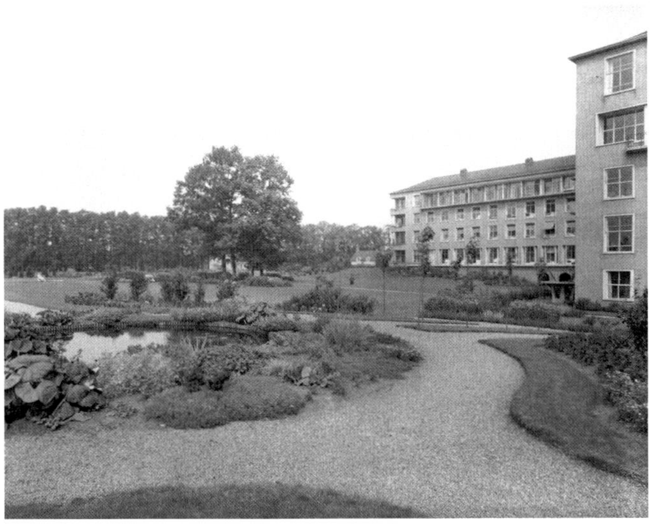

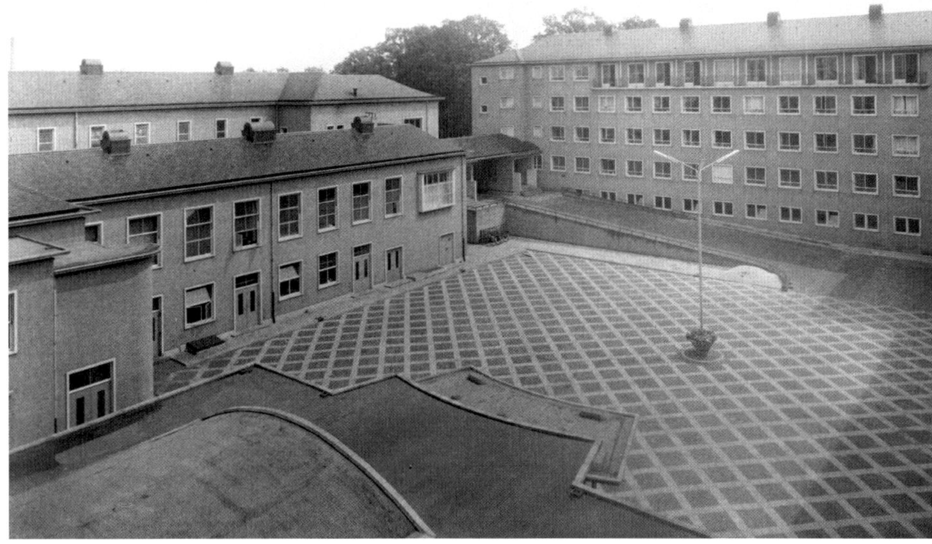

p. 87 | <
B.J.K. Cramer**, Koningin Juliana Ziekenhuis, Hengelo, 1954**

Double-corridor system after US example in the Dijkzigtziekenhuis, Rotterdam

p. 87 | >
B.J.K. Cramer**, Koningin Juliana Ziekenhuis, Hengelo, 1954**

A. Viergever**, Dijkzigtziekenhuis, Rotterdam, 1961**

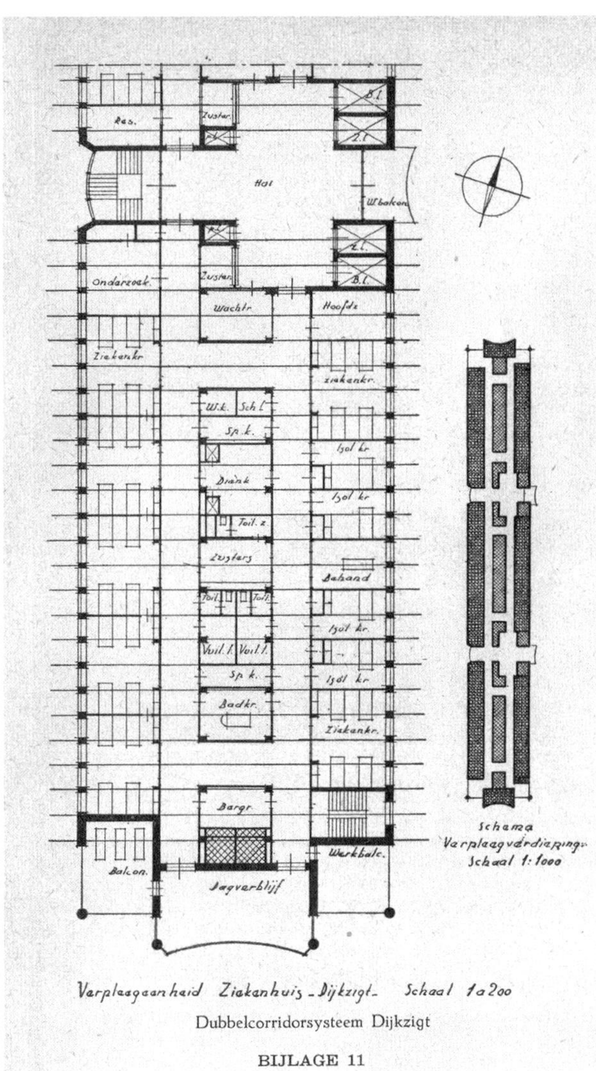

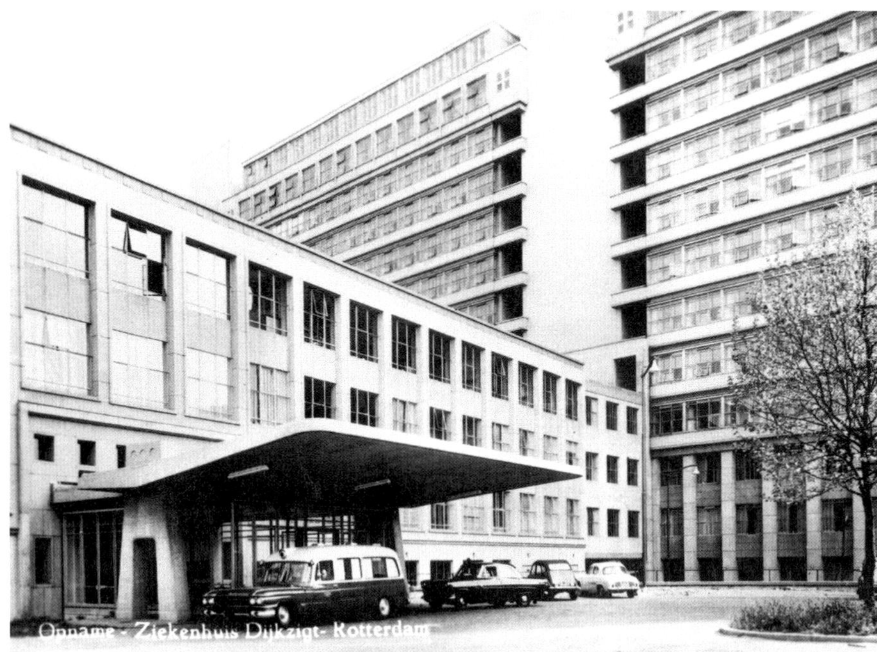

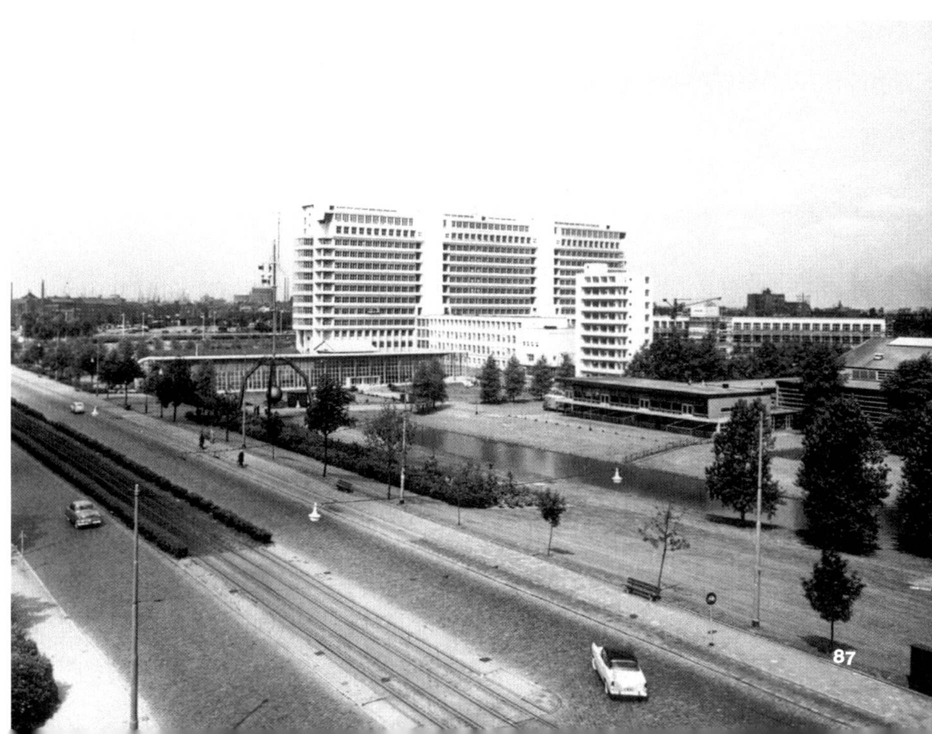

Rational hospital typology

The functioning of a hospital depends to a large extent on its functional organisation, in which the distances that the nurses have to walk should be reduced to a minimum. Care had to be taken to prevent the different traffic flows from crossing one another. Cleyndert therefore recommended that a plan should include a flow chart indicating the different routes.[16]

One of the options to reduce walking distances was high-rise building. In 1946 the interim Government Architect, H. Hoekstra, discussed a number of foreign hospitals, including the Södersjukhuset in Stockholm and the Bürgerspital in Basel, in an article in *Het Ziekenhuiswezen*. He came to the conclusion that a tendency towards centralisation and high-rise building – a centralisation that was primarily located in the height of the building – clearly prevailed abroad. Hoekstra regarded the nursing wards, treatment unit and outpatient clinic as a trinity, 'as both the nursing unit and the outpatient clinic depend on the treatment unit and as such have an influence on the elaboration of the plan'.[17] He proposed placing the treatment unit at right angles to the nursing unit, a solution frequently adopted in the 1950s that is usually referred to as the T-type.[18] The wards would be split into two equal sections, one for men and the other for women. The ground floor was for internal disorders, the first for surgery, and the second for obstetrics, gynaecology and, if necessary, a children's unit. The units in the treatment section were to correspond: the X-ray unit for diagnosis and therapy and the treatment units for cardiography, for example, on the ground floor; the operating theatres and clinical laboratory on the first floor; and the delivery rooms and corresponding operating theatre on the second floor.[19]

After a study trip to the United States, Viergever noted that a lot of experimentation with this type and with a variant, the H-type, was going on there.[20] I. Rosenfield was the first to draw up a plan using this system for the Cumberland Street Hospital in New York.

The first postwar hospitals

It was only in the course of the 1950s that typological research resulted in the first hospital designs according to the latest insights. The earliest results were hardly revolutionary, and there was little freedom of manoeuvre to give the building the desired appearance. The choice of materials was not only determined by the preference of the architect and the size of the budget, but more by the question of what was available. Iron and steel were in short supply, and there was even a shortage of reinforcing bars at first. All the same, all of the hospitals that were built in the 1950s had a concrete skeleton. Van der Laan limited its use to the first floor of the treatment unit in his Sint Jozefziekenhuis in Deventer, but that was exceptional. The hospital proved to be unsuitable for experiments with mechanised building methods, and in this respect the new hospitals did not stand out for being progressive.

Only J.P. Kloos (Juliana Ziekenhuis in Terneuzen, 1954), K.L. Sijmons (Streekziekenhuis Bennekom, 1957) and Viergever (in his Dijkzigtziekenhuis in Rotterdam, 1957) referred directly to a modern idiom of forms. The size of the skeleton articulated the walls, the windows were large and directly set between the columns to form continuous horizontal bands above brick apron walls, and the roofs were flat. B.J.K. Cramer applied much more modest windows set in the concrete frames that were characteristic of the reconstruction period in his Koningin Juliana Ziekenhuis in Hengelo; the roof was tiled instead of flat.

p. 88
Van der Laan Hermans Van der Eerden **with *P. Dijkema*, Sint Radboudziekenhuis, Nijmegen, nursing building**

p. 89
Van der Laan Hermans Van der Eerden **with *P. Dijkema*, Sint Radboudziekenhuis, Nijmegen, 1948-1965**

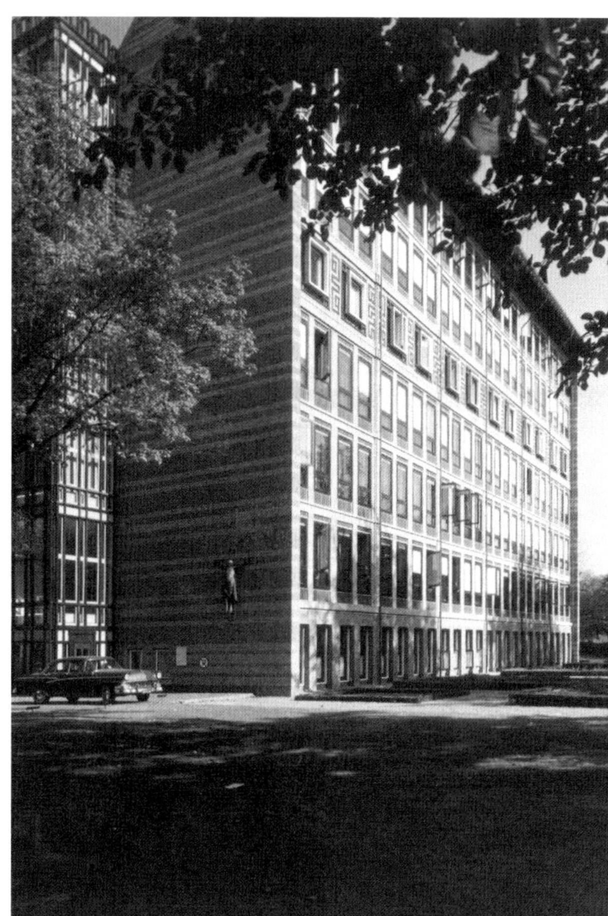

Few projects were implemented in the aftermath of the war, which makes it difficult to determine which types were preferred. Cramer grouped the units around a courtyard, Kloos designed an H-type hospital in Terneuzen in which the two long sides were for the nursing unit and the outpatient units, while the horizontal bar was for the treatment unit. This was the first time that expression was given to the triple organisation of nursing unit, treatment unit and outpatient unit. The main structure was the result of the separation of the main functions and the relation between them. This was of fundamental importance for Kloos: 'That fundamental structure is also anchored in the architectural expression in Terneuzen. No form was needed for that. It was an expression of the architecture, the organisation. And for me that is synonymous with architecture.'[21]

The Streekziekenhuis Bennekom is a pure T-type: the treatment unit is the stem, and the bar at right angles to it accommodates the wards for female patients on one side and male patients on the other. The point of intersection is where the stairs and lifts (the 'vertical ascending points') are situated. Viergever's Dijkzigtziekenhuis is dominated by an enormous ward building consisting almost entirely of nursing units; each floor corresponds to one or more medical specialisations. The treatment unit and outpatient clinics are accommodated in a separate wing, as is the fairly large home for the nurses.

After Amsterdam, Utrecht, Leiden and Groningen – four non-denominational universities – the fifth medical faculty was built for the Catholic University in Nijmegen. A medical faculty was also set up in the Protestant Vrije Universiteit in Amsterdam in 1950. Religious compartmentalisation had thus filtered through to the university training courses for physicians and medical specialists. The first of these to develop plans for a new building was Nijmegen. J.A. van der Laan started work on a plan on the basis of an urban development design drawn up under the responsibility of M.J. Granpré Molière.

Its general structure was in harmony with the park-like terrain behind Villa Heyendaal. A broad green strip separated the hospital that lay on the north side of the green boulevard, from the faculty on the south side. The (labour-intensive) treatment units were directly adjacent to the green strip and were connected with one another and with a convent complex by a long corridor. This backbone of the hospital was also the link with the nursing wards, that were built in the park on the north side. The first of them was completed in 1954. It was a robust building with attractive details in which P. Dijkema, the partner of Van der Laan and responsible for the details of the plans, applied the pattern of spatial relations elaborated by Dom H. van der Laan.

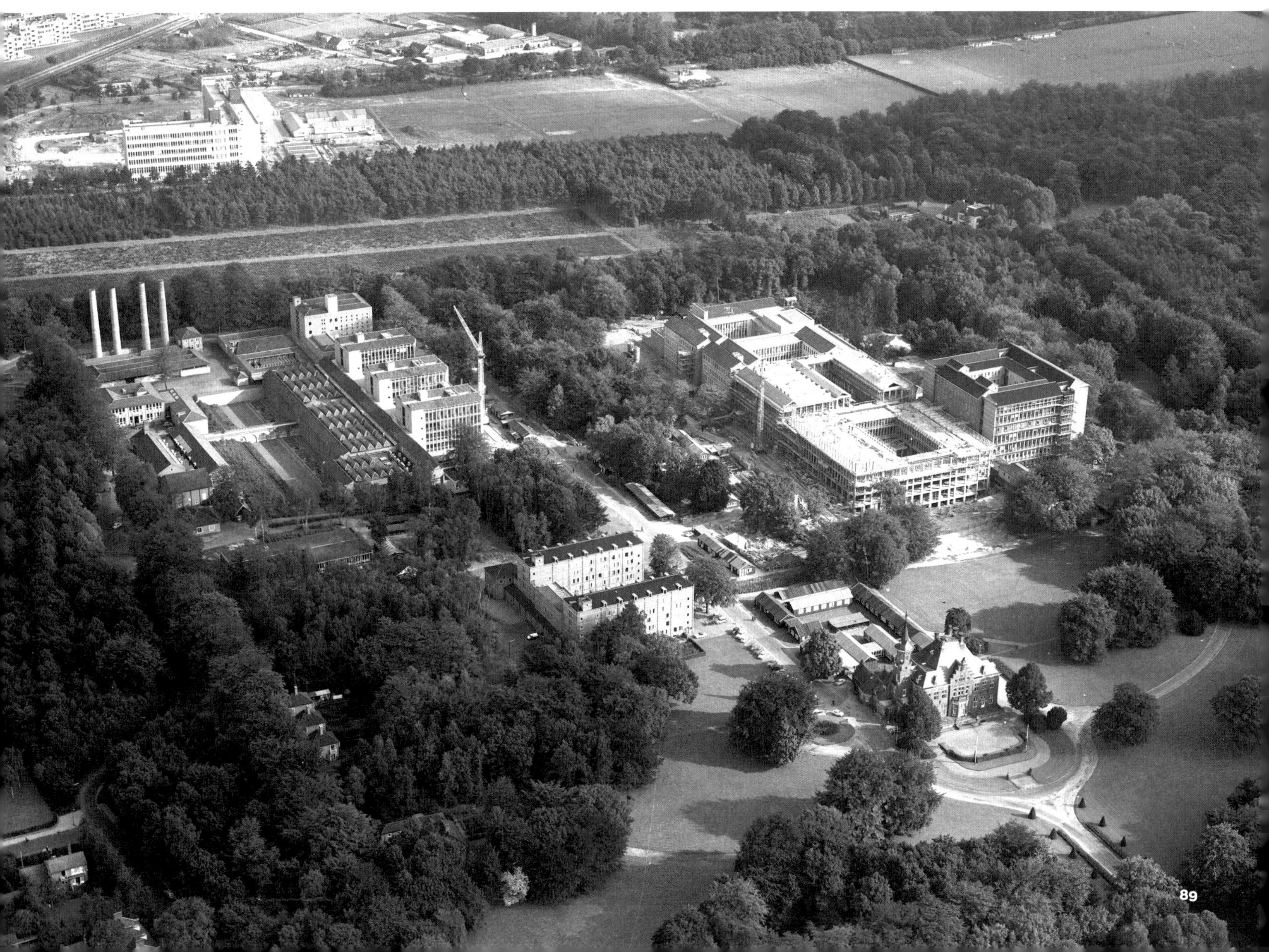

Psychiatric hospitals

After the wave of building in the 1920s and 1930s, psychiatry seemed to have entered a period of relative calm, but reality was different. At first the restoration of the many heavily damaged institutions absorbed all the attention, and the first complexes of new buildings only saw the light of day in the 1960s. In the meantime, however, a genuine revolution had taken place: psychiatric drugs put an end to the phenomenon of 'maniacal' mental illnesses. This meant major changes in the functioning of the clinics.

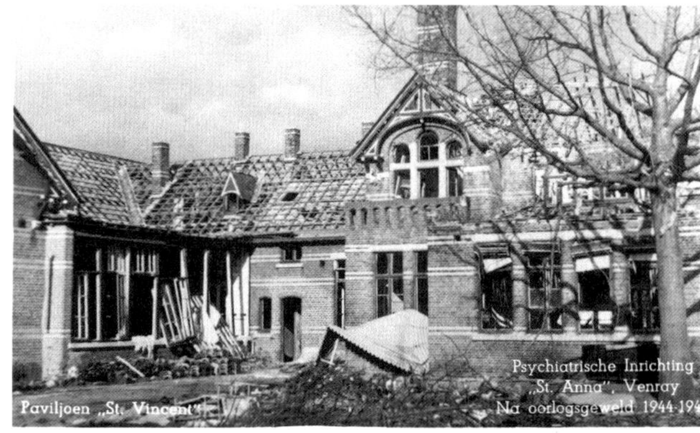
Paviljoen „St. Vincent" Psychiatrische Inrichting „St. Anna", Venray Na oorlogsgeweld 1944-1945

Reconstruction

At first there were no warning signs of the quiet revolution that was to completely change the look of psychiatric hospitals within a few decades. The damage caused during the war had to be repaired first, and even that proceeded very slowly in the first years after the liberation, when the Netherlands was confronted with the need to repair the war damage and the economic prospects were anything but rosy. The psychiatric institutions had a difficult time between 1940 and 1945. They suffered more than the regular hospitals, probably because the occupying forces attached little importance to the nursing and treatment of the mentally ill. Almost no new buildings were constructed in the 1940s except for the opening of Hulp en Heil in Leidschendam in 1949, but that was an initiative of the Dutch Reformed Church that went back to before the war. Work commenced relatively quickly on the reconstruction of the Sint Anna clinic in Venray. Some of its buildings were in ruins and only six of the eleven nursing pavilions were more or less usable. The maximal prewar capacity of 710 had been reduced by 290. Even if one disregards the destruction, the number of patients who had to be accommodated in Sint Anna after the war exceeded the maximal capacity. The former asylum was reconstructed in a new guise. The result is typical of the earliest phase of the reconstruction, which was dominated by a serene brick architecture.

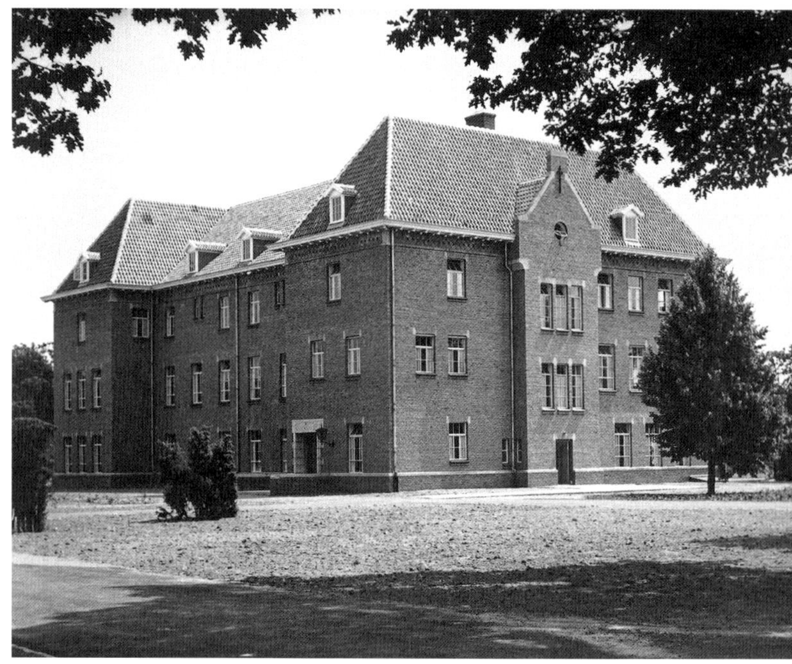

That brick could produce a different, more modern effect is shown by the reconstruction of Bloemendaal. Most of the complex was destroyed in the war. Instead of opting for new buildings, it was decided to rebuild the complex as far as possible to enable the evacuated patients to return as quickly as possible. Only ten of the eighteen pavilions were capable of being restored. Several new buildings were added to the complex, including the main building. The design was by E.J. Rothuizen, who by then had become a kind of in-house architect of the Association for the Protestant Care of Mental and Neural Disorders. In spite of the use of similar materials, the architecture is very different from that of Sint Anna in Venray: it is an exponent of the 'marriage between concrete and brick', the 'shake-hands' architecture that resulted from cooperation between the traditional and the modern movements.

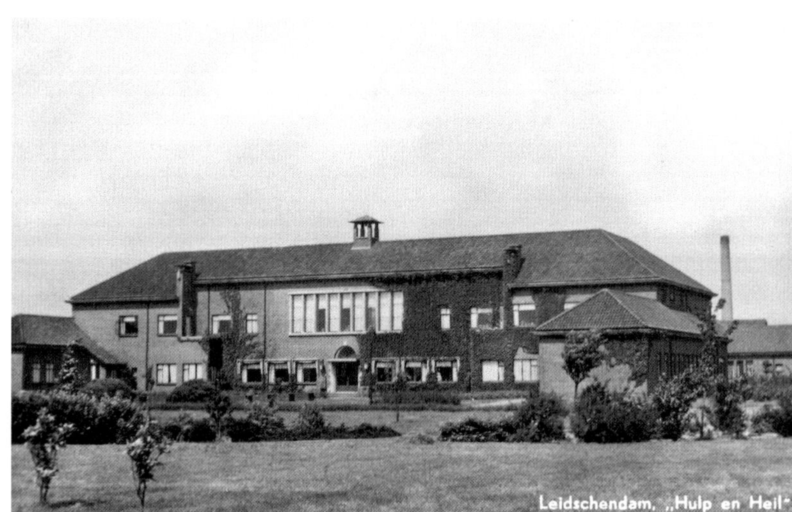
Leidschendam, „Hulp en Heil"

Expansion and new buildings

By far the largest number of buildings constructed in this period consisted of new clinics and pavilions that were added to existing structures. An example is the new observation pavilion at Maasoord in Poortugaal by E.J. Rothuizen & C. Dekker. Although it was not completed until 1960, everything about it exudes the atmosphere of the reconstruction; there are even traces of 'shake-hands' architecture. Most of all the clinic is reminiscent of the schools that were designed

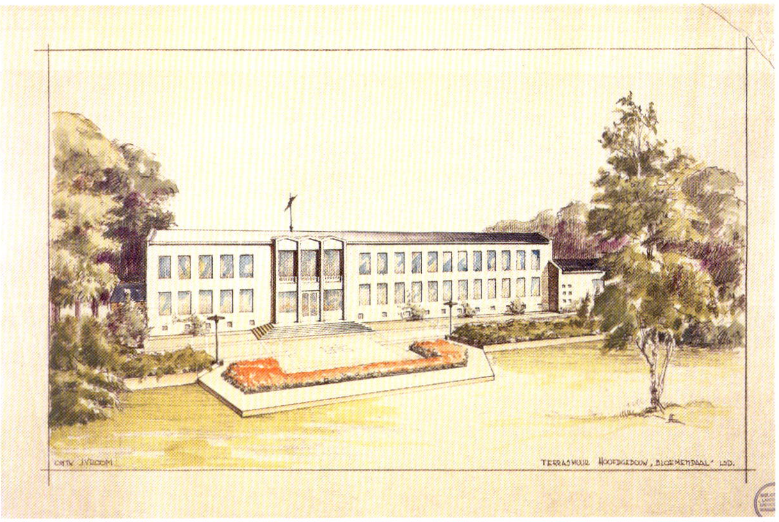

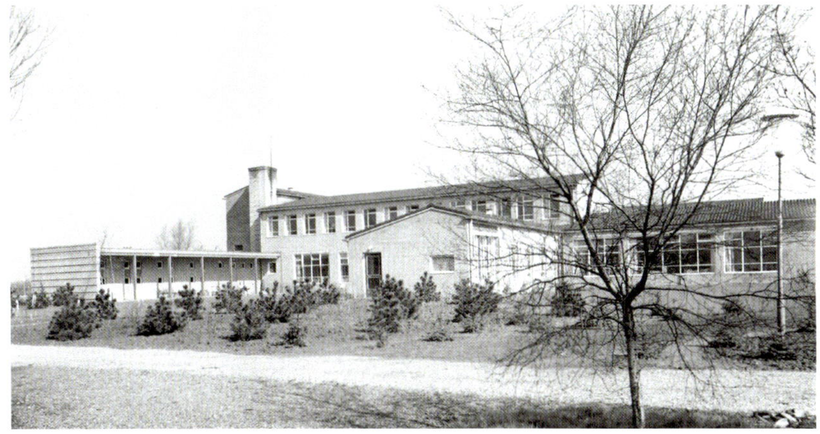

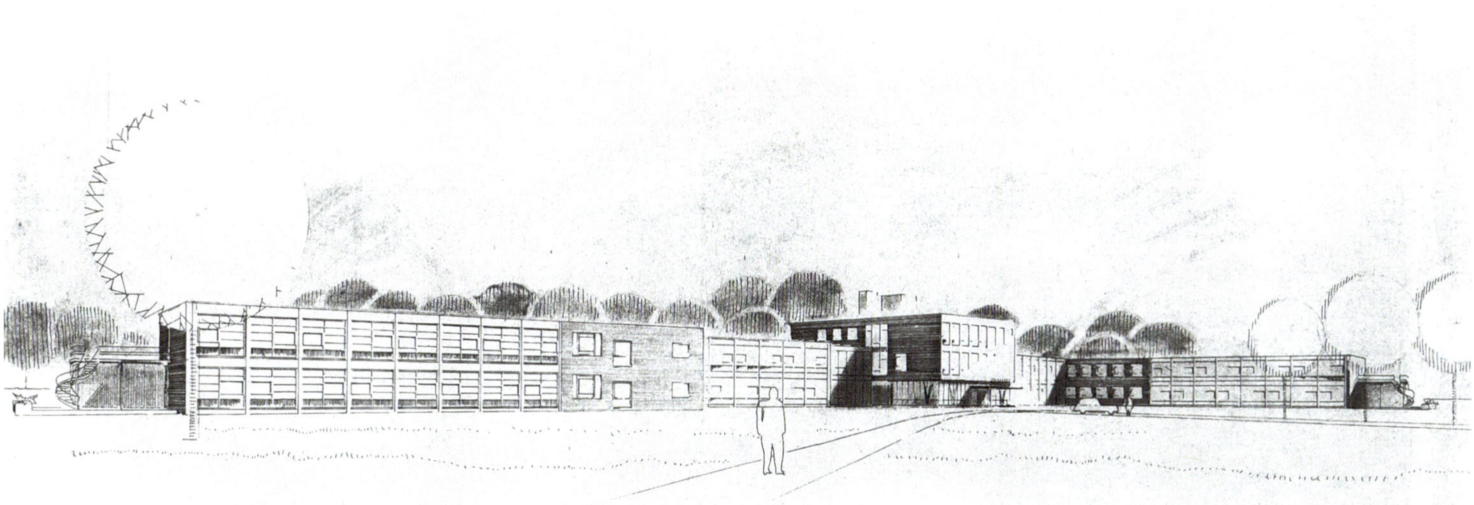

p. 90
War damage to Sint Anna psychiatric hospital, Venray

***J. van Dongen*, Sint Bernard pavilion, Sint Anna psychiatric hospital, Venray, 1949**

***Gebroeders Mensink*, Hulp en Heil, Leidschendam, 1949**

p. 91 | <
***E.J. Rothuizen*, Bloemendaal, main building, The Hague, 1954**

***C.B. Posthumus Meyjes & J.B. Narold*, Brederodekliniek, Santpoort, 1965**

p. 91 | >
***E. J. Rothuizen & C. Dekker*, Delta-ziekenhuis, Poortugaal, observation pavilion, 1953**

p. 91 | bottom
***W. Ingwersen & C.D. van Reyendam*, Vogelenzang, Bennebroek, 1958. New building for physiotherapy with situation of the building.**

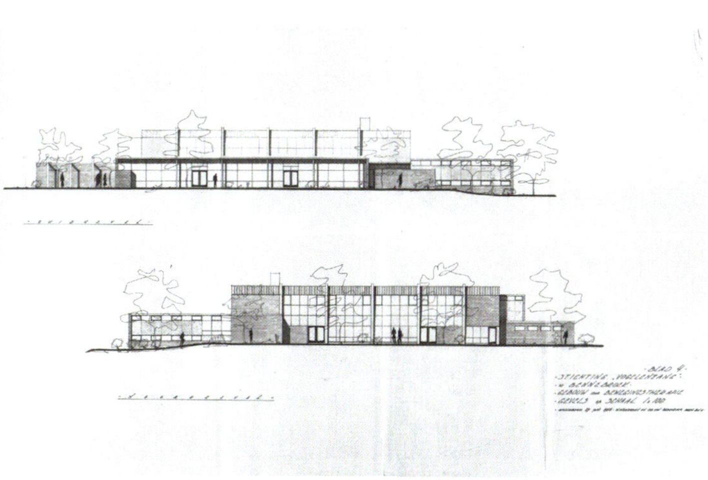

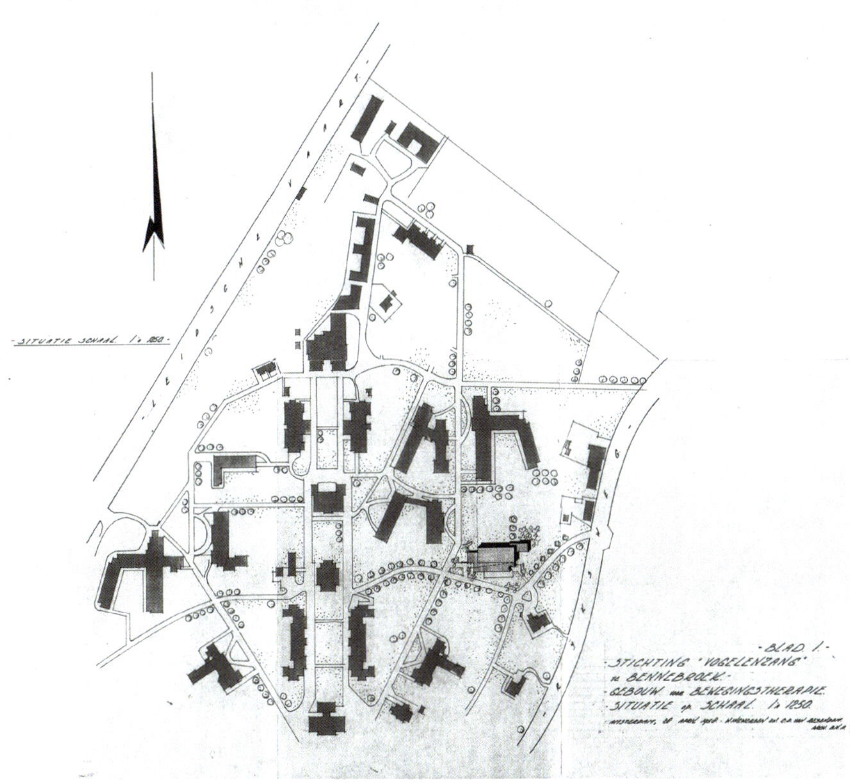

in the 1950s. Large windows, a canopy and a wing with a will of its own that simply ignores the grid on which the ground plan is based, the gentle slopes of the roof of the main volume in three layers and the canopy above the entrance mark it as a typical product of the 1950s. It was regarded as extremely modern when it opened, if only because the main building and the units for female and male patients were combined in a single building, while they had been kept strictly separate in the former Maasoord.

Another example is the Brederokliniek which was opened in the grounds of the Provinciaal Ziekenhuis Santpoort and which was also intended for the short-term treatment of patients. C.B. Postumus Meyjes & J.B. Narold received the commission for the clinic in 1958. They designed a building that derives its monumental character mainly from the central entrance, which separates the male from the female patients, and the decorative finishing of the windows in the dayrooms. There is an optimal view of the purely ornamental garden from the transparent clinic.

It often happened that the erection of new buildings on the available terrains was at the expense of the original urban planning structure and the landscape architecture. An example of this is the placing of a work therapy building designed by W. Ingwersen & C.D. van Reyendam on the Vogelenzang terrain in Bennebroek (1958).

Hardly any new building work was conducted in the immediate aftermath of the war. An exception is the Sinai Centrum in Amersfoort. This institution, designed by L.H.P. Waterman and officially opened on 18 October 1960, has a transparent, modern look. The centre was set up by the Centrale Vereniging voor de Joodse Geestelijke Gezondheidszorg (Central Association for Jewish Mental Health Care) and replaced the Apeldoornsche Bosch; the latter was put to use as a centre for the mentally handicapped by the 's Heerenloo mental institution and renamed Groot Schuylenburg. The Sinai Centrum was named after Mount Sinai in New York and built with the support of The Conference on Jewish Material Claims. The plan envisaged a psychiatric unit, a unit for the mentally handicapped, and all of the medical services that a fully fledged mental institution required; the idea of using Zon en Schild was dropped.

Housing and care for the elderly

Around the middle of the twentieth century, housing for the elderly left a great deal to be desired. Whether they were normal housing units, in which the vast majority of the elderly lived, or rest homes, most of them failed to satisfy even minimal standards. There was a serious housing shortage due to poor maintenance, the destruction of housing during the war, and ten years of inactivity in the field of social housing.

Classification of the elderly

Probably the most fundamental conclusion that was drawn in 1945 is that, irrespective of their milieu, education, standard of living and background, the elderly form a largely homogeneous group. One of the consequences was that care for the elderly may not be poor relief, but must extend to all economic categories. The only differences to be taken into account were those in the extent to which the elderly were reliant on help. There was general agreement on the existence of two categories: the elderly who needed no help at all, or only very incidentally, and the category that could not manage without daily assistance, mainly of a domestic kind. The vast majority of the elderly – ninety per cent is the estimate usually given – belonged to the first category. The remaining ten per cent – those in need of daily assistance – consisted of two main groups: valid and invalid. Not everyone who requires assistance is ill or invalid.

These distinctions formed the basis for a classification of the elderly. A second fundamental decision concerned the designation of housing as the foundation of care for the elderly. As part of social housing, accommodation for the elderly was able to reach a scale never equalled outside the Netherlands. The nursing home was excluded from the feverish activity that ensued because for a long time it proved impossible to find the appropriate funding for it. While accommodation for the elderly was incorporated in the dynamics of housing in general, the development of new types of nursing homes stagnated.

Housing study after housing study appeared and the planning and building machinery slowly but surely got under way too. A home was a primary necessity of life, but it was more. Housing was seen as the tangible expression of the social cohesion of a society and therefore determines to a large extent how that society functions. It is not just a mirror of society, but also an instrument to give it shape. The material side of housing is important, but at least equally important is the way in which it enables people to develop and to fulfil their potential. These were the principles that determined the reconstruction. They culminated in reflection on accommodation for the elderly. A better anchorage from which to combat the problems of ageing and to integrate the elderly in society seemed barely conceivable.

Different types of accommodation for the elderly

Knowledge of the different categories of the elderly was regarded as a precondition for the definition of a number of housing typologies – the concept typology refers to the tangible connection between a specific function and the building tailored to that purpose. The objective of finding the ideal match between very precisely defined categories of occupants and types of housing very precisely tailored to their demands is characteristic of functionalism.

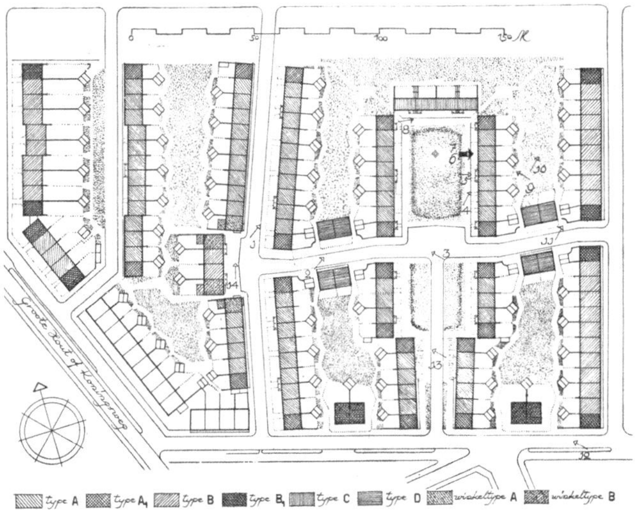

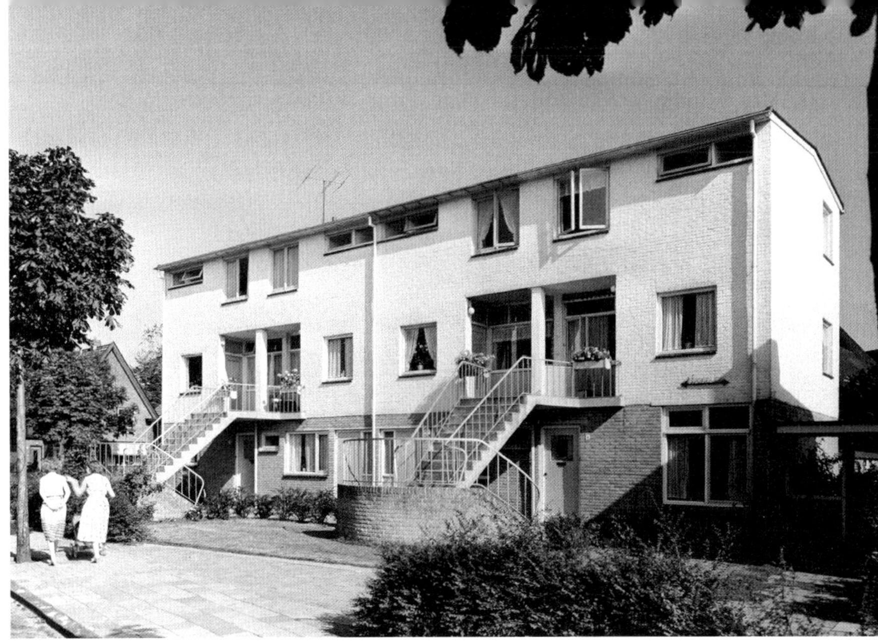

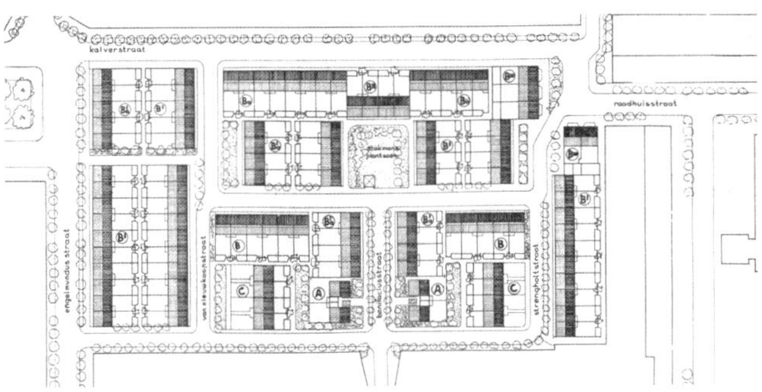

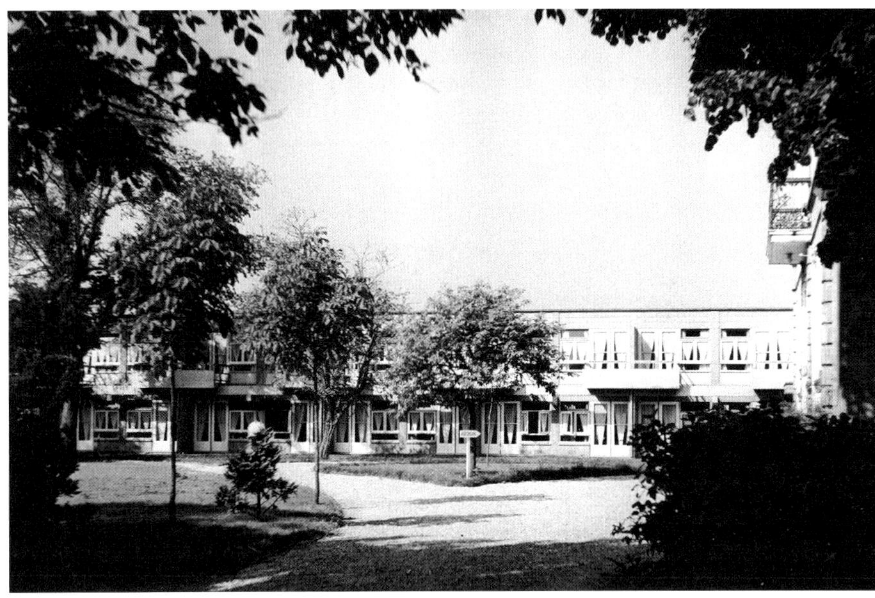

p. 93 | <

***L.A. Hoogenstraaten*, plan for residential neighbourhood with several homes for old people, IJmuiden, 1950**

***A. Staal & S. van Woerden*, plan for residential neighbourhood with several homes for old people, Velsen-Noord, 1952**

***A. van Eyck & J. Rietveld*, housing units for the elderly, Amsterdam, 1954**

p. 93 | >

***R. Romke de Vries*, housing units for the elderly, Sassenheim, 1954**

***J.P. Kloos*, Rusthuis Rozenoord, Sluis, 1952**

***M.F. Duintjer*, extension and reconstruction of the Villa Der Boede into nursing home, Koudekerke, 1953**

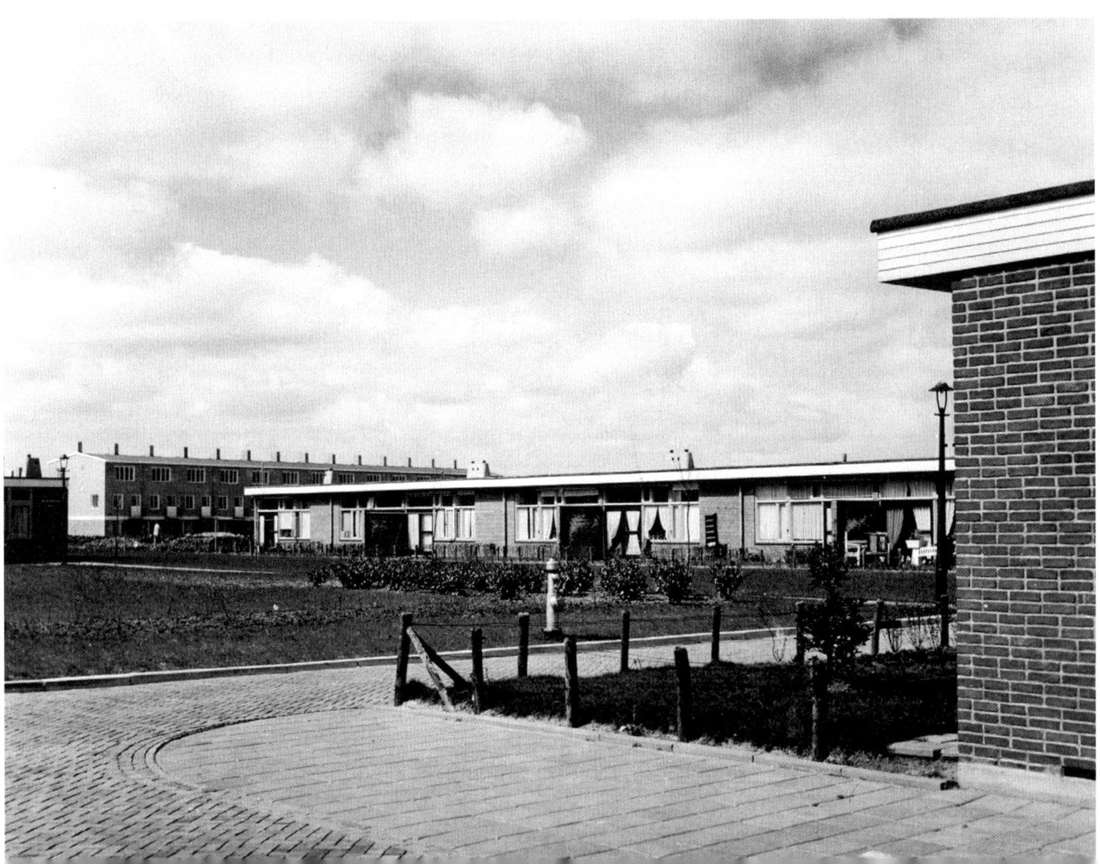

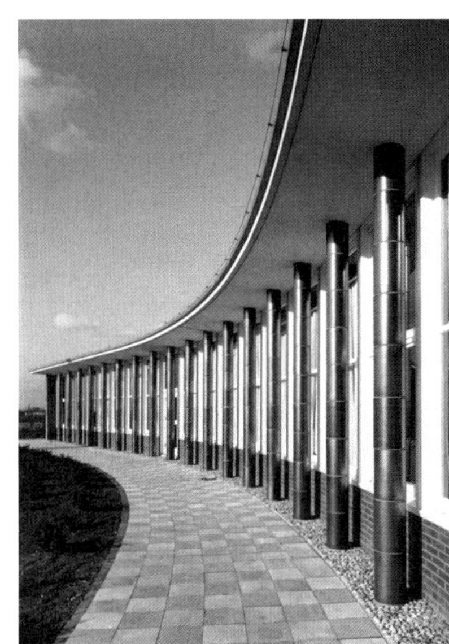

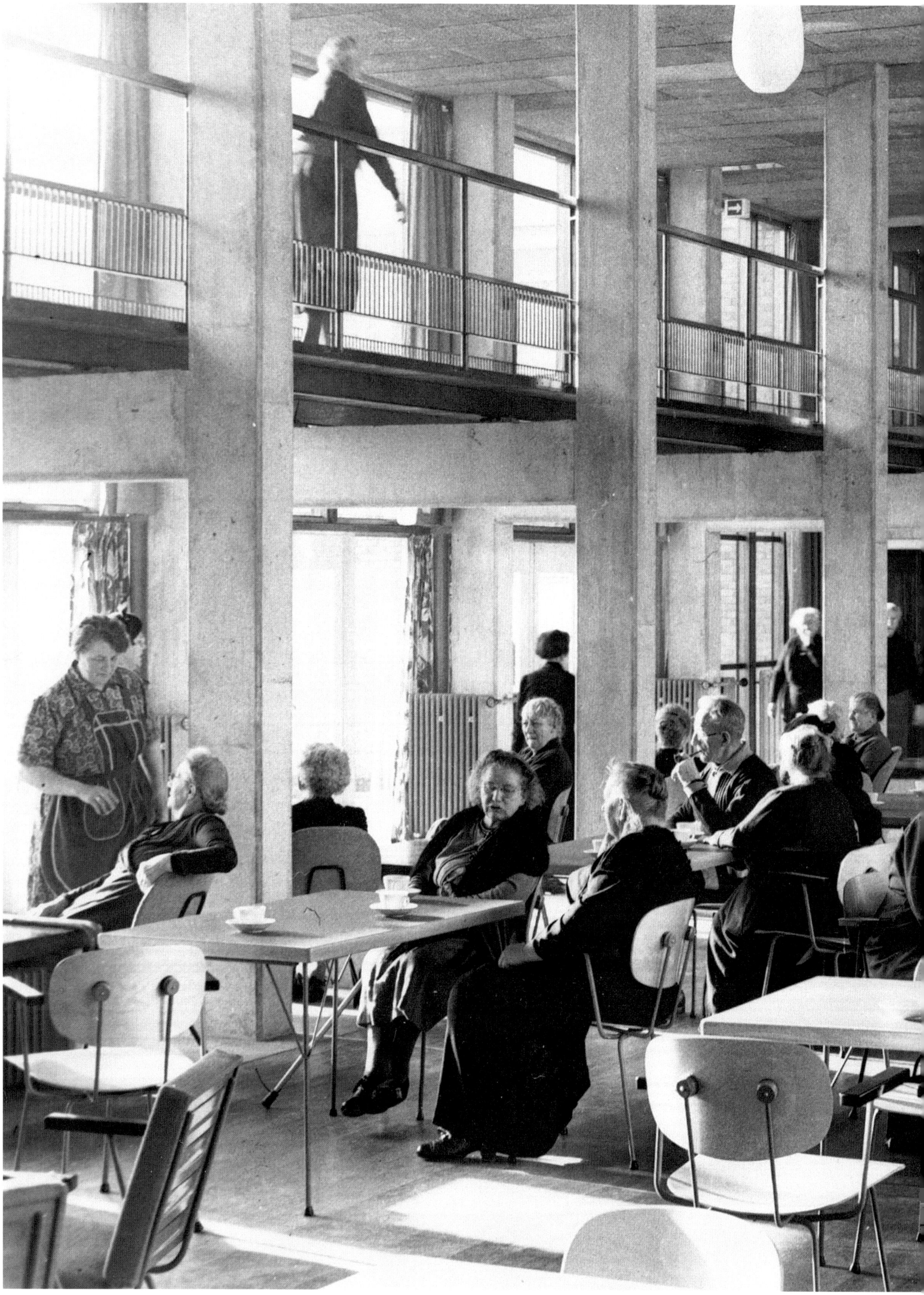

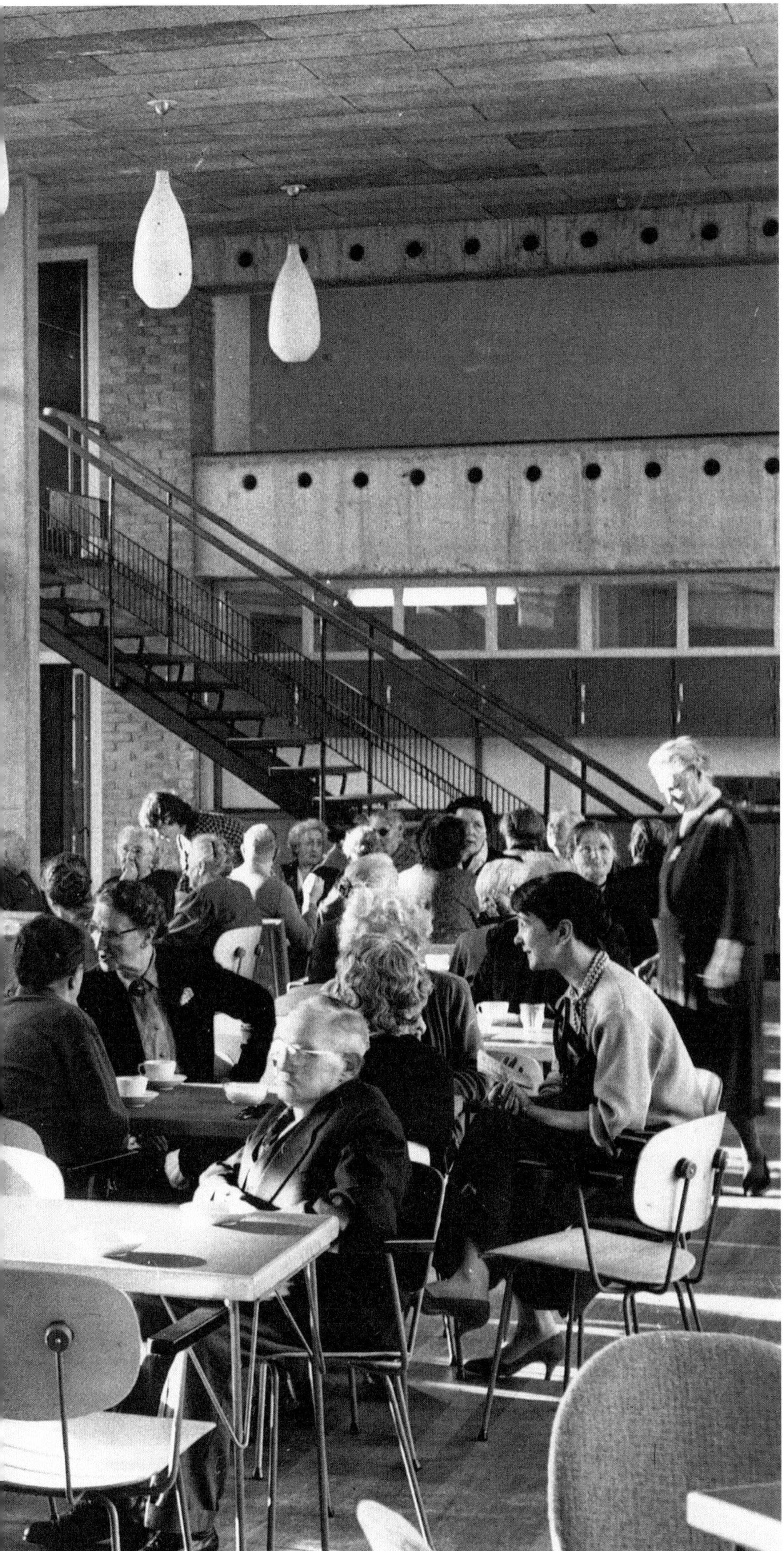

***J.A. Snellebrand & G.W. Tuynman*, Willem Dreeshuis, Amsterdam, 1957**

Housing units for the elderly
The first type was the housing unit built specially for the elderly. The only way it differed from homes for younger generations was that it was on one floor and if possible had no thresholds. Generally speaking no relation was supposed with institutions that brought assistance to the door – at the time it was still very common for the grocer and greengrocer to deliver their goods to the door and home visiting by the general practitioner was completely normal. These houses for the elderly could therefore be distributed amid other types of housing. They were intended to enable the elderly to continue to live without regular assistance, which is why they are sometimes referred to as self-sufficient housing units for the elderly.

A particularly successful example of such housing was designed in the early 1950s by Aldo van Eyck. He paid particular attention to achieving a certain scale and to relating the apartments to one another to avoid the emergence of isolated cells. Within the framework of W.M. Dudok's reconstruction plan for IJmuiden, another housing complex including a few housing units for the elderly was completed in 1950. It was designed by L.A. Hoogenstraaten. The parcellation plan with mainly streets running in a North-South direction was modified by placing the blocks at right angles to one another to achieve a more satisfactory spatial effect.[22] The housing units for the elderly were grouped in pairs and were very simple, with one floor and a sloping roof.

The housing units for the elderly designed by Romke de Vries in Sassenheim (1953-1954) have a very modern appearance. They look like ordinary one-family homes. The complex consists of twenty-two housing units, divided between two blocks each comprising eight units, and one block with 'two-on-one' units. The latter type consists of three floors and has two housing units with a living room and two bedrooms on the ground floor and four maisonettes on the upper floors, each with the living room on the first floor and the two bedrooms on the second floor. The maisonettes can be reached by two outdoor staircases.

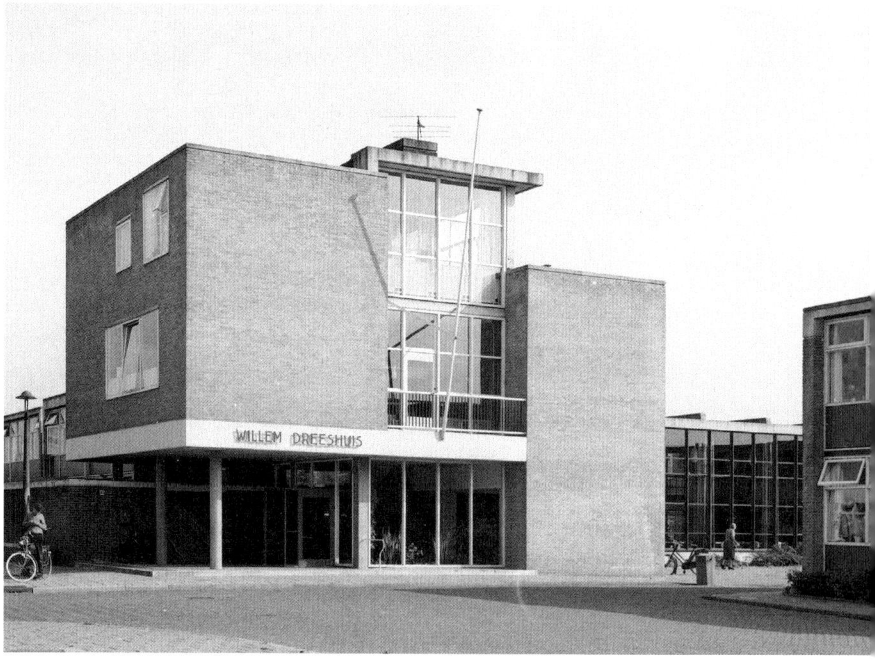

Complexes combining individual and communal facilities (pensiontehuizen)
Institutionalised homes were required for the elderly who needed some measure of help around the house. To underline the difference with earlier forms of accommodation for the elderly, the term *pensiontehuis* was used for them. Such a complex consisted of housing units for single old people, usually supplemented with a small number of units for couples. The communal facilities usually consisted of canteens, rooms for conversation and recreation (if the canteen was not used for this purpose), a central kitchen, offices, and regularly apartments for staff who lived on the premises – they disappeared in the course of the 1970s. The original idea was to have two categories: complexes with between twenty-five and thirty residents, and larger ones for between one-hundred and three-hundred.[23] There were fears that if institutions were too small, this would prevent the integration of a reasonable level of amenities and would make it difficult for the residents to form groups within which the elderly could feel at home. On the other hand, larger institutions were too big to convey the sense of a large family that was associated with smaller versions.

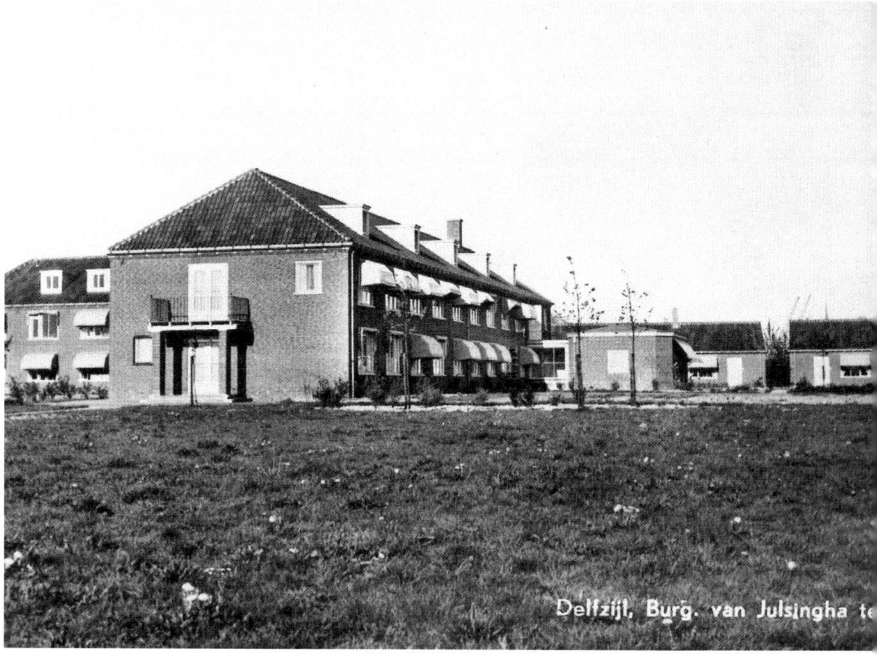

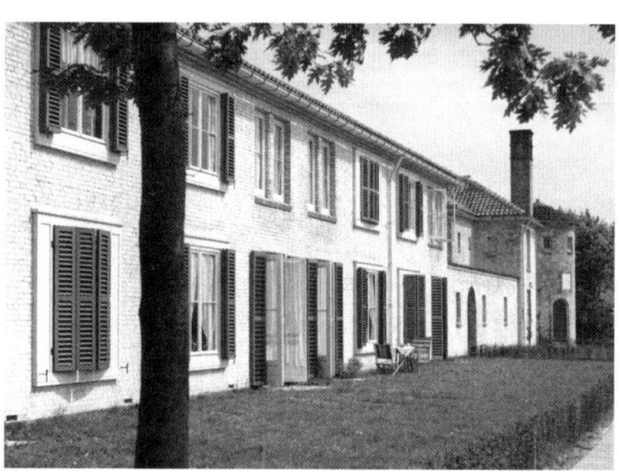

One of the fathers of Dutch functionalism, J.P. Kloos, already designed a small complex in 1946: Rusthuis Rozenoord in Sluis (Zeeland). On a small scale it contained every feature of the type: small housing units grouped around communal facilities in a building articulated in several wings. A complex designed by Auke Komter was built for 230 old people in Almelo. It is an example of 'shake-hands' architecture, a style for which Van Tijen had introduced the term 'marriage between brick and concrete' in 1939. Scandinavian architecture was a source of inspiration.[24] An old people's home was completed in Breda in 1952 that was designed in the traditionalist style by A. Evers & G.J.M. Sarlemijn. It was part of the Heuvelkwartier expansion plan, part of which was designed by M.J. Granpré Molière. A site for the home had been reserved on the corner of this small neighbourhood. The complex refers to the old cluster of almshouses type by projecting four wings around a large square enclosed garden. Parallel to the wing where the entrance is situated there is a further wing on the other side of the street, which articulates the complex with the rest of the neighbourhood. This old people's home was built in accordance with the Housing Law, which laid down at that time that the combined volume of living rooms, bedrooms and care rooms should not exceed 75 m^3 per person.[25]

Jos Bedaux designed the Pensiontehuis Sint Jozefzorg in Tilburg (1946-1954). This complex too refers to the old clusters of almshouses for the elderly. It consists of an elongated volume with a comb-shaped ground plan of four identical wings and three courtyards between them. On the closed side of the comb behind the first courtyard is a rectangular part of the building that encloses a large courtyard. At right angles to this are a chapel on one side and a part of the building with several kitchens on the other side. The building comprises fifty-two housing units for couples. Each unit is very small and has its own entrance at the front and an entrance at the rear. The latter opens into a corridor connected with the communal facilities, such as a canteen.

Willem Dreeshuis in Amsterdam, designed by J.A. Snellebrand & G.W. Tuynman, is an old people's home that forms part of the Jeruzalem garden village from the 1950s. Its scale matches the blocks of apartments in the district. The building consists of two two-storey L-shaped wings which are connected to one another by an intermediate part where the recreation room is situated. The complex includes single and double rooms, which are very simply furnished and only have a washbasin. Toilets and bathrooms are communal, and there is a central kitchen and canteen.

Nursing homes

Finally there were the nursing homes. These were in fact hospitals for chronic patients and were subject to virtually the same regulations as the regular hospitals. The main difference lay in the level of medical services, which was considerably lower and attuned to the character of the target group: too infirm to be able to live on their own, but not ill enough to be constantly in need of sophisticated medical care. Although intended for the sick and built under the same regime as normal hospitals, they differ from the H-type, K-type and T-type that were common in those days. While the architecture of the hospital was determined at the time by the distinction between three main functions – treatment unit, outpatient clinic and nursing unit – the latter prevailed in the nursing homes. They had no outpatient clinic, and the

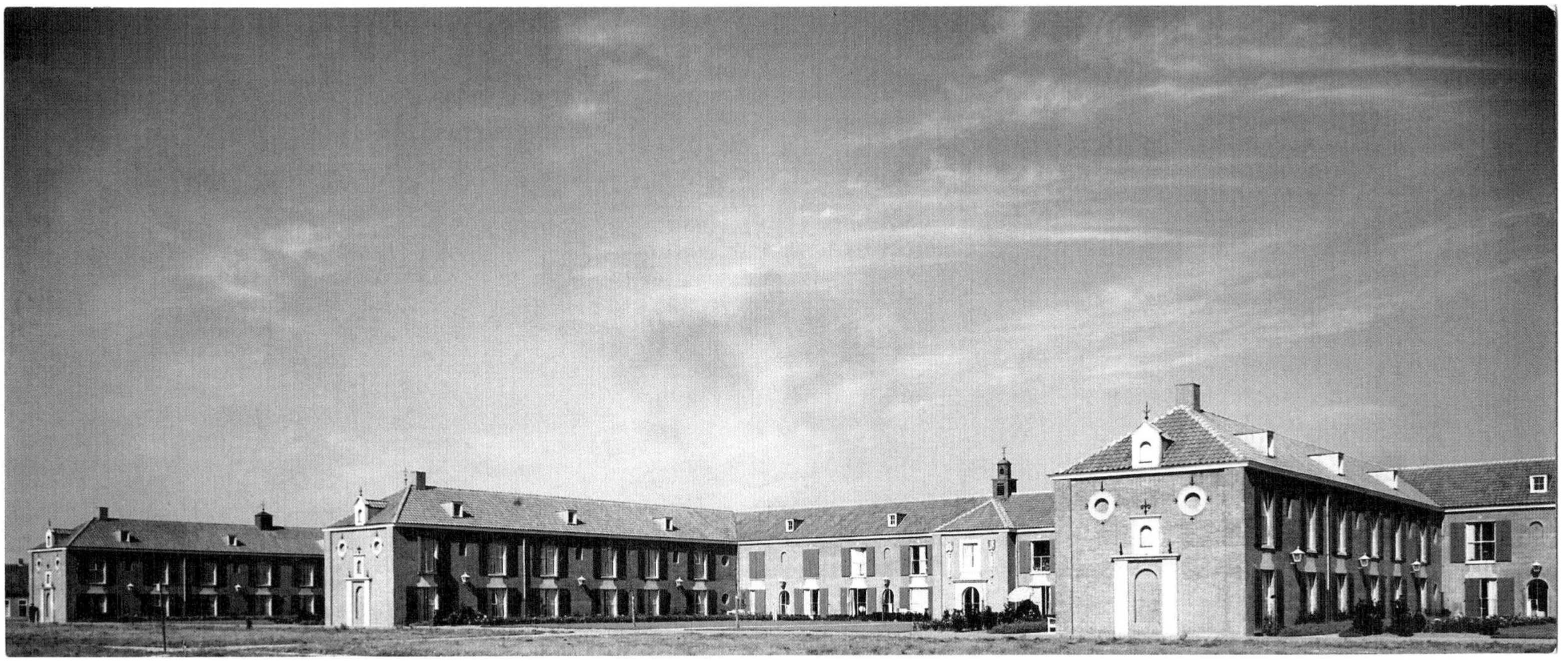

p. 96
***J.A. Snellebrand & G.W. Tuynman*, Willem Dreeshuis, Amsterdam, 1957**

***P. Oom & J. Kuipers*, Burgemeester van Julsinghatehuis and 28 housing units for the elderly, Delfzijl, 1955**

***A. Evers & G.J.M. Sarlemijn*, old people's home, Breda, 1952**

p. 97
***Jos Bedaux*, Pensiontehuis Sint Jozefzorg, Tilburg, 1954**

***A. Baart*, housing units for the elderly around the Colleheim old people's home, Kollum, 1949**

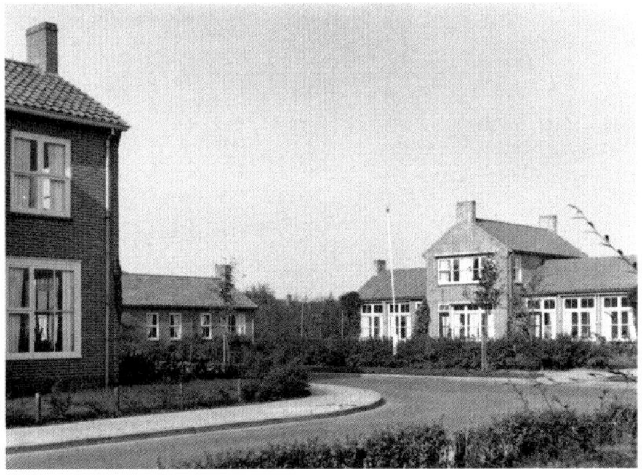

treatment units were relatively simple and usually integrated in the main volume. The construction of nursing homes on a large scale did not begin until the 1960s. The first to result from a combination of new buildings and expansion during the reconstruction period was Der Boede in Koudekerken. It was also the first nursing home to be built according to the approval procedures of the Hospital Commission.[26] The current Villa Der Boede was restored and expanded with two curved wings.

Combination of complexes combining individual and communal facilities with self-sufficient housing units for the elderly

One of the most frequent solutions was the combination of two types: the complex with individual and communal facilities and the self-sufficient housing unit for the elderly. In such cases the communal part – the service centre integrated in the former – could also serve the latter.

A. Baart produced a design for housing units for the elderly with the Colleheim old people's home in Kollum (1949). Another example is the Burgemeester van Julsinghatehuis in Delfzijl with twenty-eight self-sufficient housing units for old people. While these housing units are completely separate from the home, in other cases they often form a part of it. This solution is found in various forms. In Sint Servatius in Maastricht, designed by J.H.A. Huysmans, the self-sufficient housing units are accommodated in a separate wing that is parallel to the care area. The two parts are connected by a section containing the communal facilities.

Service flats

Besides housing units for more well-to-do old people, private initiative also produced the service flat: blocks of apartments with communal facilities paid for by the residents. This was not an entirely new type; inspired by the United States and Great Britain, Jan Wils and Frans Lourijsen had introduced the 'residential hotel' (*woonhotel*) in the Jozef Israëlsplein in The Hague in the 1920s. This was a block of flats with all modern conveniences: central heating, a central kitchen, lifts, an intercom, and separate rooms for guests.[27] The first real service flats for old people were built in Amersfoort. Designed by C.B. van der Tak for De Terp cooperative housing association, the block contained a total of 84 apartments with nine different floor plans for 156 residents. There was a service building with five rooms for personnel next door.

With the exception of the nursing home, these types that were defined in the reconstruction period were built in unprecedently large numbers from the end of the 1950s. The following chapter deals in more detail with the building boom which was part of the expansion of cities, towns and villages. It led in the Randstad urban agglomeration to a phenomenon that was new for the Netherlands: the suburb.

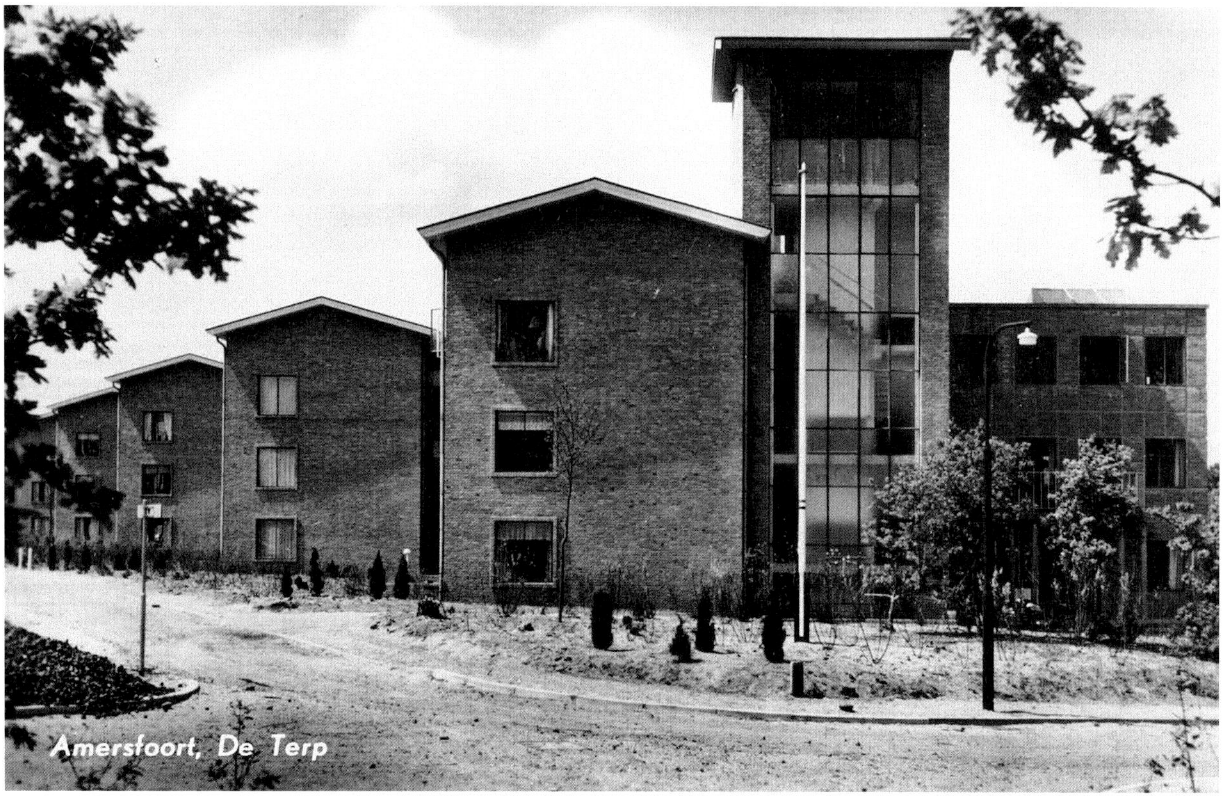

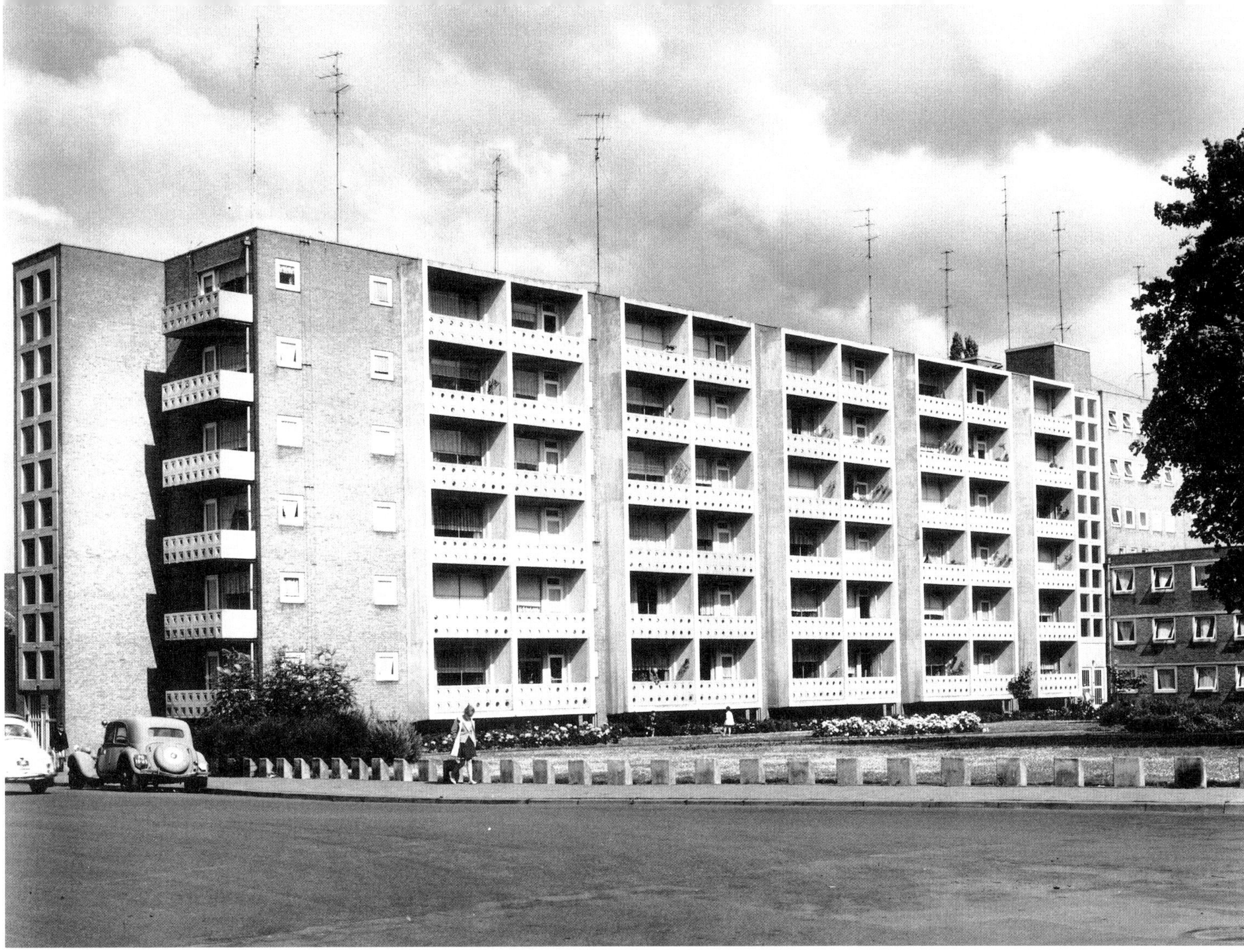

p. 98
***C.B. van der Tak*, De Terp service flat, Amersfoort, 1954**

p. 99
***J.H.A. Huysmans*, Sint Servatius (Aldenhof) old people's home, Maastricht, 1957**

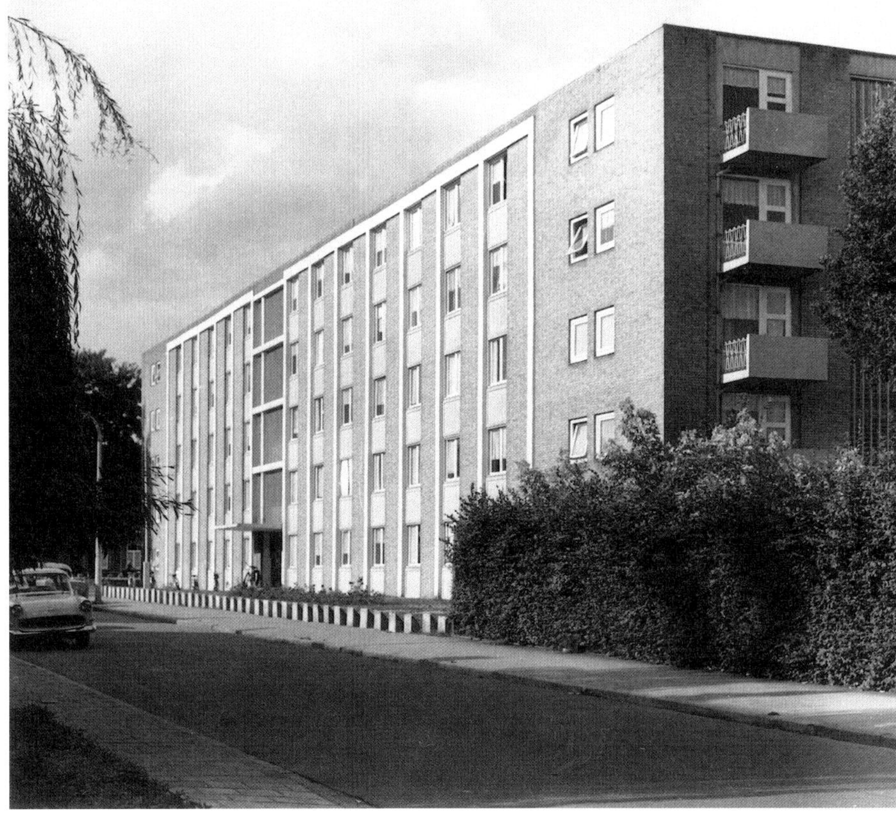

Clarity

J.P. Kloos

Juliana Ziekenhuis
Terneuzen
1947-1954

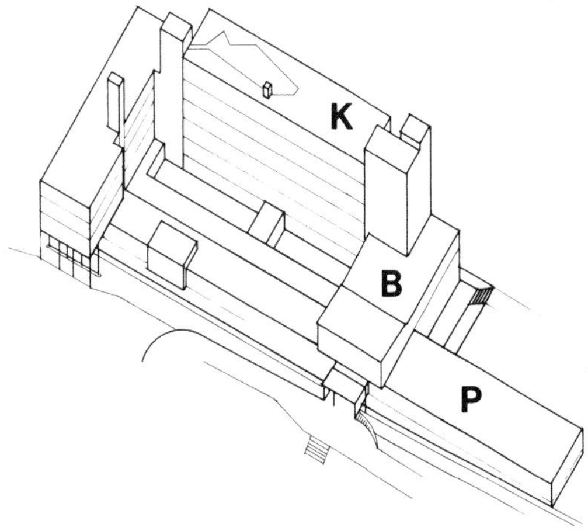

Main structure
K *clinic (ward)*
B *treatment department*
P *outpatient department*

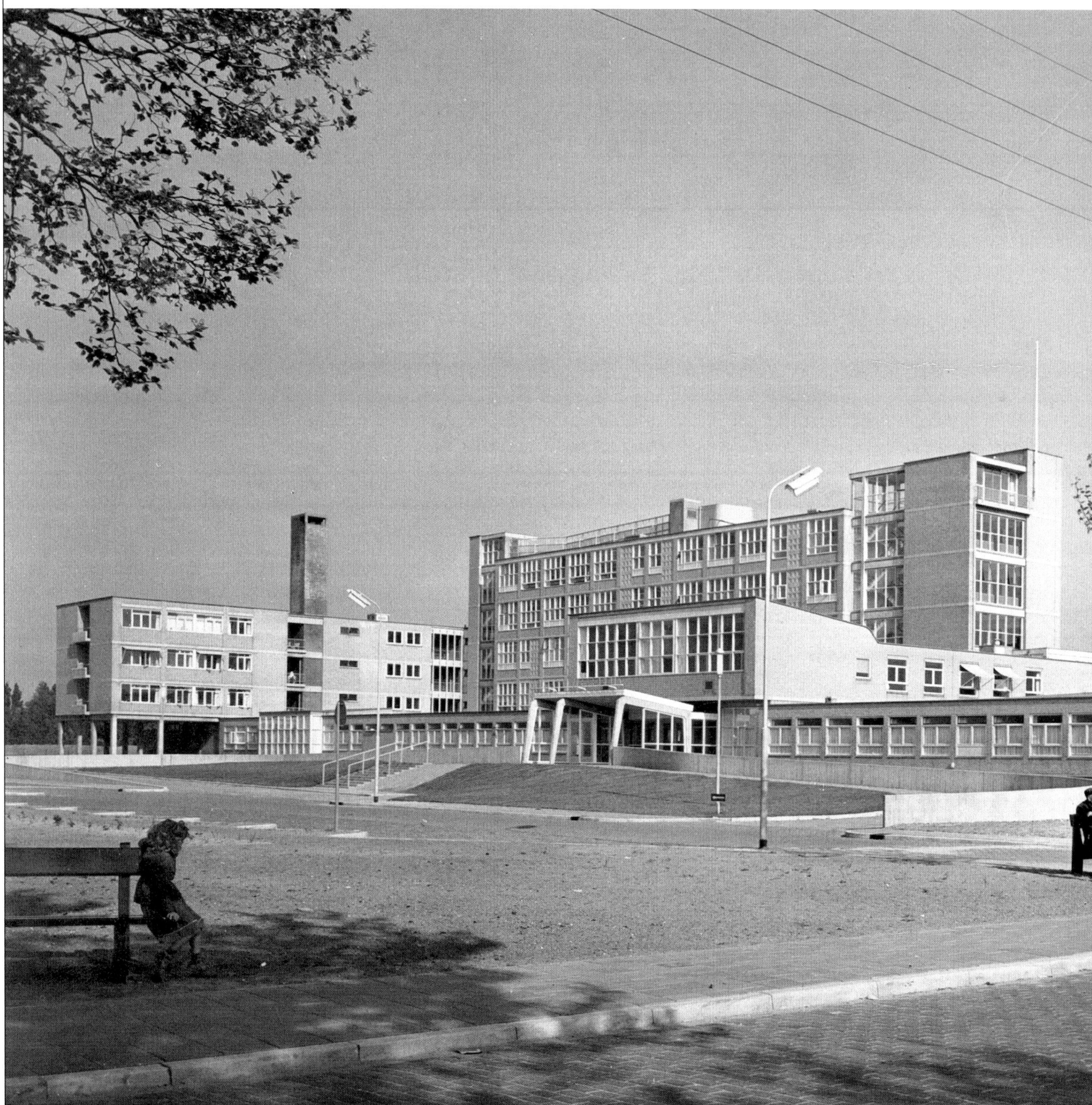

One of the first hospitals to be built after the Second World War is the Juliana Ziekenhuis, a Protestant regional hospital. Kloos, one of the most rigorous representatives of functionalism, tried to bring the separate parts to life. The architect characterised the structure of this hospital as the H-type because the ground plan resembles the letter H if the house for the nurses is disregarded. The most salient feature is the five-storey ward block (clinic). As in most hospitals of the time, it faces south. The general facilities in the nursing units are given a central position to reduce the walking distance of the staff to a minimum. A postwar innovation is the introduction of rooms for four or six patients, which are luminous and airy thanks to the large windows. On the west side the ward block adjoins the nurses' home, on the other side the treatment unit, where the main entrance is located. The operating theatre is positioned above the striking canopy of the entrance and is guaranteed daylight by the large windows. Wedged between the nurses' home and the operating theatre and parallel to the ward block is the administration wing that closes the courtyard. The outpatient clinics lie beyond it and at right angles to the treatment unit, with the X-ray unit as the link. Kloos took expansion of the outpatient clinics into account and designed the complex so that this would not involve complications for the other parts. Separate and at an angle from the outpatient clinic is a pavilion for (contagious) tuberculosis patients. The building has a concrete skeleton. The façades are of yellow-grey brick, interrupted by bands of concrete. The frames, windows and doors are wooden.

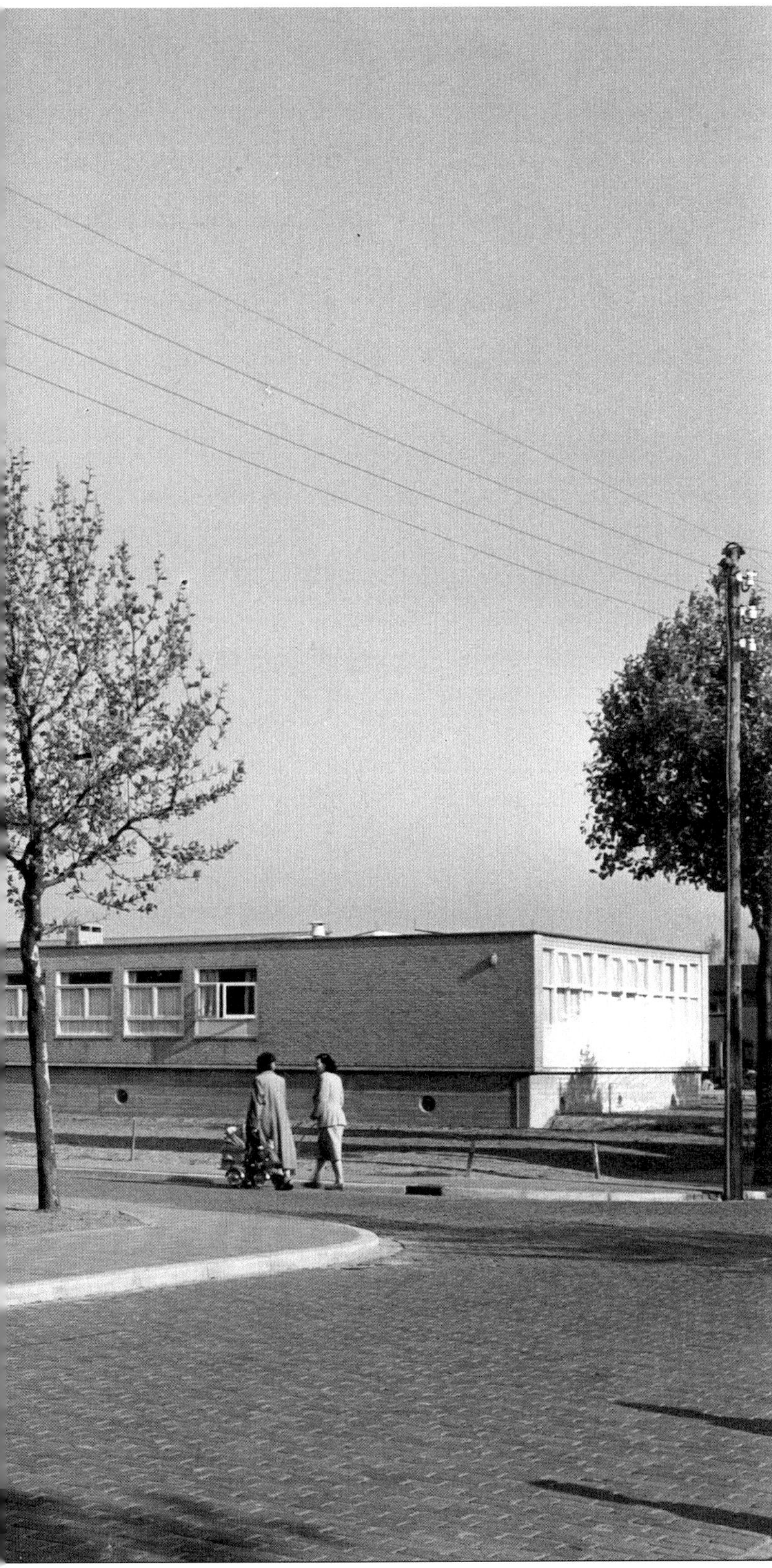

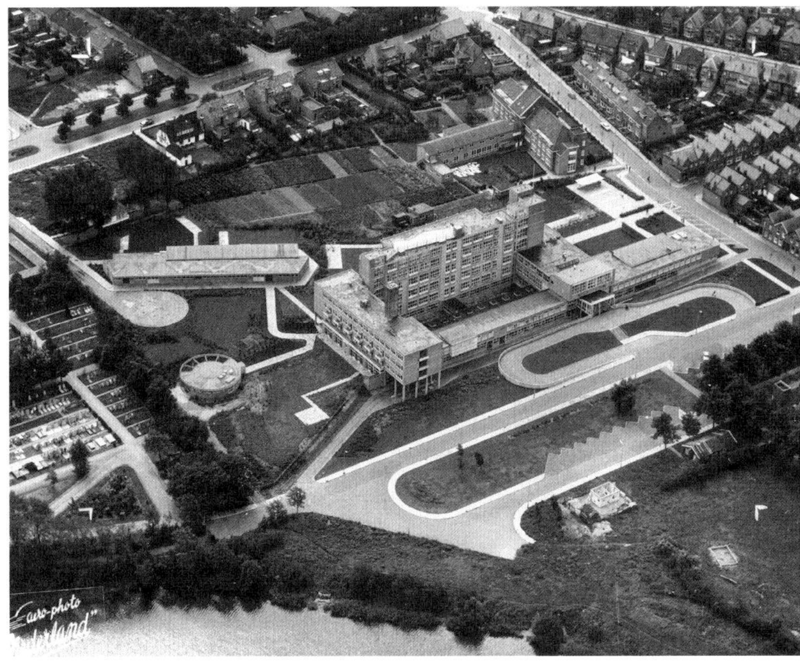

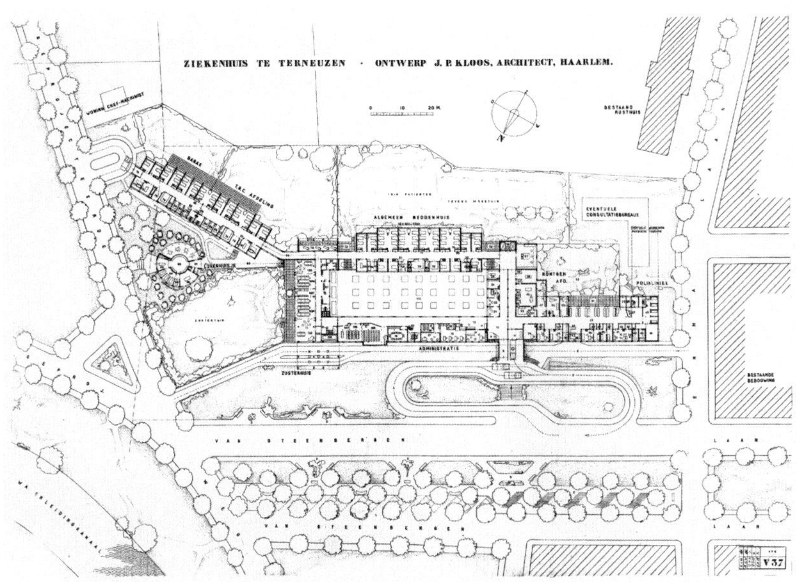

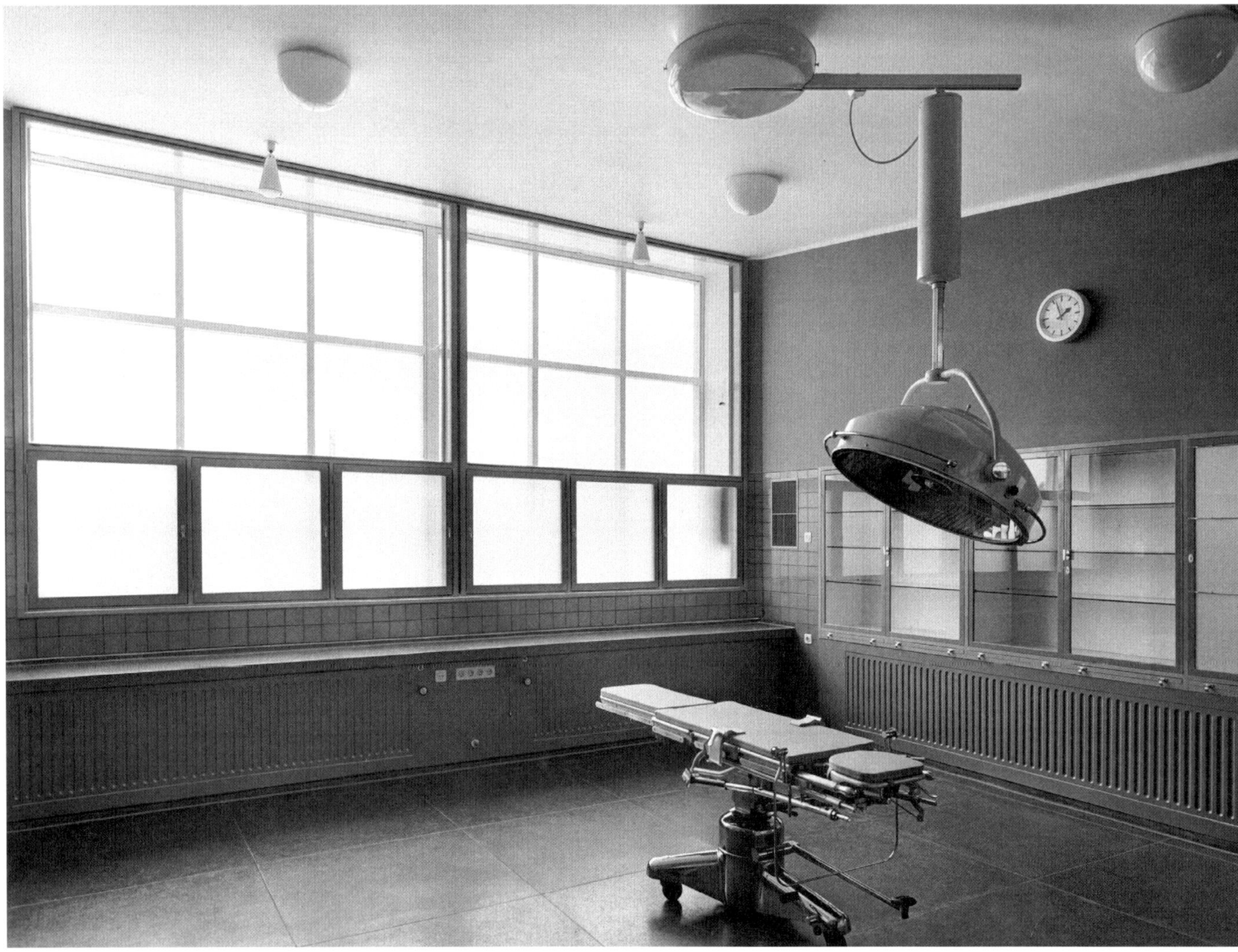

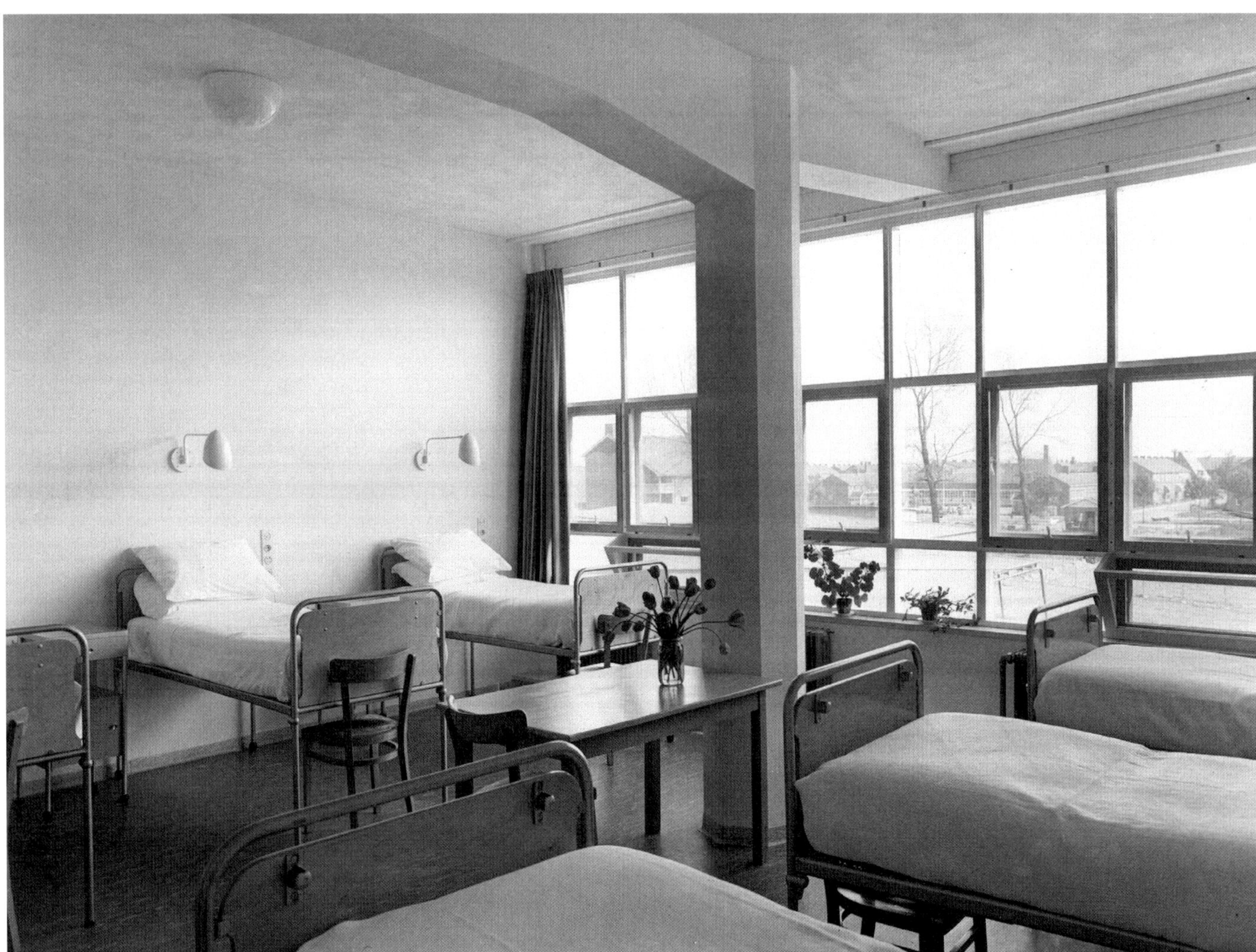

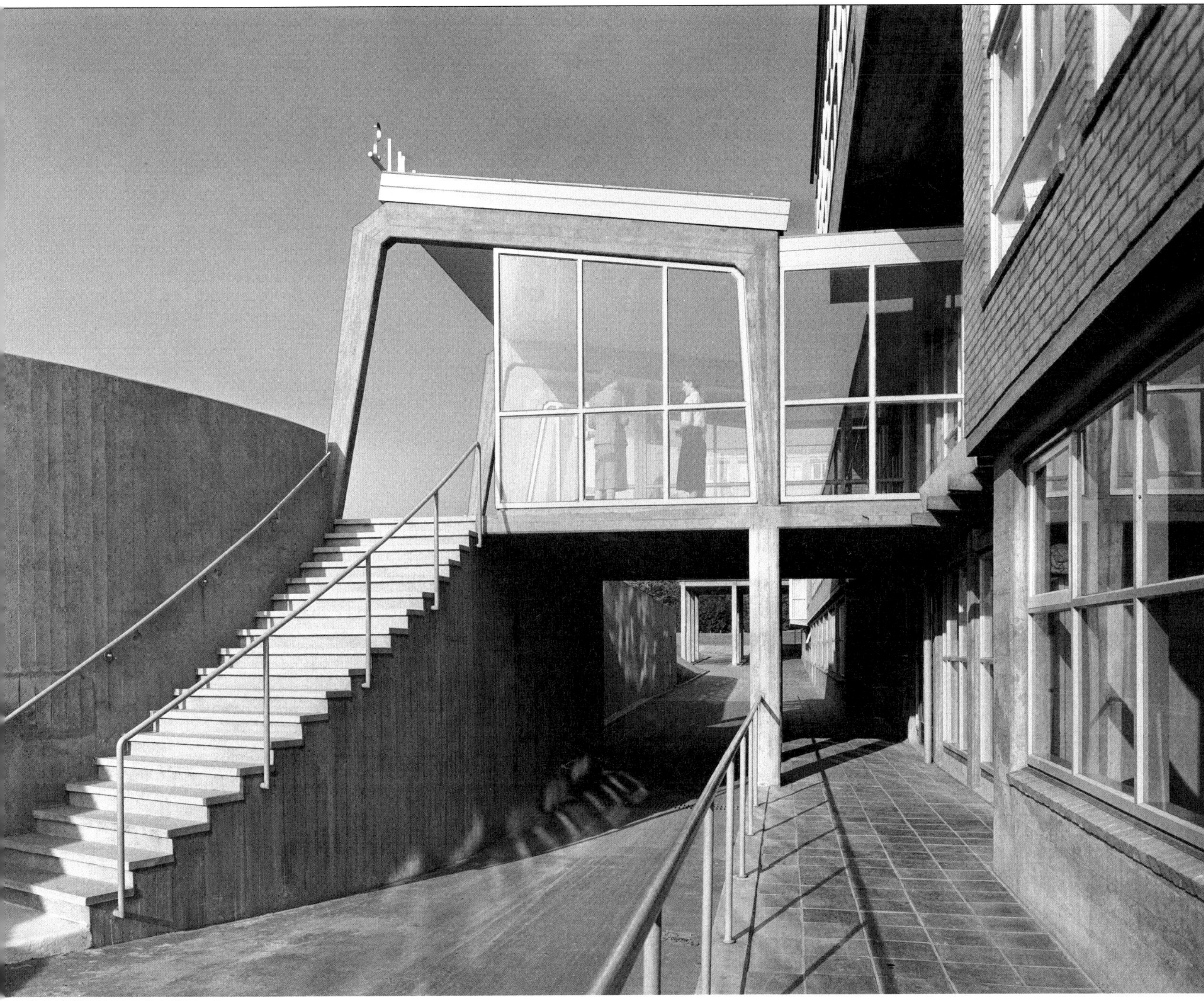

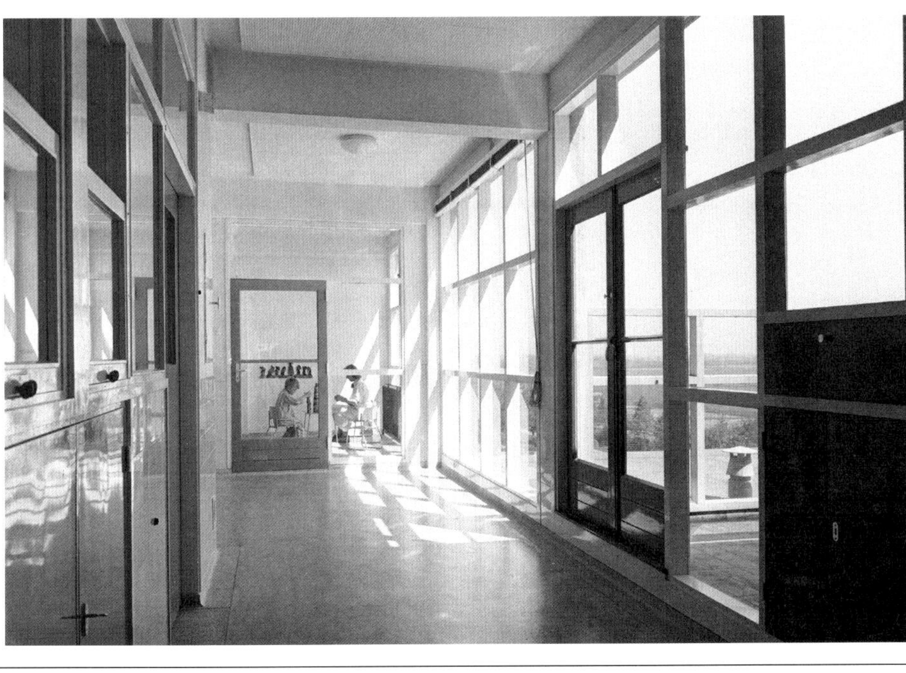

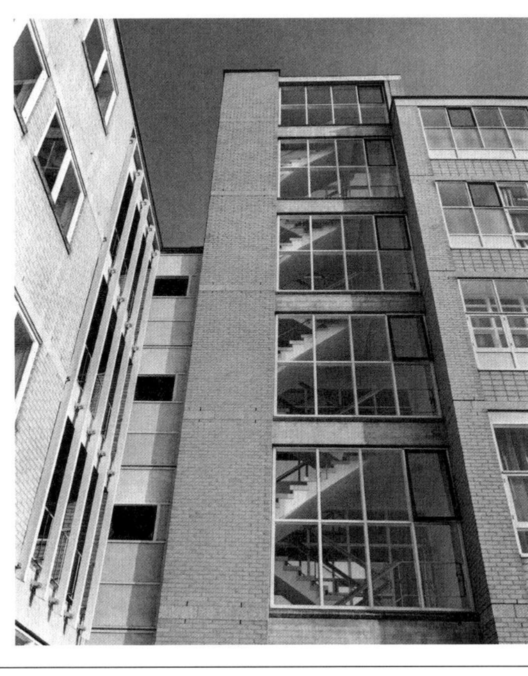

‘Shake-hands’

Auke Komter

De Klokkenbelt old people’s home
Almelo
1947-1952

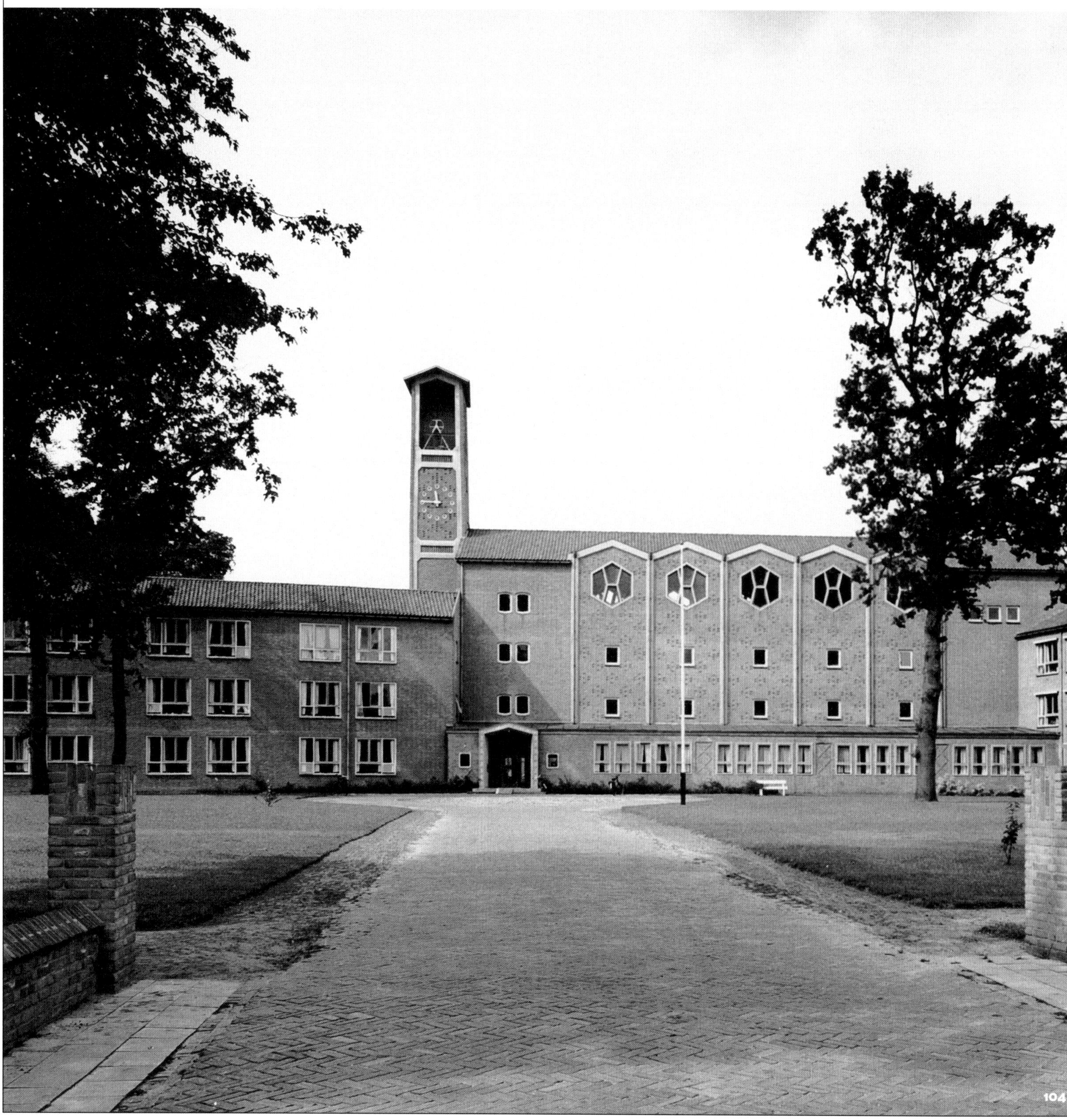

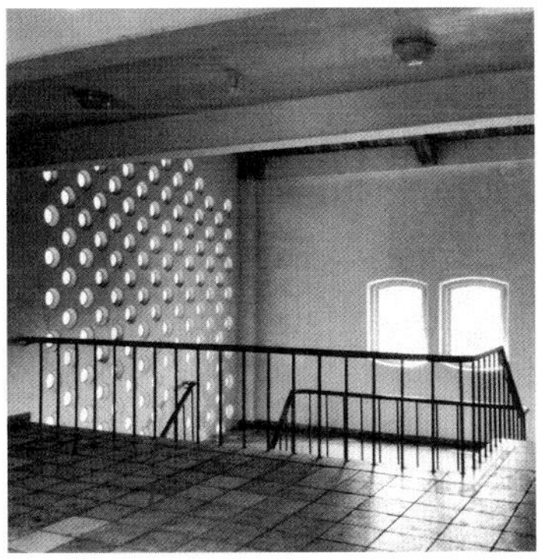

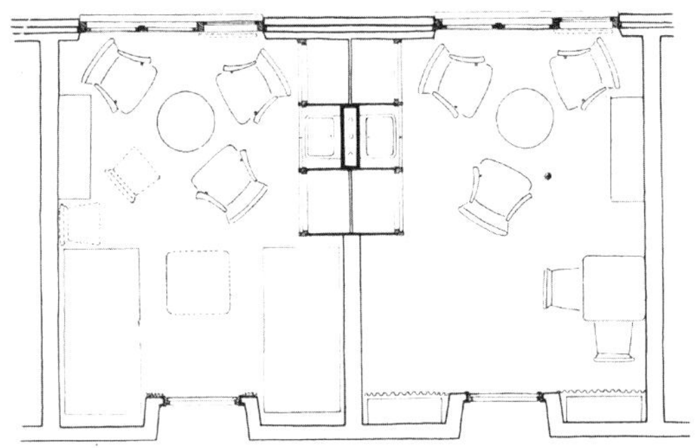

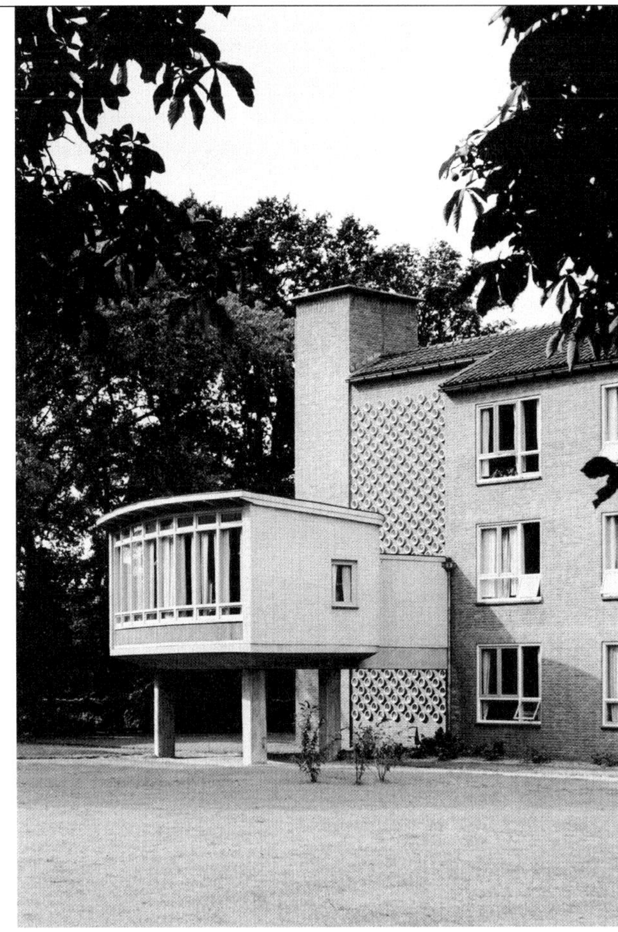

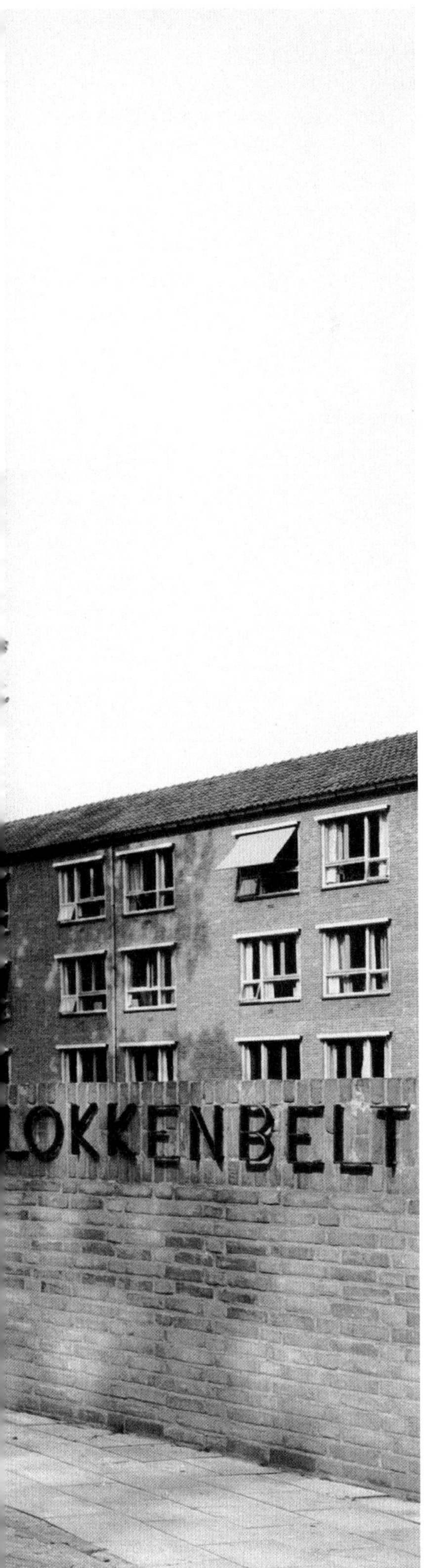

In 1947 the Dutch Reformed Church commissioned Auke Komter to design a home for some 230 elderly people. He was to take into account a large differentiation among the residents, as both rich and poor were destined to live there. De Klokkenbelt, twenty-five hectares of park-like grounds on which the country house had been demolished, were purchased for the purpose.

The complex consists of a large square part that is open on the south side and which is flanked by residential wings. It comprises a main building, a service wing and sick bay, and a wing for the staff who live on the premises. The main building, which includes a chapel, is flanked by a clock tower. The main building has four storeys, the other buildings three. The shorter residential wing for the more well-to-do patients has housing units on one side of a corridor. The longer wing is a double one with housing units on both sides of a corridor. The recreation rooms are situated at the ends of the wings. The recreation room of the double wing is an eye-catching volume that is somewhat detached from the building and placed on columns.

The building is an example of 'shake hands' architecture, a blend of functionalist and traditionalist styles. The main building, the tower and the service wing have a concrete skeleton that has been left visible in the chapel and in the outside walls. The façades are filled with brick and decorated with pentagonal windows.

Situation
A *main building*
B *service wing*
C *wing with staff dormitory*
D *wings with housing units*

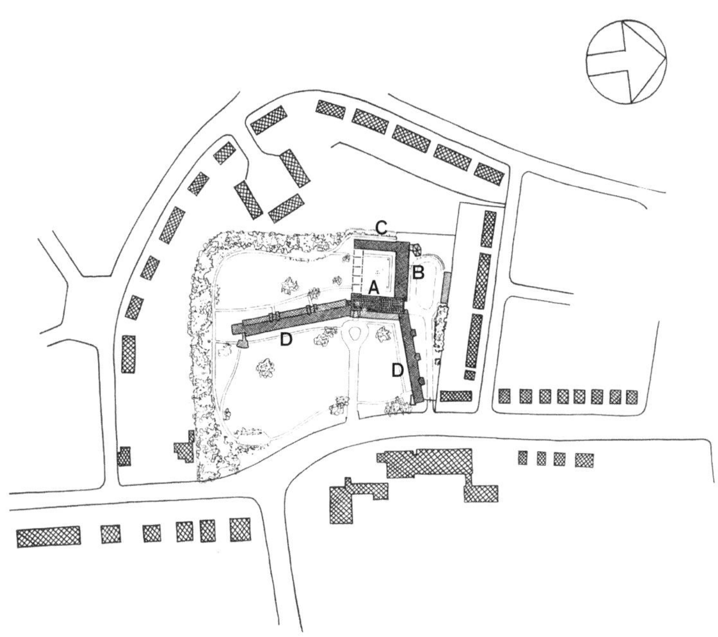

Rest

Van Tijen en Maaskant

Huis in de Duinen
Zandvoort
1952-1955

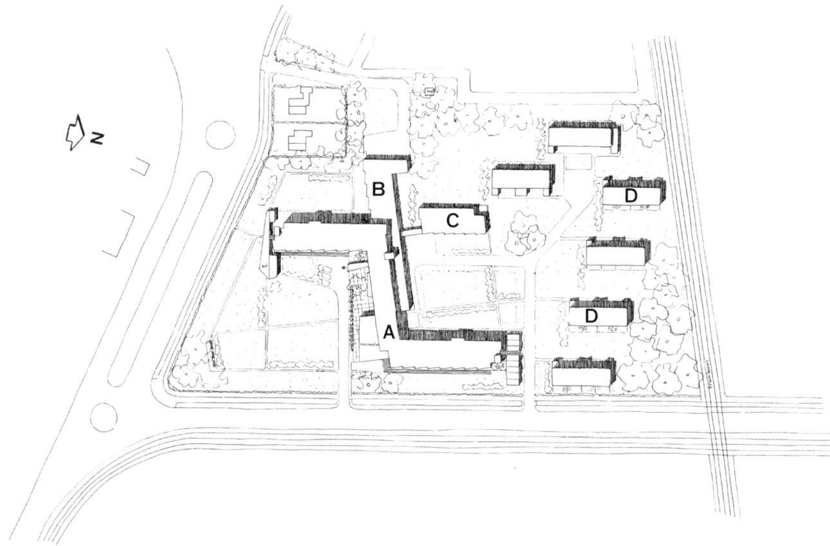

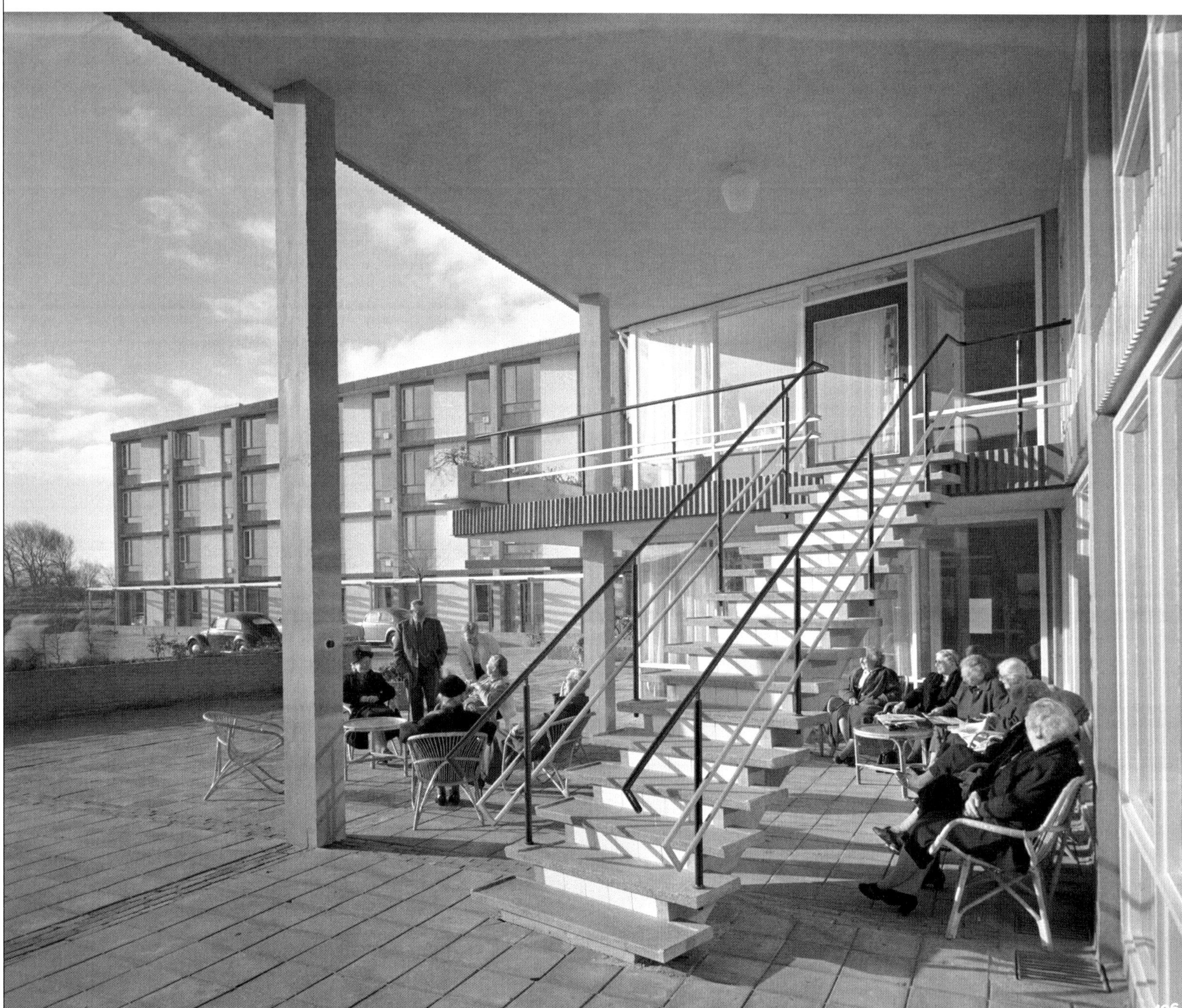

Situation
A *recreation*
B *sickbay*
C *nurses' dormitory*
D *housing units for independent elderly people*

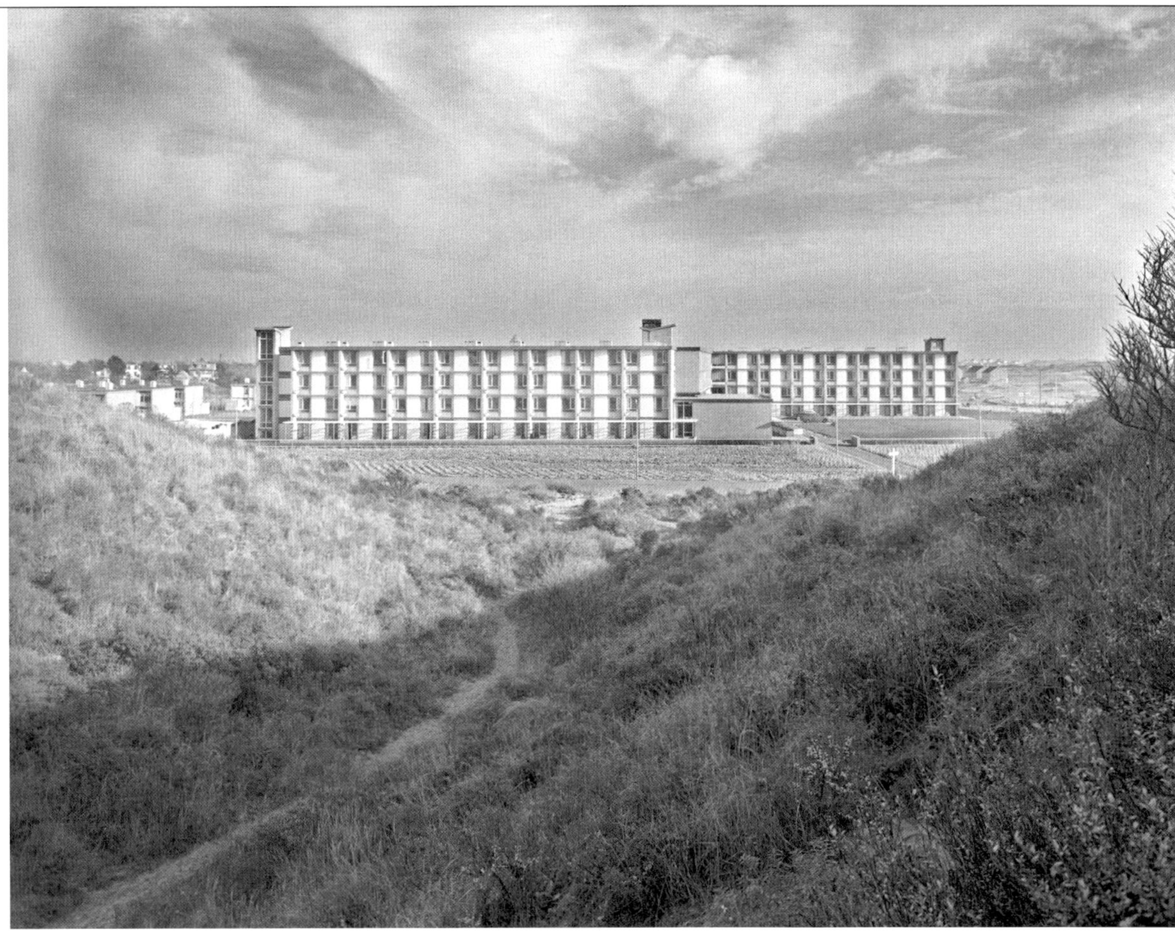

In the early 1950s Van Tijen and his assistant M. Boom designed this Huis in de Duinen as the first in a series of old people's homes for The Netherlands Centre for Housing of Old People (NCHB). The NCHB is an organisation set up to build and manage old people's homes on a non-denominational basis.

The modern old people's centre consists of a care building with 279 beds and 48 self-sufficient apartments. All of the central facilities are accommodated in the care building such as administration, the recreation room, the kitchen, the sick bay, etc., as well as the rooms for those residents who require daily care. It comprises both one-storey and four-storey volumes and has four wings: two for the elderly residents, one for the sick bay, and one for the nursing staff. There are 164 small single rooms (4.10 x 2.70 metres), 24 double rooms (5.90 x 4.60 metres), 16 rooms for couples (5.50 x 4.10 metres), 29 rooms for staff who live on the premises, and a number of sick rooms. The dimensions are based on the regulation that lays down that an old people's home in its entirety may not exceed 80 m³ (roughly 30 m²) per occupant.

At a distance from the care building are six small apartment blocks for the elderly who can take care of themselves.

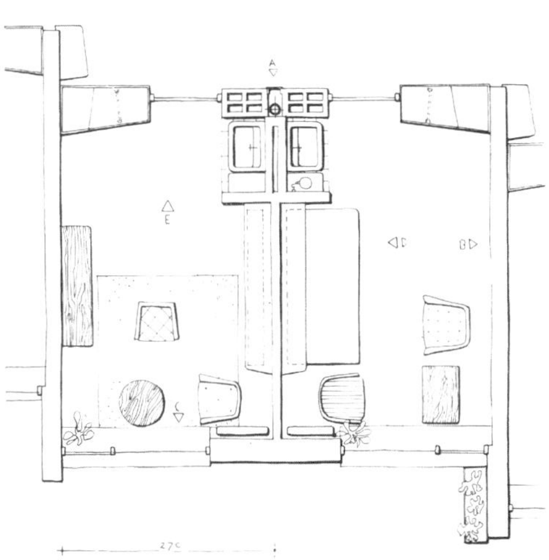

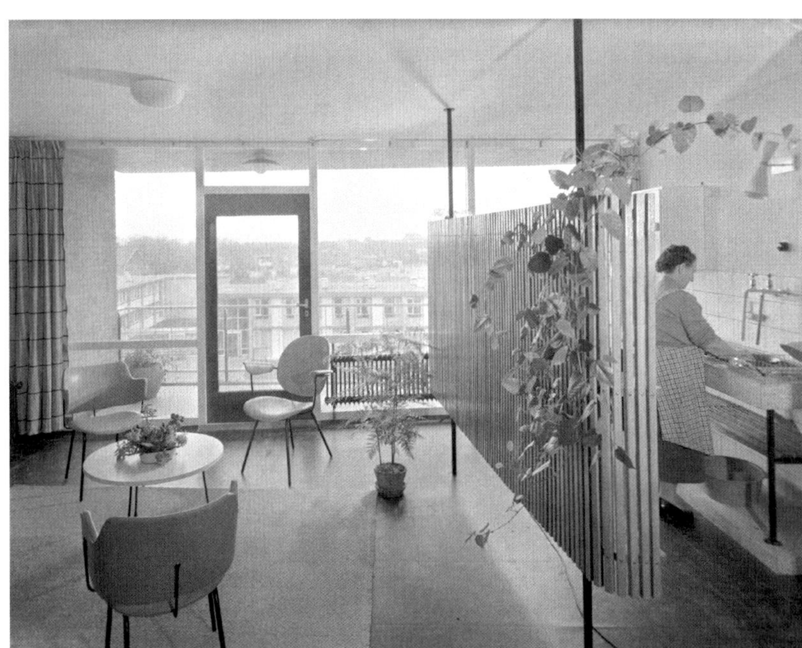

H

J.M. Luthmann

Rode Kruis Ziekenhuis
The Hague
1950-1960

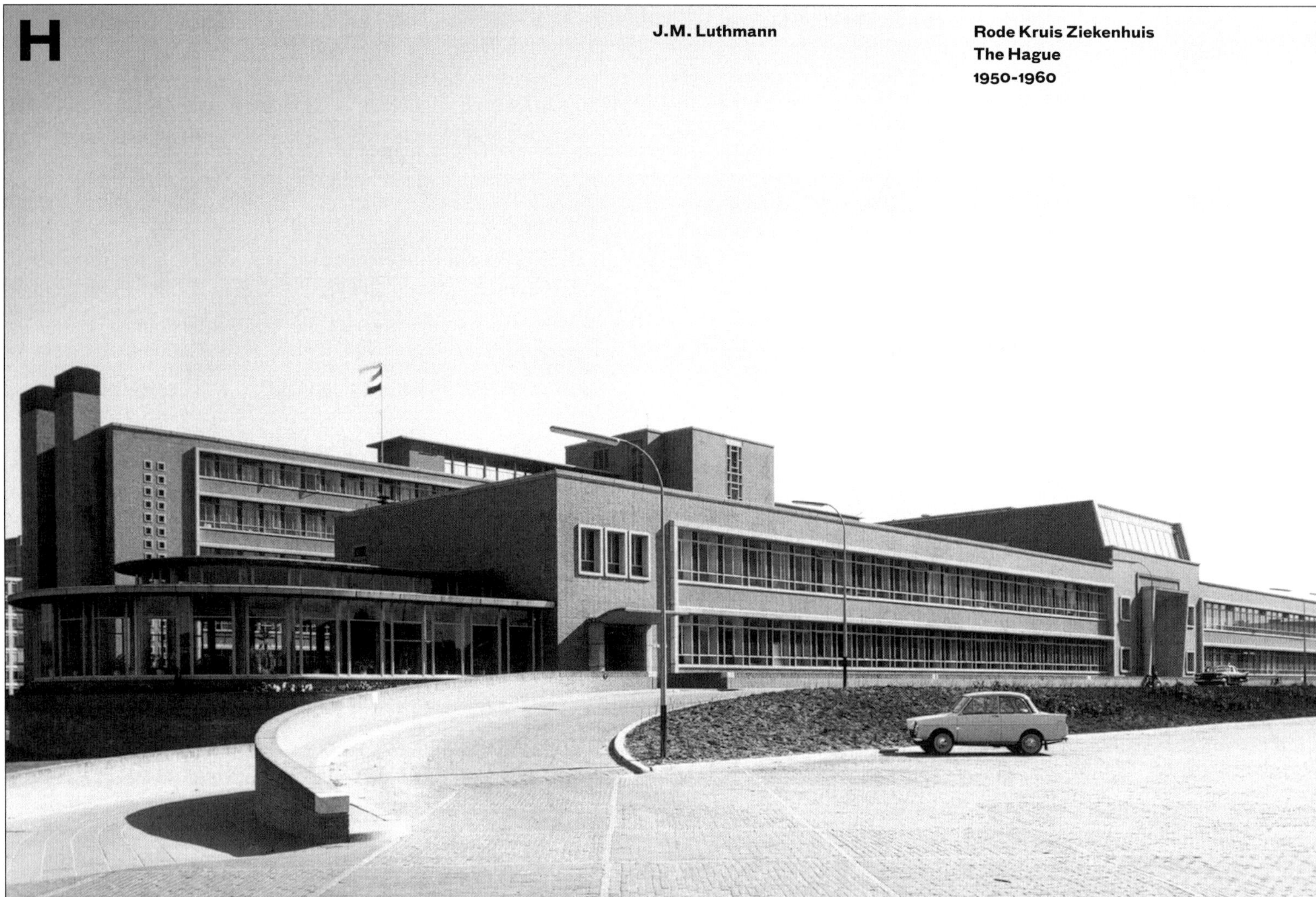

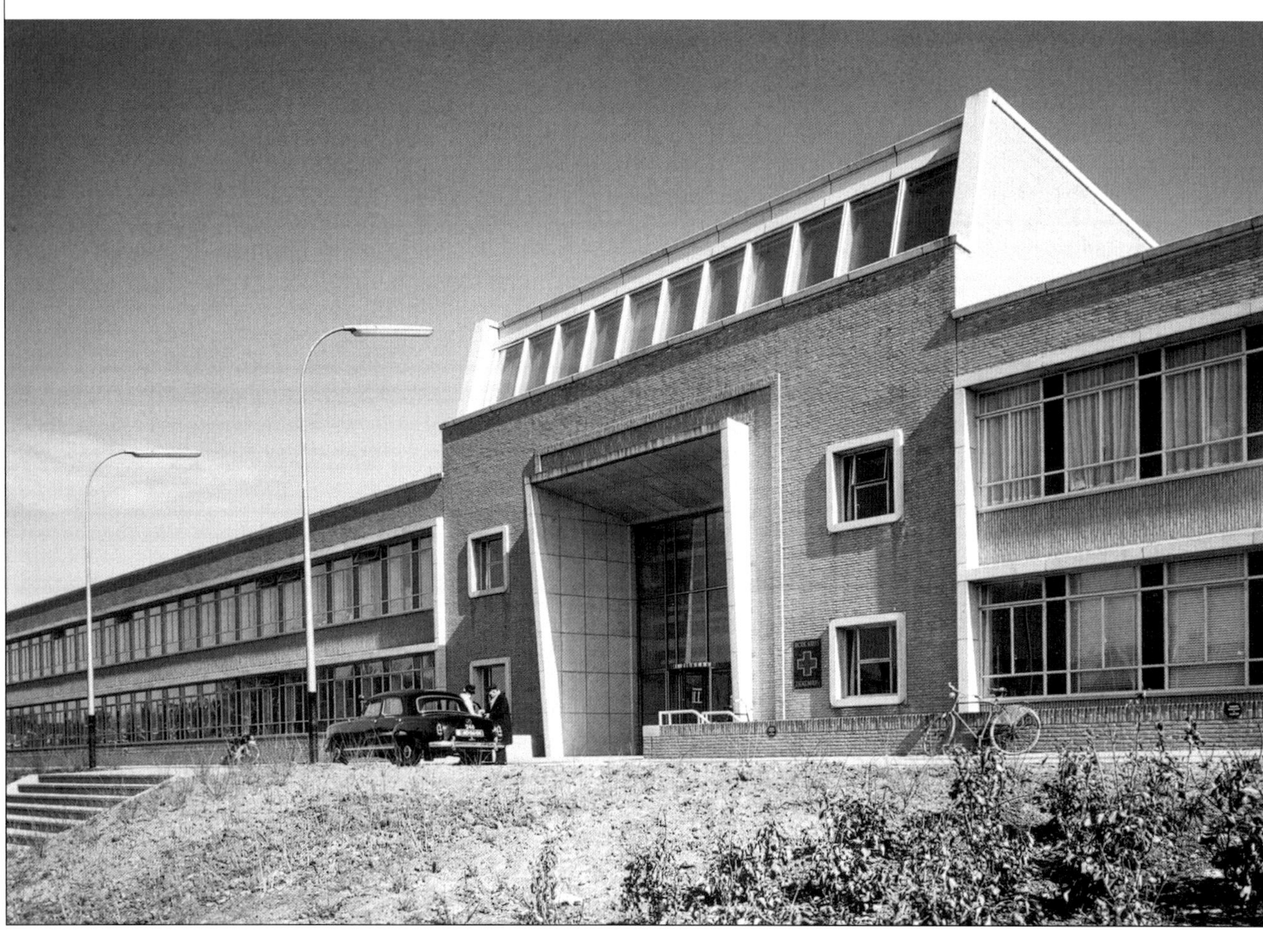

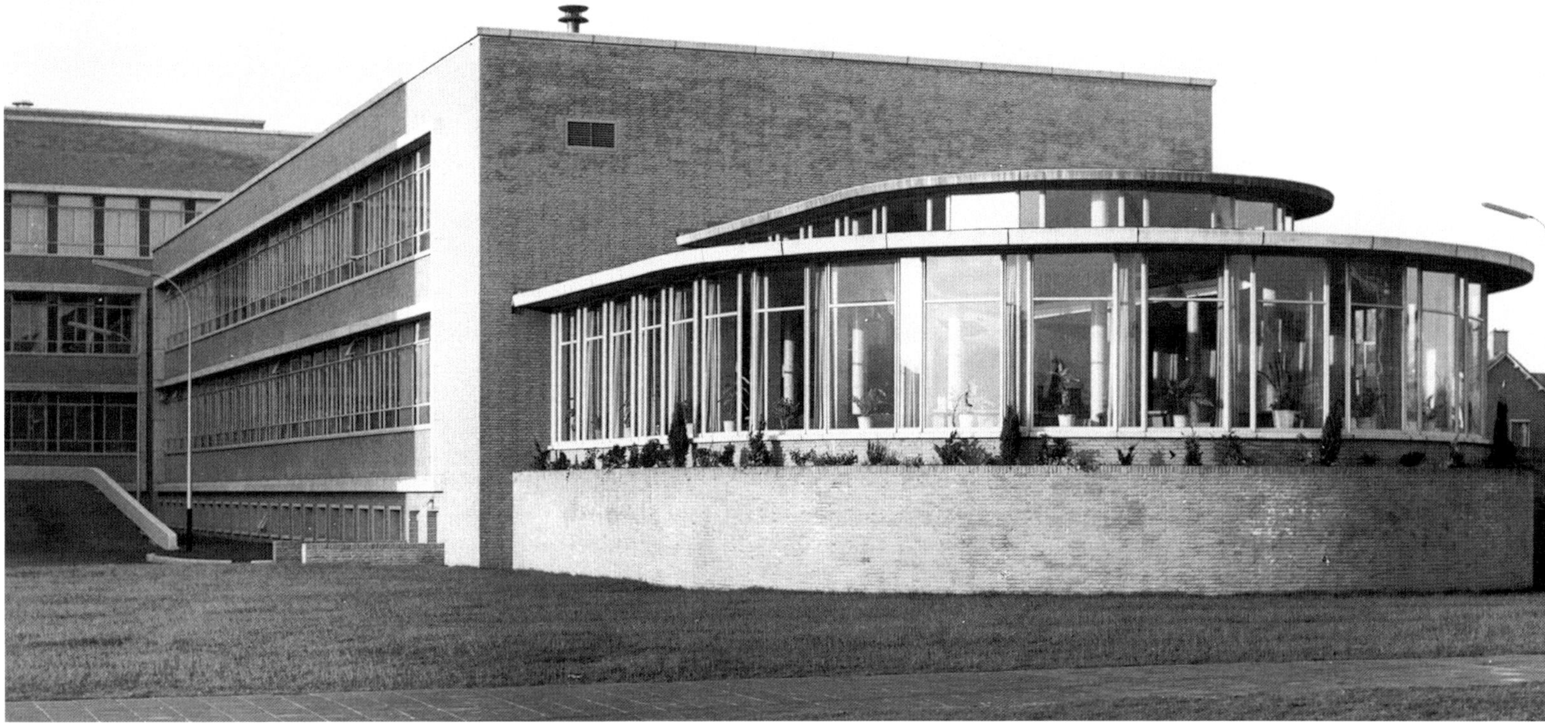

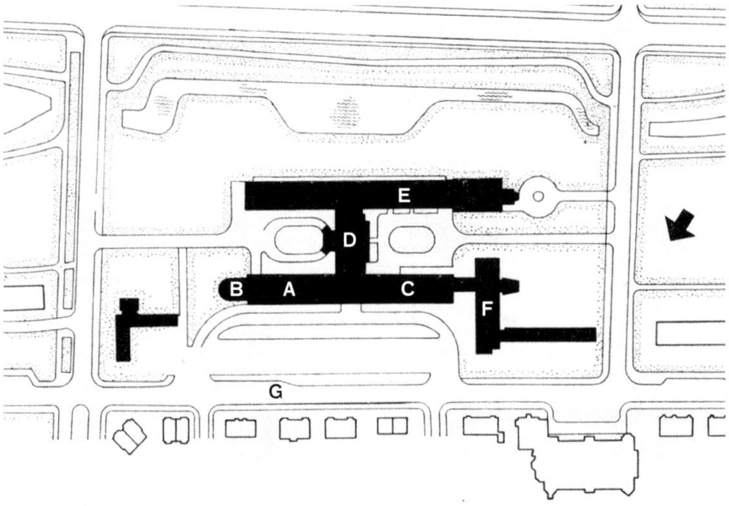

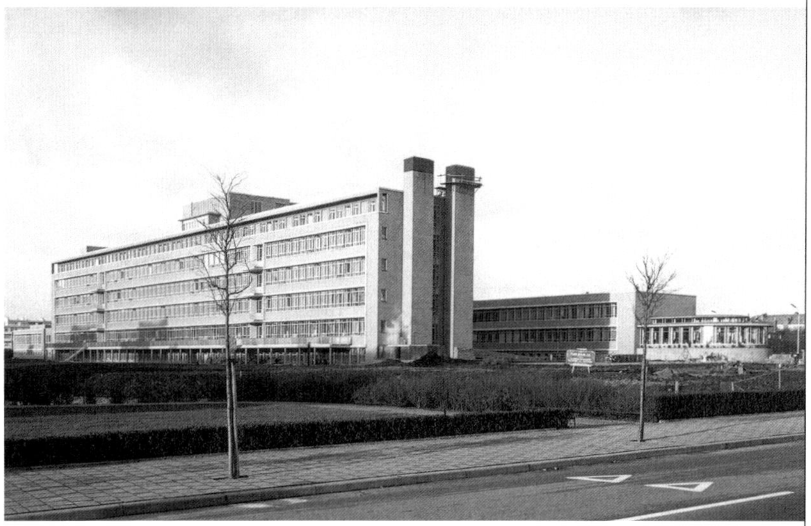

Situation
A *treatment department*
B *outpatient department*
C *board and administration*
D *laboratory*
E *clinic (ward)*
F *nurses' dormitory*
G *Sportlaan*

The Rode Kruis Ziekenhuis was built on the location of the building that had been demolished in 1942, within the reconstruction plan of W.M. Dudok. A delegation of the board and the medical superintendent went on a study trip to the United States in 1946. Luthmann visited Switzerland, Sweden and France before presenting his plan in 1947.

The hospital has 386 beds including 18 for babies. The structure of the building follows the H-type. The five-storey ward block is on the south side, while there is a low volume on the north side to accommodate the outpatients clinic, administration, laboratories, storage rooms and the main entrance. The semicircular outpatients waiting room is situated at one end of this volume.

Those functions are concentrated in the connecting part for which a central location is considered important because they have to be accessible from both sides. This is where the kitchen, admission and management rooms and operating unit are situated. Because of the height required for operating theatres, they are situated on the top floor above the main entrance hall. They are visible from outside through the horizontal strip of sloping windows that guarantee enough daylight.

The building construction is a concrete skeleton. The external walls are clad with a cream-coloured imitation brick. The window strips are set in concrete frames – a characteristic feature of the reconstruction period. Luthmann aimed at a sober architectural style that is tempered by the meticulous detailing. This and the design of the outpatients waiting room betray the influence of Swiss models.

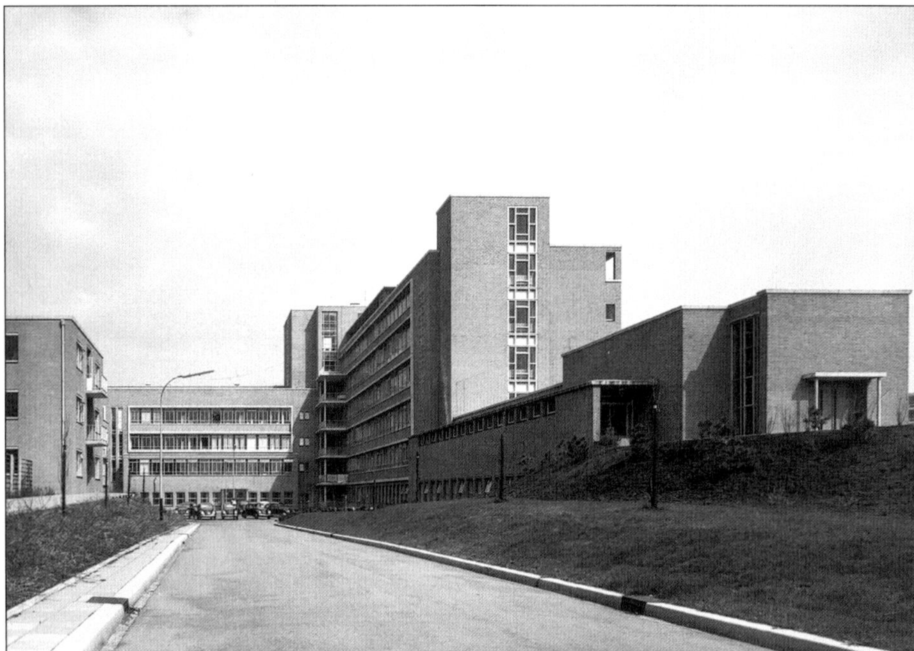

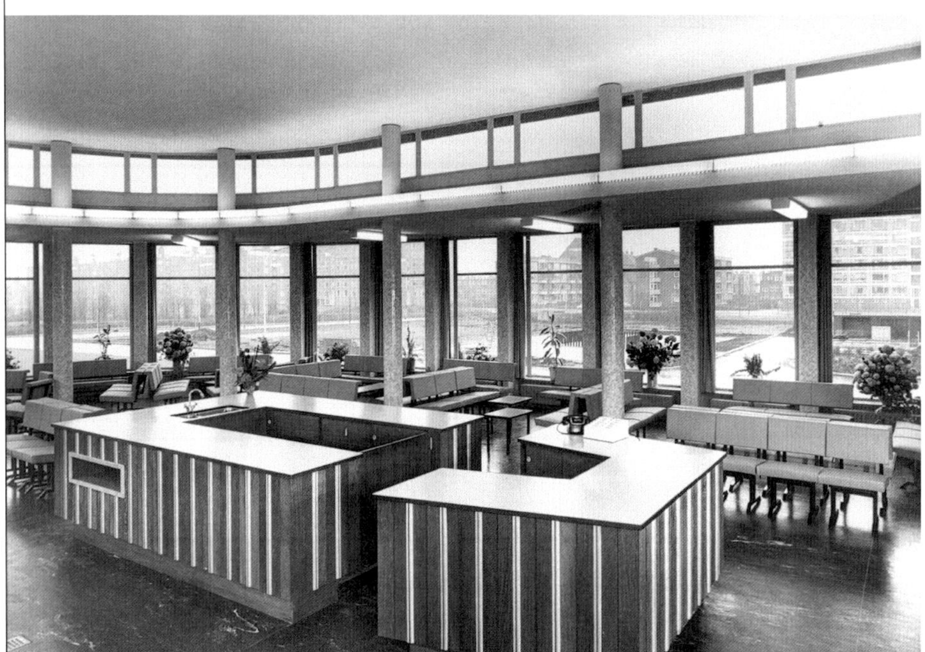

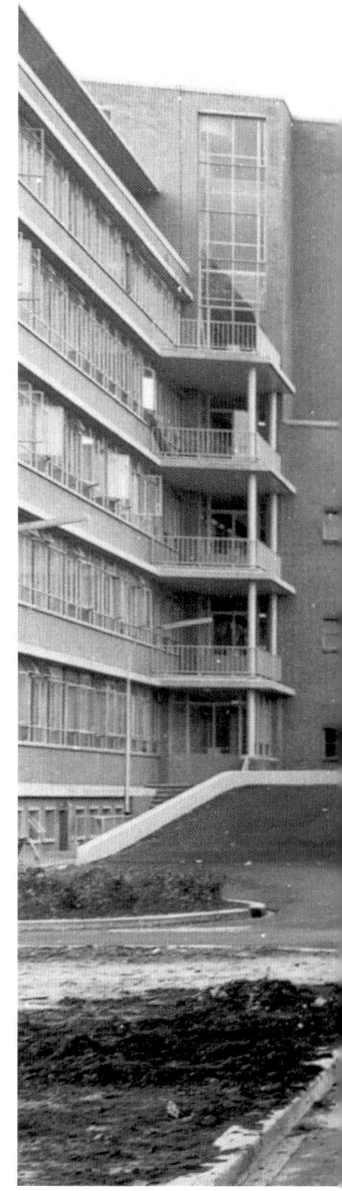

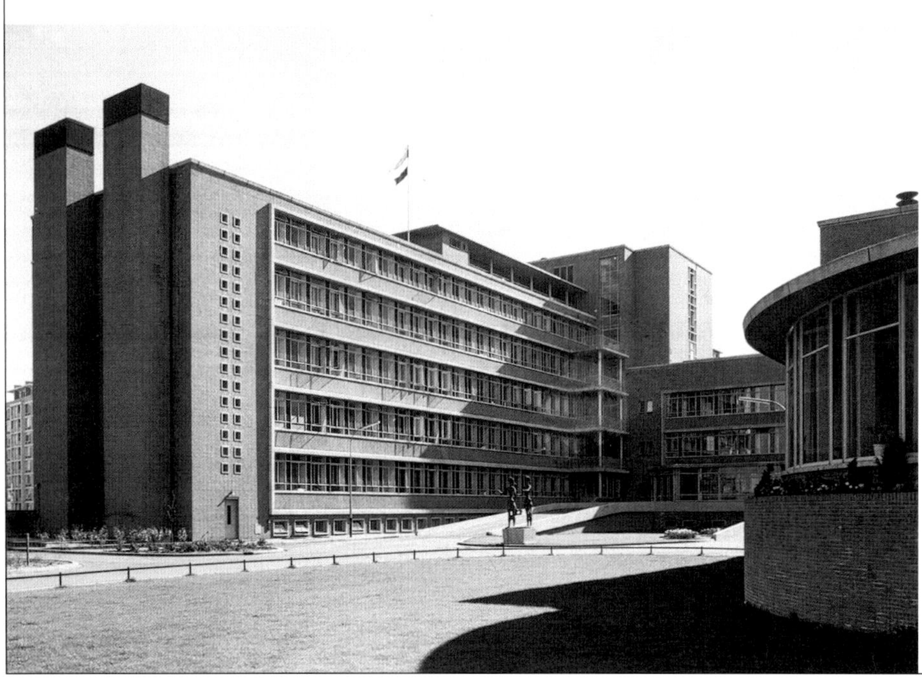

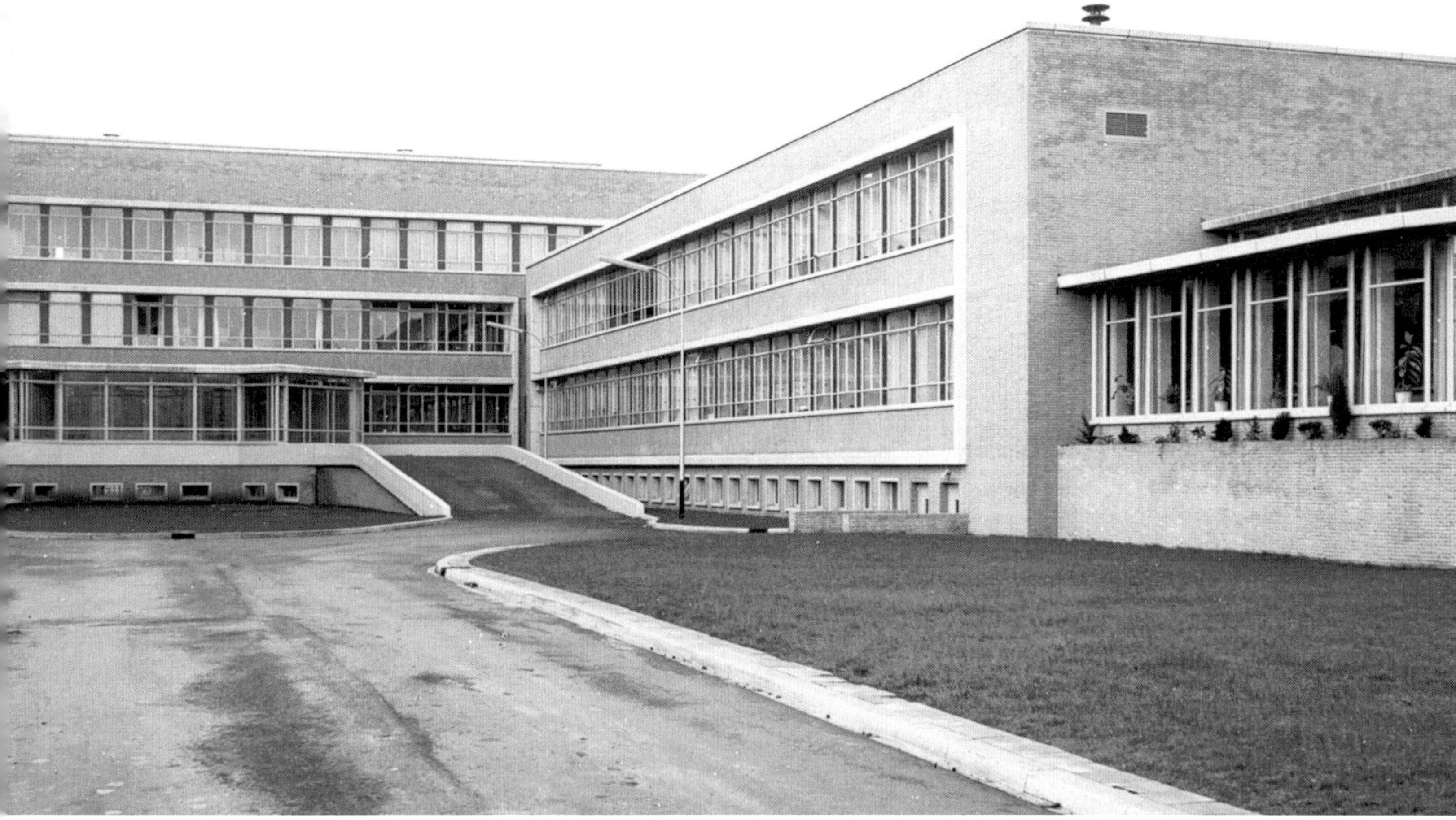

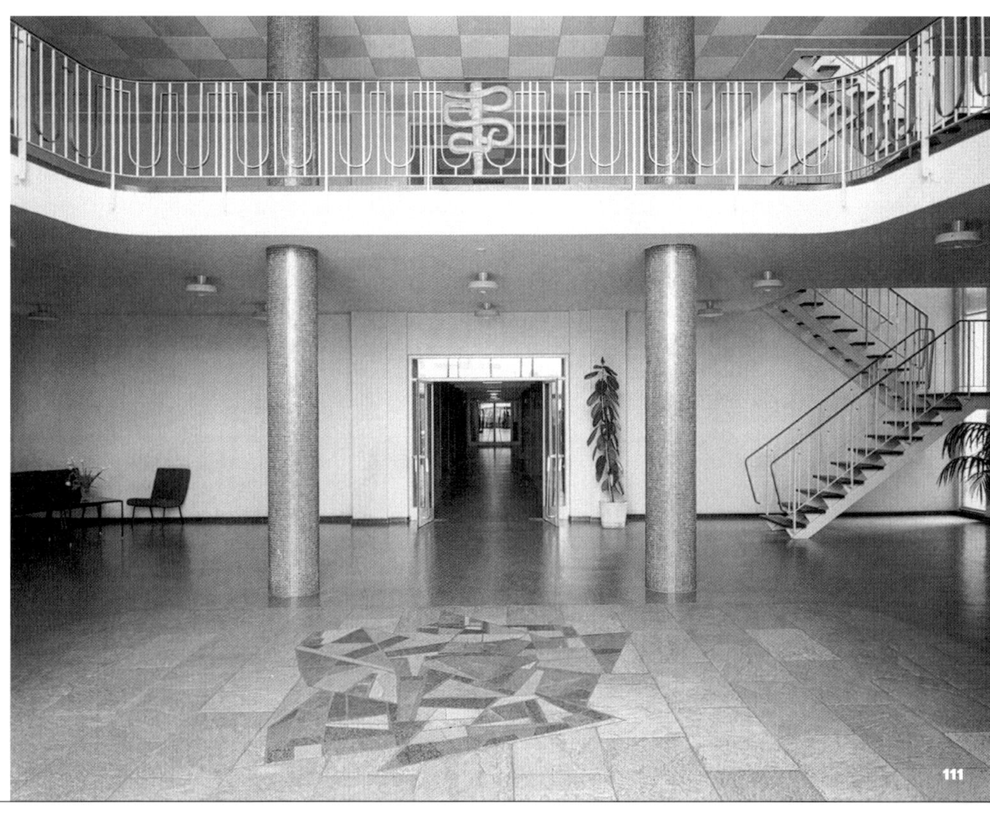

Oasis

L.H.P. Waterman

Sinai Centrum
Amersfoort
1955-1960

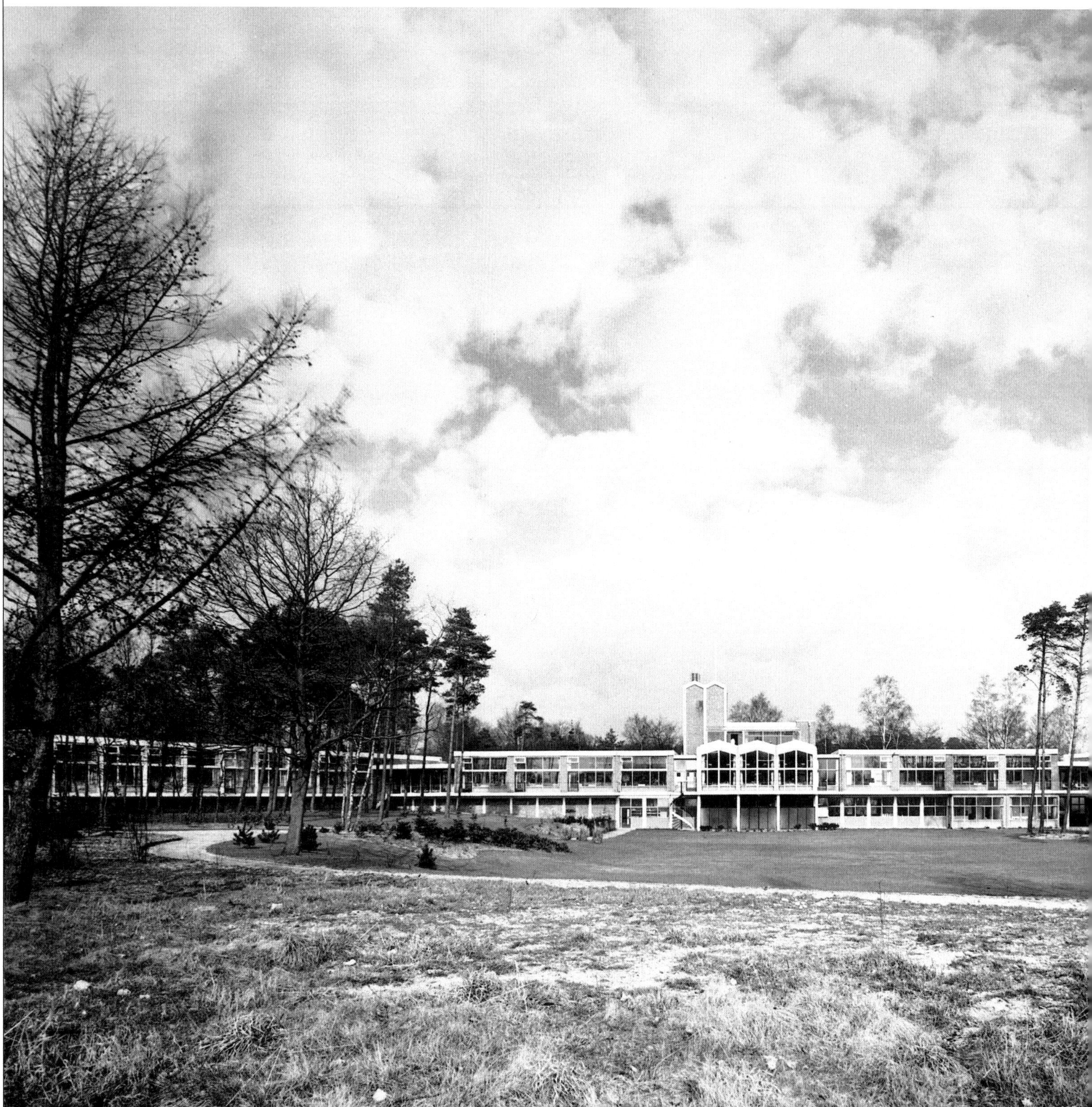

The Sinai Centrum was set up by the Central Association for Jewish Mental Health Care and replaced the Apeldoornsche Bosch with its grim wartime past; the latter was put to use as a centre for the mentally handicapped by the 's Heerenloo mental institution and renamed Groot Schuylenburg.
L.H.P. Waterman's design for the Sinai Centrum is decidedly modern. It is a safe oasis in an exuberant green setting. The programme is a response to the major changes that were taking place in psychiatry at that moment. All the patients are accommodated in a single building and distributed among smaller nursing units to provide differentiated nursing for different categories of patients. The design assumed an intake capacity of 76 patients, later increased to 82. The building has a T-shaped central section with two L-shaped volumes at the ends which are angled slightly outwards. These are the residential blocks for the female patients on one side and the male patients on the other. The T-shaped central section contains the general services, administration, kitchen and treatment units with consultation rooms. The complex was officially opened on 18 October 1960.

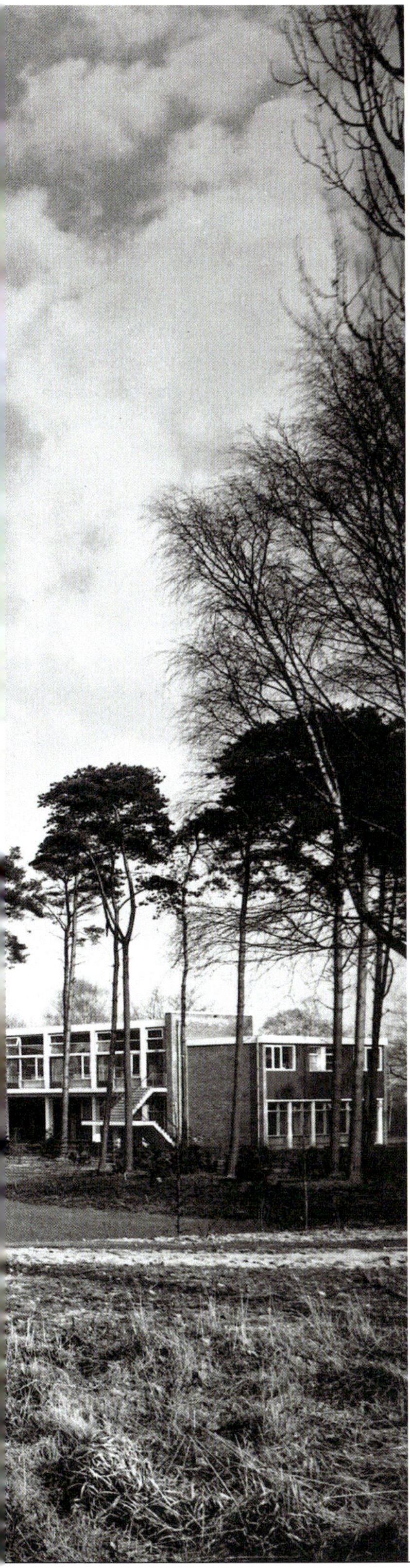

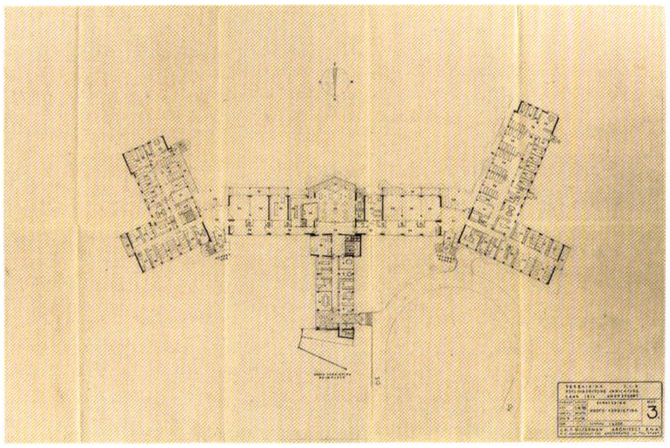

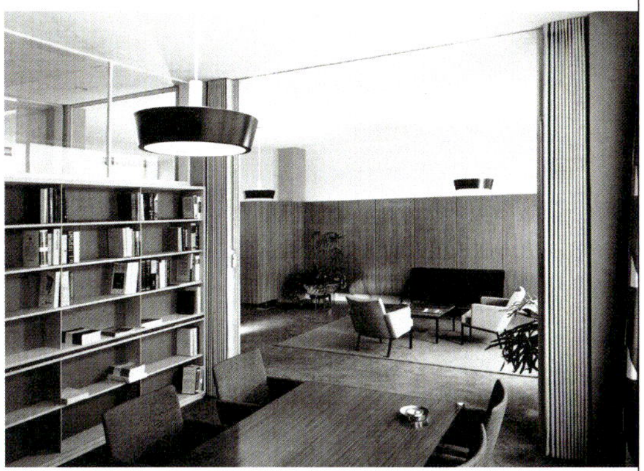

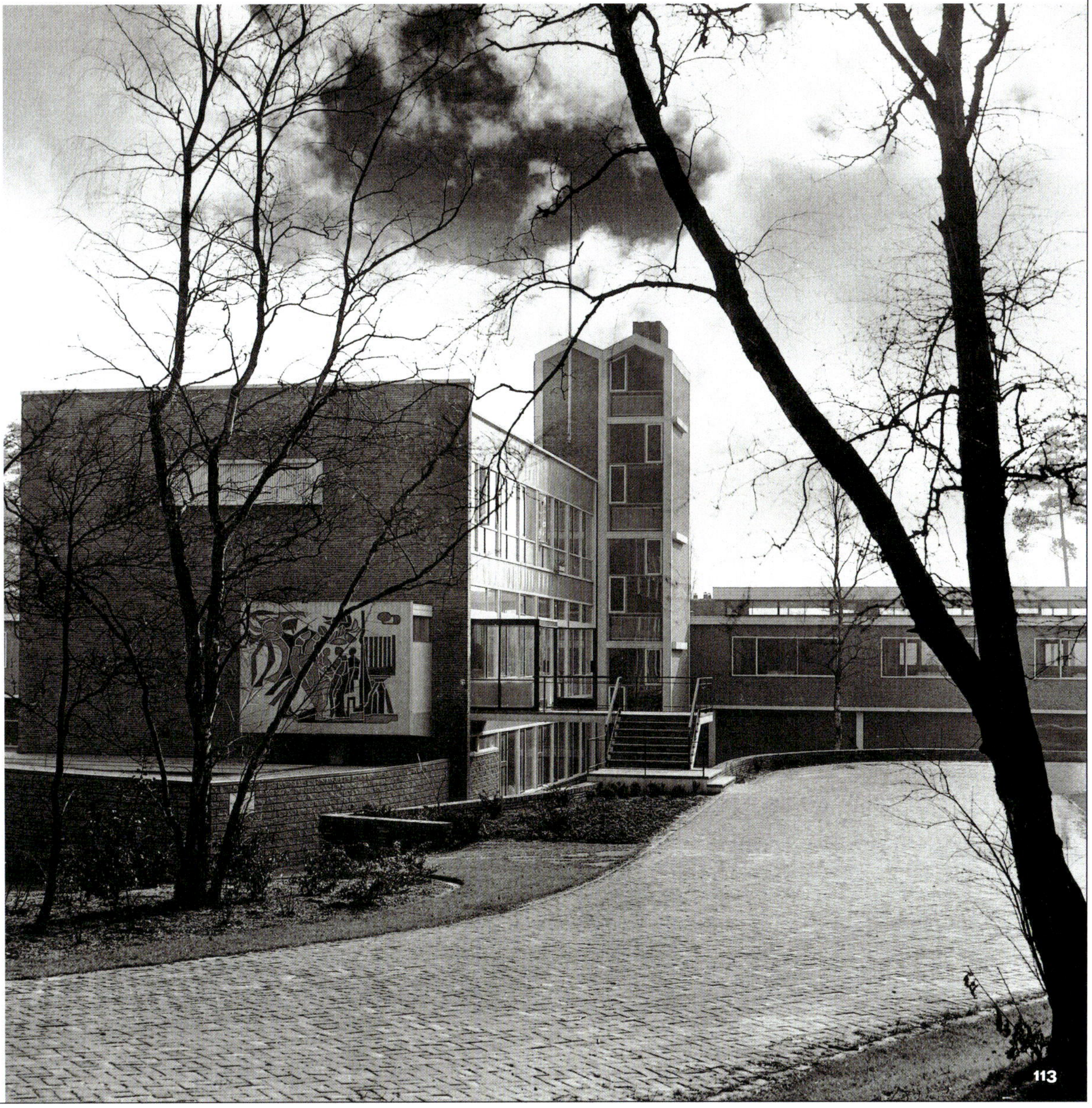

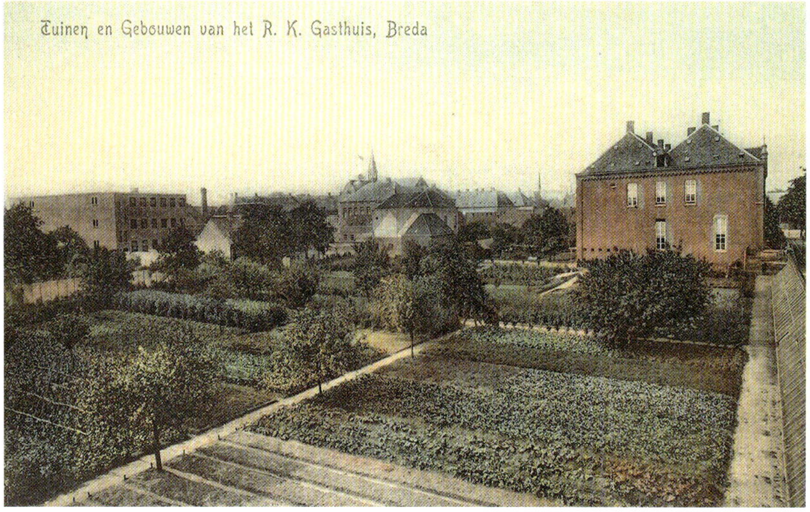

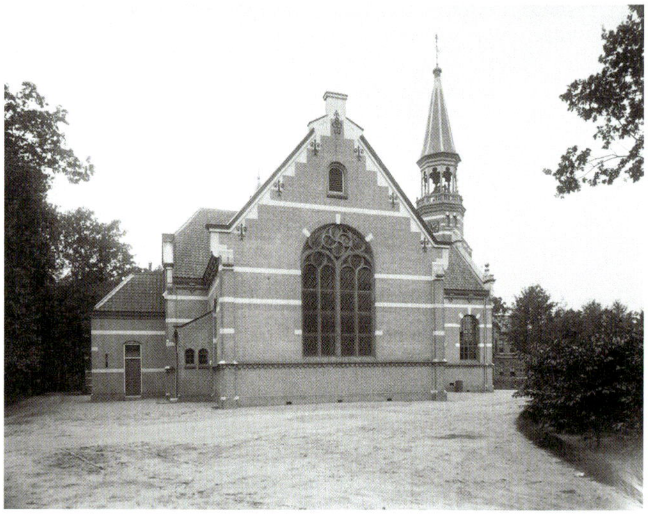

Compartmentalisation

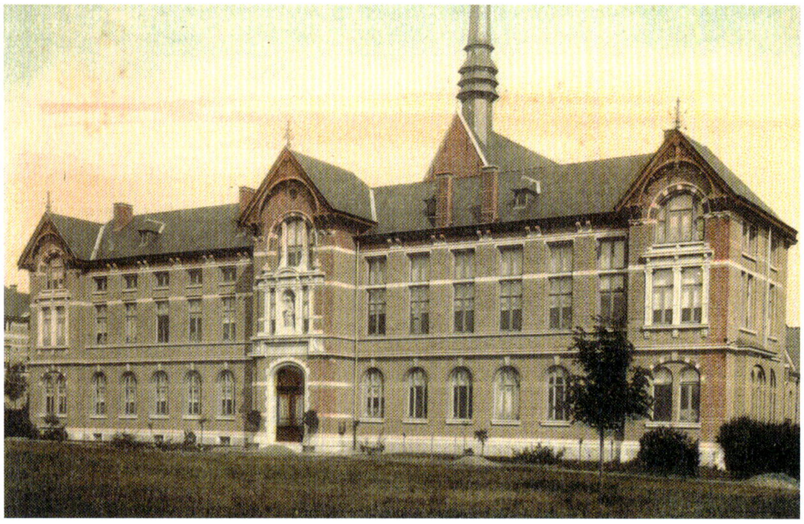
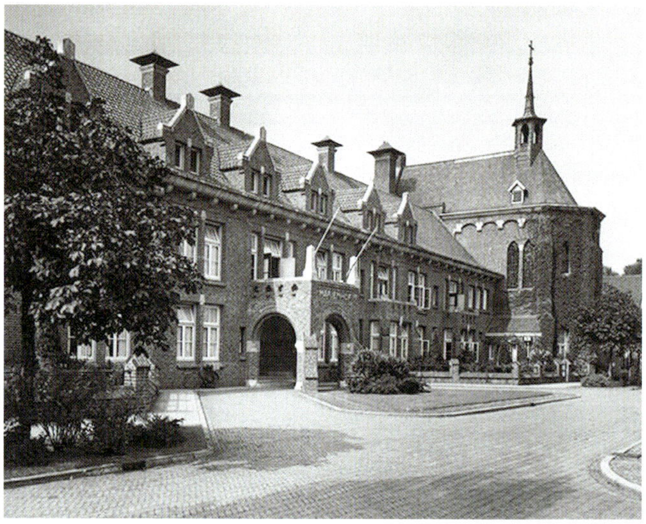

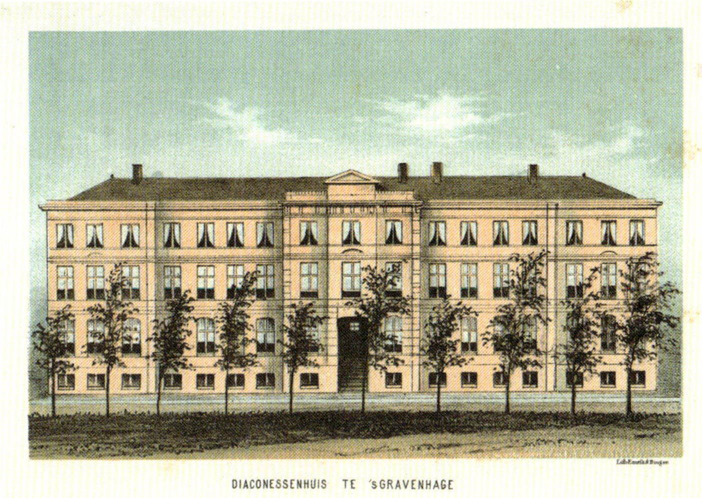

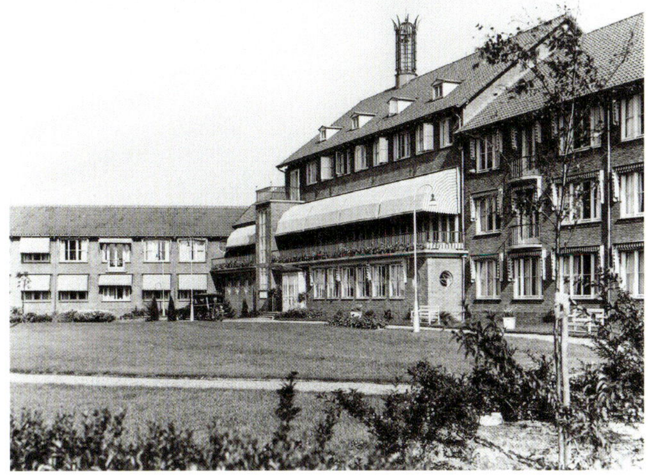

In the last quarter of the nineteenth century the contours of a phenomenon came into sight that was to be characteristic of Dutch society down to the 1960s: compartmentalisation. Compartmentalisation was a more or less spontaneous phenomenon firmly rooted in the nineteenth century, but it was formally ratified in 1917 with the resolution of a conflict that had been dragging on for years: in exchange for the introduction of universal suffrage, the Social Democrats accepted that Protestant or Catholic schools would be treated in the same way as non-denominational schools. This meant that from now on the state would fund them in the same way as the regular schools. This not only guaranteed the survival of the denominational schools, but it also formalised the compartmentalisation and the relation between state and society. There were three main schools of thought: the Roman Catholics, the Protestants, and the 'neutrals'. The latter comprised liberals, who considered that the public tasks of the government should not be performed by institutions of a particular denominational persuasion, and the Social Democrats. They had their own newspapers, their own schools, and a diverse range of associations that covered virtually every form of leisure activity there was. The Protestant and Catholic blocs also managed to set up their own universities. After the creation of the various political parties around 1900, these parties formed the apex of these blocs and joined in shifting coalitions to govern the country.

One of the most important fields in which the different blocs wanted to express their own identity was health care. The first Catholic hospital – R.K. Gasthuis – was already established in Breda in 1823, followed by many others in the provinces of Brabant and Limburg in the successive decades. A Catholic building boom got under way all over the country after 1850. The Protestants also began to build their own health care facilities, so that within a short time there was a widespread network of denominational institutions. Of course, both the Catholic and the Protestant hospitals were intended as charitable institutions. The Catholic ones were run by religious congregations with resounding names like the Congregation of the Sisters of Love for Our Lady, Mother of Mercy, while their Protestant counterparts were in the hands of laymen who were mainly paid from the proceeds of the collection. In 1884 the Dutch Reformed Church established the Association for the Protestant Care of the Insane and Neurasthenics in the Netherlands.

The inspiration for change in this quarter came from Theodor Fliedner, who had launched the order of deaconesses (*diaconessen*) in Germany in 1836. The association wanted to achieve for the mentally ill what he had achieved for the poor who were physically ill: to dispose of its own institutions based on a shared religious conviction. The aim of the association was 'the promotion of Protestant care in accordance with the Word of God for the insane and for neurasthenics'. One of its instruments to achieve this was the setting up of institutions for that purpose. The first result was the establishment of the Veldwijk institution in Ermelo, which opened in 1886, only two years after the foundation of the association.

From the beginning of the twentieth century, and thus somewhat later than the Protestants, the Catholics also entered the field of mental health care with their own newly built institutions. They were run by two Belgian congregations that were both based in Ghent: the Brothers of Love and the Sisters of Love. St. Servatius opened in Venray in 1907, followed in the next year by St. Anna in the same place. The only Catholic asylum outside the southern provinces was St. Bavo in Noordwijkerhout (1913).

Top
R.K. Gasthuis, Breda, 1823

E.G. Wentink, Veldwijk, chapel, Ermelo, 1884

Diaconessenhuis, The Hague, 1865

W. Bruin, De Rusthoeve, Purmerend, 1936

Bottom
J.C. Haché, Sint Anna, Venray, 1908

A.J. Kropholler, Mariënhof, Vught, 1939

Diaconessenhuis, Utrecht, 1844

A.J. Kropholler, Pension Mariëngaarde, Tilburg, 1935

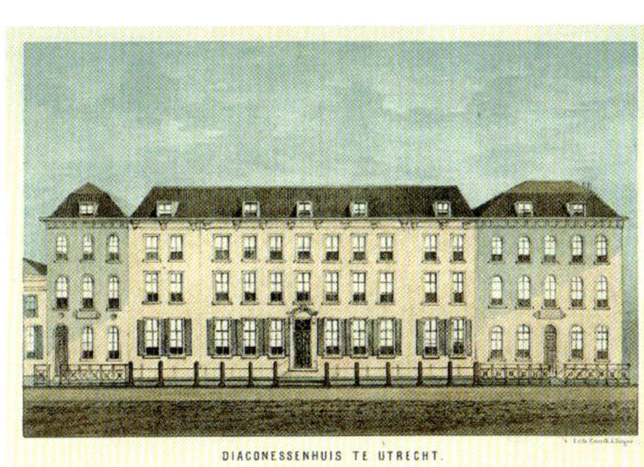

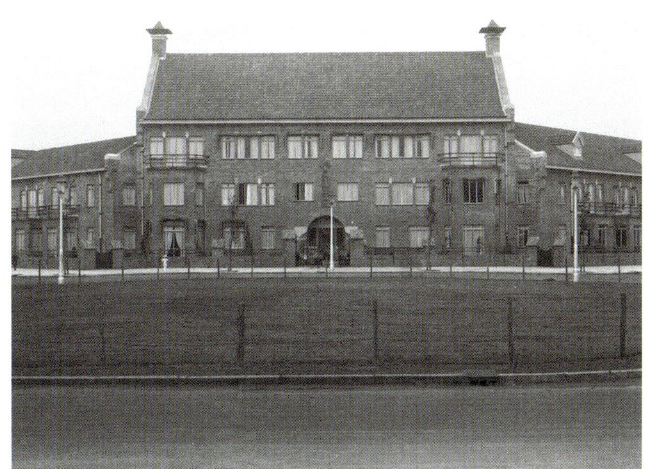

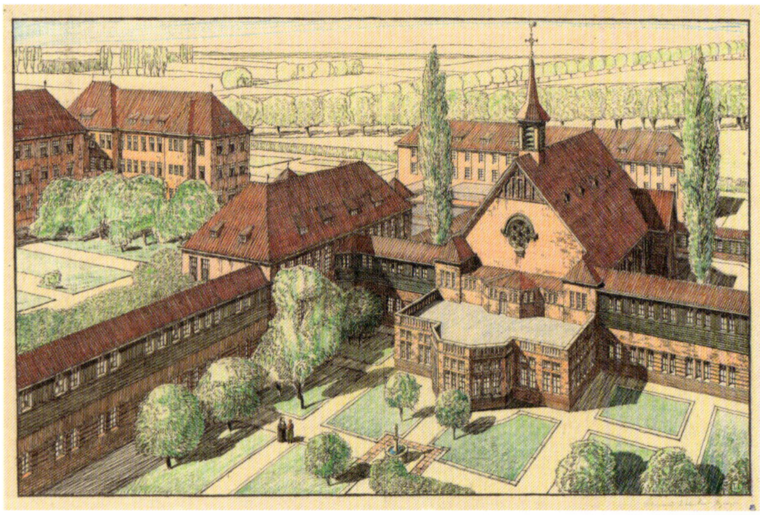

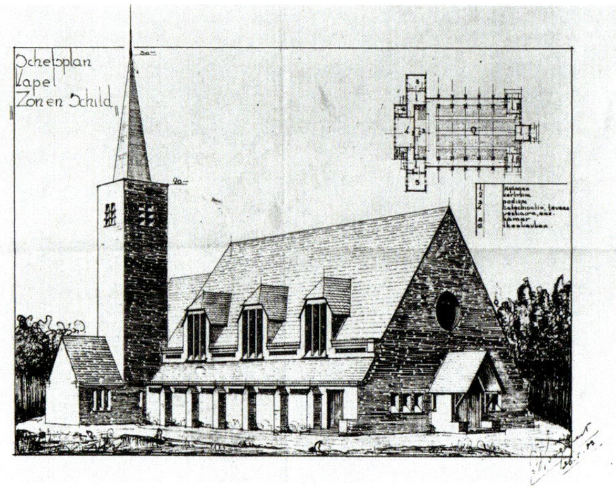

Fliedner's order of deaconesses was particularly influential in promoting the establishment of Protestant hospitals. The first of these was opened in Kaiserswerth near Düsseldorf in 1836; the first Diaconessenhuis in the Netherlands was inaugurated in Utrecht in 1844, followed by a second in The Hague in 1865, and many more in the 1880s. Of the 108 hospitals built in the nineteenth century, 19 were Protestant, 45 Catholic, and 44 non-denominational.[1] Only 19 of the 142 hospitals built before the Second World War were Protestant, as against 76 Catholic and 47 non-denominational ones. In the province of Groningen, where only 6 per cent of the population was Catholic, there were still 485 Catholic beds as against 290 Protestant ones in 1950.[2]

The result was a further extension of the blocs, partly stimulated by state aid. The building of various types of accommodation for the elderly who shared the same religious conviction began in the first decades of the twentieth century. Here too the Catholics were the most active. They established many homes for the poor and the more well-to-do elderly, especially in Brabant and Limburg. A major source of inspiration was the monastery or convent. Splendid examples are several buildings designed by A.J. Kropholler such as Pension Mariëngaarde in Tilburg (1935) and Mariënhof in Vught (1939). Craftsmanship and representative qualities played an important role in projects of this kind. The Protestants targeted the less well-endowed elderly. The Association of Reformed Deaconries in the classis of Edam established De Rusthoeve, a rest home designed by Wieger Bruin, in Purmerend. It was intended for old people who could not afford the expense themselves and for their more well-to-do peers, a distinction that was clearly expressed in the design of the building too.[3]

Architects usually built for their own bloc and became specialised in the design of hospitals and sanatoria. The Catholic architect Ed. Cuypers, for example, built hospitals in The Hague, Eindhoven, Nijmegen and Tilburg. W.A. Maas was another important architect in this field in the period between the wars. He designed several sanatoria and hospitals. His Sint Maartenskliniek was opened in Nijmegen in 1936. The building is sober and functional; aspects such as light and fresh air play an important role.

Such a complex often included a church or chapel, as in the Catholic hospitals designed by Cuypers. He usually observed a strict symmetry, with the chapel in the middle of the complex. The chapel also occupied an important position in Dutch Reformed institutions such as the Zon en Schild psychiatric hospital.

In the face of the common foe, initiatives were undertaken during the Second World War to put an end to the traditional ideological schizophrenia of Dutch society, but after liberation the blocs proved to be too strong for this ideal to have much effect. Compartmentalisation even reached a climax in the 1950s. Institutions with a pronounced Social Democratic character now appeared on the scene as well, including the Willem Dreeshuis in Amsterdam (1954-1957) designed by J.A. Snellebrand & G.W. Tuynman.

Each bloc built its own churches, hospitals, old people's homes, apartments for the elderly and psychiatric hospitals all over the country. At first the style of the Protestant institutions was somewhat more modern than that of the Catholics. For instance, Architectenbureau Wiegerinck en Van Balen's St. Lambertusziekenhuis in Helmond and Van der Laan Hermans Van der Eerden's Sint Jozefziekenhuis in Deventer were built for the Catholic bloc. K.L. Sijmons designed the Protestant Streekziekenhuis in Bennekom, and M.F. Duintjer en D.J. Istha implemented the Diaconessenhuis in Breda. In the course

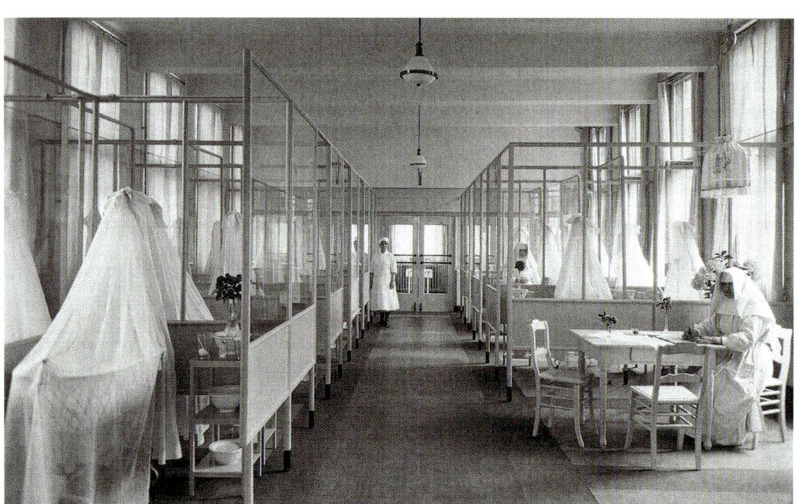

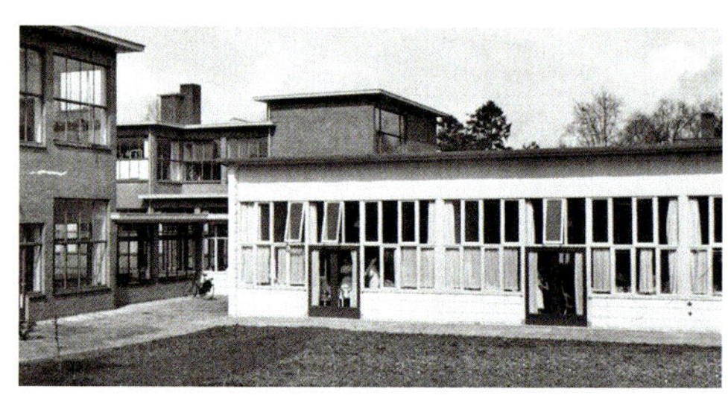

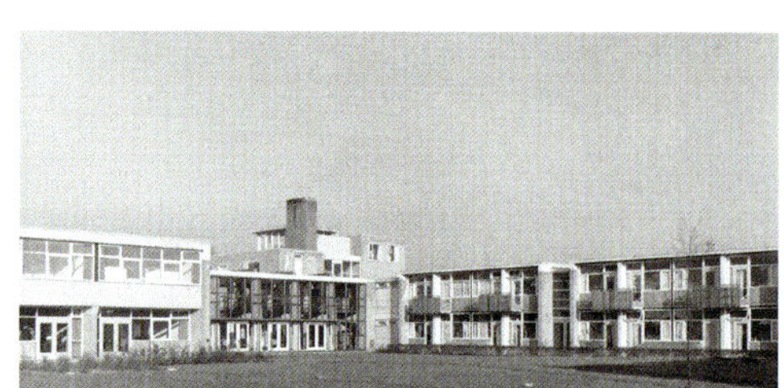

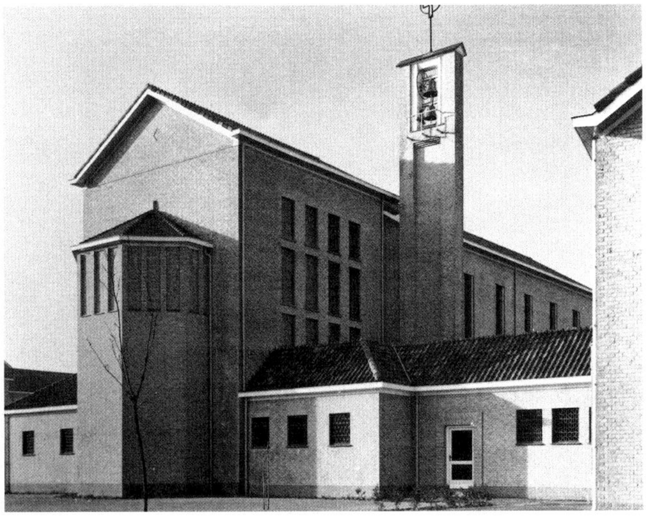

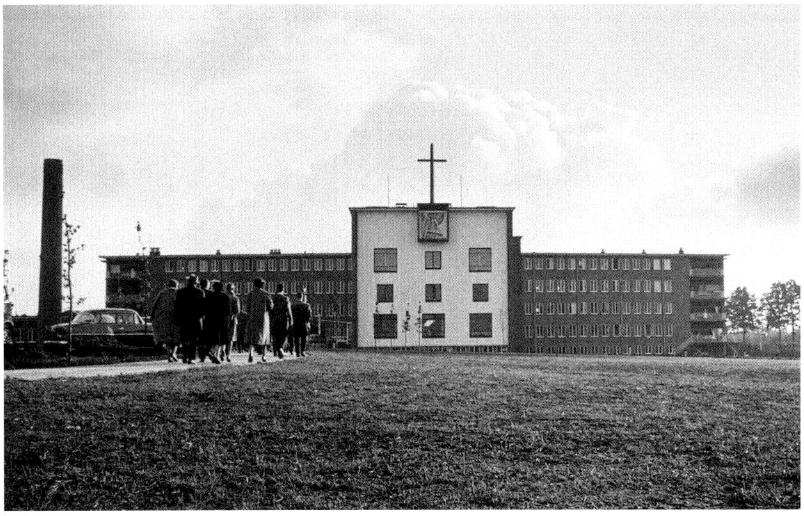

of the 1950s a modern style was generally adopted because it matched the function of the building better. For instance, the Sint Lucas Ziekenhuis in Amsterdam designed by F.P.J. Peutz and the Sint Gregorius Ziekenhuis in Brunssum by A. Swinkels en B. Salemans have a much more modern look than earlier examples.

The anti-authoritarian rebellion of the 1960s challenged the authority of the blocs. The media – especially television, but also the radio and the alternative culture that it disseminated (particularly pop music) – played a decisive role, which is why they were viewed with suspicion by the establishment. A consequence of the dismantling of the bloc system was the simultaneous fragmentation and clustering of the different movements. Protestants and Catholics even managed to form a joint political party and many denominational associations decided to revise their statutes. Apart from a few persistent enclaves, there are now hardly any traces left of the old blocs organised as parallel societies that were closed off from the outside world. The clear-cut, transparently structured but also extremely paternalistic compartmentalisation has been replaced by a highly diverse landscape of an almost infinite number of subcultures. The disappearance of compartmentalisation has also brought major changes to the world of health care. The desire to achieve a certain balance between provisions made available by different denominations had often led to redundancies in the past; nowadays a more efficient distribution is possible. This sometimes takes the form of a merger between institutions that belonged to different denominations and preferred not to have anything to do with one another in the past.

Top
Ed. Cuypers, Sint Canisius Ziekenhuis, Nijmegen, 1922-1926

G. van Hoogevest, Zon en Schild, design for the chapel, Amersfoort, 1933

Architectenbureau Wiegerinck en Van Balen, chapel Sint Lambertus Ziekenhuis, Helmond, 1958

M.F. Duintjer en D.J. Istha, Diaconessenhuis, Breda, 1960

Bottom
Ed. Cuypers, Sint Elisabeth Ziekenhuis, Tilburg, 1926

W.A. Maas, Sint Maartenskliniek, Nijmegen, 1936

J.A. Snellebrand & G.W. Tuynman, Willem Dreeshuis, Amsterdam, 1957

Van der Laan Hermans Van der Eerden, Sint Jozefziekenhuis Deventer, 1956

F.P.J. Peutz, Sint Lucas Ziekenhuis, Amsterdam, 1968

Ir. A. Swinkels en ir. B. Salemans, Sint Gregorius Ziekenhuis, Brunssum, 1961

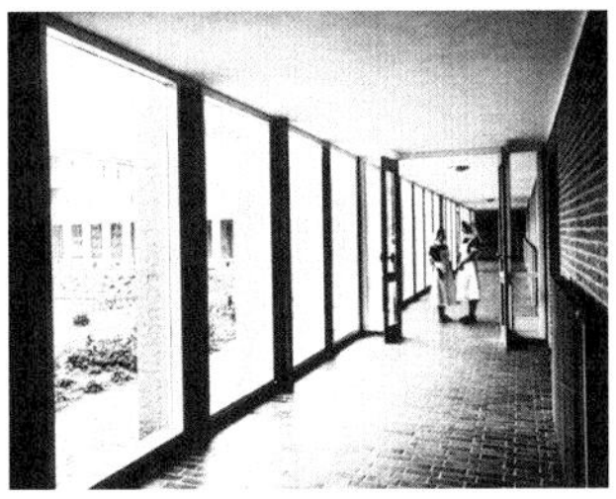

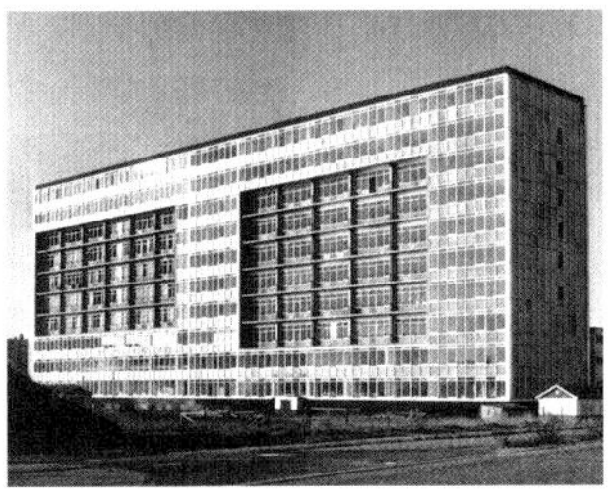

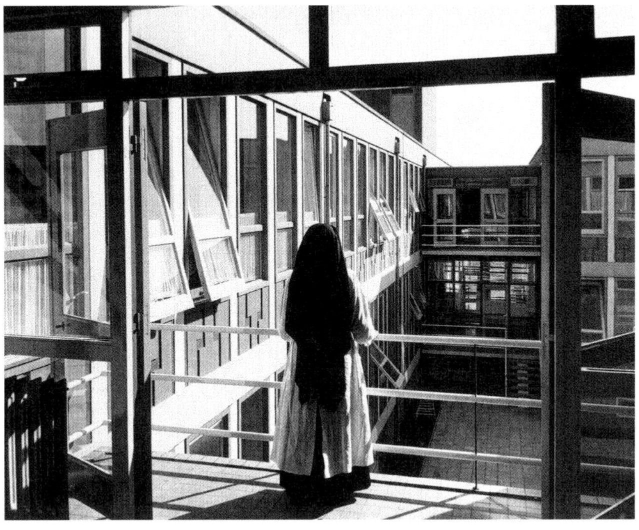

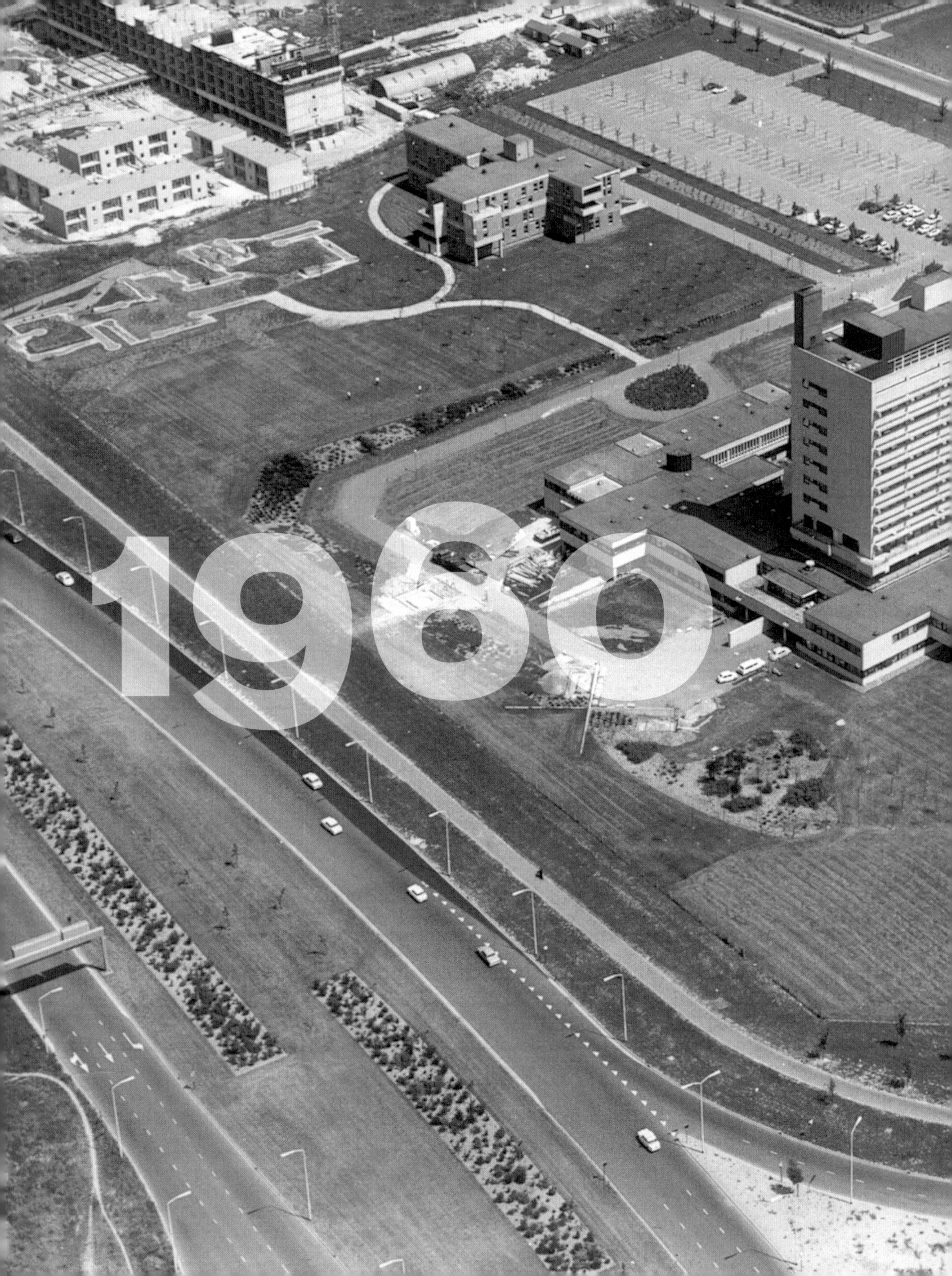

1960

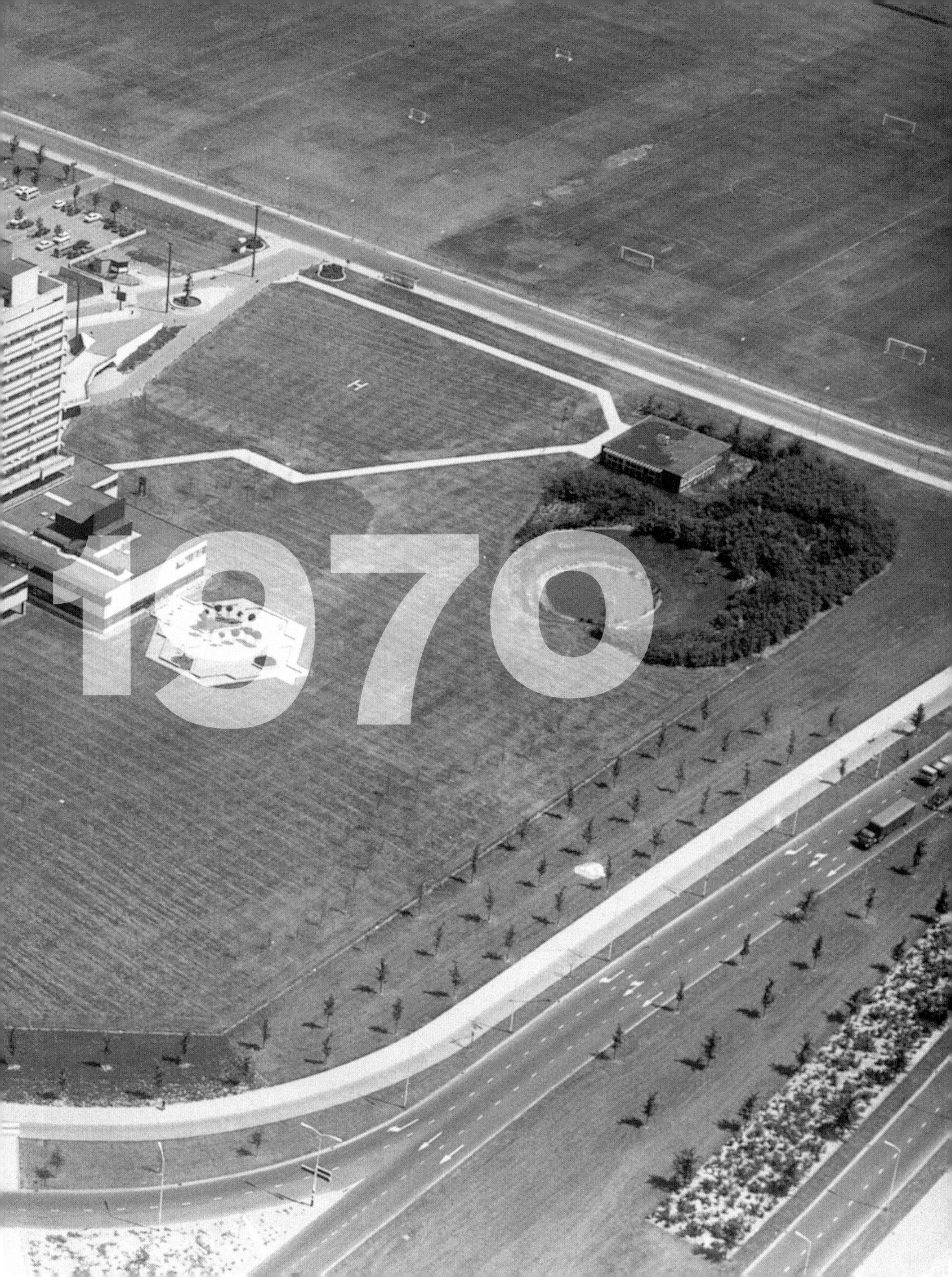
1970

Building boom

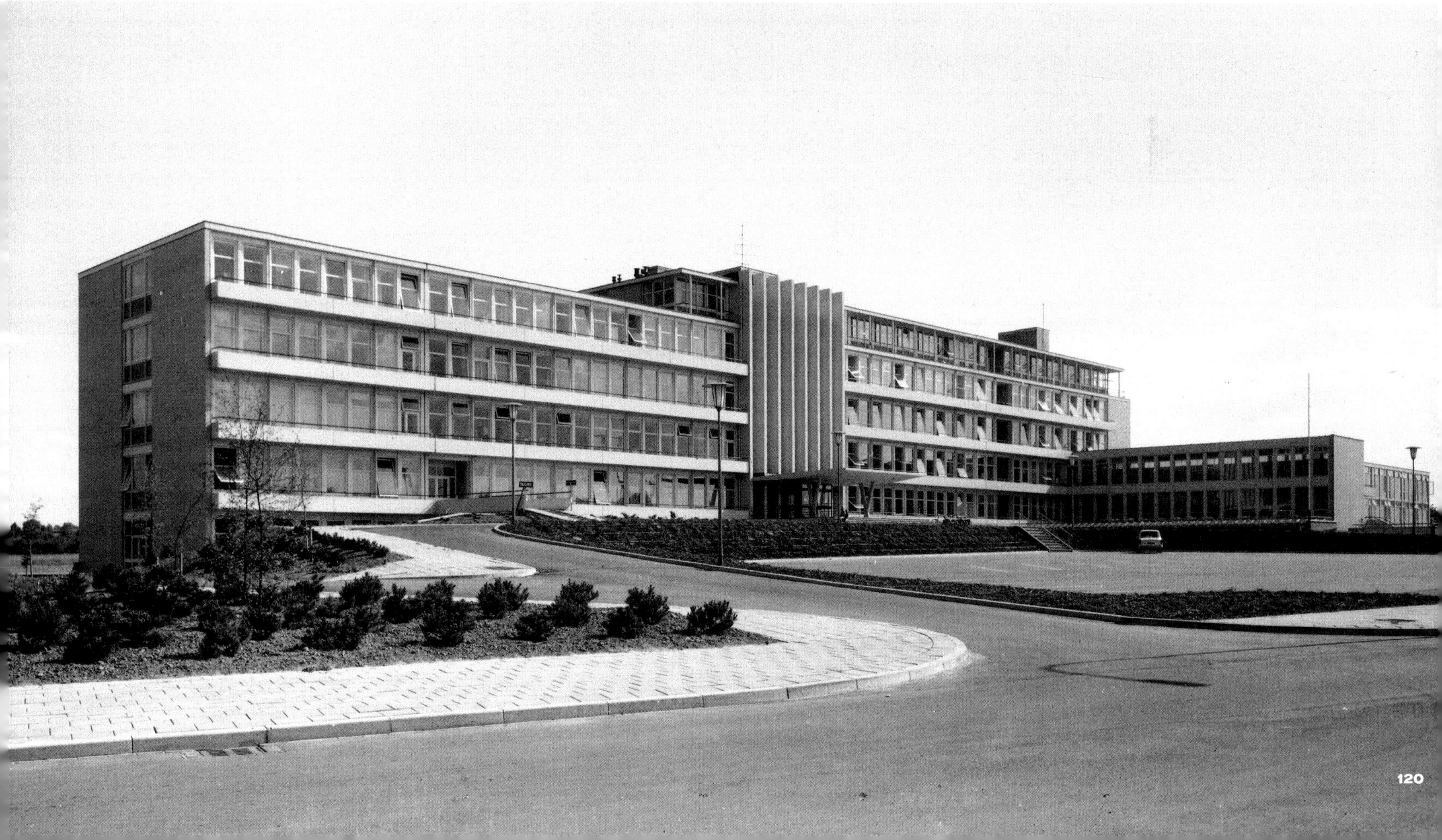

Care for all

It is a frequently heard cliché: the appearance of the Netherlands changed more drastically in the twenty years after the Second World War than in the preceding two hundred years. The population grew as never before. The industrialisation that was given every encouragement created new social and economic relations. The country became divided into economic core regions and backward regions where special incentive measures were barely able to prevent a further regression. There was an exodus from the backward regions to the promising areas in the West of the country, where it was not the larger cities that absorbed the demographic growth, as they had done in the past, but the smaller centres on the periphery. In the jargon of the urban planners, the city was fragmented and lost its traditional qualities as a clearly demarcated socio-economic unit within clearly identifiable physical borders. Probably the effect on the open polder landscape in the Randstad was more important. J.J.P. Oud, the celebrated Dutch pioneer of Modernism in architecture, even spoke of a 'housing bomb'.[1] The rapid increase in car ownership stimulated the emergence of commuter villages. The Netherlands became suburban.

It is only natural to suppose that these stormy developments had consequences for health care. In the first place, the number of services had to at least keep up with the population growth. Hospitals and housing and care amenities for the elderly would have to be incorporated in the new settlement patterns. That meant that most new institutions were created in the commuter towns and the rapidly growing suburbs. An additional advantage that was particularly important for hospitals was ease of accessibility via an expanding network of main roads and motorways. In psychiatry an attractive landscape setting in woods or dunes was still preferred.

Naturally enough, the new residential and work environment that was created in record time had an effect on health. Prosperity-related complaints and stress took their toll and provided material for a growing volume of criticism (see Chapter 5). The most important effect on the elderly was considered to be an increasing alienation. C. Lijnzaad, director of the Opbouworgaan Noord-Holland (North Holland Provincial Institute of Social Work), claimed: 'There must be few periods in history in which such great changes have taken place within a lifetime as in our time. You do not have to be old to have experienced the development from petrol lamp and gas flame to electric light – probably soon generated by nuclear energy. Traffic has evolved from the horse-drawn tram and cart to the racing car, jet plane and rocket-propelled plane. The means of communication have become so refined and intensive that you can see and hear the world in your living room.'[2] The best way to tackle these specific problems of old people would be to create a residential environment specially attuned to their needs. This led to a building boom of facilities for the elderly that was unparalleled in any other country.

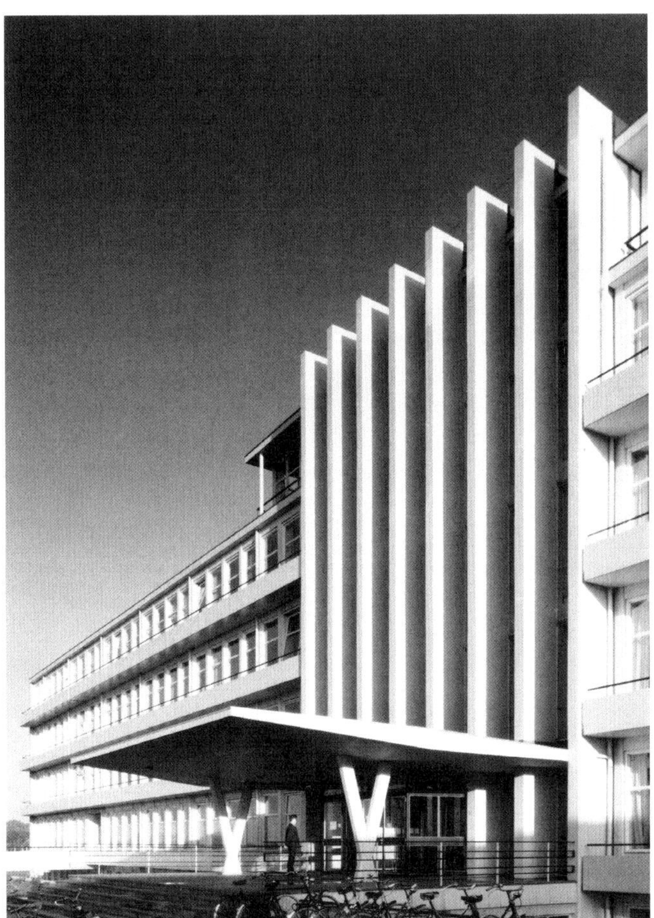

p. 118
W.F. Lugthart,
Diaconessenhuis,
Eindhoven, 1966

p. 120 and 121
Ir. A. Swinkels en
ir. B. Salemans,
Sint Barbara Ziekenhuis,
Geleen, 1964

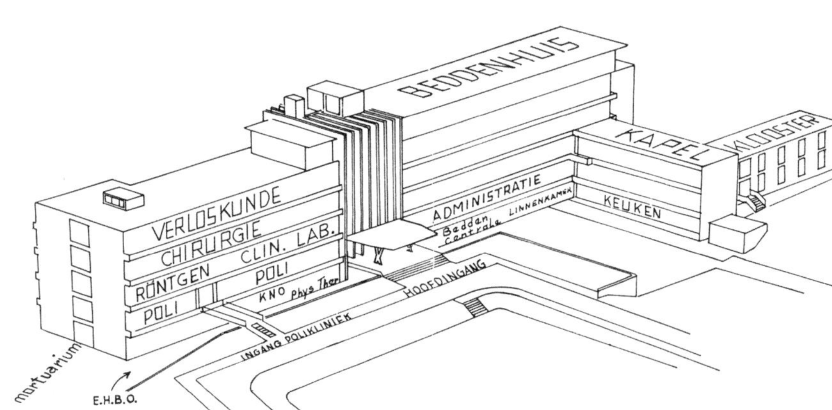

Hospitals

Hardly any hospitals were built during the first years after the liberation. The existing buildings had to cater for the rapidly growing demand, no matter how outdated they sometimes were. Afterwards the first signs of growth became visible. The number of beds grew from 42,000 to 58,000 between 1950 and 1960, and the number of medical interventions doubled; the number of nursing days per 1,000 insured rose by sixty per cent.[3] Between five and ten new hospitals were opened each year in the second half of the 1960s. The number of patients who were treated in hospitals rose even faster than the number of beds. Not only was every bed immediately taken into use with an inflexible regularity – 'a bed built is a bed filled', a US hospital researcher remarked in 1961 – but the use of the beds was intensified as well because the nursing period was reduced.[4]

The growth in the number of hospital beds speeded up in the 1960s. There were various reasons for this. Probably the most important was the inclusion of health care in the networks of the welfare state. Expensive hospital care now came within reach of the entire population. It is therefore natural to suppose that the expansion of existing hospitals and the building of new ones reflected the demographic growth, which was considerable; in fact, the 1960s were referred to as a period of demographic explosion. So even if medical expertise had remained at the same level, it would still have been necessary to build. Medical science and technology, however, did not remain still. On the contrary, major progress was made that caused the range of treatments to expand rapidly.

It is noteworthy that this growth was totally unplanned. Denominational compartmentalisation was a major obstacle to planning, and was in fact an extra incentive to build a lot. Hospitals sprang up like mushrooms. R.G. Greve, head of the department of the Ministry of Social Affairs and Public Health responsible for the supervision of the building volume in health care, remarked: 'It was the heyday of the 5/1000 norm. It was not a question of whether more hospitals should be permitted, but of whether the next one should be a Catholic, a Protestant or a non-denominational one'.[5] For instance, if a local authority had a well equipped Catholic hospital with enough beds, it was always possible that a Protestant mayor would want a Protestant hospital too. If it proved impossible to meet this demand by allowing a Protestant nursing home, for example, then there was no way of avoiding expensive duplication of facilities.[6] Sometimes hospitals of different religious persuasions were built very close to one another, usually on new estates far from the centre.

A wave of mergers began in 1967, reaching a peak in 1970.[7] An unmistakable trend towards increase of scale could be discerned as smaller hospitals closed down. Mergers afforded a way of maintaining the level of the 'medical stock'.

Block types

How did architects try to meet the new demands? What were the main trends? In the first place there was a spectacular growth of outpatient units. This was partly due to the ongoing revolution in medical technology. As more advanced equipment became available, more specialists preferred to accommodate it in the outpatient units and to have it maintained by the technical staff of the hospital. As a

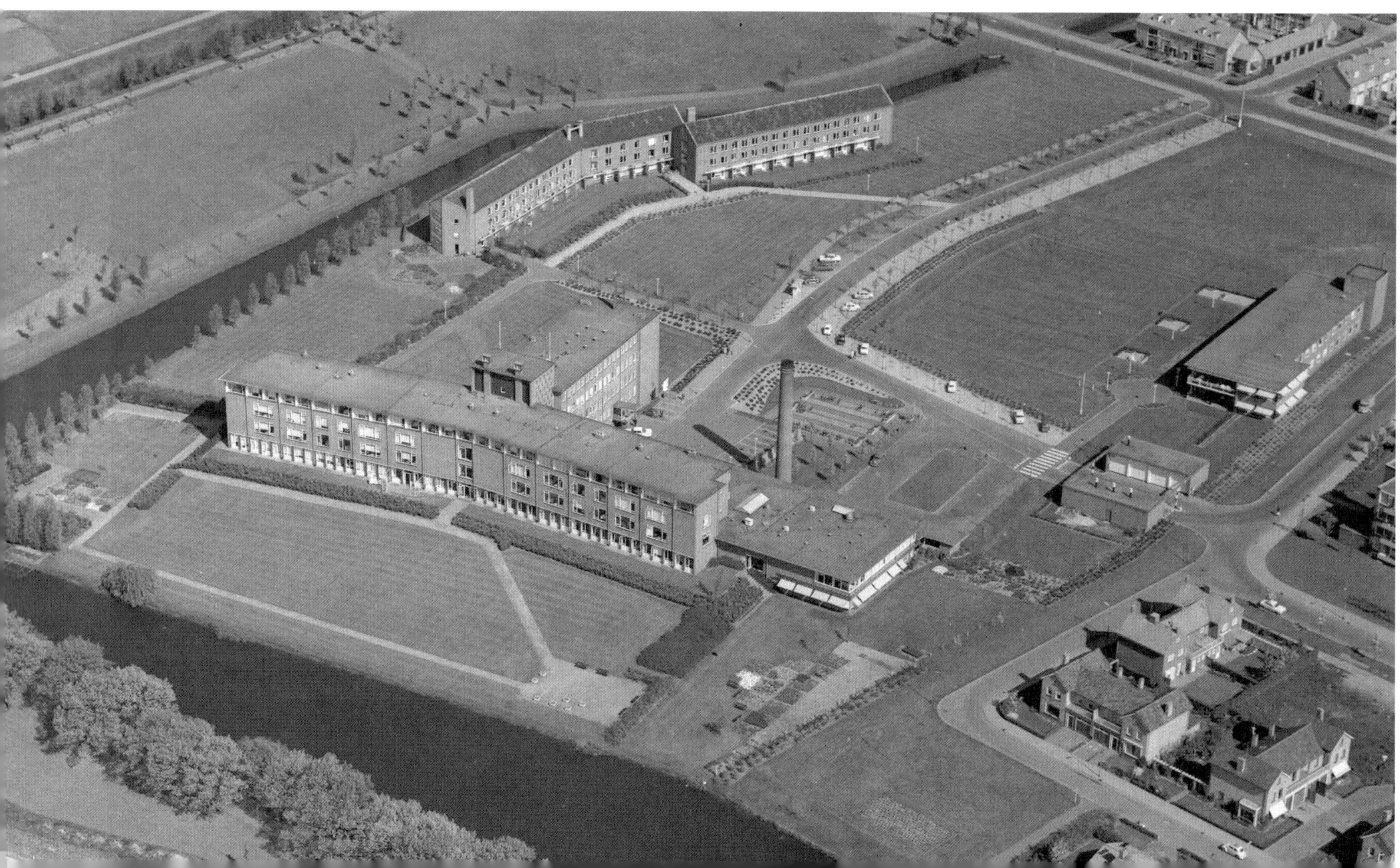

result, the latter developed to become a facility maintenance service for medical specialists who worked there as self-employed entrepreneurs. The outpatient units proved to be veritable traffic machines that could process many patients – who rarely made the journey to the outpatient unit on their own.

The same medical technology had other consequences too. An increasing number of technologies became available, and as progress advanced the machinery went more quickly out of date, which in turn made it necessary to replace it sooner. Above all the speed at which the technology became outdated caused many a specialist to protest that the new buildings were still designed for yesterday's technology. They complained bitterly: 'The hospital that is finished today is qualitatively the hospital of five to ten years ago. The hospital that will be finished in five or ten years' time is today's hospital'.[8] Constant renovation was unavoidable. 'For years every hospital has been trying to keep up with the lightning development by demolition and building.'[9] The fastest developments took place in the operating theatres, the X-ray units and the laboratories. 'Development here is proceeding at such a pace that it can be stated without exaggeration that even in our brand-new hospitals these units are no longer up to date the moment they are opened'.[10] Technological progress forced the hospitals to renovate all the time; it was not rare for renovation to start even before the hospital was properly opened. Hospitals had to be capable of anticipating these constant adjustments.

Medical progress went hand in hand with increasing specialisation. Internal medicine was divided into special heart, lung and respiratory units, while surgical specialisations included orthopaedic, plastic and neurosurgery. New disciplines called for new rooms that often had to satisfy certain requirements. Expandability and flexibility became more important than ever. The strategy to achieve this was a continuation of Synthetic Modernism. Each of the three main units of the hospital – wards, treatment unit and outpatient unit – had its own dynamics. By being separated from the others, it could serve those dynamics without interfering with the activities of the other units. Until the mid-60s most architects looked for ways of perfecting the T-type and the H-type, with both of which they had considerable experience by then. The firm of M.F. Duintjer en D.J. Istha preferred the T-shape.

A good example is the Diaconessenhuis in Breda, which was completed in 1960. The outpatient units were situated on the ground floor of the four-storey treatment block, which had a striking wall at the end: nine large windows set in black frames interrupted the light-coloured masonry, while in the middle the edge of the roof was broken by a heavy black cartouche around a work of art. Above this deep niche that leaned forward a mast in the form of a cross had been set slightly to the rear. The wards formed an angle with the treatment units, and the detached home for the nurses displayed the same boomerang-shaped ground plan. The architects provided the outside walls with a clear, rhythmical articulation that gave the complex – one of the smaller hospitals with 208 beds – a distinguished appearance.

A fairly small hospital, the Sint Barbara Ziekenhuis in Geleen (150 beds), was designed by F. Knibbeler from the firm A. Swinkels en B. Salemans as an elongated block that allowed for later extension to form a T-shape. A striking central part with a series of vertical concrete elements and a canopy mark the main entrance and the staircase. The wards

p. 122
***M.F. Duintjer en D.J. Istha*, Diaconessenhuis, Breda, 1960**

p. 123
***A. Swinkels en B. Salemans*, Sint Gregorius Ziekenhuis, Brunssum, 1961**

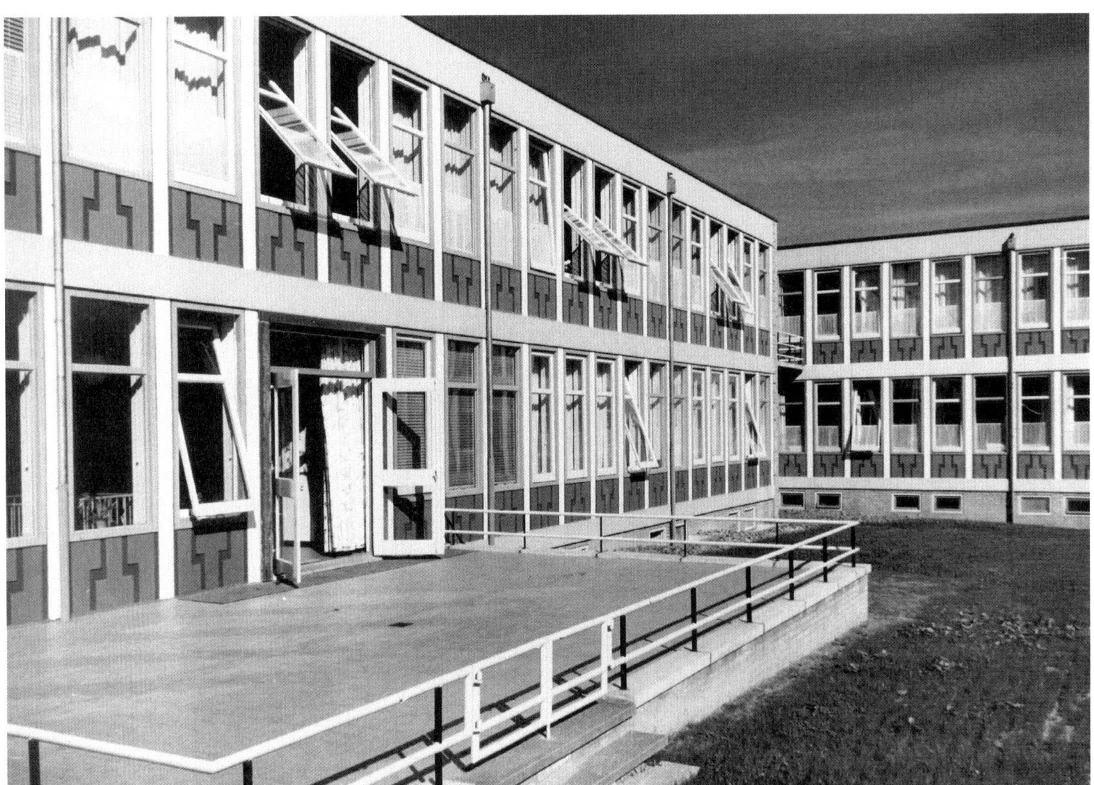

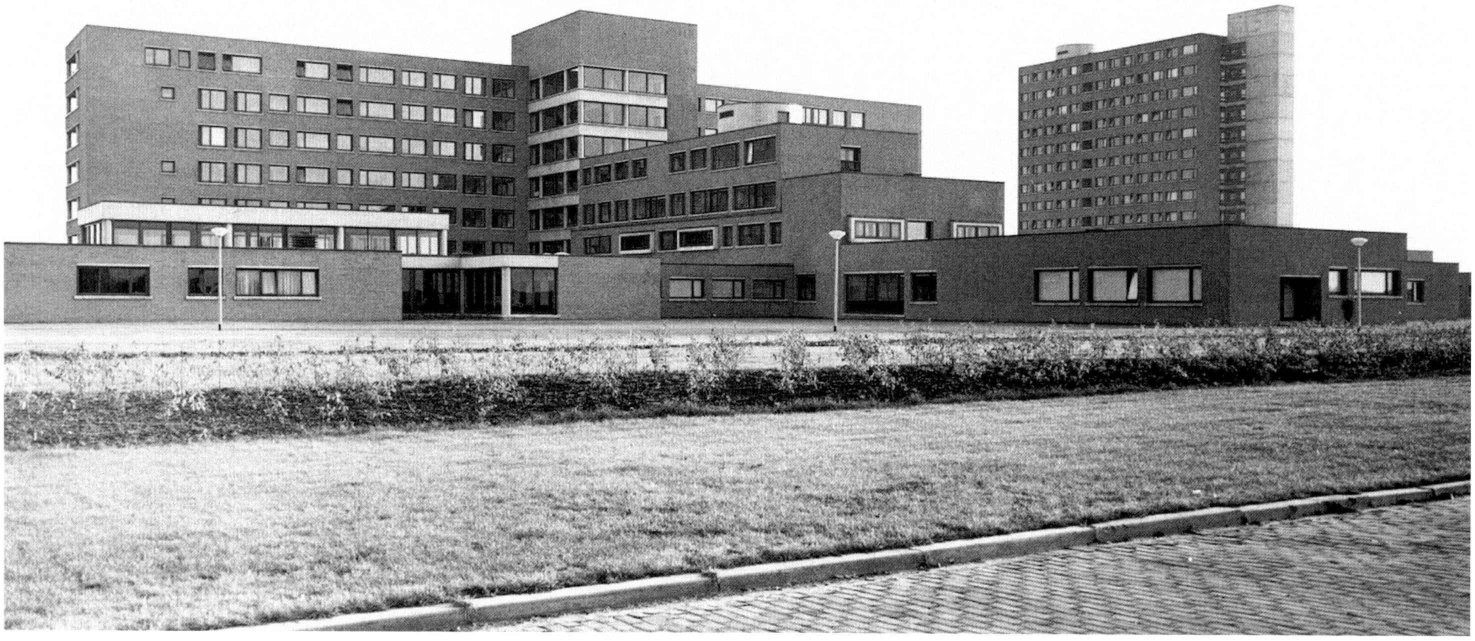

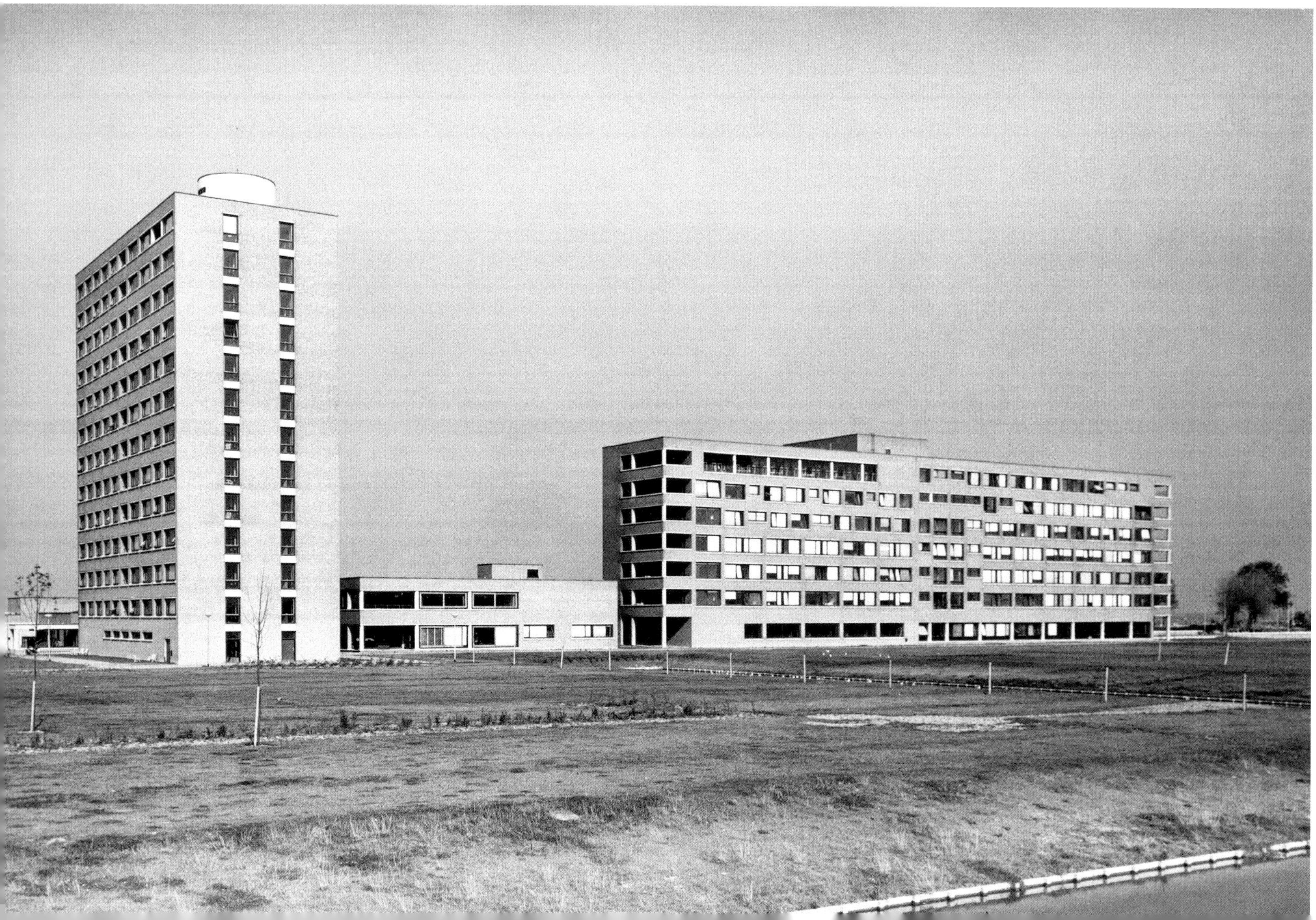

are on one side, while the treatment unit and outpatient unit are on the other side.

The Sint Gregorius Ziekenhuis in Brunssum, designed by the same firm, was a striking exception. With its 180 beds it was a small hospital too, but it was unique in that it consisted almost entirely of two floors. One of the advantages was the possibility of building and opening it in stages. As was common in Catholic hospitals at the time, the opening ceremony held in 1961 was accompanied by an episcopal consecration of the chapel.

A variant on the H-theme was the K-type. Examples of this type are the Diaconessenhuis designed by J.P. Kloos in the De Wijert urban expansion district of Groningen and the Diaconessenhuis in Leiden by Cramer en Kruisheer that was completed in 1963. The difference from the H-model was the bend in the wards. In Leiden Kruisheer placed the main entrances beneath the chapel, which he situated next to the middle of the treatment unit. The most unusual feature was not the type, but the severe, clear design that displayed a certain bravura.

Kloos turned his back on what he later called 'show business' in his K-hospital in Groningen and followed the programme closely. If that did not lend itself for showpieces of studied design, he did not try to force it. All the same, the results of this self-imposed discipline were no less impressive. The Diaconessenhuis in Groningen opened in 1965: a medium-sized complex with 360 beds and a large outpatient unit with its own entrance to one side of the main entrance and directly connected with the treatment unit.

New types

Although considerable experience had been acquired with the familiar letter types, there was nevertheless a demand for new types. The Holy-ziekenhuis in Vlaardingen, a design by J.W.C. Boks, W. Eijkelenboom, A. Middelhoek architecten, was one of the most eye-catching to be built in this period. As in the projects of Istha, Kruisheer and Kloos, for example, it was based on a clear architectural conception of design, but was elaborated in a manner closer to urban planning. The basis was the classic T-shape, but this was by no means obvious in the final complex. A seven-storey ward block with attractive French balconies at the ends was built at right angles to a treatment block, while the single-storey outpatient units were at right angles to the latter. The unusual feature was to accommodate several functions in separate, low volumes. At the same time it was a strategy in order to be able to build the complex in stages, to allow each part to be expandable without disturbing the total structure, and to enable an aesthetic design. The designers regarded the latter aspect as the core of their assignment: 'In the implementation, converting all of the functional hard requirements into matter, the architect as artist also has the task of using form, materials and colour to give it such a form that the result is a whole; a whole in which each part, each function fits and has a place of its own', as W. Eijkelenboom put it.[11]

While the Holy-ziekenhuis was so specific that it can hardly be considered a type, a new solution was introduced from the United States in the 1960s that was soon to grow

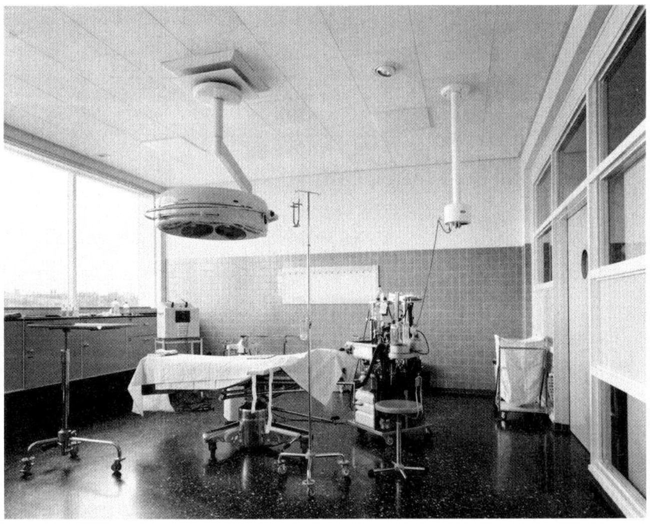

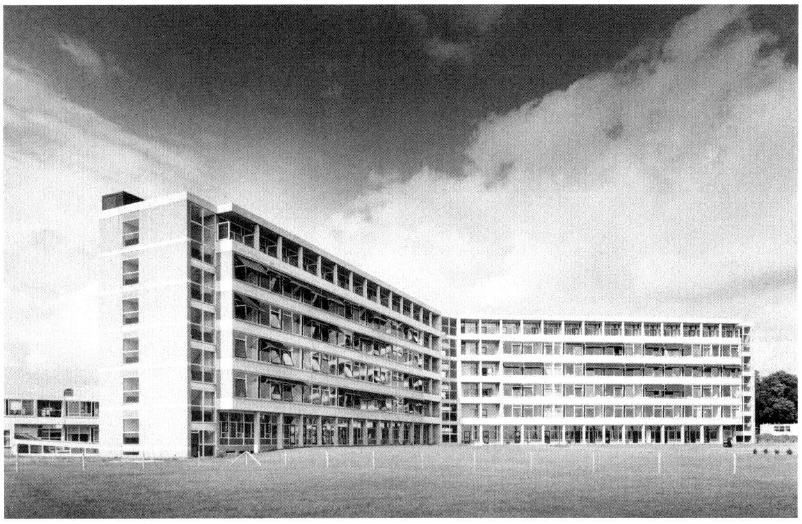

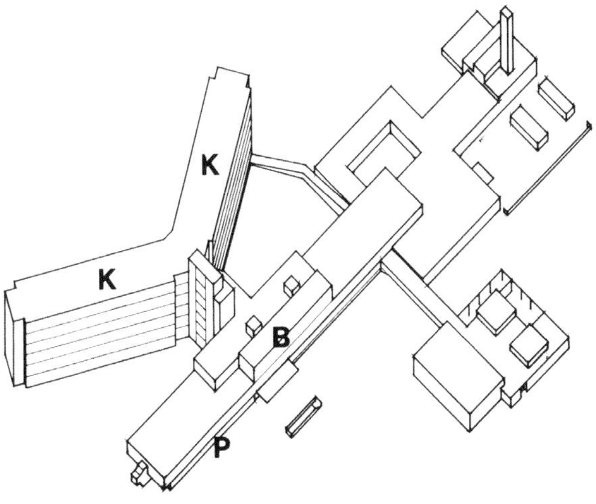

p. 124
***J.W.C. Boks, W. Eijkelenboom, A. Middelhoek architecten,* Holy-ziekenhuis, Vlaardingen, 1964**

p. 125
***J.P. Kloos*, operating theatre at the Diaconessenhuis, Groningen, 1965**

***J.P. Kloos*, Diaconessenhuis, Groningen, 1965**

***J.P. Kloos*, Diaconessenhuis, Groningen, lay-out**

K = clinic (ward)
B = treatment department
P = outpatient department

J.P. Kloos,
**Diaconessenhuis,
Groningen, 1965**

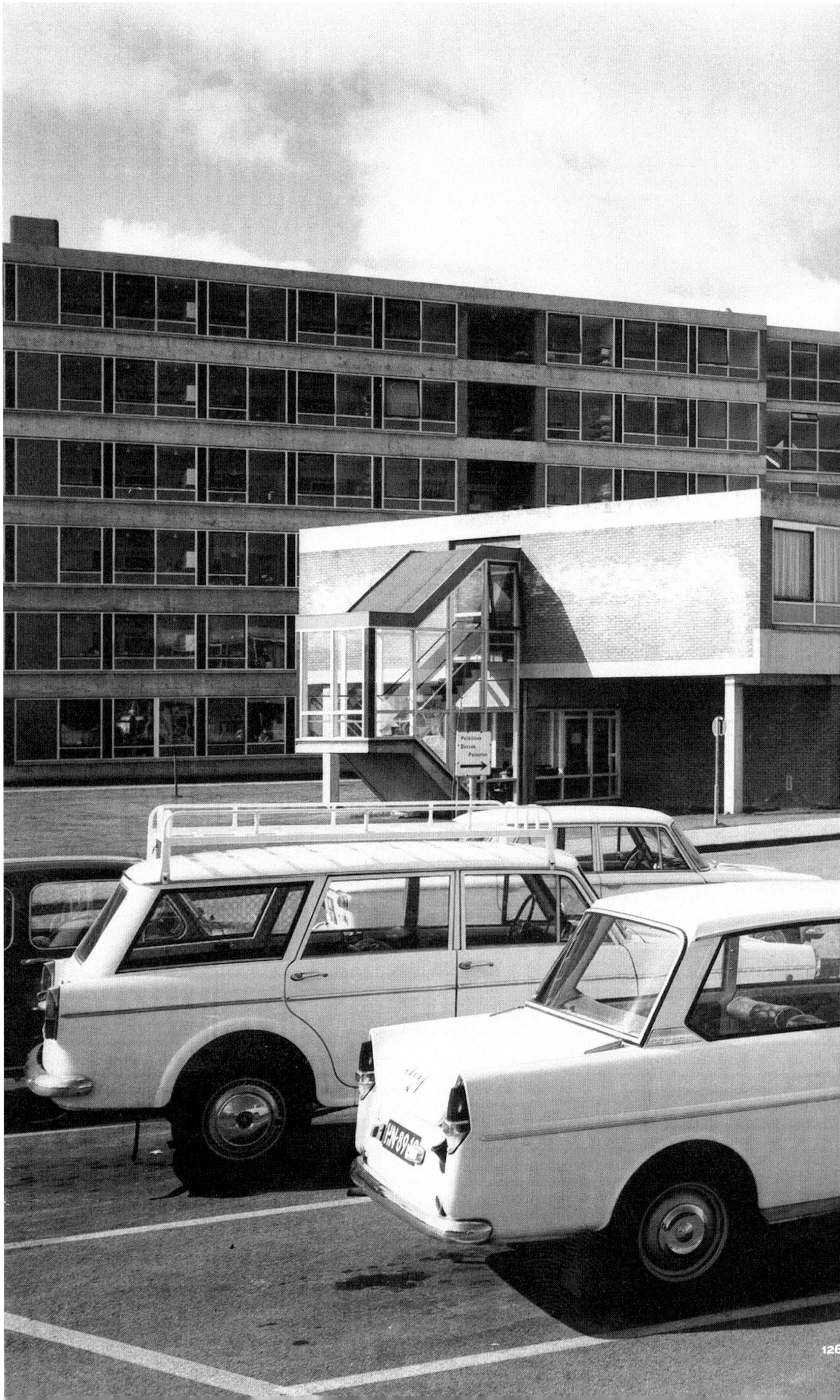

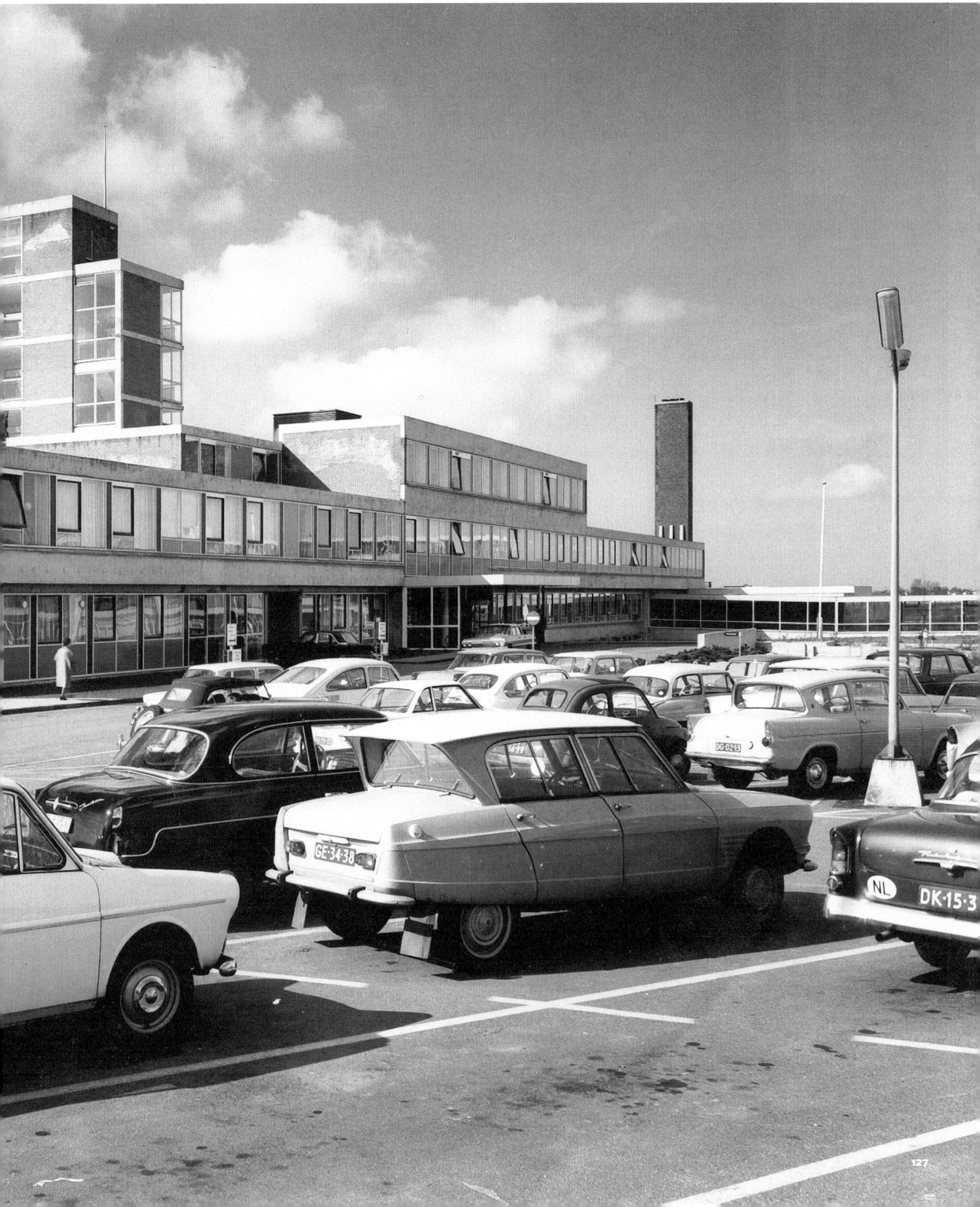
GE-34-38
NL
DK-15-3

and become the most common model all over the world. Its name varied from country to country: 'tower on podium type' or 'matchbox on a muffin' in the English-speaking world, 'socletour', 'hôpital arbre', 'mono-bloc sur galette' in French, 'Breitfuß' in German, and 'piastra-torre' in Italian.[12] P. Nelson, whom we have already come across as a pioneer of high-rise hospital buildings in Europe, designed the first example in France: the famous Hôpital Mémorial France-États-Unis in Saint-Lô, which opened in 1956. Fernand Léger supplied the colour scheme.

The essence of the tower on podium type is the accommodation of the treatment unit and the outpatient unit, where the medical technology is concentrated, in a broad low-rise volume. This made it relatively easy to introduce new and to replace existing equipment. The high-rise block of wards was built on top of this low-rise block; developments in this sector were less dominated by technology so that the need for renovation was less urgent.

The first hospital of this type in the Netherlands was the Diaconessenhuis that W.F. Lugthart built in Eindhoven between 1962 and 1966; the most spectacular was the Leyenburgziekenhuis in The Hague by K.L. Sijmons. 'A hospital complex is in the first place a utilitarian building. However, if it fails to rise above that level, it becomes a health factory'.[13] The ten-storey block of wards towered above a two-part low-rise building that fanned out broadly and in which all of the clinical, outpatient and auxiliary units were included. Prefab concrete elements blended with the construction and gave the different parts a monolithic character: the ward block and the low-rise building seemed to consist of a single block and to have been set down in a grand gesture. An enormous canopy marked the entrance, to which a V-shaped, sloping plateau led. The situation of the complex was unusual: it was right next to an old district of the city.

Most of the hospitals of this type were implemented on the outskirts of cities, often close to a ring road. That was also the case with the Sint Franciscus Gasthuis in Rotterdam, a design by Kraaijvanger architecten together with Hendriks Campman Tennekes, which was only completed in 1975. The medical block has three floors and includes two large inner courtyards. Above it towers the ten-floor block of wards, whose open south elevation contrasts with the more closed character of the low-rise building. While the design bears the hallmark of the 60s, when this kind of somewhat clean, streamlined high-rise building was frequently applied in hospital architecture, the interior unmistakably radiates the atmosphere of the 70s.

The ward block was not always built on top of the treatment and outpatient units. In some cases the different elements were juxtaposed, as in the Sint Elisabeth's or Groote Gasthuis in Haarlem (Kruisheer + Hallink), or placed in a row, as in the Sint Franciscusziekenhuis in Roosendaal (Margry en Jacobs).

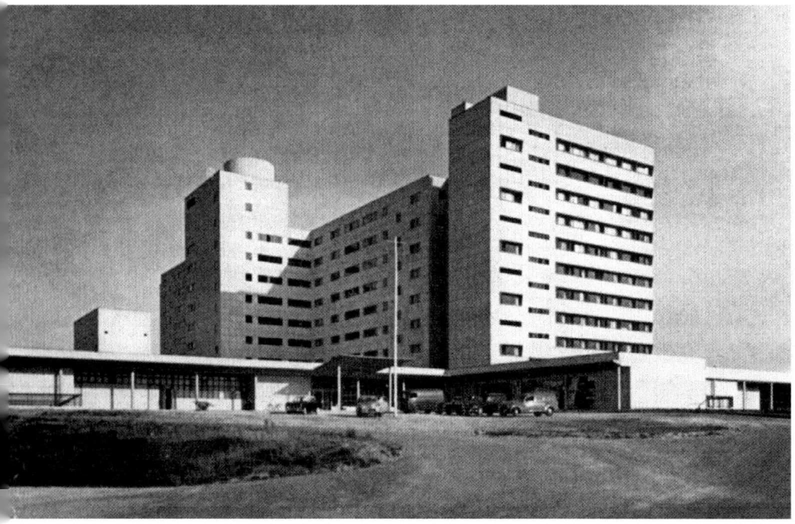

p. 128
***P. Nelson*, Hôpital Mémorial France-États-Unis, Saint-Lô, 1956**

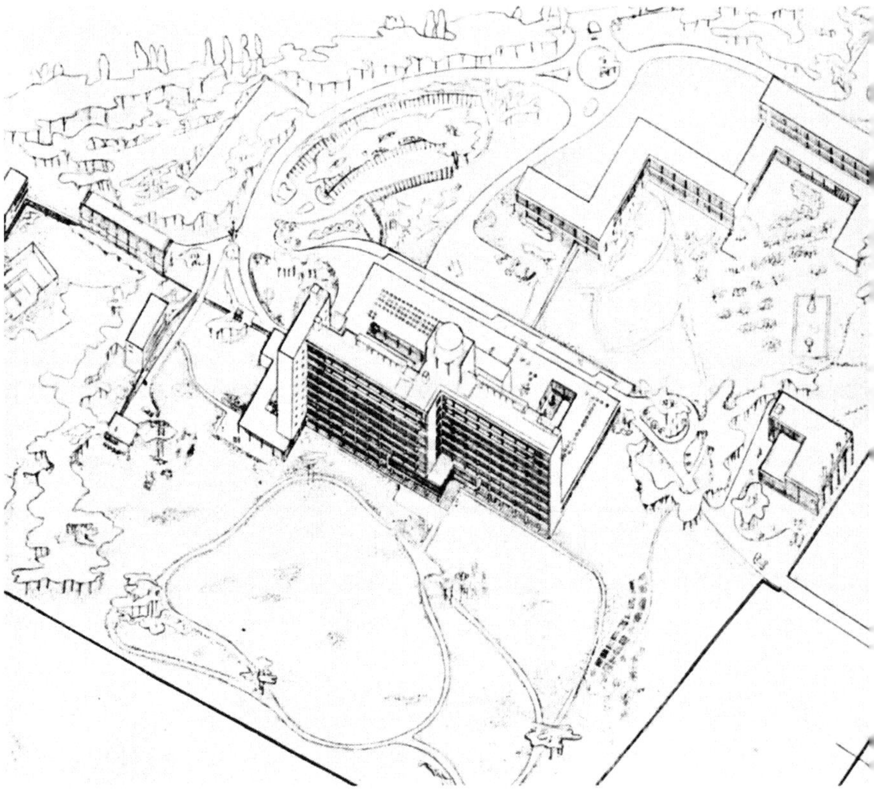

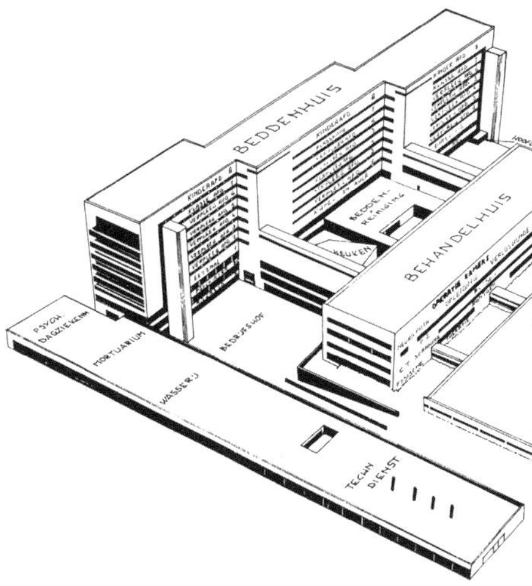

p. 129 | <
***Kruisheer + Hallink architecten*, Sint Elisabeth's or Groote Gasthuis, Haarlem, 1971**

***Kruisheer + Hallink architecten*, Sint Elisabeth's or Groote Gasthuis, Haarlem, 1971**

***Margry en Jacobs*, Sint Franciscusziekenhuis, Roosendaal, 1968**

p. 129 | >
***K.L. Sijmons*, Leyenburgziekenhuis, The Hague, 1971**

***Kraaijvanger architecten with Hendriks Campman Tennekes*, Sint Franciscus Gasthuis, Rotterdam, 1975**

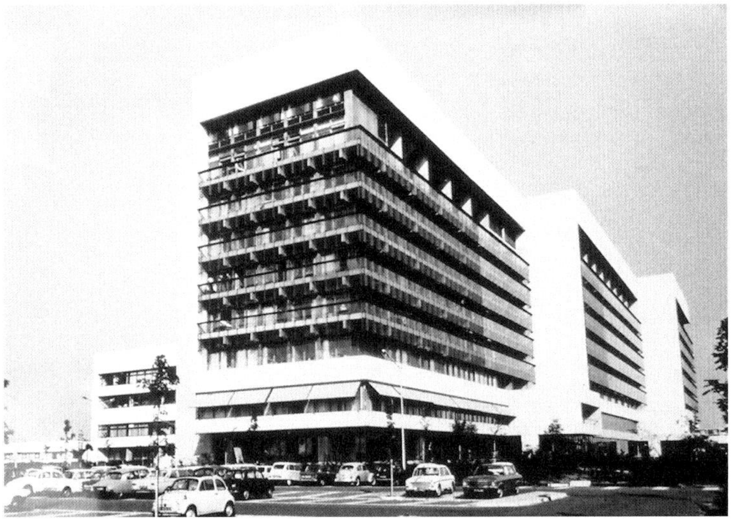

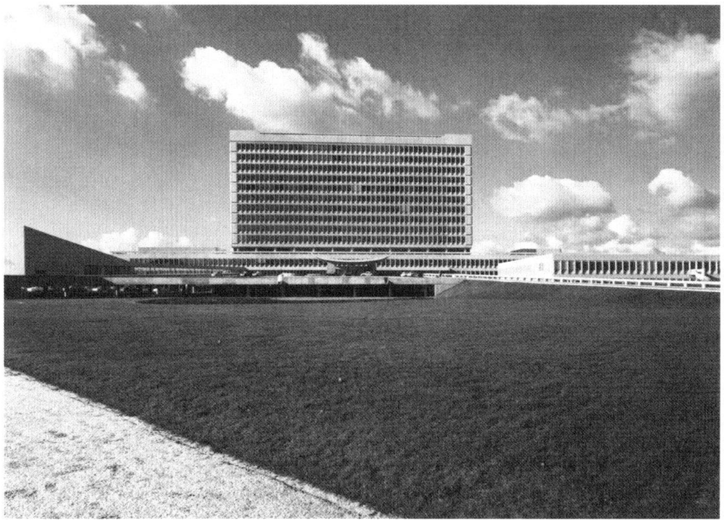

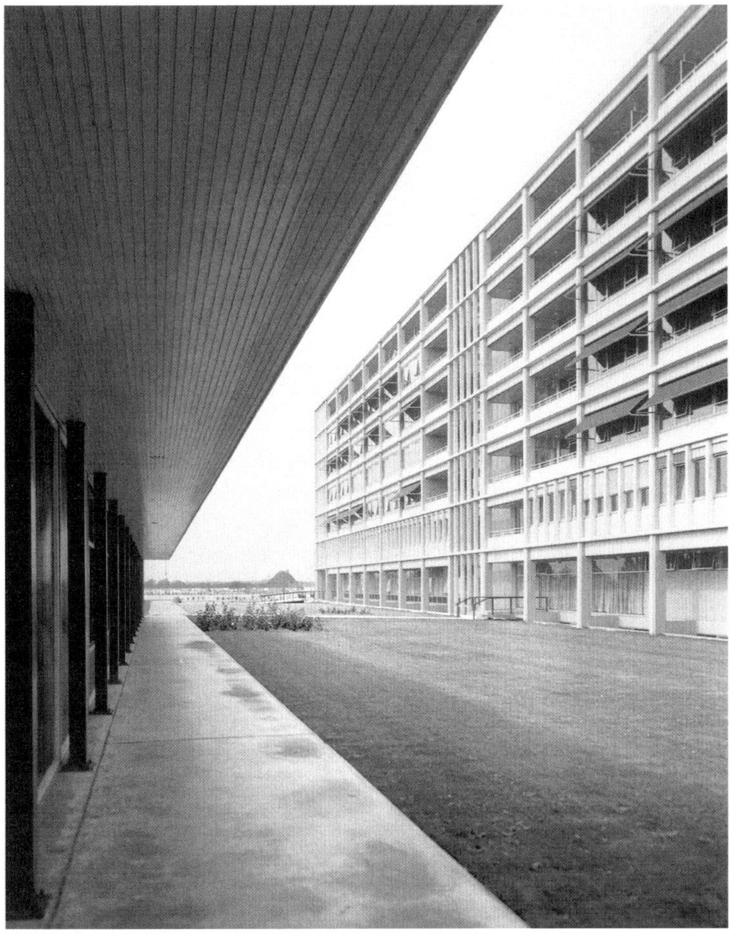

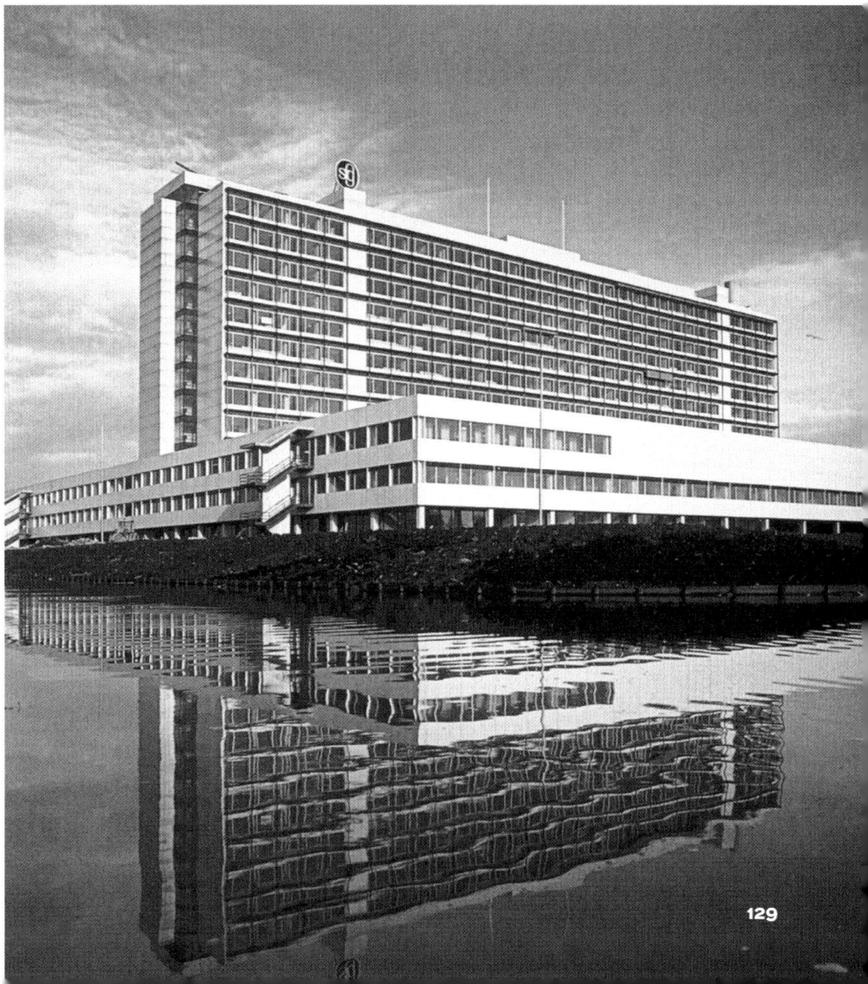

Psychiatric hospitals

A boom of new buildings got under way in psychiatry too, though on a more modest scale than in the regular hospitals. The main advantage of the pavilion architecture that was still the common model for these buildings was the opportunity it offered to add, modify or replace buildings. Perhaps the most important innovation was the introduction of psychiatric drugs, which put an end to the problem of restless and 'maniacal' inpatients. Another breakthrough was that of psychology. This breakthrough coincided with a certain psychologisation of the entire postwar society, encouraged by the need to discover the deeper motives for the kind of behaviour that was held responsible for the horrors to which the Western world had been exposed around the middle of the twentieth century. That was, after all, no natural catastrophe but a completely manmade one. The idea that 'ordinary' society too fell prey to unknown and uncontrolled instincts seemed to call the hard distinction between institution and outside world into question.
A second innovation that was partly due to the psychiatric drugs was the attempt to bring the community inside the institution in line with 'ordinary' society as far as possible. The first complex in which these ideas were embodied was the Sint Franciscushof in Raalte, which opened in 1967. Equally radical in the attempt to key into ordinary postwar society was Vijverdal in Maastricht, which opened in 1973. While Vijverdal is a robust institute that does nothing to camouflage its scale, the social homes in Wolfheze are completely absorbed in the neighbourhood. De Viersprong in Halsteren gave form to the concept of the therapeutic community, another important innovation of these years.

Four exemplary new building projects

The Sint Franciscushof bears witness to a revolution in psychiatry that took place partly when the design process was already fully under way. In the words of the designers, Van den Bosch and Hendriks, in 1968: 'The changed view that a person whose mind is ill is unable to help it himself and so can no longer be treated as inferior by the community has contributed to the fact that we have been able to design rooms in the new hospital and institutions that would have been unthinkable ten years ago'.[14] The Sint Franciscushof consists of several pavilions, but is unlike the classic pavilion hospital. Instead, a village was created in which the buildings are grouped around a number of squares, while in the centre they are linked with one another by a shopping street. Each pavilion is different from the rest and specially adapted to its specific function. The era in which patients were distinguished in terms of controllability was gone for good; the new criteria were age category and the nature of the therapy.

Besides the availability of an ultramodern medical complex, one of the exemplary aspects of the Sint Franciscushof was the modern psychological treatment centre, but most important was the ambition of the designers to create a complex that was as close as possible to 'normal' society. This accounts for the lack of monumentality, the attempt to make the rooms for patients as normal as possible – there are even bungalows – and the opening of what was originally intended as a complex only for female patients to male patients as well in 1969. This was a fairly big step for a Catholic institution, and was partly connected with the growing laicisation of social life in the 1960s, as could also be seen from the 'ecumenical' character of the meeting

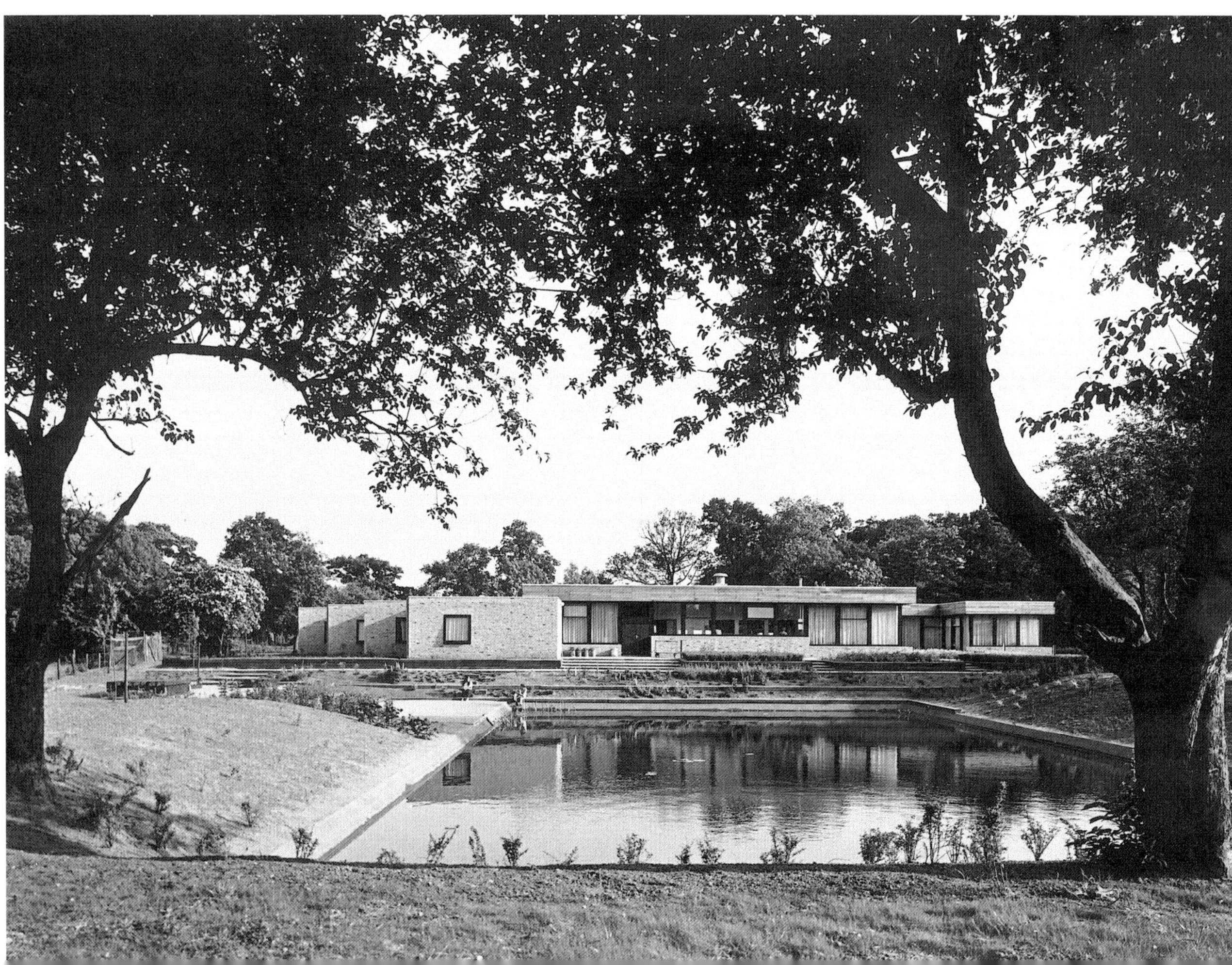

p. 130
***O. Greiner*, De Viersprong, Halsteren, 1971**

p. 131
***E.J. Rothuizen & C. Dekker*, regular housing units for groups of patients, Wolfheze psychiatric hospital Wolfheze, 1961**

centre: 'There is room for everyone in the community centre. The Catholics hold their services there, while there is a meditation area for the Protestants. At other times it is used for beat music, theatre, song and dance. It is nobody's stronghold'.[15] The Sint Franciscushof illustrates how psychiatry may have changed more in the two decades after 1945 than in the preceding two centuries and also makes clear that many of the post-1965 'revolutions' were already in the offing beforehand.

Vijverdal, which is unique for several reasons, was built in Maastricht between 1968 and 1973. The complex, designed by Swinkels en Salemans, looks modern and seems to bear the signature of the International Style, but justifies the choice of a fairly hard high-rise building with arguments that seem closer to the contrary movement: high-rise fits in with the urban atmosphere which is, after all, characterised by modern flats. This reduces the gap between city and institution.

Probably the most far-reaching form of turning psychiatric institutions into communities was tried out in Wolfheze, where the first experiment was made with social homes. These were simple terraced homes that were identical to the standard social housing of the reconstruction period, and were intended for small groups of patients who could lead their lives there as normally as possible. The background was the idea of the socio-therapeutic community, the social model that harked back to the ideals of the neighbourhood on the scale of the small local community. Almost 300 of the 820 patients were accommodated in double homes in groups of six persons.

Finally, De Viersprong in Halsteren is based on the same idea, but in this case a specific architectural form was found for it. The function itself, that of the therapeutic community, is an expression of the great progress in methods of treatment. A therapeutic community is after all *the* social model and in that sense the pinnacle of the quiet revolution in psychiatry in the 50s and 60s. The architecture is revolutionary thanks to Onno Greiner's attempt to keep the building as simple as possible. 'It is so simple, so acceptable, by no means eye-catching architecture', the designer claimed. 'Everything is based on the division of the space and above all on the right proportion between space and use of materials'.[16] However 'ordinary' it may have been, the complex won him international recognition. And precisely the ambition to be ordinary makes De Viersprong prophetic of the following stage in the development of the psychiatric institution.

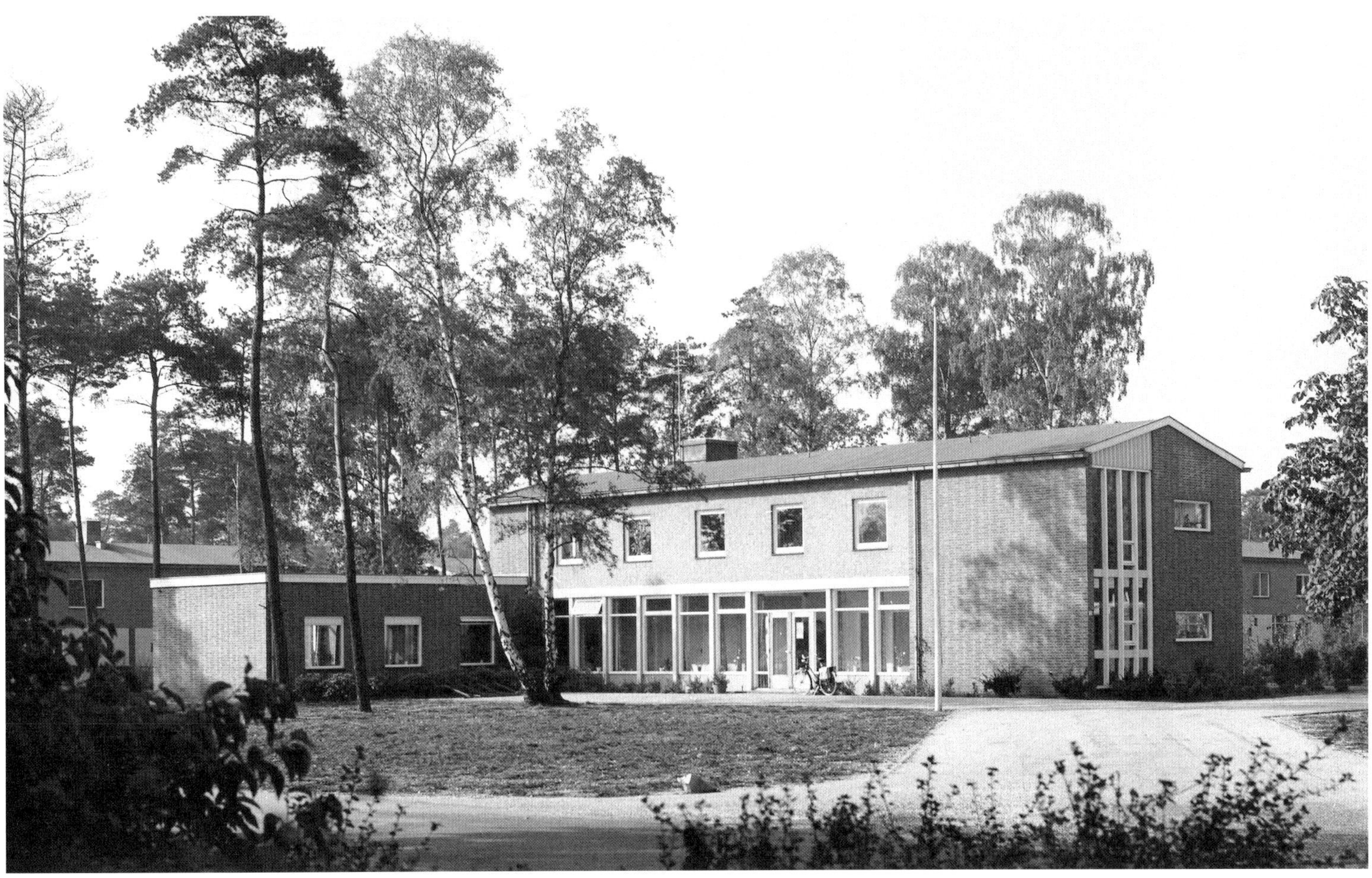

Housing and care for the elderly

The 1960s were golden years, and that is true of housing for the elderly too. The lion's share of housing for the elderly was subsidised by the government. Whether that was done on the basis of the Housing Law or by appealing to other regulations, the government assumed responsibility for funds and organisation. The result was a building boom which even put the building explosion in the hospital world in the shade. Since policy on the elderly targeted the whole age category and not just the poor among them, this entire group was to be accommodated in homes that satisfied their specific needs. That implied new or renovated homes for all of the elderly whose needs had not yet been satisfied. No other country entertained such a high ambition, and nowhere was so much built for the elderly as in the Netherlands. The contours of a veritable population shift came into view. Within ten years 3,967 specific housing units for the elderly were built and 126 clusters with communal and individual facilities; 12,729 old people had found appropriate accomodation.[17] It was impossible to keep up with the demand; there were three candidates for every vacancy in an old people's home in 1958.[18]

So building proceeded apace. Between 1945 and 1964 25,006 housing units for the elderly were built; since they were usually occupied by couples, it is reasonable to assume that a maximum of 50,000 belonging to this age category could be accommodated in them. The 364 combined individual and communal clusters opened in the same period had a total capacity of 35,069 beds. A paradox of the situation was that for a long time the chronically ill and those with a mental disorder, the group most in need of care, were disregarded. Self-sufficient homes and rest homes fell under the regime of the Housing Law and benefited from the planning and funding machinery at its disposal. Nursing homes, on the other hand, had to be funded from elsewhere. It was not until the completion of the system of social security with the Exceptional Medical Expenses Act (AWBZ) of 1968 that building commenced, but within a few years the backlog had been cleared away.

Nursing homes

Since being nursed is not the same as having a home, the nursing home was excluded from the regulations that stimulated the boom of new rest homes, self-sufficient housing units and communal/individual complexes. The legislation drew a sharp distinction between the care that was provided in rest homes and the medically orientated care that was characteristic of the nursing home. Rest homes provided domestic help for the healthy elderly, while nursing homes offered light medical support for patients whose complaints were often of a chronic kind. The nursing home was thus a hospital, but lay outside the system of funding on which the building of the hospitals was based. The construction of nursing homes only became possible after the passing of the Exceptional Medical Expenses Act (AWBZ) in 1968. On the basis of the AWBZ, a rapid start was made to clear away the backlog that had existed for decades because of the almost total failure to provide any facilities for the chronically ill. If the AWBZ was the financial and administrative keystone of the welfare state, the nursing home was the crown on the architecture of the welfare state.

The period between 1969 and 1976 saw the addition of 25,000 beds in nursing homes. The nursing home for the

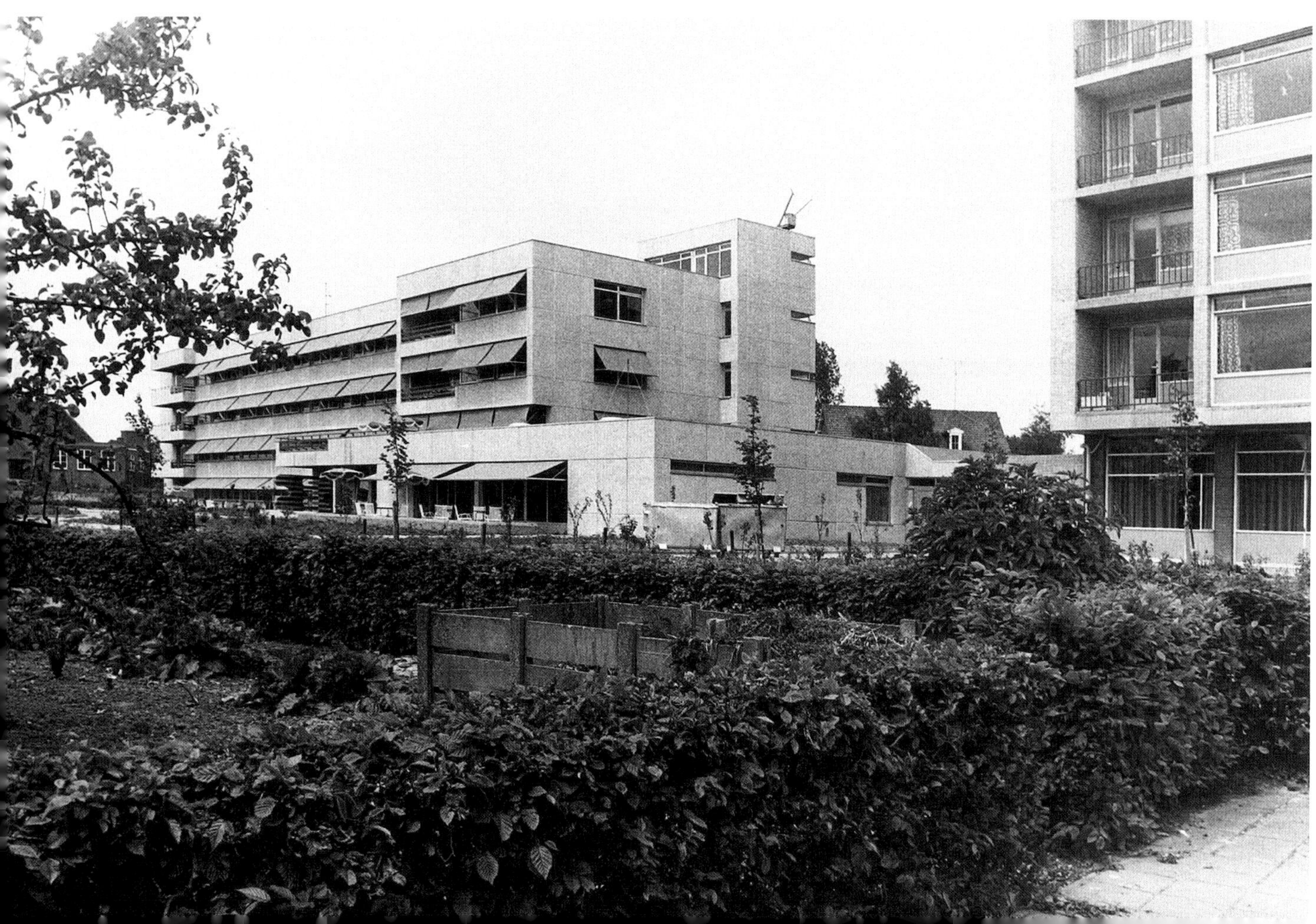

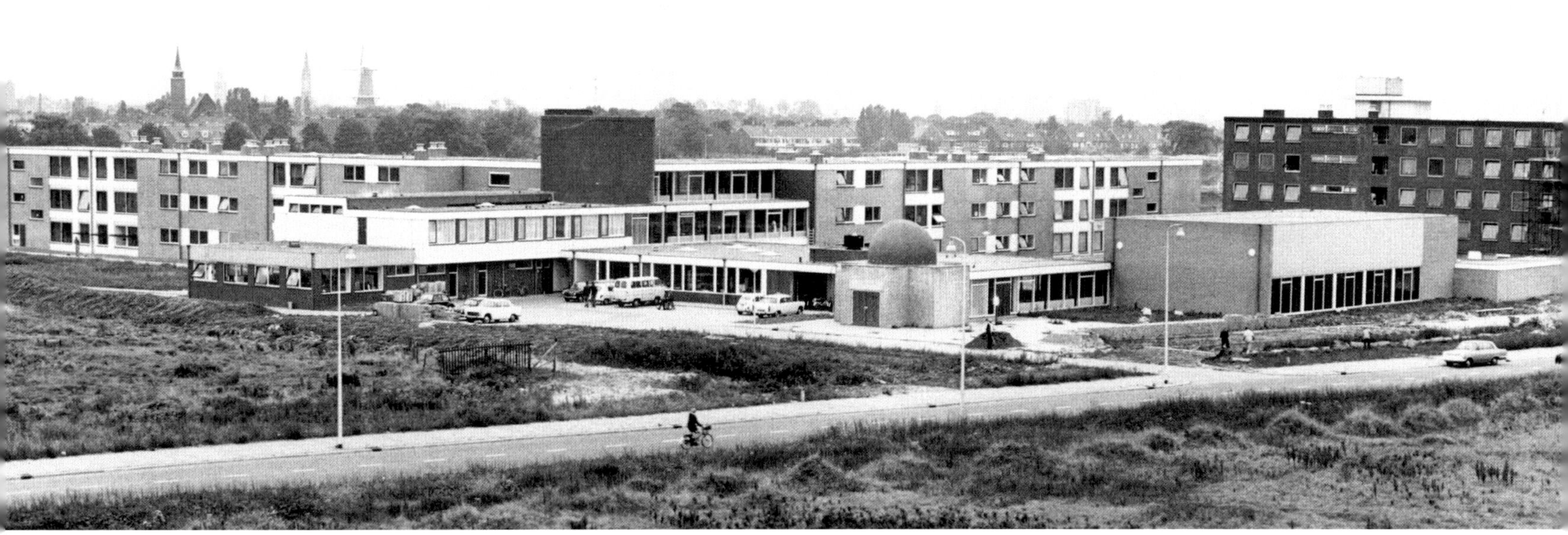

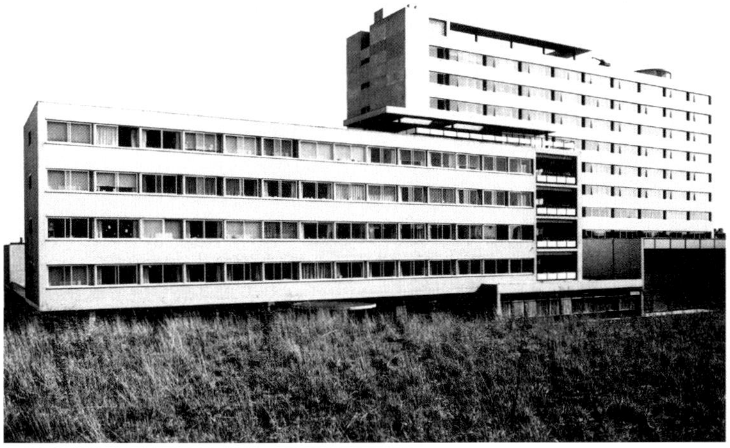

p. 132
***Bureau voor architectuur en stedebouw ir. J.J. Margry*, Sancta Maria nursing home, Zevenbergen, 1970**

p. 133
***R.H. Fledderus*, Het Zonnehuis, Vlaardingen, 1971**

***Architectenbureau Margry en Jacobs*, nursing and rest home, Amsterdam-Buitenveldert, 1969**

***G. Gerritse*, Crabbehoff nursing home, Dordrecht, 1964**

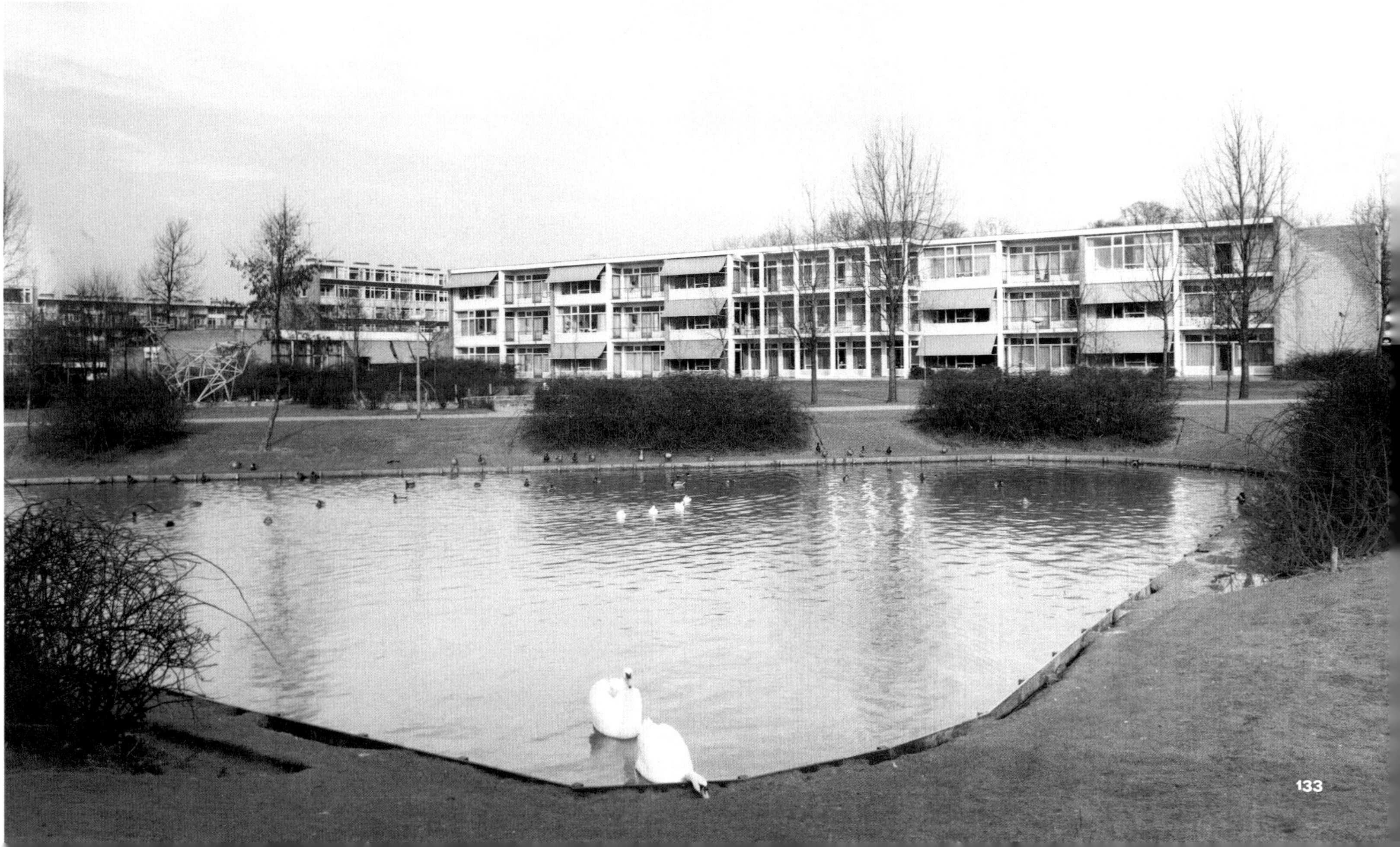

elderly is the latest newcomer on the care scene. The first in the Netherlands, Zonnehuis in Beekbergen (1929), initially targeted young people with a handicap. The number of nursing homes slowly increased in the years leading up to 1968, but by 1950 there were still less than ten of them; the total number of beds available was 1,500. Most of these nursing homes were small; only a few had between 100 and 200 beds. Only thirty years later the situation had changed completely: by then there were 47,000 beds in 330 homes; between 55 and 60 per cent of them had gone up in the seven years between 1969 and 1976.[19]

Initially the nursing home was primarily for somatic patients, old people with physical complaints who as a result were no longer capable of successfully performing the Activities of Daily Living (ADL) required for normal functioning without nursing. Psychogeriatric cases – elderly people with a mental disorder – formed a minority and hardly any specific facilities were provided for them. It was only in 1966 that that the Central Council for Public Health recommended separating the two categories: those with a mental disturbance should not be put in a nursing home. They required special homes, and if they did happen to stay in nursing homes, separate areas would have to be partitioned off for them.[20] Nursing homes were mainly wards with six or four persons and a few double or single rooms with a fairly small range of therapies aimed to reactivate the patients (reactivation was a key term in the 40s and 50s). What was the function of the nursing home? Like the hospital, it provided medical care, while like the rest home it was for residents who often spent a long time there. The first nursing homes corresponded to the hospital model with the emphasis on the reactivation of the patient. This resulted in adapted copies of the regular hospitals in this period. Wards dominate the picture; at first the nursing home was far more of a place for sleeping than the hospital was. The treatment units were relatively modest, and there were hardly any outpatient units at all. While the regular hospital of this period usually consisted of three clearly distinguished zones – wards, treatment unit and outpatient unit – the nursing home had only the first two, and the wards were dominant. Because the nursing home was still in its infancy, designing a nursing home was often preceded by wide-ranging study.

An example is the design by G. Gerritse for the Crabbehoff nursing home in Dordrecht.[21] The complex comprises not only the nursing home for 174 long-term patients but also the Vijverhof rest home, 24 self-sufficient housing units for the elderly, and a home for the nurses. The nursing home itself consists of three floors, each with two or three nursing units containing thirty beds on average. The situation of the nursing units was determined by the fact that the patients' rooms should face south and the walking distance to the centrally located general facilities should be short.[22]

In his design for Het Zonnehuis in Vlaardingen, R.H. Fledderus stated: 'It is of economic and social importance to demonstrate that the formation of the programme and the development of care for long-term patients should move in the direction of a very limited increase in the space allocated per bed. The current maxima make it very difficult for the architects to design a spatially and architecturally well-conceived building. The norms that apply at the moment lead to a time-consuming tug of war between "dream and action".'[23]

The architect pointed out that a nursing home is not a hospital, but a building in which a community is accommodated. That calls for a domestic atmosphere.[24] The nursing home has a capacity for 200 long-term patients, including 30 demented old people. There are six nursing units, five with 34 beds and one with 30 beds. Each unit also has a dayroom (living room), and there is a living room-dining room for every two units (per floor). In some nursing homes meals were served in the dayrooms, in others in the dining rooms.

As a follow-up to a rest home that had been built several years earlier, J.J. Margry designed a nursing home in Zevenbergen with a capacity of 100 beds distributed over three nursing units. The ground-floor building also contains the general facilities here.

The firm Margry en Jacobs was commissioned to design a nursing and rest home in the Buitenveldert district of Amsterdam in 1962. The second to the tenth floors of the eleven-storey tower block contain the nursing units. Each of these has 36 beds, mainly in 5-bed rooms. The treatment units are on the first floor, administration and management are on the ground floor. The rest home function is accommodated in the low-rise building around the tower with single and double room apartments, a chapel, recreation rooms and the kitchen.

The Netherlands Centre for Housing of Old People (NCHB) commissioned J.P. Kloos to design the Eduard Douwes Dekkerhuis in Amsterdam. The nursing home for 120 mentally disturbed elderly patients is separate from the rest home. Two groups of fifteen patients are accommodated on each of the four floors. The services building with administration, management, the kitchens and suchlike has only one floor.

These projects were the prelude to the major building boom that began at the end of the 60s.

Homes for the elderly

The vast majority of investments in housing for the elderly were spent on old people's homes (rest homes, centres for old people), often in combination with self-sufficient housing units that in such cases were called sheltered homes. These institutions were regarded as monuments of progress. They must give the elderly who lived there a reassuring environment amid a modernising world – of which these complexes were at the same time striking symbols. Like the self-sufficient housing units, they fell under the regime of the Ministry of Public Works and Reconstruction, the precursor of the present Ministry of Housing, Spatial Planning and Environmental Hygiene.

Financial support was not provided unless the building plans met strict criteria; after the liberation these were laid down in the well-known *Voorschriften en Wenken* (Regulations and Guidelines), which were revised at regular intervals. This guaranteed a thorough quality check for accommodation for the elderly that was implemented within the terms of the Housing Law. In 1966 these regulations and guidelines for the building of old people's homes were detached from those for regular social housing. The aim was 'to raise the housing level appreciably and to promote industrialisation and prefabrication by standardisation'.[25]

The size of the apartments remained very small: a bed-sitter for a pensioner could not be more than twelve square metres, a bedroom was set at six square metres, a living room for two pensioners at fourteen, and a double bedroom at ten. An apartment measuring twenty-four square metres was thus quite large by these standards. Only ten per cent of the rooms were for couples. If the apartments did not have their own bath or shower, there had to be a communal bath for every twelve units. Each floor had to have a balcony of at least five square metres unless the rooms had their own balconies. In spite of the minimal dimensions of the housing units – the term that became fashionable in the second half of the 60s – the complexes could be quite considerable because of the large concentration of apartments and the shared facilities. The total size of an old people's home, however, was limited to the number of beds times forty square metres.[26]

In terms of typology, there are similarities to the hospitals of the reconstruction period. The early and generally speaking smaller examples often consist of a combination of various wings in the form of a T, an H, a U, or grouped around a courtyard and variants of this. The general functions were generally given a central position, while the old people's apartments and the nursing units were in the various wings. Larger homes were often high-rise, with the tower block placed on top or next to a flat building (the tower on podium type). The rooms were located in the tower block and the general functions in the flat building.

The Schoorwijck old people's centre in Leidschendam (1962-1964) designed by W. & W.H. Verschoor consists of a rectangular main building of six storeys, with two low-rise wings at right angles to one of the ends. The shorter wing on the west side contains a ward for patients and a mortuary. The longer wing accommodates the main entrance, which leads to a wide corridor flanked by the service areas and rooms for management and administration. At the end of this wing are the dining and recreation room and the kitchens, followed by a row of five blocks of apartments, each with three housing units for the elderly.

Work on designing the old people's centre in Zwanenburg (1950-1965) began in 1950 by J.P. Kloos with Brakel en Buma. Sixteen bungalows and a block of eight gallery access apartments were built for self-sufficient old people. The home consists of a wing with gallery access apartments

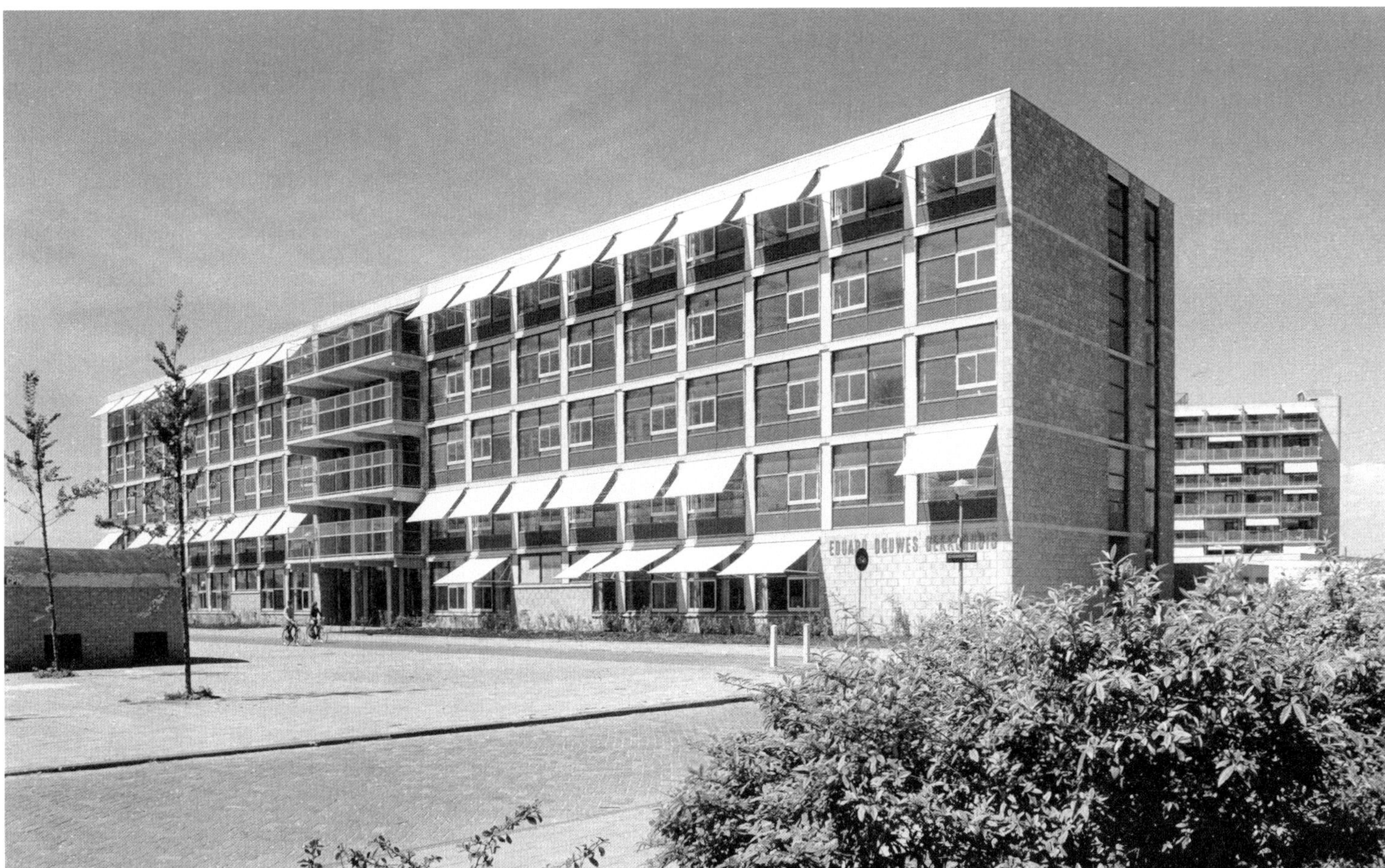

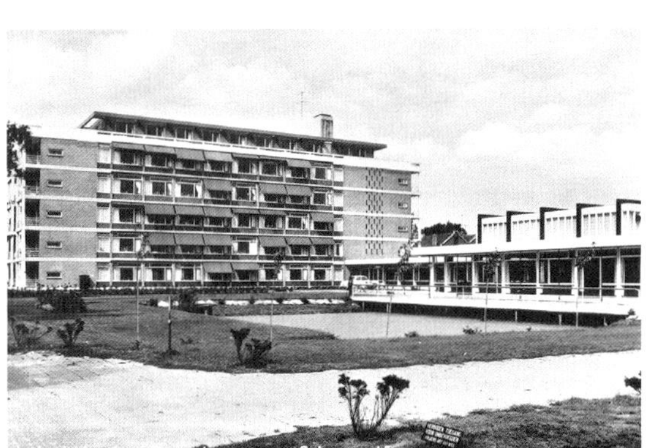

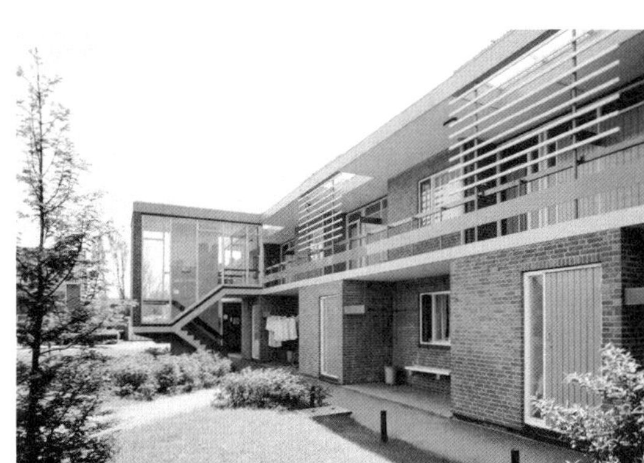

***J.P. Kloos*, Eduard Douwes Dekkerhuis, Amsterdam, 1975**

***W. Verschoor & W.H. Verschoor*, Schoorwijck old people's centre, Leidschendam, 1964**

***J.P. Kloos with Brakel en Buma*, old people's centre, Zwanenburg, 1965**

and a patients wing. The recreation room and the kitchen complex are wedged in between these wings. This central position entails a reduction of service distances to a minimum.

The Dutch Reformed Transwijk centre for old people in Utrecht (1959-1966) by Architectenbureau H.A. en ir. G. Pothoven was designed for three categories of elderly people: those who were fit but could not take care of themselves, those who were less fit, and those who were fit and could take care of themselves. The structure was determined by the first and largest category in the old people's home. This had an East-West orientation so that, by building the rooms on either side of a corridor, every room would have sun at some time of the day. There is a wing on either side of the home, one with nursing units for the less fit elderly and general amenities, and one with apartments for self-sufficient residents.

De Nudehof old people's home in Wageningen (1959-1966) designed by the Rietveld, Van Dillen en Van Tricht consists of three wings arranged in a U shape: a short wing with flats for self-sufficient pensioners, and two other wings with single and double rooms, the personnel rooms, recreation and conversation rooms, a sick bay, kitchens and other service areas.

De Golfslag old people's home (1966-1970) was designed by A. Bonnema in a Modernist style that refers to the architecture of Le Corbusier. A high-rise block on seven-metre columns is placed at right angles on top of a low-rise block. The high-rise block contains the apartments for the elderly, which are accessed via a corridor on the north side that widens out at some points to form a bay. The north and south wings have continuous strips of windows. The low-rise building contains the main entrance, a recreation room, facility maintenance services, a nursing unit and personnel areas. At one end of the high-rise block is a roof construction with a relaxation area and a roof terrace.

It is noteworthy that the complex with individual and communal facilities and the high-rise old people's home offered ideal urban planning accents. High-rise buildings were a welcome change in the new residential areas dominated by one-family homes and gallery access flats. One of the first examples appeared in Gorinchem. Designed by S.J. van Embden, it was built between 1954 and 1961. The pioneer was the local authority, which wanted to underline its forward-looking image.

***A. Bonnema*, De Golfslag old people's home, Emmeloord, 1970**

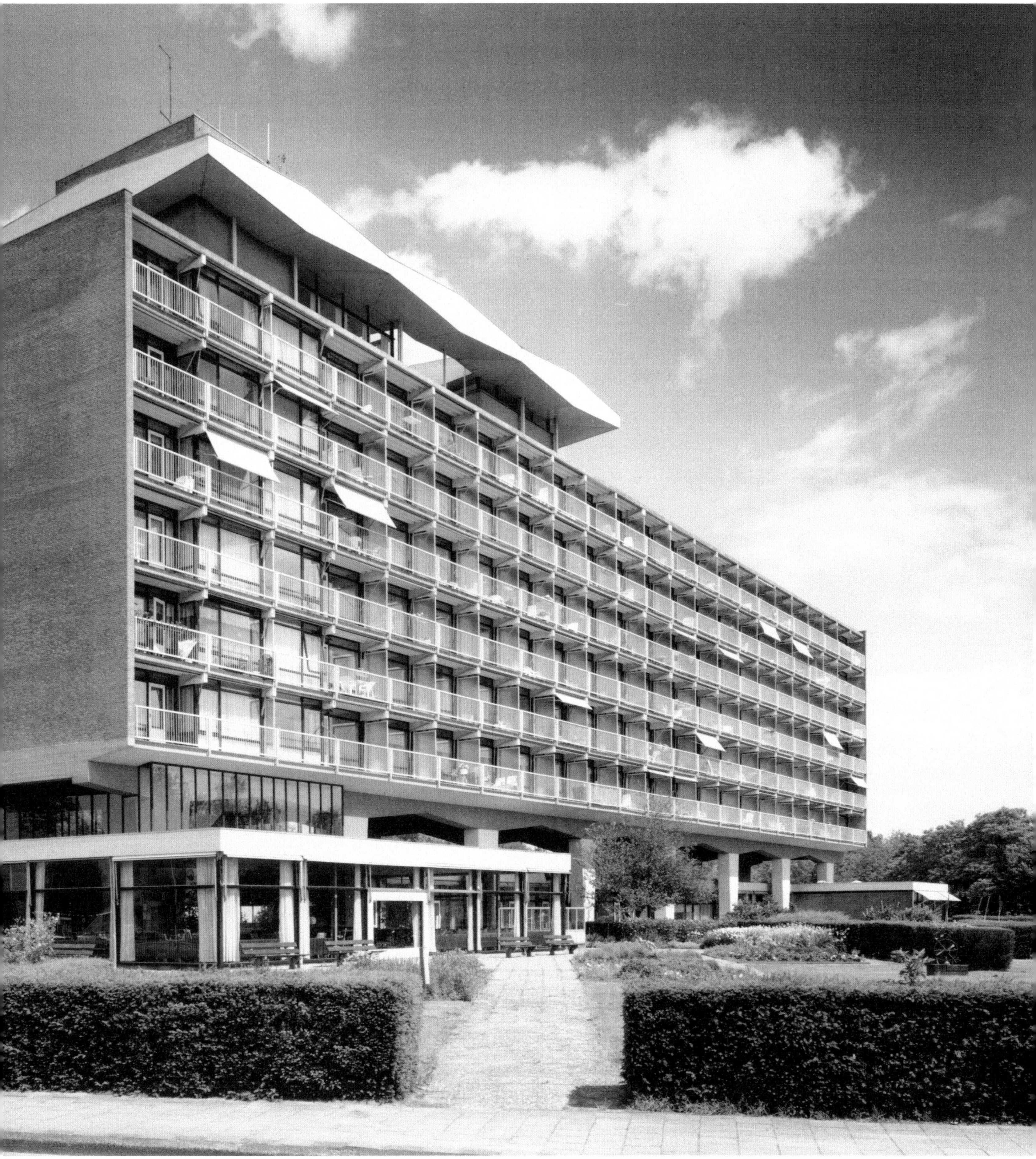

Skyscraper

S.J. van Embden

Old people's home
Hagemuntstraat
Gorinchem
1954-1961

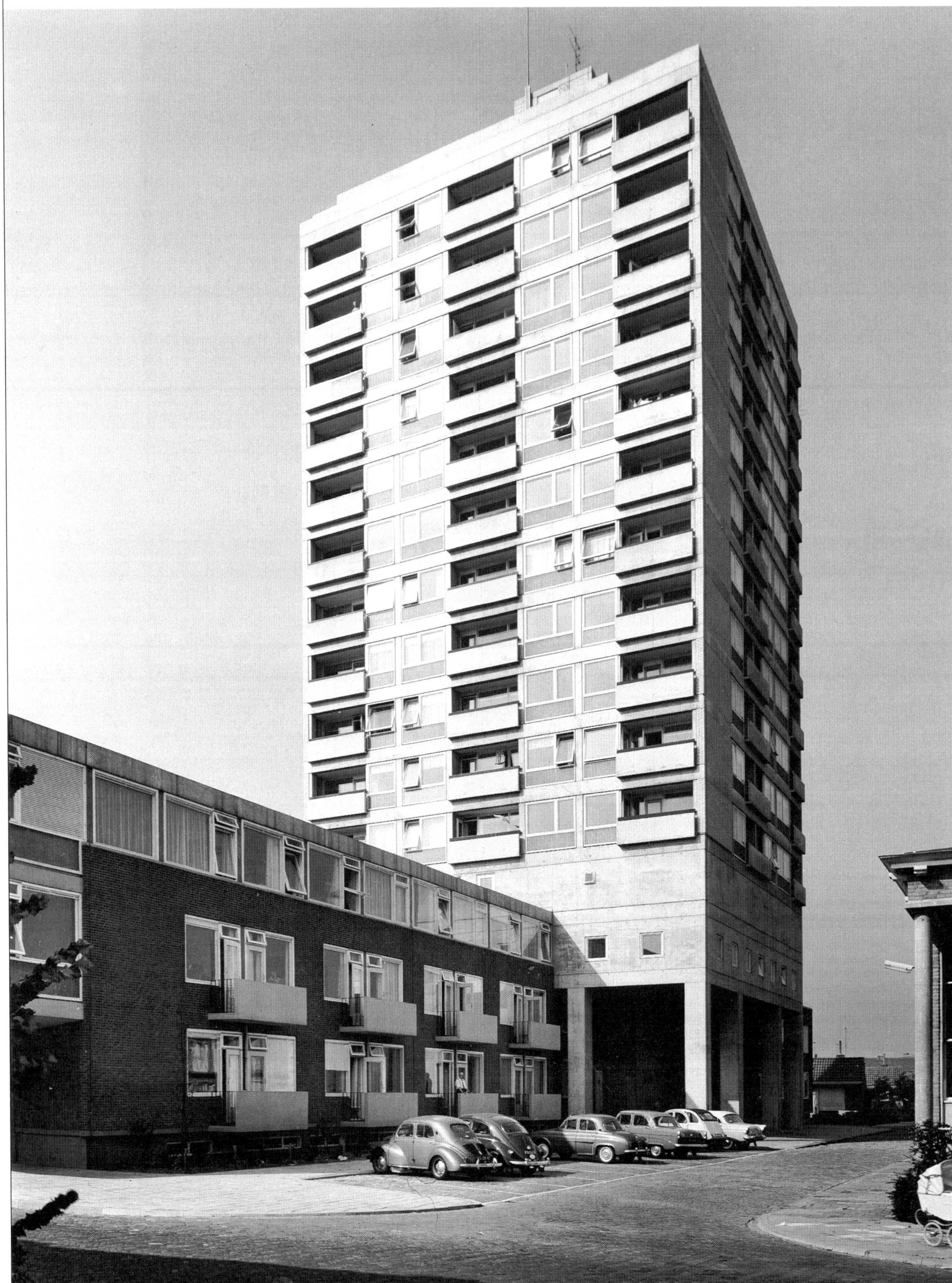

In 1954 S.J. van Embden was commissioned to design a residential district (Haarwijk plan) in Gorinchem. The Housing Inspectorate imposed the condition that an old people's home must be added. The local authority also wanted to include the 'Skyscraper' in the plan. The result was an old people's home consisting of three wings and a 51-metre tower block at the point where the three wings meet. The lower south wing of the home has three storeys and comprises fifty single and four double rooms. The one-storey wing on the east side of the tower block accommodates the main entrance, a restaurant and kitchen. The short two-storey wing on the north side contains living quarters for the director and concierge, the sick bay and the mortuary.

The tower block situated at the point where the three wings meet has a total of fifty-five apartments on the fifth to the fifteenth floors. This part has a central well with the staircase and the lifts. They provide access to the galleries on the floors leading to the apartments. There are two 4-room and two 3-room apartments at the corner of each floor. There is a 1-room apartment between the 4-person rooms on the south side. The fourth floor accommodates the storage areas for the flats, and the sixteenth floor, which is set slightly back, has a restaurant with kitchen.

The core of the upper floors is a shaft of reinforced concrete that is connected with the columns via an intermediate construction (also of reinforced concrete). The reinforced concrete floors rest on these columns in the external walls. They are not equidistant from one another; their distribution follows the arrangement of the apartments.

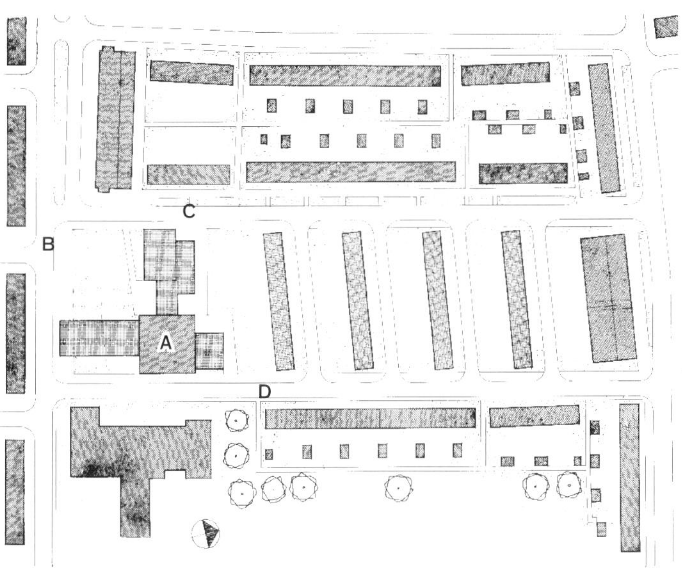

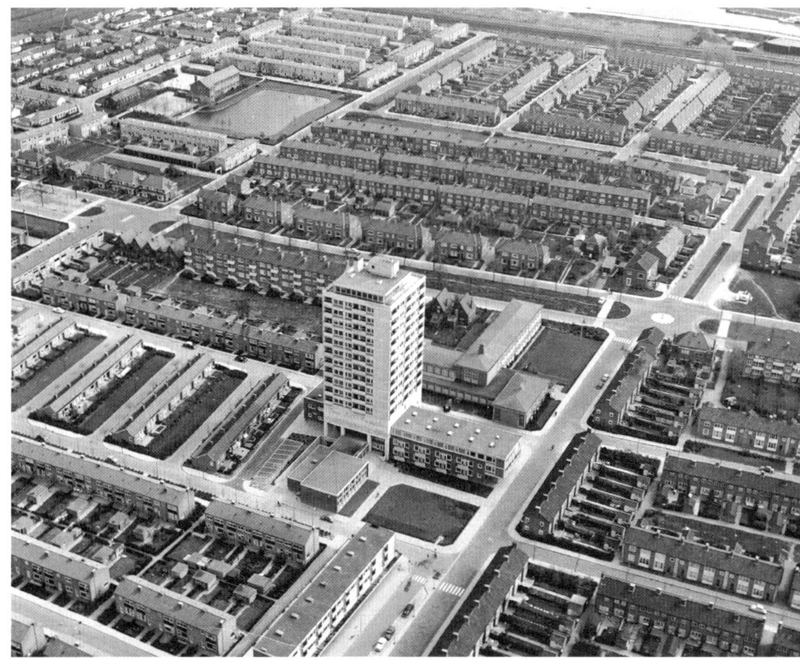

Situation
A *home for the elderly*
B *Koningin Wilhelminalaan*
C *Hagemuntstraat*
D *Don Antoniostraat*

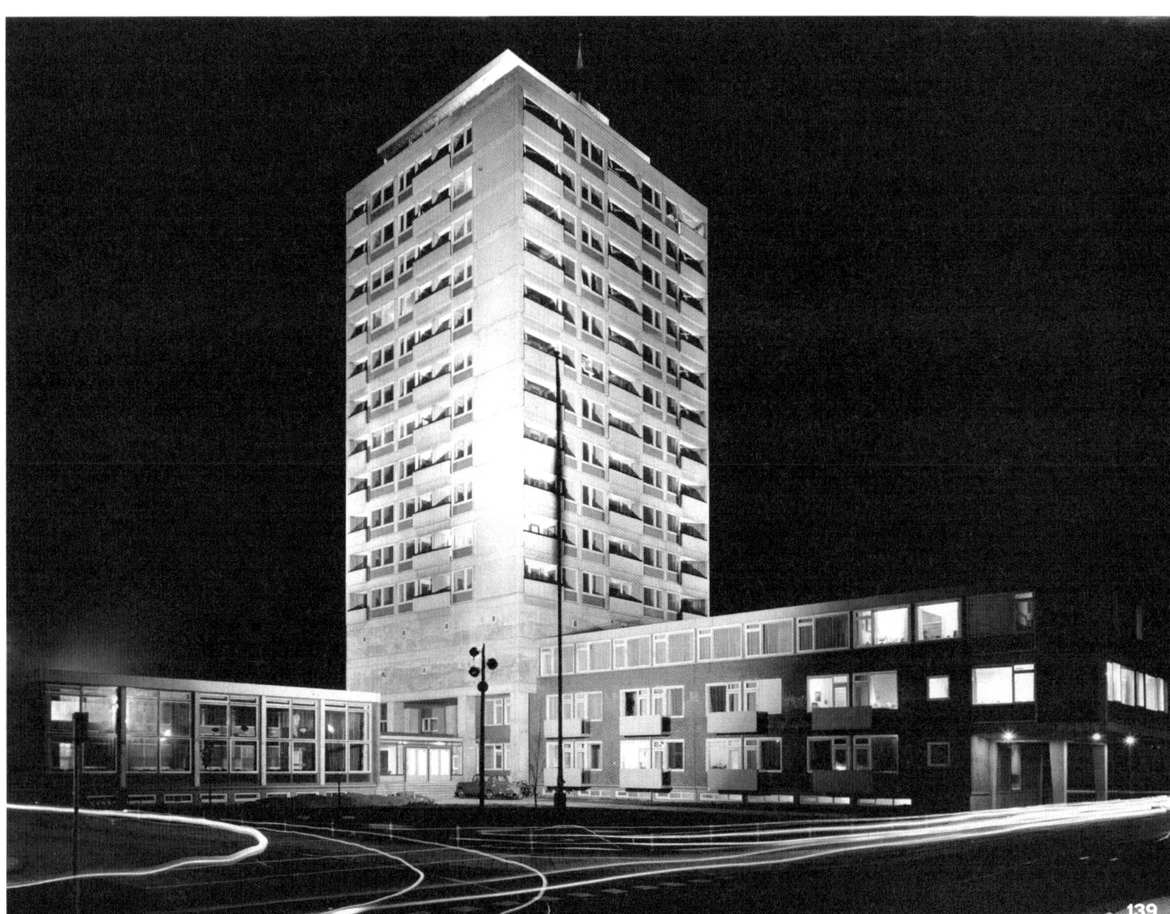

K

Architectenbureau B.J.K. Cramer
en J.E. Kruisheer

Diaconessenhuis
Leiden
1952-1963

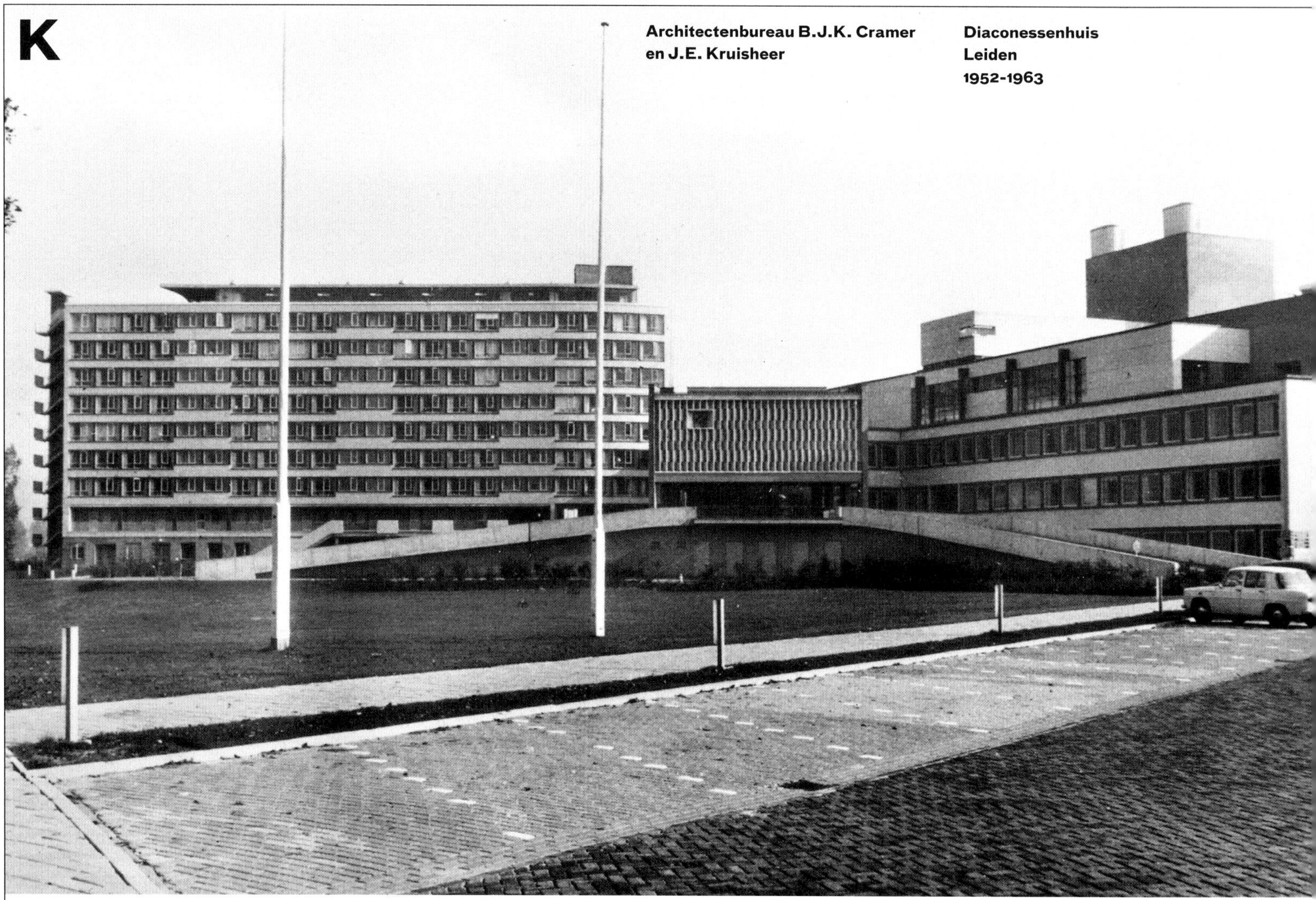

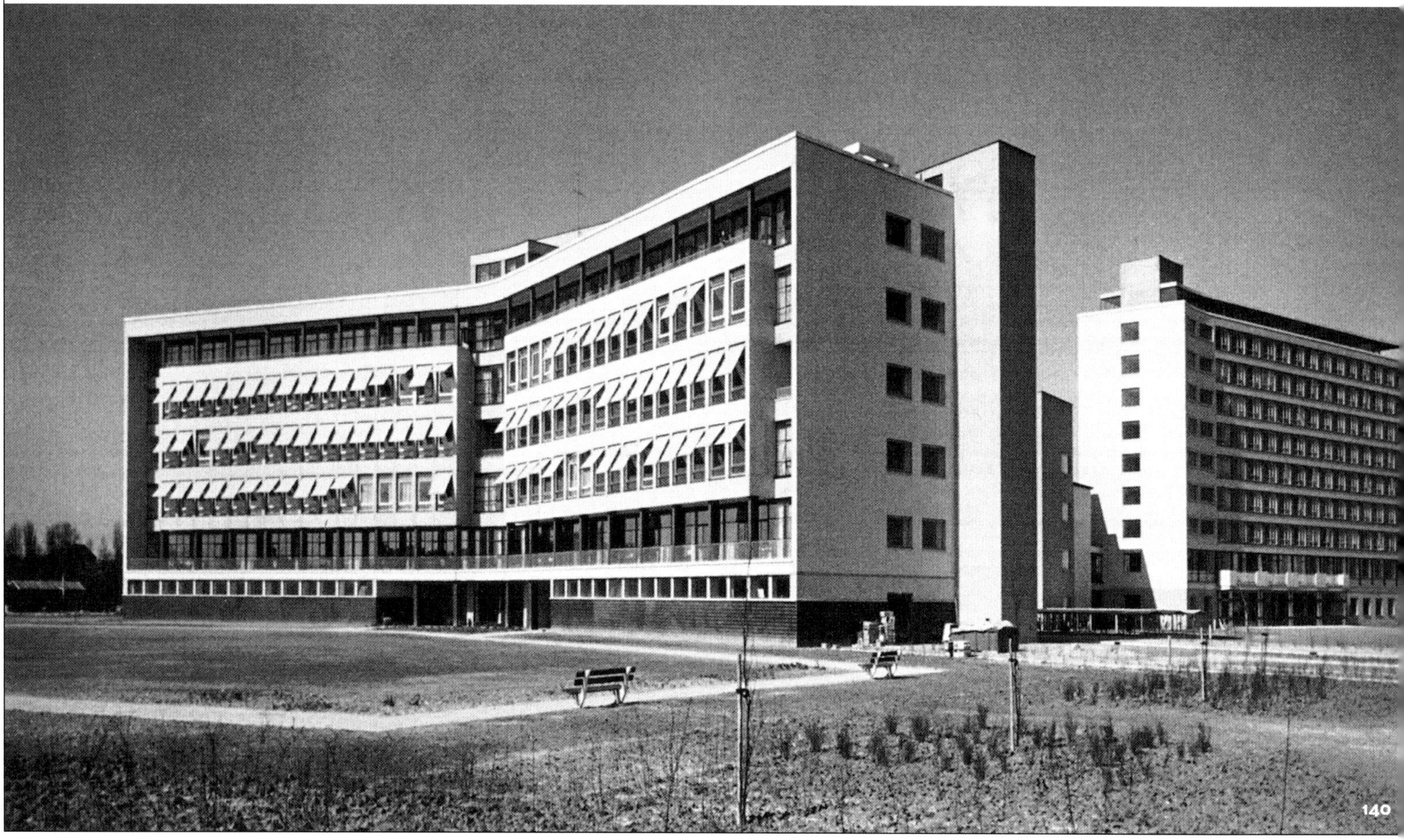

With their design for the Diaconessenhuis, the architects demonstrated that a hospital could still be a representative public building in the 1950s and 1960s. The design is rich in details and has a pronounced modern, monumental appearance. The most striking is the central entrance in front of the treatment unit. It is situated on the first floor beneath the chapel, which stands on pilotis. The main entrance is reached by car via a ramp, beneath which storage depots are situated.

The complex follows the K-type structure, a variant of the H-type, both of which are also known as the block type. The functions such as nursing, treatment and general functions are accommodated in separate volumes. The composition of the building elements is explicitly derived from the organisation of the hospital. In the case of the K-type, the two wings of the ward unit display a slight bend in relation to one another.

In the Diaconessenhuis the treatment unit at the front is linked to the ward unit by means of a central connecting corridor. This runs from the chapel through the treatment unit to the ward unit and accommodates the central services such as the outpatient units, the X-ray unit, the operating unit, the administration, and the kitchens. Besides the bend in the ward unit, which produces more space and light, the articulation of the façade is striking. It is set in a broad surround. On the second, third and fourth floors the façade juts out slightly at the level of the wards, thereby creating space for balconies on the first and fifth floors.

The block of nurses' flats is parallel to the ramp. Like the chapel, this building is set at a slight angle to the treatment unit, which the block smoothly joins via a curved bend. An attractive canopy crowns the ten-storey nurses' block, which is the largest building of the complex.

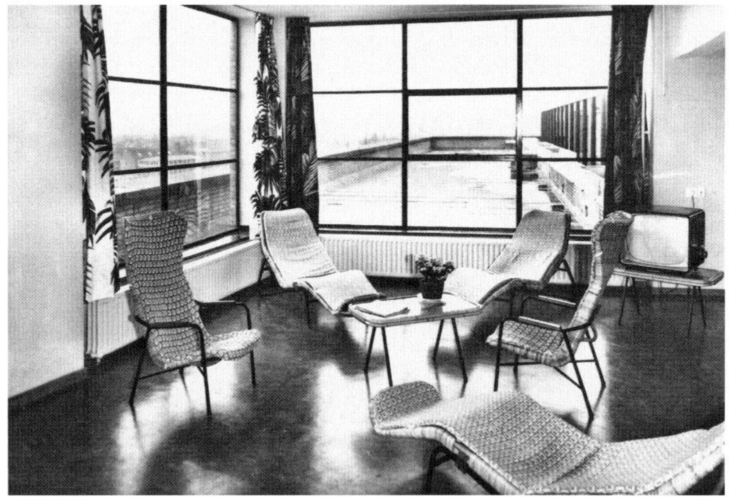

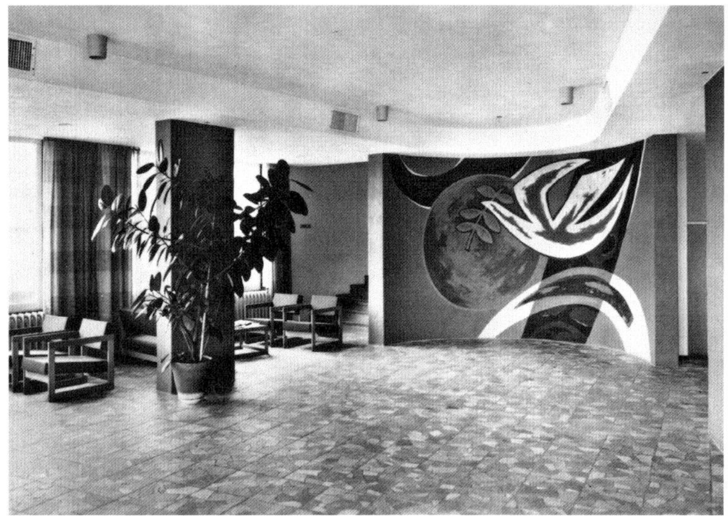

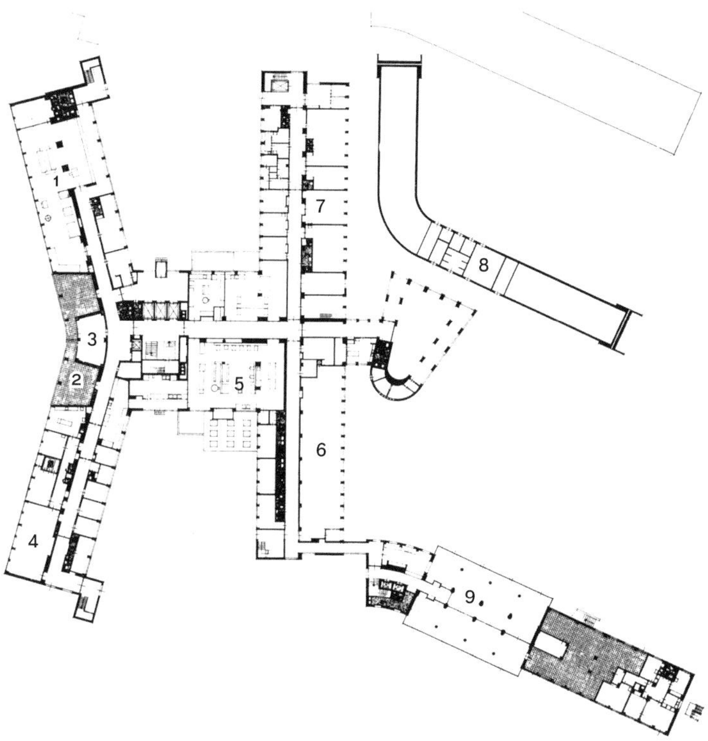

Ground floor
1 *laundry*
2 *loggia*
3 *classroom*
4 *auditorium*
5 *kitchens*
6 *storage*
7 *technical services*
8 *storage*
9 *dining and living room for nurses*

Structure
A *main entrance*
B *treatment area*
C *ward*
D *chapel*
E *nurses' dormitory*

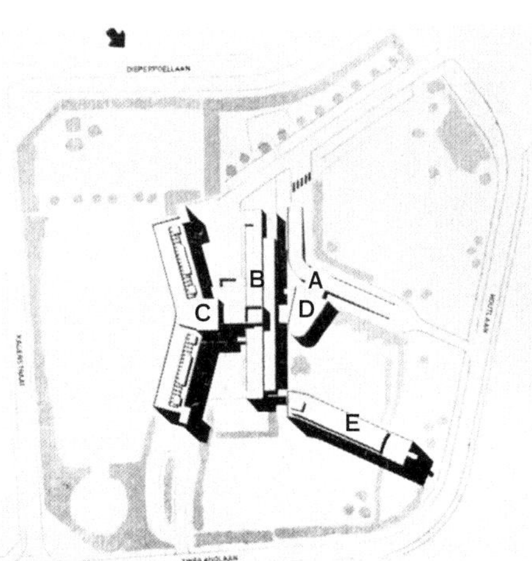

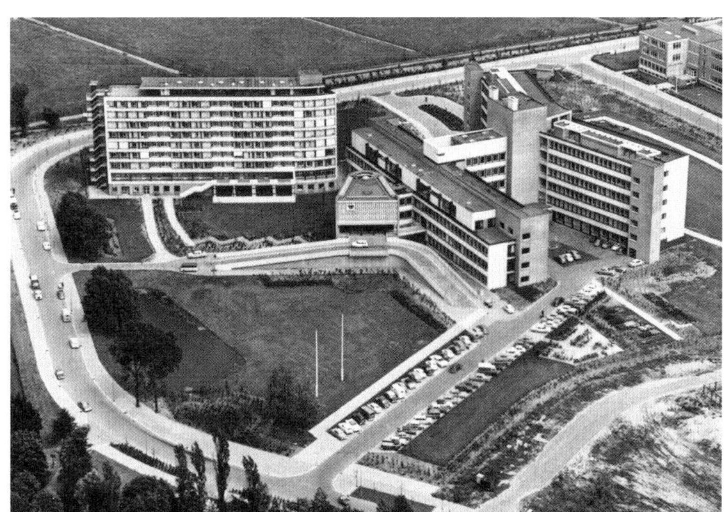

Tower on a podium

W.F. Lughart

Diaconessenhuis
Eindhoven
1956-1966

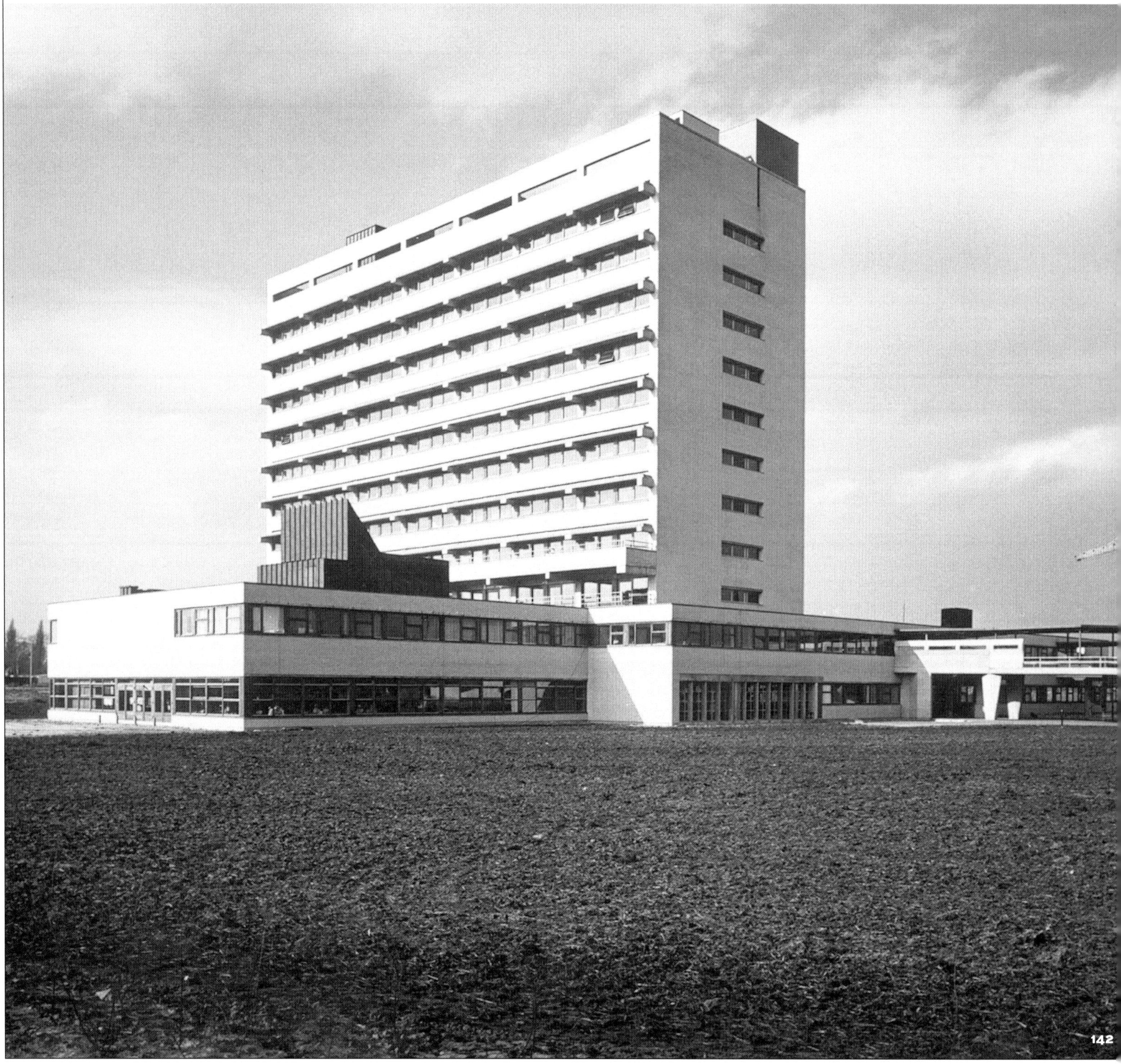

The Diaconessenhuis in Eindhoven is regarded as the first example of a tower on a podium hospital in the Netherlands. From the 1950s on this became *the* hospital type and was widely applied both in the Netherlands and abroad. Characteristic of this type is the distinction between the dynamic units, which are in need of constant modification and extension, and the more static treatment unit.

The Eindhoven Diaconessenhuis is exemplary of this type. A nine-storey ward block is placed on top of a two-storey flat and broad wedge. The ground floor accommodates the administration, management, kitchens, entrance and technical unit. The medical floor above accommodates the research and treatment unit, the outpatient clinics, the hospital admission desk and first aid. The main entrance is on a raised forecourt immediately in front of this medical floor. It is accessible for ambulances by means of a gently sloping ramp, a common feature of hospital architecture in the 1960s.
In accordance with the assignment, the hospital capacity can be expanded from 300 to 600 beds, provided that the structure of the building is not fundamentally affected as a result. Traffic flows to and from the clinical and outpatient units should be kept separate from one another as much as possible, and walking distances must be short.

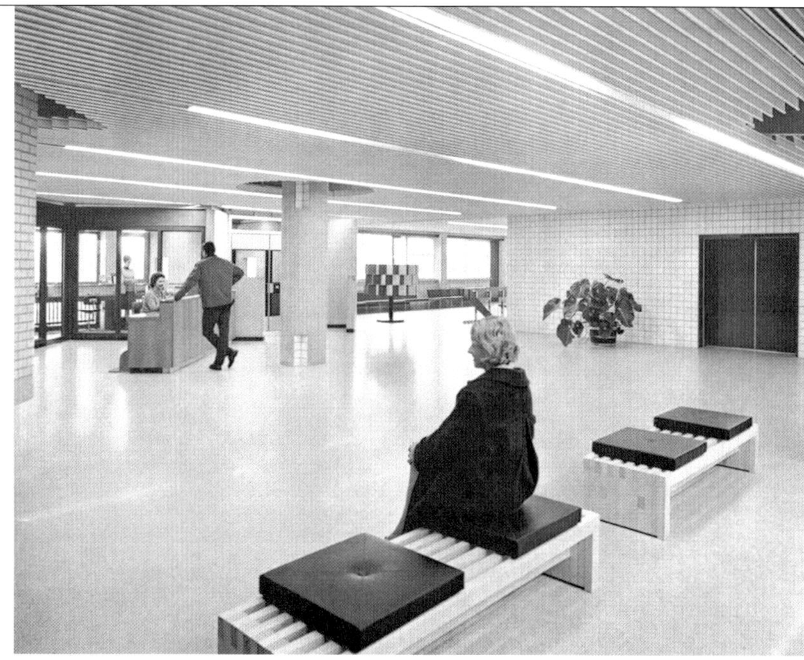

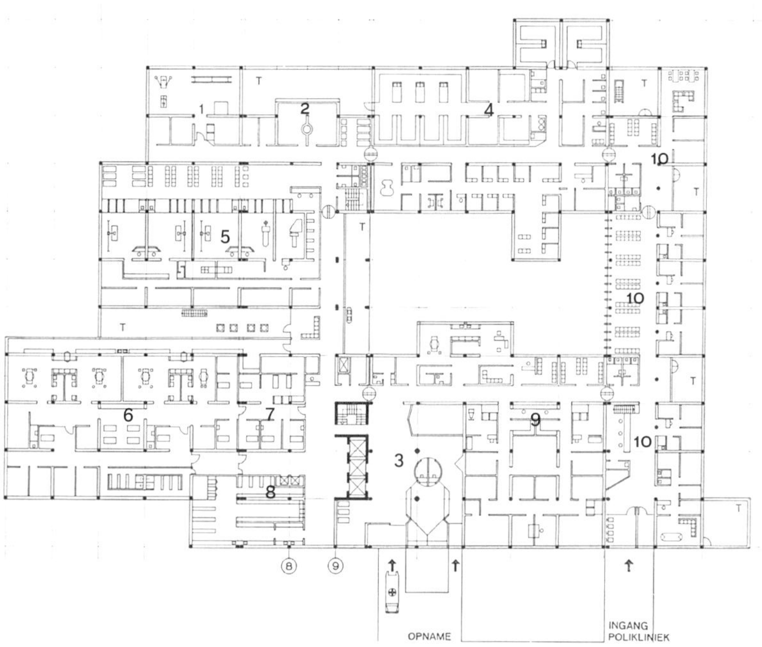

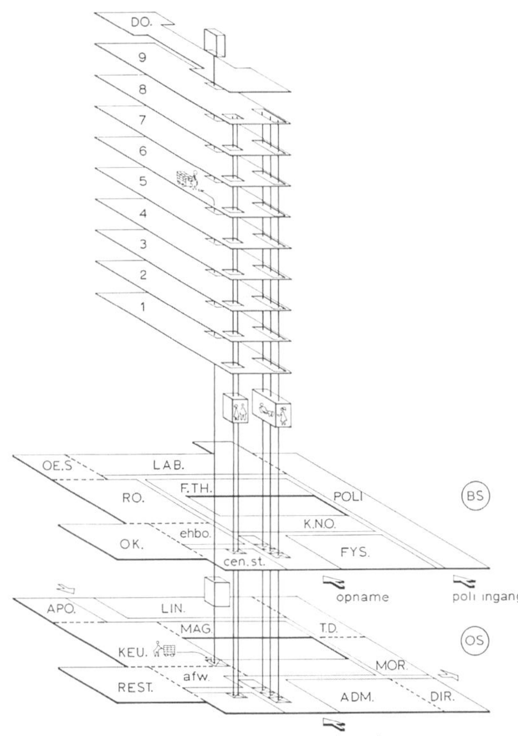

First floor
1 *fysiotherapy*
2 *clinical psychologist*
3 *reception with elevators leading to the ward*
4 *laboratory*
5 *X-ray unit*
6 *operating room*
7 *first aid and transfusion*
8 *central sterilisation*
9 *throat, nose and ear department*
10 *outward patient departments*

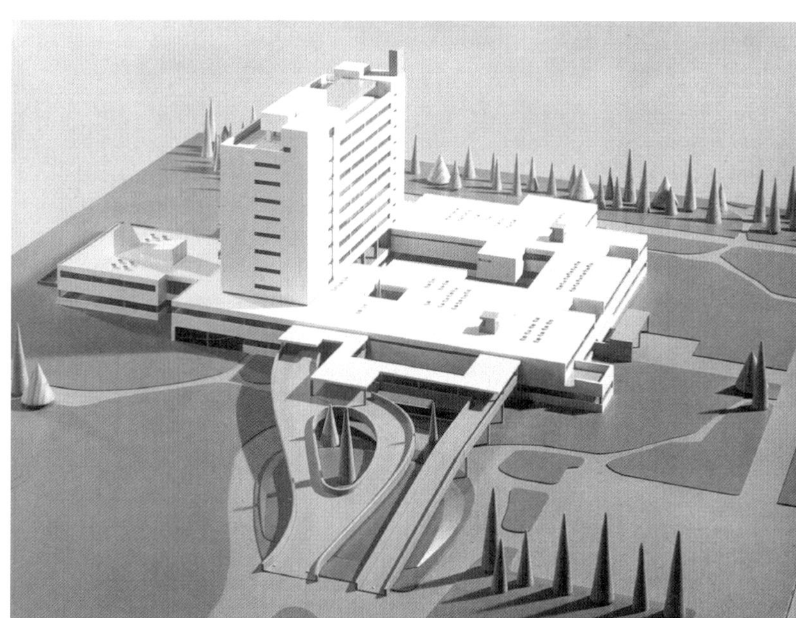

Glass

Rietveld, Van Dillen en Van Tricht

De Nudehof old people's centre
Wageningen
1959-1966

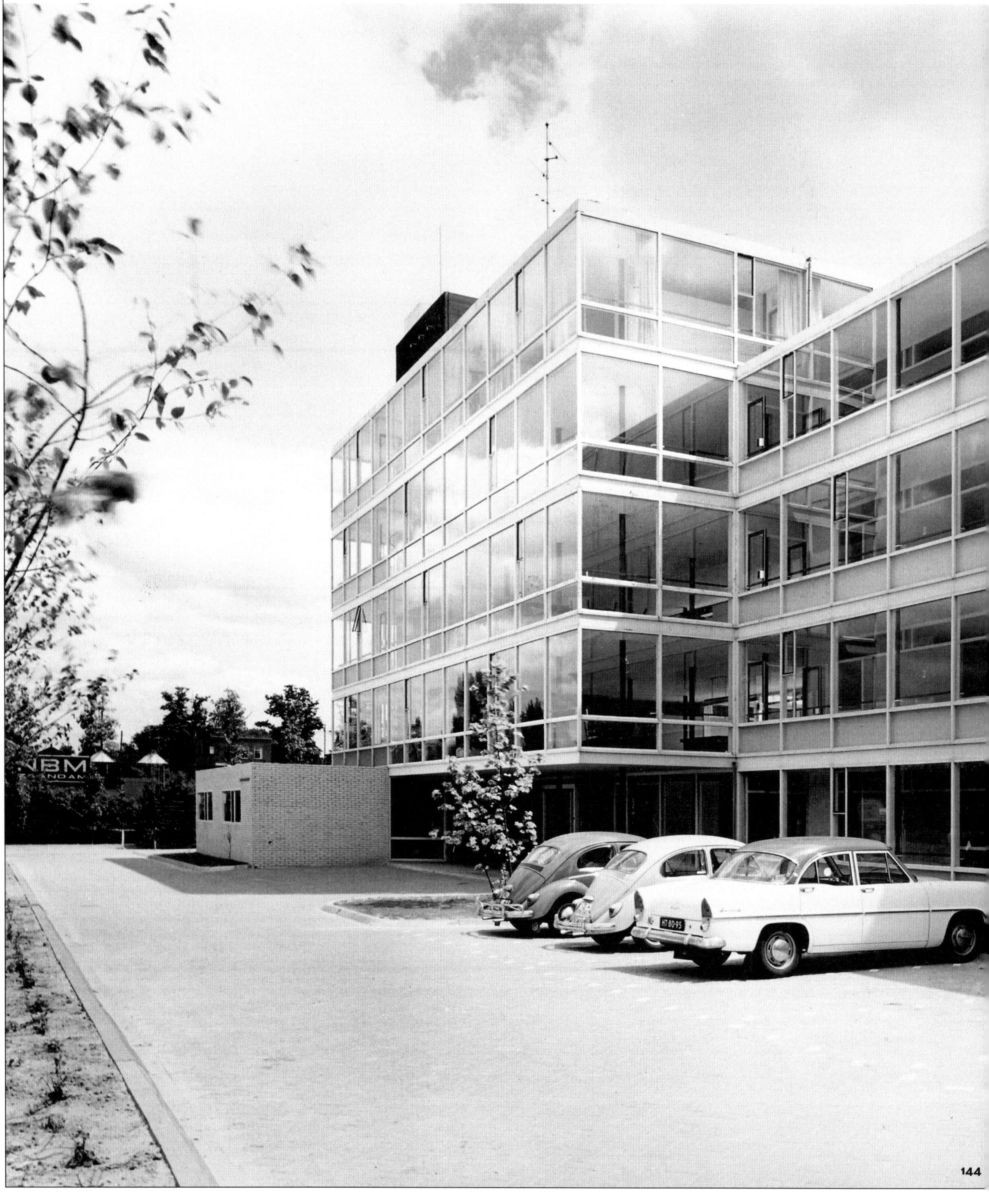

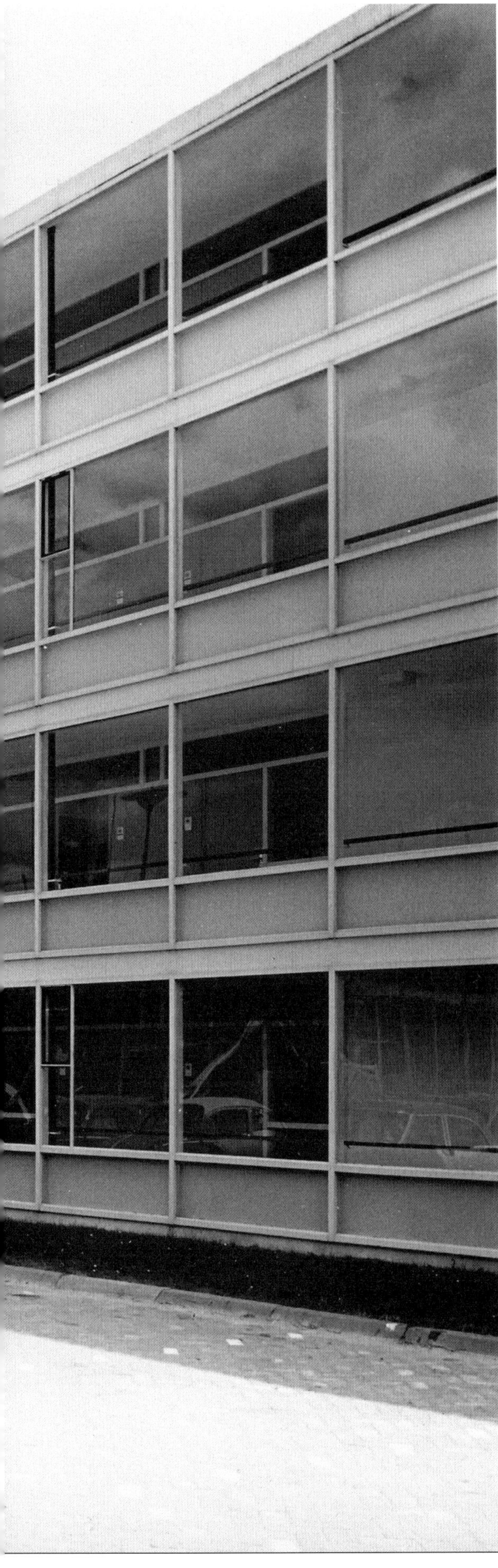

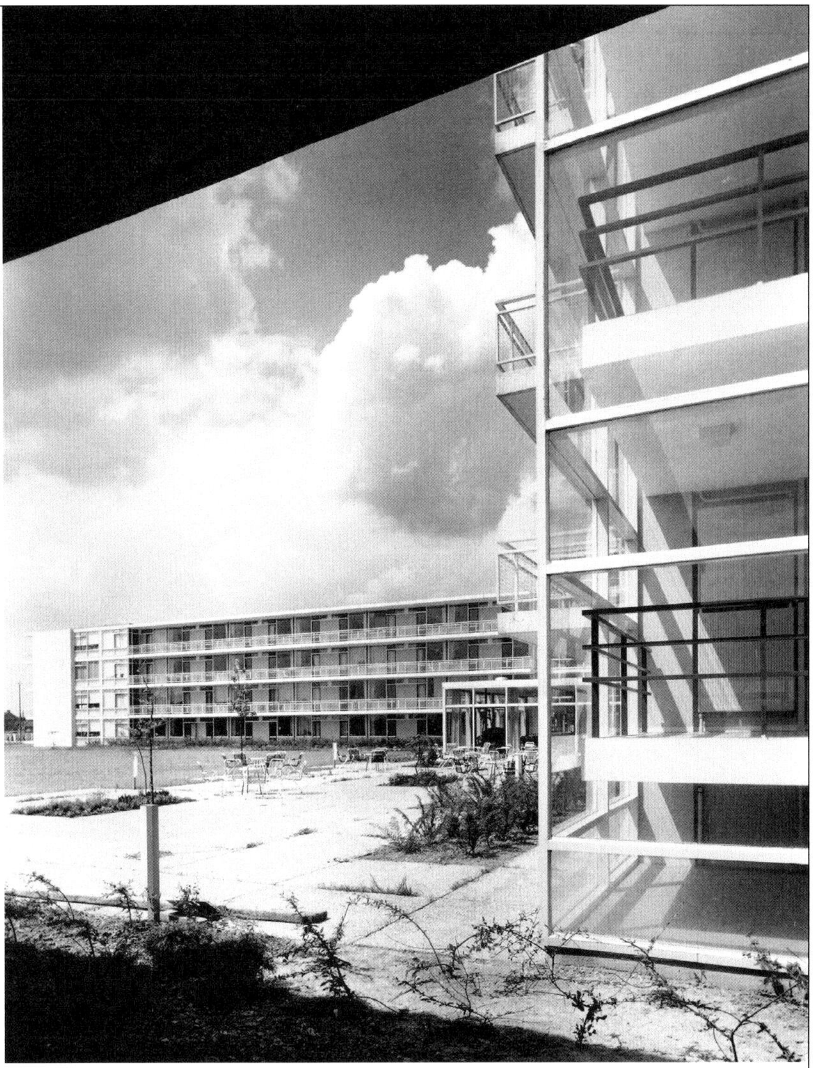

The complex, designed to house 127 elderly people, consists of three wings that combine to form a U-shape: a short two-storey wing, a five-storey wing in the middle, and a long four-storey wing. The short wing comprises twelve apartments for elderly people who are able to live by themselves. The other two wings contain the single and double rooms, the staff rooms, recreation and conversation rooms, sick bays, kitchens and other service areas. There is a slightly higher central section at the point where these wings meet. This accommodates the main entrance and the vertical connections.

The façades have a predominantly horizontal articulation. They are of white and dark blue brickwork and have wooden frames with a relatively large glass surface. These elements give the building a fresh and modern look.

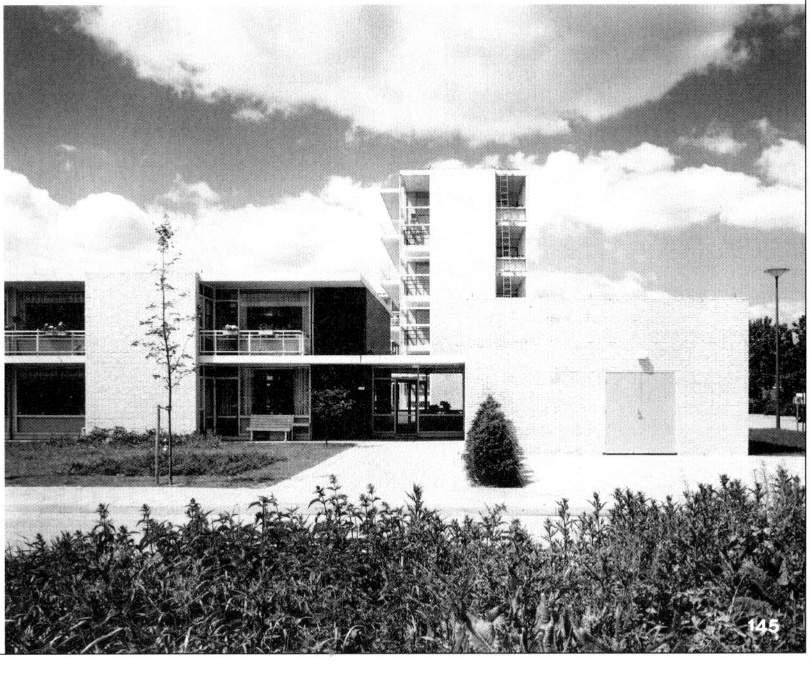

Circuit

L.A. van den Bosch
& J.P.L. Hendriks

Sint Franciscushof
psychiatric hospital
Raalte
1952-1970

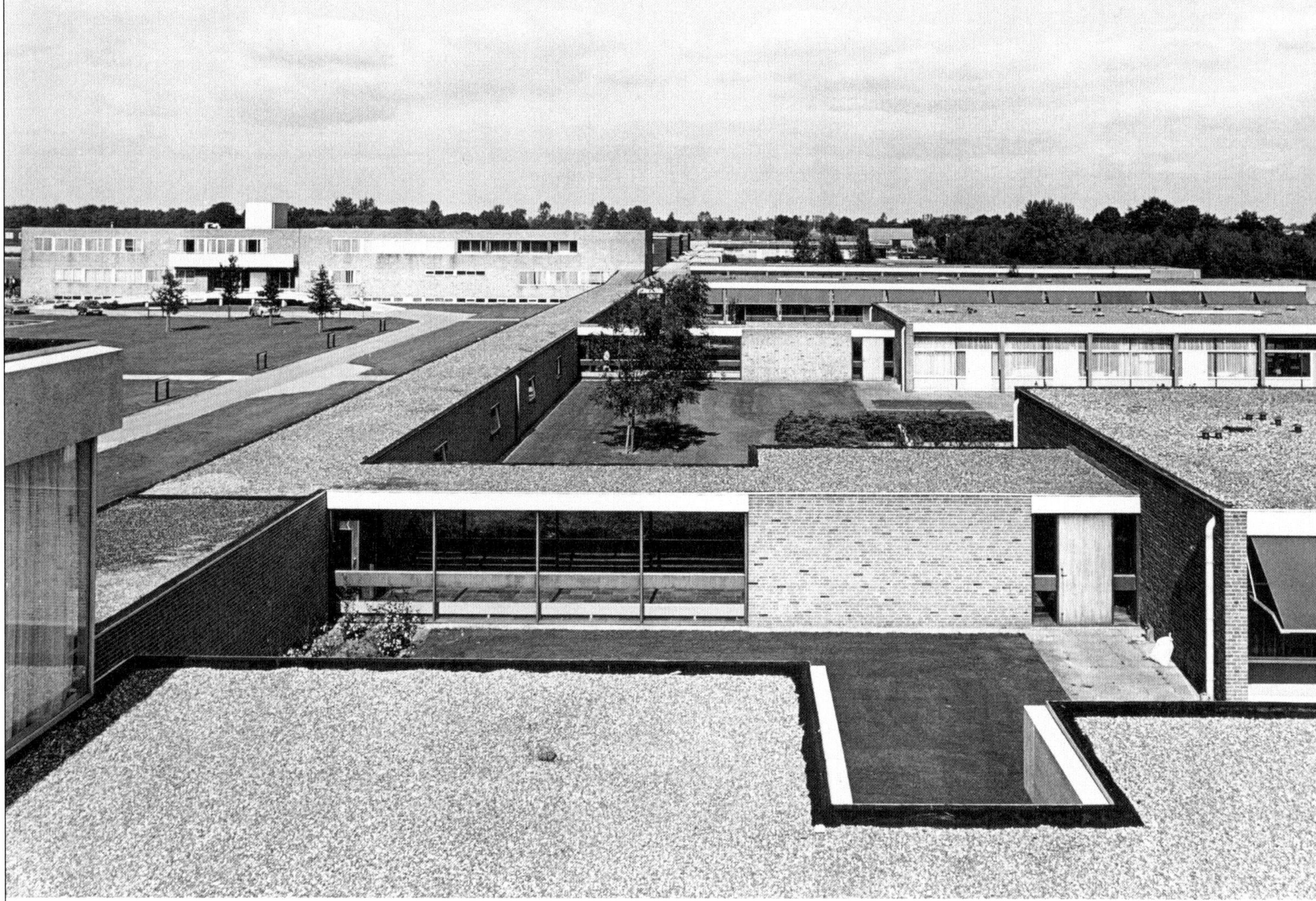

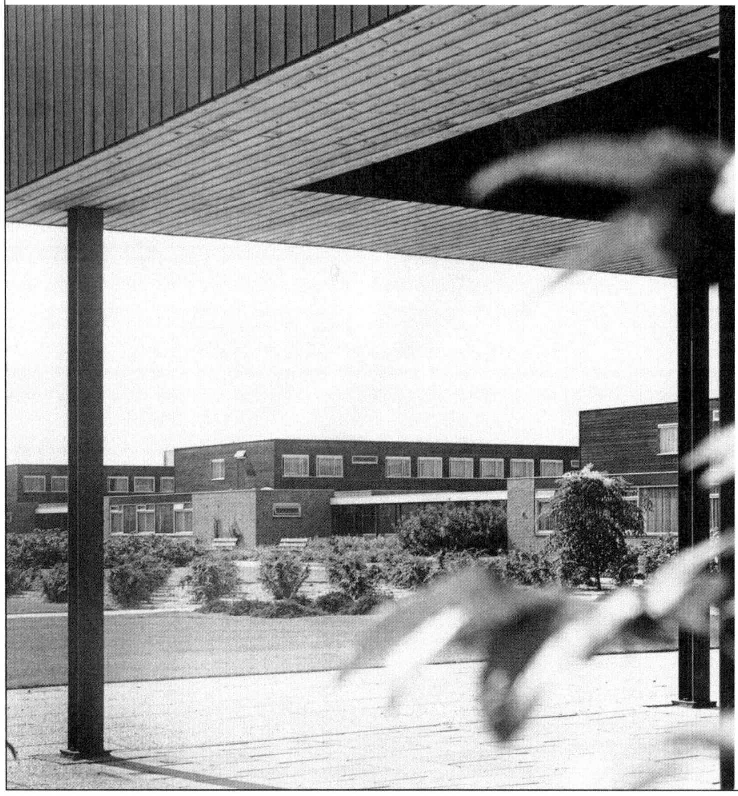

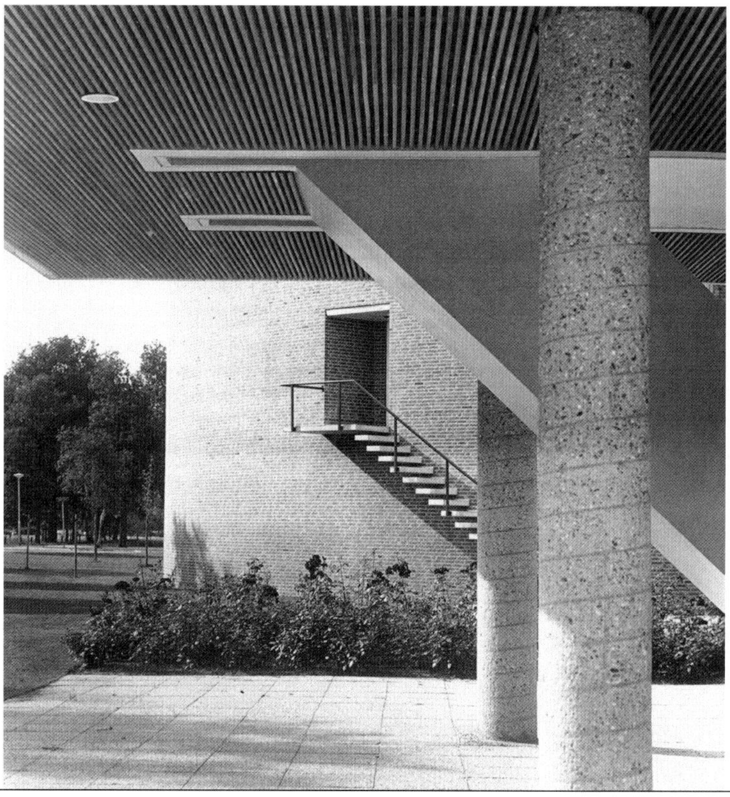

The Sint Franciscushof is distinguished by the assignment to create a community that hardly differs from life outside the hospital. The pavilions are arranged in a circuit behind one another and are arranged according to the stages of the healing process. A long corridor with a glass wall on one side forms the link between the pavilions. At the start are two nursing pavilions for patients with a physical complaint and two observation pavilions. Each pavilion is intended for four groups of eight patients. These are followed by the residential pavilions, each of which can accommodate thirty-two patients. They are two-storey buildings with four living rooms with corners for sitting and eating, a television room, a kitchen, a laundry and ironing room, an area for work therapy and an isolation room all on the ground floor. Between the residential pavilions there is a one-floor pavilion for forty geriatric patients.

In the middle of the connecting corridor is the medical administrative centre on two floors. This is where the outpatients unit, the treatment rooms, the offices of the specialists and the administrative staff, the dispensary, the laboratory and the X-ray unit are to be found. At the start of the connecting corridor is a community centre. The library, hairdresser, manicurist, kiosk and meditation room are grouped around a light well.

The paramedical centre with buildings for work, movement and creative therapy is located on the opposite side of a large lawn. The technical centre with the central kitchen, boiler house, storage depots, transformer kiosk and technical service are also situated there.

On the edge of the terrain are four bungalows where the patients can prepare for their return to society.

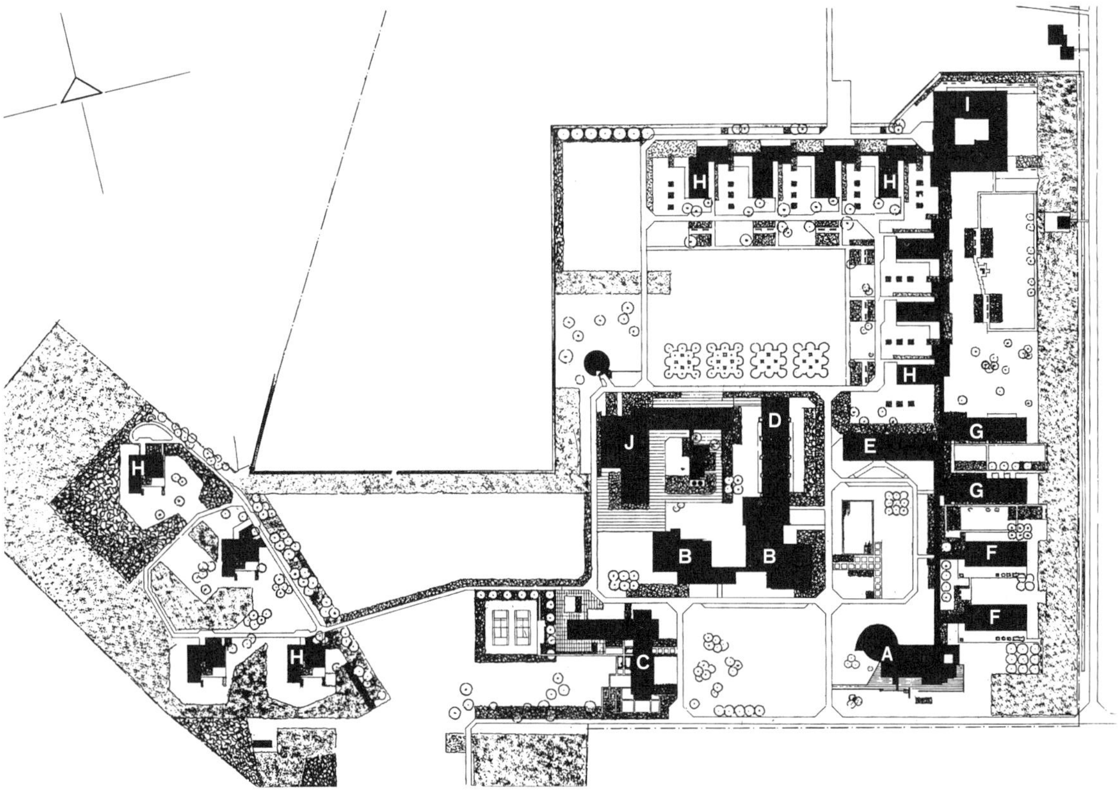

Situation
A *community centre*
B *building for physiotherapy and labour therapy*
C *nurses' dormitory*
D *labour therapy*
E *medical admistrative centre*
F *pavilion for ill patients*
G *observation pavilion*
H *housing pavilion*
I *pavilion for geriatric patients*
J *service buildings*

Ground floor community centre

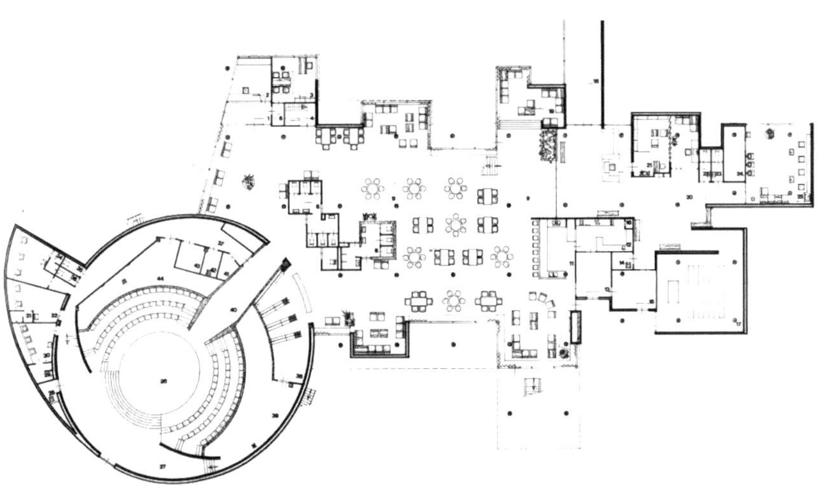

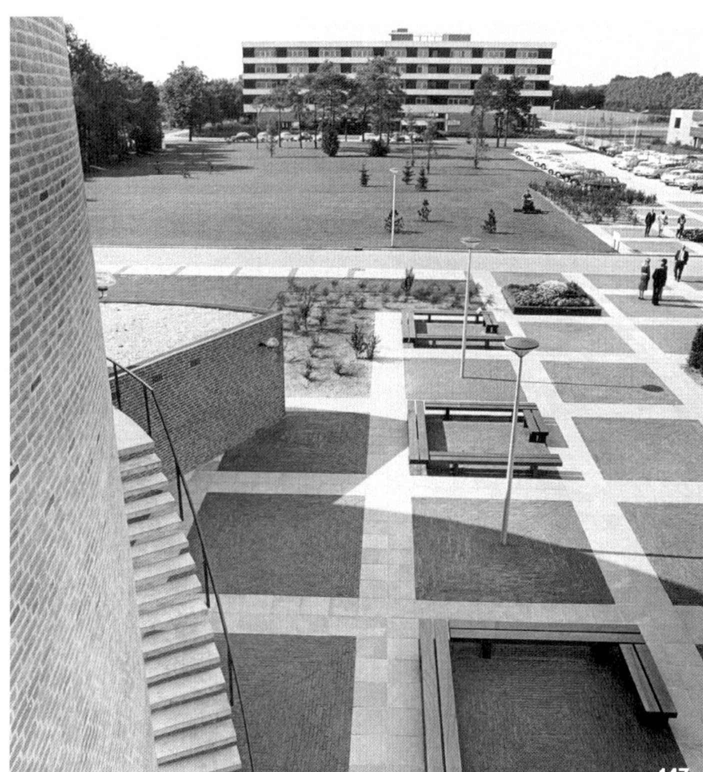

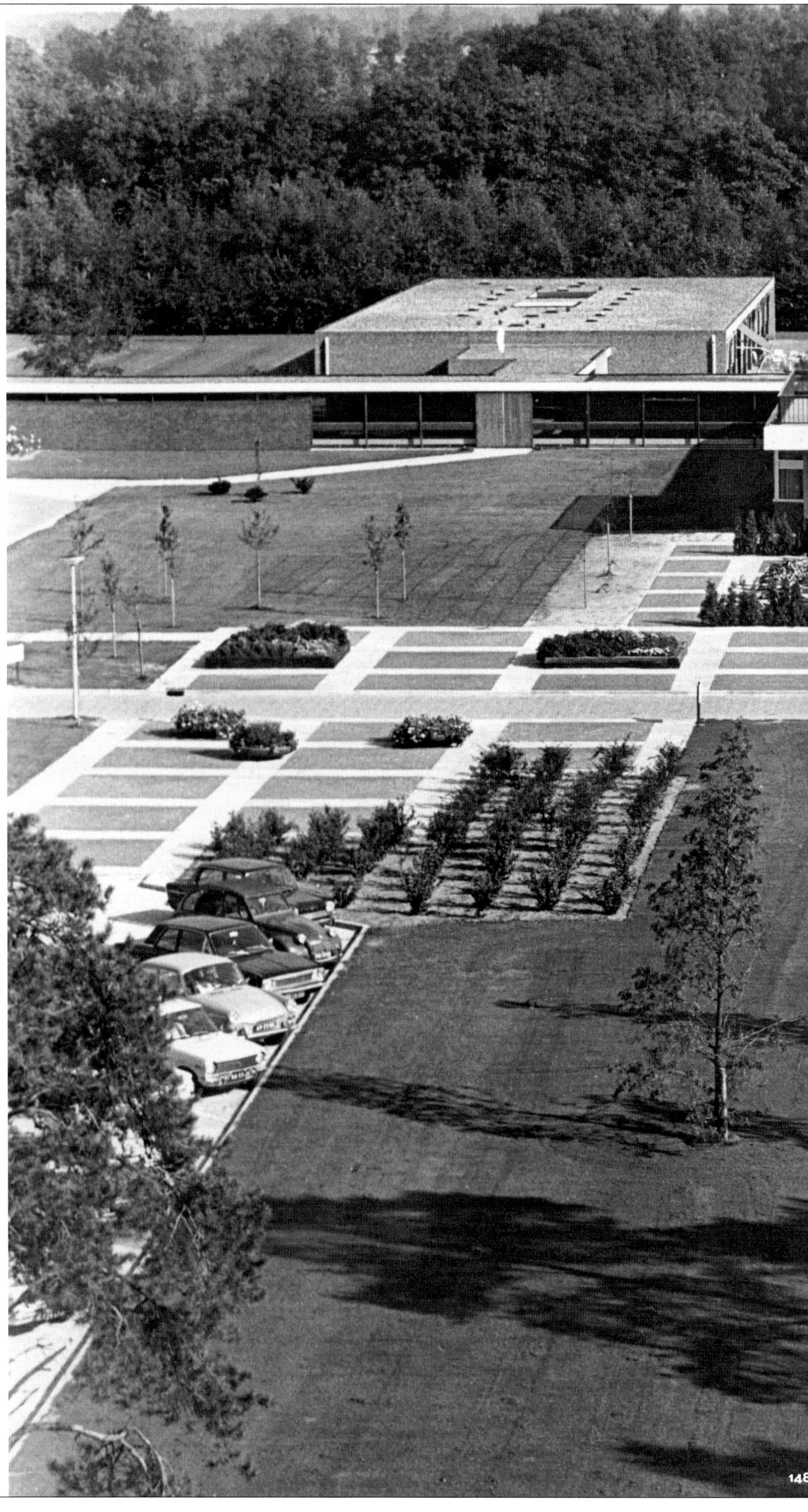

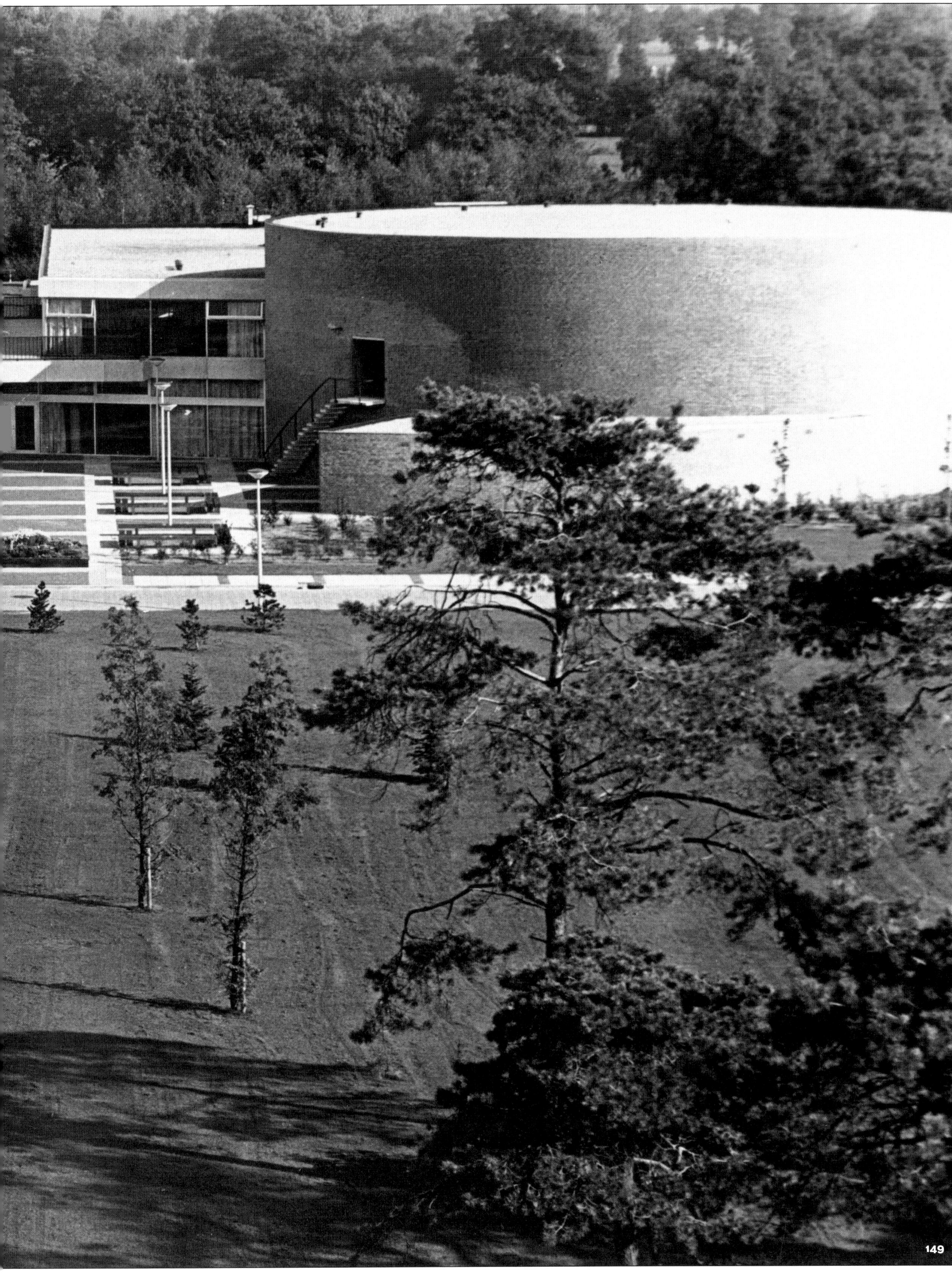

Tower

Architectenbureau Swinkels en Salemans

Vijverdal
Maastricht
1968-1973

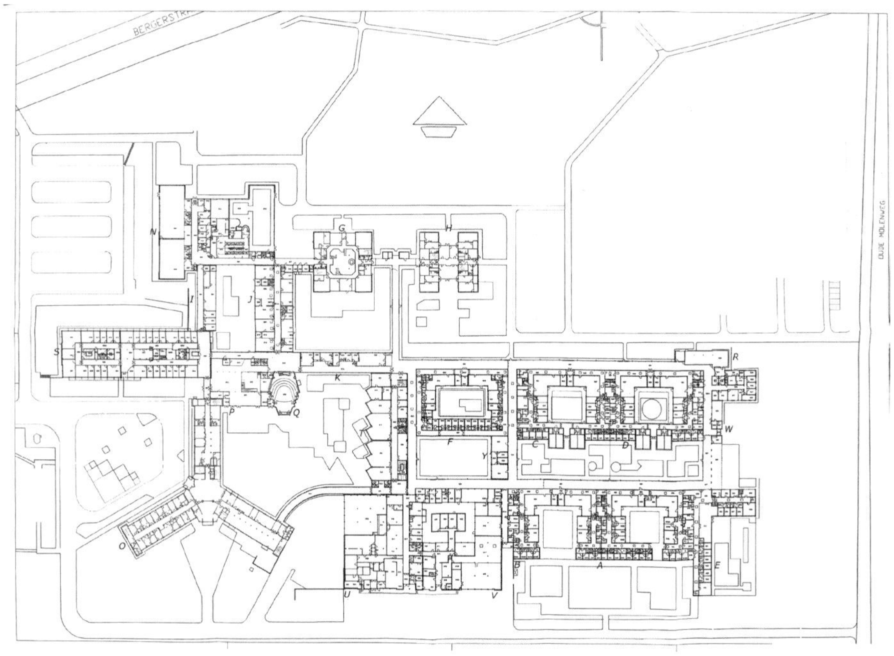

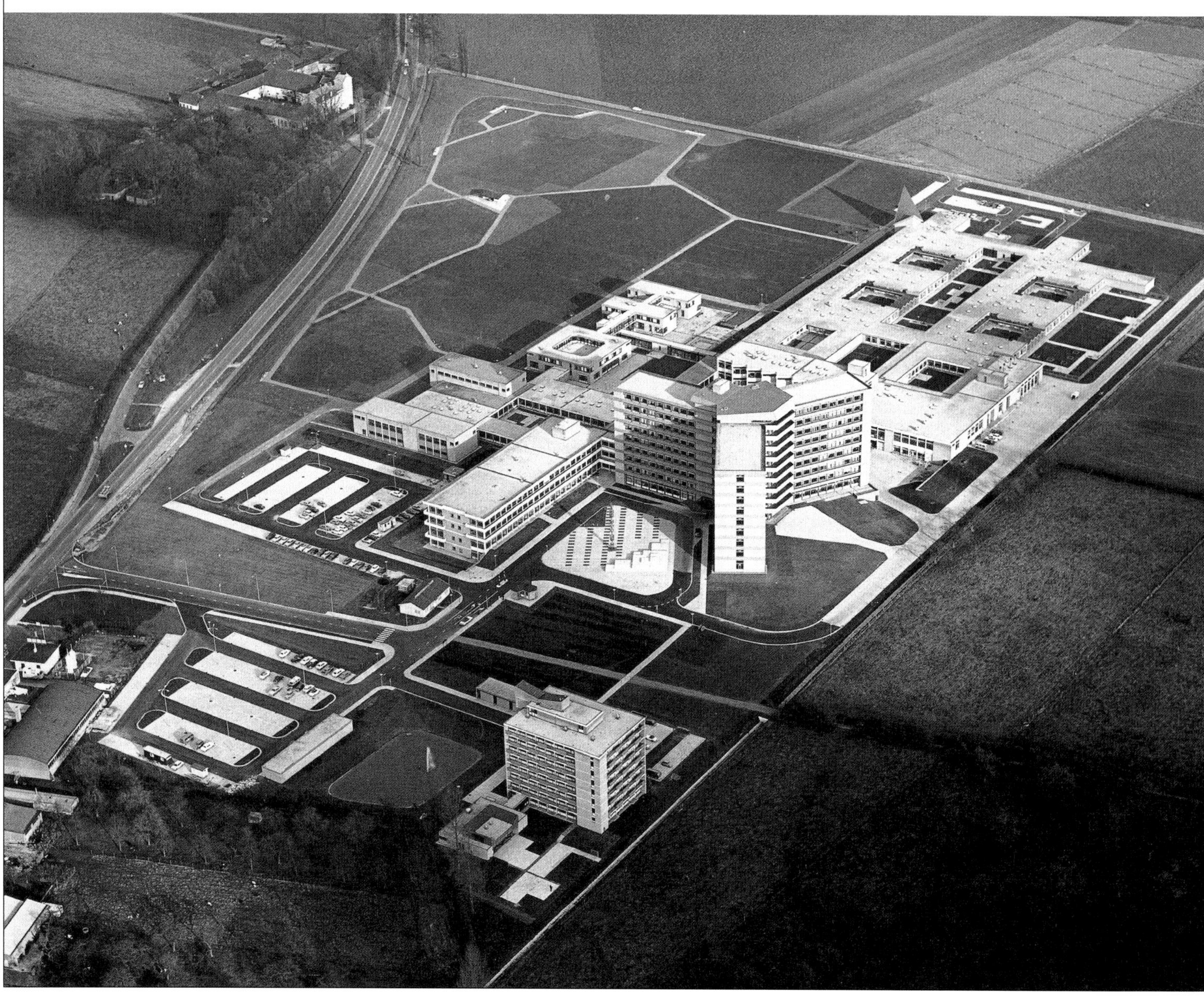

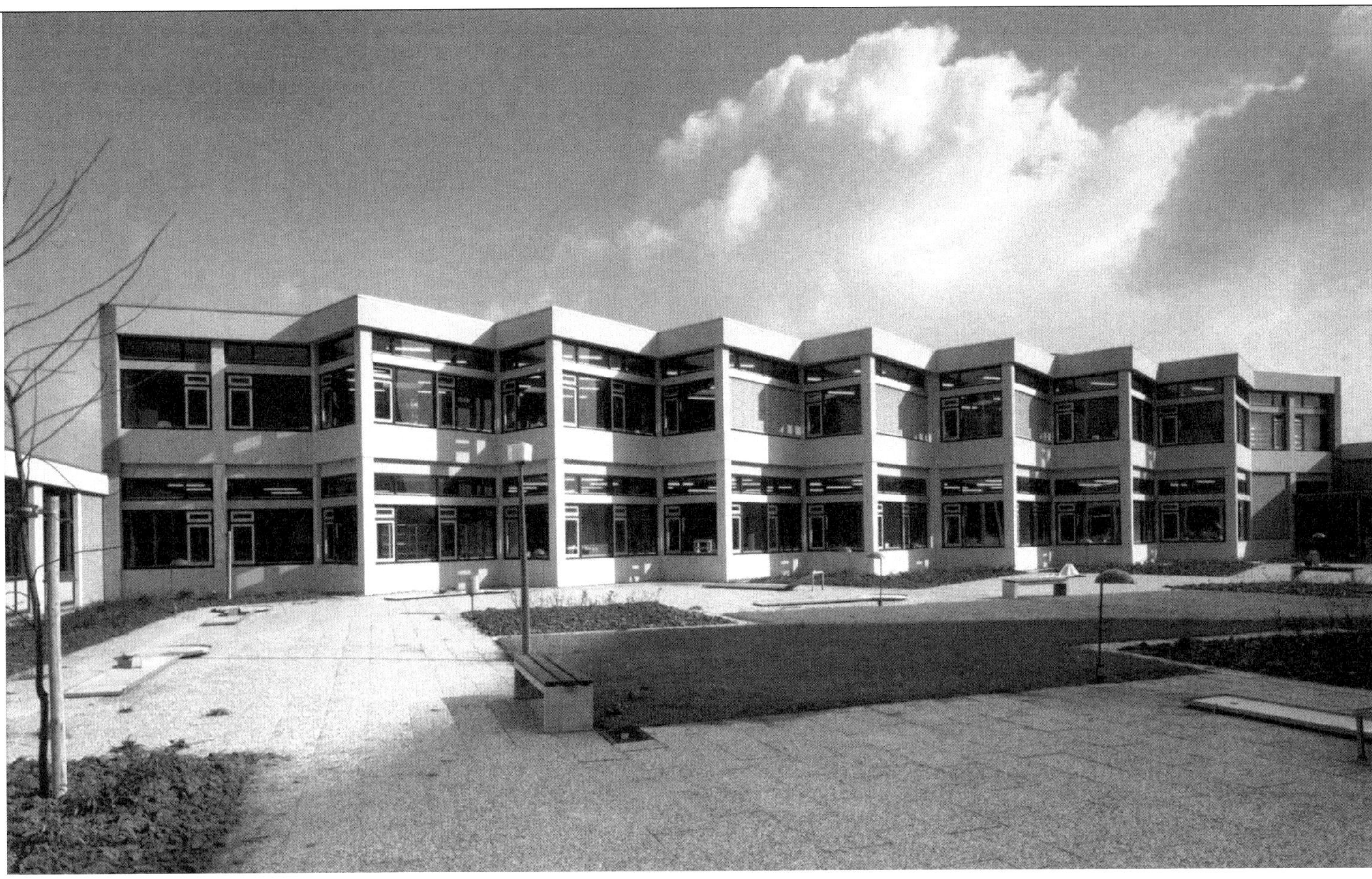

Department for labour therapy

bottom left
Sitting area in the flat for the personnel

bottom right
View from the sitting area at the promenade in the low-rise building

This design by Swinkels en Salemans breaks with the notion that psychiatric institutions should be built far from the inhabited world. Vijverdal was the first such institution in the Netherlands to accommodate a large number of patients in a block of flats. Only a part of the complex consists of low-rise building. The low-rise building contains the units for the elderly and for long-term residential patients. The therapy areas and the general and technical services are situated between these two units. The lowest two floors of the star-shaped nine-storey tower block are for the medical and administrative services. Above them are the admission and resocialisation units. Three groups of twelve patients are accommodated on each floor. Each group has its own wing comprising bedrooms, a day room and an isolation room. The three wings meet at the 'village square'. Each floor has its own dining room where the patients from the three groups can eat together.

A curved loggia connects the main building with the central kitchen, the domestic service and the staff dining room. The meeting point is the link between the main building and the various therapy areas, the outpatient unit and three three-storey Concorde building. The theatre next to the meeting point is intended not only for the patients but also for locals. The two youth pavilions occupy a rather isolated position within the complex and are furnished as an up-to-date youth club. The pavilions for long-term patients are arranged around patios. The chapel with the striking spire is situated on the east side of the complex.

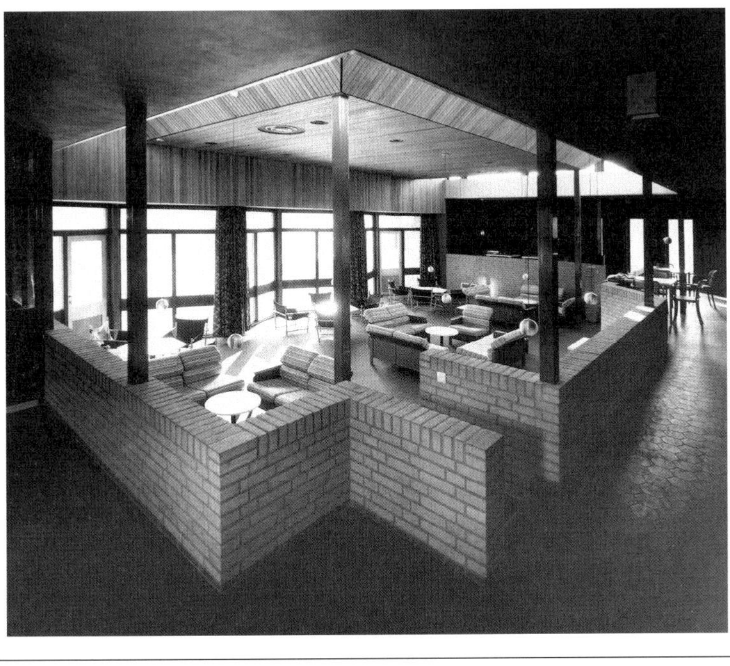

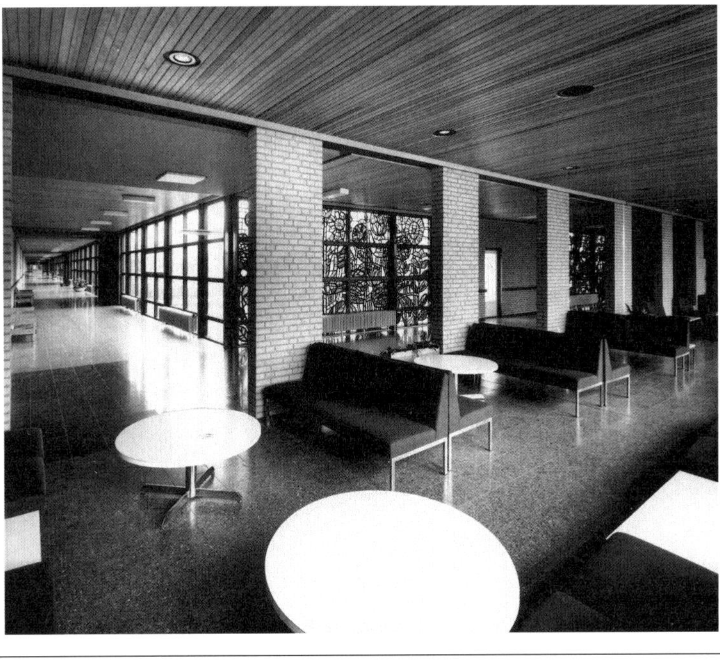

Conversation pit

Onno Greiner

De Viersprong psychotherapeutic centre
Halsteren
1966-1971

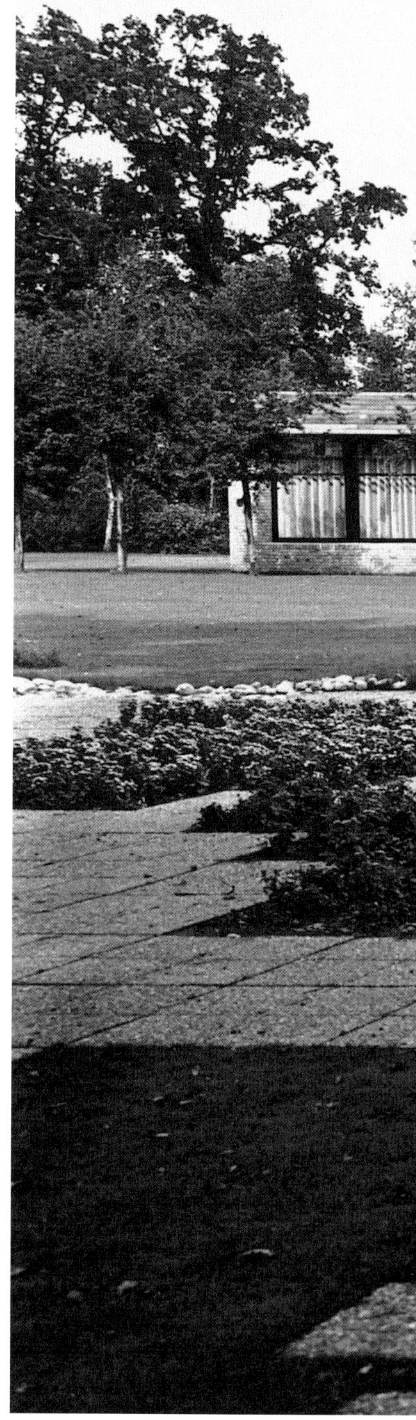

De Viersprong in Halsteren is a neuro-sanatorium for clinical psychotherapy. In 1966 Onno Greiner was commissioned to extend the villa in which the parent organisation, Vrederust psychiatric hospital, had initially accommodated this institution. The design is based on a structure that charts the route of the patients through the institution. Greiner managed to design a building in which there are hardly any corridors. Adult residents are accommodated in the villa and the modernised annex, while young patients have a residential building of their own on the other side of the terrain, near the building for movement therapy. The therapy buildings and the outpatients unit are situated between the residential buildings. The residential unit for young patients is designed to accommodate twenty patients of either sex. They are only strictly separated from one another in the sleeping quarters. Each of the two outermost blocks has a patio. Each bedroom sleeps four, and the bedrooms are completely symmetrical to avoid any form of privilege. The bedroom wings can be closed off.

As in the outpatient unit, all of the rooms in the therapy building are arranged around a patio; the consultation rooms and group therapy rooms are grouped on two sides, the rooms for creative therapy such as music and handicraft are grouped on the other two sides. In the new adult therapy building the space that functions as a patio in the other buildings is used as a recreational hall, resulting in what amounts to a very large conversation pit. De Viersprong is the second neuro-sanatorium in the Netherlands to have been consistently organised as a therapeutic community.

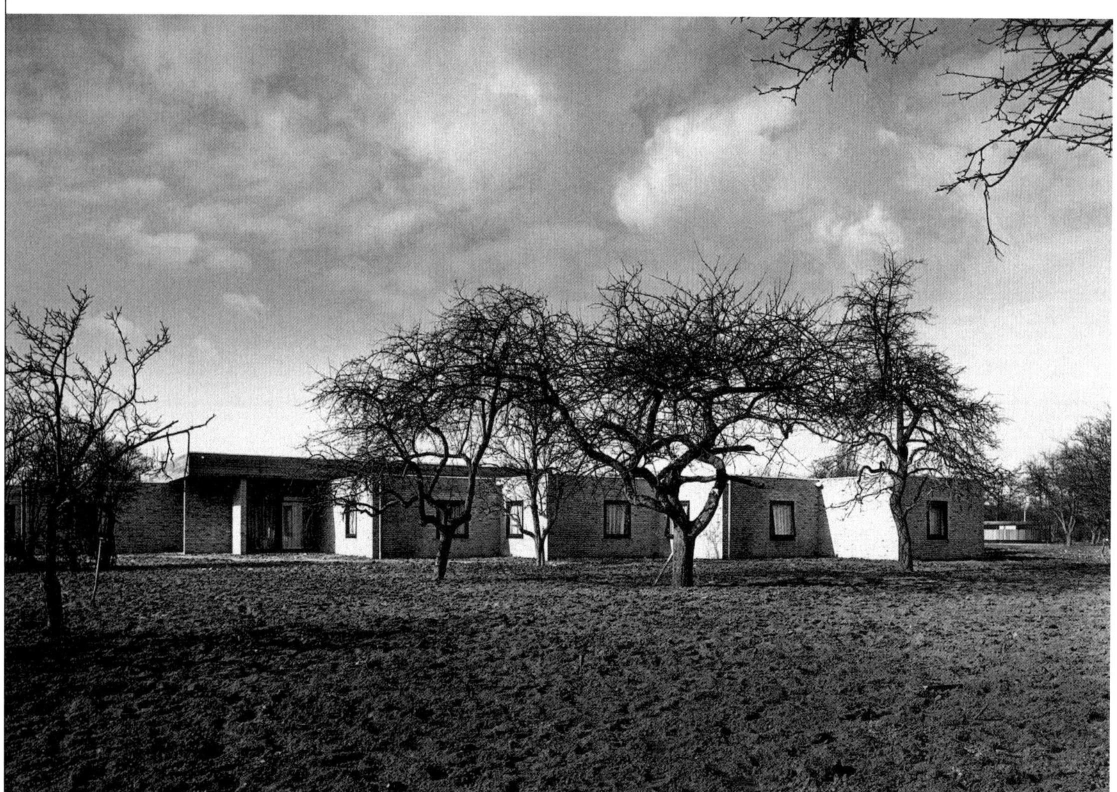

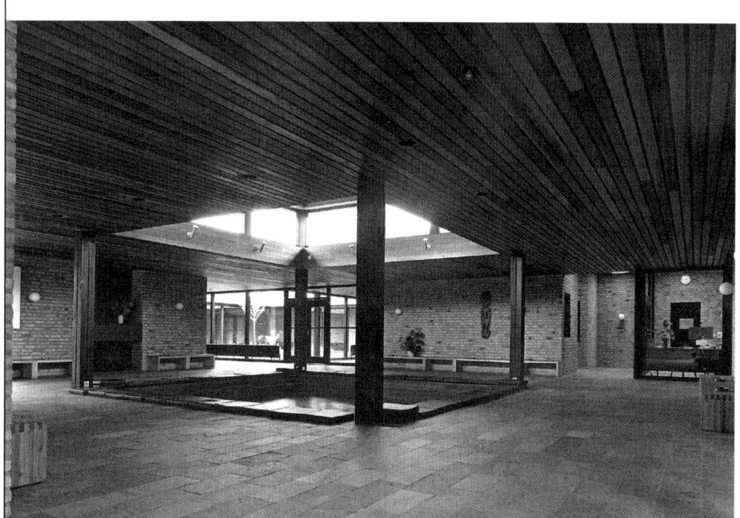

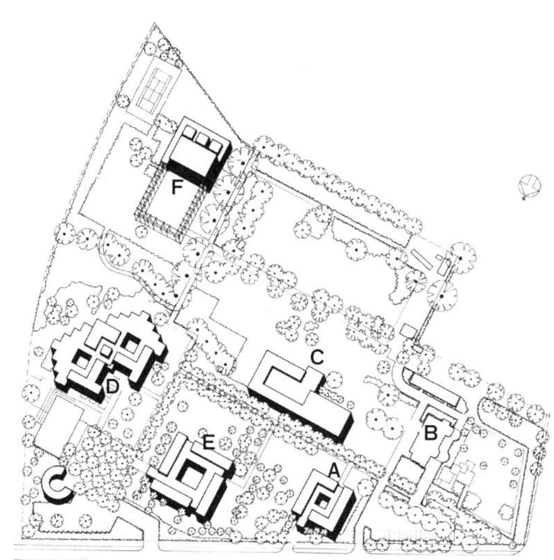

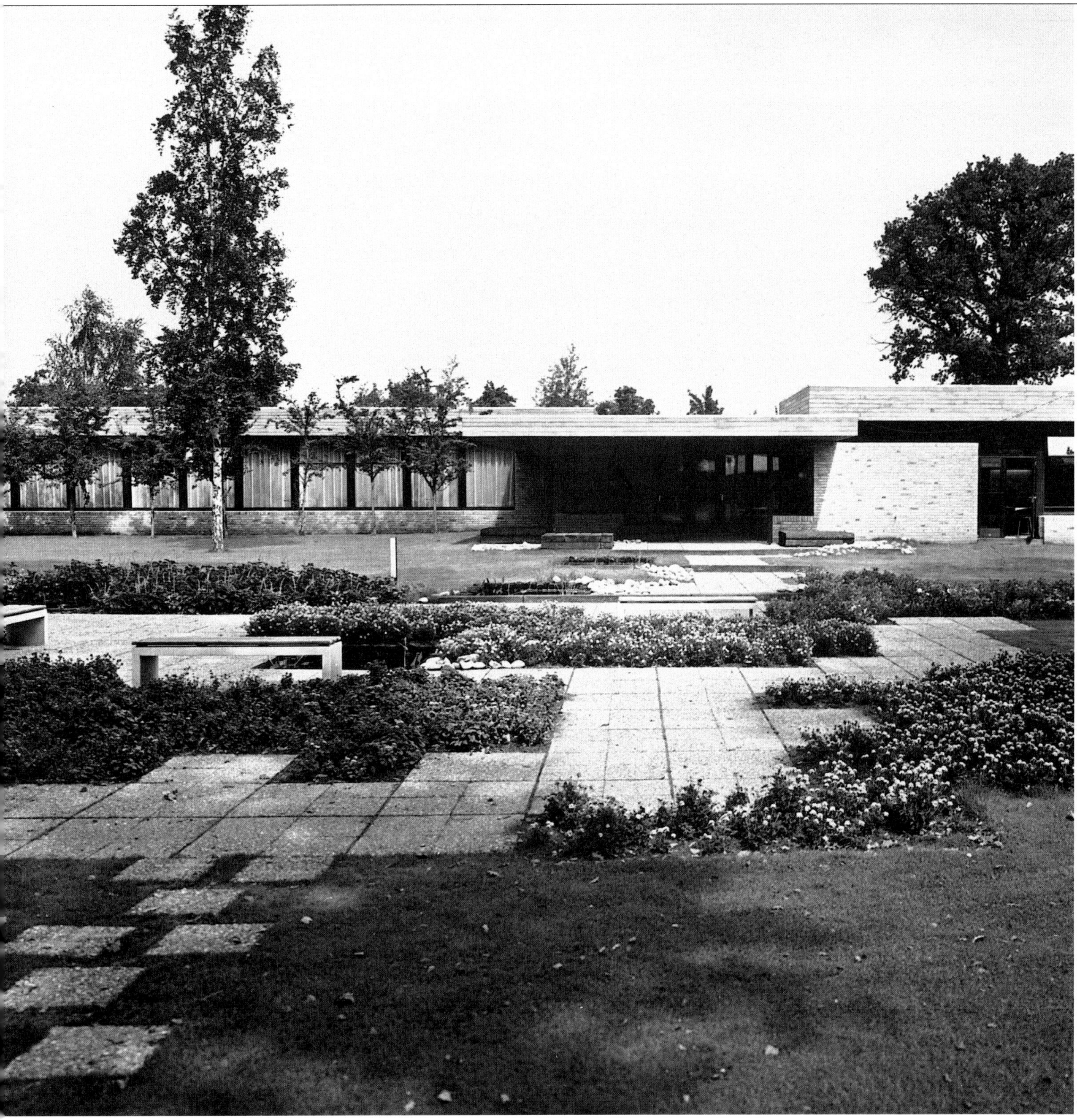

Situation

A *outward patient department*
B *housing for grown up patients*
C *therapy building for grown up patients*
D *housing for adolescent patients*
E *therapy building for adolescent patients*
F *physiotherapy*

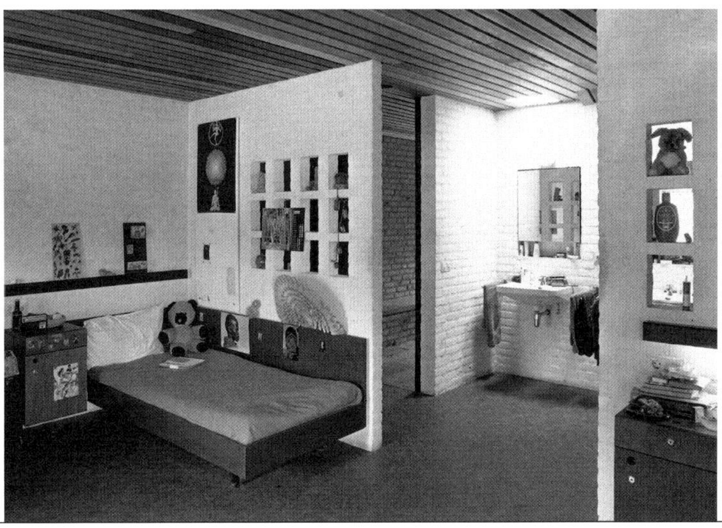

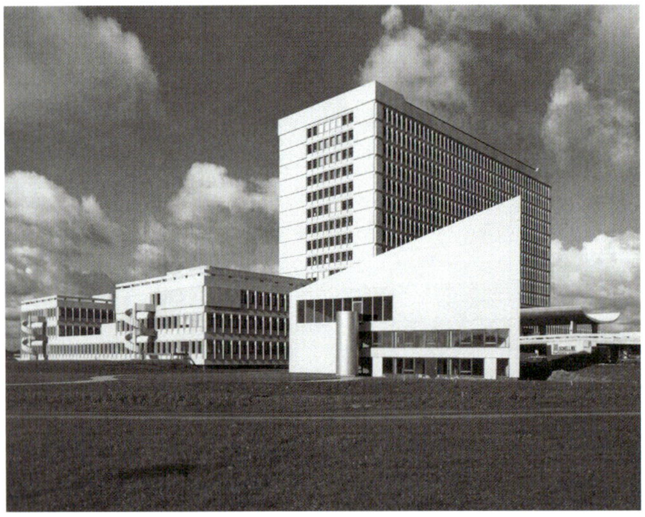

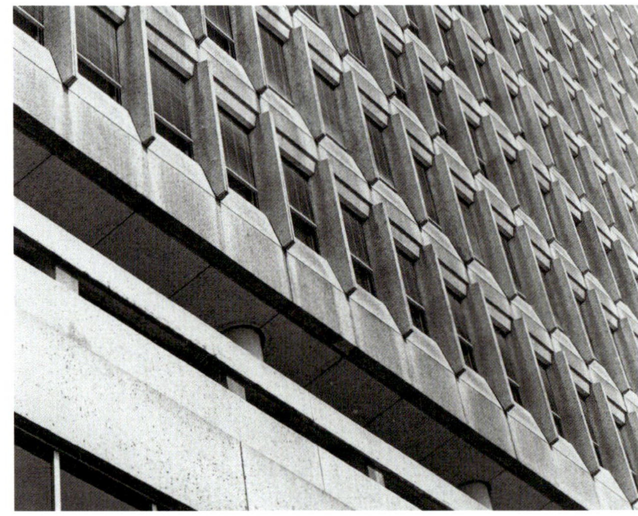

Standardisation

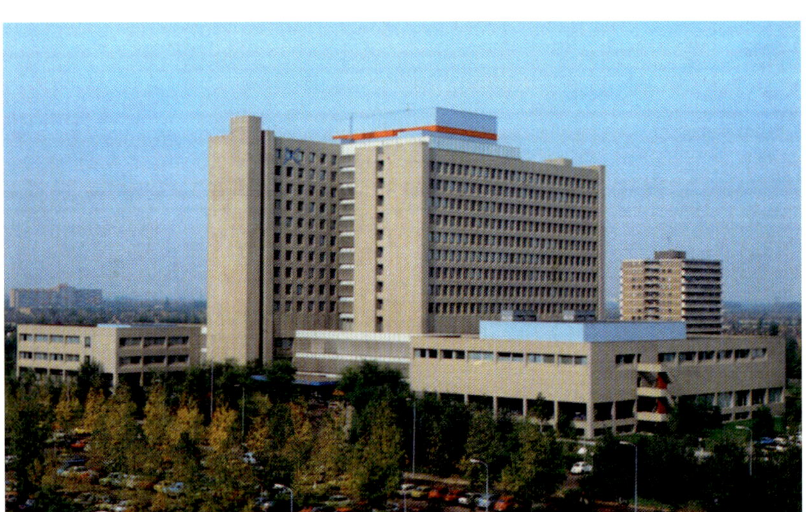

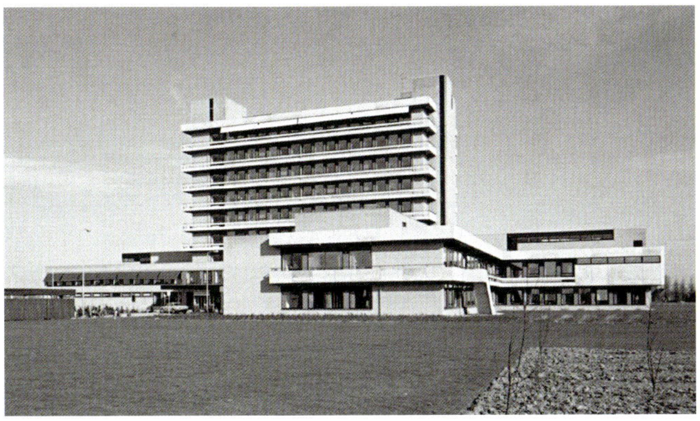

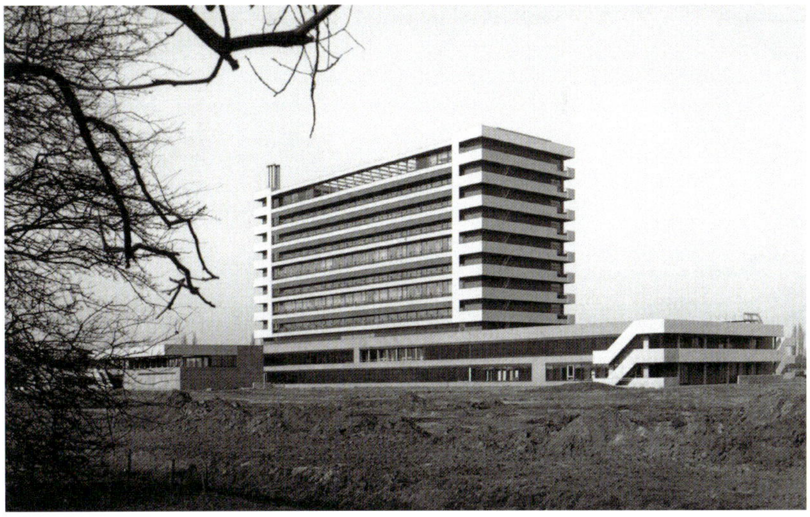

The modernisation of the Dutch building industry proceeded at full pace during and after the Second World War. That led to experiments in the mechanisation of building, the design of standard types, and more generally the goal of a more factory-like production. Standardisation can take place in various ways. Many experiments were carried out with building systems during the reconstruction period. These were construction methods based on standardised, usually prefab elements, almost always combined with a fixed system of dimensions. The main reasons for these sometimes cumbersome and always expensive experiments was initially the shortage of skilled labour. Later the emphasis shifted to the faster pace at which (predominantly) housing could be built according to this modern method. Another form of standardisation was the prefabrication of complete components of the building. This method was used mostly for showers, toilets and kitchens, which were fittings rather than a part of the building. Finally, it was possible to standardise entire buildings. This had been common practice in social housing for years, but except for petrol stations, bus shelters and other motorway architecture it proved to be barely feasible for other types of building.

Standard elements were also used in health care buildings. Irrespective of how the results of designing standardised components according to a fixed system of dimensions were explained, in practice they had one thing in common: they pointed in the direction of further increase of scale and the combination of large numbers of basic units that were to a great extent identical. Consequently, hospitals, care homes (which were already larger than their counterparts abroad) and blocks of flats for the elderly grew even larger in size.

The application of prefab façade elements gave the Leyenburgziekenhuis in The Hague (designed by K.L. Sijmons) a pronouncedly modern look. It is a paragon of modern building technology and of a hard monumentality reminiscent here and there of Niemeyer's Brasilia or Le Corbusier's Chandigarh. Prefab concrete elements were also applied on a large scale to the Catharina Ziekenhuis in Eindhoven designed by L.L.J. de Bever & L.J.H.F. de Bever with Kirch Hermans van der Eerden.

The standardisation of buildings presupposes that the functions that take place inside them – the programme – are repeatable. Local peculiarities and the personal preferences of the clients do not play any role. The number of programmes is limited for housing, but this is much less the case for almost any other function. Completely identical hospitals have never been built, but hospitals that make use of a standard programme have. The best-known are the five Wiegerinck hospitals in Utrecht, IJmuiden, Heemstede, 's-Hertogenbosch and Oosterhout. They are tower on a podium hospitals with the treatment unit in the low-rise building and the outpatient units, with their own entrance, at right angles. The application of the double corridor system has resulted in an exceptionally compact ward block.

Although the five Wiegerinck hospitals are not entirely identical, they do illustrate the ideal of the universal hospital building package, of the hospital that paid as little heed as possible to its surroundings and could be placed on any arbitrary location.[1] In that respect, however, they were not essentially different from other, non-standardised complexes that just as often seemed to have fallen from of the sky and been built without any spatial or social relation with their environment. The idea that standardisation was a way of saving a lot of money proved to be unfounded. For some researchers the major advantage was the low level of influence of the medical staff on the design process.[2]

Top
K.L. Sijmons, Leyenburgziekenhuis, The Hague, 1971. South elevation and detail of façade.

Architectenbureau Wiegerinck Van Balen Meurkens Dorigo Architects, standard hospitals ('Wiegerinck hospitals') in Oosterhout and 's-Hertogenbosch

Bottom
L.L.J. de Bever & L.J.H.F. de Bever with Kirch Hermans van der Eerden, Catharina Ziekenhuis, Eindhoven, 1974

J.E. Kruisheer, Duintjer en Istha, and Architectenbureau Wiegerinck Van Balen Meurkens Dorigo, study for the hospital of the future, 1969

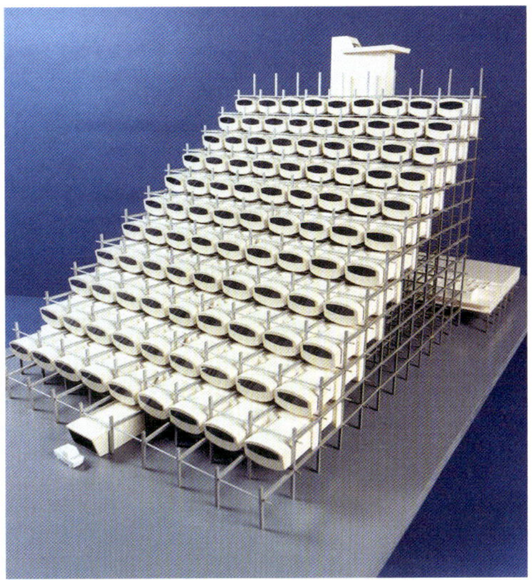

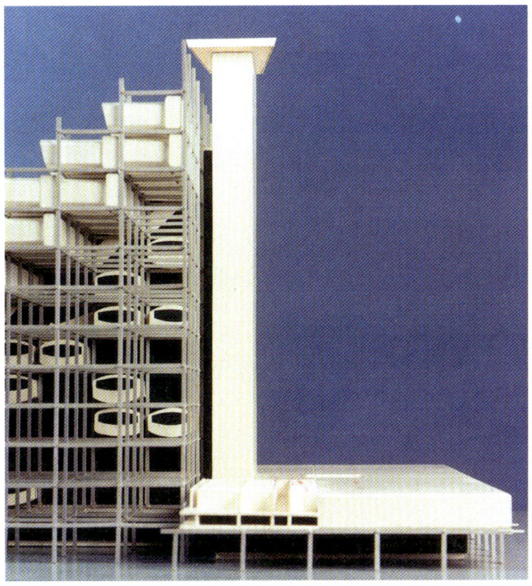

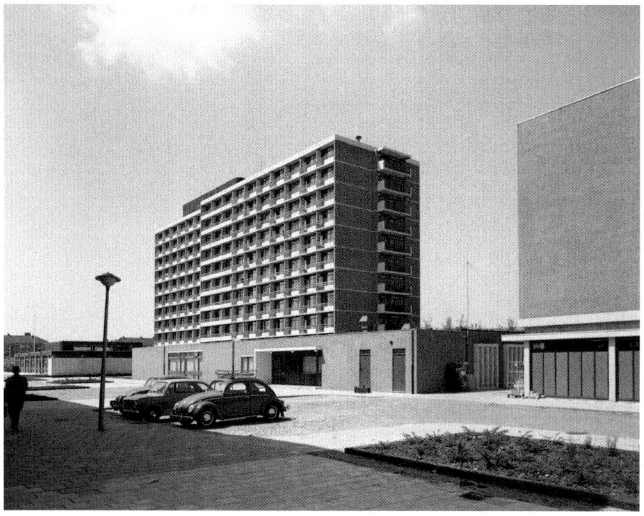

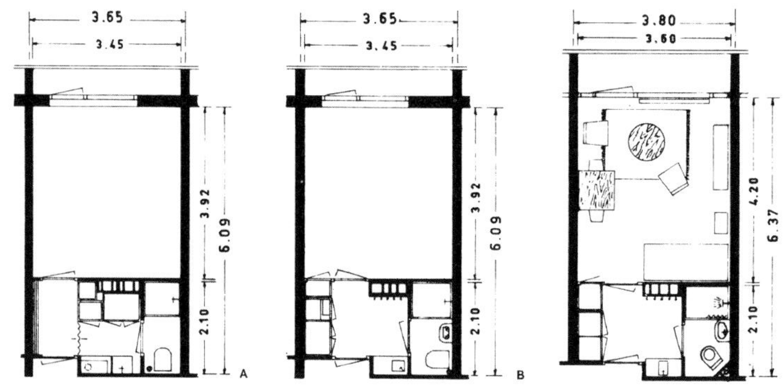

2 Bejaardenunits 1 : 100

The standardisation of programmes of requirements or of complete buildings presupposes the possibility of being able to produce them in large quantities, but this seldom proves to be the case. Would it not be possible to identify the properties that all building types have in common, irrespective of their location or function? In that case the Achilles' heel of standardisation – the need to take local peculiarities and personal preferences into account –would no longer create any difficulties. This offered unprecedented prospects for the industrial manufacture of very large numbers of identical elements to literally form the skeleton that could then be made suitable for a specific function by means of infill packages. The advantages were obvious: the infill package could be replaced quickly, which rendered this building method flexible. Optimal profit was derived from industry without the usual disadvantages. Uniformity, monotony and the negation of individual preferences were easy to avoid; industrial mass production and possibilities of individual expression were reconciled with one another. The constructional framework was a grid that resembled the parcellation of old cities, a structure that was equally capable of combining a large variety of functions with an even greater diversity of individual form elements. J. Habraken was the pioneer of this philosophy, which was elaborated by the Foundation for Architects Research (SAR) based in the Eindhoven Polytechnic (now Eindhoven University of Technology). Architecture and urban planning were one in the world of the SAR. From now on designing would be tantamount to devising structures. That makes this method an industrial variant of Structuralism. Its social dimension stems from the potential to fulfil the individual needs of the modern 'urban nomad'. Within the industrially produced load-bearing structure, he could choose his own infill package.

This procedure seemed extremely suitable for the building of hospitals, where the infill packages had a high turnover speed. At the Medica exhibition held in the Jaarbeurs in Utrecht in 1969, three firms of architects – J.E. Kruisheer, Duintjer en Istha, and Wiegerinck Van Balen Meurkens Dorigo – presented a study of the hospital of the future. The requirements that they demanded of it were: a short preparatory and building period, it must not be already outdated by the time it is completed, and must be simple to adapt to the inevitable changes. Separating the support from the infill could be the solution here too. The support consisted of a constructional grid with fixed dimensions that bore the weight of the building and also offered room for gas and water pipes and electric cables. This fixed core was the basis within which the infill packages were placed; the latter were easy to replace and met the specific (individual) demands. The separation of support and infill also offered major advantages to the suppliers of medical infill packages (operating theatres, X-ray units, dialysis equipment). Provided the dimensions of the medical machinery matched those of the constructional grid, one of the major obstacles in the introduction of new technology would have been removed. The inevitable dismantling and demolition would become a thing of the past; if a piece of equipment was out of date – and it soon was – it could be replaced quickly and without much fuss by a more recent model.

The separation of support and infill seemed to be an ideal strategy for the hospital, and also offered an opportunity to give it a more humane face.[3]

A separation between support and infill was also applied during the building of the Rotterdam medical faculty. As the size of some parts of the new faculty was still not known while the building was going up – the information on the distribution of

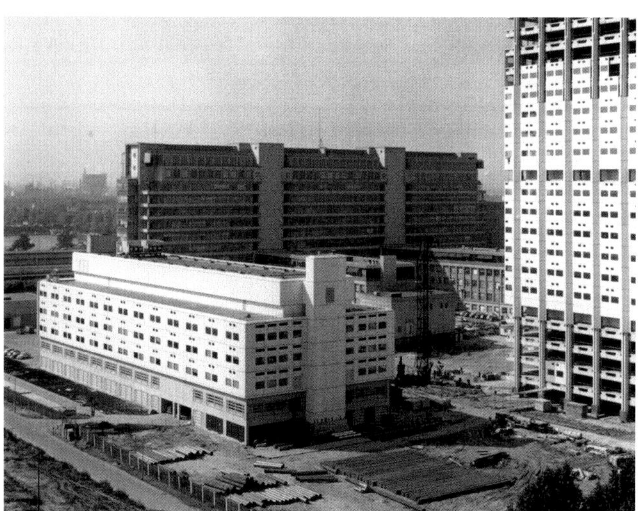

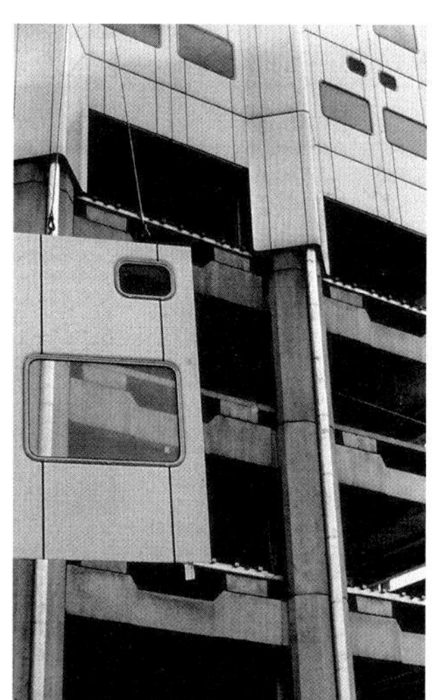

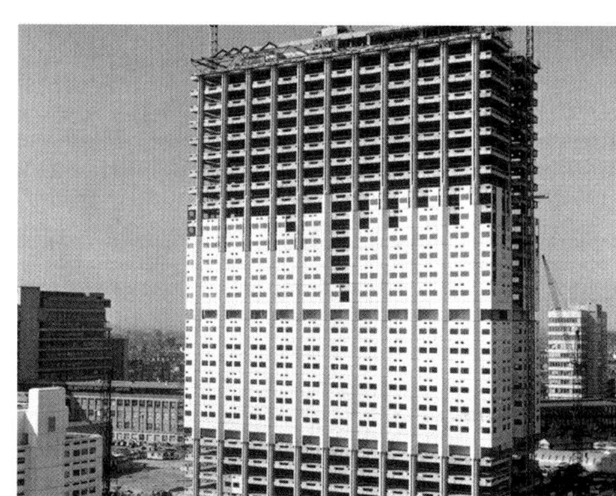

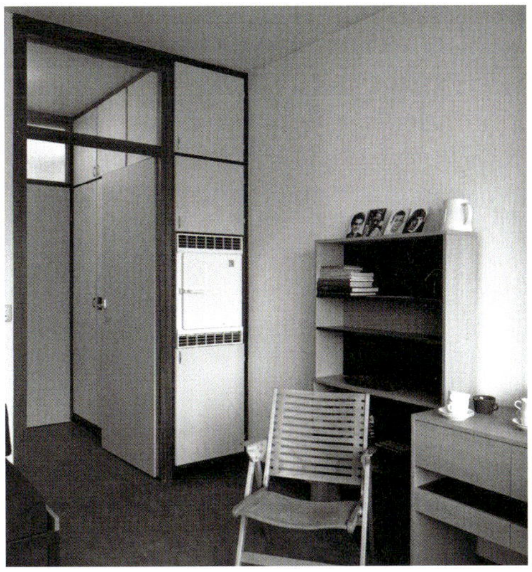

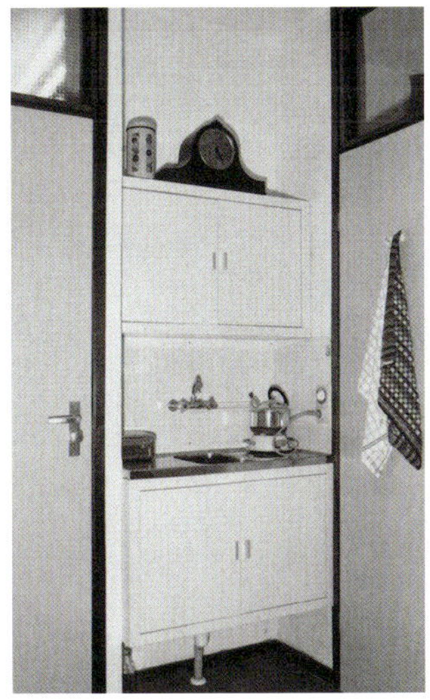

Top
De Kimme care home, Amsterdam, 1969

Building team care homes Amsterdam, ground plans of the housing unit, 1968

De Kimme care home, Amsterdam, 1969

Bottom
OD 205, Medical Faculty, Rotterdam, 1972. Façade panels designed by J. Prouvé.

Burger Grunstra architecten adviseurs, Martini Ziekenhuis, Groningen, 2007

space was only made available a few months before the opening – a method of construction had to be used that would leave the eventual distribution of space in the building open. The central laboratory with a floor area of 25,000 m² was incorporated in the 26-storey tower block. It comprises a core shaft (9.6 m wide) extending the full length of the building, around which the prefab concrete elements, columns, beams and floor plates have been assembled. The French constructional engineer Jean Prouvé designed the façade composed of self-supporting panels 8 cm thick consisting of a core of polyurethane foam coated on the outside with white varnished aluminium panels and on the inside with steel sheeting. These façade elements, in which the windows were set without frames as in a passenger train, were the building's most striking features.. The parallel is not fortuitous: Prouvé was working for a manufacturer of railway material. The interior is extremely flexible: it consists of movable metal partitions in which the pipes and cables are incorporated. The designer, A. Hagoort from the OD 205 firm of architects, compared the tower to a stranded spaceship made like a Junkers airplane.[4]

Experiments were carried out with complete prefab components of a building in a series of old people's homes. At the end of 1963 an old people's home building team was set up with four firms of architects: Peters senior & junior, Pot & Pot-Keegstra, Van Woerden & Schneider, and Zwiers & Westerduin. The Bataafse Aannemingsmaatschappij supplied the expertise from the building world, and civil servants from the municipal departments for housing, urban development and the building and housing inspectorate together with their colleagues from the social housing and architecture board of the province of North Holland completed the team. The uniformity that they aimed for was confined to certain elements: the housing unit, staircases, lifts, boilers, radiators. In spite of the standardisation, it should still be possible to come up with designs with a character of their own. 'Thus no repetition of externally uniform old people's homes, but a repetition of their component parts.'[5] What was standardised at any rate was the system of dimensions, otherwise the uniform building elements would simply not have fitted. Eight new old people's homes was the minimum number required for the Amsterdam experiment to be economically feasible. These were the De Kimme care home in Nieuwendam-Noord, a home for the Reformed Remonstrant religious community in the Rivierenlaan, an old people's home in Osdorp, Nieuw Amstelhof in Buitenveldert, an old people's home in Buikslotermeer, the second Willem Dreeshuis in Buikslotermeer, a complex for old people in Oostzaan-West, and a home for the Humanist Architecture Foundation for Care of the Elderly in Osdorp.

The Martini Ziekenhuis in Groningen designed by Burger Grunstra that was completed in 2007 made use of the Industrial, Flexible and Demountable (IFD) building system based on standardisation. The building skeleton, which consists of uniform building blocks, the façade panels and system walls, and the shafts for pipes and cables are all fully prefabricated. Thanks to the standard dimensions, the outpatient units are suitable for different specialisations. The advantage of IFD building is that it enables new building or extension work to be carried out quickly.[6]

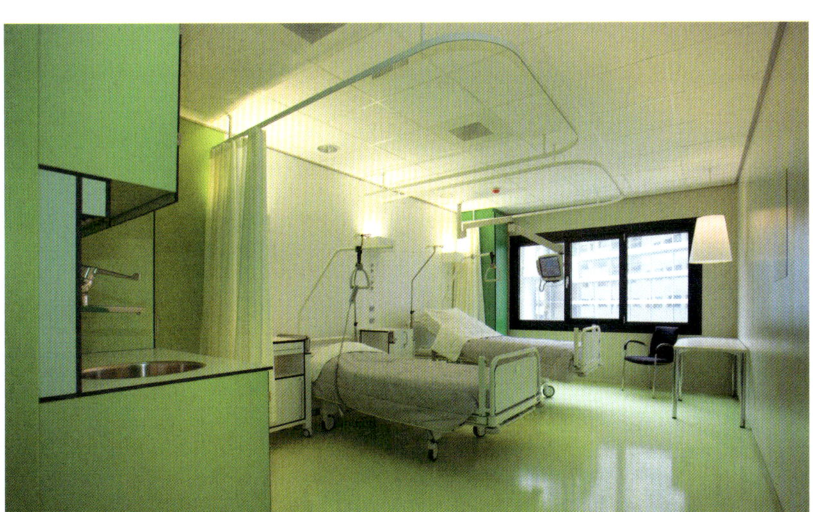

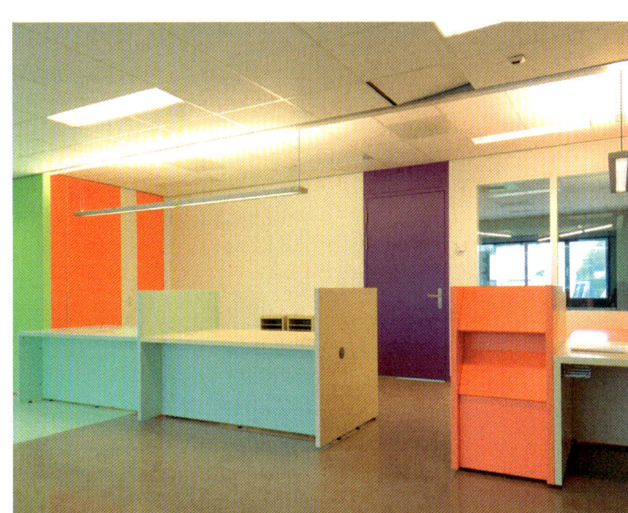

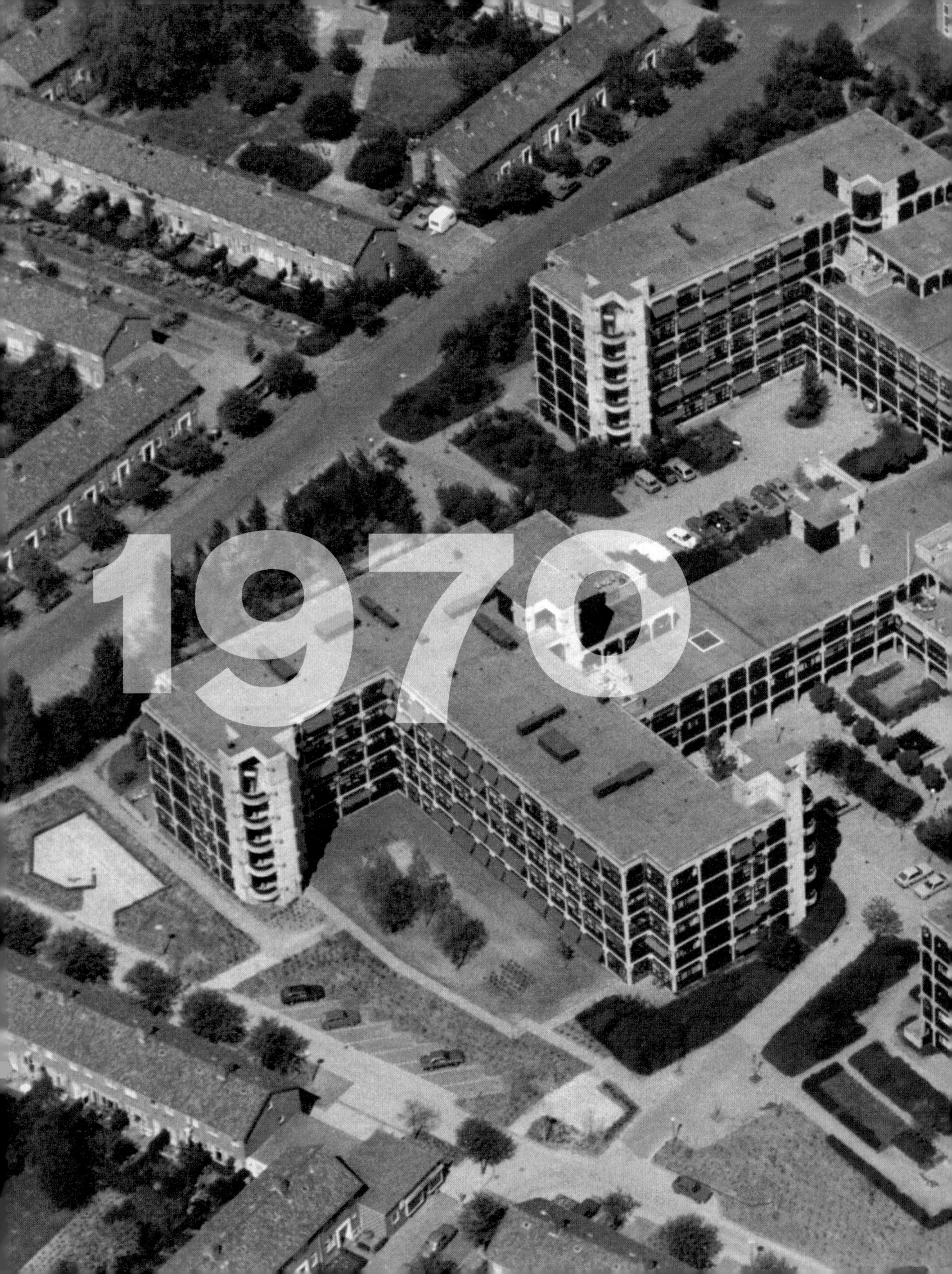
1970

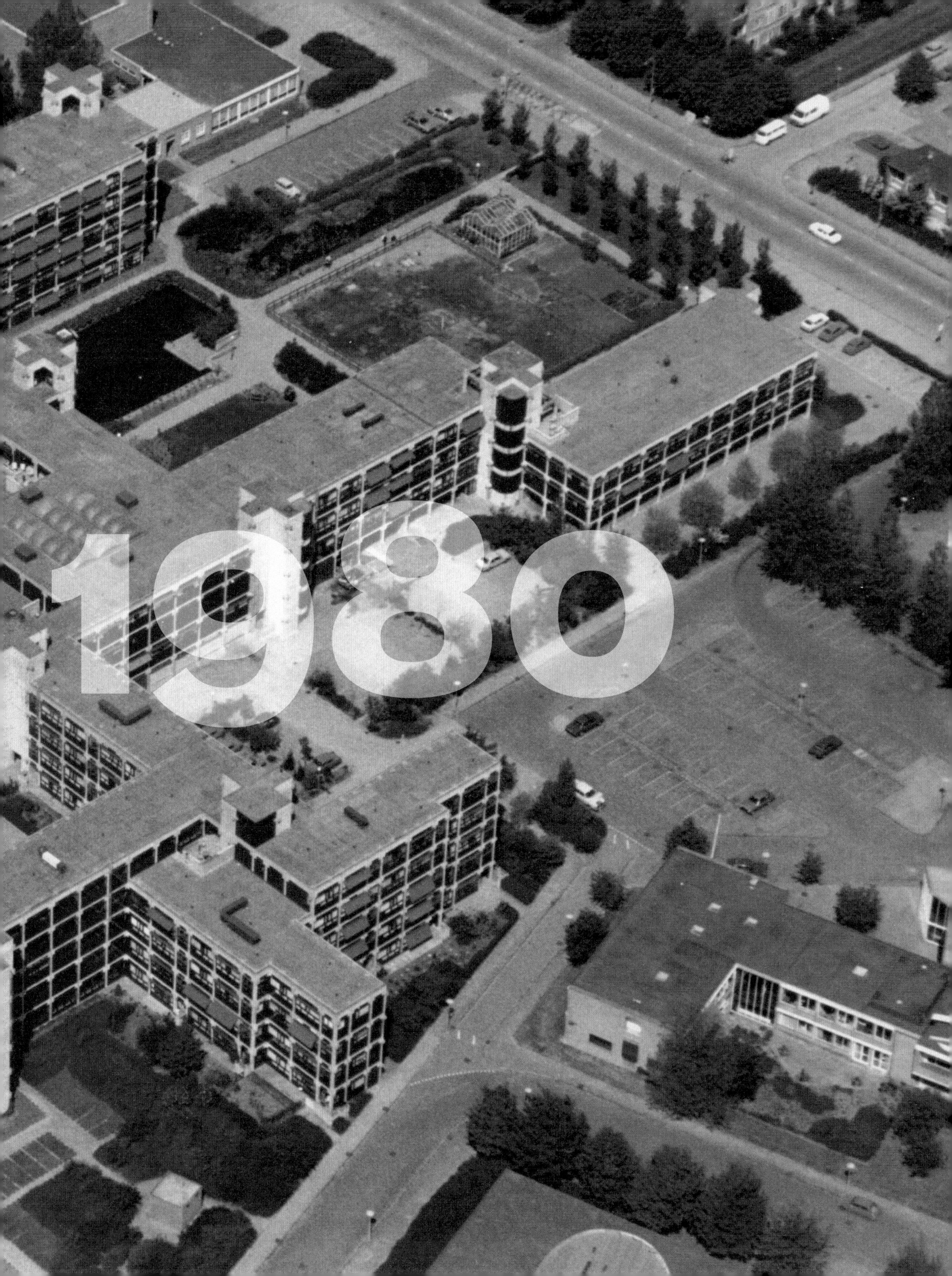
1980

The critical Seventies

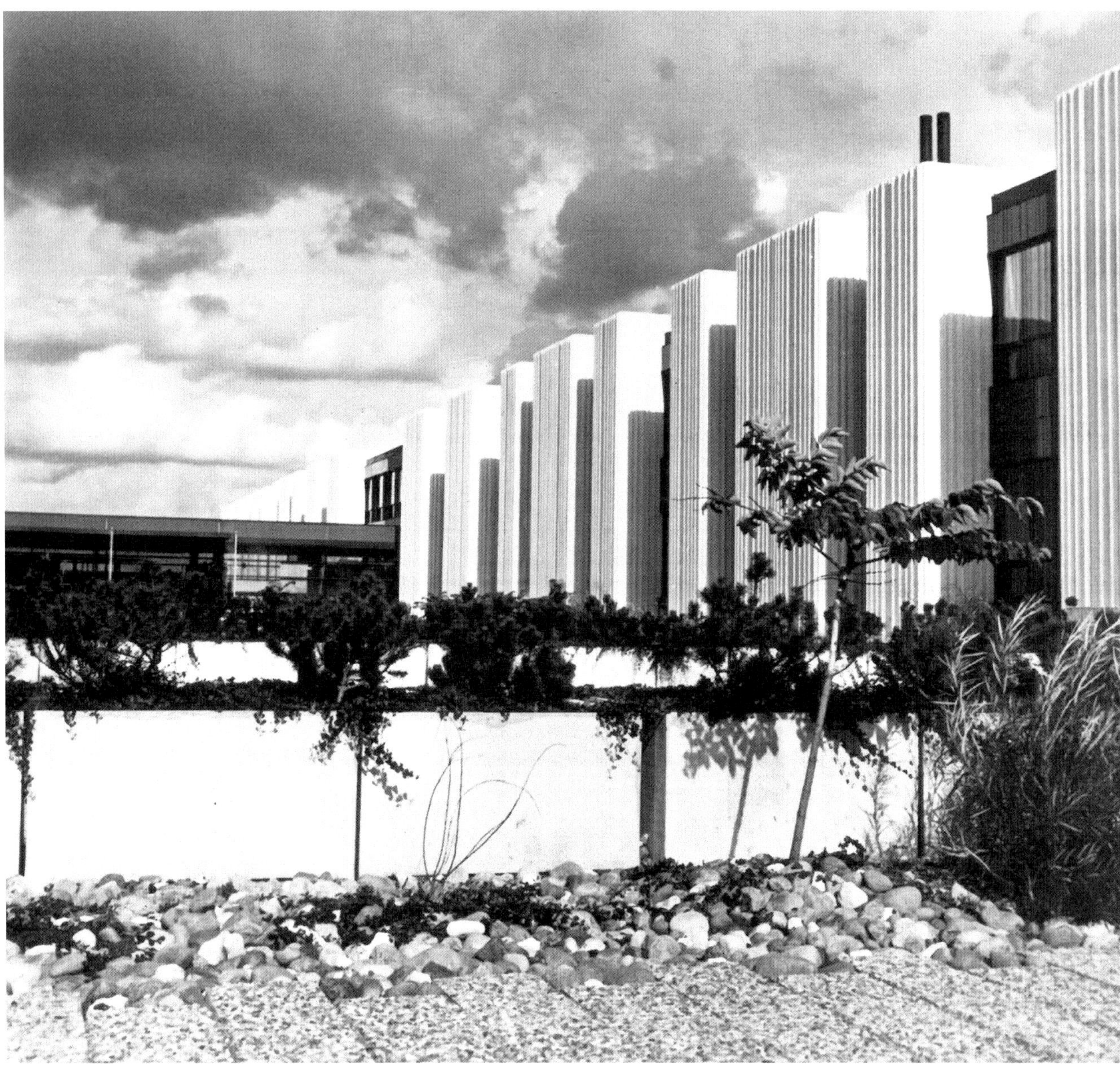

The end of growth

The economic upsurge that had commenced with the reconstruction reached a climax in the early 1970s. The tempo at which the care sector developed proved to be considerably higher than the average growth, and the percentage of the gross national product (GNP) increased rapidly. This was particularly true of the hospital world and housing for the elderly. Critics complained that the improvement of the level of health care did not keep pace with this disproportionate growth – care became more expensive and comprehensive, but not better. Although there were enough funds for the time being, this criticism caused questions to be raised about the path that had been followed. Besides, funding was not the only or even the most important economic criterion: if the care sector continued to grow at the same tempo, there would soon be a shortage of staff, particularly nursing staff, to supply all the new institutions with personnel. So a stop had to be called to the unlimited growth anyway. Restraint became a major theme, especially in the hospital world and in care for the elderly, but also in psychiatry.

The second major theme concerned criticism of the functioning of health care institutions. They were accused of being total institutions that made the patients and the elderly dependent and meek. According to J.C.M. Hattinga Verschure, Professor of Hospital Science at the University of Utrecht, for decades the structure of health care and of the hospital had been determined by the dominant position of the doctors. Hospitals were organised not around the patients but around the specialists. Almost everything and everyone had to make way for the doctors. 'They are the key figures. The doctor has an equally dominant position in relation to the patients; he knows what is good for the patient'.[1] This criticism coincided with the growing protest against the welfare state in general. Nowhere was this protest as vociferous as in psychiatry – which was always the sector that was influenced most directly by opinions regarding people and society.

The impact of this criticism was expressed without delay in the emergence of new architectural concepts. The key concepts were small scale, security and warmth. There should be social spaces where people could spontaneously form small, temporary communities. Modern functionalist urban planning was accused of frustrating this by declaring the narrow streets, alleys and squares of the past to be out of date. Premodern urban planning now became the major source of inspiration. This also applied to one of the most widely discussed architectural and urban planning concepts of these years: the principle of support structure and infill or

p. 158
***H. Hertzberger*, De Drie Hoven, Amsterdam, 1974**

p. 160
***Krohn & Hartvig Rasmussen*, Hvidovre hospital, Copenhagen, 1975**

p. 161
***Krohn & Hartvig Rasmussen*, Hvidovre hospital, Copenhagen, 1975. Section.**

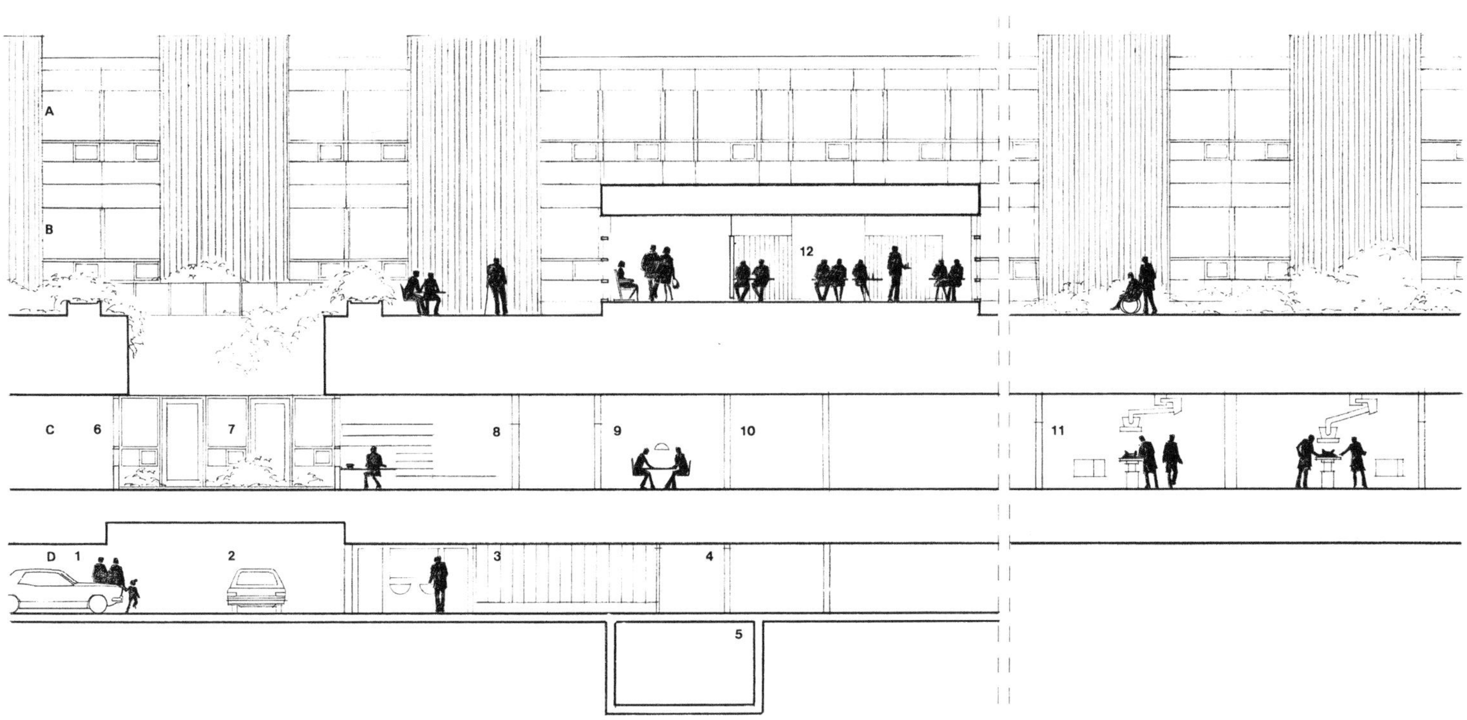

interior fit-out developed by John Habraken with his Foundation for Architects Research (SAR). Historical cities evolved on the basis of permanent elements (the street pattern and parcellation of plots that taken together formed the urban fabric), and semi-permanent elements (historic monuments), but by far the largest part of them consisted of a floating stock of buildings. By separating the industrially manufactured support from an infill package designed to meet the needs of the user, the SAR hoped to harmonise personal freedom with modern industrial society. This distinction between a permanent structure and a flexible interior had already formed the basis for *Aspecten van het ziekenhuis van de toekomst* (Aspects of the hospital of the future) in 1969. While most of the alternative, fabric-like plans for hospitals generally proved to be impracticable, the building of small-scale group facilities did take off in psychiatry. These group areas were incorporated within the structure of the existing institutions. As for accommodation for the elderly, the building of large complexes divided into pleasant smaller units by numerous small streets and squares became popular.

Hospitals

Although the ideologically motivated assault on the 'medical bulwark' caused quite a stir in the 1960s, the roots of the criticisms went further back in time. In the 1950s the view had been expressed at many a medical congress that the modern society that was taking shape during the reconstruction period involved major health hazards. Architecture and urban planning played an important role in this respect. The impressive *Medizin und Städtebau. Ein handbuch für gesundheitlichen Städtebau* (Medicine and City Planning. A Handbook for City Planning in Relation to Health (1957)) is characteristic. This encyclopaedic study carried out by the most prominent German experts was at the same time a diatribe against modern civilisation and the metropolis and a eulogy of city planning as an instrument to combat its drawbacks. The first chapter already explained how the confrontation with modern culture resulted in a catastrophe for 'primitive' societies.[2] The same threat now faced the modern dwellers in the new cities. Life in the big city was accused of causing 'damage to civilisation' and providing a lot of work for ear, nose and throat specialists, ophthalmologists, dermatologists, psychologists, orthopaedists, paediatricians and specialists in internal medicine.

While initially it was mainly physicians who expressed their concern, in the 1960s and 1970s their criticisms were effortlessly absorbed in a much wider resistance to modern society. In a certain sense the hospital was a typical

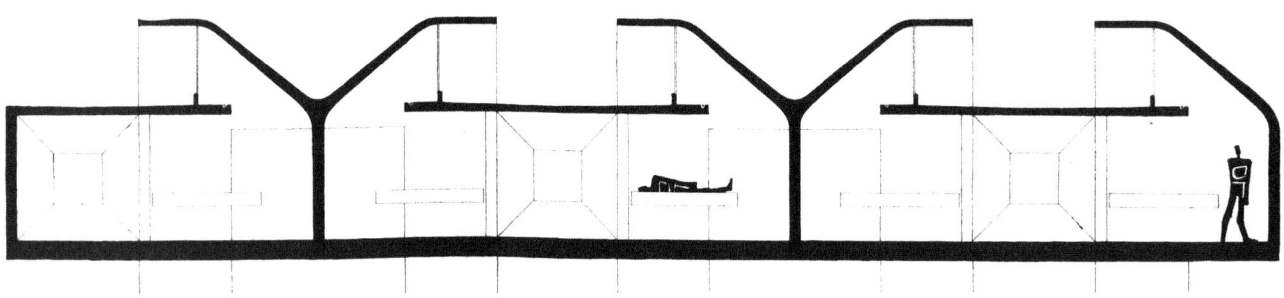

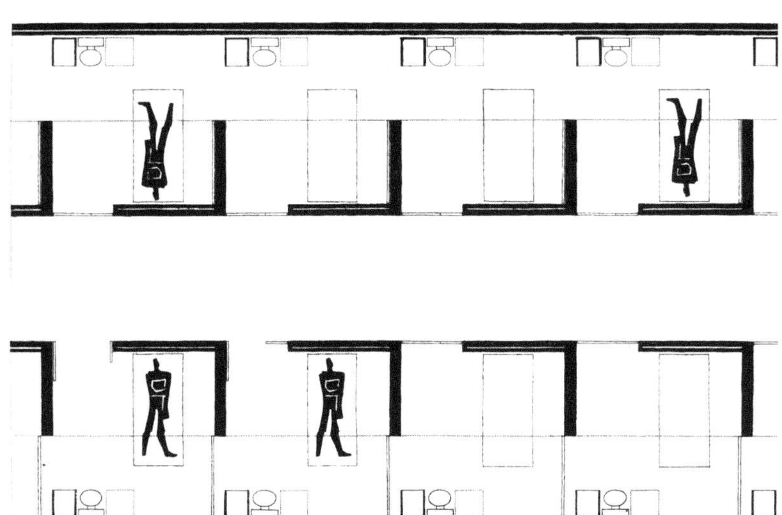

p. 162
***Le Corbusier*, design for a hospital in Venice, 1964. Section of the rooms and ground plans of the rooms.**

p. 163
***Le Corbusier*, design for a hospital in Venice, 1964**

phenomenon of that society: huge, technocratic, authoritarian, clinical, cold and autonomous: no one could really get a grip on it, least of all the patient. The criticisms of the massive scale and impersonality of the hospital started to grow from the mid-1960s. In 1960 P.A. Heeres already remarked that the nurses only had time to learn to deal with technology. He saw the terrifying vision of the hospital factory looming up, and was not the only one.[3] Bureaucracy and technology seemed to push the patient into the background. Treatment should not be confined to combating illness, but should target the 'whole man' including his personality.[4]

The famous examples of the past now became the nightmares of the future. What had first been seen as paragons of progress were now criticised for being the built expression of inhuman medical processes. Organisation, technology and logistics, not the welfare of the patient, were taken to determine the architecture. The desire to reduce unnecessary traffic led to a recurrent theme in the hospital world: the short walking routes for nursing and medical staff. The easiest way to achieve that was to make the building as concentrated as possible. Most of the block types satisfied that criterion, but the other side of the coin was that these complexes looked like 'medical bulwarks' – the criticism ran – in which the medical staff cut themselves off from the outside world and created their own hermetically sealed domain. An alternative to the concentrated 'bulwarks' was low-rise building.

Already in the mid-1950s one of the authors of a well-known handbook, Hassenpflug, had demonstrated that a less compact form with more low-rise building was also quite possible.[5] The criterion of distance became less important as more mechanical transport facilities were integrated; pneumatic dispatch was especially popular. The largest stir was caused by a design by the Danish firm Krohn & Hartvig Rasmussen for a hospital in Hvidovre in Copenhagen: a long corridor on the ground floor linked five three-storey pavilions with one another that could accommodate a thousand patients. Tunnels completed the traffic system. The treatment units were beneath the wards, where they could be expanded at will without altering the character of the design.[6]

In his well-known project for a hospital in Venice, the last that he would complete and his first experiment in health care, Le Corbusier also opted for a low-rise solution. Like the Danish design, his hospital had a capacity of a thousand patients, who were accommodated in a three-storey complex that was articulated by streets and squares. The most original part was the bedroom (*unité lit*) with reflecting sunlight but no view of outside.[7] Each nursing unit had twenty-eight of these one-person rooms. Le Corbusier hoped to solve the problems of the relatively large distances by automating, mechanising and rationalising the means of transport.[8] The project was embedded in the urban fabric on the edge of the historic city centre. Some see the influence of Structuralism in it.[9] Early experiments with low-rise double comb structures were also carried out in Finland. Swedish research, in which a traditional high-rise building,

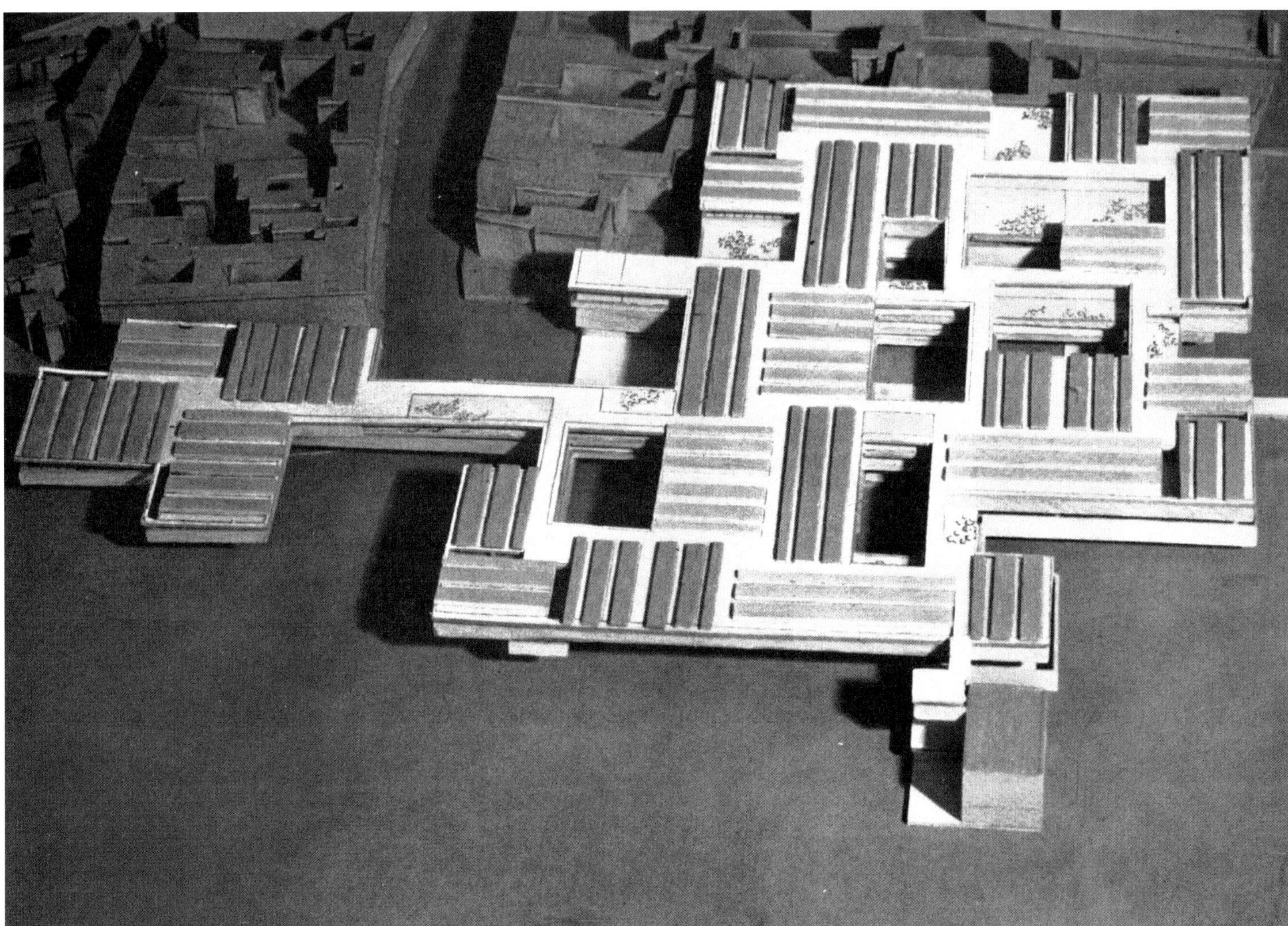

p. 164 | <
***Kruisheer + Hallink*, developmental plan for the Academisch Ziekenhuis Groningen, 1976. Covered street.**

The Humane and Modern Hospital, integration of the hospital in the urban fabric

p. 164 | >
***Kruisheer + Hallink*, developmental plan Academisch Ziekenhuis Groningen, 1976**

p. 165
The Humane and Modern Hospital, four bed ward with for every patient his own corner.

The Humane and Modern Hospital, scheme 'zones'. Integration of the functions living and working within the hospital.

The Humane and Modern Hospital, floor plan of a ward with the walking range of the patient after surgery. Black: the first days; dark grey: one step closer towards recovery; light grey: preparation for going home.

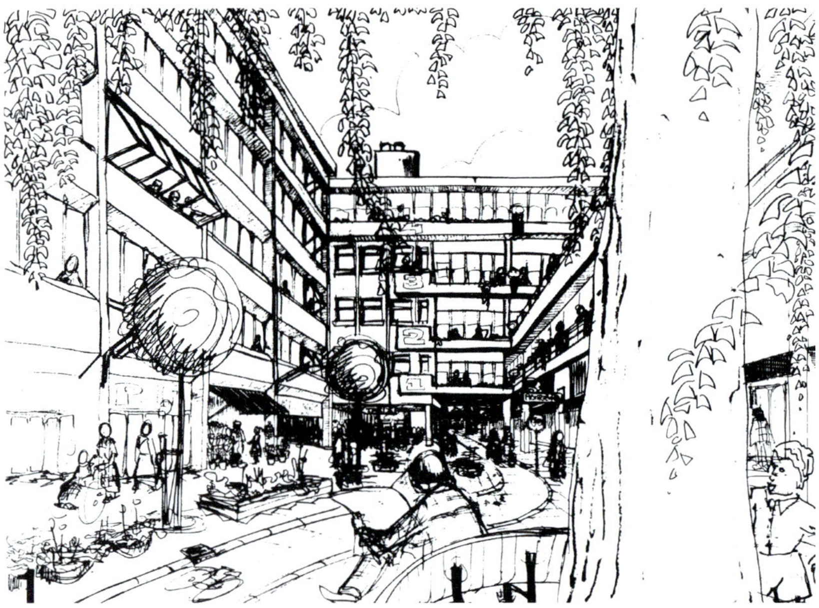

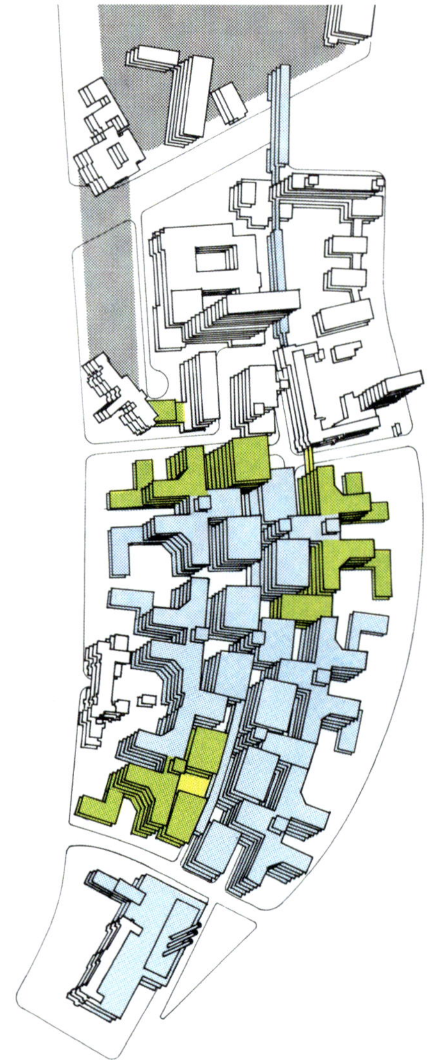

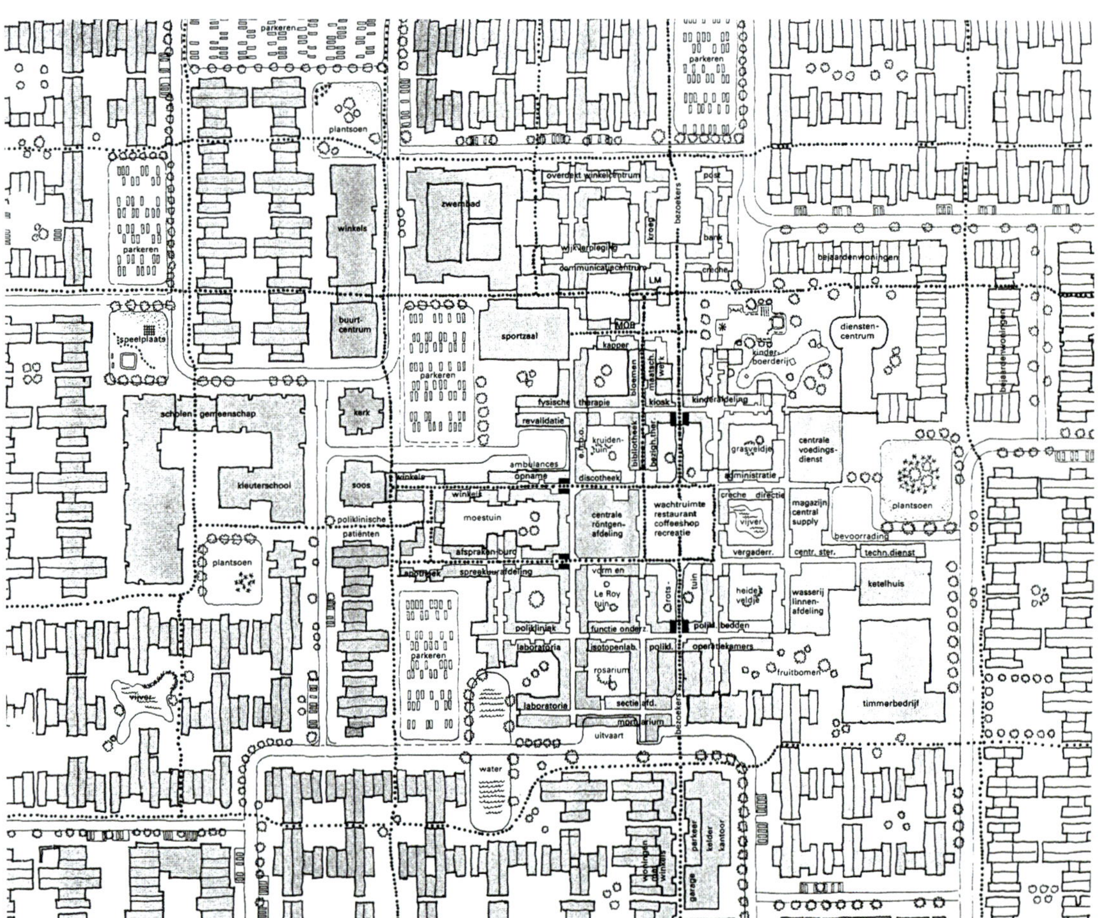

a low pavilion hospital like the Hvidovre and a hybrid form were designed for a given programme, demonstrated that the high-rise building was the least efficient: the distances and the time wasted in transporting goods and patients were by far the largest.[10] Even I. Rosenfield, who had advocated high-rise building all his life, later showed more appreciation for low-rise solutions: 'it's better to go out than up'.[11]

As for hospitals in the Netherlands, although their quality was not called into question, a study trip organised in 1970 by the International Hospital Federation (IHF) concluded that they were certainly not pioneering in the exploration of new possibilities. The programme included visits to a large number of projects.[12] Before the study trip had begun, J.B. Stolte wrote in *World Hospitals*, the organ of the IHF, that the design of Dutch hospitals was conservative, 'consisting often of separate, but linked ward, diagnostic and service blocks, with in most cases the diagnostic and treatment block arranged in such a way that expansion is possible, but the ward block designed as if no change in that area is to be expected'.[13] It soon proved to be the case that it was difficult to adapt these hospitals, which had only been completed very recently, to changing demands.

The regulation of hospital construction

The cost of health care went up by almost a factor of ten (from 797 million to 7388 million guilders) between 1953 and 1970. The share of national income that was spent on health care rose in the same period from 3.3 to 6.4 per cent. The share of hospital health care (excluding treatment by specialists) rose from 32.8 to 43.8 per cent.[14] The rising costs were mainly due to the increase in the number of general hospitals and of the number of beds. By the spring of 1969 there were 220 general hospitals with a total of 66,000 beds, amounting to 5.1 per 1,000 of the population. Even the most optimistic economic predictions did not alter the fact that health care was well on the way to becoming unaffordable. To prevent that from happening, the system of regulations on supply was overhauled. If regulations were imposed on hospital construction, it was hoped that hospital use would decrease too. This approach was embodied in the Hospital Provisions Act of 1971. This envisaged the setting up of a Hospital Provisions Board to look into the desirability of new buildings and to draw up a national hospital plan to that end. This resulted in a regional distribution plan that soon proved to be unfeasible. The Board had more success in drawing up criteria to be met by the building plans. The research was contracted out to the hospital specialists united in the Foundation for Architects Research on Health Care Buildings (Stagg).

At first the Stagg tried to develop a standard programme, but that turned out to be overambitious. Instead, under the leadership of Central Project Head J.P. Kloos, the Stagg investigated the optimal dimensions of the various parts of a hospital. Another important step in regulating supply was the Structural Memorandum presented by the state secretary of health J. Hendriks in 1974. It combined two strategies: the introduction of a ladder structure (which meant that expensive equipment could only be installed in hospitals) and regionalisation (geographical distribution in accordance with the aims of the Hospital Provisions Board). An important feature of the Memorandum was the curbing of access to hospital provisions: from now on, before they could be admitted to a hospital, patients had to be referred by their general practitioner; the latter acquired the function of a gatekeeper.

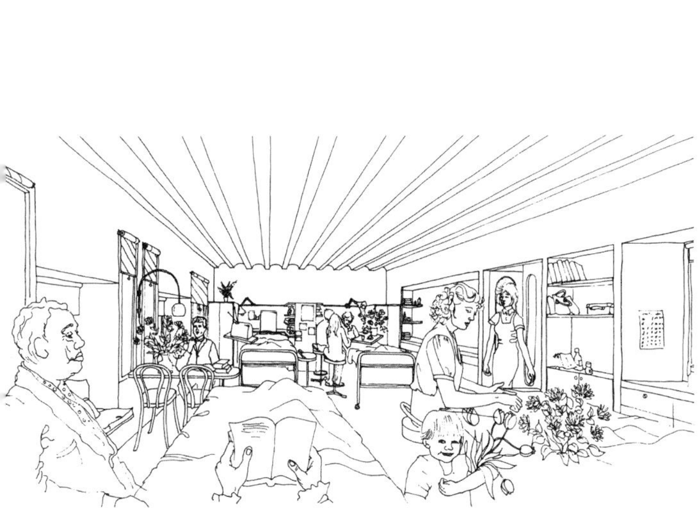

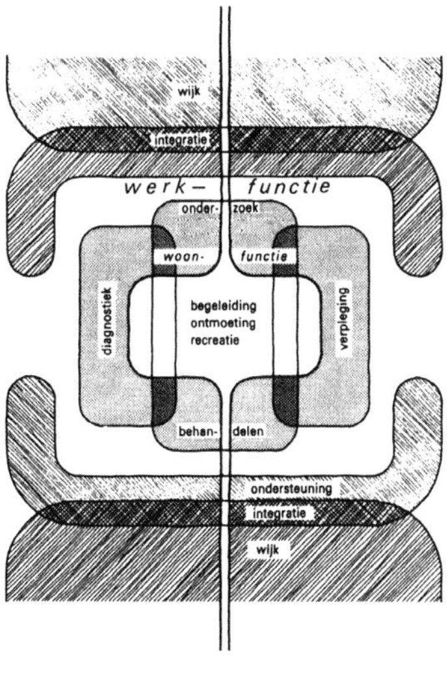

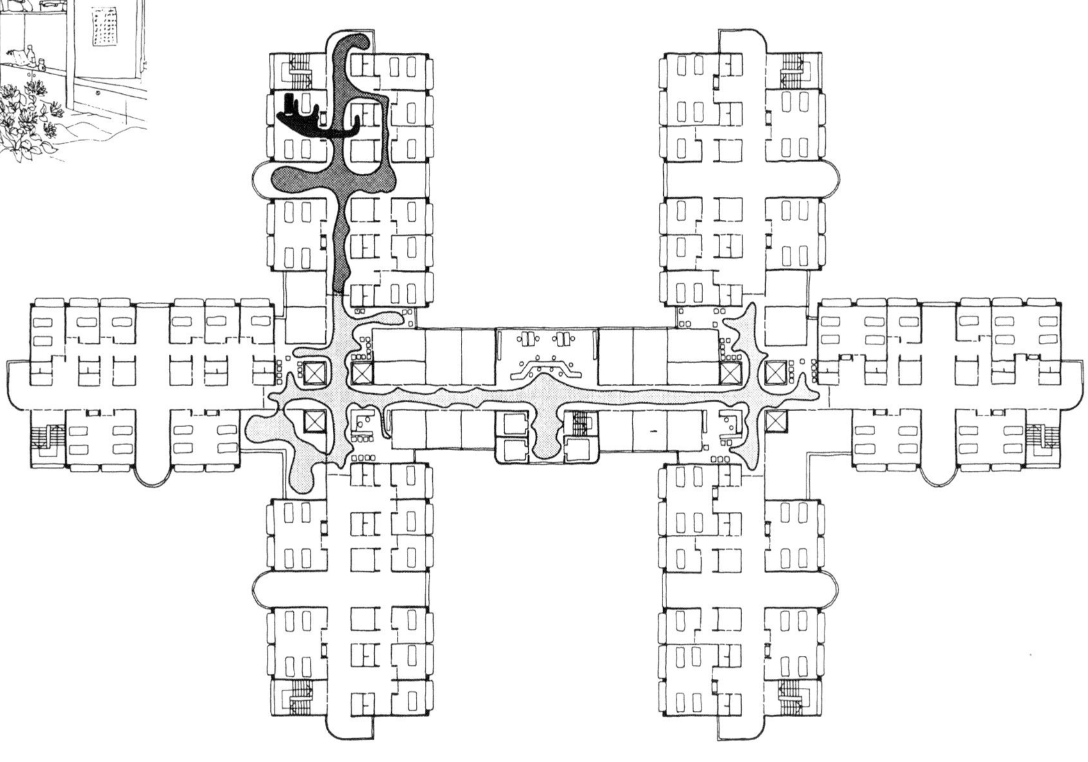

A direct consequence for architecture of the regulating of supply was a sharp increase in the standardisation of the basic components of a hospital. The Board considered research on 'building criteria' to be inevitable. Apart from the surface measurements that R. Nicolaï had been making since 1969 for the National Hospital Institute (NZI), there were few hard facts on the dimensions required for the various departments, except for the surface area per bed, which was still regarded as the main criterion and had increased between 1953 and 1968 from 53 to 79 m^2, and the fact that most of this increase had been caused by the outpatient units.[15] Nicolaï's studies compared the surface areas of the different parts of a hospital, but did not relate the results to the actual functioning of these parts, so the Board wanted further research to be conducted. Besides, Nicolaï confined himself to charting existing hospitals, and the Board believed that that would lead to outdated information: 'The basing of assessment criteria on these historical numbers for guidance alone seems a risky enterprise because precisely now, when health care should have to function in a stringency model, most of the recent buildings were developed during an economic boom.'[16]

However, years passed before the norms and guidelines, later referred to as 'architectural functional assessment criteria', were drawn up, partly as a result of the increasing complexity. Moreover, patients were calling for more and more attention. In 1979 the Board noted that there was now a tendency to view the 'carrier of the illness with which the specialists are primarily concerned increasingly as a person'.[17] The designing of 'building modules' was entrusted to the NZI in 1979 to draw up generally elaborated standard elements. The Board saw no future in the design of a complete standard hospital; in the building of the five Wiegerinck hospitals, which were created on the basis of the same standard programme, major changes in the design had proved to be inevitable, and designing without a standard was already difficult enough.[18]

The Humane and Modern Hospital

The attempts of the Stagg to work on innovative hospital concepts led to reflection on new principles. These were directly influenced by the criticisms of the so-called 'white elephants' and reflected alternative views about a different way of organising society. The Stichting Ziekenhuis Menselijk en Modern (The Humane and Modern Hospital Foundation) played a large role. Increasing emphasis came to be put on the welfare of the patient in the early 1970s on the part of the government, the medical world and designers. Magazines such as *Het Ziekenhuis* were full of articles with phrases about 'putting the patient at the centre' and 'humanity' in the hospital. This theme played a major role in the Werkgroep 2000 (Working Group 2000), under the inspired leadership of A.J.H. Thiadens, which occupied itself from 1965 on with the position of the patient amidst the rapid developments in the field of medicine.

The Humane and Modern Hospital Foundation was an initiative of this working group. It consisted of a number of experts in the field of health care who were drawn from the world of design, architecture and medicine. They included A.H. Wiebenga and J.C.M. Hattinga Verschure, who were both Professors of Hospital Science. Among the architects was W. Eijkelenboom from the Rotterdam firm Eijkelenboom Gerritse Middelhoek. Modernism had come under increasing fire since the 1950s, and those criticisms had an impact on the issues that the working group tackled: 'Is a modern hospital still humane? Is a humane home for the sick always a modern hospital?'[19] This resulted in the publication *Ziekenhuis Menselijk en Modern*. This handbook, which was published as a loose leaf system between 1969 and 1975, gives an accurate picture of the views that were held in the 1970s.

'Humane' was associated with a small-scale entity in which it was easy to find one's way and the creation of organisational and spatial structures that guaranteed the largest possible degree of self-determination. This was taken to be in accordance with 'natural' human living conditions; if social conditions obstructed that, people would become alienated. 'Modern' stood for the technological and economic progress whose positive effects could not be denied; moreover, it now also benefited those strata of the population who had previously been denied it. But 'modern' also meant cold, aloof, immune to the influence of the individual, authoritarian, a machine that was not directed by people's needs but was fully autonomous and at the service of a politico-economic system that was exclusively orientated towards the generation of prosperity and the maintenance of the existing power structures: 'The mass of products, materials, technologies, building physics, increase of scale and dimension, the entire production of housing and working, is increasing brought into the sphere of the economic principle. This has led to alienation, reduced contact, irritation, aggression and more. If you add the alienation between housing and work, the result is the monocultures of the dormitory towns, industrial estates, commercial and shopping centres, etc.'[20] The objective of the foundation was to bring the beneficial effects of modern technology and science into line with the 'natural' demands of human existence. Could the hospital as a 'fortress of science and human intelligence' ever become a home for the sick in which the humane and the modern were reconciled with one another?[21]

What was wrong with the hospitals was more than the design: the very principles on which they were based were fundamentally wrong. There was therefore a need for a new basic philosophy. What must change, at any rate, was the literal division of the hospital into specialised units. According to Draaisma, the representative of the National Hospital Council (NZR), the work of the Humane and Modern Hospital Foundation resulted in nothing less than a basic philosophy. Its most important aspects were: equality of the patient and members of staff, respect for everyone's need for privacy, and the vision that treatment and counselling were inextricably interrelated. Patients should be enabled to play an active part in their own and one another's healing and to be able to continue their personal lifestyle as much as possible. The accommodation and work function of every area should be integrated and the hospital should be given a 'human scale' and embedded in the built-up environment. The hospital was viewed as a large therapeutic community.

It was the job of the architect to create the spatial conditions in which this community could be created and function. And that was something different from 'designing an efficient healing factory with a quasi-humane touch such as shops in the reception area and a reproduction on the wall'.[22] The architect was expected to create a humane environment in which the technological perfection of medicine and health care would coincide with care for the wellbeing of the patient. It was thus the search for a synthesis between humane and modern in the design of the building as well.

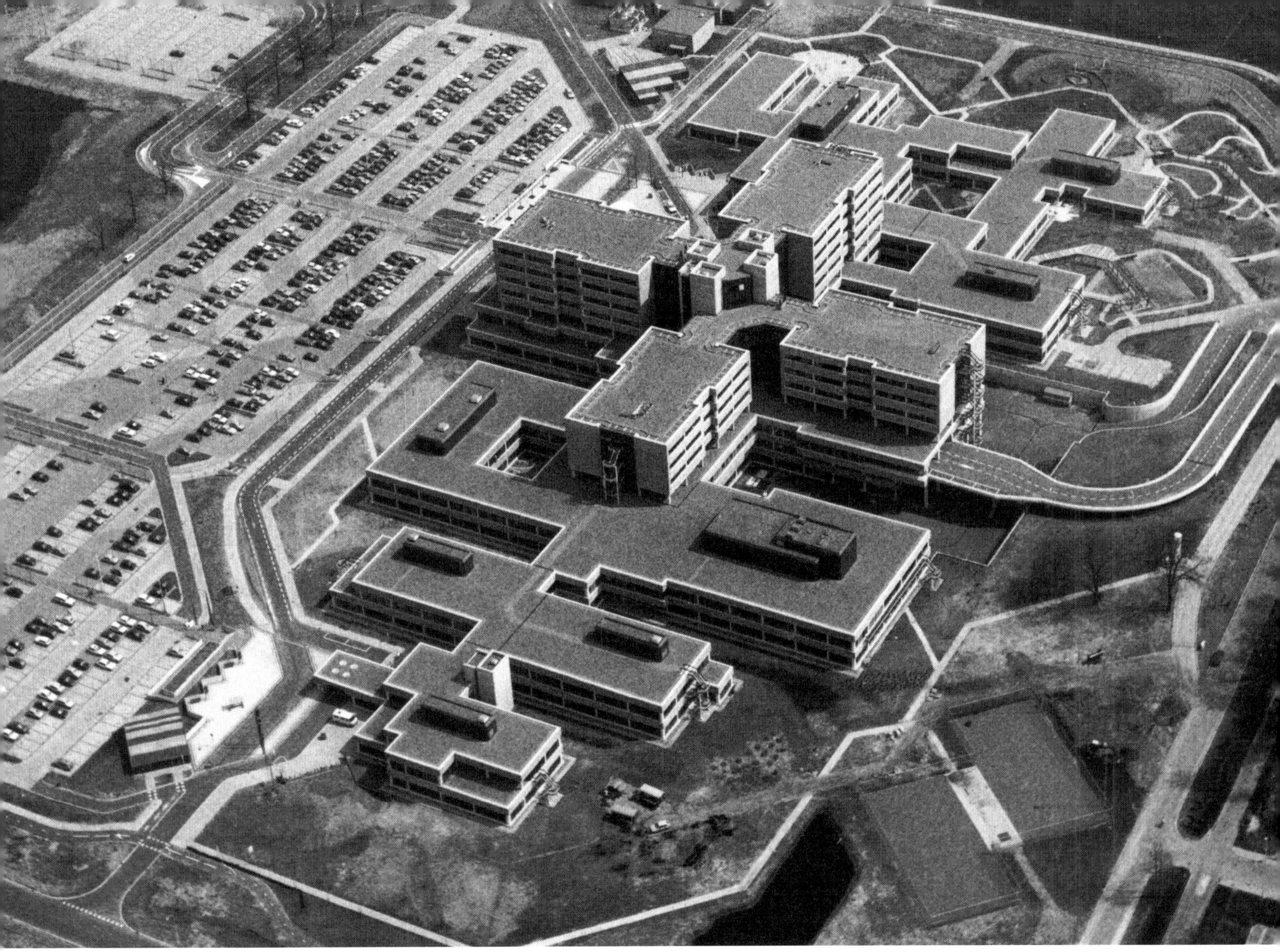

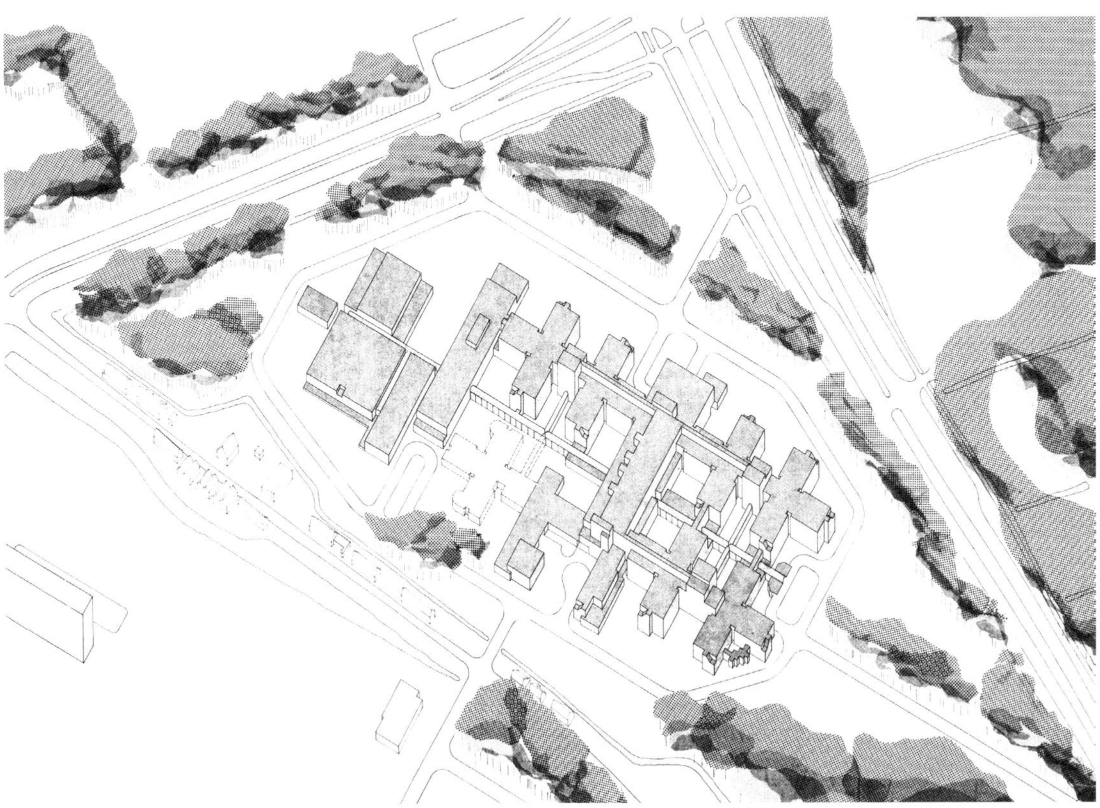

Architektenburo Roelofs Nijst Lucas, Streekziekenhuis, Almelo, 1984

Eijkelenboom Gerritse Middelhoek architecten, design for the Dordwijk Ziekenhuis, Dordrecht 1973

Architectural protest

Philosophising is one thing, architecture is another. How were the alternative visions expressed in buildings? A few designs were made in the 1970s that, even though some of them were only implemented in a radically revised form if at all, are nevertheless exemplary of the ideas that were developed in the 1970s. In 1973 Eijkelenboom was commissioned to design the Dordwijk Ziekenhuis in Dordrecht (the later Merwedeziekenhuis), a medium-sized hospital with 530 beds. The immediate motivation for the commission was Eijkelenboom's account of the views of the Humane and Modern Hospital Foundation, which went down well with the board of directors.[23] Those views were taken fairly literally as the premises of the design. High tech medical provisions such as operating theatres were placed in a high 'rib', the intensive care and nursing units were close to this rib, and the wards for more ambulant patients were further away. The most striking feature was the design of the wards, whose ground plan was shaped like a leaf of clover in which the three petals were the nursing units and the space in between functioned as a subcentre. A small meeting point was created here, entirely in accordance with the social ambitions of the foundation. The subcentres of the two wards were connected with a main centre that was located underneath the central rib. The nursing units were intended to represent the residential home in terms of nursing, care, counselling and individual initiative.[24] Eijkelenboom conceived this design as a small town – this too was in line with the philosophy of the foundation.[25]

Dordwijk is typical of a way of working that was specific to the 1970s. It implied doing away with the hegemony of the specialists. The plan itself was not implemented, but some of its features, such as the clover-shaped wards, can be seen in the definitive design for the Merwedeziekenhuis.

Another design that was never implemented is J.E. Kruisheer's 1976 design for the new university hospital in Groningen. It was separate from the trio of designs for university hospitals in Amsterdam, Leiden and Utrecht, for which a joint programme of criteria was developed. In 1975 the hospital decided to invite Kruisheer as head architect to elaborate an almost complete replacement of the old pavilions. This was based on a study by the Institut für Krankenhausbau that had indicated that the grounds were large enough for this operation to be possible. The ambitions were high: the new complex was to offer 1,733 beds, later to be expanded to 1,896 if desired – a good 75 per cent more than, for example, the Amsterdam university hospital (AMC).[26] Kruisheer presented his development plan in 1976. This plan too completely radiated the atmosphere of the period in which it was conceived. The context of this plan was unusual: it was one of the few new hospitals to be projected on the existing site on the outskirts of the historic city centre. This gave Kruisheer a unique opportunity to implement his ideal of integration with the urban fabric.

An extra stimulus for this was undoubtedly the pioneering Groningen inner city plan of 1972, one of the first official policy memoranda in the Netherlands to advocate transparency, warmth, small scale and combining of functions. One of the expressions of this was the Traffic Circulation Plan, which removed through traffic from the city centre. Kruisheer's plan was a collage of relatively small-scale pavilions. They had a rational logistical organisation in the form of underground corridors, but were otherwise orientated towards the scale and structure of their built-up surroundings. The public area of the city continued virtually

p. 168
***Hendriks Campman Tennekes*, Sint Antonius Ziekenhuis, Nieuwegein, 1983**

p. 169
***Buro Wiegerinck Architekten*, Sint-Maartensgasthuis, Venlo (Tegelen), 1983**

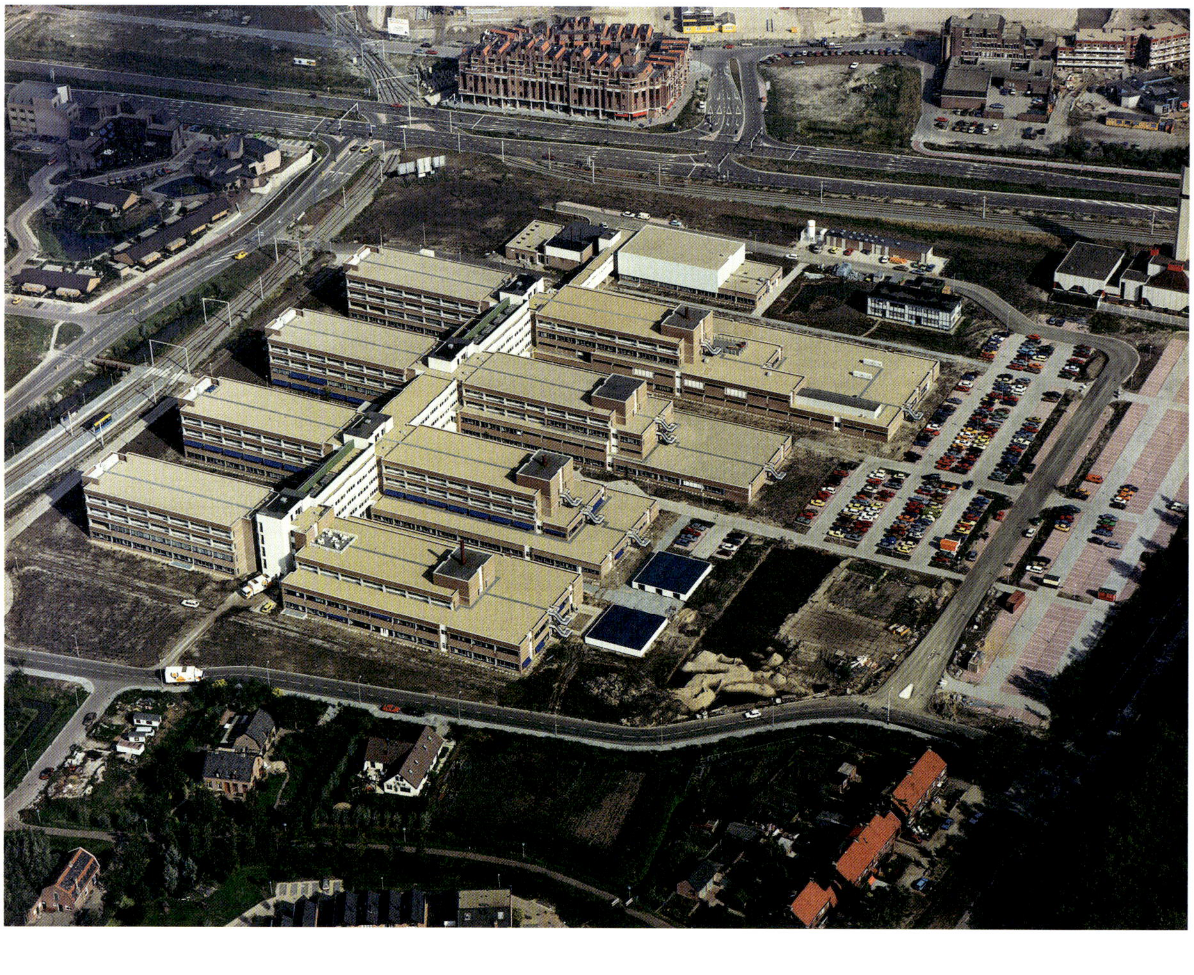

uninterrupted on the site of the hospital, and the services that it offered would also be available to local residents. Each pavilion had its own entrance. If extension outside the hospital grounds were to prove necessary in the future, the small-scale structure would avoid the presence of harsh contrasts. A completely transformed version of this plan, a typical product of the 1970s, was eventually implemented in the 1990s.

Open-end structures

While the lofty social ambitions of institutions like the Working Group 2000 and the Humane and Modern Hospital Foundation were only rarely incarnated in implemented plans, a lasting memory of the 1970s was the requirement that a hospital should be amenable to change once it had been completed. That had always been a theme, but now everything seemed to focus on maximising flexibility. Roelofs Nijst Lucas designed the Sint Elisabeth Ziekenhuis in Tilburg and the Streekziekenhuis in Almelo in the second half of the 1970s. Both hospitals were laid out in accordance with the double comb structure. One of the reasons for adopting this type was that it was optimally expandable and the division into small units was believed to result in a human scale. The various units at right angles to the main axis can be expanded as necessary, and each unit could be given a design of its own. A somewhat higher ward building was placed on top of the comb structure. The designers wanted to combine the advantages of low-rise with those of high-rise building, reminiscent of the tower on a podium type of hospital. The wards were somewhat articulated and raised slightly above the building below to produce a less closed effect. The switch from high-rise to low-rise building could also be seen in the activities of Hendriks Campman Tennekes in this period, where the open-end structure was introduced too. The Sint Antonius Ziekenhuis in Nieuwegein was built at the same time as the Sint Elisabeth Ziekenhuis in Tilburg and also had a double comb structure. According to H.J. Tennekes, apart from the kitchen and laundry there was no other organisation that applied to the hospital organisation in its entirely.

The design for the Sint-Maartensgasthuis in Venlo, a project by Buro Wiegerinck Architekten, was preceded by three-hundred pages of basic philosophy and basic programme. It contains all the standard ingredients: integration into the neighbourhood, communal use of as many facilities as possible by both the neighbourhood and the hospital, and, finally, the striving for flexibility. A geometrical grid determines the structure of this double comb type, each tooth of which was theoretically extendable. After thirteen years of planning and talking, the hospital finally opened in 1983, by which time the basic philosophy had almost become a historical document.

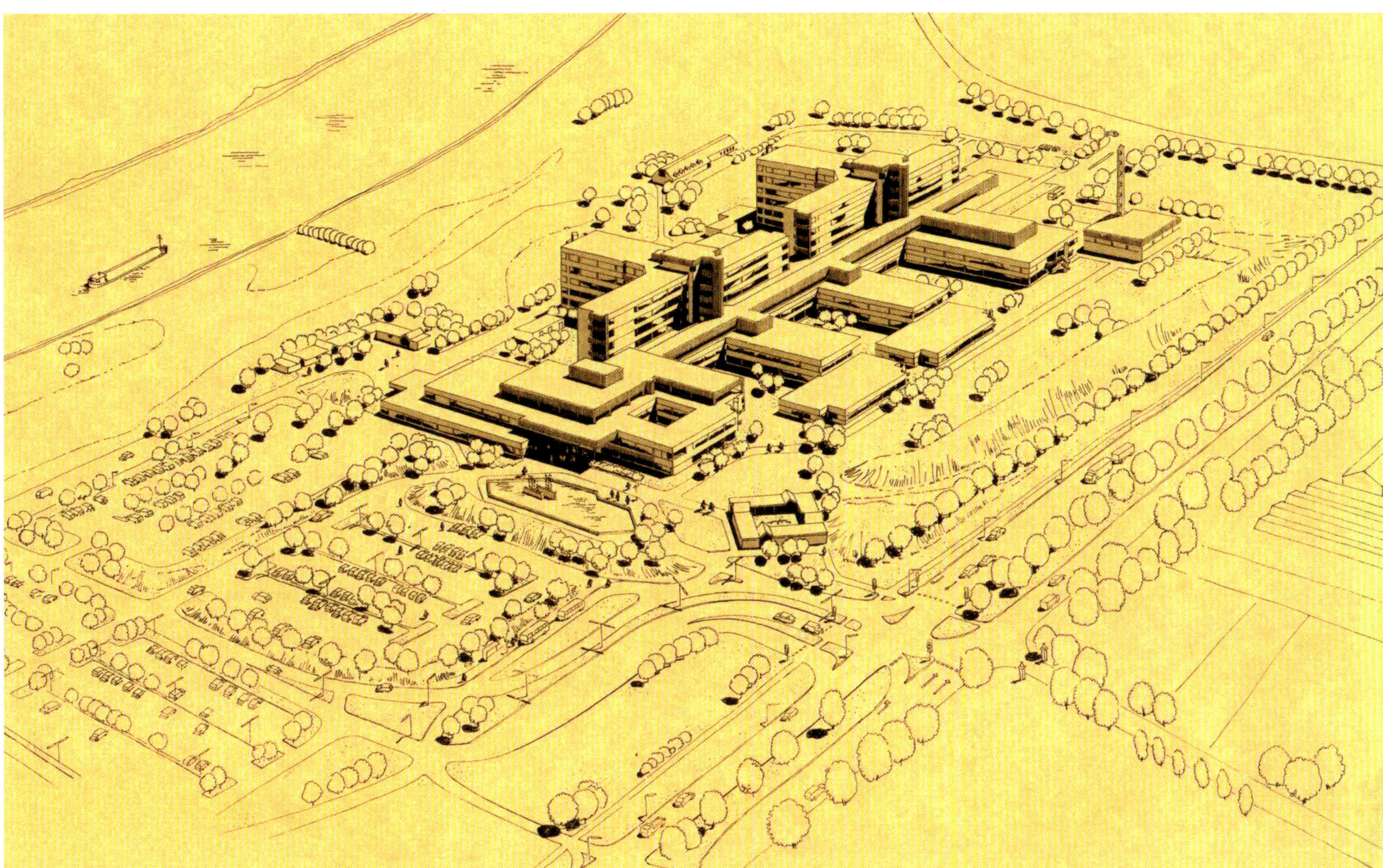

Psychiatry

Unlike in the world of the hospitals, the striving for standardisation and regulation did not play a large role in psychiatry. After the introduction of psychiatric drugs, the strong growth in the importance of all kinds of forms of psychotherapy was the next influential innovation, and since many of these therapies worked best with small groups, they confronted the institutions with a process of reduction of scale. Often the different therapies were accommodated in specially designed small buildings that were set more or less at random between the existing buildings. If the different therapies were taken as the basis for the accommodation of the patients – a process known as categorisation – this led to far smaller groups than had been the case previously on the basis of the commonly applied rough division into categories of controllability. The existing buildings were often too large to meet the new demands. The same was true of the classic pavilions, which had expanded to become complete small hospitals, especially in the later complexes. One short-term solution was to divide up the existing buildings, but the ideal was to demolish them and replace them with new ones. Paradoxically enough, this sometimes led to plans for large buildings on the principle of small scale in large scale. As in the hospitals this ran up against opposition, though this was much heaver in psychiatry, and threatened the very foundations of psychiatry as such. In the wake of this development, the raison d'être of the institutions was called into question.

Around 1970 the psychiatric hospitals were the theme of a frontal assault on the status quo. Many of the institutions were run by governing bodies whose composition was hardly different from what had been common practice for centuries. That made them all the more vulnerable to charges of being total institutions in which the ruling class removed recalcitrant citizens from its midst and kept them under control. At any rate it seemed out of key with the demands of a modern, efficient organisation and that met with increasing opposition that was apparently supported by more than just a few psychiatrists, psychologists and therapists from the counterculture. Anti-psychiatry originated in Italy, where it was championed by the psychiatrist Francesco Basaglia. Under his influence, institutions in the cities under Communist control were closed down.[27]

The campaign of the countermovement within psychiatry and the changes in the conception of the architecture of the psychiatric hospital were motivated by the desire to conform more closely to the wishes of the patient. The child psychiatrist Sjef Teuns caused a big stir at the Leids Medisch Opvoedkundig Bureau (Leiden Child Guidance Clinic) around 1970. A conference held in that year, 'Te gek om los te lopen', (the title, literally 'too crazy to be on the loose', is a pun on the Dutch expression meaning 'too ridiculous for words') focused attention on abuses in psychiatry. The Dennendal conflict of 1971 drew attention to the mental asylum and various publications kept the institution in the public eye in the following years. Carel Muller, who was not a psychiatrist but a therapist, regarded those with a mental disability as fully fledged citizens from which many 'healthy' people caught up in the modern rat race could learn a thing or two.

The architect Frank van Klingeren, famous at the time for his multifunctional complex De Meerpaal in Dronten, was prepared to translate Muller's ideals into design. He first proposed closing down the asylum and integrating its residents in a normal urban environment, but when that plan proved too ambitious, he came up with a proposal to build homes for healthy occupants in the grounds of the institution. This second plan eventually came to nothing. What was at stake in all this was the normalisation of the psychiatric patient, which was popularised in various quarters. Besides Jan Foudraine's famous bestseller *Wie is van hout* (published in English as *Not made of wood*), they included E. Tellegen's *Waar was de dood nog meer* (Where else was death) and C. van Eijk's *Laat ze het maar voelen* (Just let them feel it).[28]

Although it was all about the interests of the patients, they played no role of significance for a long time. The Pandora Foundation had been set up in 1964, but it kept psychiatric patients on the sidelines too until the early 1970s. The initiative for Pandora came from A.L. van Amerongen, a prosperous businessman who had emigrated to the United States, where he was inspired by the mental health movement that was supported by the Kennedy administration.[29] At first Pandora made every effort to remove the stigma from psychiatry. Posters were produced (Waarom 'gek' – omdat hij anders is? (Why 'crazy' – because he's different?) from 1969, for instance) and excursions were organised to the Willem Arntsz Foundation and elsewhere. The aim was to create a positive image and to remove old prejudices. Pandora's most famous poster came out in 1973 with the text by Simon Carmiggelt 'Ooit 'n normaal mens ontmoet? En...,

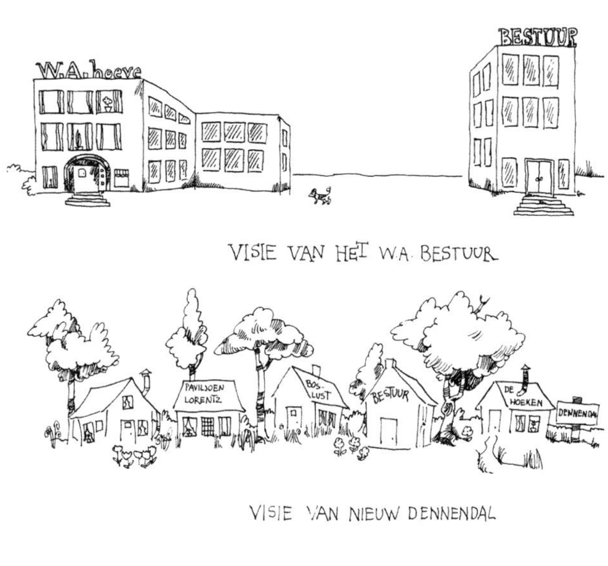

p. 170
Cartoons on the Dennendal conflict in 1971. The vision of the board of the Willem Arntsz Hoeve confronts that of the Nieuw-Dennendal mental asylum.

p. 171
***Swinkels Salemans Knibbeler Swinkels architekten en ingenieurs*, De Welterhof, Heerlen, 1971-1974. Situation and facades.**

***A. Evers, G.J.M. Sarlemijn, C.F.M. Sarlemijn, R. Scheltema*, substitute new building project for the Sint Willibrordusstichting, Heiloo, 1980**

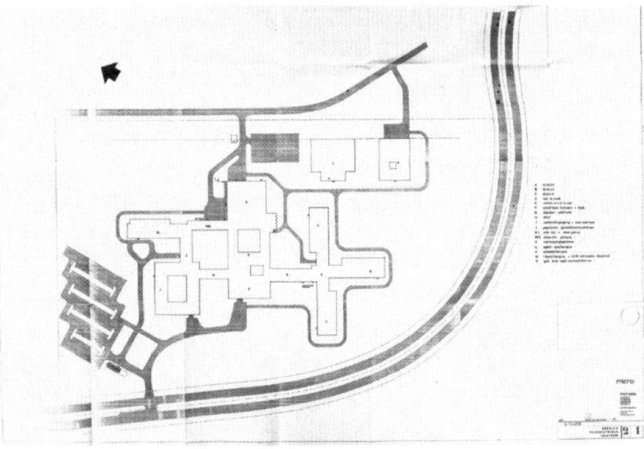

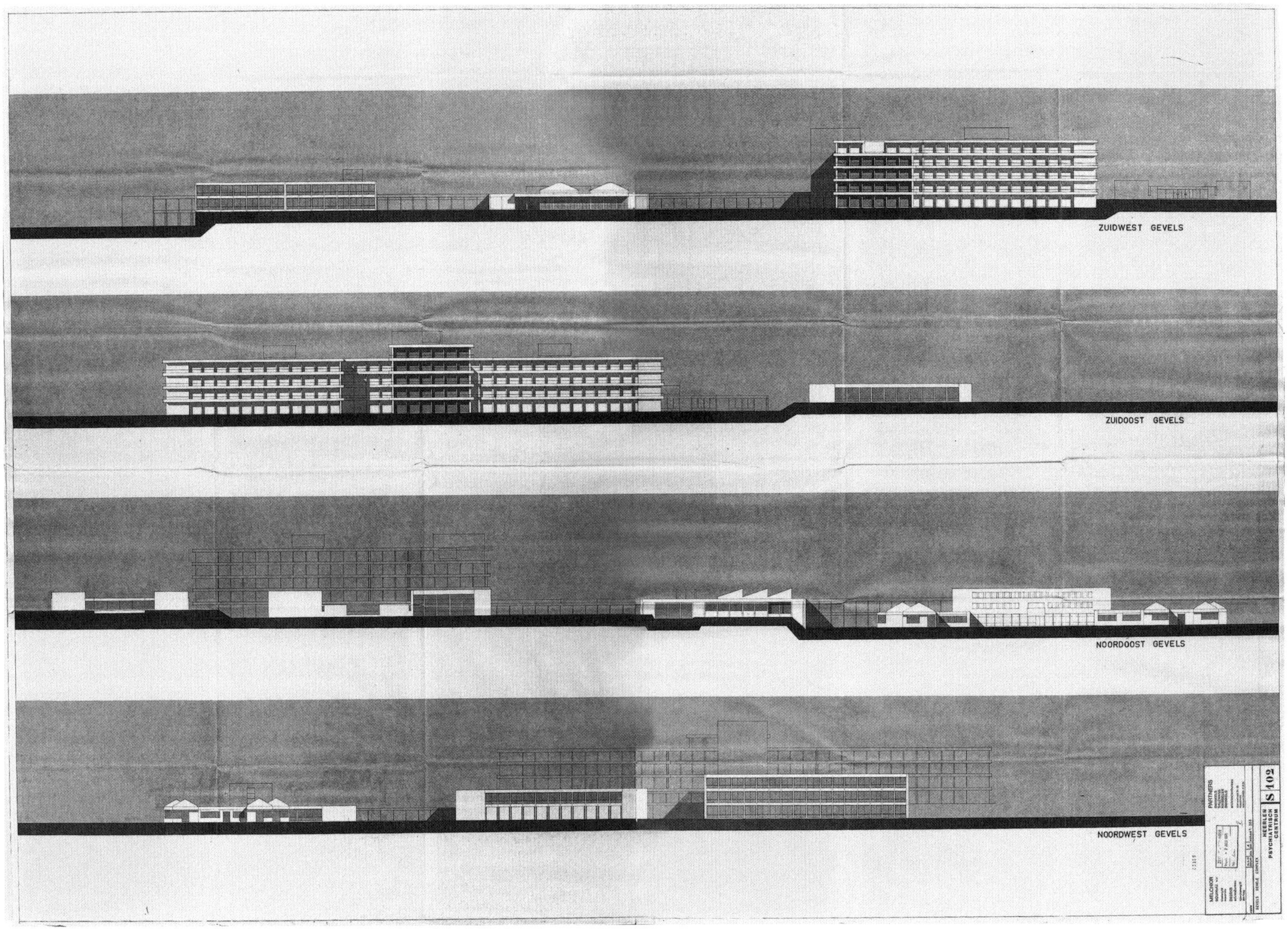
ZUIDWEST GEVELS
ZUIDOOST GEVELS
NOORDOOST GEVELS
NOORDWEST GEVELS
S 102

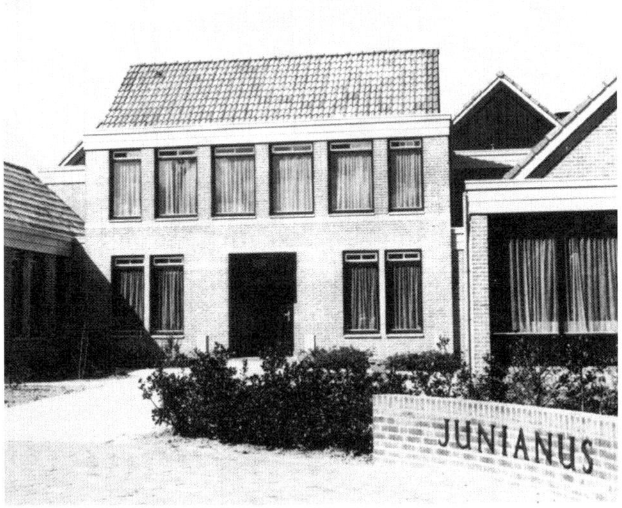
JUNIANUS

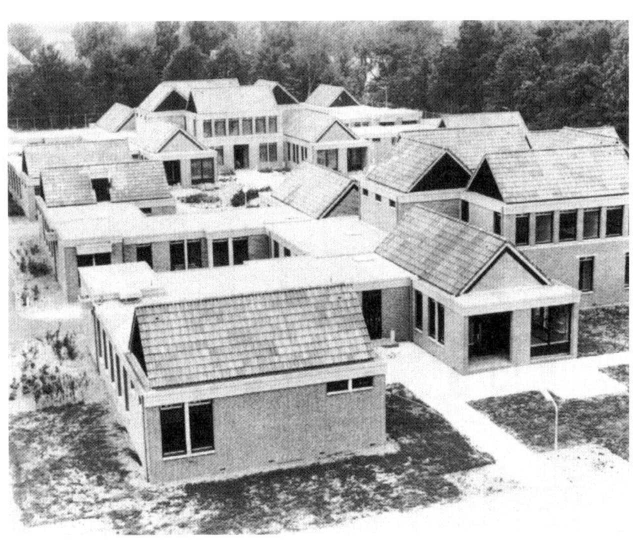

beviel 't?' (Ever meet a normal person? And... what was it like?). That year also witnessed the publication of the first issue of *De gekkenkrant*, the most direct mouthpiece of (former) patients in mental health care until its disappearance in 1981. The patient was rarely more at the centre of things than in this paper.

The pinnacle of the normalisation of the psychiatric patient was ideally the abolition of psychiatry, but no matter how influential this anti-psychiatry was for a while, this extreme consequence was never drawn in the Netherlands. Instead, the institutions became the theatre of a large-scale operation aimed at reduction of scale and favouring giving a higher priority to accommodation than to therapy. Accommodation was usually in groups: this operation led to the building of large numbers of small communities, entirely in accordance with the group thinking that became so popular at this time.

The big renovation

Small scale was the winning card in psychiatry, just as low-rise building was in hospitals. An example of the new insights is the decision of the Sint Willibrordusstichting in Heiloo to commission new buildings. This led in 1975 to a plan based on small groups of eight persons. The first tangible result was completed in 1980, relatively soon after the initial idea.

Typical of many new building projects is the wordy and often philosophically tinged justification for them. An example is the plan for expansion that Swinkels en Salemans drew up for the St. Josephstichting in Apeldoorn in 1977. Although the design envisages no more than a number of solidly designed, well detailed residential buildings, T. Swinkels could not resist carrying out a lengthy analysis of the role of the architect vis-à-vis the principal. Drawing up a plan, Swinkels argued, is to a certain extent nothing more than making a translation. The designs for the St. Josephstichting were to facilitate and promote the objectives of the institution. The purpose was clear: the asylum must no longer be an asylum, relations between the two sides of the institution walls must be intensified, and the hospitalisation of patients reduced. Swinkels wanted to avoid harsh confrontations with cold new buildings and spared natural features and historic buildings as much as possible. The renovated hospital should promote social contacts and should thus, in the terminology of Humphrey Osmond, be sociopetal. On the other hand, everyone wanted a certain measure of privacy (sociofugal). The programme for the new building was based on this analysis of the problem. The solution was a specific form of housing.

Whereas Swinkels en Salemans managed to turn their theoretical reflections into an actual design, this proved more difficult for the 'Kenniscentrum voor de humane en ambulante behandeling van gedrags- en persoonlijkheidsstoornissen' (Knowledge centre for the humane and ambulant treatment of behavioural and personality disorders) Jan Wier in Tilburg. The basic philosophy of this new institution left no doubts about the intentions: 'Jan Wier is based on the premise that people manifest themselves as a unity on the basis of their psychological, somatic and social components or capacities. Human beings maintain or develop themselves in constant interaction with their surroundings. Inroads on that development cause disturbances. If the damage is in the field of human feeling, desire or action, they are psychological disturbances. It is those disturbances that psychiatric care tackles.'[30]

p. 172 and 173
***G.A. Heldoorn*, Lankwert, Groot Lankum psychiatric hospital, Franeker, 1971**

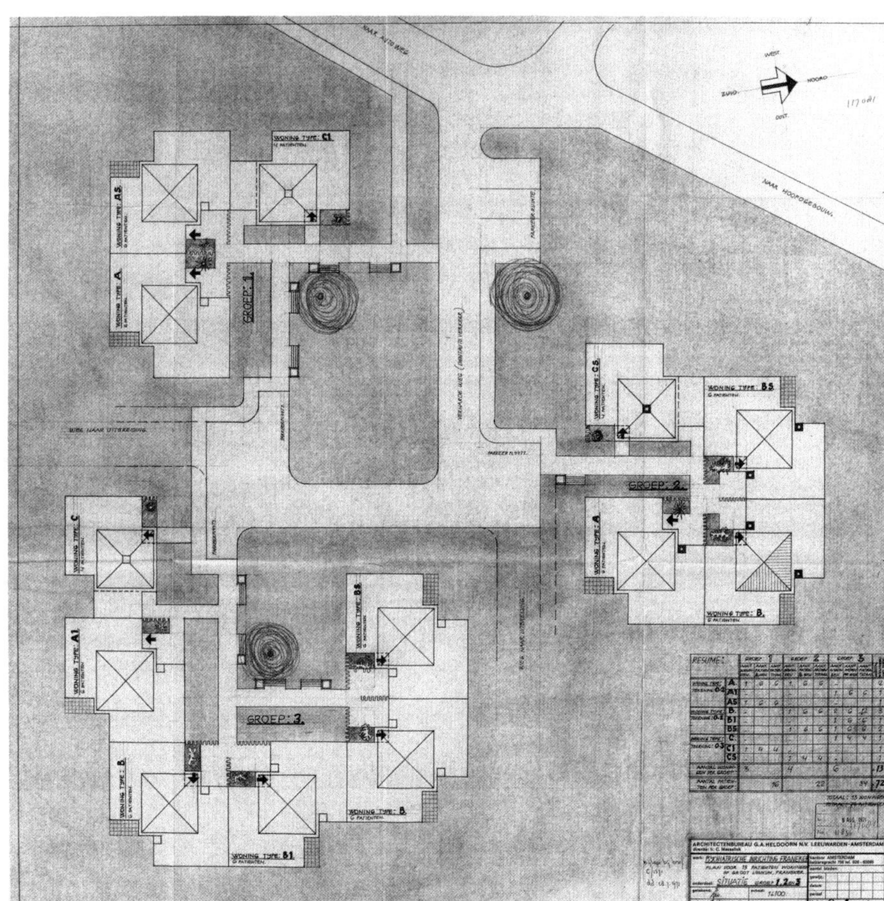

No plan was drawn up in these years that did not envisage a community centre, meeting point or social space. They form the public forums of the psychiatric hospitals and are intended to act as a catalyst of social contacts. Everybody Join In, as Camiel van Winkel sums it up, was the motto.[31] The ultimate form of this ideal was of course the therapeutic community, but it was on the way up outside that community as well.

In the Welterhof in Heerlen, another project by Swinkels en Salemans, there was a cosy bar and alcoholic drinks were on sale in the supermarket. This new complex was a tangible symbol of the abandonment of the medical model.[32] The premise was the concept of the therapeutic community. The patients were divided into categories according to where they came from and accommodated together on one floor. Each floor consisted of six 12-person units and was treated by a multidisciplinary team. The whole was composed as an urban development plan, in which the apartment block and the treatment building were the main elements and a covered street between them was the most striking feature. The architects drew inspiration from the Lijnbaan in Rotterdam and the Kalverstraat in Amsterdam, two examples held in high esteem by the rebel avant-garde within the modern movement. The designers admitted that they had also taken a good look at the Sint Franciscushof in Raalte. An attempt was made to reduce admission as much as possible in line with the desire to break down the barrier between institution and society. Five social psychiatric community centres formed a cordon around the new clinic; only those who could not be treated by those centres could spend some time in the Welterhof.

It should be clear by now that the main trend of the 1970s was to imagine alternative forms of housing. They were usually an alternative not just to the usual way of accommodating patients in psychiatric hospitals, but at the same time to how people lived in society outside the institutions. Everything in this period seemed to be about reconstructing on a small scale a social milieu that was intended to counter alienation, anticipating a complete overhaul of modern society in all its manifold aspects. However, as at the end of the eighteenth century, it turned out to be easier to create niches in the existing society as a prelude to this ideal situation: social and spatial ideal models on the scale of the residential group within and outside the psychiatric hospital.

An example of the latter, a 'village' that, although related to an institution, was nevertheless fairly autonomous, illustrates the enduring renewal that had been maturing since the 1950s but took shape in this period. In 1974 the Groot Lankum psychiatric hospital in Franeker opened a new village. It consisted of thirteen homes intended for seventy patients of different categories. With the hospital only a stone's throw away, they could lead their own lives here in relative independence, able to count on assistance when necessary, but in theory as autonomous as possible. In all its modesty, Lankwert is a symbol of the main trends of the 1970s, when the aim was to abolish the distinction between normal and abnormal, to no longer see 'madness' as deviance nor deviant behaviour as a symptom of madness, to stop hospitals from manifesting themselves as medical bulwarks but to integrate them in the urban fabric – all in the name of dehospitalisation.

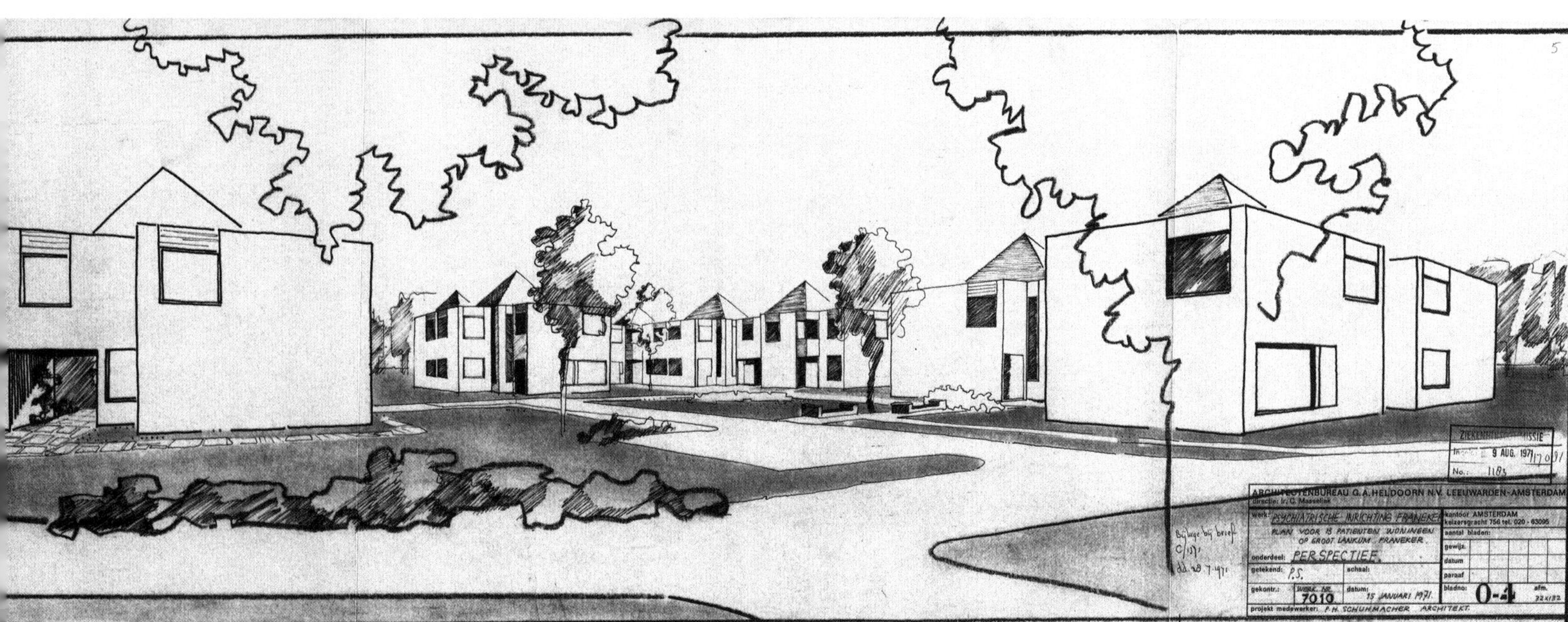

Housing and care for the elderly

Like the hospital world, housing for the elderly was also exposed to attempts to bring the explosive costs down by regulating the supply of expensive institutions. At the same time more radical voices were heard in this sector as well. In the meantime the building of nursing homes accelerated, but while this upsurge of building activity was taking place, the character of the nursing home changed from a simple hospital to an institution that gave priority to how people lived and spent their time there.

What opportunities were there to reduce the costs of accommodation for the elderly? The original intentions of the policy that had been launched in 1945 remained intact. In principle appropriate housing should be offered to every elderly person. However, this was not an open cheque. The nursing home was by far the most expensive of the various forms of home. A cheaper option was the self-sufficient housing unit, and finally some of the regular housing stock was suitable for the elderly without any extra investments. Research demonstrated that many old people stayed in a more expensive type of accommodation than was justified by the nature of their demand for care. This led to what was known as a substitution policy: the demand for more expensive forms must be drastically reduced in favour of cheaper alternatives.

Two complementary strategies were implemented in the 1970s for this purpose: the building of extra self-sufficient housing units, and the promotion of service centres that provided facilities to make it easier for the elderly to avoid institutional care. The promotion of the building of self-sufficient housing units was mainly paid for by reducing the building of old people's homes. When that did not seem to yield results quickly enough, it was decided to invest more money in accommodation for the elderly; of course most of this was spent on housing. The Policy on the Elderly Memorandum of 1970 envisaged the production between that year and 1974 of at least 60,000 self-sufficient housing units, as well as fifty service centres a year. This involved an extra investment of 359 million guilders from the national budget. The government anticipated an increase in the number of old people between 1965 and 2000 of no less than eighty per cent: 'The demographic structure of our country is thus changing drastically and the problem of the elderly will thereby become an issue that includes every facet connected with changes in that structure and their social, economic, cultural and health consequences for our society'.[33]

To make it easier for the elderly to continue to live at home, the government stimulated the building of service centres. Since they would not have to leave their own neighbourhood for the services provided by the centre, this measure would remove the need to move to an institutional home for the elderly. All the old people in the neighbourhood were to be serviced by the centre, irrespective of their living conditions. In its mature form, the service centre can be considered as a communal complex without living quarters.

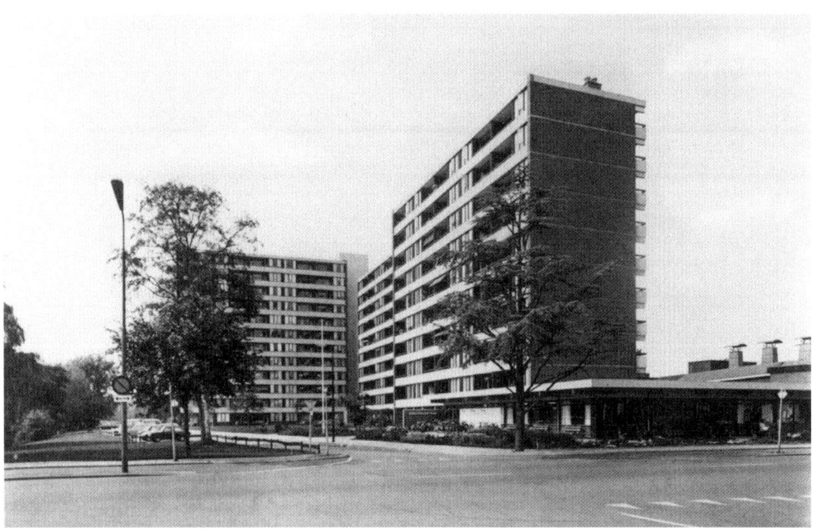

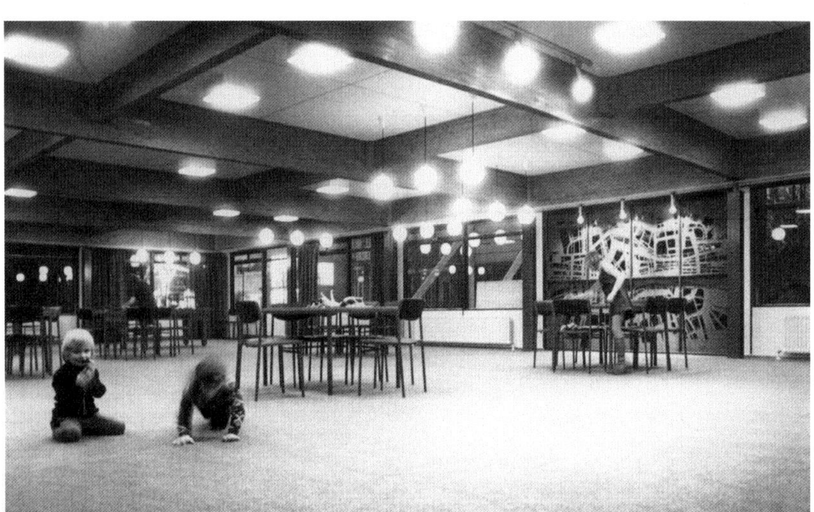

p. 174
Duivenwal service centre, Veenendaal, 1970

p. 175
***M. Gerbenzon*, service centre, Menaldum, 1970**

***Architectenbureau Postma*, service centre, Delft, 1972**

The elderly live elsewhere, either in housing not specifically built for that purpose, or in old people's homes that are scattered among the ordinary stock of housing or placed near the service centre and then offer similar facilities as in the combination of communal facilities and individual residential units. There was usually a central kitchen; a central bathroom facility and a central launderette. The following service centres were implemented: Duivenwal in Veenendaal (1970), a service centre with 112 residential units in the Schalkwijk district of Haarlem and designed by Brakel en Buma, a service centre in Delft (1972) designed by Architectenbureau Postma, and one in Menaldum (1970) designed by M. Gerbenzon.

The version of the service centre as a separate building did not really get off the ground, which is why the number is fairly limited; if integrated in the communal complex with individual residential units, it offered similar compositional possibilities to the latter. The less well-to-do elderly proved in practice to make hardly any use of the central kitchen, central bathroom facilities could never replace a bath or shower at home, and laundering could just as easily be done at home. There was also little enthusiasm to combine the service centre with a communal complex with individual residential units; it must be clear that the latter could not assume responsibilities for all the elderly persons in the neighbourhood, and that they in turn had no right to make use of the facilities of the complex.[34] The substitution policy was not very successful at first. In 1977 it was therefore decided to impose strict admission requirements on acceptance in an institution that combined communal facilities and individual residential units. Only those who really needed care were welcome.

Nursing homes: from medical model to home model

The first generation of nursing homes were hospitals without high-quality medical facilities. Although much was done to reactivate the residents, they nevertheless spent a large part of the day in shared bedrooms. That laid the nursing home even more open than the care home to the charge of being a total institution.

When they were not undergoing all kinds of therapies in the rest units, the patients spent their time in the equivalent of the nursing units in a regular hospital. A large number of those in for nursing stayed in bed, but there were also social rooms for chronically ill old people who were not permanently bedridden. As they often stayed in nursing homes for a long time, the way they spent their time was the equivalent of what in normal circumstances is regarded as being at home. In nursing homes, however, a real feeling of being at home was frustrated by the failure to satisfy its primary conditions: there is little privacy, there are no opportunities to arrange your interior as you would like, and the possibilities of dividing up your time as you choose are limited by the inevitable institutional regime, which dictates not only the treatment periods, but also the times when visitors are allowed and mealtimes. In fact the institutional

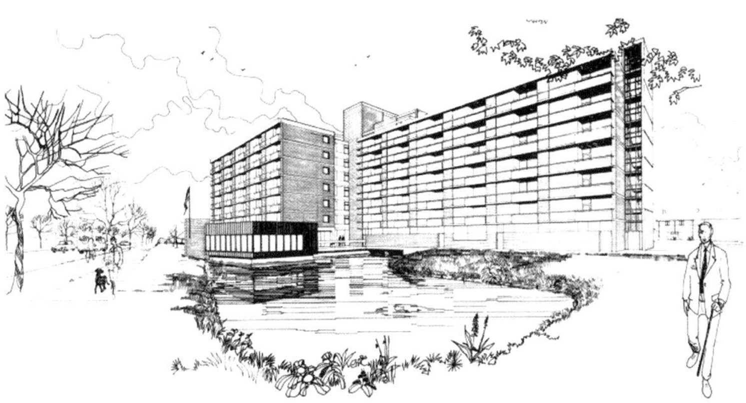

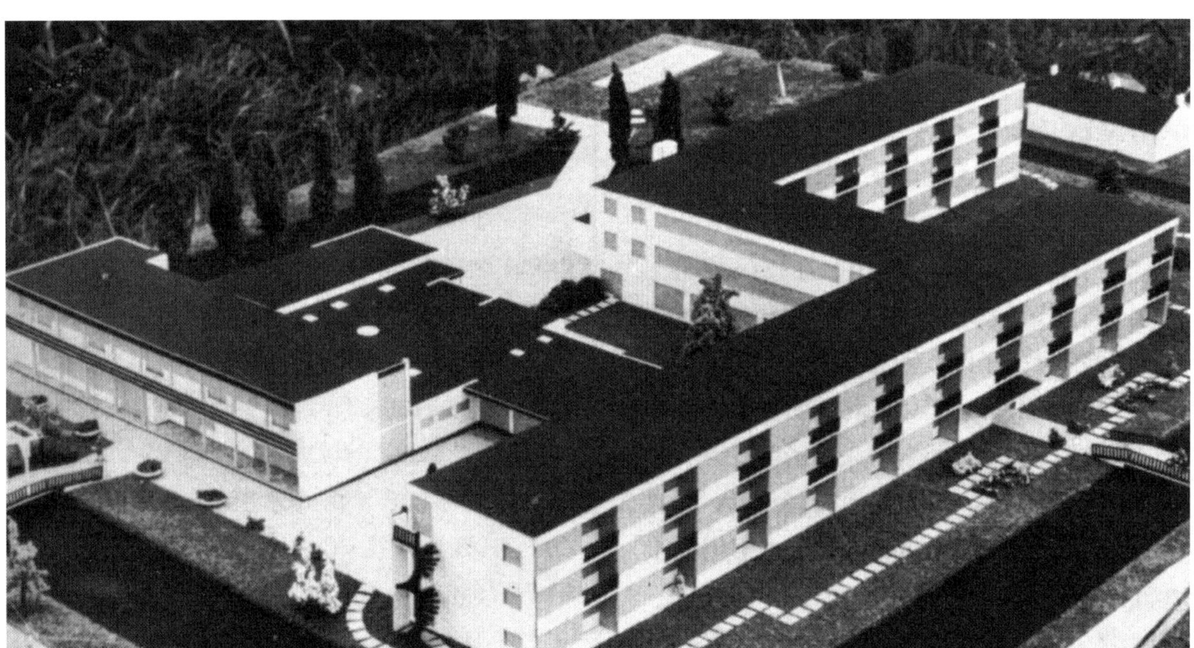

regime determines almost everything and leaves hardly any scope for the residents to develop their own initiatives. Somatic patients who are perfectly fit mentally will feel this as a burden that probably is not compensated by the benefits of what may be necessary therapies. The home model was intended to change this situation. The Stagg called for a change of direction as early as 1976: the nursing home as hospital institution was criticized as an expression of views on society that were fundamentally incorrect.

This implies in the first place trying to offer patients much more privacy, if possible by means of at least a bedroom of their own. Shared bedrooms should be avoided, and ideally eligible patients should also have a dayroom of their own at their disposal (usually they have to share it with other residents). However, the Hospital Provisions Board warned of overoptimistic expectations in 1981: 'The nursing home will necessarily fall short and never be able to satisfy every wish'.[35] In the following year the Hospital Board was positive about the attempt to increase the number of single rooms as far as possible, but added that 'developments in this direction will have to be limited for the time being in the light of the financial consequences'.[36] The practical consequence was that the home model would still have to be implemented within organisational frameworks that only admitted its most natural basis, an individual (bed)room for each resident in the nursing home, on a limited scale.

The Pronsweide nursing home in Winterswijk (1976-1981), designed by Hendriks Campman Tennekes, was intended for 202 patients, of whom 112 psycho-geriatric and 90 somatic. A separation of these two groups was an important premise in the layout of the building. In addition the architect wanted to create a domestic environment in reaction to the nursing homes where the emphasis had usually been on nursing. The nursing units are all composed following the same spatial concept, with a clear-cut subdivision into sleeping and living quarters. A connecting street leads from the front door into a hall with a corner for sitting, the central sister's post and two living rooms (with a corner for eating and sitting). Just beyond the sister's post are the sleeping quarters with a corridor around the centrally located sanitary facilities. On the other side of the corridor are the rooms for one, two and four persons.

The Beth Shalom centre for the elderly in Amsterdam (1969-1978) was built to replace two homes in the Plantage district of Amsterdam. A suitable location was found on a triangular plot outside the city in Osdorp. Salomonson Templeman Egberts (Hein Salomonson with Rik Egberts) designed the complex, that consists of a care home of six to seven storeys and a two-storey nursing home. The latter comprises two rectangular building volumes set adjacent to and partly overlapping one another. They are wide and low and have the double corridor system. The rooms that do not need daylight such as storage rooms and kitchens are in the middle where the buildings overlap and can be reached from both sides via a corridor. The residents' rooms are on the outside. The low-rise building connecting the nursing home with the care home is a corridor that encloses a garden on all sides. This is where areas for general use are situated such as the reception area, a shop, a cosy bar, hairdresser, library, a large recreation room and an area for handiwork.

Criticism

Like the hospitals, psychiatric clinics and nursing homes, accommodation for the elderly also met with considerable opposition. Several aspects recur in that criticism.

Mismatch

The most commonly built type of accommodation for the elderly, the complex with communal facilities and individual residential units (rest home or old people's home) was designed for the elderly who needed a certain form of domestic assistance, irrespective of their origin or income. However, it became partly filled with old people who were

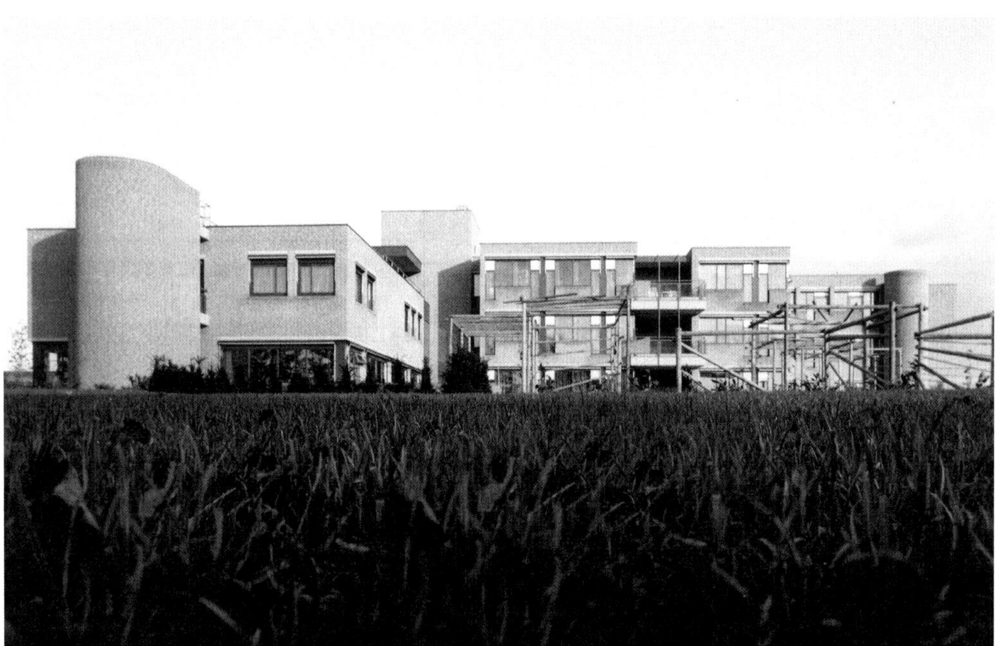

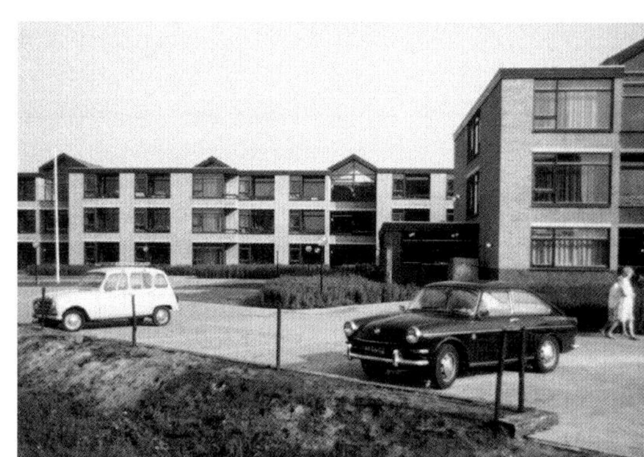

p. 176
***Hendriks Campman Tennekes*, Pronsweide nursing home, Winterswijk, 1981**

***J. Lengkeek*, De Esdoorn home for the elderly, Zwolle, 1972**

p. 177
***Salomonson Templeman Egberts*, Beth Shalom centre for the elderly, Amsterdam, 1977**

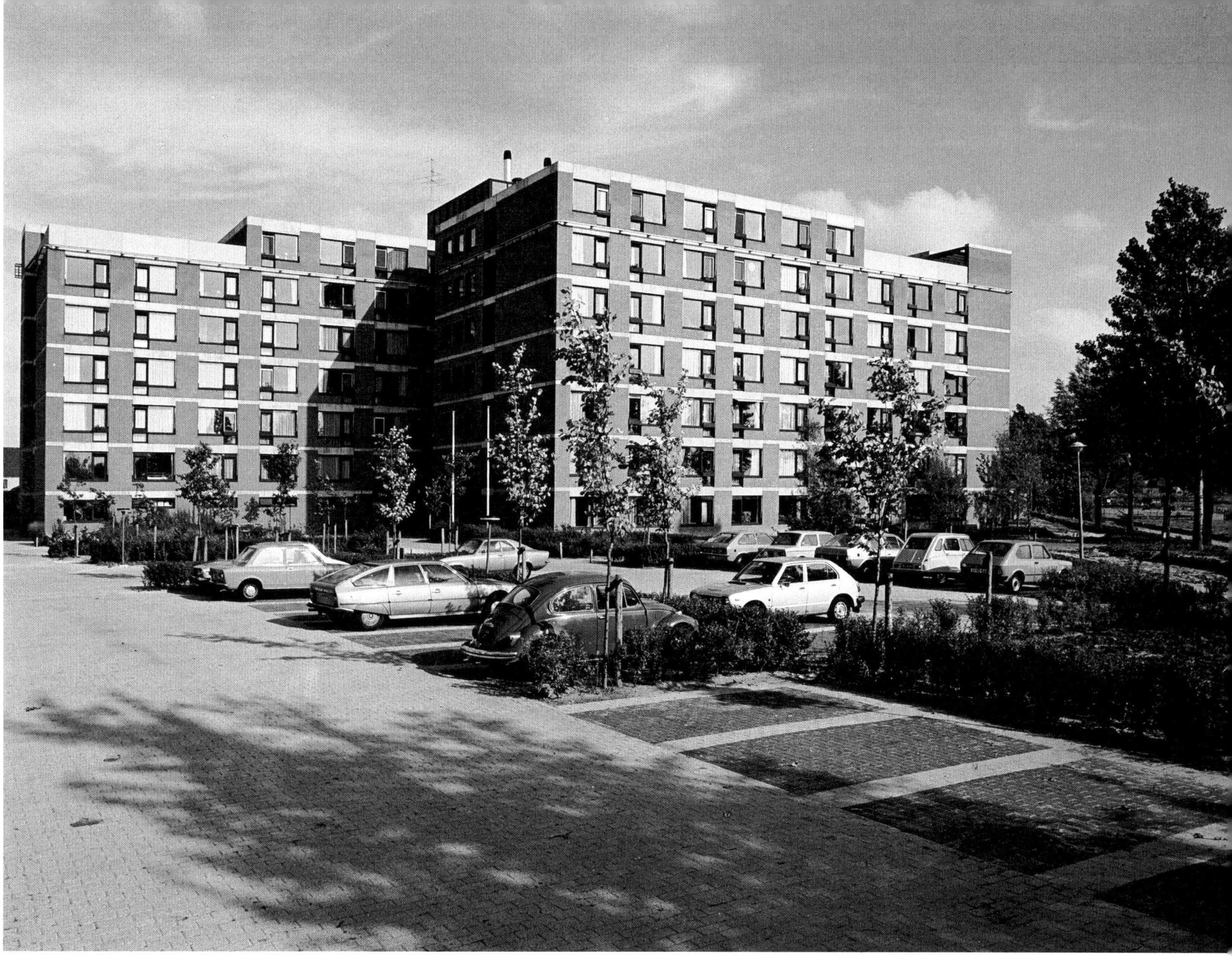

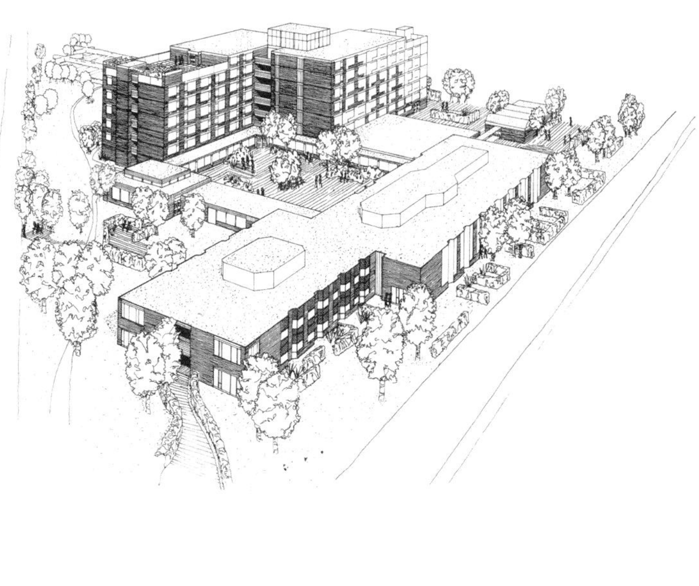

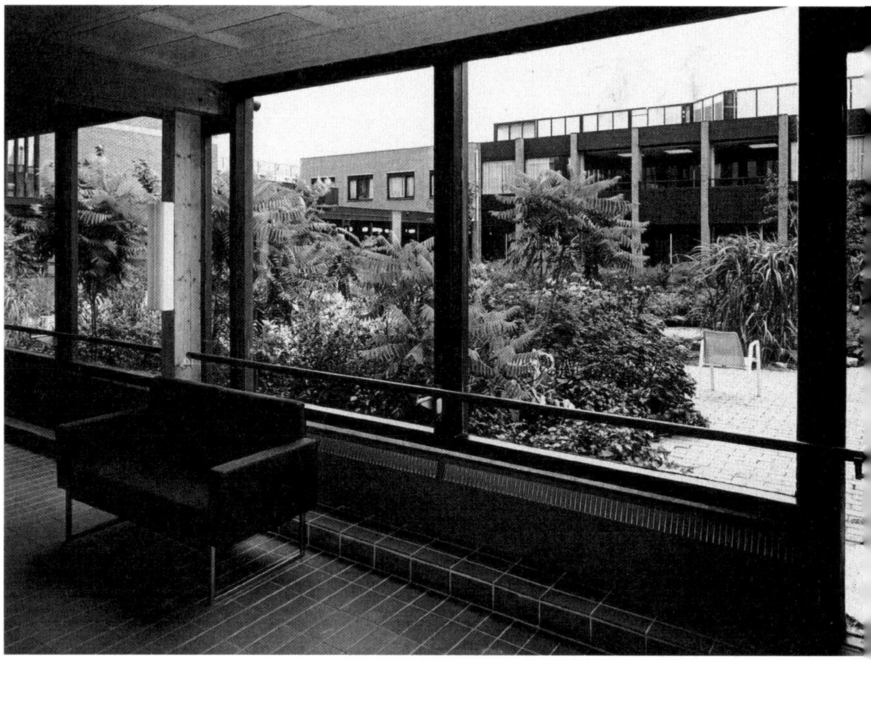

able to take care of themselves and could just as well have continued to do so at home. Some of them hoped that this would be a way of escaping admission to a more restrictive institution in the future. In principle elderly persons who were ill were not eligible for admission to one of these complexes. Their destiny was the nursing home and, in serious cases, the hospital.

Paternalism

The residents in an old people's home had to conform to the rules of the institution. This led to reflection on old people 'as people'; not the apparatus of the home, but personal encounter should be given priority.[37] L. van der Meer, head of Geriatric Care of the Ministry of Culture, Recreation and Social Work, connected the omnipresent paternalism with the persistence of old traditions, which was hardly surprising among 'a people so intensely infected by social work as we are'.[38] The care home was regarded as a total institution, to use the term introduced by Ervin Goffman that was current at the time.

Isolation

What had been intended to contribute to the integration of the elderly in everyday society had led to the opposite result: concentrated in big, hospital-like buildings, they had been literally isolated. 'In our hygienically thinking age we place them tidily apart in an "incubator for pensioners" and have then neatly solved the problem', a critic remarked in 1958. Similar views were expressed by others: 'We should never forget that putting our old people into separate homes specially built for the elderly is a blot on our society'.[39]

Architecture

Apparently this criticism referred more to the content than to the form of the accommodation for the elderly, though both aspects came under attack. High-rise buildings in particular were viewed with disdain: the idea gained ground 'that those monuments of care for the elderly towering high above everyday cares' were in fact nothing but 'waiting rooms of the Grim Reaper'.[40]

Rejection

What did the elderly themselves think? For a long time virtually nothing was known about that. However, surveys conducted among the elderly who lived independently outside the social safety net of the specific accommodation for old people indicated that the vast majority of them preferred to keep things that way. Research in Groningen revealed that two-thirds of the elderly who were eligible for admission to an old people's home were not attracted by the idea. The figure in Rotterdam was even higher: 88 per cent preferred to continue to live on their own; 10 per cent preferred to move in with their children rather than make the transition to an old people's home.[41]

The building as an improved city

The 1970s witnessed an about-turn in architecture. Accommodation for the elderly played a major role in this. Many of the disadvantages attributed to the classic, specific and therefore fairly isolated forms of accommodation could be avoided by conceiving of large buildings as small towns, and no longer demolishing existing urban structures but making use of the flexibility that they offered in contrast to new buildings.

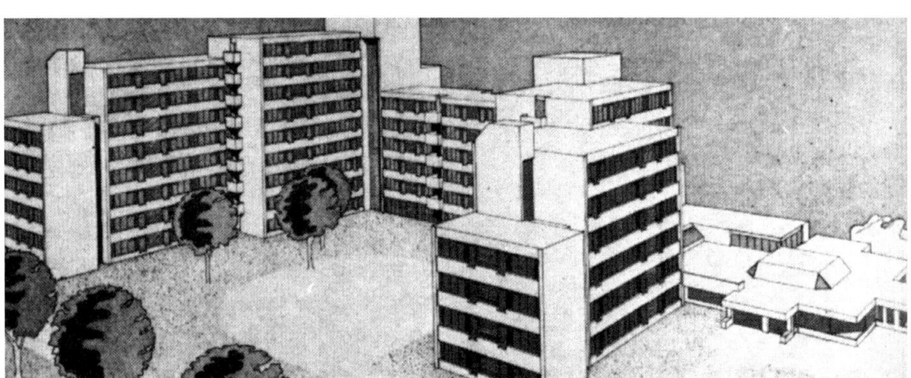

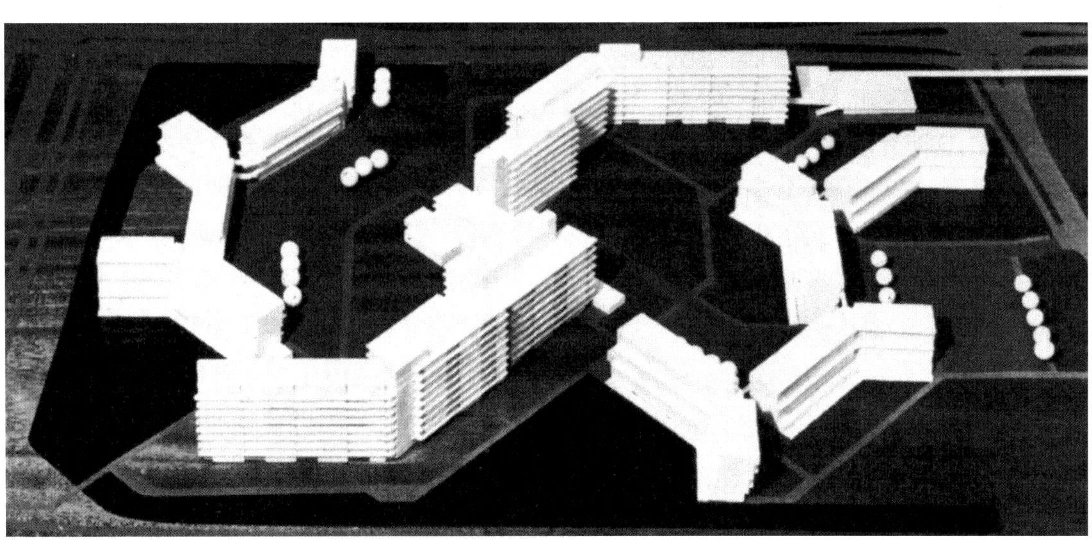

p. 178
***Architectenbureau Olsmeijer*, care home for the elderly, Enschede, 1974**

***Van Tijen, Boom en Posno*, centre for the elderly, Capelle aan den IJssel, 1970-1975**

p. 179
***Hoogstad, Schultze, Van Tilburg*, homes for the elderly, Zoetermeer, 1977**

An early example of a large-scale old people's complex as an urban facility was designed by Van Tijen, Boom en Posno in Capelle aan den IJssel. It was commissioned by the regular principal of this firm, the Netherlands Centre for Housing of Old People (NCHB). Characteristic of this project is the way in which the accommodation for the elderly nestles in a fairly colossal housing complex that also houses other age categories: the mixture seems to be purely organisational in this case and is barely expressed in the architectural and urban planning design. The relatively anonymous structure of the complex includes a service centre, a care home with 200 beds, 202 service flats, 48 gallery access flats, 235 maisonettes, and 29 garages; public transport is provided by the metro, and urban vitality by a shopping centre to be built in the future.[42]

There was no end to the number of small streets and squares in care homes in the 1970s. In De Esdoorn everyone lived next to their own little square, the residents in a home in Enschede even had a 'main street' at their disposal, and the homes for the elderly project that Hoogstad, Schultze, Van Tilburg implemented in Zoetermeer was accessed by a system of internal streets too. These small streets led to a centre with shops, a travel agency and recreational facilities – in other words, a small city centre.[43] Moreover, a covered pedestrian street ran right through this complex to connect the old village centre with a new housing estate.[44] It pointed to a different use of all these internal streets and squares: even the traffic outside the complex could promote integration in the surroundings. In some cases general public amenities were so integrated in a building that the routes to it functioned as normal (pedestrian) streets for the public. An example of this was the Anne Frank Centrum in Waddinxveen, which included not only a service centre for the target group but also a children's library, schools and a theatre: 'In this way everyday encounters take place that do not have the character of visits, but of chance encounters'.[45] This strategy was later applied to psychiatric provisions that returned to the city, as in the Psychiatrisch Centrum Amsterdam built by Onno Greiner en Martien van Goor Architekten between 1989 and 1994.[46]

De Drie Hoven is probably the most pronounced example of this new direction. This project by Herman Hertzberger was completed in 1976 and is viewed as an autonomous link in the series extending from the neighbourhood via the district to the city as a whole – the reminiscences of the neighbourhood idea of twenty-five years earlier are evident. De Drie Hoven consists of a care home for 190 residents, a combined nursing home for 250 patients and accommodation for nursing personnel and technical staff. They combine to form a community in which the care personnel 'can be regarded as temporary or permanent fellow residents'.[47] Although there were calls to limit resident personnel as much as possible, here it was deployed as a contribution to the formation of a community, an argument that was often heard to defend resident staff.

Since the building of self-sufficient housing units and care homes was classified as housing, it was difficult to deviate from the regulations that applied in that sector. Exemption was necessary if experiments were to be possible and since experiments cost money, a call for extra funds would be inevitable. Both conditions were met on 14 May 1968 by allowing experiments by law, but only after a qualified jury had been able to assess their value on the basis of a preliminary design and explanatory comments.[48] Some of the most interesting experiments concerned accommodation for the elderly. Probably the most exotic of these was

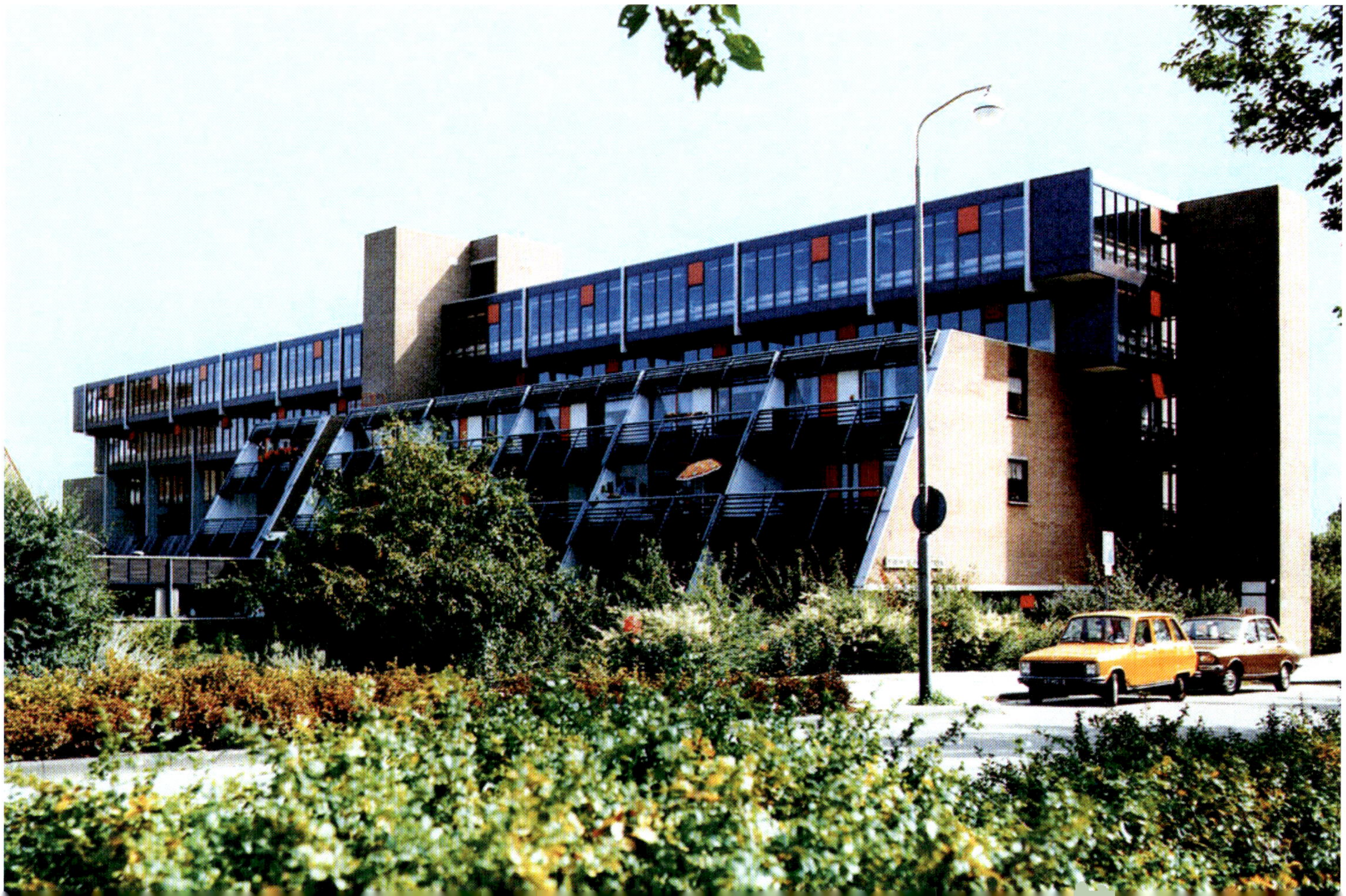

connected with the fiftieth anniversary of the famous Vreewijk district of Rotterdam; building there had commenced in the 1920s on the initiative of well-to-do Rotterdam private parties.[49] Four firms were assessed by the jury. The project submitted by E. Hartsuyker & L. Hartsuyker-Curjel under the motto 'Zonnetrap' was unanimously proposed for further elaboration as an experimental project and was built ten years later. Characteristic is the construction with different components that are staggered to create a large terrace for each apartment. It is noteworthy that the designers presented their plan as the fragment of a new city. 'Dissatisfied with urban planning practice since 1945, since 1960 we have been intensively concerned with such questions as What is a city?, How does a city of this century work?, What difference is there between a city of the past and a city of the post-industrial era?, What are the connections between a home, a building and a city?'[50]

De Zonnetrap does indeed prove to be the offspring of a much larger project, an urban development proposal for Hydrobiopolis, projected in the sea off the coast of Wassenaar and intended for 20,000 residents. De Zonnetrap included 180 residential units in receipt of a government grant, 69 smaller residential units, 1,200 m² of office space, some of it to be used by the Lombardijen Housing Foundation, 400 m² of studio space for artists, and a service centre. The complex was to derive its urban quality from a principle that was diametrically opposed to the separation of functions that had been sometimes taken to extremes in the urban development of the reconstruction period: here it was the mixing of functions and groups of residents that was intended to lead to the emergence of a fragment of the city.

What all these experiments had in common was the need to design alternatives to forms of accommodation that apparently did not function satisfactorily. That this was the case could be seen not only from the criticisms levelled by the counterculture. More important were the results of surveys among residents. Both tendencies – experimentation and the conducting of resident surveys – were to take off in the 1980s.

p. 180
E. Hartsuyker &
***L. Hartsuyker-Curjel*, De Zonnetrap apartment block, Rotterdam, 1980**

E. Hartsuyker &
***L. Hartsuyker-Curjel*, Hydrobiopolis urban development proposal, off the coast of Wassenaar, 1968**

p. 181
E. Hartsuyker &
***L. Hartsuyker-Curjel*, De Zonnetrap apartment block, Rotterdam, 1980**

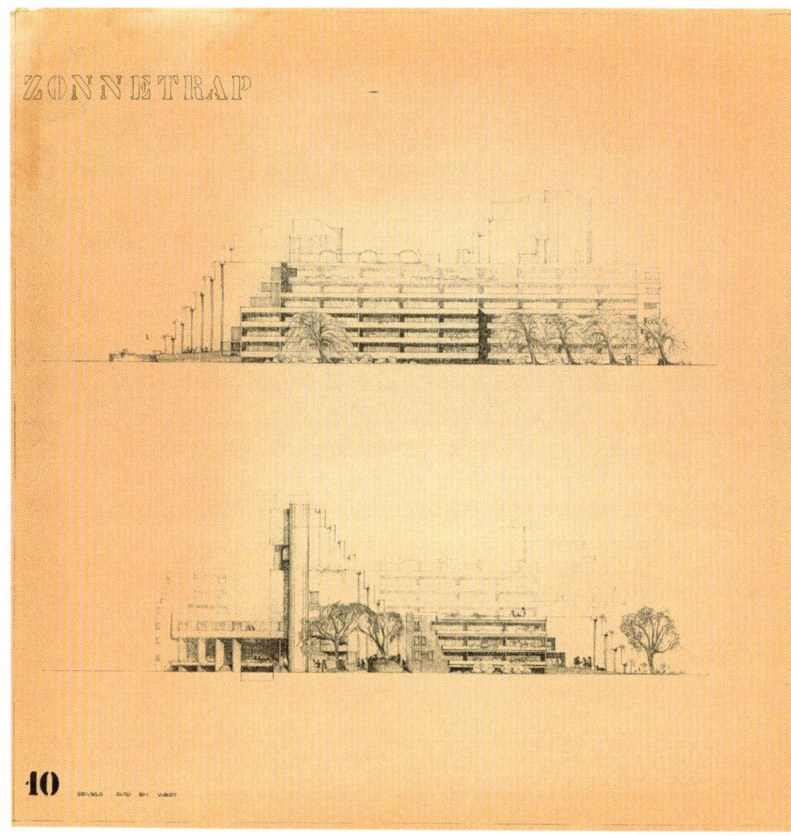

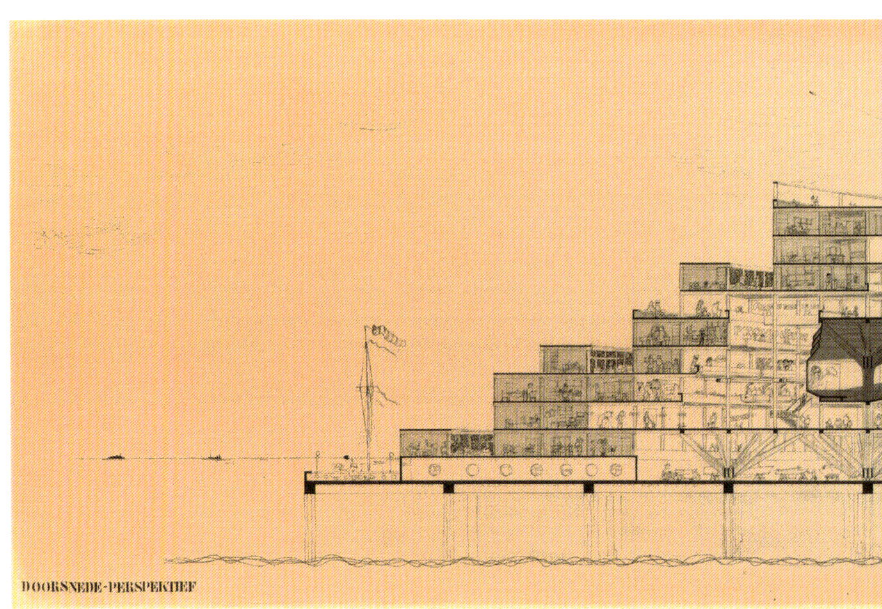

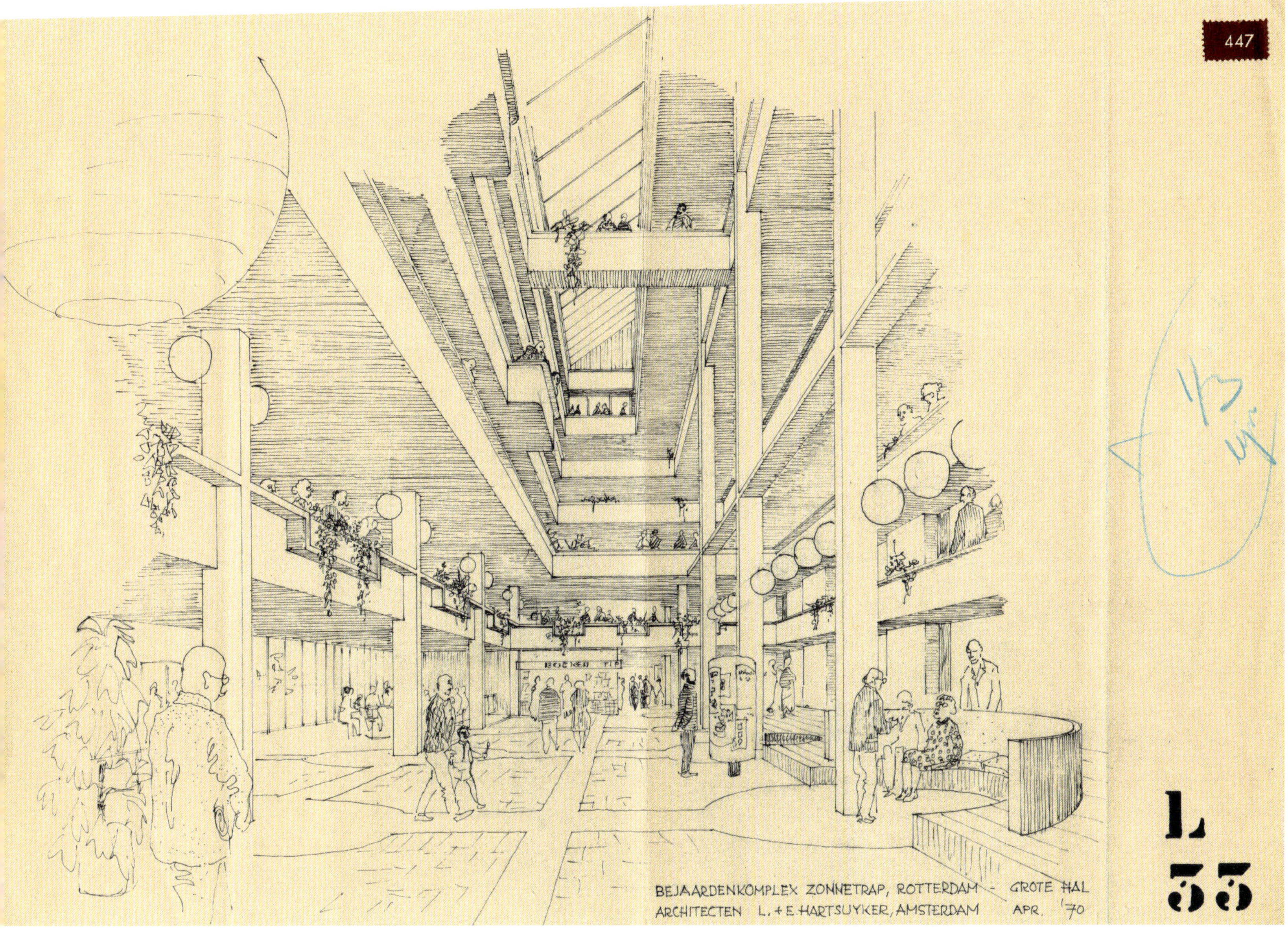
447
BEJAARDENKOMPLEX ZONNETRAP, ROTTERDAM - GROTE HAL
ARCHITECTEN L. + E. HARTSUYKER, AMSTERDAM APR. '70
L
33

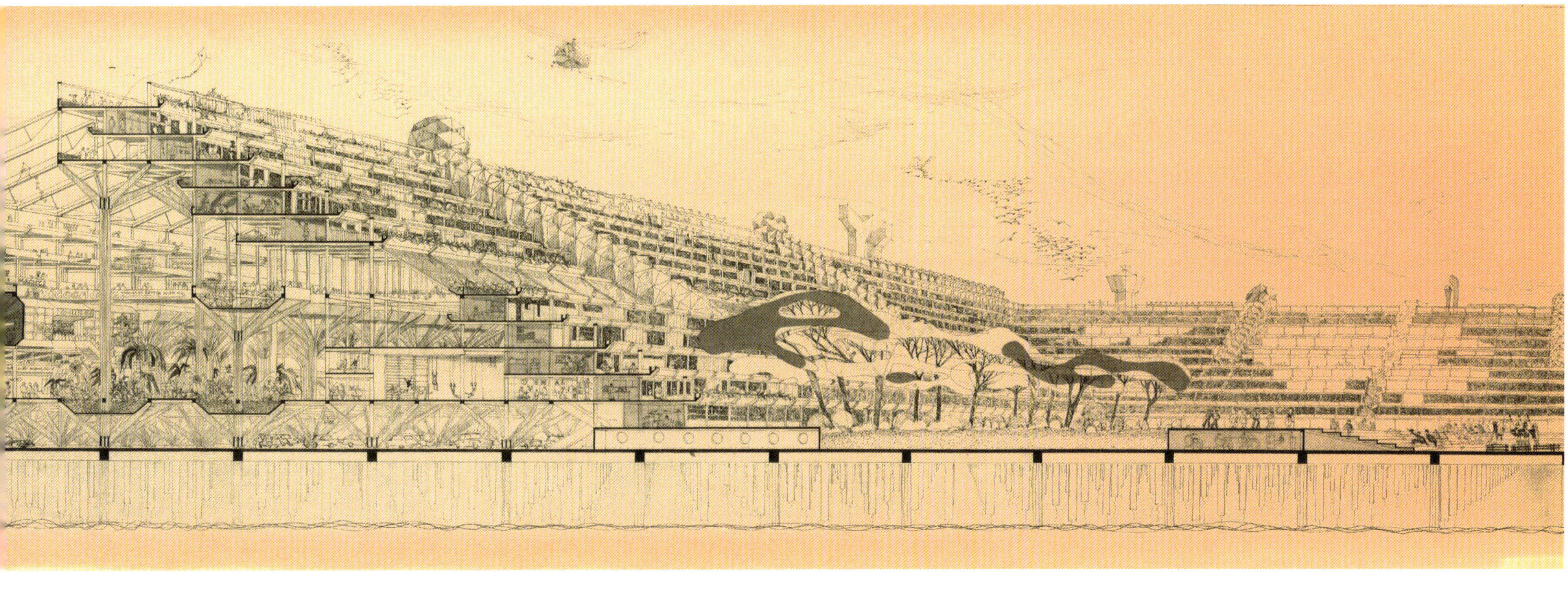

Village square

Herman Hertzberger

De Drie Hoven
Amsterdam
1964-1974

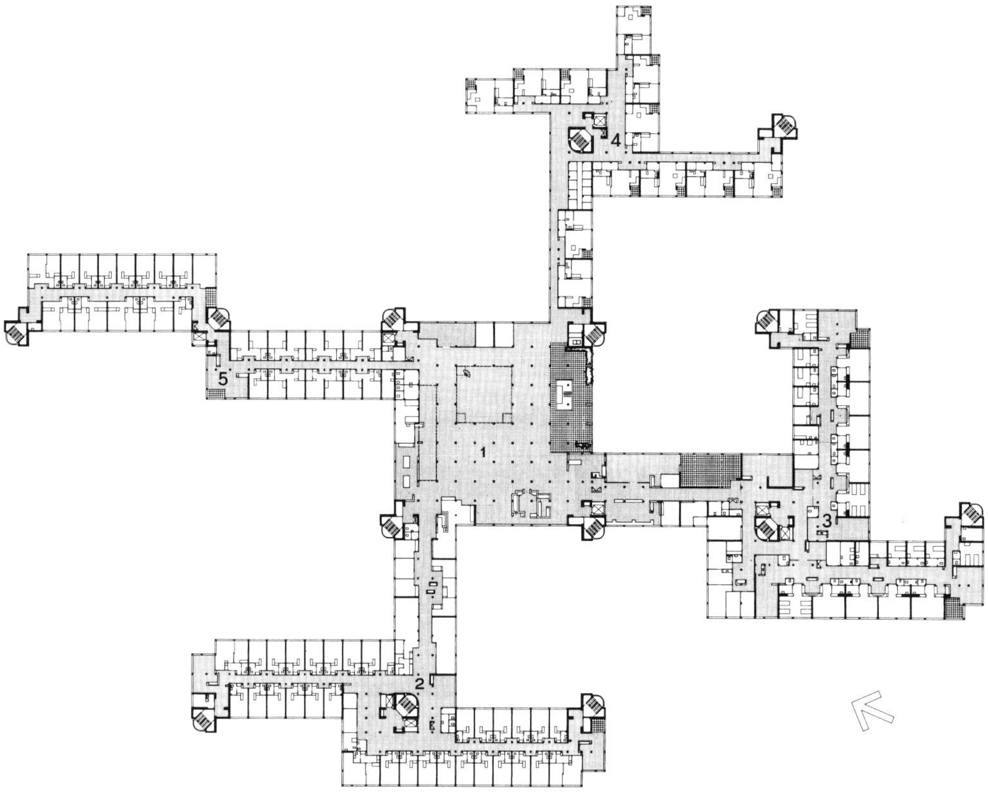

Second floor
1 *central hall*
2 *old people's home*
3 *nursing home*
4 *housing for married couples*
5 *dormitory for personnel*

p. 183
Schemes
From left to right: site, programme, grid with theoretical location for towers, juxtaposition, final scheme

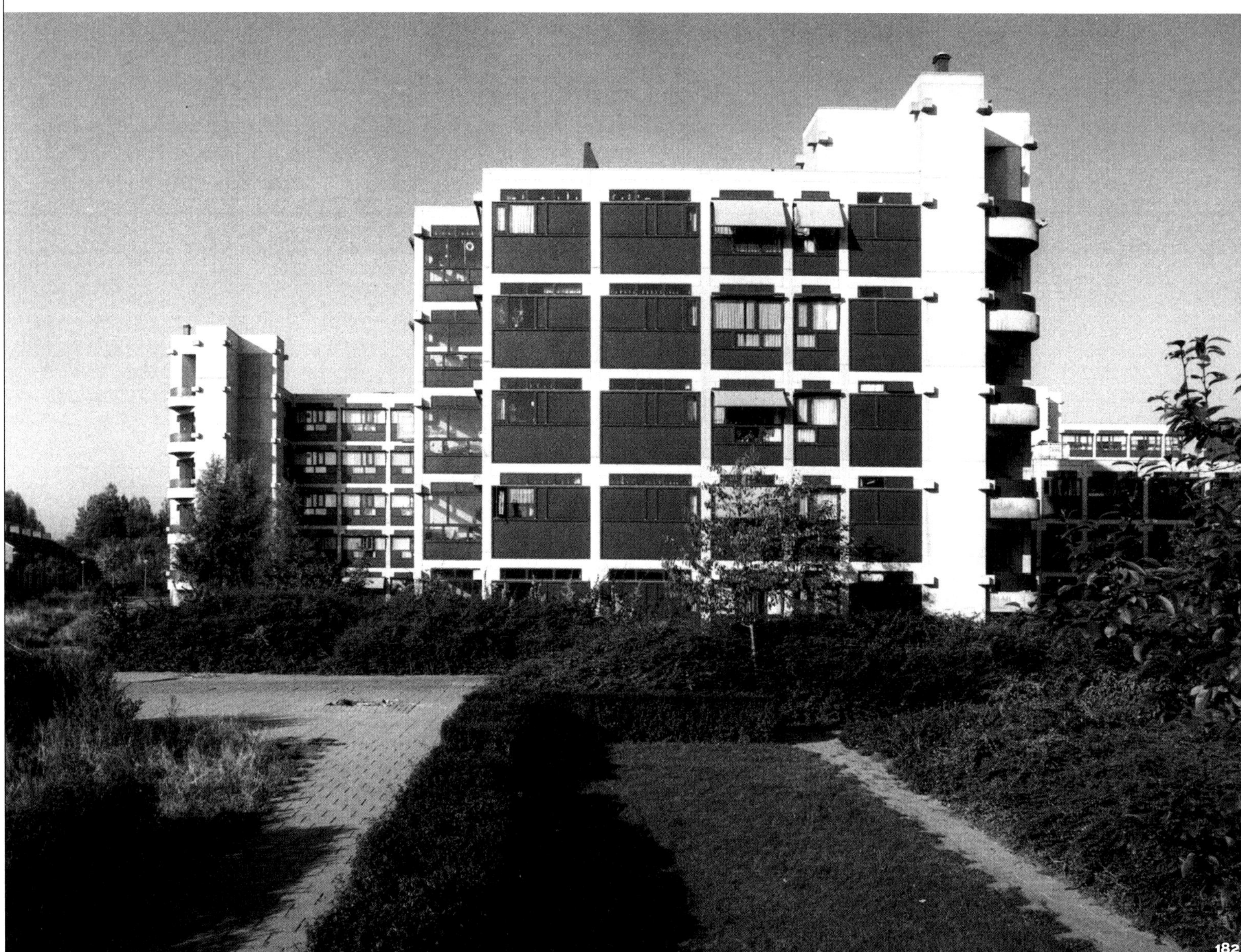

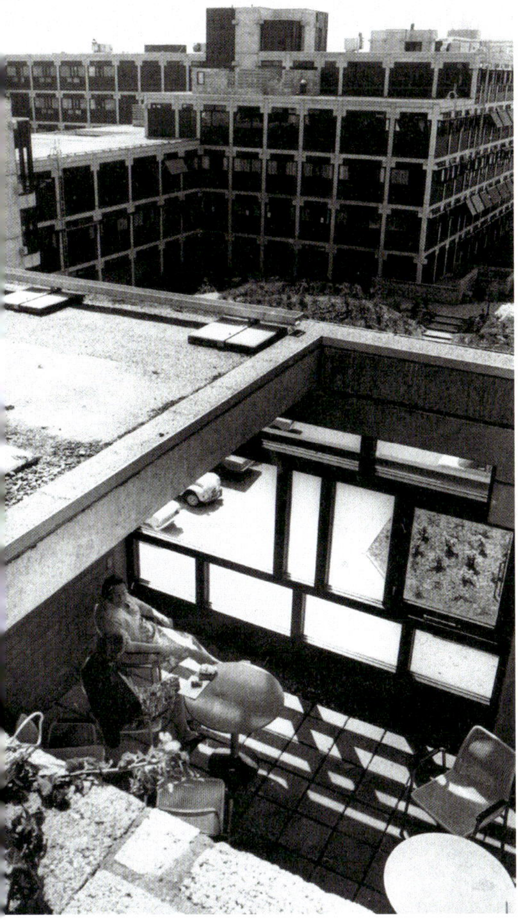

De Drie Hoven is intended for old people with a physical and mental handicap. The complex consists of a central building with four volumes fanning out from each corner. The first comprises 55 residential units for couples. The second is a care home with 171 units for 190 persons, in which each unit consists of a room with sanitary fittings and a corner for cooking. The third is a nursing home with 250 beds for long-term patients with a physical and mental disorder; it is composed of 25-bed nursing units divided up into bedrooms for one, two or four persons. The fourth is the staff building with 21 two-room flats with a corner for cooking, three guest rooms, ten flats for managerial staff, sixteen rooms for nurses, board rooms, and an apartment for the head of the technical service.

The central building, where the different volumes converge, accommodates all kinds of central functions such as a multifunctional meeting area, shops, a bar, library, billiards room, hairdresser, laundry, kitchens, workshop and storage depots. The central hall functions like a village square, the system of corridors like a system of streets, to facilitate encounters and counter loneliness. The streets are wider near the entrance to the residential units to create a forecourt that belongs to both the residential unit and the public street.

The entire complex is based on a system of dimensions whose smallest module is a unit of 92 cm. The staircases in the various volumes are on a grid based on a multiple of 92 cm. A building system of prefab concrete elements – columns, supports and floors – was used. Their dimensions too are based on the same system of module.

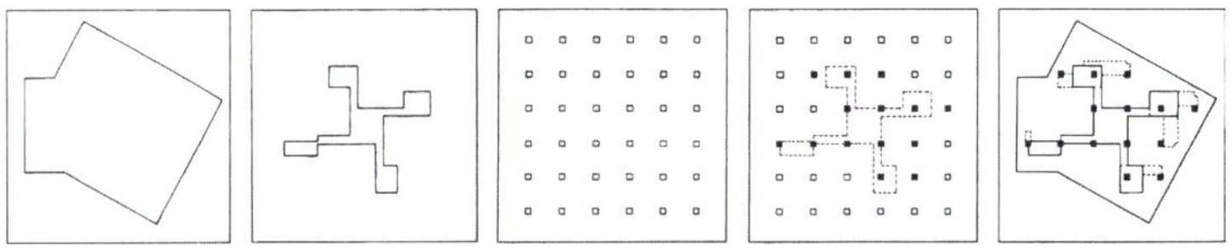

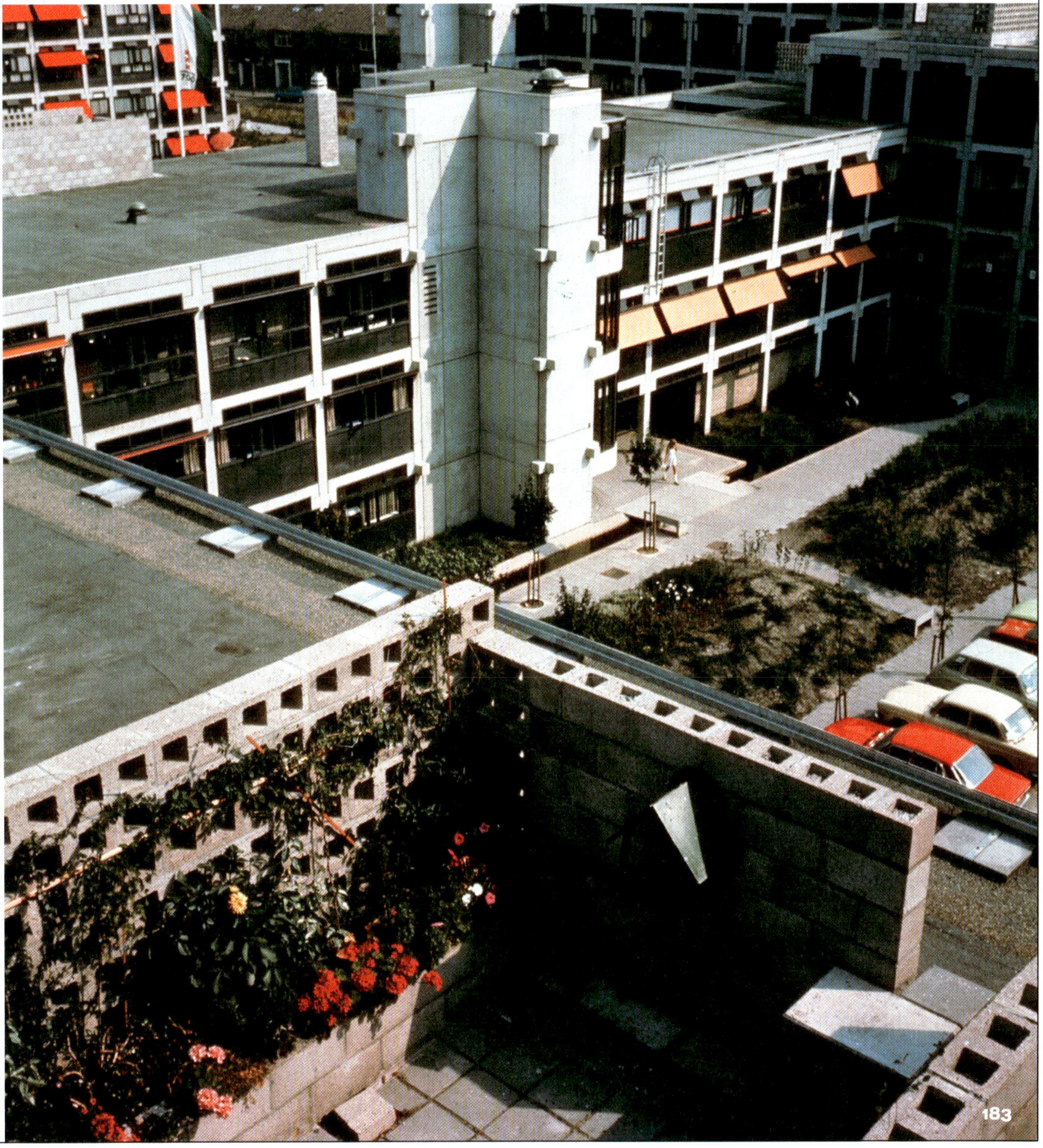

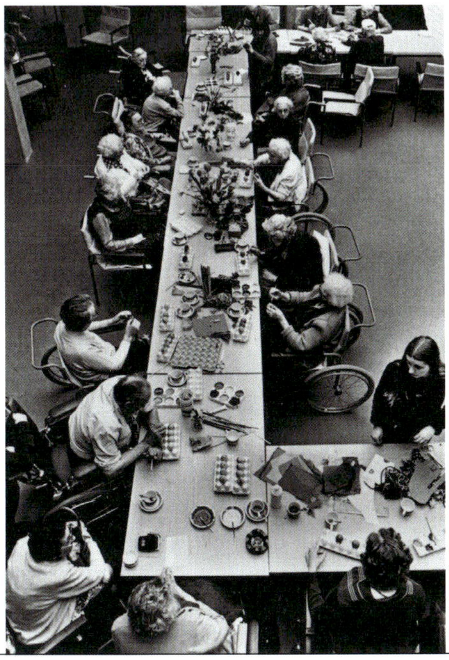

Terraces

Enrico Hartsuyker &
Luzia Hartsuyker-Curjel

De Zonnetrap residential building
Rotterdam
1970–1980

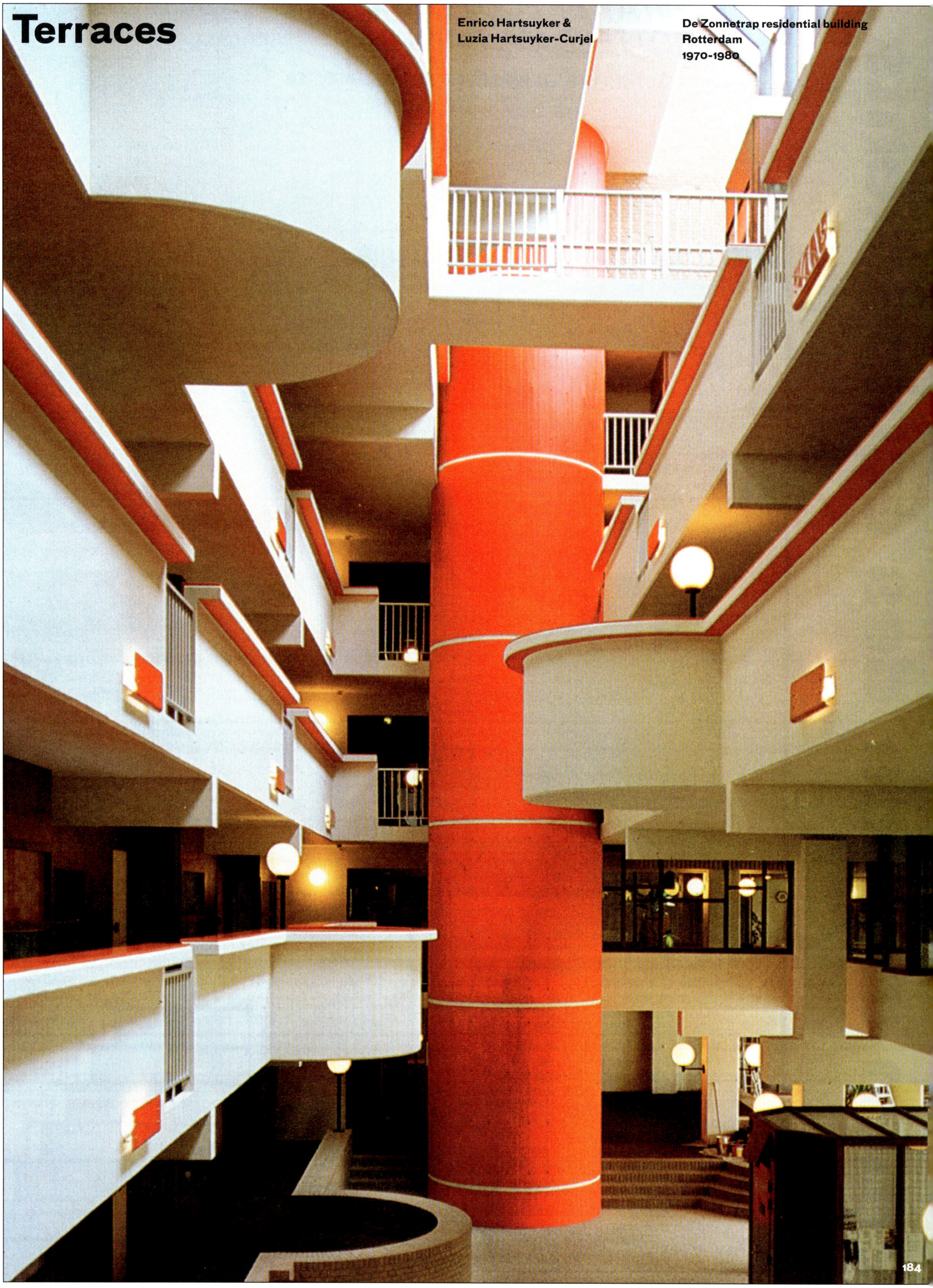

The complex has a staggered structure with terraces for the apartments and a covered hall in which all kinds of communal functions and offices are accommodated. It consists of three interconnected sections. A five-storey south wing whose height matches that of the surrounding buildings, a seven-storey central section with a north-south orientation, and a ten-storey north wing whose height corresponds to that of the buildings behind it. In the north wing and the central sections are two halls at right angles that are connected with one another and reach up to the seventh floor. The offices, communal and neighbourhood facilities adjoin these halls. The relatively comprehensive package of provisions consists of a service centre for the elderly, two recreational halls, a toddlers' playroom, an after school facility, a billiards room, a library, laundrette, hobby areas and workshops. The apartments are situated in a shell around them and in the south wing. They have a staggered structure per floor, which creates room for large terraces. The main entrance with a sheltered forecourt is on the west side.

Of the total of 179 apartments, there are 110 three-room apartments, 9 corner apartments, 69 two-room apartments, and an apartment for the manager. The apartments are of the 'walkaround' type: the living room and bedrooms and the kitchen are built around a closed core which includes the bathroom facilities. If required, (sliding) doors can be used to close off areas.

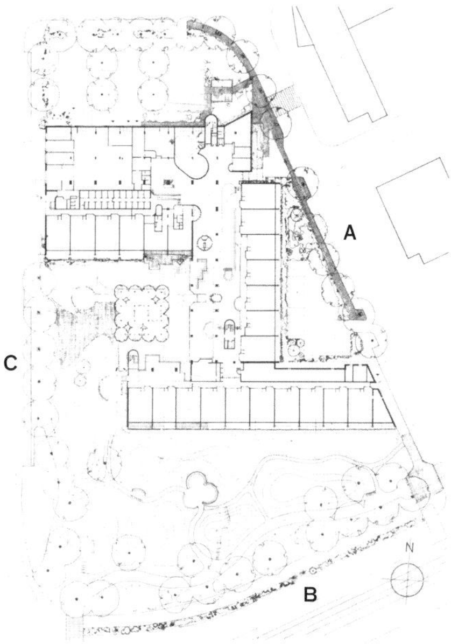

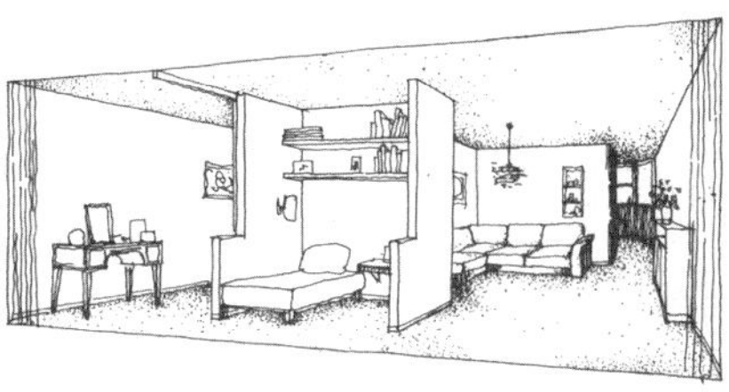

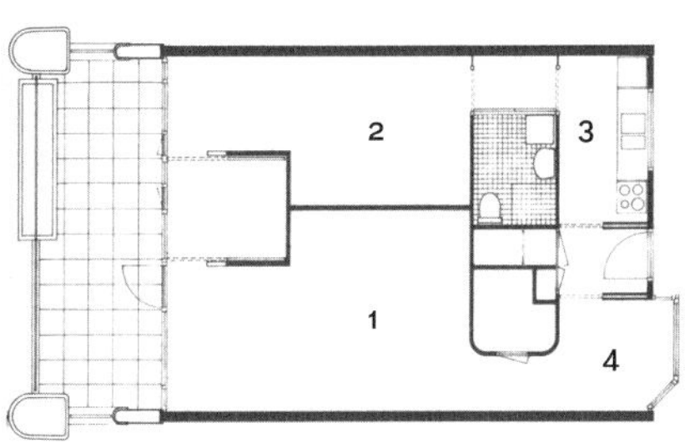

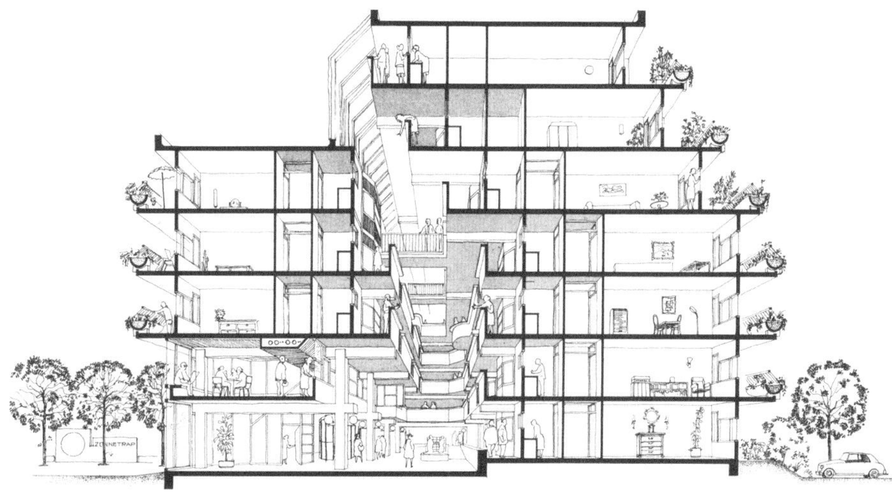

Floor plan housing unit
1 *living*
2 *sleeping*
3 *kitchen*
4 *dining*

Situation
A *Pythagorasweg*
B *Spinozaweg*
C *Molenvliet*

Section

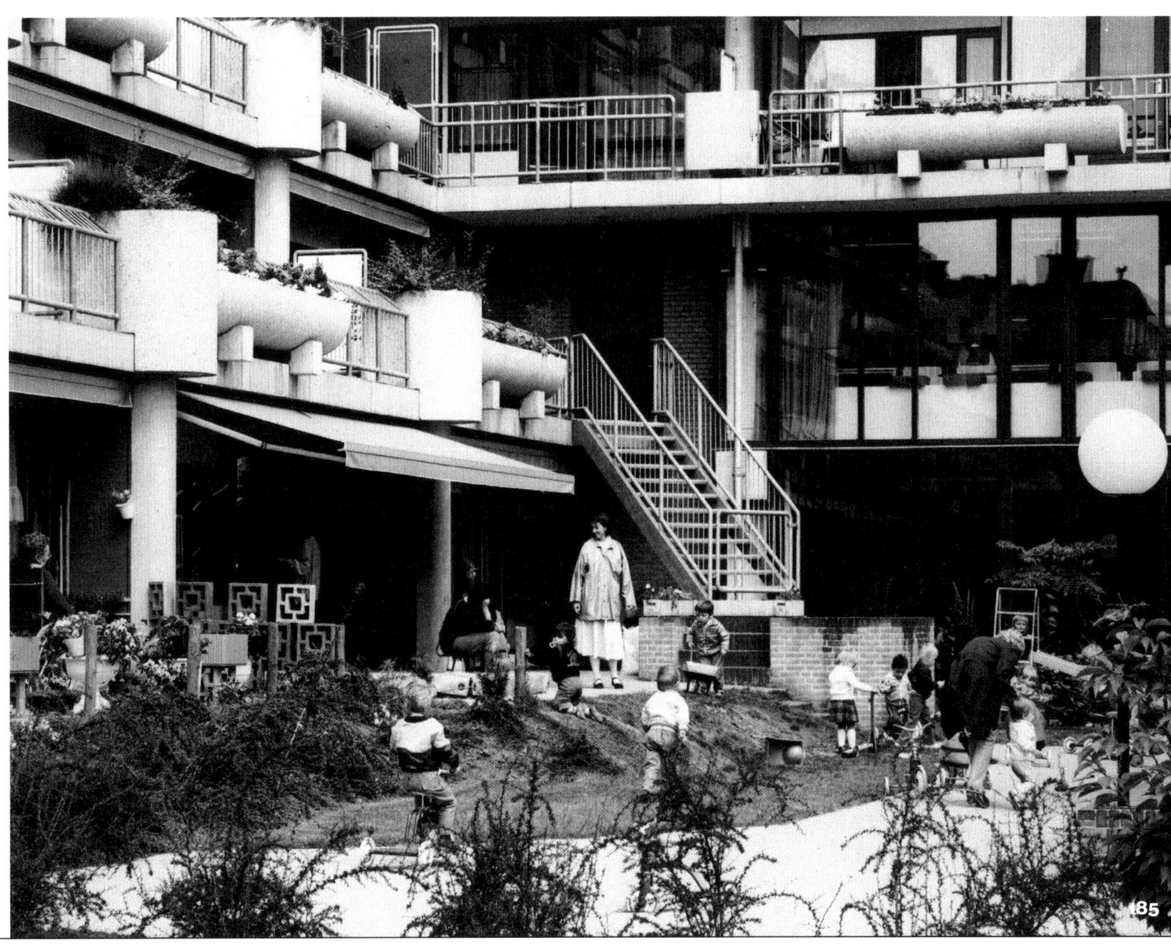

Comb

Architektenburo Roelofs Nijst Lucas

Sint Elisabeth Ziekenhuis
Tilburg
1973-1982

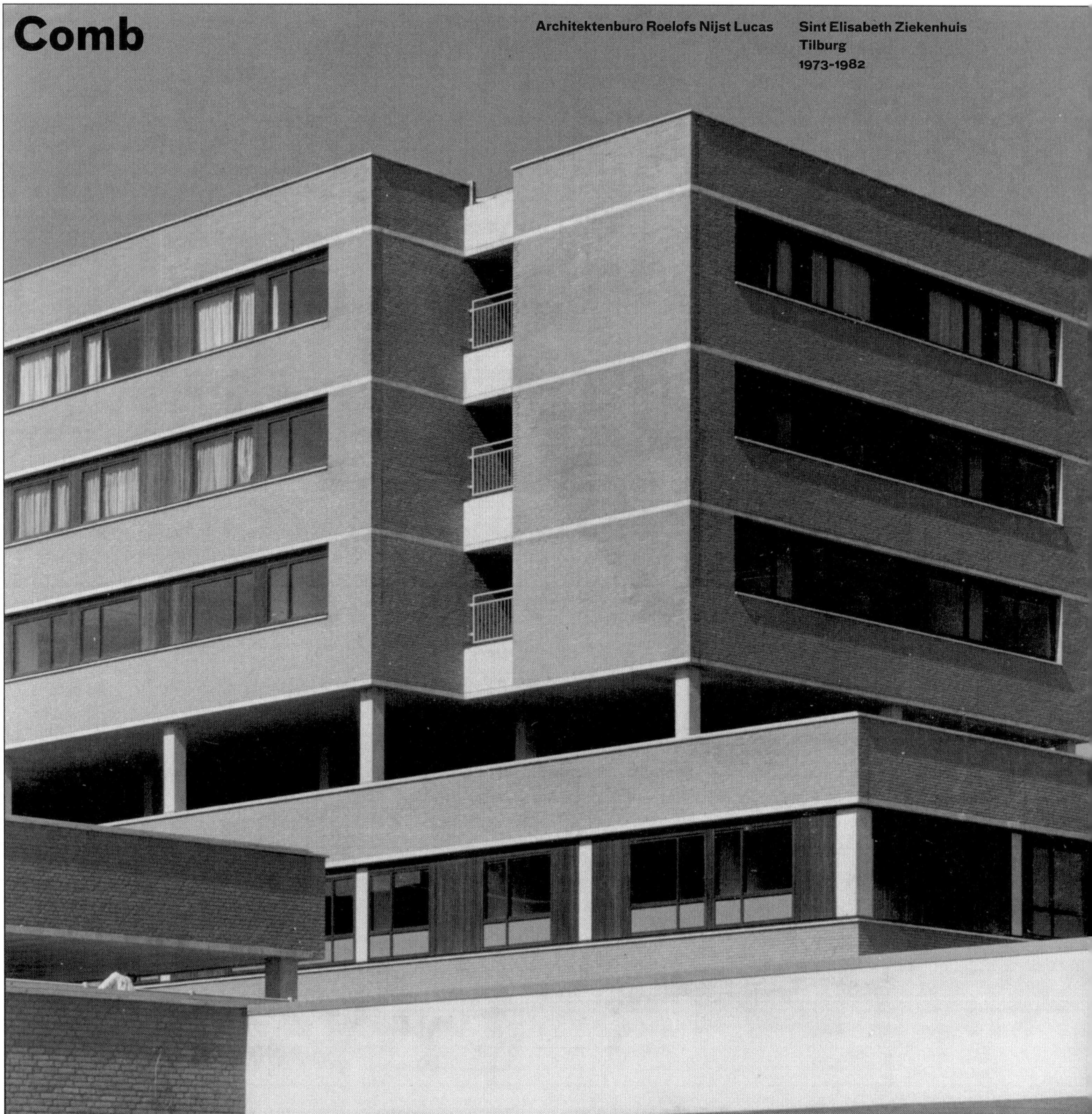

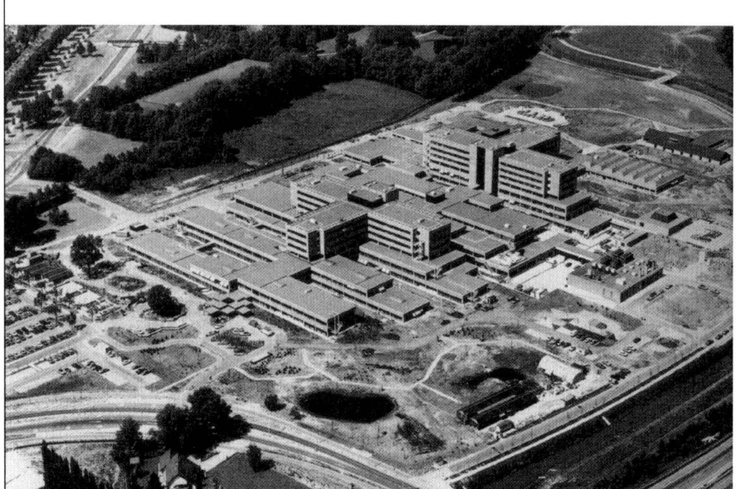

Although the Sint Elisabeth Ziekenhuis (750 beds) is one of the biggest, it is organised on a relatively small scale. This is a result of the double comb structure on which the design is based. The division of the whole into small volumes guarantees the preservation of the human dimension. Light can easily enter between the low 'teeth' of the comb, and the green strips in between ensure a pleasant view. Moreover, the comb structure is flexible so that the different research and treatment units can be expanded if necessary.

The main traffic axis forms the backbone of the design. It links the parallel blocks, which are almost equal in length. The entrance is situated in the first block, which contains some of the outpatient clinics, and provides access to the main axis. The widest block houses the main concentration of the treatment units. The two symmetrical T-shaped wards are situated on the blocks on either side of this central treatment area. The façades are clad with reddish brown brick. The continuous strips of windows give them a decidedly horizontal character that emphasises the small scale for which the designers aimed.

The colour scheme is characteristic of the 1970s and early 1980s: peaceful basic colours for the floors, walls and ceilings, bright accents in orange, yellow and purple for the reception desks, furniture and frames.

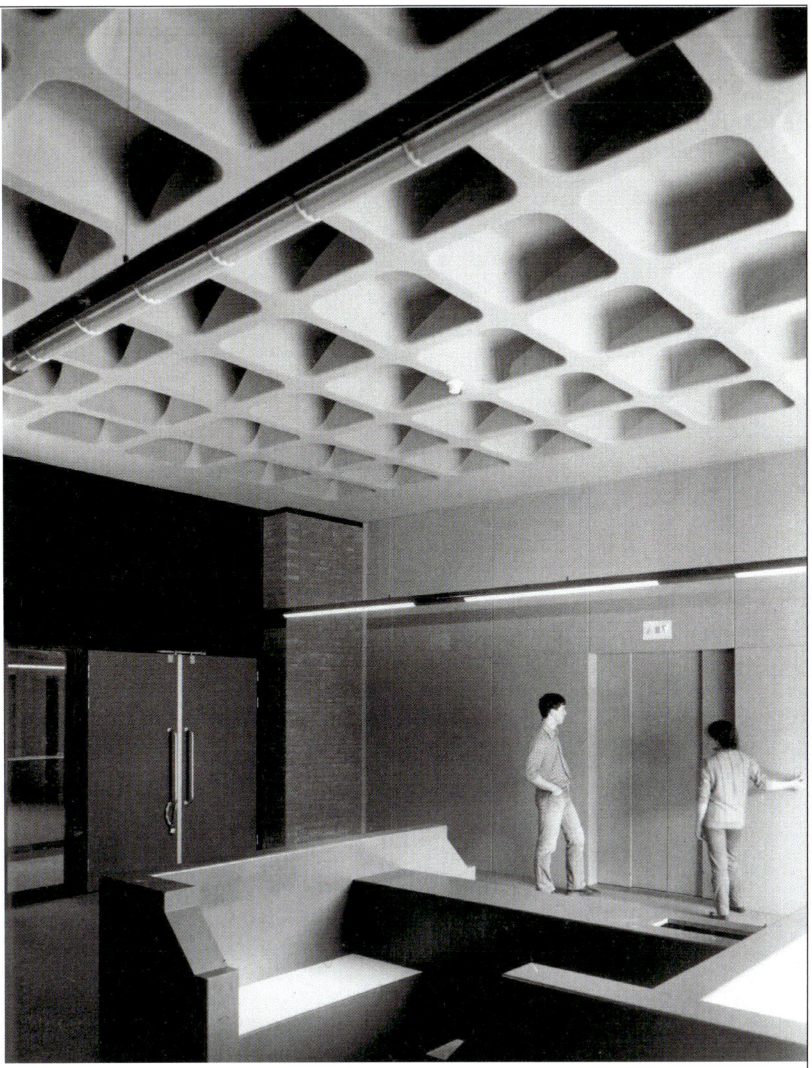

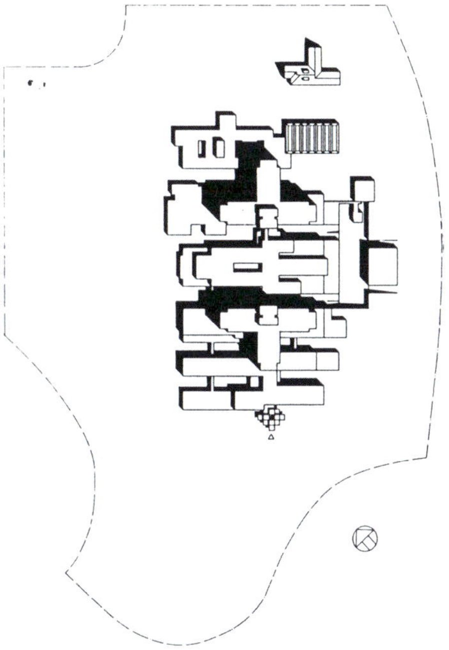

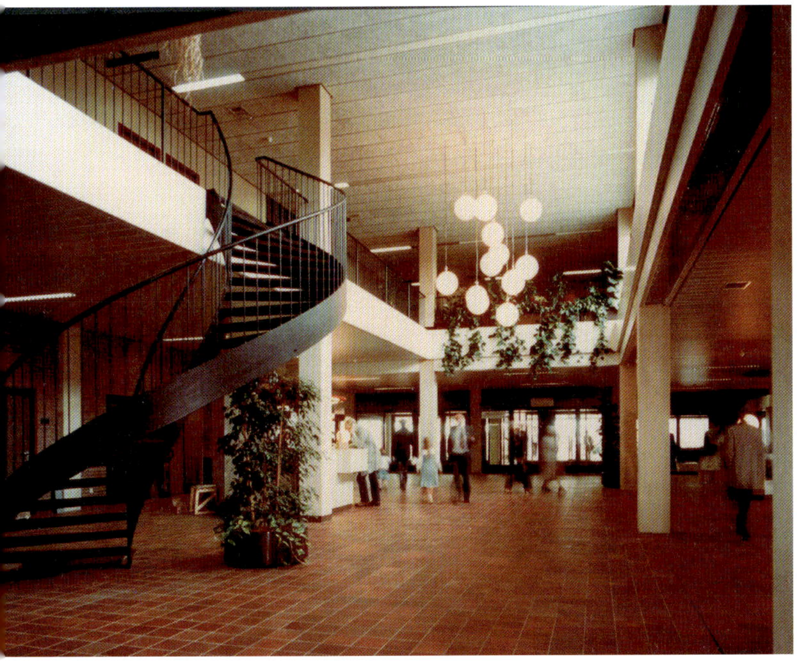

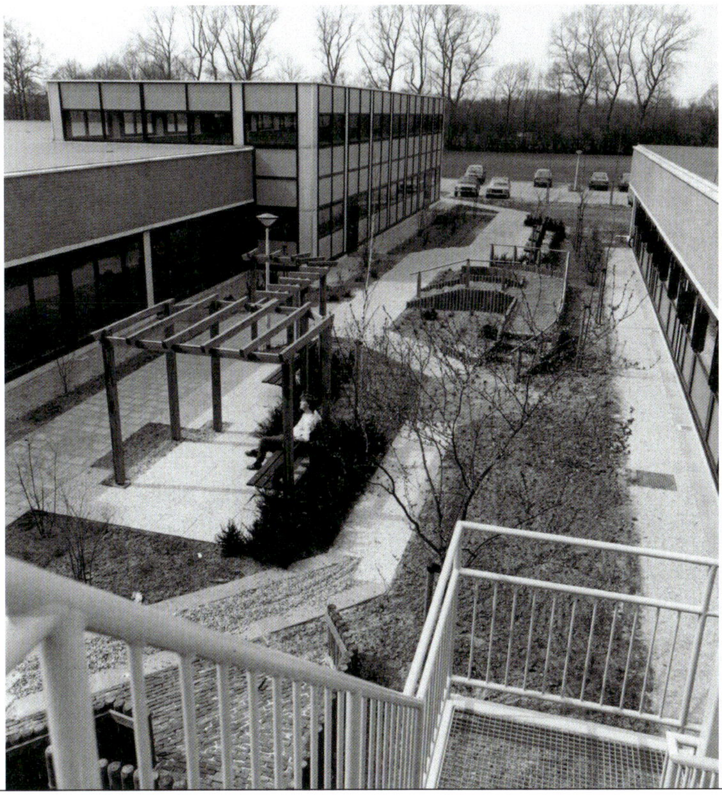

Community

Architectenbureau Swinkels Salemans

Clinic for acute psychiatry and socio-therapeutic community of Sint Joseph de Wellen
Apeldoorn
1971-1982

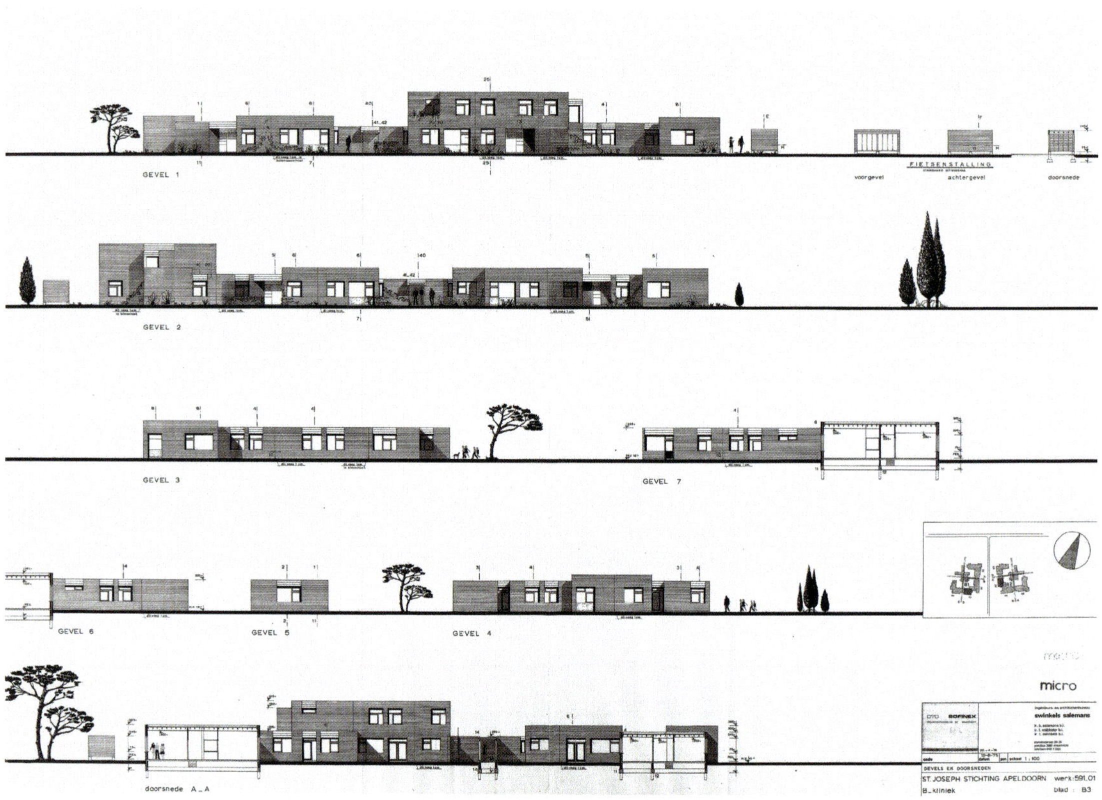

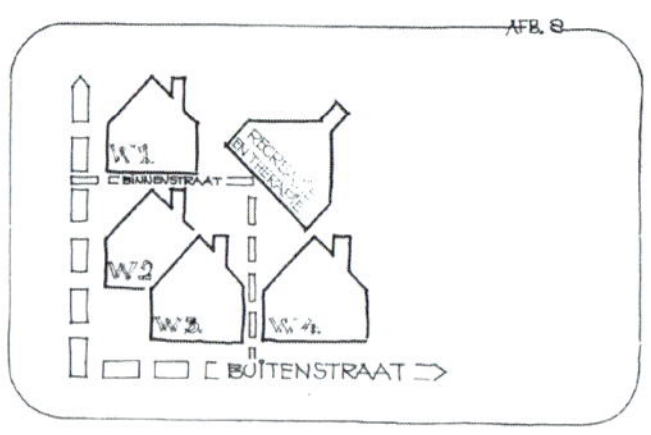

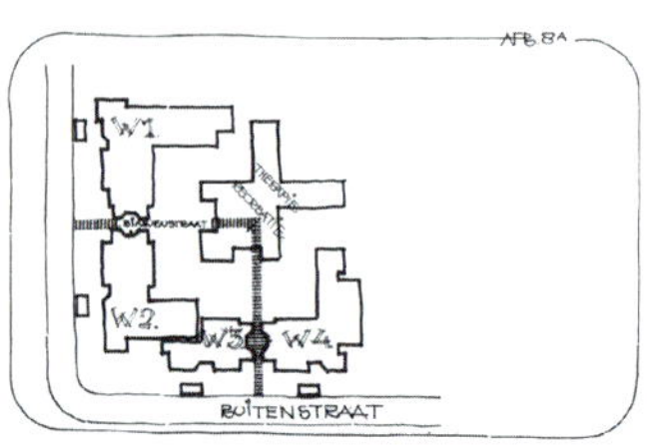

bottom
P.A.M. Buys & B. van der Vliet, garden design for the inner courts

The integral psychiatric centre Sint Joseph de Wellen is based on the principle that patients move on from the clinic for acute psychiatry to follow-up clinics such as the resocialisation unit and long-term nursing. In the designs for the clinic for acute psychiatry and the resocialisation unit, T. Swinkels chose a middle course between normalisation and therapeutic specialisation. The clinic for acute psychiatry consists of a residential unit and a treatment unit, which are connected with one another by two corridors. The residential unit has two wings set at right angles to one another, while the treatment unit consists of three wings that fan out. The residential unit has two open and two closed sections. The resocialisation unit consists of a socio-therapeutic community with an area for recreation and therapy. The socio-therapeutic community is accommodated in two identical pavilions facing one another, each of which can house 48 patients. Each pavilion comprises four residential groups of twelve patients each. Each group has a large and a small living room, a multifunctional room, a serving kitchen, a room for the group leader, a four-person room, two double rooms, a few single rooms, and an isolation room.

A corridor – Swinkels refers to inner streets – leads from two wings to the communal area for recreation and therapy. Because the residential units are grouped around it in a square, it does not immediately draw attention to itself. The areas for therapy consist of a communal area with a conversation pit, a hobby area, and rooms for the team members. Because the patients are treated in what looks like an ordinary setting, it is easier for them to return to society.

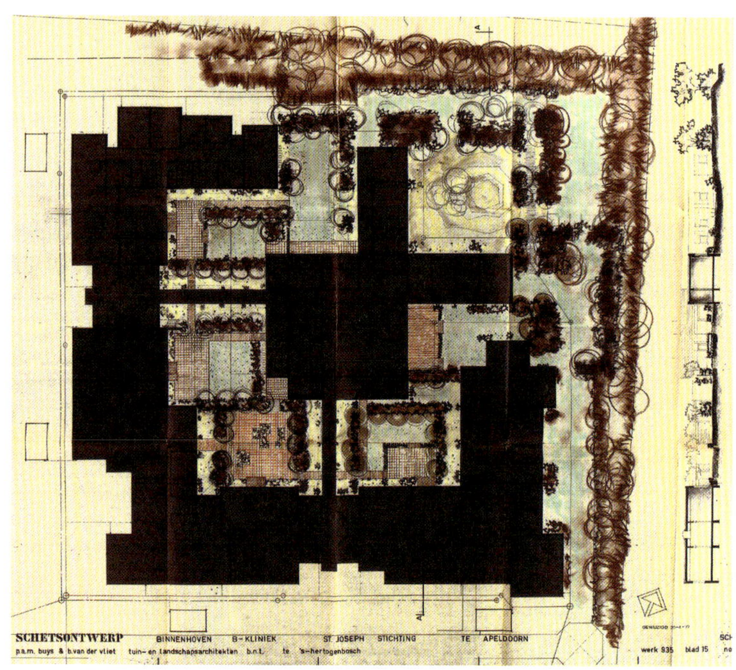

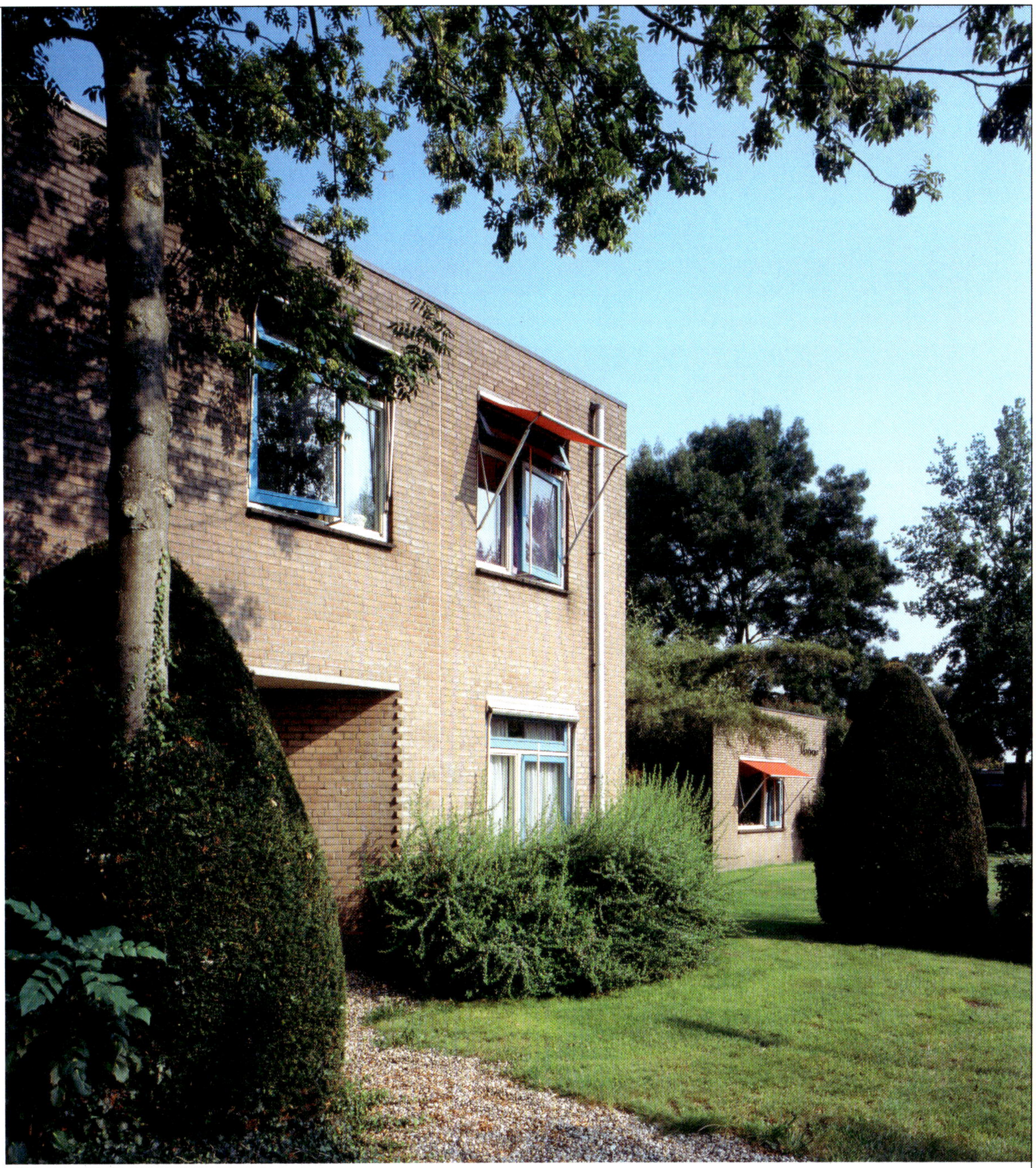

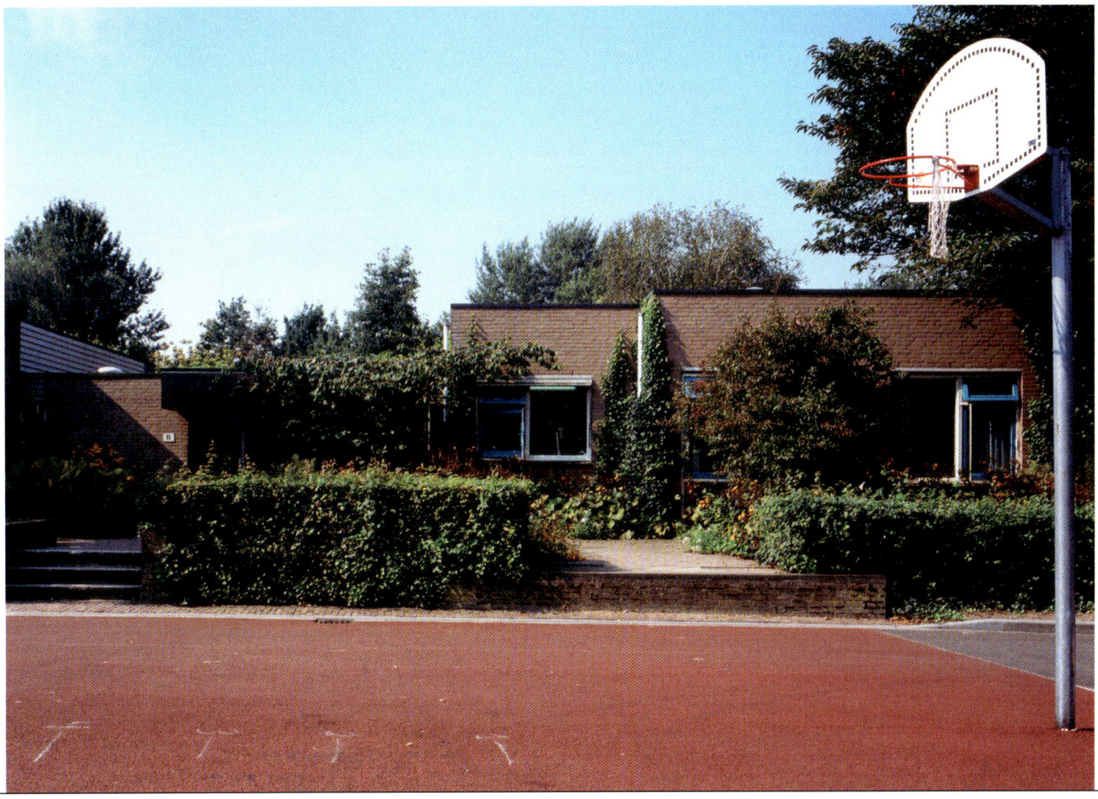

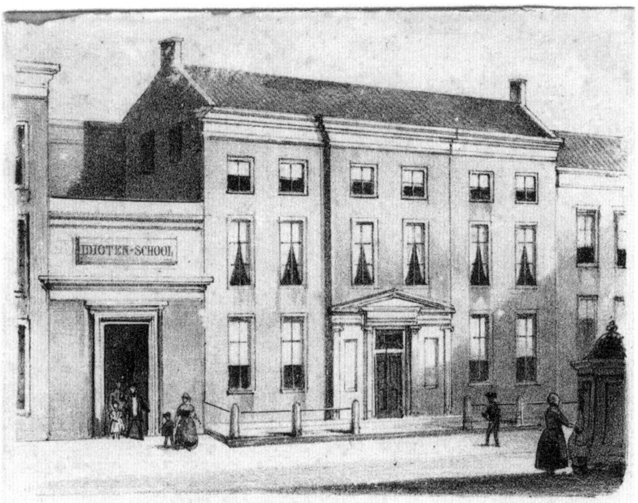

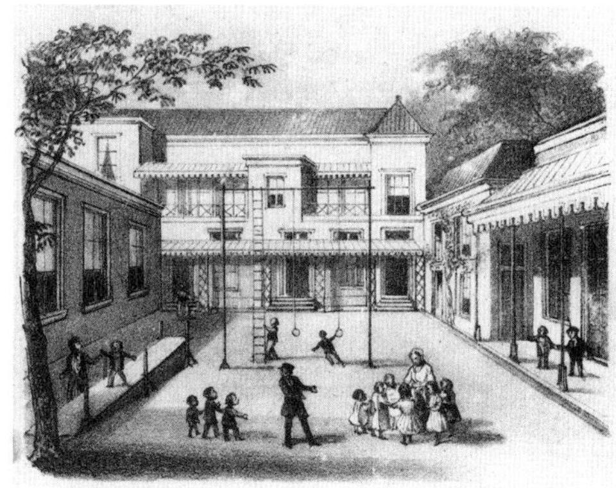

Top
Medical Asylum for Juvenile Idiots, The Hague

J. Heykants, Huize Assisië, Udenhout, 1904

J.E.W.G. Kortlang, 's Heerenloo, Lozenoord, Ermelo, 1911

Bottom
Bethesda, Wagenborgen, 1904

J.E.W.G. Kortlang, 's Heerenloo pavilion, Ermelo

Ed. Cuypers, Boldershof, Druten, 1914

Architectenbureau Leo de Jonge, 's Koonings Jaght, Schaarsbergen, 1968

Housing for the mentally handicapped

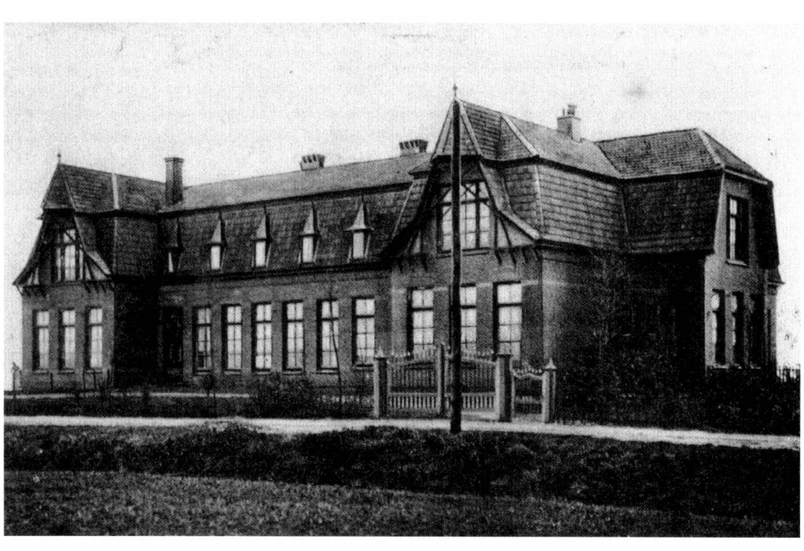

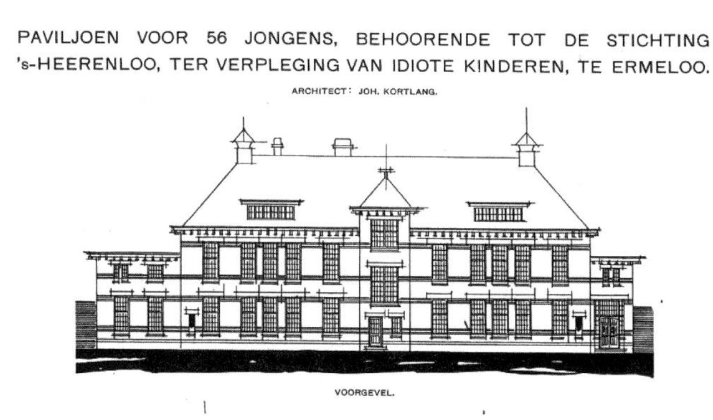

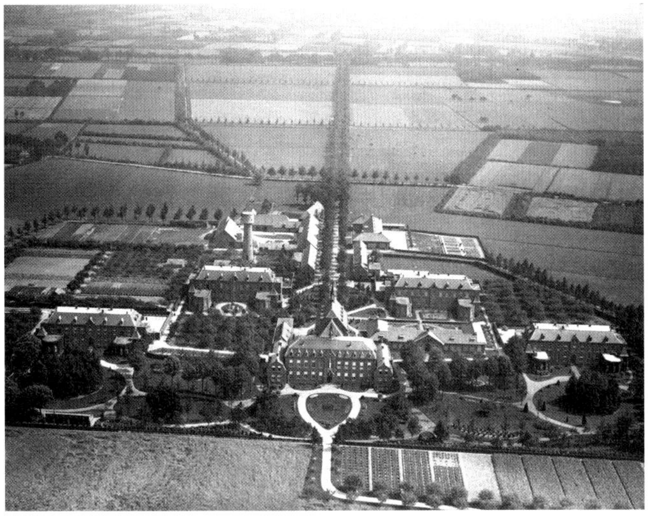

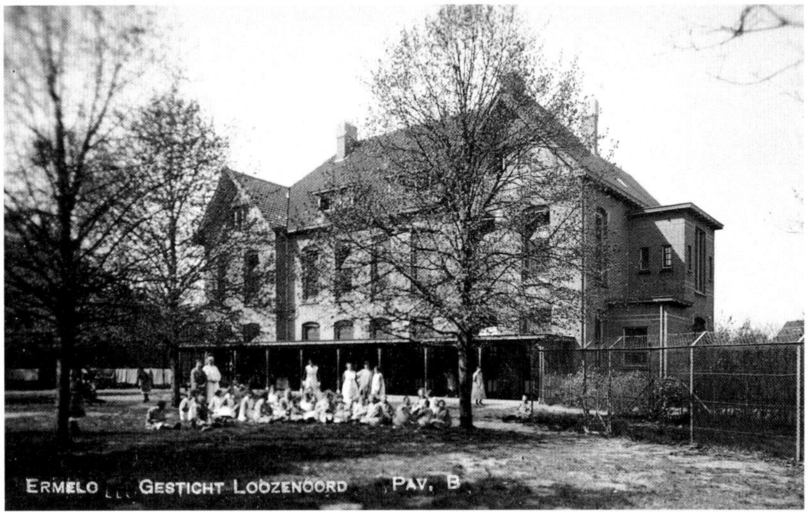

Those with a mental handicap (they were called idiots at first, later the term mentally deficient came into fashion) form a separate group. They are not patients and they are more in need of care than of medical treatment. Ideas about caring for and accommodating this group have changed over the years.

Until the middle of the nineteenth century, institutional care for those with a mental handicap was limited. Usually they continued to live with their family. If this was impossible, they generally shared the fate of the insane and were shut up in asylums, homes and sometimes even in prisons. Their situation improved in the nineteenth century. Those with a mental handicap were regarded as insane – as psychiatric patients were called – and fell under the Law on the Insane (1841). They usually ended up in psychiatric hospitals. Admission of a person with a mental handicap was only possible on the authority of a magistrate and treatment took place amid the psychiatric patients, which was not felt to be satisfactory. It was in the interest of the mentally handicapped to be treated in separate institutions or at least in separate units. The first school for 'idiots' was set up in the Meerenberg provincial asylum in Santpoort in 1853. A private school was opened in the Hague for children who were mild idiots and lived at home in 1855. Children were also adopted by the teacher's family. This Medical Asylum for Juvenile Idiots, founded in 1857, moved to premises in the Westeinde in 1858. Its main goal was to bring up the children. Voorburg in Vught opened a separate unit for idiots in 1890, followed by Huize Padua in Boekel in 1902. A special unit for the free treatment of the mentally deficient was opened in Huize Padua in 1916.

The Netherlands was fairly late in introducing separate provisions by comparison with Germany, the United Kingdom or the United States. In 1888 the Dutch Reformed Church decided to create an association for 'the education and nursing of idiots and backward children'.[1] It purchased the 's Heerenloo estate in Ermelo for this purpose in 1890, and extended it with several pavilions in the following years. The architect was J.E.W.G. Kortlang, the son of the first director of the institution, Fokko Kortlang, who had given up his career as an architect to care for the mentally handicapped. This was followed by an asylum in Wagenborgen (Bethesda) in 1904. The Catholic Huize Assisië was founded in Udenhout in the same year. Like most psychiatric hospitals of this period, the design (by J. Heykants) applied the pavilion system. It is a symmetrical plan with the administration building and chapel located on the central axis, flanked by the pavilions and service buildings. A Catholic asylum for female mental patients designed by Ed. Cuypers was built on the old Boldershof estate in Druten between 1906 and 1914. It was a large, symmetrical building with a chapel and main entrance in the middle and a pavilion on each side. The facility in 's Heerenloo was split in 1911: the girls were accommodated in a separate asylum (Lozenoord) designed, as the first one had been, by Kortlang. Otherwise many of those with a mental handicap were kept in psychiatric hospitals until the Second World War.

It was not until after the war that care for the mentally handicapped was definitively separated from care for psychiatric patients, though sometimes still in the same grounds. Many new institutions were built, others were extended. The first of these were large-scale complexes, followed by a reduction of scale as a reaction to them in the 1960s. Leo de Jonge designed a home for patients with a severe mental handicap on the 's Koonings Jaght estate in Schaarsbergen. The scattered pavilions house compactly composed residential groups.

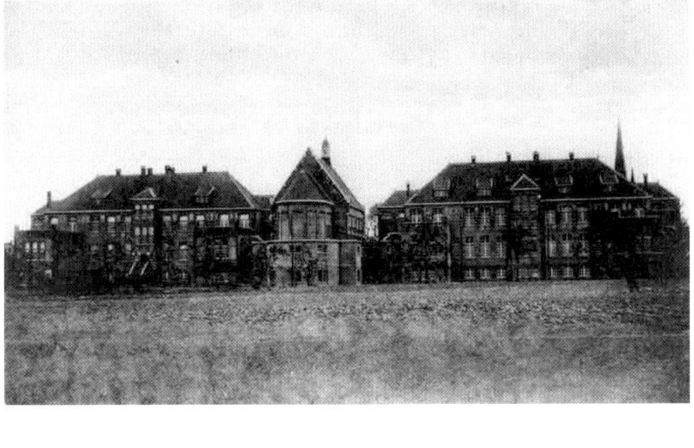

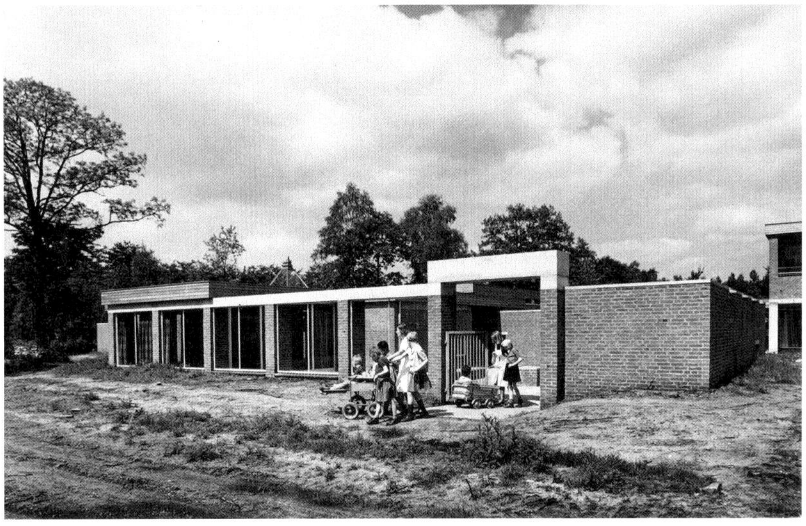

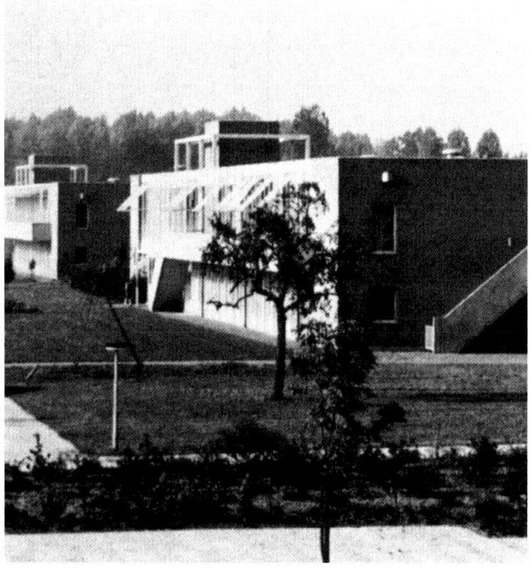

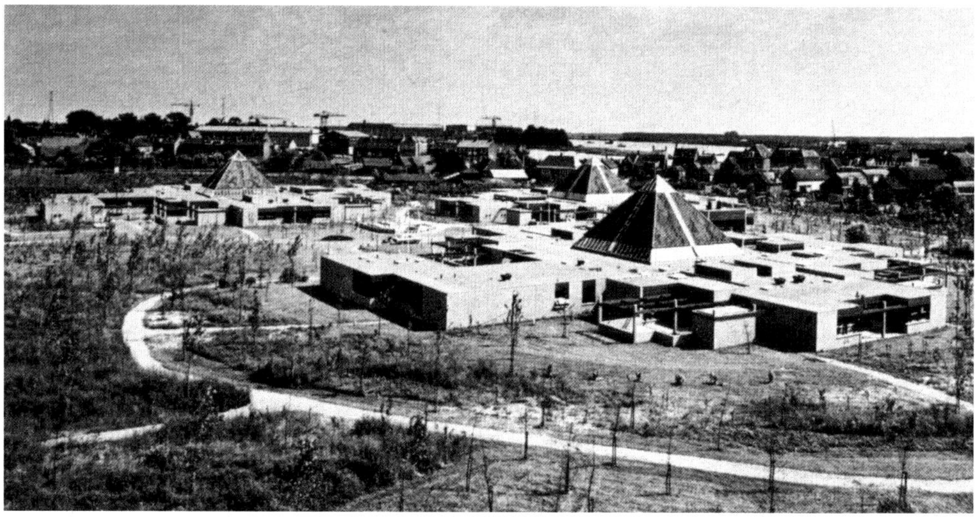

A service corridor runs around the general facilities on the inside; the residential quarters are distributed around it next to patios.

In its early years, the Foundation for Architects Research on Health Care Buildings (Stagg) studied the possibilities of a reduction of scale.[2] This shifted the accent from institutional care to housing. Residential pavilions for groups of eight to ten persons were often grouped around inner courtyards or patios. Tjeerd Dijkstra (Architectengroep Verster Dijkstra Loerakker) designed De Merwebolder in Sliedrecht in 1969. It was intended for 480 persons, and could be expanded to accommodate 600. The pavilions consist of residential units, each for nine persons, that are arranged in a circle around a central zone in an attempt 'to strengthen the feeling of being together under one roof and still to give each unit a different orientation with a different view and different natural lighting to avoid a sense of massiveness'.[3]

The Boldershof buildings in Druten were no longer up to date by the early 1960s and were gradually replaced by new ones. A plan was drawn up by the Jos Bedaux together with the landscape architect P.A.M. Buys. A central axis was projected in the middle of the grounds with pavilions for the residents on either side: two for children, five for adults. The former, which were the first to be built, consisted of four residential groups for six patients and three for twelve patients. Five housing units were built for more independent patients. On the outskirts of the grounds is a block of flats that can accommodate 200 nurses.

The attempt to integrate those with a mental handicap as much as possible in society and to allow them to live as normal a life as possible resulted in the building of housing for working adults in this category (GVTs). They were viewed with scepticism at first and large institutions remained the commonest form of care, but after the government's official recognition of the GVTs in 1976, their number grew explosively.[4] Ordinary housing units (*sociowoningen*) were also built on the outskirts of grounds in the 1960s. A whole series of homes were implemented on the initiative of the Philadelphia Foundation, which was set up by parents. The aim was to integrate small-scale facilities in normal society. Housing and daily activities were kept separate.

Hernesseroord, designed by Van den Broek en Bakema, was built in Middelharnis between 1964 and 1975. The main structure of the complex comprises a steel corridor 3.5 metres wide and 5 metres above ground level. Beneath this corridor are the pavilions for residents and the general facilities, above it are the sister units (prefab 4x7 m cabins that can be attached, removed or moved as required).

The development model came into prominence in the 1970s, which meant that care was increasingly focused on the development of skills and group activities.[5] The groups became smaller, and old buildings were renovated or replaced. This trend was also followed in Dennendal, the institute of the Willem Arntsz Hoeve in Den Dolder for those with a mental handicap. The psychologist Carel Muller introduced a number of reforms there to accommodate the patients in small residential communities. Fired by the ideals of the alternative culture of the 1960s, Muller went a step further: he regarded the mentally handicapped as people who had escaped from the corrupting influence of modern capitalist society, which made them in a certain sense saner than 'normal' people. He commissioned F. van Klingeren, famous for his multifunctional Meerpaal in Dronten, to draw up a plan to build homes for 'normal' people in the grounds of Dennendal. This policy of dilution was intended to reduce the concentration of the mentally handicapped and to enable ordinary citizens to learn from

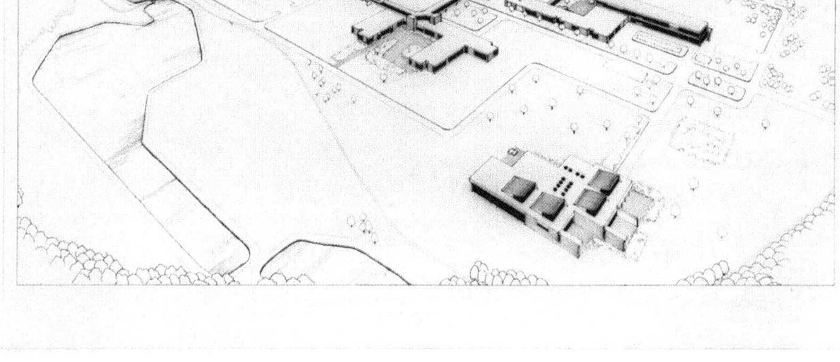

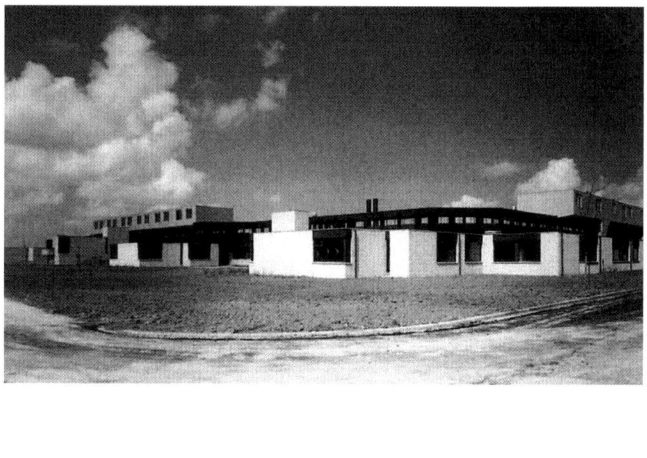

Top
Jos Bedaux, substitute new premises Boldershof, Druten, 1966-1971

Architectengroep Verster Dijkstra Loerakker, De Merwebolder, Sliedrecht, 1969

Reigersdaal, Heerhugowaard, 1976

Bottom
Van den Broek en Bakema, Hernesseroord, Middelharnis, 1975

Marlies Rohmer, De Zeester, Willem van den Bergh care centre, Noordwijk, 2007

Van den Berg Architecten, Druivenhof, Willem van den Bergh care centre, Noordwijk, 2007

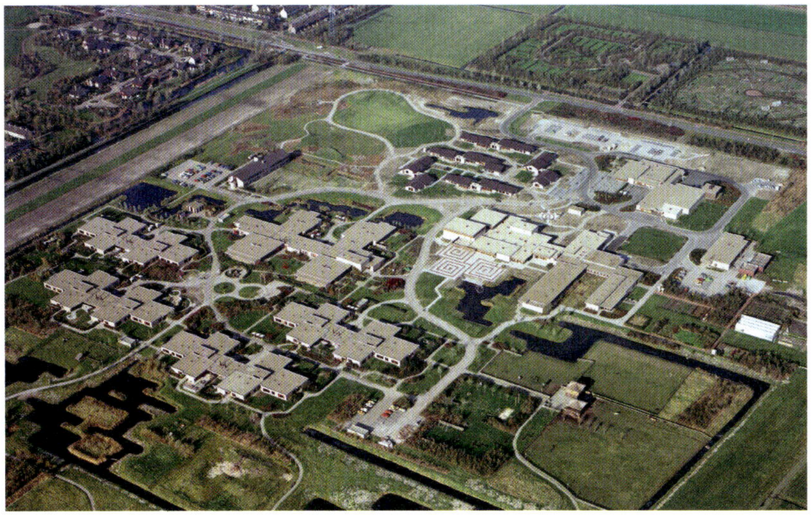

them. The plan was thwarted by the commotion that Muller's alternative views provoked. The police were called in to evacuate Dennendal in 1974, dealing a hard blow to Muller's alternative utopia.

Reigersdaal in Heerhugowaard was opened in 1976. This was an initiative of the board of the Sint Willibrordus psychiatric hospital in Heiloo. The complex looks like a small village, with meandering streets and scattered pavilions. All kinds of amenities are available on the location. The idea was that people should feel comfortable, sheltered and secure here. Most of the homes have four-person rooms, a structure to match the focus on functioning within the group. The landscape architecture of the site, in which the water structure plays an important part, was designed by the garden architect Mien Ruys.

The individual needs of those with a mental handicap came to the fore in the 1980s. More attention was paid to privacy. Besides a further growth in the number of GVTs, more day provisions were created in this period as well. Since the 1990s the emphasis has come to lie more on citizenship and the related right of those with a mental handicap to have their say. This support model gives pride of place to the individual's choice of the appropriate type of housing. Needs in the field of housing, activities, training and treatment are laid down in an individual care plan. Care is demand-orientated instead of supply-driven. The modern institution consists of branches scattered in the region.[6]

These trends have gradually led to the emptying of many of the large institutions. As in the case of psychiatric hospitals, where the same trend can be seen, sites are restructured. Some two-thirds of the original residents of the Willem van den Bergh care centre in Noordwijk, an institution of the 's Heerenloo organisation, were moved to housing in the neighbourhood. Claus en Kaan drew up an urban development plan (2004-2005) for the redevelopment of the site to enable reverse integration. Van den Berg Architecten in Houten designed 84 housing units in the Druivenhof, consisting of five apartment buildings grouped around an inner courtyard. Marlies Rohmer implemented a day centre for the mentally handicapped, De Zeester, between 2003 and 2007. Besides some 200 housing units with corresponding facilities for the remaining residents, 500 more housing units were built on the site for people from 'outside'. So the ideal that Muller and Van Klingeren had wanted to implement in Dennendal in the 1970s has finally been put into practice. This strategy, which has been applied on a larger scale in the last few years, is now referred to as reverse integration.

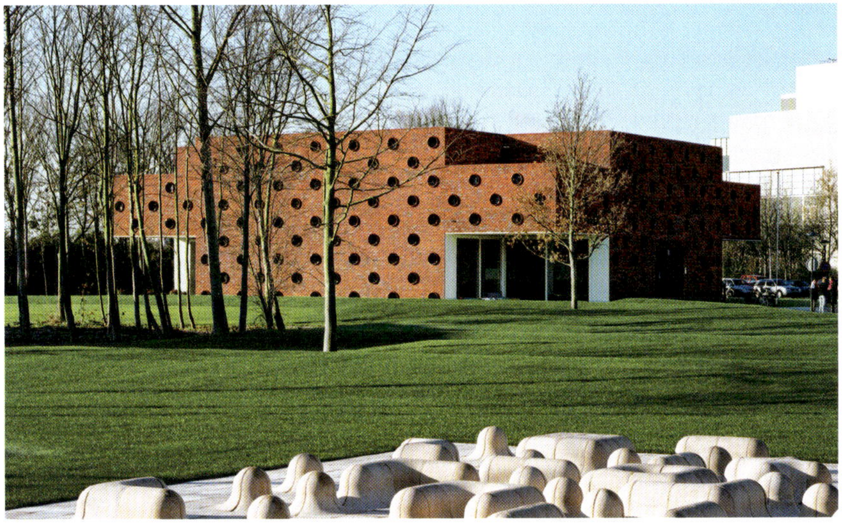

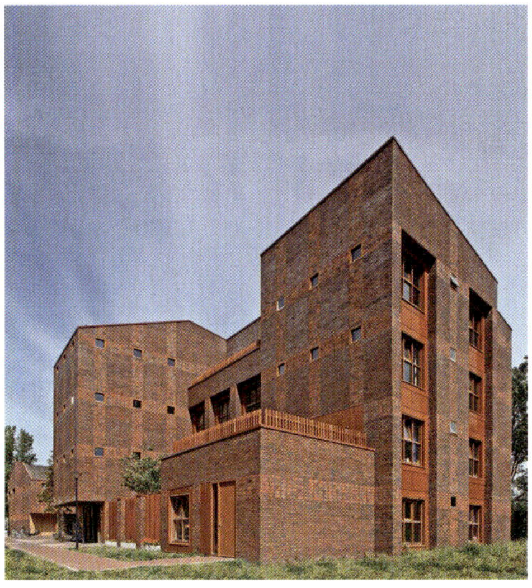

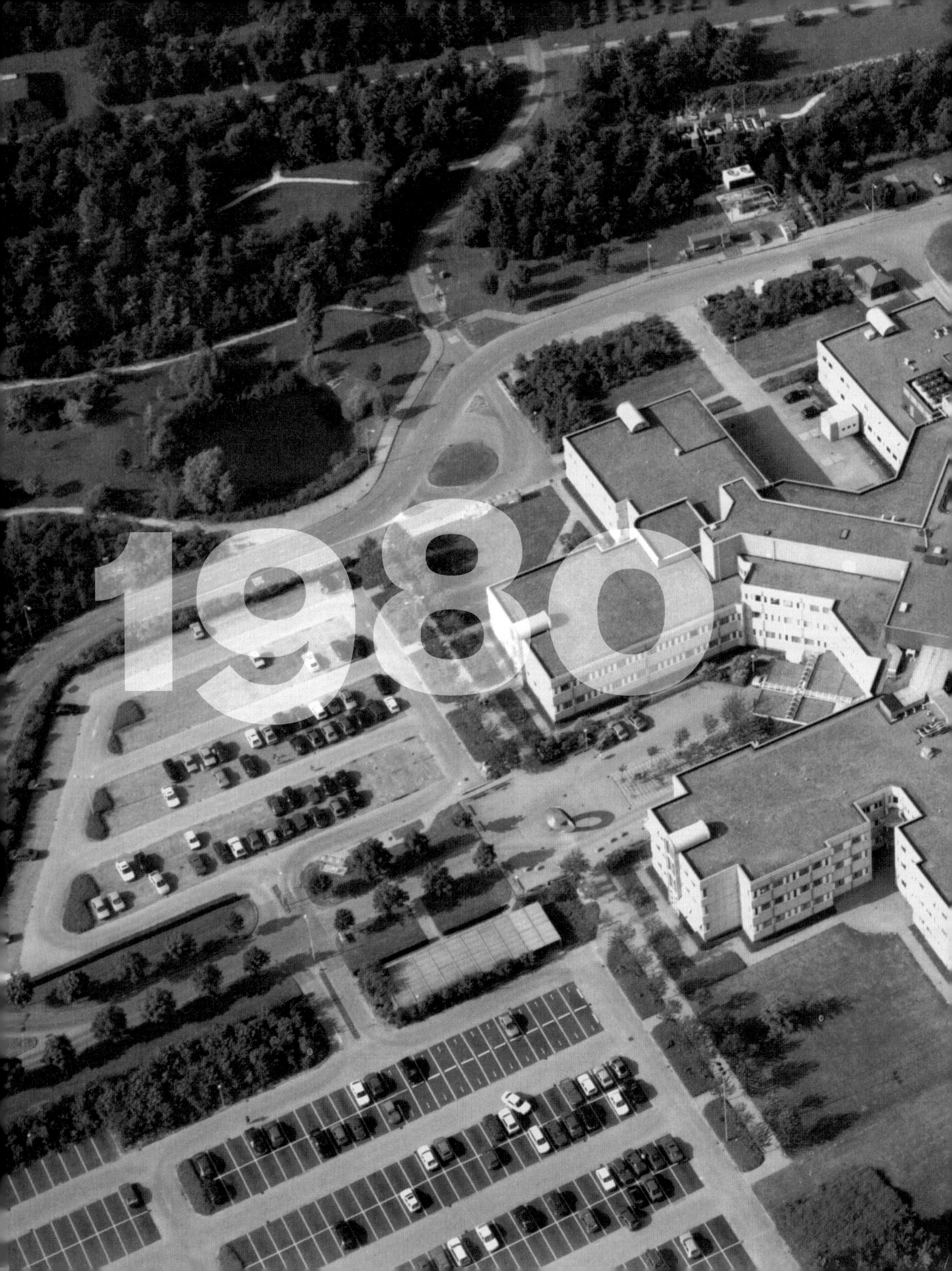
1980

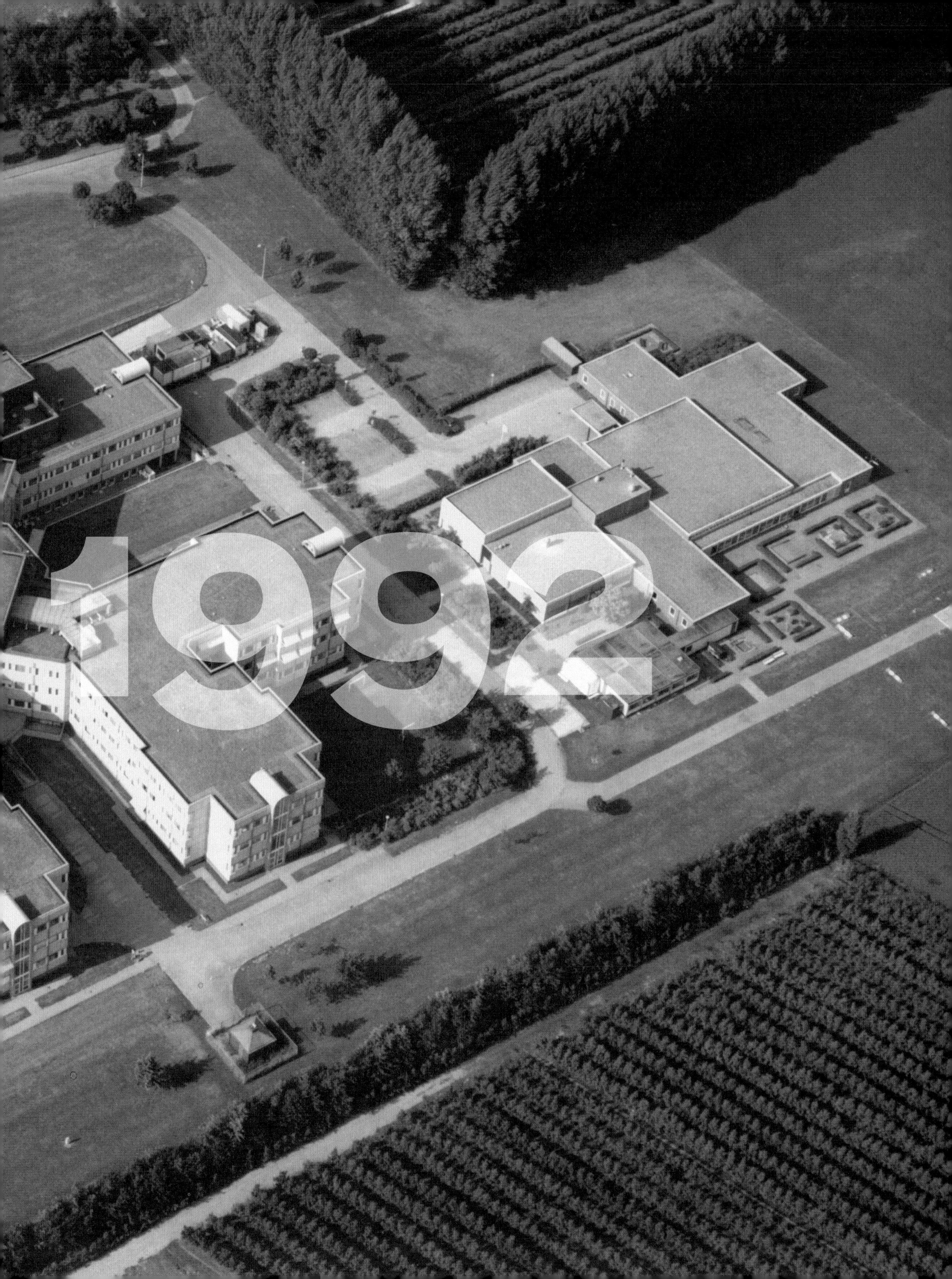
1992

Flexibility and urbanity

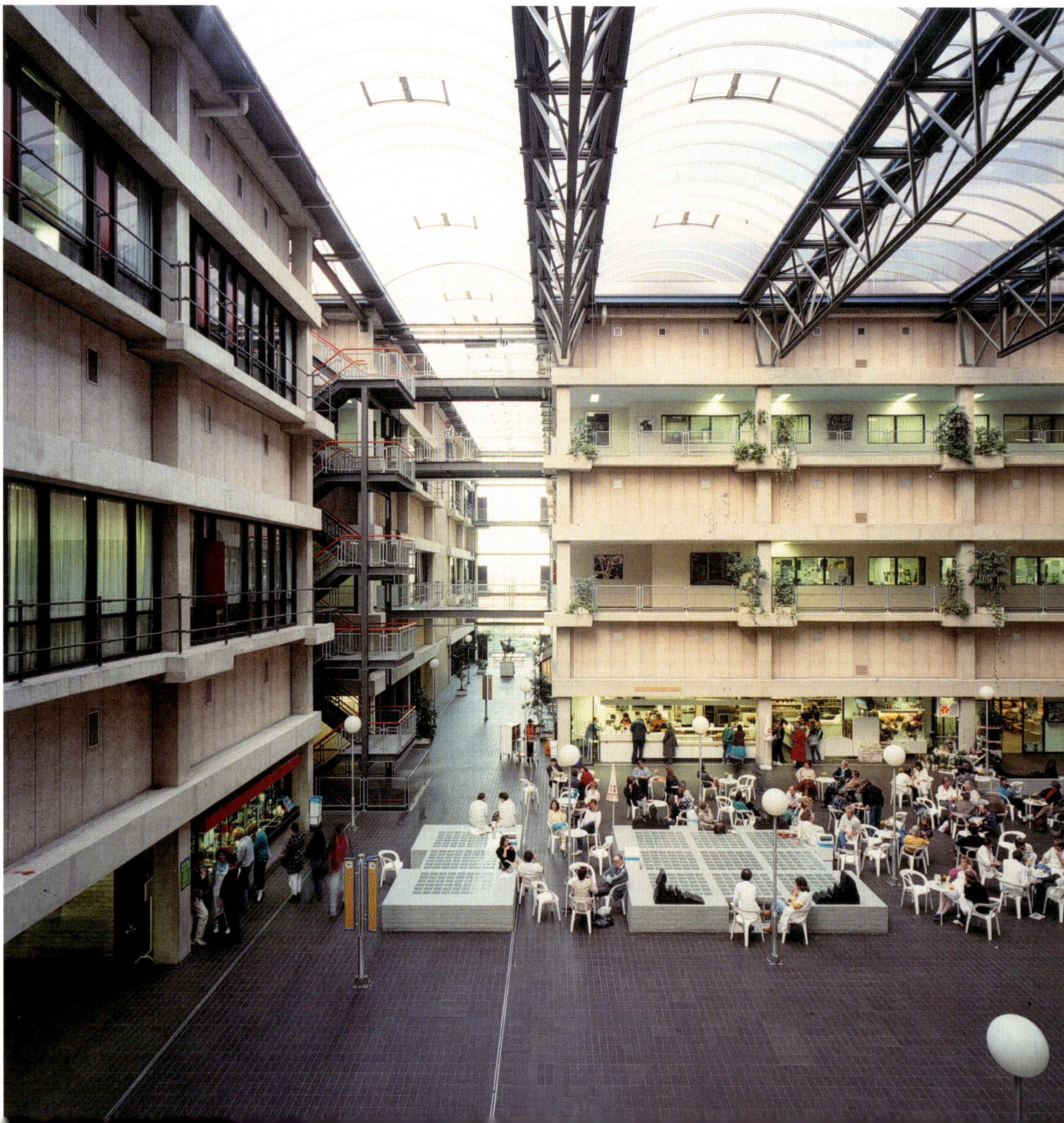

Health care dismantled?

The 1980s were a decade of farewell to utopias, and architecture was no exception. No-nonsense policy was initiated that was to eliminate the 'soft' edges of the caring state and eventually to call the whole welfare state model into question. The redistribution of wealth was replaced by the promotion of economic potential. In the hospitals that led, on the one hand, to a combination of technological and logistical strategies to guarantee more flexibility, and on the other hand, a reappraisal of the cultural impact of architecture on the design and shape of the environment we live in. Those aspects found particular expression in the public areas of the buildings. Psychiatry gave up the utopias of anti-psychiatry, though they continued to resonate in a very radical transformation in which the big old institutions were largely abandoned and replaced by clinics integrated in the city. Once this substitution policy was complete, many a former institutional site was left forsaken in the woods.

The substitution policy that was already being applied to care for the elderly continued unabated. Initially targeting the care home, it now turned its focus on self-sufficient housing units for the elderly. The ideal became to enable as many old people as possible to make use of the regular housing market, which should ideally be made suitable for that purpose in its entirety. Although the concept of the service centre was not abandoned, more importance was now attached to the phenomenon of unpaid care for the elderly. In the meantime nursing homes slowly but surely left the hospital model further behind, which found expression, for instance, in a reinforcing of their domestic character.

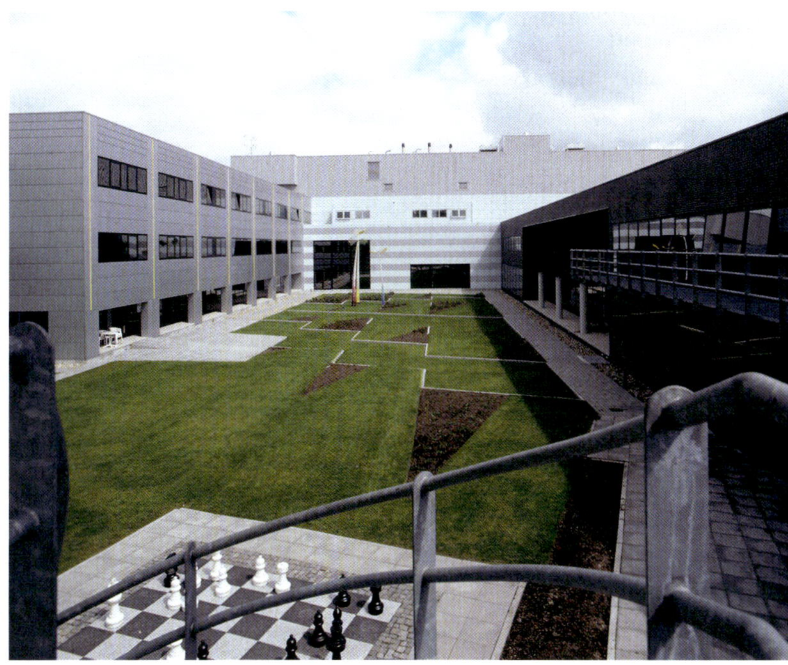

p. 194
***Kruisheer Hallink Arends architecten*, Oosterschelde-ziekenhuis, Goes, 1987**

p. 196
***Architektenburo Duintjer Istha Kramer Van Willegen, with D. van Mourik*, Academisch Medisch Centrum (AMC), Amsterdam, 1981/1985**

p. 197
***Tuns + Horsting Architecten*, Wilhelmina Ziekenhuis, Assen, 1990**

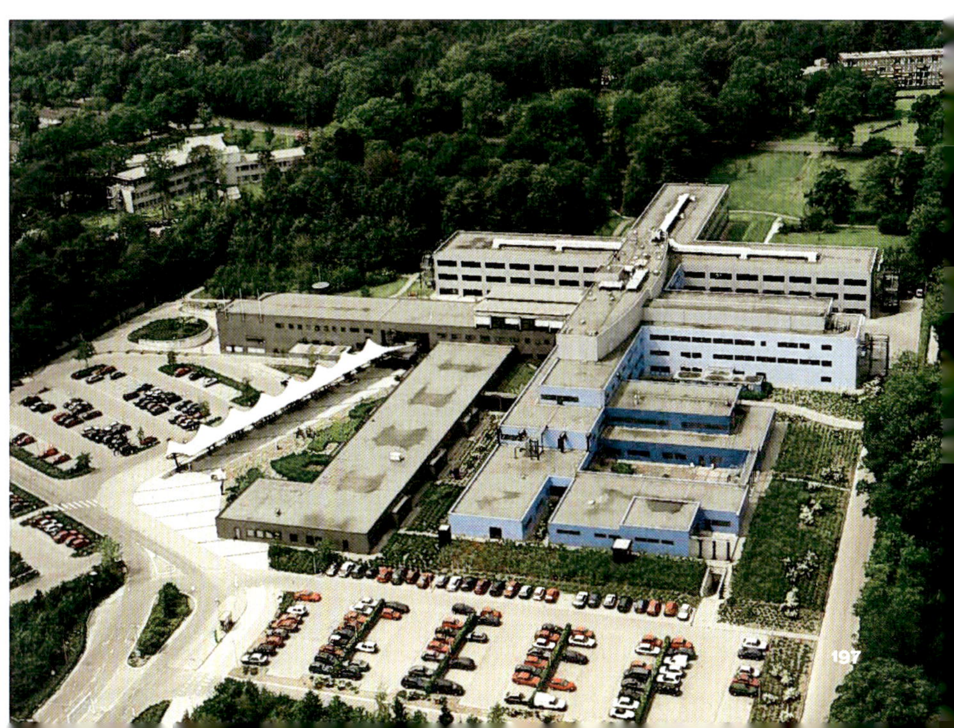

Hospitals

Investments in the building of hospital provisions in the 1980s were determined by a series of lists of hospitals to be closed, (provincial) alternatives to them, and lists of priorities that indicated which building projects had first priority to be selected from the pool and led to the stage in which, sometimes many years later, they could actually be implemented. The first list was already published in February 1978, though the plan to issue a new edition each year came to nothing.[1]

A lot of commotion arose when the minister M.H.M.F. Gardeniers announced the bed reduction plan in 1982. 'Although the intention of substantially reducing the number of hospital beds (...) was not a surprise, the actual proposal produced a serious shock and provoked large unrest in many places because, besides the general principles to arrive at a reduction, it also already presented a specific elaboration in the form of twenty-five regional visions.'[2] No less than twenty-five hospitals were to close down, and one or more departments in another seventy-seven were to follow suit. The reaction of the hospital world was one of consternation. The list included institutions in which the paint of recent renovations was barely dry.[3] The norm applied by the minister was 3.7 beds per 1000 residents, while at that moment the target of 4.0 per 1000 had not even yet been reached. All regions that were expected to have more beds in 1990 than this norm allowed would have to cut the surplus of beds within four years.[4]

A plethora of alternative plans was the result, with proposals to close less institutions down entirely and to distribute the cuts more evenly by closing down departments in a larger number of hospitals. However, this had a negative effect on longer-term planning: the more outdated buildings remained in use, the larger was the share of the total building budget that was drained from the necessary new building projects, and the longer it took before a rational, planned distribution pattern emerged. The lack of a consensus on the plan for closures and the resistance of the institutions under threat prevented it from being much of a success.

The hospitals that were built in the 1980s were structures rather than buildings. They were solutions not to formal architectural problems, but to brakes on the inevitable process of adaptation and expansion. They were complexes that did not stand as buildings in the city, but retreated to the centre of the plot allocated to them, ready at any moment to take over the whole plot. The need arose to design hospitals in such a way that they could be adapted to the constantly changing demands without too much difficulty or expense. Buildings whose fabric could still last for years soon became functionally outdated; flexibility could prolong their lives. Patios, inner courtyards and entrance halls, to which more flexible rules apply than to the treatment and nursing units, offer the architect more room for manoeuvre. Virtually expelled from the design of the hospital proper, the designers could find compensation elsewhere.

Three types of hospital that were developed with a view to flexibility offered scope for the upgrading of the public areas: the cross type, the square type, and the linear type (with variants). It is characteristic of these types that in each of them the traffic structure determines the plan, and that the units linked to it can be expanded individually (open-end structures). Sometimes a particular articulation of the various units might result in an open or roofed patio, for example, where public amenities such as a restaurant and shops could be added. The goals of the humane and open hospital of the 1970s could thus be given a contemporary twist here. J. Rentes de Carvalho remarked on a visit to the Academisch Medisch Centrum (AMC): 'I enthusiastically discovered a real square and a transparent roof further on. A bank and a post office, both with helpful, smiling personnel. Telephone booths undisturbed by vandals. A bar, a book shop, a florist's, a kiosk, restaurants. (...) But because work called I had to go and at that moment, as I was about to enter the revolving door, I was overwhelmed by an inexplicable aversion to the grey, cold world outside. I suddenly realised that I had the absurd desire to stay here for ever (...).'[5]

On a smaller scale, the same transformation took place in the general hospitals as well. In the Streekziekenhuis Waterland in Purmerend (1988) designed by Campman Tennekes De Jong, the public space with all kinds of amenities has been magnified to become the main feature of the building. The hospital consists of an enormous central passage flanked by a T-shaped segment on each side with the base of the T pointing away from the building. The outpatient clinics are on the ground floor, the services, laboratories and operating unit on the first floor, while the nursing wards are on the second and third floors. There is a technical layer between the first and the second floors.

In the Merwedeziekenhuis in Dordrecht, W. Eijkelenboom turned the hall into the dramatic centre. 'Every emotion from birth to death is experienced here. Such a hall must be restful and not cause extra stress. But it must also be usable, you must also be able to get to the hairdresser there.' The

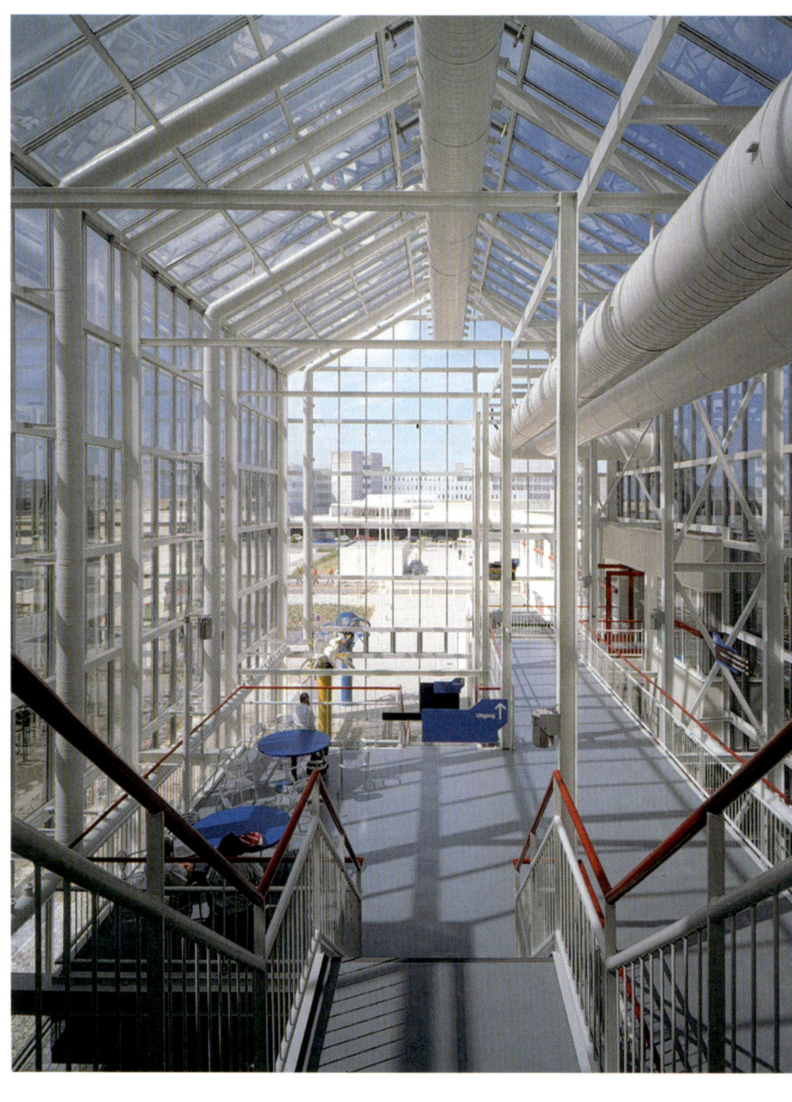

central hall is the core of the design and everything else is reached from there. The circulation pattern is very clear and easy to grasp. The architecture accentuates the open ends where the hospital can expand further. In the interior it is not just the central hall that is eye-catching: everywhere special attention has been paid to the waiting rooms and traffic areas. Bright colours brighten up the pavilions, while the application of works of art adds life to the hospital.

Designers pounced on the potential of the public areas to make architecture again. In the 1970s architecture and urban planning had become a form of social critique in concrete; in the 1980s they were rediscovered as disciplines that had an artistic and cultural task on top of their practical and social functions. The number of public events, urban design competitions with exhibitions, lectures with slides and debates focused on design rapidly increased. The consensus on what architecture was changed. Instead of being just a tool to serve a particular purpose, it was also a visual image, a sign in the city.

A. Tuns devised new solutions by taking trends that had already pointed in the same direction for decades further architecturally and reacting to the differentiation between wards and treatment units. The ward, which had been dominant for years, decreased in significance. What was more natural than to subordinate it to the treatment unit and outpatient clinic?[6] What was more natural than to divide the hospital into its different constituent parts? And why should they not be allowed to display high tech refinement in their design?

The Wilhelmina Ziekenhuis in Assen is based on these ideas: a showpiece of Deconstructionism with the image of de luxe design. Tuns separated the three main functions and provided, making use of the possibility of designing the treatment units and wards in accordance with a different basic pattern, each with its own dimensions, texture, colour and details. The advantage is that not every part of the hospital had to be implemented for the same high costs. It also has urban development implications: it was easier to integrate the complex in its surroundings. Tuns' creation is an immediate eye-catcher – but not as a hospital.

The division of the hospitals into smaller units can be seen in other new building projects too. Tennekes set the trend in his designs for Purmerend and Almere, although there the separate elements were connected with one another by the roofing.

p. 198 and 199
***Campman Tennekes de Jong architecten*, Flevo Ziekenhuis, Almere, 1990**

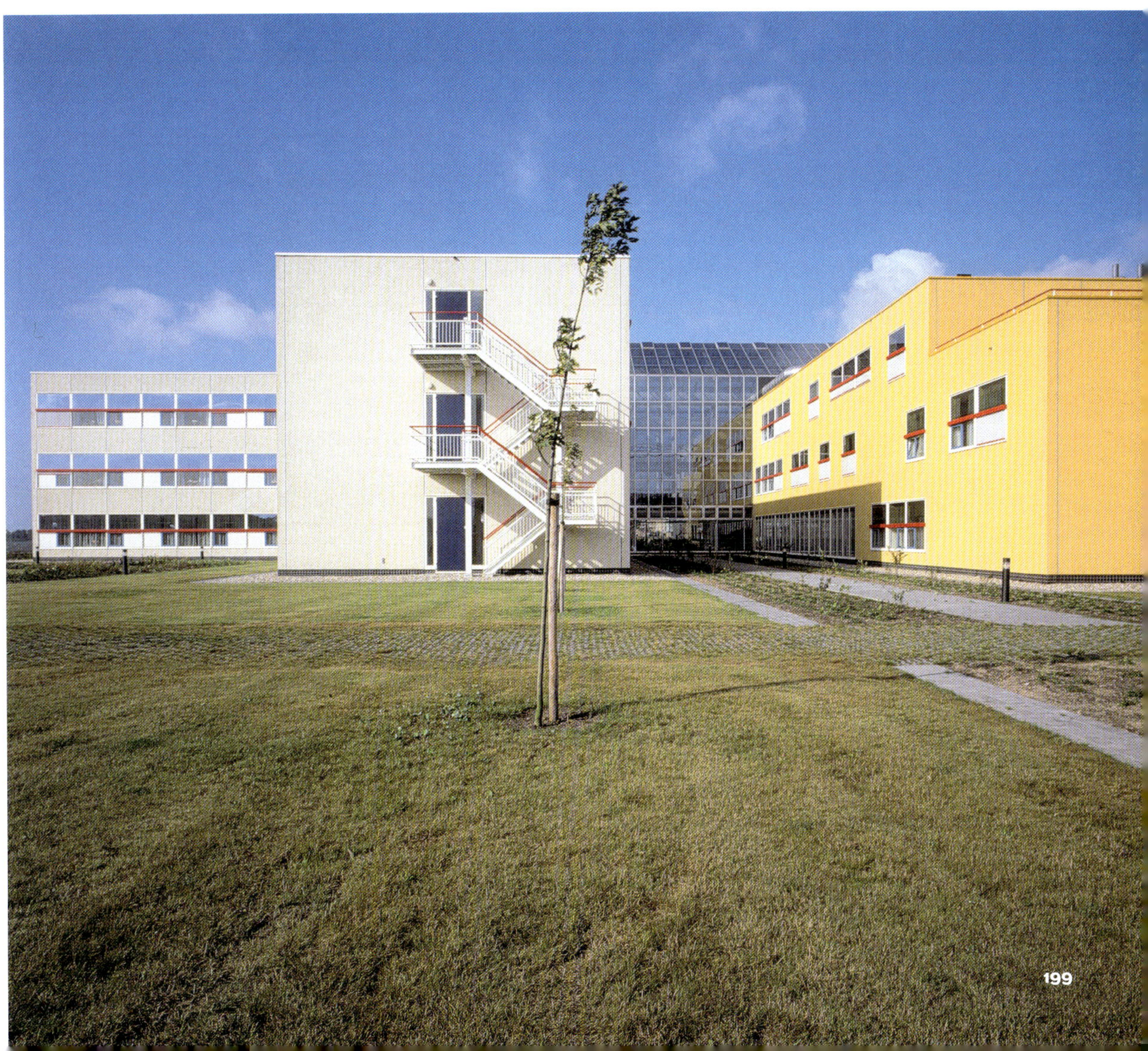

Psychiatric hospitals

While the revolutionary attempts within psychiatry absorbed all attention in the 1970s, fundamental changes were going on behind the scenes. All the same, the proposal to set up a new institution in Nijmegen in the 1980s provoked a brief revival of the rebellion against the asylum: prominent authorities in psychiatry called for the postponement of this project – which threatened to be affected by spending cuts anyway – to be made permanent. 'They call institutions "redundant, useless and harmful to the residents", characterised by coercion, lack of liberty and punitive measures.'[7] This countermovement ran parallel to the moratorium action that, paradoxically enough, marked the end of anti-psychiatry in the Netherlands. From then on the no-nonsense search for a new psychiatry offered more prospects of success.[8]

The only lasting result of the anti-psychiatric assault on the establishment was the wish to abandon the classic asylum. This motive was a guiding principle of the moratorium action in 1982 and has been a thread running through government policy ever since. The government determined the course. The New Memorandum on Mental Health of 1984 had a great influence, in which the government reaped the fruits of the moratorium action and pressed for scattered small-scale provisions for clinical and ambulant psychiatry. The setting up of the Regional Institutes for Mental Welfare (RIAGG) in the 1980s was one of the results of this policy.[9] The multifunctional unit (MFE) that was to radically change the landscape of psychiatric care also goes back to this memorandum. The Memorandum 2000, which was issued in April 1986, was also of great importance. It detached thinking about health care from thinking in terms of such institutions as hospitals and psychiatric clinics. Prevention became a major theme, and the line between health care and environmental hygiene became a fluid one. It was thought that making society healthier might well have a more positive effect than just pumping money into health care.[10]

Substitution – replacing as many psychiatric beds as possible in the classic institutions by provisions elsewhere that were integrated into the urban fabric – became the core of the new policy. In the end, all that remained of the classic asylums were places to keep chronic patients. While there had been experiments in the 1970s with more or less autonomous housing facilities on or in the immediate vicinity of the psychiatric hospitals, a further step was now taken as attempts were made to integrate these forms of housing in ordinary, everyday new housing estates. Such units maintained only organisational links with the institutions to which they belonged. Some of the housing functions of the classic asylum were transferred to institutions for sheltered forms of housing; these too were integrated in residential neighbourhoods and the counselling was reduced to a minimum.

More radical than the decentralisation of part of the institution was the building of an entirely new psychiatric hospital without a central main branch. That was the essence of new building plans in Dordrecht that were entirely dominated by the principle of deconcentration. A fundamental shift in thinking about social therapy had taken place. While the 1950s, 1960s and 1970s concentrated entirely on the residential group, in other words, the collectivity, in the 1980s more importance was attached to the individuality of the patient. In the meantime it had become clear that spending twenty-four hours a day in the same residential group had its disadvantages too. Instead of learning self-reliance, there was a danger that the patients would become

p. 200
***Architectenmaatschap Cannegieter*, Helmerzijde psychiatric hospital, Enschede, 1985. Medical centre.**

***Architectenmaatschap Cannegieter*, Helmerzijde psychiatric hospital, Enschede, 1985. Dwelling.**

p. 201
***Architectenbureau Rothuizen en 't Hooft*, Psychiatrisch Ziekenhuis Zeeland, Goes, 1990**

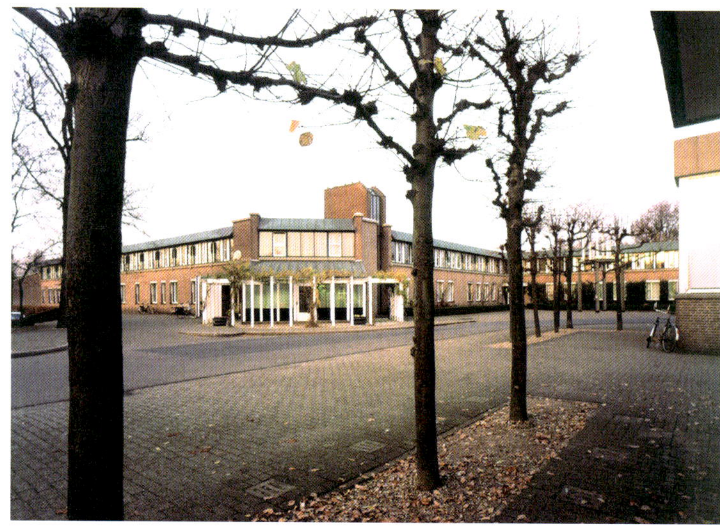

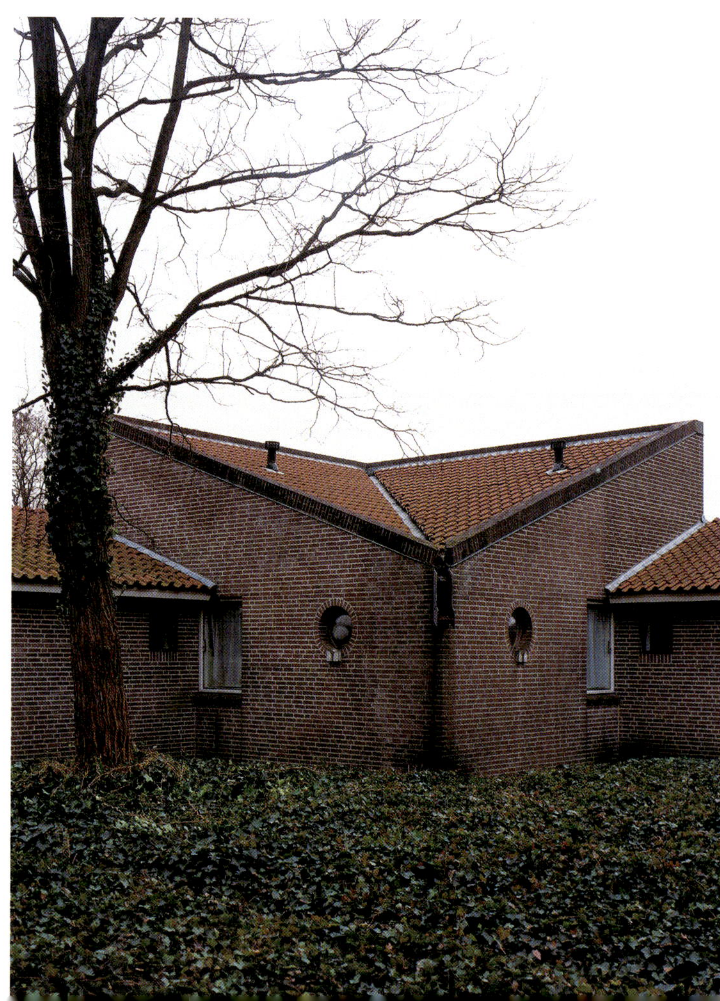

totally dependent on one another, often leaving no alternative but to endlessly extend their stay in a residential group. And that, of course, had not been the intention. The Boston model, which was introduced in the Netherlands around the middle of the 1980s, seemed to offer an alternative. Nowhere in the USA had the replacement of ordinary psychiatric beds by sheltered forms of housing and day treatment centres been taken further than in Massachusetts, where the Massachusetts Mental Health Center played a pioneering role. Study commissions from the Valeriuskliniek in Amsterdam and elsewhere visited this institution and drew their inspiration from the US model.[11]

The core of the Boston model was a split between treatment and housing, which were also physically accommodated in different buildings. The advantages were obvious. The collective part of the treatment was relegated to the treatment units, after which the patients returned to their private world. The treatment units were not only for the residents themselves; they would also be used as outpatient clinics or day treatment units for patients from outside. The clear division of functions that this structure entailed was to leave its mark on new building projects from the late 1980s on.

The last traditional psychiatric hospitals

Hardly any new psychiatric hospitals were built in the 1980s. Those that were built were usually to fill gaps and were relatively small complexes. An exception is the psychiatric hospital Helmerzijde in Enschede, designed by B. van den Bos and J. Cannegieter between 1979 and 1982. With 204 beds it exceeds the usual scale of new building projects in this period. Helmerzijde is a fully fledged clinic with all of the corresponding departments and functions. All the same, the designers were asked to strip this hospital of the traditional institutional character. It was to be somewhere between a hospital and a normal residential neighbourhood, and the relation between the residents in the institution and those outside was to be kept open.[12] That explains the decision to group the general amenities beside a small square adjacent to the access road, and the decision to intersect the grounds with a cycle and pedestrian route accessible to all. Its use was stimulated by the way in which the grounds related to the structure of the new housing estate: the more people used them, the more successful the desired integration would be.

One of the consequences of leaving the grounds entirely open – there are no walls or fences shutting them off from the surroundings – is the design of the closed areas: the open spaces required for them were found in the form of patios inside the building volumes, which could therefore remain relatively closed on the outside. The design was intended to promote the emergence of an urban environment and to integrate the hospital in a normal social setting. This presupposed that the anxiety of the 'average citizens' about having psychiatric patients in their midst would have to be removed. The building of the centre is in line with the objective of regionalisation: it aims to satisfy the real demands of the region without attracting patients from elsewhere.[13]

Normalisation of the institution was also the aim of Rothuizen en 't Hooft in their plan for the Psychiatrisch Ziekenhuis Zeeland in Goes. That dictated the structure: 'The general arrangement of the buildings was to create the idea of a village with a central square of which the part closest to the social centre will increasingly function as a meeting place'.[14] The low-rise complex with 200 beds is organised around a central square where the obligatory

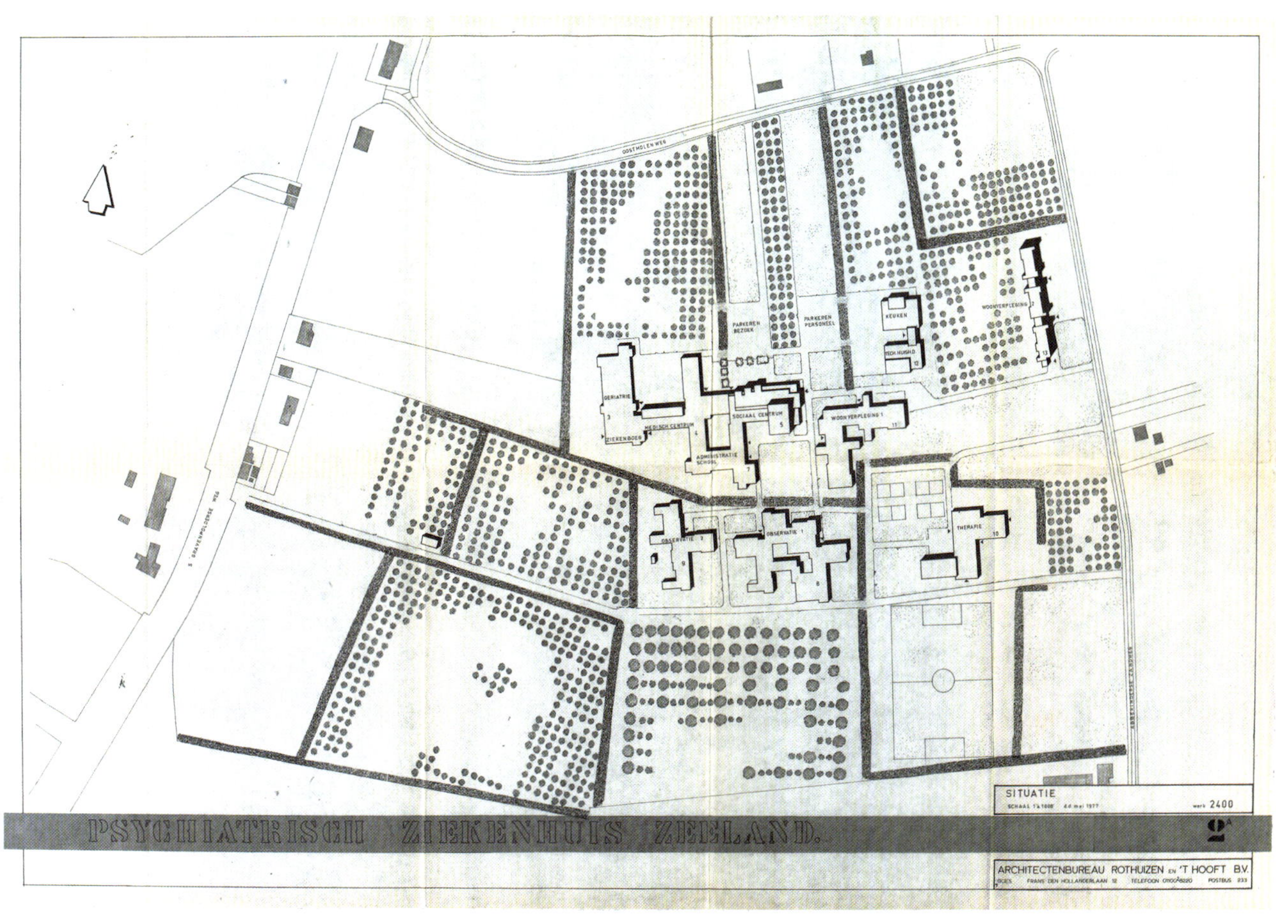

social centre is also located. The four wings orientate the residents towards this social heart. So the concept of the community which was gradually abandoned in the succeeding years still determines the programme in this hospital, and the breaking down of the barriers between society and institution is concentrated in the simulation of a purified form of community within the context of the institution modelled on 'normal' society. The completion of the hospital marked the conclusion of a planning procedure that had begun in 1969.

A number of small pavilions were opened in the grounds of Huize Padua in Boekel in 1989. They were designed by Aldo & Hannie van Eyck and attracted considerable attention. After all, it was not often that a famous architect was tempted to design health care buildings. Aldo van Eyck, who had been one of the leading figures in the protest of architects against the International Style in the 1950s and 1960s, seized this assignment to criticise the system from within. The small-scale complex that he and his wife designed has a modest look and is somewhat set back on the extensive grounds of the hospital. The pavilions, for which the commission had already been placed in 1980, stand out for their far-reaching use of detail, their carefully conceived logistics, and the striking use of materials and colours. Some critics regarded this as the Achilles' heel of the design: 'That is what makes it terribly vulnerable at the same time; everything is deliberate, nothing can be left out, a very high intensity of ideas and attention permeates every fibre of these buildings'.[15]

Van Eyck translated the programme, which envisaged both open and closed units, into low-rise buildings that radiated openness in all directions. A gently curving corridor provides access to the clusters of single rooms, which are arranged around a central patio. The rooms correspond exactly to the regulations of the time, but the way the designers have achieved this seems to be wanting to make fun of the bureaucracy. The maximum size for a patient's room was nine m^2, so Van Eyck designed simple rectangular rooms that far exceeded this maximum and then cut a round section out of them. Some commentators saw this as a 'solution that pitilessly exposes the absurdity of the dogmatic regulations'.[16]

The end of the psychiatric institution

Joyce Smook-Noach designed the first completely new psychiatric hospital to be structured in accordance with the principles of deconcentration and small scale in 1989. De Grote Rivieren psychiatric centre has its main branch in Dordrecht, where two satellites were also built; a third satellite was built in Gorinchem. The main branch could accommodate fifty-four patients, distributed among three open and two closed units. Each unit had its own accommodation block and the institution also had a treatment block that was made to look like an office block. The architecture of both blocks matched that of ordinary apartment and office blocks. The complex does not look like a psychiatric hospital and thereby satisfies one of the aims: a non-institutional design that looks as normal as possible. Life in the new institution was to refer to that of 'normal' society. This implied 'a daily rhythm based on domestic activities (sleeping, eating, hobby, relaxation), on the one hand, and activities outside the home (work, recreation, sport, shopping, walking, etc.), on the other'.[17] Living and working were to be kept apart and if at all possible the traffic between them should be over the public road. The separation between home and work, in other words between the living quarters of the patients and the treatment units where the range of therapies was concentrated, was one of the innovative aspects of De Grote Rivieren and is reminiscent of the Boston model, which was introduced at roughly the same time.

Since the beginning of the 1980s the sheltered forms of housing have come to play an increasingly prominent role within mental health care. Unlike the housing innovations within the psychiatric clinics, the priority is to minimise

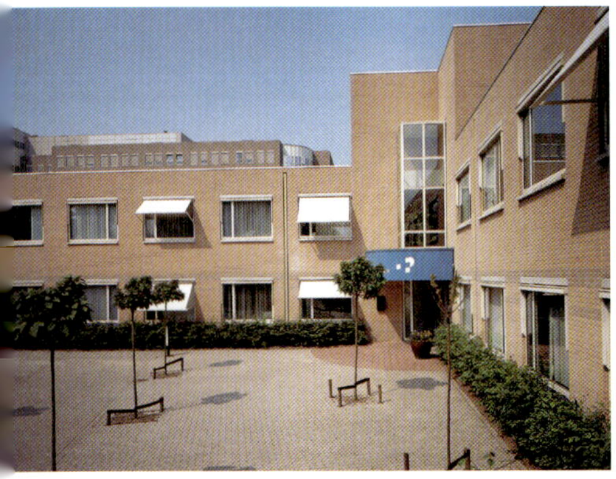

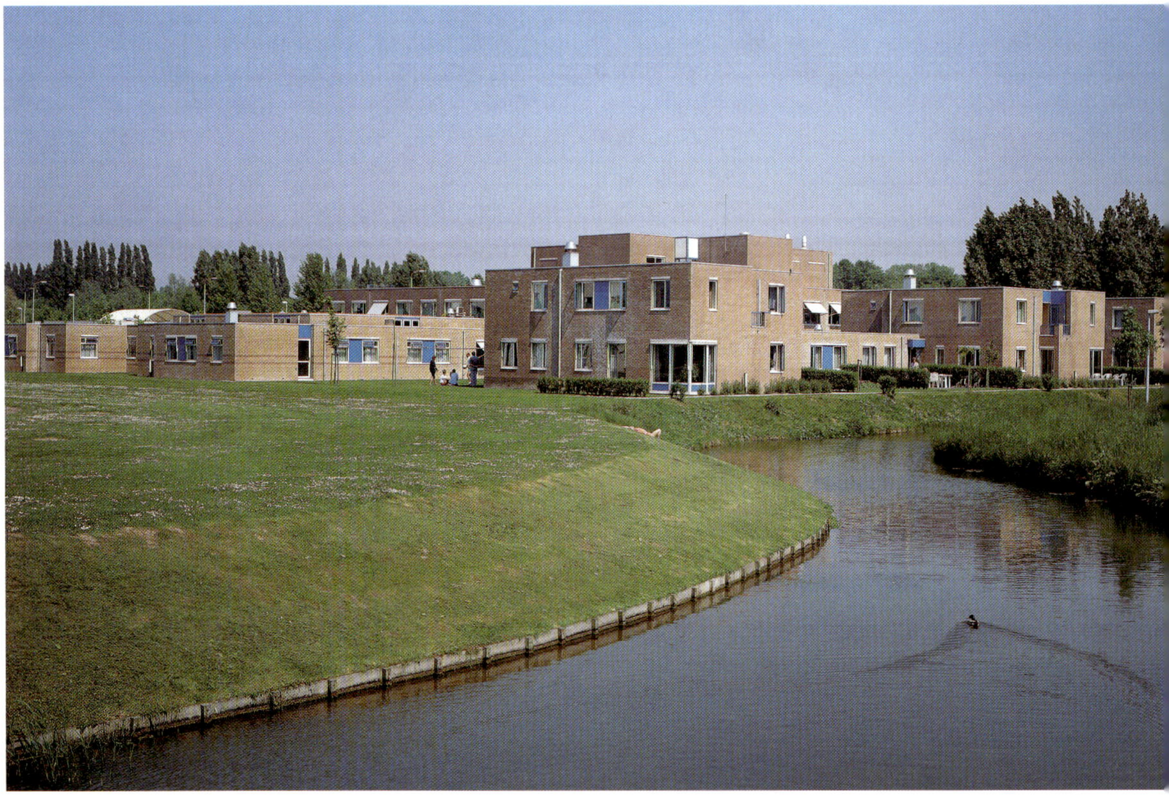

therapeutic counselling with the aim, where possible, of resocialising the patient. If that proves overambitious, the forms of sheltered housing can form a good alternative to a continuous stay in a psychiatric hospital. The first Regionale Instelling voor Beschermende Woonvormen (RIBW) (Regional Institution for Sheltered Forms of Housing), was set up for the Oost-Veluwe region in Apeldoorn in 1980 and was an initiative of the Psychiatrische Tussenvoorziening Apeldoorn (Psychiatric Intermediate Provision Apeldoorn). The integration within mental health care was not formalised until 1989; since then RIBWs have sprung up everywhere.

Back to the city

Building for psychiatric patients became increasingly concentrated on the city in the 1980s. In the meantime this had major consequences for the classic institutions in the countryside, which were partly or completely bereft of their function. That fate befell the first model institution in the Netherlands, Meerenberg in Santpoort, usually simply referred to as Santpoort. No matter how picturesque a stay in the classic asylums often situated in beautifully laid out grounds may have been, they had serious disadvantages as well. One negative side-effect was the severing of the patient's social ties, which in the worst case made return to regular society impossible. That was the background of a movement away from the idyllic countryside and back to the city. Santpoort had its own outpatients unit, but the idea arose in the 1980s that it would be more logical to move it to the neighbouring cities of Haarlem or Alkmaar.[18]

Santpoort did in fact set up three outpatient units outside the hospital grounds in 1985. They were in Amsterdam, a location much closer to the home base of many of the patients. That proved to be the start of a much more ambitious plan: the decentralisation of the entire institution and the transfer of most of its facilities to the capital. This Amsterdam model was to cause considerable debate in the following years. A facility was opened in Amsterdam in 1989 – the Vlaamse Passage designed by Greiner en Van Goor in the Sloten district of the city– for the category of chronic patients who had traditionally been sent to Santpoort. In this case there was no alternative admission to a traditional institution, as the corresponding institution, Santpoort, was evacuated at the end of the 1980s. The Vlaamse Passage seemed to blend imperceptibly with its surroundings. It accommodated seventy chronic patients in housing units whose front door opened onto the street. The project completed a building block intersected by a public pedestrian route which had to be maintained. The block on the north side has two floors, that on the opposite side three. The day activities centre is close to the street and was made to look like an ordinary shopping centre like the ones on the new housing estates.

The complete closing down of Santpoort, which played such a prominent role in the history of psychiatry in the Netherlands, was the most radical expression of the new policy that the government launched in 1984. Not a single institution escaped the integration policy, which eventually transferred all patients for whom it was possible to the city. Where this substitution had been completed, it often left the sites of the classic institutions partly empty, giving some of them a desolate, forsaken look.

p. 202
***Smook Architekten*, De Grote Rivieren psychiatric centre, Gorinchem, 1992**

***Smook Architekten*, De Grote Rivieren psychiatric centre, Dordrecht, 1989**

p. 203
***Smook Architekten*, De Grote Rivieren psychiatric centre, Dordrecht, 1989**

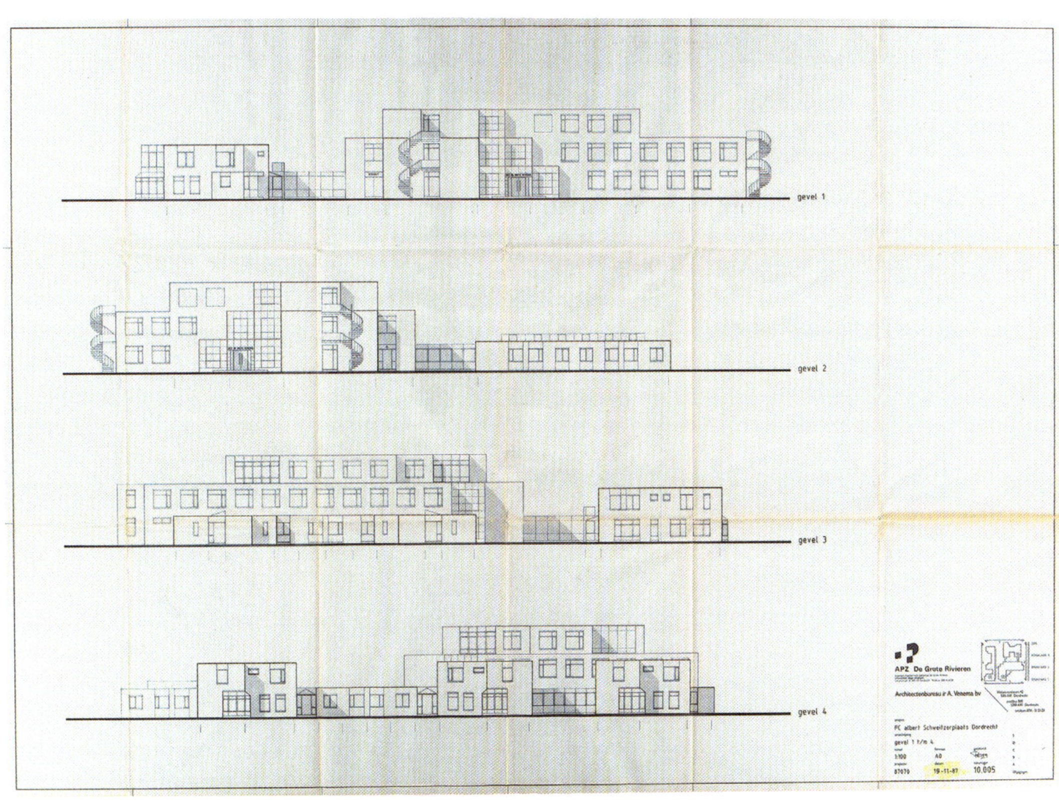

Housing and care for the elderly

The question was raised again at the beginning of the 1980s of whether the original principles of accommodation for the elderly could still be maintained. The answer to this question in the 1970s had been in the affirmative, unless alternative forms were devised, but now several fundamental principles of the early years were relinquished. What had initially been the backbone of care for the elderly – specific forms of housing for the elderly – was gradually abandoned. This did not mean that no more building activities for the elderly were carried out – on the contrary, investments involving billions of guilders were planned. What distinguishes this building boom from that of the 1950s is that this one focused on housing without integrated care facilities. It seems to have given shape to the second wave of emancipation: if the first delivered the elderly from the aura of poverty, the second now shook the aura of needing care for twenty-four hours a day. On the housing market, the elderly 'housing consumer' was no different from any other.

The nursing home

Care for the elderly retreated into the nursing homes. They had emerged in the 1970s out of the blue, and now seemed to be the most durable sector of accommodation for the elderly.[19] The nursing house proved to be a particularly dynamic type that turned out to be full of potential as soon as it freed itself from the original hospital model. As soon as a stay in a nursing home began to seem more like living at home, care could be organised as an independent function. Nursing homes therefore went over to a different form of organisation. Even partial extramural care was given a try. It was a slow but apparently unavoidable development.

T. Swinkels and P. Boelen built a home for psycho-geriatric residents in Hillegom, a meandering low-rise building that takes over the grounds and disguises the fact that it can accommodate 180 residents. Architectenbureau G. Geluk en J.G. Treurniet implemented a three-storey nursing home in Rotterdam for 150 psycho-geriatric patients that is organised around an atrium and three patios. In the course of the 1980s the value of separating psycho-geriatric and somatic residents from one another was called into question.

The nursing unit – an element of the hospital that was modified for the nursing home – can be regarded as the basic component of every nursing home. D.J.M. van der Voordt and D. Terpstra distinguished a total of nine types, defined on the basis of the number of floors and the number of nursing units per floor. These types determine the volumes and the logistical main structure. Other parameters that they mentioned are the position of the amenities, the main access (line, loop, star and network), the structure of the individual nursing units, the form of the walking circuit, internal access, the dayrooms, the bedrooms, and finally the sanitary facilities and the staff areas. Various design solutions, partly connected with the preferred model of care, were available for each of these parameters. It is hardly surprising that the range of possibilities shows a strong resemblance to that of the regular hospitals and the psychiatric clinics. Unlike the latter two forms of care architecture, however, in the further course of its development the nursing home tends to gradually dissolve, coincide with the architecture of the care home, and subsequently become assimilated to regular housing architecture. This trend applies to the whole genre except for a few specific types for specific groups of patients, although here too the model of a residential community was increasingly often assumed as the guiding principle.

Substitution completed: ordinary housing for the elderly

It sounds simple and plausible: housing as many old people as possible in homes that are nothing out of the ordinary. However, this ambition required drastic modifications of the existing housing stock and the drawing up of rules for new buildings. Ideally, the whole housing stock should be suitable for every category of occupier, or capable of being adapted at very little expense. The Experimental Housing Foundation (SEV) played a key role in both fields.

The SEV broke the existing housing stock down into four categories on the basis of their suitability as housing for the elderly. The first group was suitable for fit old people, with minor adjustments the second could be made suitable for old people with a slight disability, the third entailed more drastic interventions and could then be maintained in use by wheelchair patients, for instance. The fourth and last group consisted of housing that was unsuitable even for fit old people. For each of the three themes – accessibility, visitability, usability – the SEV developed three 'upgrade packages': prevention, minor and major adjustments, and came up with a label. This label was based on an analysis of the existing housing stock and contained instructions for a renovation that would enable housing to remain suitable for the elderly, but equally important was the ambition to take the label into account in the building of new homes as well.

The renovation of apartments without lifs, the commonest type, was an expensive business, but the gallery access flats, which had been built in large numbers too, proved to be very suitable for conversion into flats for old people. All that was needed was to introduce an alarm system, handgrips and railings where necessary, and the glazing of the galleries, so that there was no longer any need to go out into the open air to make the journey between the lift and the front door. An experiment with an old flat in Overschie revealed that the main entrance required attention too, because many old people were afraid of strangers in their flat.[20] Gooioord in Amsterdam, one of the blocks of flats from the 1960s on the Bijlmermeer housing estate that had been built for families, was now made suitable as housing for the elderly. The Rochdale Housing Corporation brought in Bruins Soedjono and Valtos. The interventions were mainly directed at matching the wishes and needs of older residents better by improving access, increasing the feeling of security, and expanding the provision of services.

The SEV also played a pioneering role in flexible building. This was 'one of the most comprehensive and complicated experiments of the SEV programme, but also has potentially major consequences for building and housing in the Netherlands', the steering committee stated in 1991.[21] The investigation of flexibility resulted in various products, including a senior label, a nationally accepted and standardised list of requirements for housing for the elderly.[22] Numerous home tests and manuals appeared in the course of time, all intended to chart and improve the suitability of homes and residential environments for the elderly.[23] The Ministry for Housing, Regional Development and the Environment (VROM), the National Housing Council, the Association of Netherlands Municipalities (VNG) and the Council for the Handicapped also targeted flexible building, often in cooperation with the SEV.[24]

Renovation with a view to the elderly means carrying out interventions afterwards, which would often have been unnecessary if a different way of designing had been adopted. This awareness led to the life-cycle resistant home, in which a certain measure of flexibility was already built in. This proved to be a successful approach. The Woonzorg Nederland housing corporation commissioned IAA Architecten to design the Zorghuis Dichteren in Doetinchem. It comprises 120 apartments, 95 of them rented by Zorginstelling Sorgsaem, 45 extramural on the basis of the law on old people's homes, and 45 extramural nursing units. All of the apartments satisfy the criteria of the senior label.

Residential groups

The concept of the commune for the elderly, which goes back to the 1960s, was revived in the 1980s. The Landelijke Vereniging Groepswonen voor Ouderen (National Association for Communes for the Elderly) was set up in 1984; five years later thirty residential communities, as they were called in the 1980s, had already joined.[25] The renewed popularity was triggered by a television documentary about the Altersheim Christiansfelde in Bad Segeberg, Germany, broadcast in 1981.[26] The common factor of these residential groups was 'the search for safety and security, the search for ways of countering loneliness, wanting to remain active, the search for ways to avoid dependence on institutional forms of accommodation and care'.[27] About 900 old people were living in residential groups in 1989, and many new initiatives were in preparation. By 1993 the number of affiliated groups had risen to 147; 79 of them had suitable housing, 11 were under construction, and 57 were still at the initial stage.[28]

Most residential groups are small. They usually consist of between five and fifteen households. They share communal

***T. Swinkels and P. Boelen,* home for psycho-geriatric residents, Hillegom, 1983**

***Architectenbureau G. Geluk en J.G. Treurniet,* nursing home for 150 psycho-geriatric patients, Rotterdam, 1986**

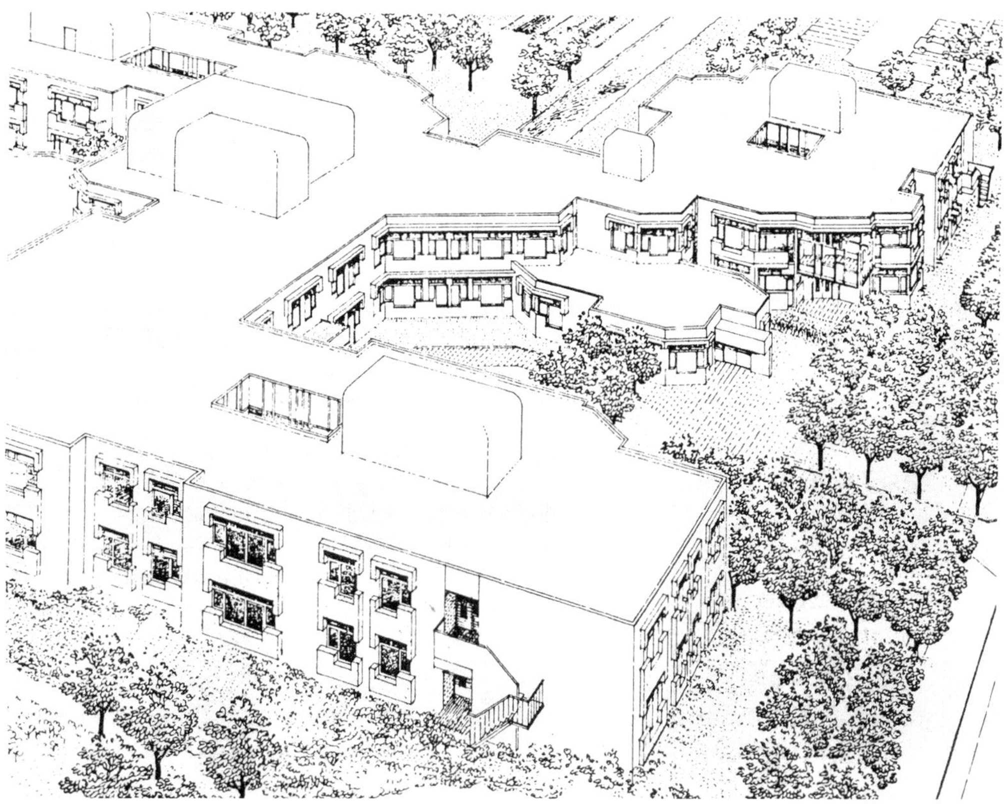

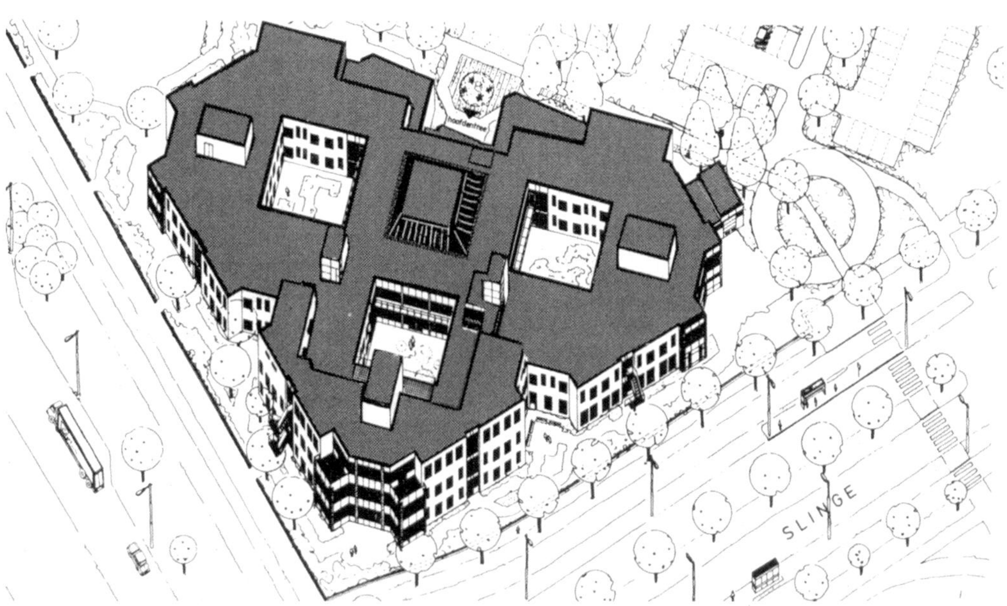

facilities such as a living room, kitchen-diner, hobby room and guest room.[29] An example of such a small residential group is the Oude Schans project in the Nieuwmarkt district of Amsterdam designed by Architektenburo Joh. Nust. The complex consists of thirteen residential units and a limited number of communal facilities spread over six floors. The combination of several units made it possible to include a lift.

Besides these small groups, much larger ones were created as well. A complex of 111 housing units was implemented in the Oog in Al district of Utrecht. After the closure of the Welgelegen rest home had been announced, a nurse and a social worker took the initiative of developing a plan with and for the residents from the surrounding neighbourhood for the renovation and extension of the home with self-sufficient housing units for old people.[30] Op ten Noort Blijdenstein Architecten was brought in to draw up a design. The Neo-Classical Welgelegen villa was renovated and made suitable for the communal facilities. For the housing units, a curved three-storey wing was built on each side and a four-storey rectilinear wing at right angles to the rear. There is also a separate block of apartments on the north side of the park.

On the initiative of residents in IJsselmonde in Rotterdam, who were organised in the Vereniging Anders Wonen voor Ouderen (Alternative Housing for the Elderly Association), a building was implemented with communal facilities 'where they could voluntarily share the responsibility for one another's wellbeing'.[31] The building, designed by Wytze Patijn, consists of two parallel four-storey apartment blocks on either side of a communal atrium. The complex has a total of 67 housing units that are accessed from the galleries adjacent to the atrium.

Unpaid care

This normalisation of housing for the elderly was intended to proceed in parallel with the normalisation of care. Instead of being provided by professionals, it should be provided as far as possible by neighbours, acquaintances and relatives (*mantelzorg*). This idea was introduced in the 1970s by J.C.M. Hattinga Verschure, a specialist in internal medicine and a champion of the social model in medicine. It illustrates how the need to cut down spending on care for the elderly could also be a welcome pretext to alter the contents of that care. When the machinery of accommodation for the elderly in the Netherlands was running at full speed it proved impossible to stop it again. As a result, the share of Dutch old people in homes remained much larger than in the neighbouring countries. It amounted to 14.5 per cent in 1980, as against 5 per cent in Belgium and France and only 4.5 per cent in Germany.

Hattinga Verschure turned out to be a fervent and efficient advocate of an essentially different system, in which the centre of gravity of state-organised care returned to taking care of oneself, aided by relatives, neighbours and acquaintances. The balance had been lost. 'Care for oneself and unpaid health care shrank to a very low level, but professional care developed at an unprecedented pace. The hospitals flourished. In these bastions of curative health care, the provision of professional care took giant strides forwards.'[32] It looked so wonderful, all that professionally organised care, but what proved to be the case? "The better you took care of the elderly and the less they needed to do, the more their behaviour seemed to regress!'[33] So the austerity measures could have a beneficial effect by pruning excessive care. Hattinga Verschure had little difficulty with it, because it would lead to 'a shift of emphasis from an anonymous, collectively financed solidarity that threatens to become unaffordable because of the budgetary situation and the demographic evolution, to a solidarity based on relations between people, experienced individually and in the human community, and put into practice practically'.[34]

Voluntary care – the provision of services by one's own circle –, which could count on increasing interest since the 1980s, was a key concept in the thinking of Hattinga Verschure. *Zelfredzame ouderen* (Elderly who are able to cope for themselves) reads like a manual in which old people learn to cherish their self-sufficiency at every stage of the ageing process and to stay out of the familiar institutions as much as possible. It presupposes an informal network that is located in the neighbourhood and is thus in line with the old ideal of the neighbourhood concept. That the institutions were apparently necessary all the same was probably connected with a development that was already noted at the beginning of the 1980s: the reduced sense of neighbourhood resulting from a changing demographic composition.[35] It would appear that the growth of individualism slowed down the full development of informal assistance. Its essence, however, the reduction of institutional care, was to form the core of the new definition of policy that took shape in the 1990s.

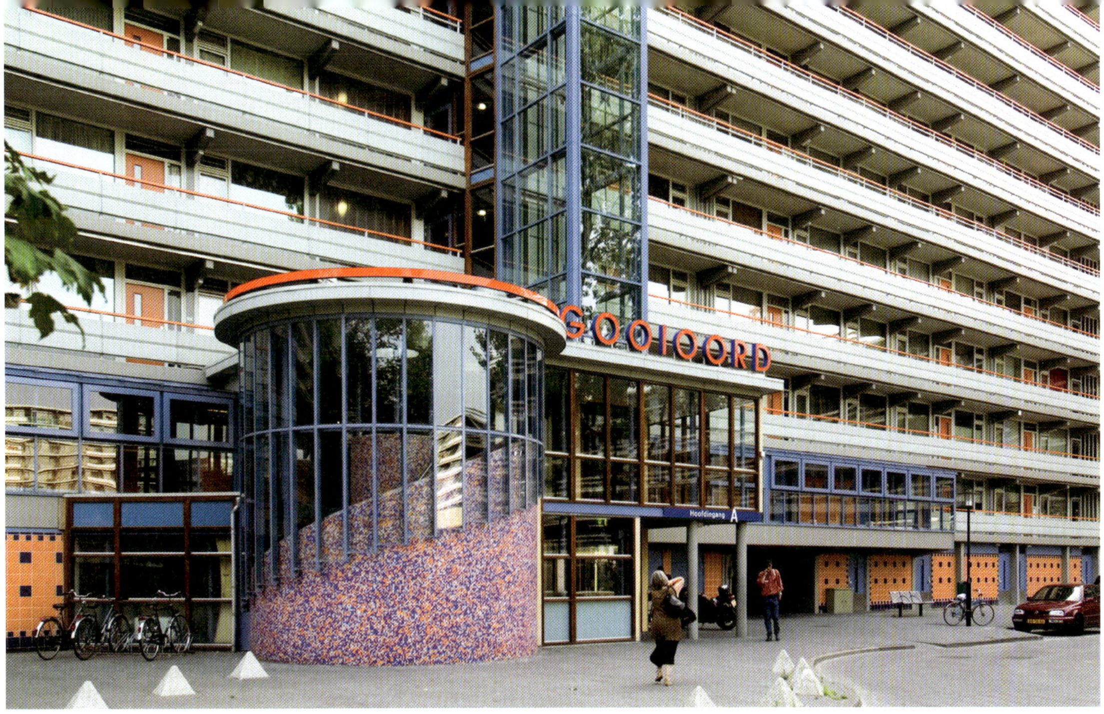

***Architectenbureau Bruins Soedjono and Valtos Architects*, renovation of Gooioord, Amsterdam-Zuidoost, 2001**

***IAA Architecten*, Zorghuis Dichteren, Doetinchem, 2002**

***Architectenbureau Op ten Noort Blijdenstein*, renovation and expansion of Welgelegen, Utrecht, 1992**

***Architectenburo Joh. Nust*, Oude Schans residential group, Amsterdam, 1987**

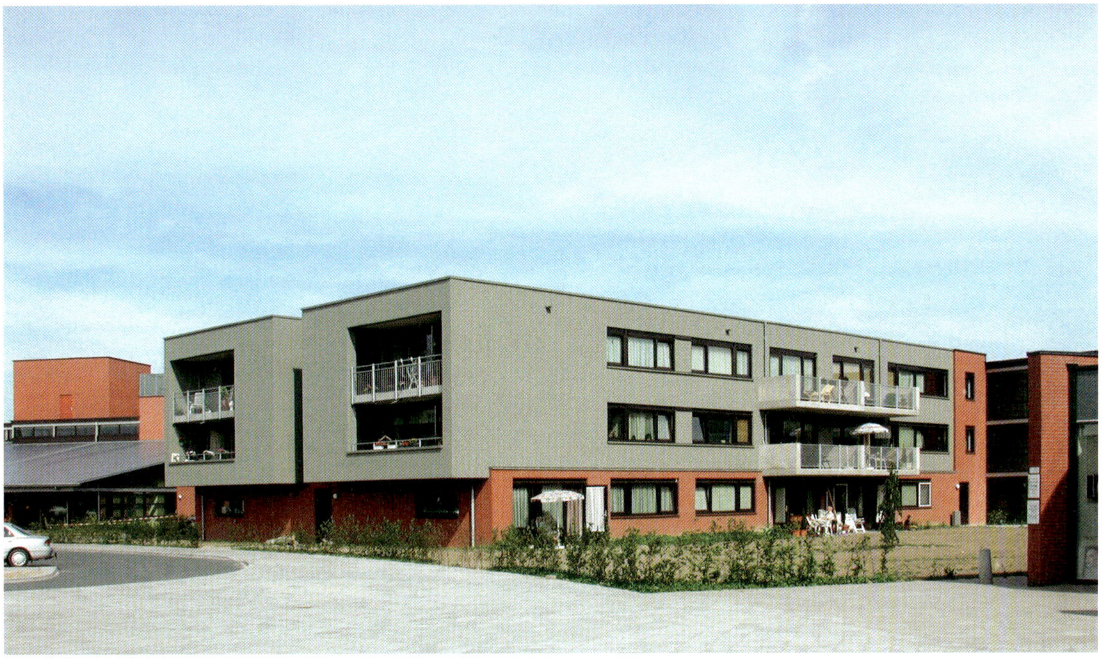

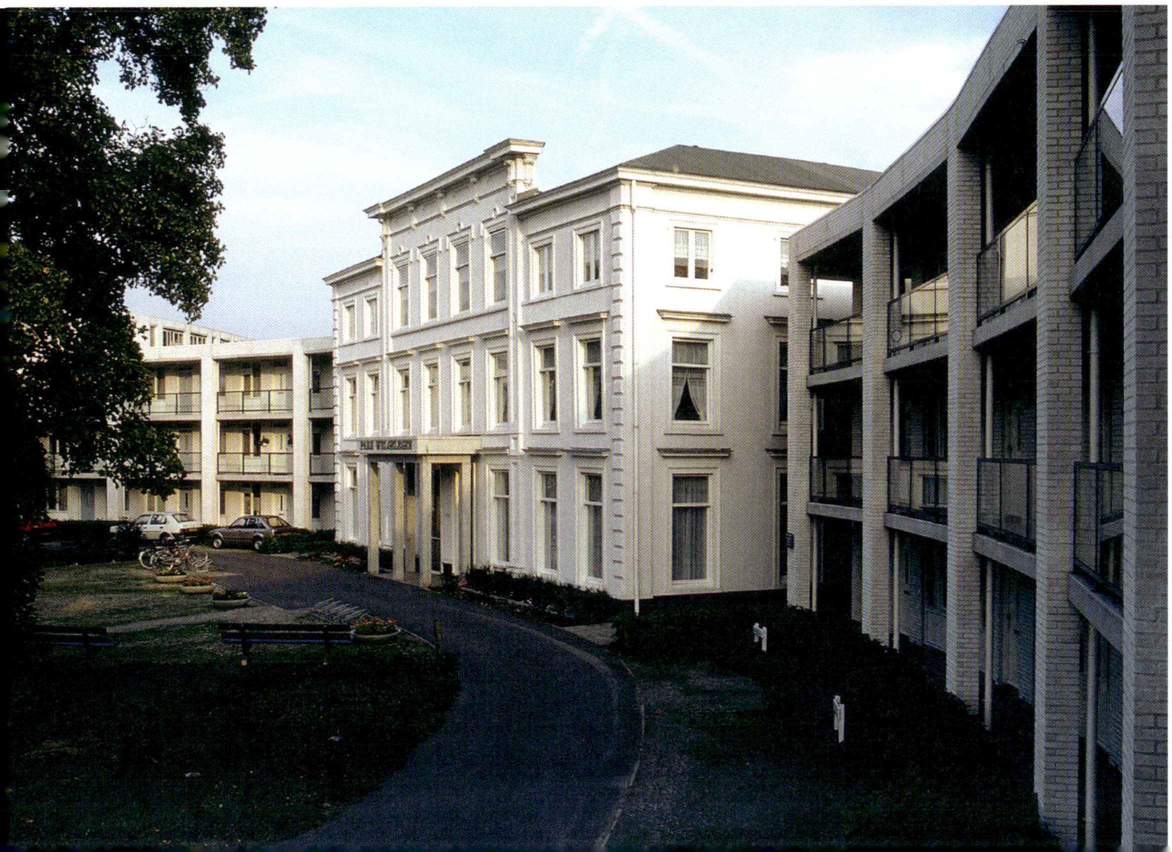

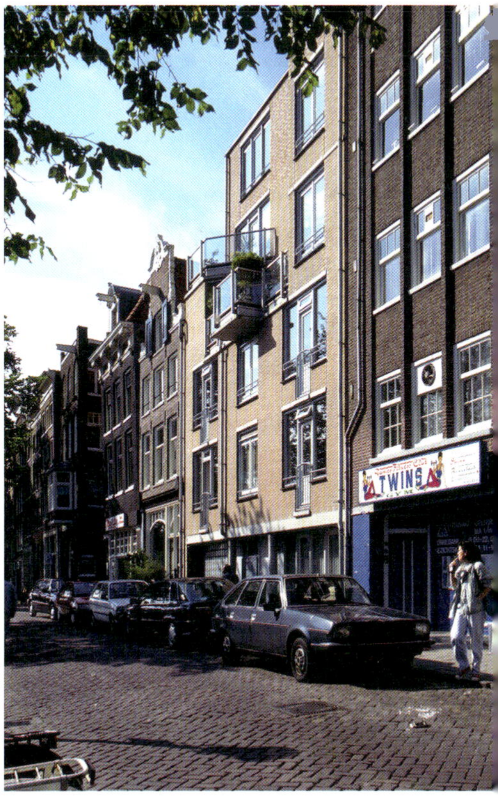

Enclosed garden

Herman Hertzberger

De Overloop old people's home
Almere
1980-1984

Situation
A *care home*
B *homes for two persons (sheltered homes)*
C *pond and pergola*
D *Veluwemeerdijk*

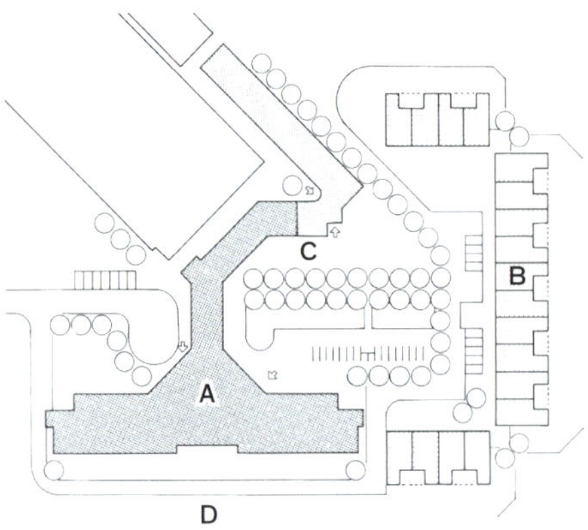

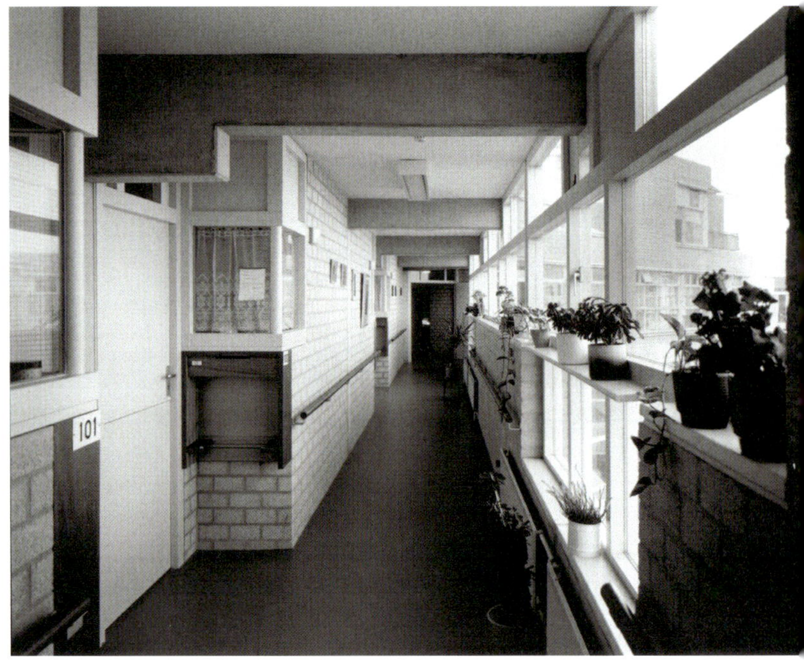

This old people's home is wedged between a car park, a school and a road that leads to a dyke and offers a view over the Gooimeer. The complex is built around an enclosed garden to protect it from the wind that comes from the water. The central middle section of the building on the west side of the terrain has five storeys and is flanked by three-storey wings on each side. At right angles is a third wing of the same height, but much longer and narrower. It is bent at three points and folds itself around the car park. The middle section contains a central hall. The service rooms and communal areas are adjacent to this hall. The three wings have a total of 84 single and eight double residential units. Detached from the main building, a one-storey U-shaped wing on the south side contains eighteen double residential units.

The residential units in the main building have balconies with large glass bays with square panes for every two or four units. The central part is set slightly back on the fourth and fifth floors to create room for terraces. A large circular disk on the roof provides the canopy for the top-floor units.

The double units form symmetrical pairs and each pair encloses the two adjacent gardens. The living rooms are on the garden side, while the entrance, kitchen, storage space and shower are at the front of the unit. Beside the front entrance there is a modest little roof over a bench to encourage contact with the neighbours and passers-by. Spots like this have also been created at various points in the main building: on the ground floor near the entrance to the residential units, and on the upper floors by means of windows between the kitchen and corridor and sitting areas beside the front door.

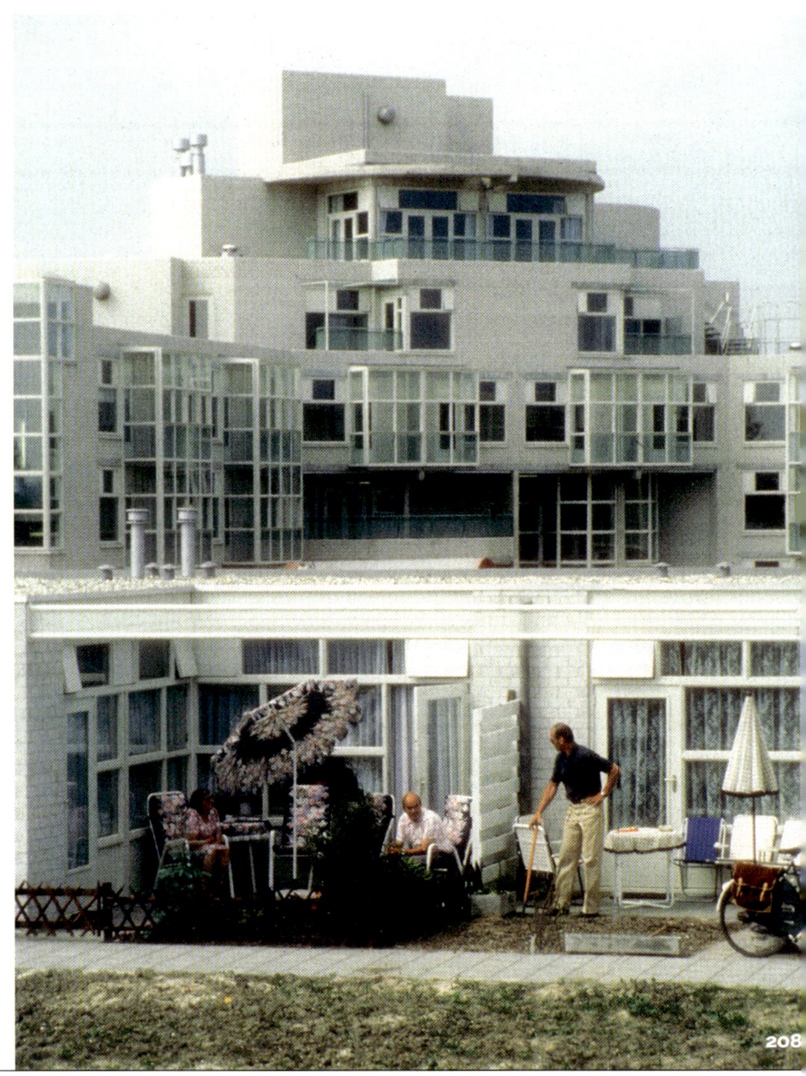

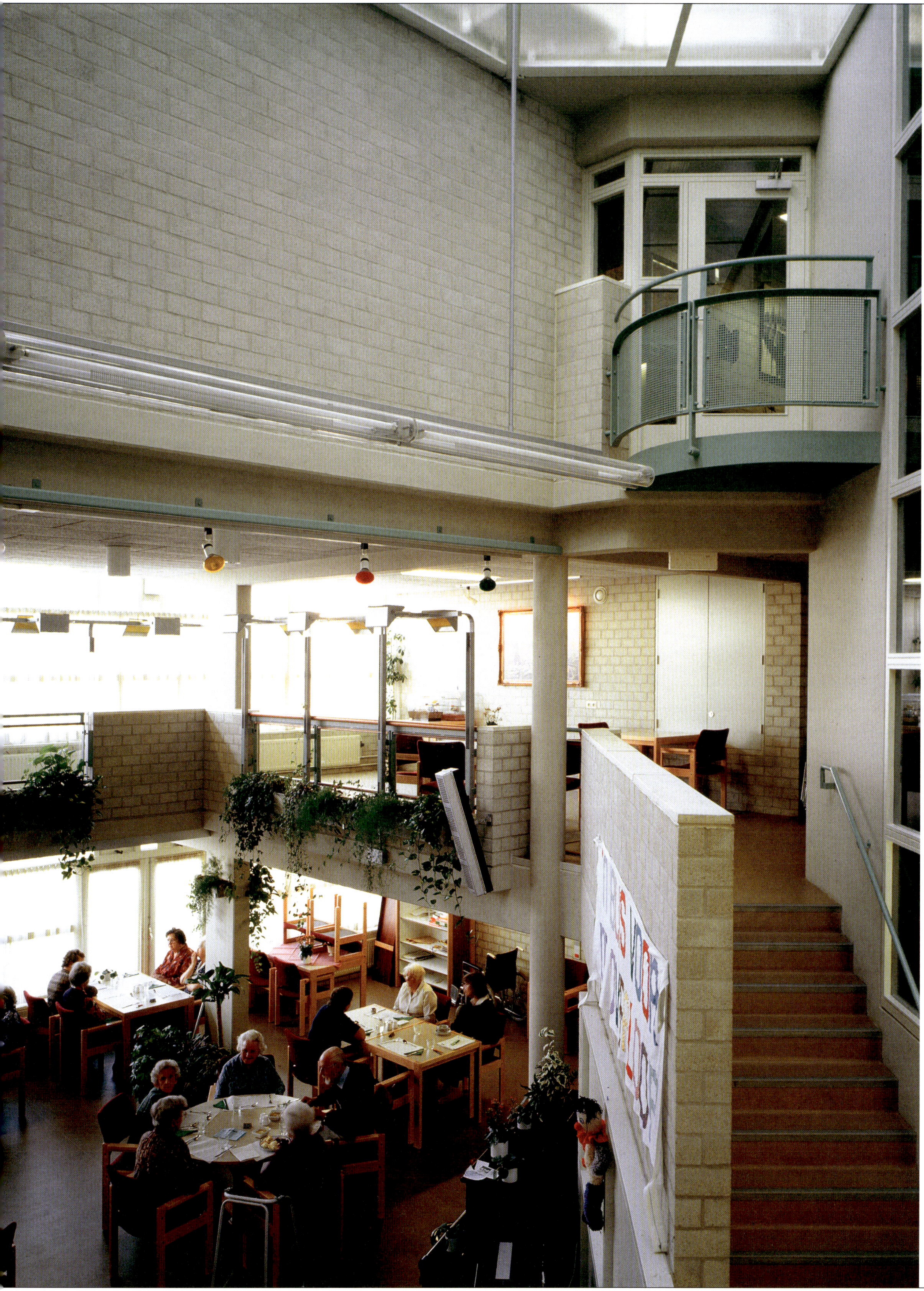

Squares

Duintjer Istha Kramer Van Willegen
in cooperation with D. van Mourik

Academisch Medisch Centrum
(AMC)
Amsterdam
1966-1981/1985

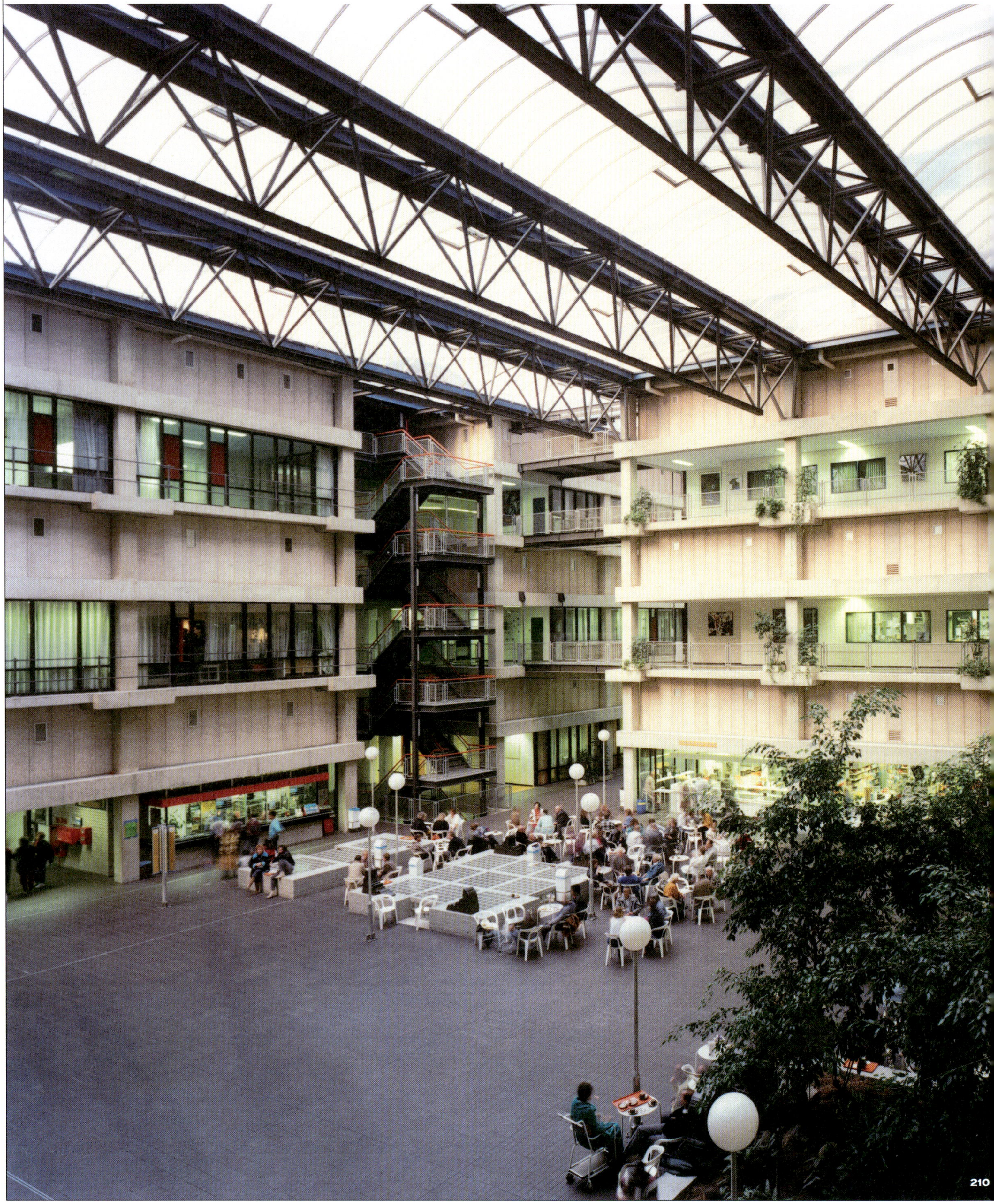

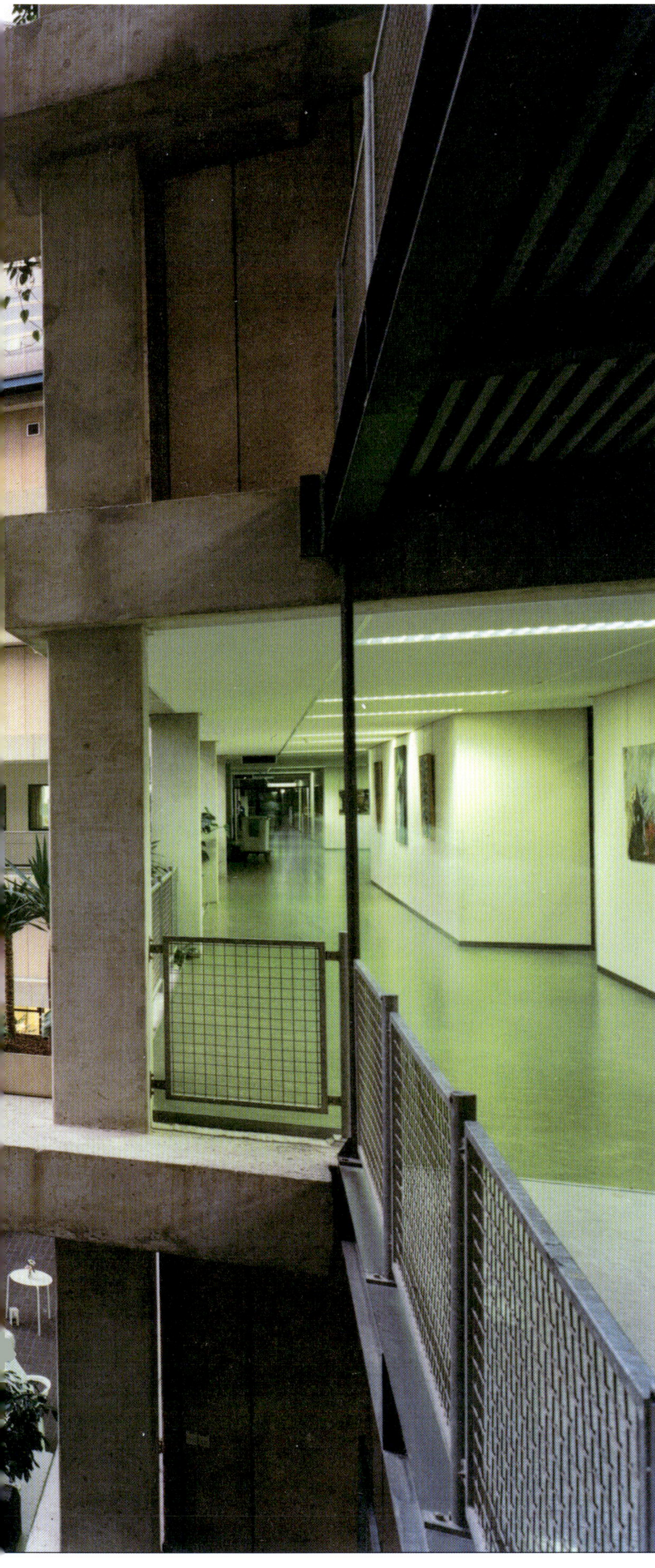

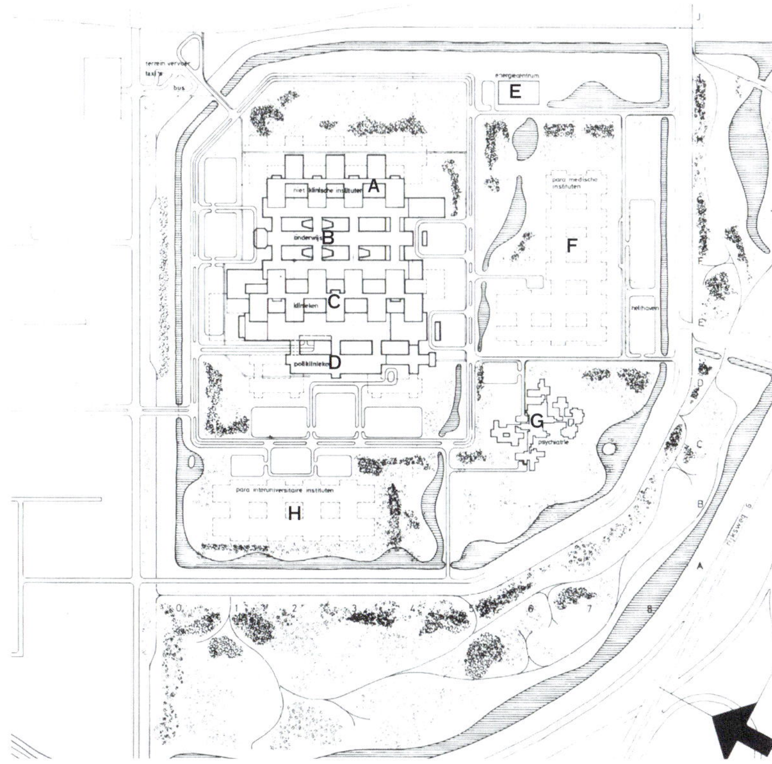

Situation
A *non-clinical institutes*
B *teaching*
C *clinics*
D *outpatients*
E *energy centre*
F *para-medical institutes*
G *psychiatry*
H *para-university institutes*

The new premises of the Academisch Medisch Centrum Amsterdam (AMC) formed part of a building project on an unprecedented scale: the replacement and transfer of the old university hospitals of Amsterdam, Leiden and Utrecht. The principal was the Ministry of Education and Science, which regarded the hospitals as a first step towards moving the universities to a campus on the outskirts of the city. The AMC was relocated on a site in the south-east of the Bijlmer housing estate. Situated close to a motorway and a metro line, the complex has excellent accessibility. The idea that the three hospitals had much in common led to the appointment of J. Wester, the medical adviser to the ministry, to draw up a joint programme. The basic concept of the AMC has four parallel zones: the outpatient clinics, the research and treatment units, the staff, and the non-clinical institutes. There is also a triple division into internal medicine, surgery, and neurogenous disciplines. The nursing units are on the top floors above the staff wing. The ground floor of the staff wing contains one of the main traffic routes of the AMC, the second provides access to the outpatient clinics. Transversal connections link up the whole and provide access to the various covered courtyards and lively shopping streets that determine the character of the interior of the AMC. On the outside it is above all the exorbitant size that is striking: the footprint is large enough to accommodate St. Peter's, the Escorial, the Houses of Parliament in London, Stockholm Town Hall and the Paris Opéra. The Pentagon is roughly the same size.

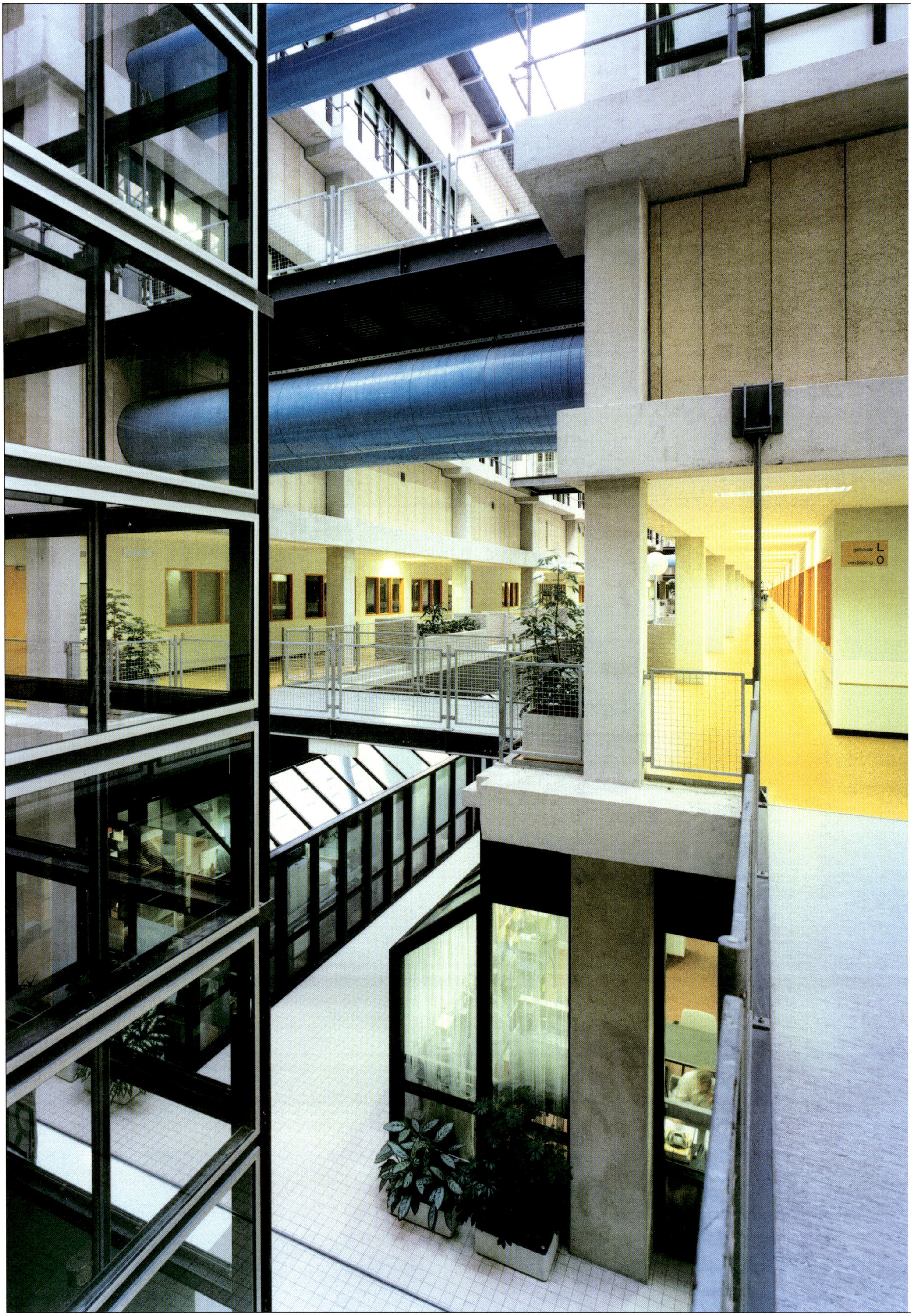
gebouw L
verdieping 0

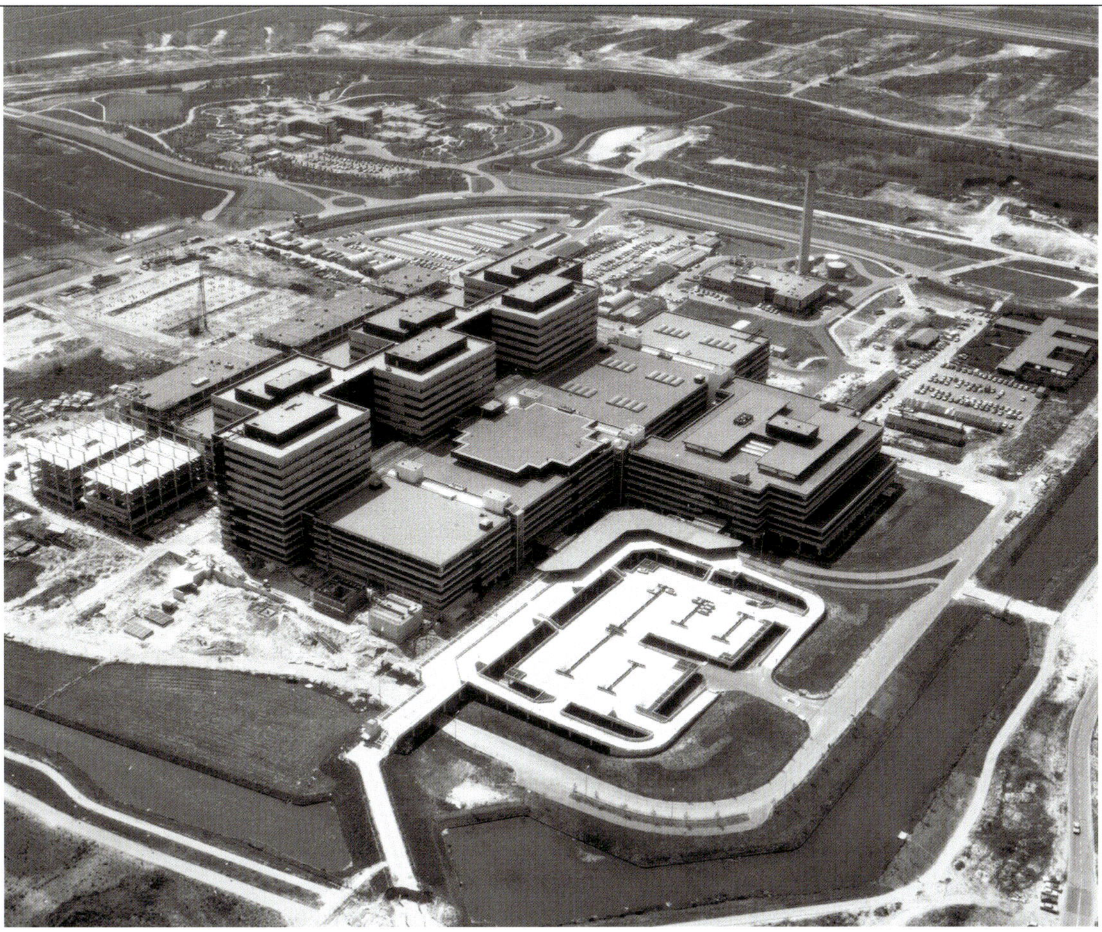

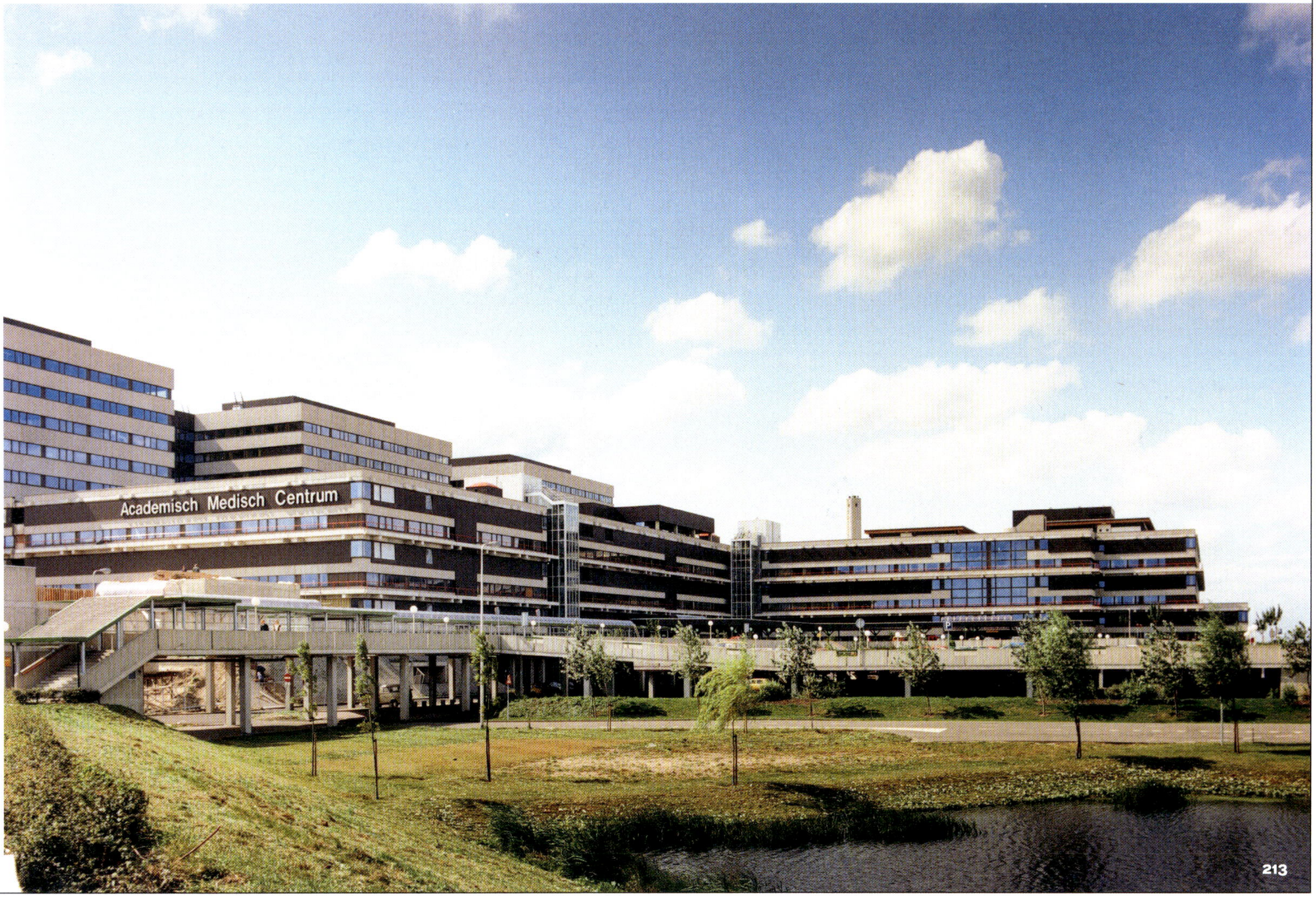
Academisch Medisch Centrum

Passage

Campman Tennekes de Jong
Architecten

Streekziekenhuis Waterland
Purmerend
1980-1988

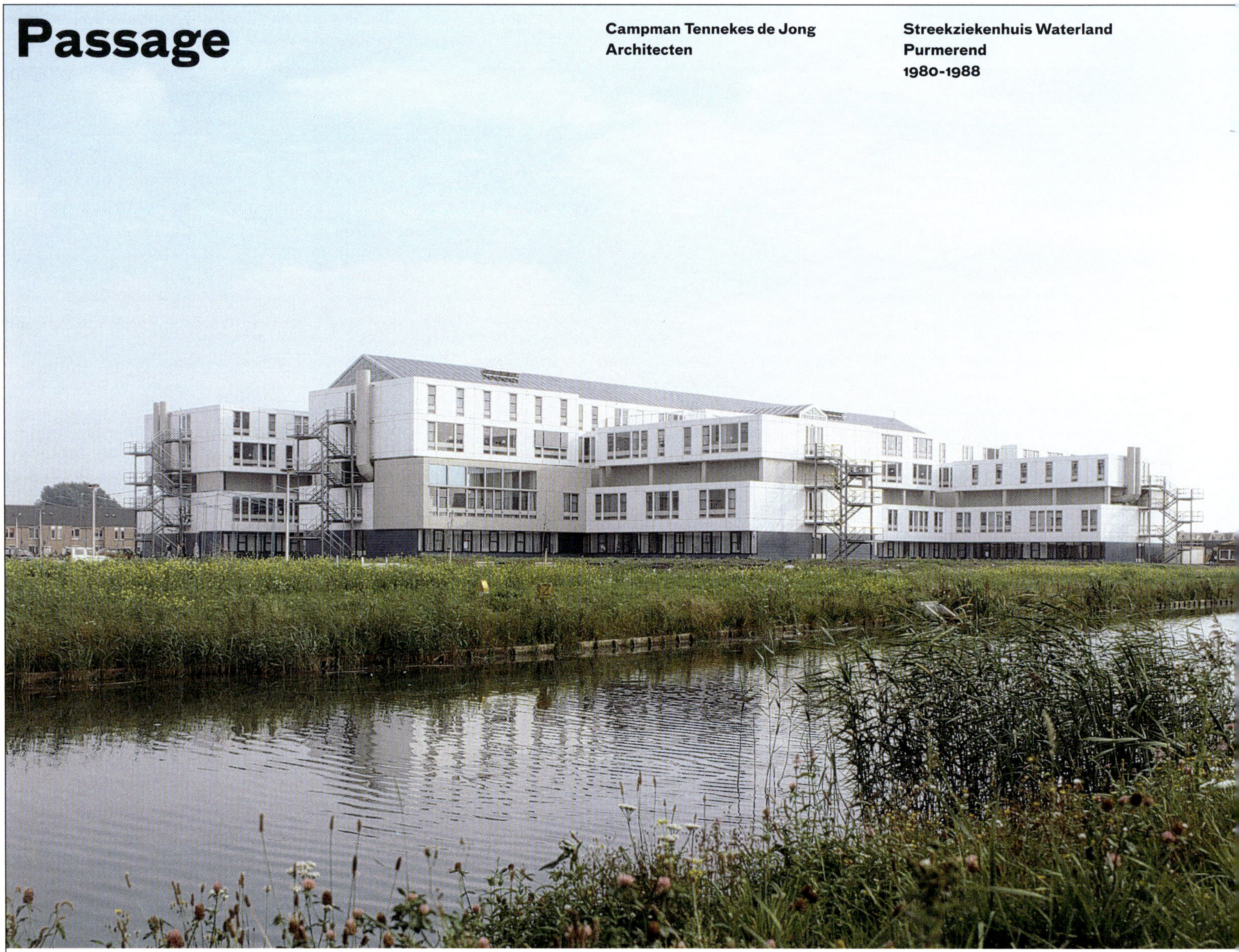

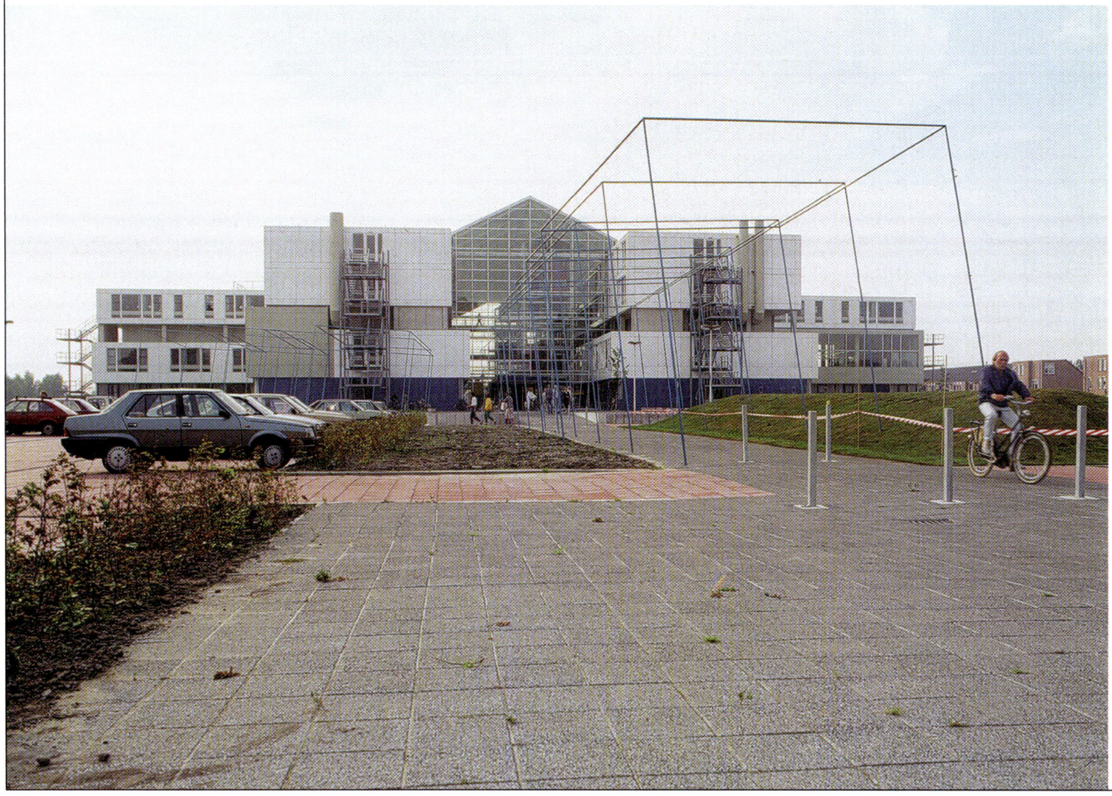

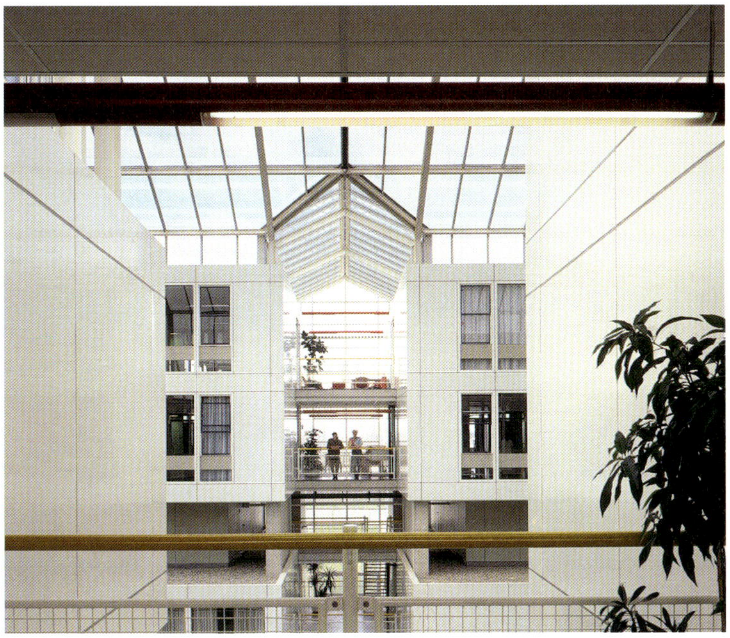

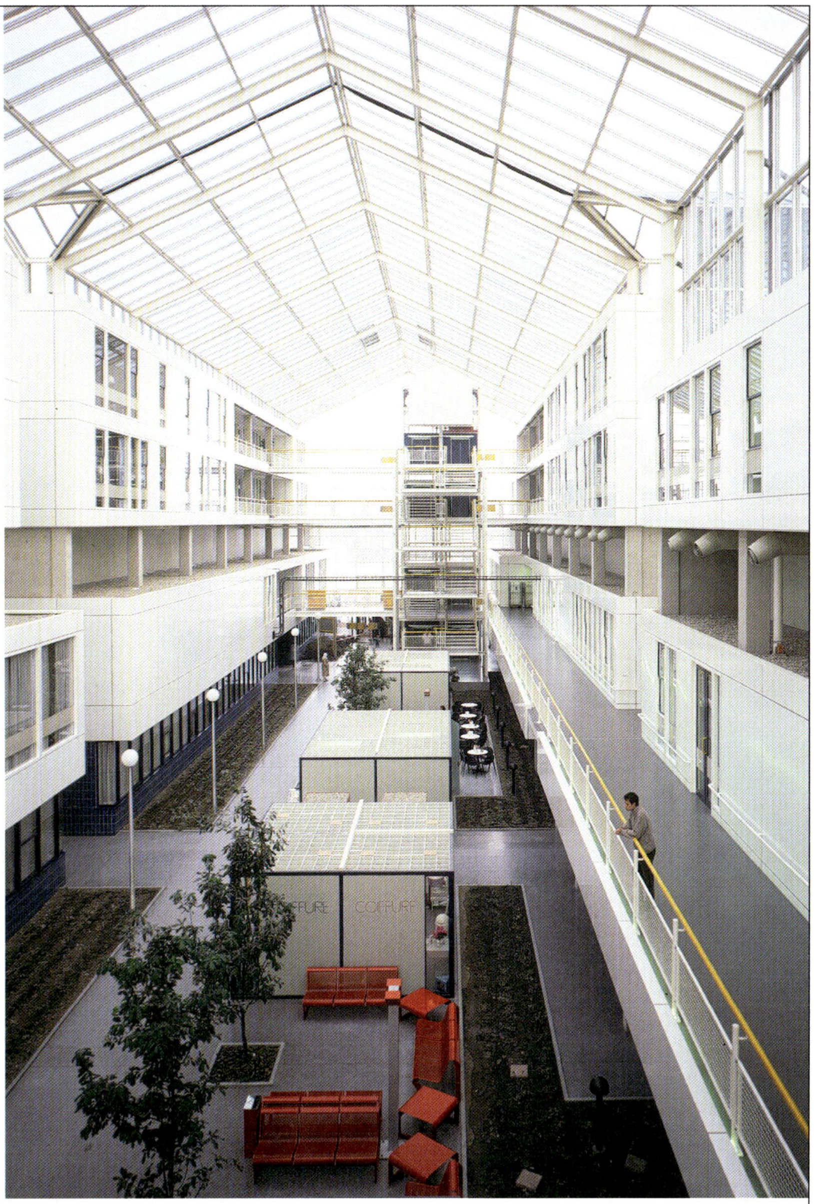

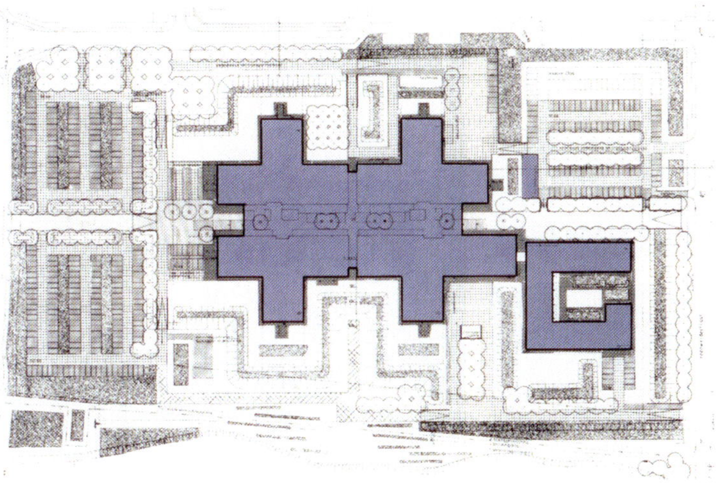

Situation and ground plan second floor with general nursing wards and intensive care

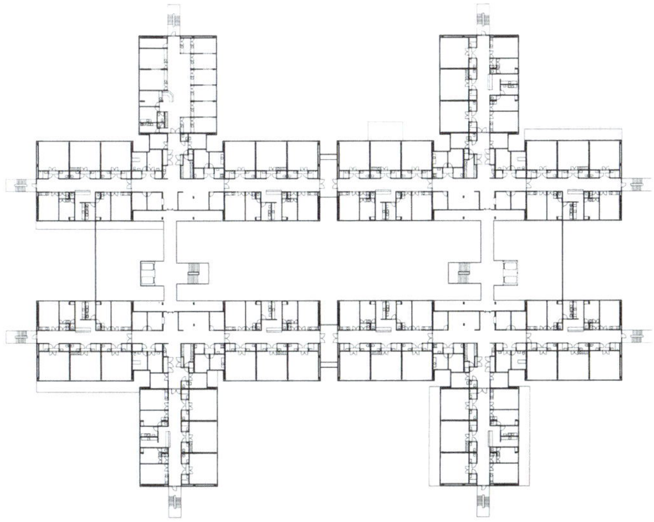

The passage hospital was a new addition to the hospital typology of the early 1980s. It entailed breaking the building down into distinct, clearly defined parts (four in this case) and separating them from one another by a wide, covered inner passage.

The outpatient units are on the ground floor, the services, laboratories and operating unit on the first, and the nursing wards on the second and third floors. The first floor is separated from the second by a technical layer. The passage includes public amenities such as small shops and a cafeteria. Access to the upper floors is from points at either end of the passage. Walkways connect these points with the T-shaped parts of the building on either side of the passage. These walkways lead into the intersection of the T-shape, from where the three limbs of the T are clearly visible.

Flexibility was a priority in the design of the Waterland regional hospital. This is partly provided by the method of construction: a concrete skeleton with a precast slab floor and infill with assembly elements. The infill package consisted of partition walls, steel indoor frames and a system ceiling. The engineer and architect produced assembly elements for the façades in which the construction, insulation, inner and outer skin form a single prefab whole. The use of these materials and techniques meant that the building work could be done very quickly.

The use of colour is fresh and simple: the ground-floor façades are in blue, the façades behind which the technical installations are situated are light grey, and the other façades are white. Colour accents have been applied to such features as handrails, lamps and routing.

Simplicity

EGM architecten

Merwedeziekenhuis
Dordrecht
1981-1989

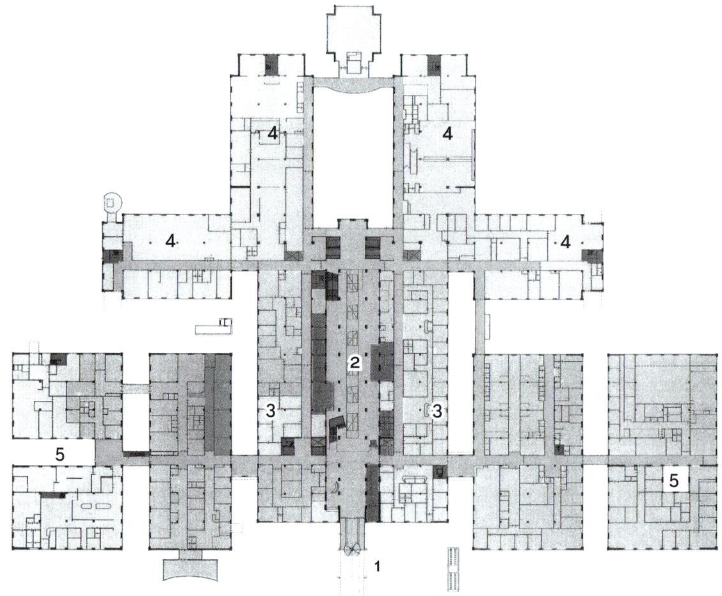

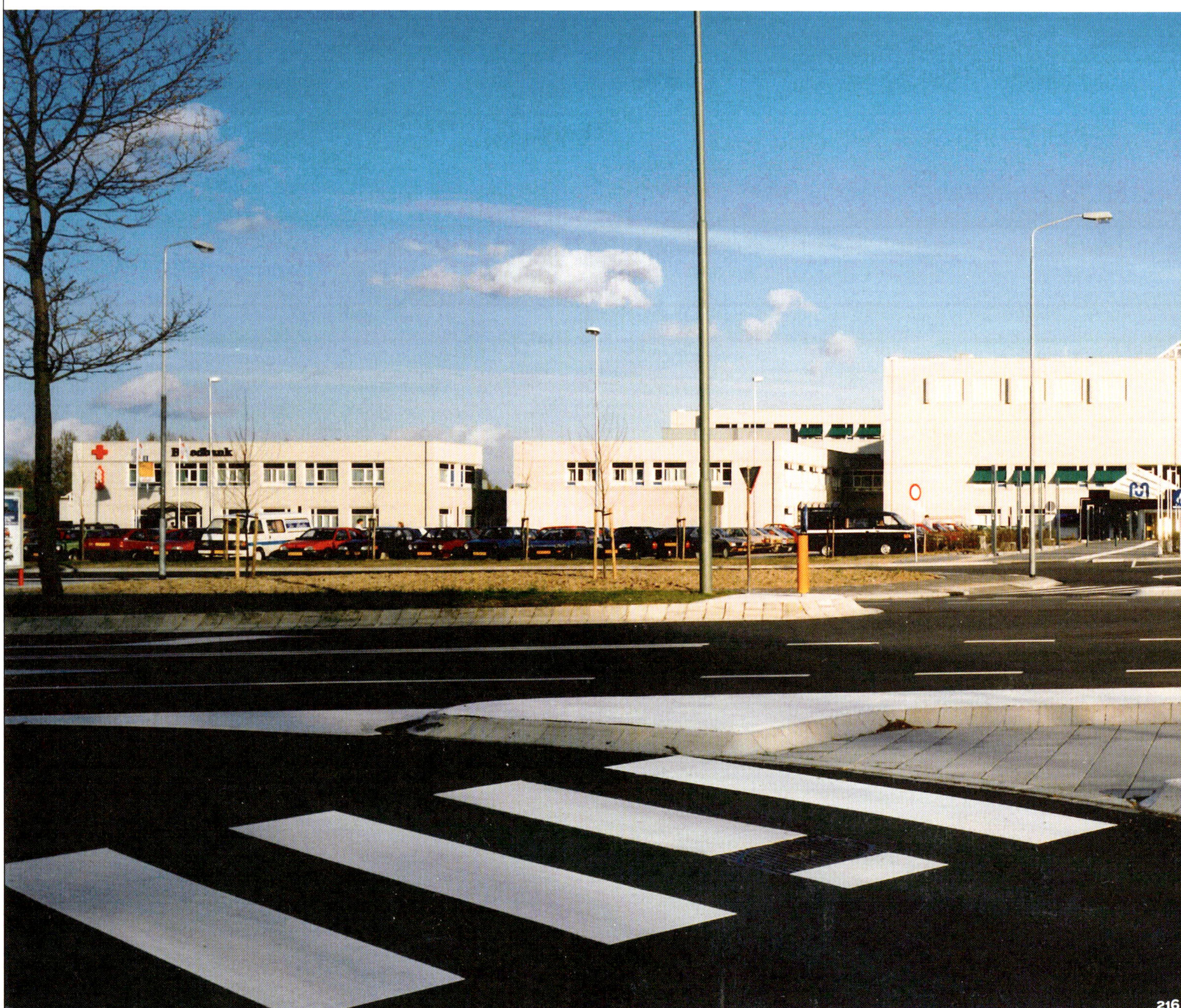

Ground floor
1 *main entrance*
2 *central hall*
3 *examination and treatment unit*
4 *nursing ward*
5 *other functions*

The design of the Merwedeziekenhuis was based on flexibility, short walking distances, maximal daylight, and low energy consumption. The hospital was to have 430 beds. The structure of the building is practically symmetrical and is composed around a central street or mall. This central area has the main entrance at one end and the lifts and stairs at the other. Two four-storey volumes containing the research and treatment units flank the central street. The other functional groups are accommodated in two two-storey volumes on either side of the central street and linked with one another by another street at right angles to it.

The nursing wards, accommodated in four detached wings and stacked in four layers, are situated at the end of the complex. The short and wide wards have a central traffic and service area surrounded by the bedrooms which have a view of outdoors. The wings form pairs at right angles to one another. The lifts and staircases are situated at the point where they meet.

The use of materials and colour is sober: light grey concrete stone with blue and green colour accents on the outside.

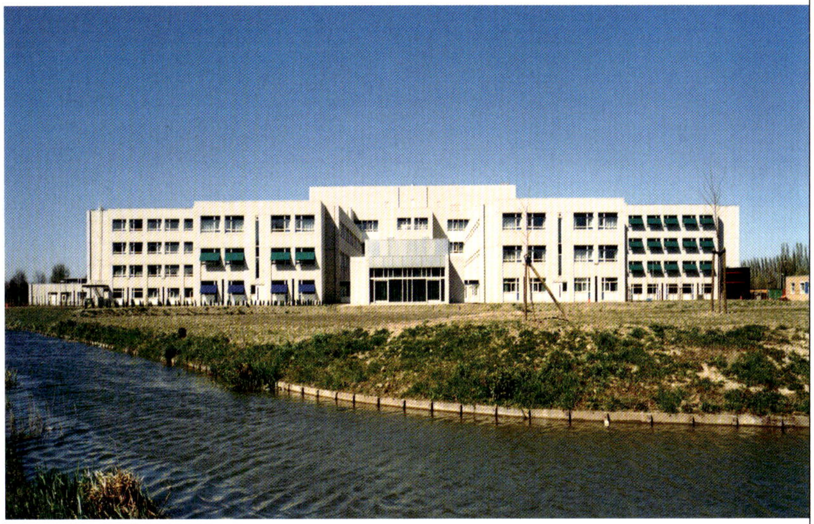

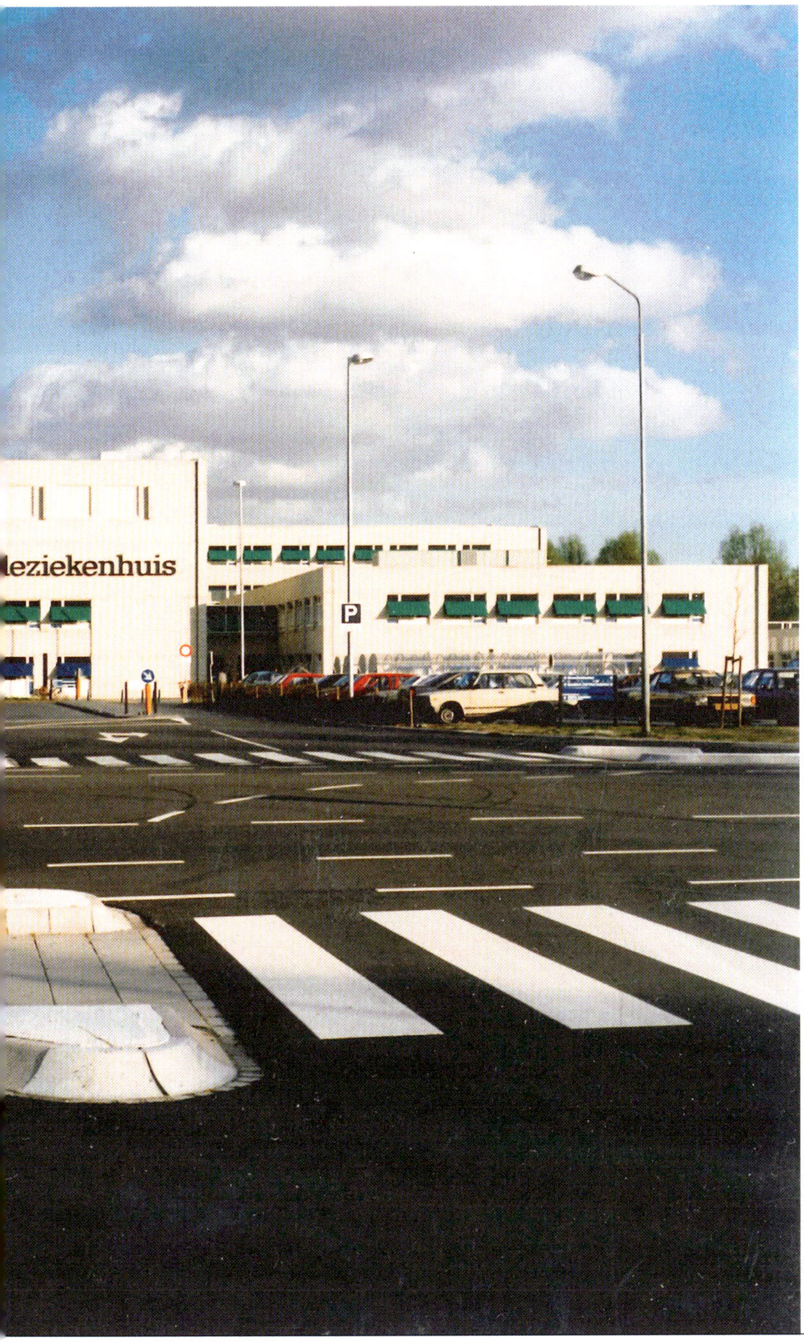

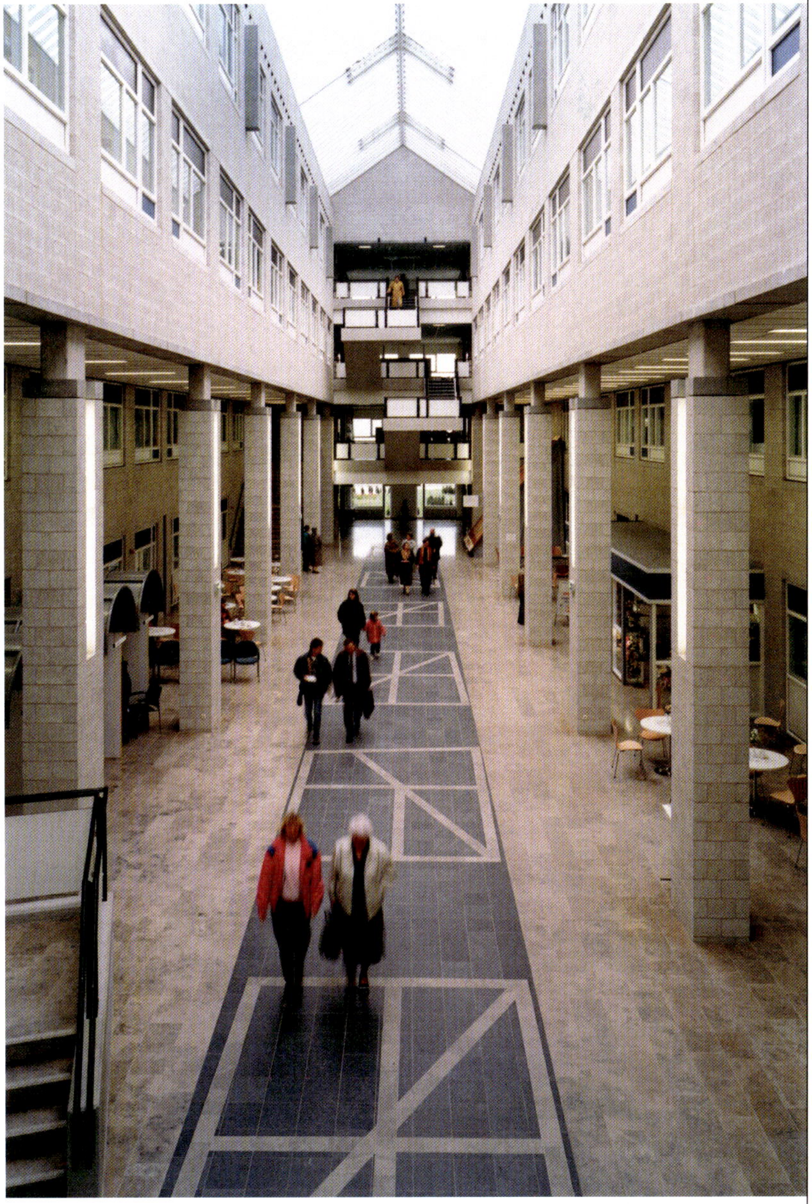

Open

Aldo & Hannie van Eyck

Eikenheuvel pavilions, Huize Padua
Boekel
1980-1989

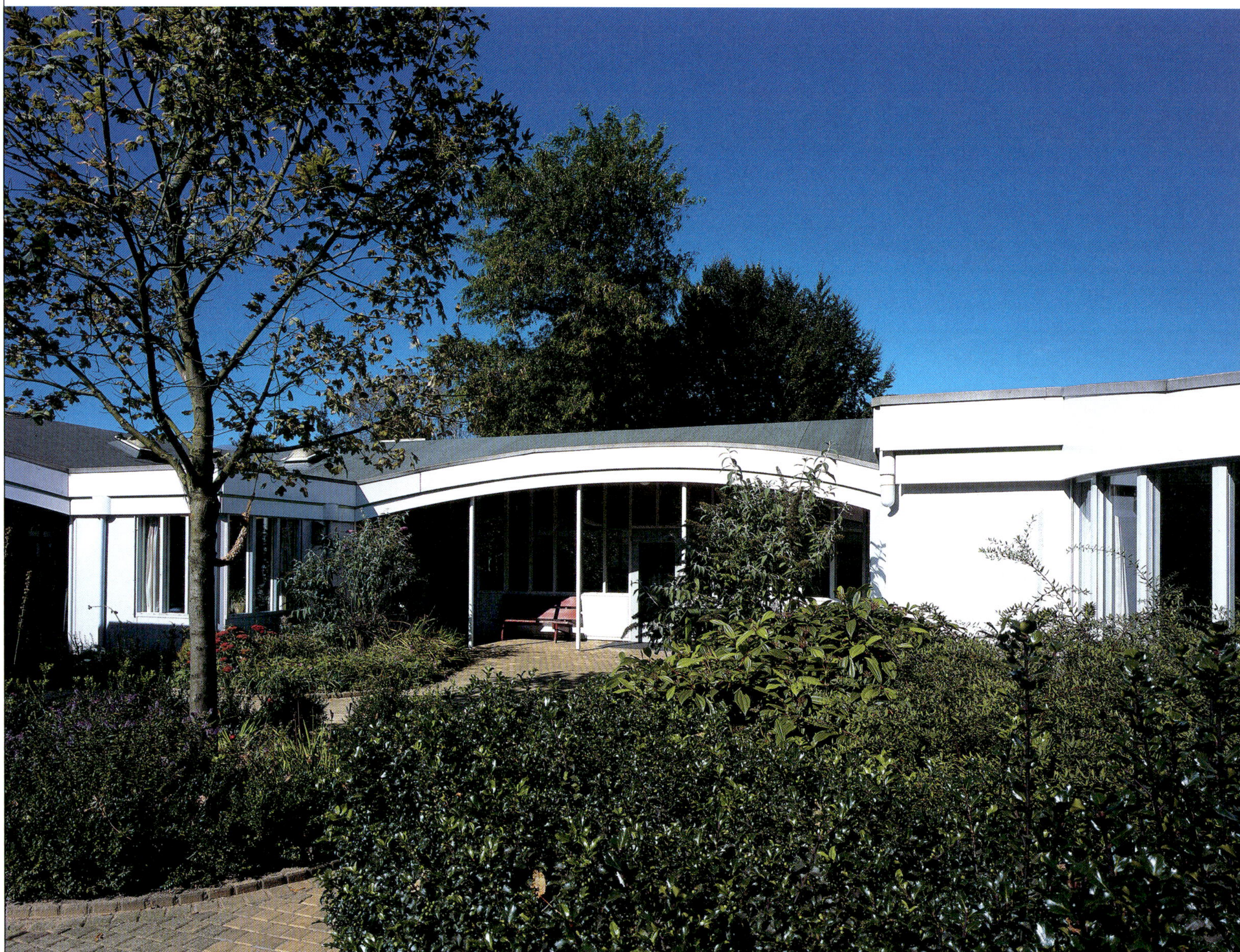

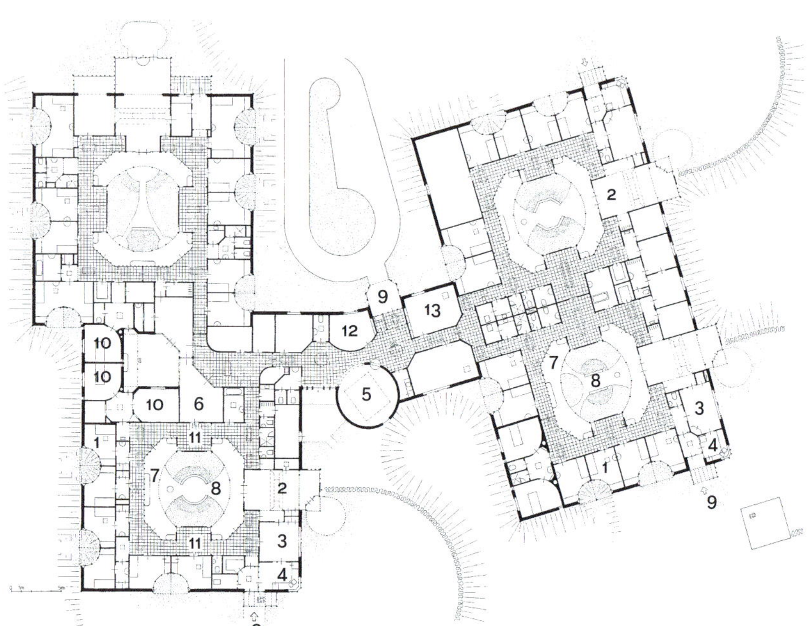

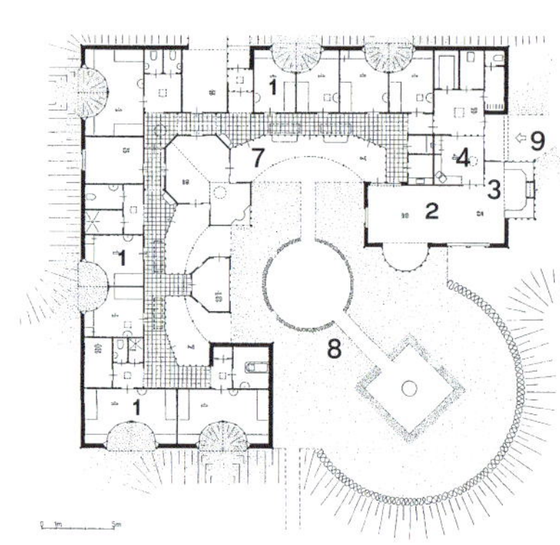

In 1980 the architect duo Aldo & Hannie van Eyck was commissioned to extend Huize Padua with three new ground-floor pavilions. The strict conditions imposed by the government on functions, surface dimensions and connecting passages usually led to endlessly long corridors and a string of cells. Aldo & Hannie van Eyck designed square ground plans with clusters of single rooms. In the pavilion for the open category they designed rooms for two or three persons which are grouped with the day lounges, recreational area and dining room around a patio with a curved corridor. In this way hardly any space was wasted on corridors.

The two L-shaped pavilions for the open category accommodated two groups of twelve patients. The patients' rooms were situated along the outside of the L, while the day lounge, kitchen and dining room were located at its tip, next to the entrance to the pavilion. The curved corridor and the half-open patio with a verandah were situated on the inside of the L.

The closed category consisted of two pavilions connected with one another by a wing. This connecting wing contained the area for visitors, the conference room, the superintendent's room and the psychologist's room. Each pavilion had two patios with a curved corridor giving access to the single and double rooms. The clusters with rooms alternated with a day lounge, a kitchen and a dining room. The patios were closed off from the corridor by a glass partition.

All of the patients' rooms and even the isolation rooms enabled them to maintain visual contact with the world outside. The raised sections of the roof above the communal areas and the corridor were furnished with a large number of small skylights.

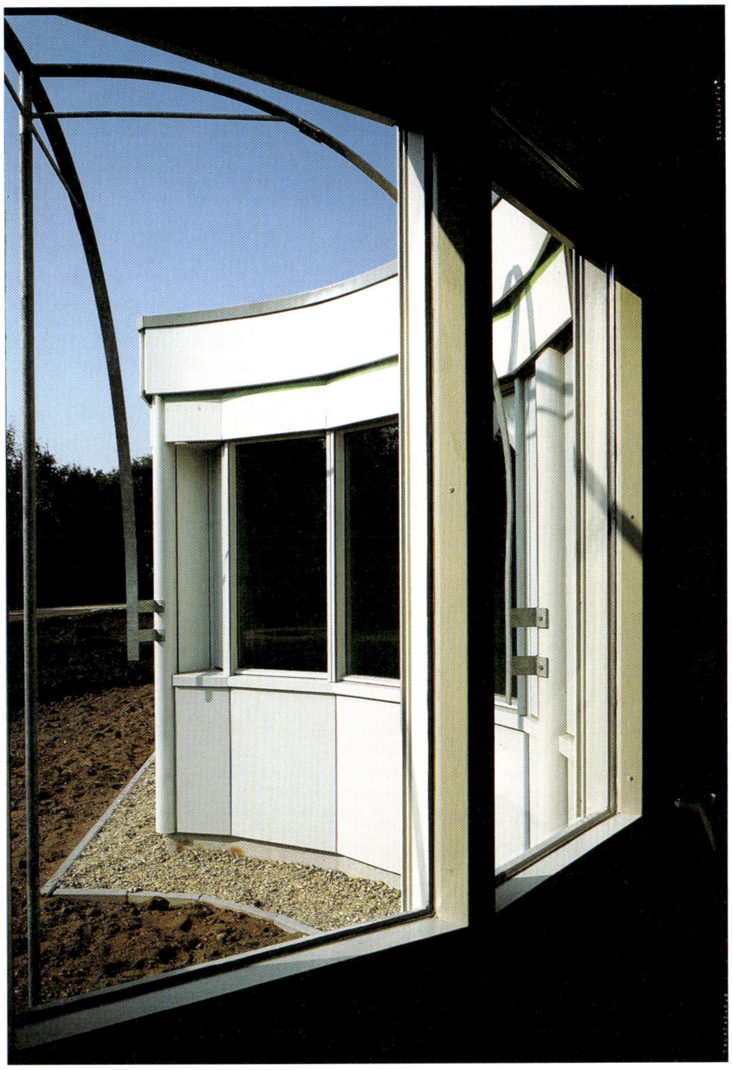

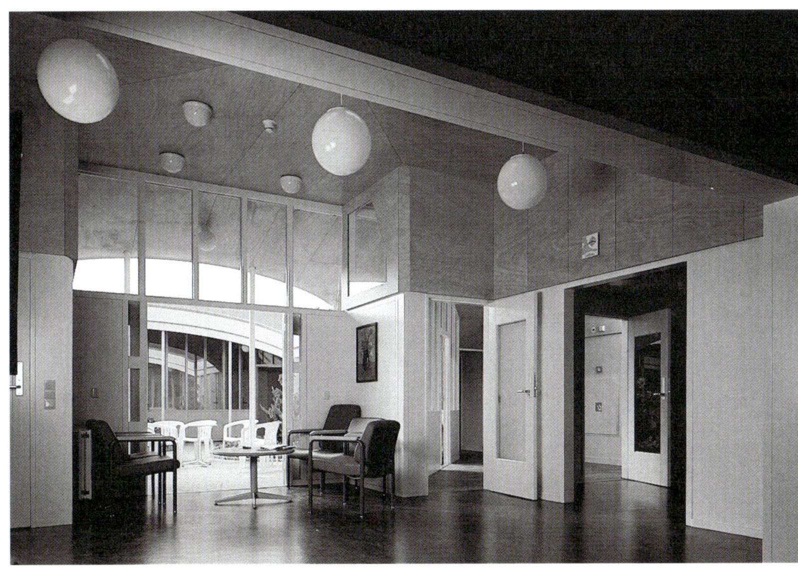

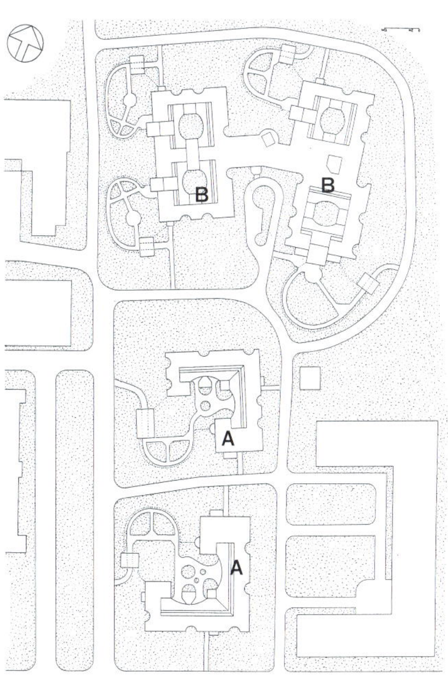

Ground plan closed units and semi-closed unit

1 *bedroom*
2 *day lounge*
3 *dining room*
4 *kitchen*
5 *visitors*
6 *staff*
7 *roofed patio*
8 *patio*
9 *entrance*
10 *isolation area*
11 *recreation*
12 *superintendent*
13 *psychiatrist*

Situation

A *closed units*
B *semi-closed unit*

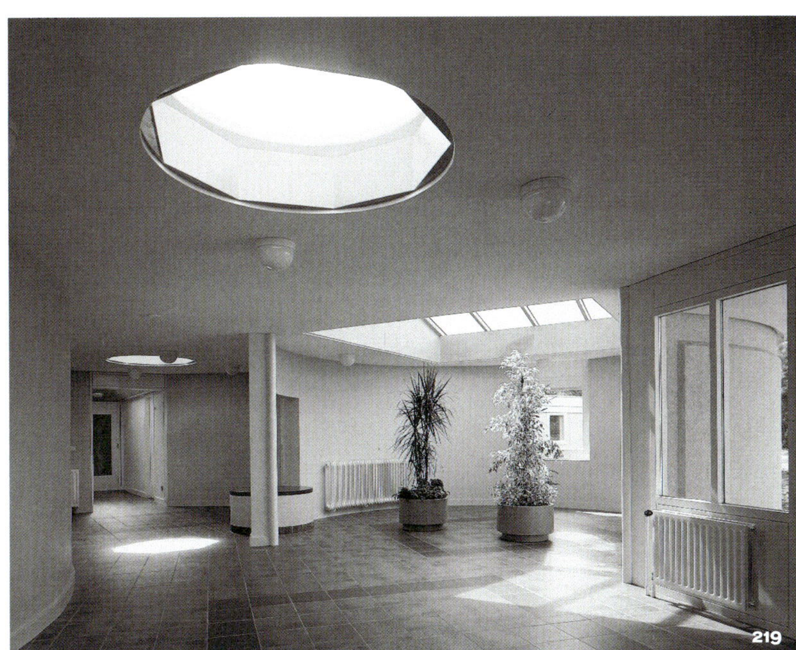

Atrium

Wytze Patijn architecten

Kreilerburcht apartment block
Rotterdam
1991-1993

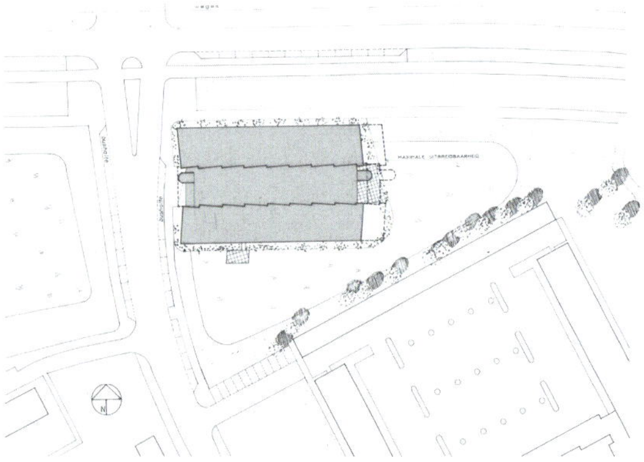

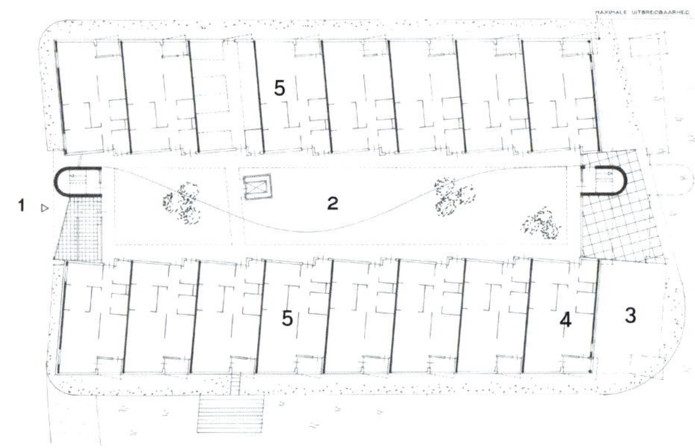

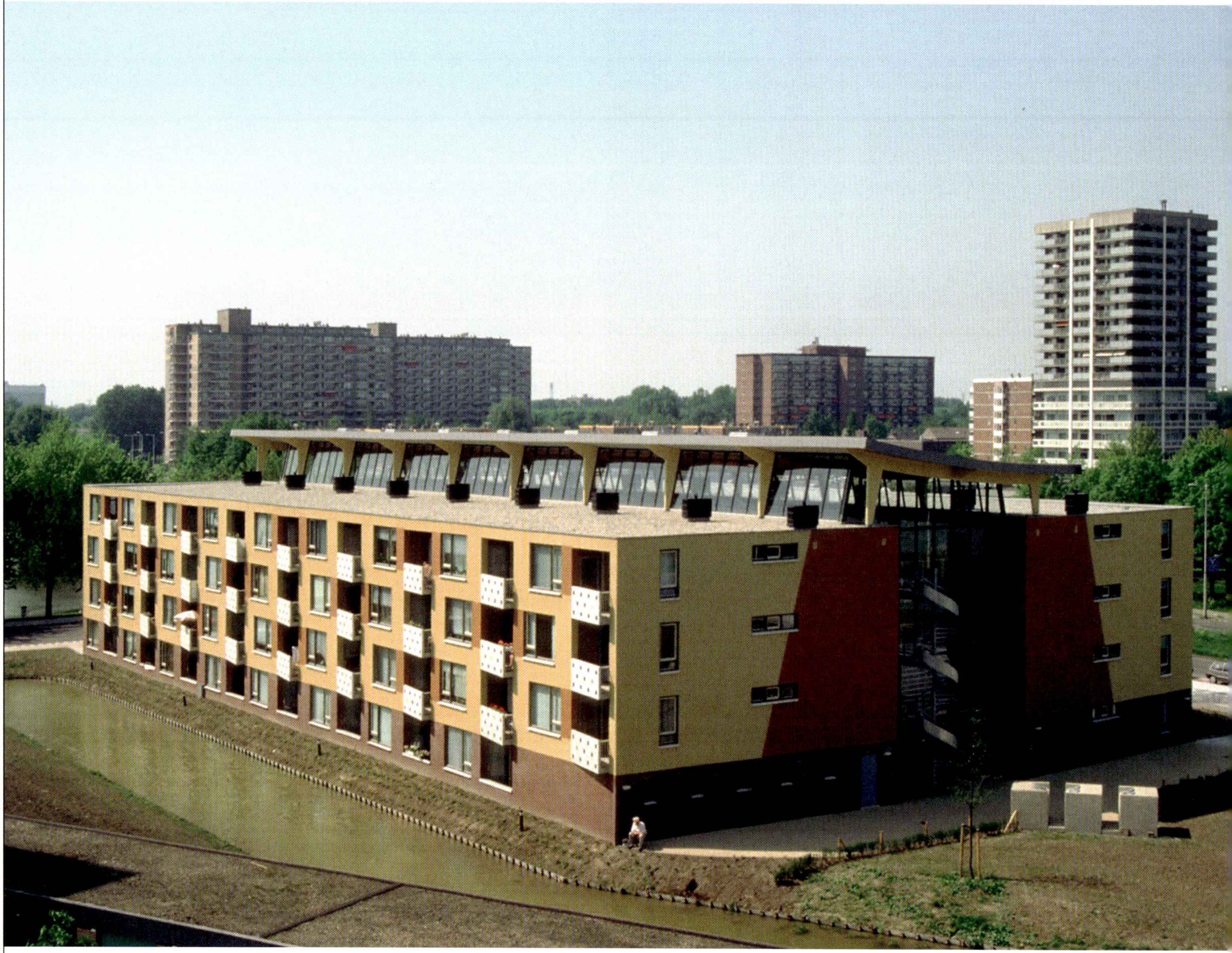

Situation

Ground floor

1 *entrance*
2 *atrium*
3 *cycle shed*
4 *communal area*
5 *residential unit*

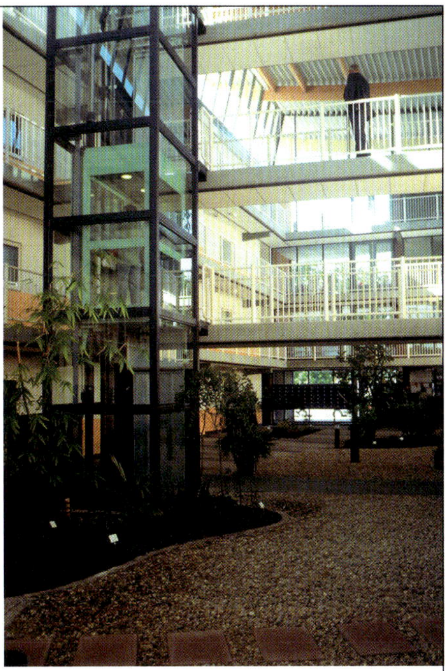

This apartment block for residents above the age of 55 was built on the initiative of the inhabitants who had organised themselves in 1987 in the Alternative Housing for Old People Association. The rectangular building consists of two blocks of four floors that flank a communal atrium. A curved steel roof above the atrium rests on wooden columns. Daylight enters through the sloping windows below the raised roof and through the side walls. The entrance, located in the side wall on the west, is set slightly back from the blocks. The three-room apartments (67 in total) are accessed from galleries that can be reached via two staircases and a glass lift in the atrium. There are communal areas on every floor: a guest room, washing and drying areas, a lounge, and on every floor, next to the semicircular staircase at the front, a communal balcony. The atrium is decorated with subtropical and tropical plants. The plastered façades of the upper floors are in two colours (white and yellow), with black masonry on the ground floor.

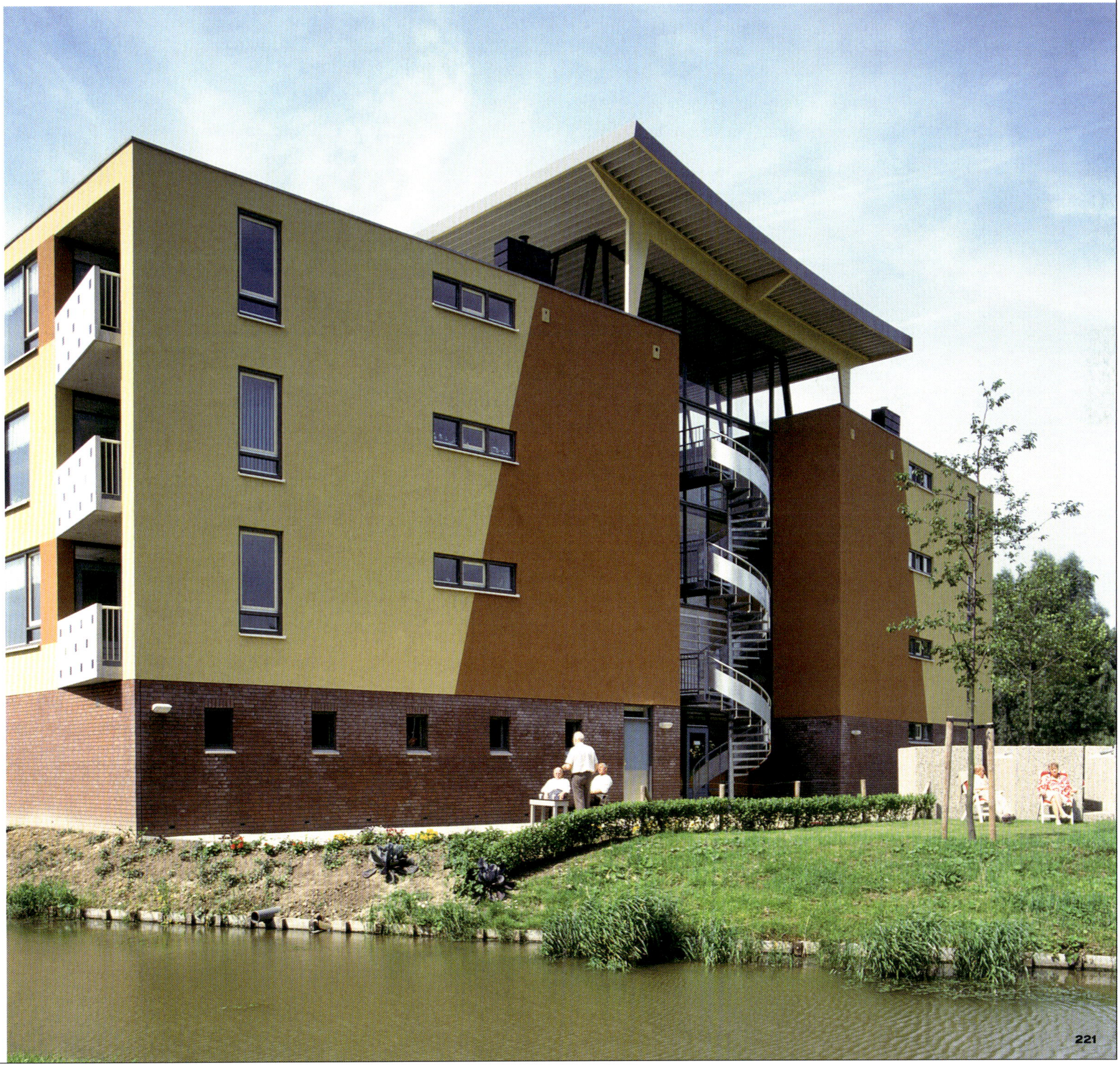

Neighbourhood

Greiner Van Goor Architecten

Psychiatrisch Centrum Amsterdam
Amsterdam
1989-1994

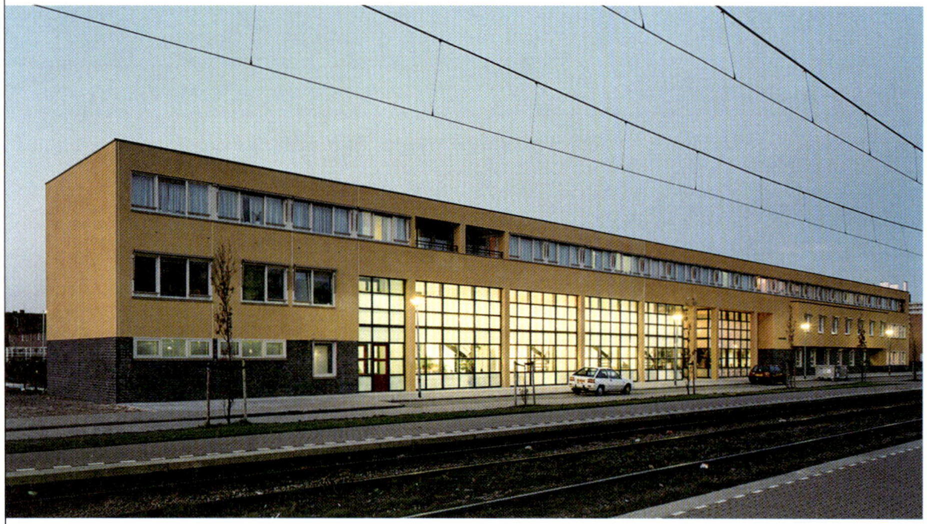

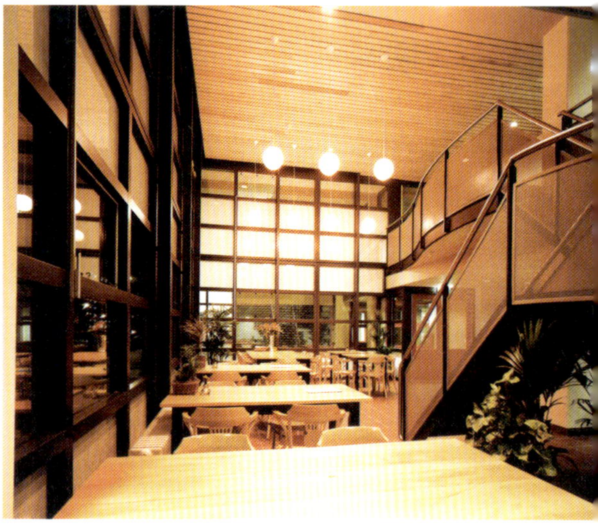

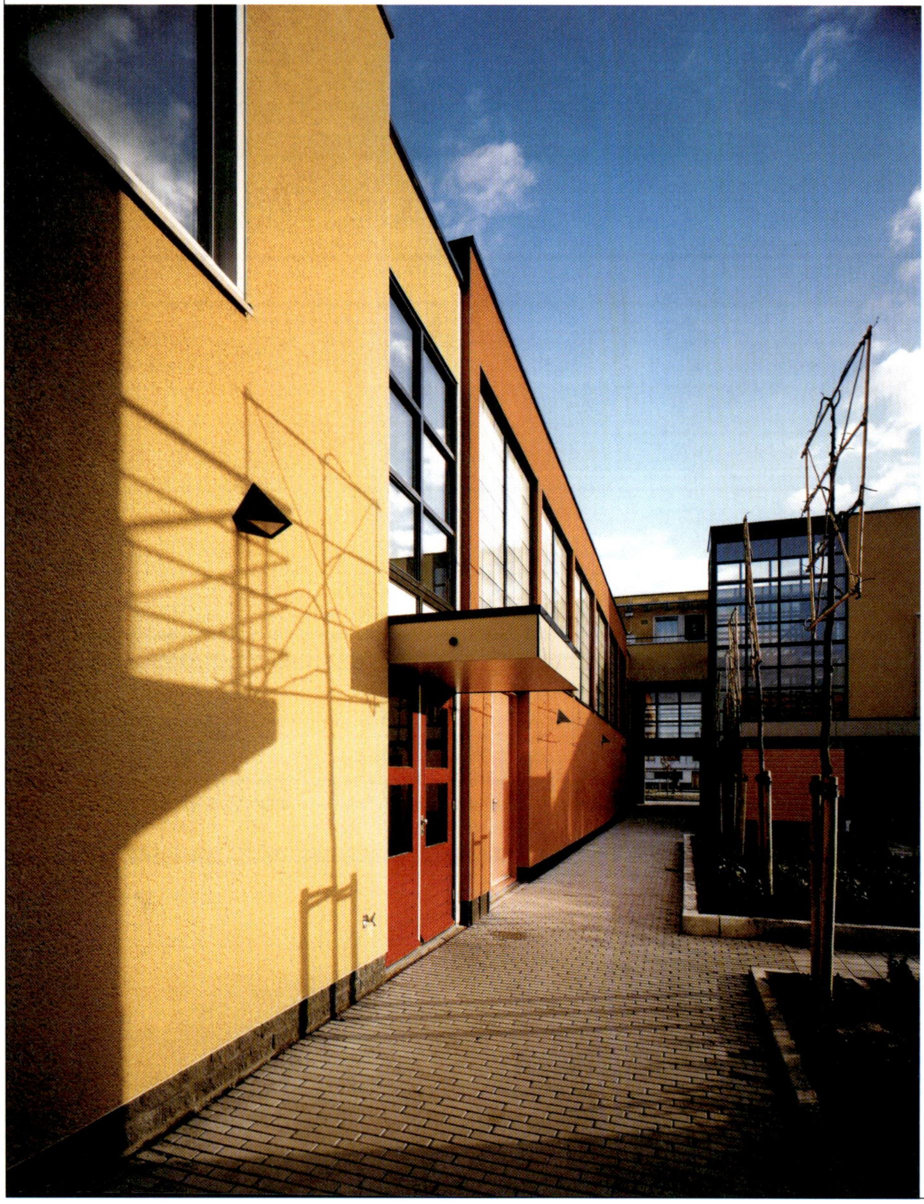

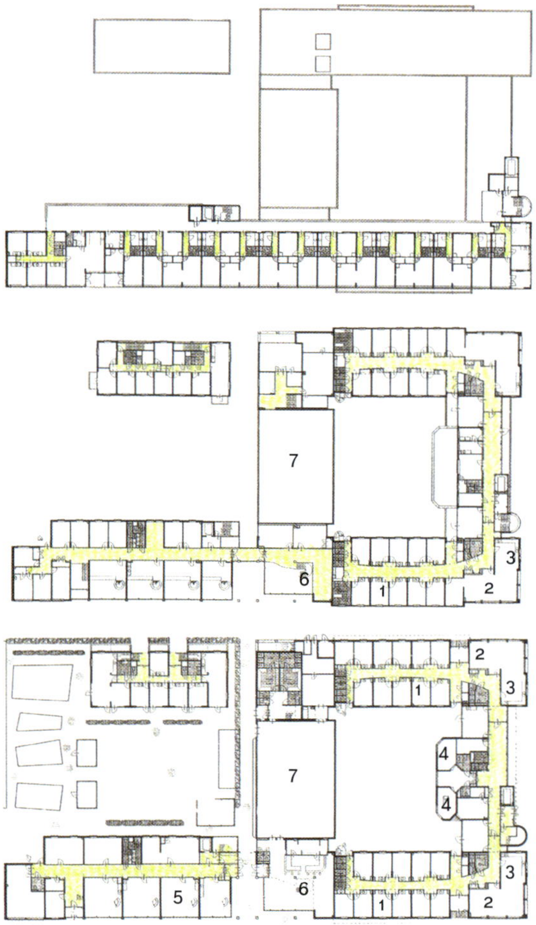

Second floor with flexible residential units, first floor with open unit and ground floor with closed unit

1 *single room*
2 *day room*
3 *kitchen*
4 *isolation room*
5 *creative therapy*
6 *meeting area*
7 *sports facility for psycho-motoric therapy*

Psychiatrisch Centrum Amsterdam is one of the institutions that have replaced the Provinciaal Ziekenhuis Meerenberg in Santpoort. The principal wanted a residential building that would blend with the surroundings, with patient units in the form of apartments with their front doors opening onto the street and favourably situated with respect to community facilities and public transport. Housing and treatment had to be kept separate.

Nieuw-Sloten was to match the style of the buildings in the neighbourhood. Van Goor divided the terrain into two. He designed a block with a square ground plan around an enclosed garden on the one side, and two rectangular blocks on the other. A public footpath divides the Psychiatrisch Centrum in two. The footpath is intensively used by the locals because it is the shortest route between the homes and school on the north side and the tram stop on the south side of the centre. The patients of the centre also make intensive use of the footpath, because not only the main entrance but also the entrances to the areas for creative therapy, the meeting centre, the sports hall and the staircase and lift to the first and second floors are situated beside the footpath.

The closed block accommodates groups of ten patients on each floor. The communal lounges with a kitchen-diner are located at the corners, while the single bedrooms of the patients are on the front side and at the rear. Opposite the residential block are the therapy building, the staff offices, and the rooms for the technical service. The second floors have single rooms for the patients who do not require much care, and guest rooms. A detached block contains the apartments of the autonomous residential group.

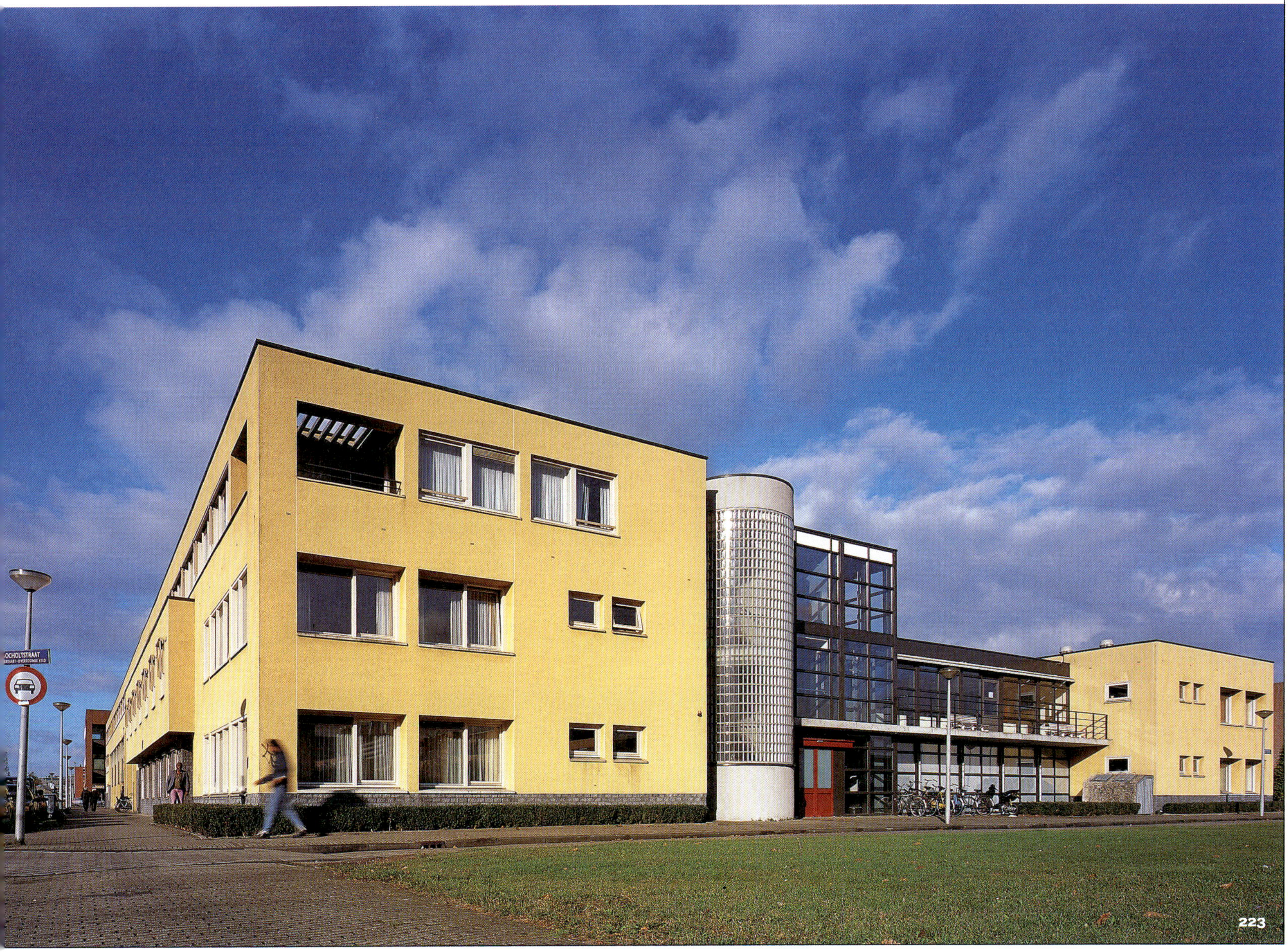

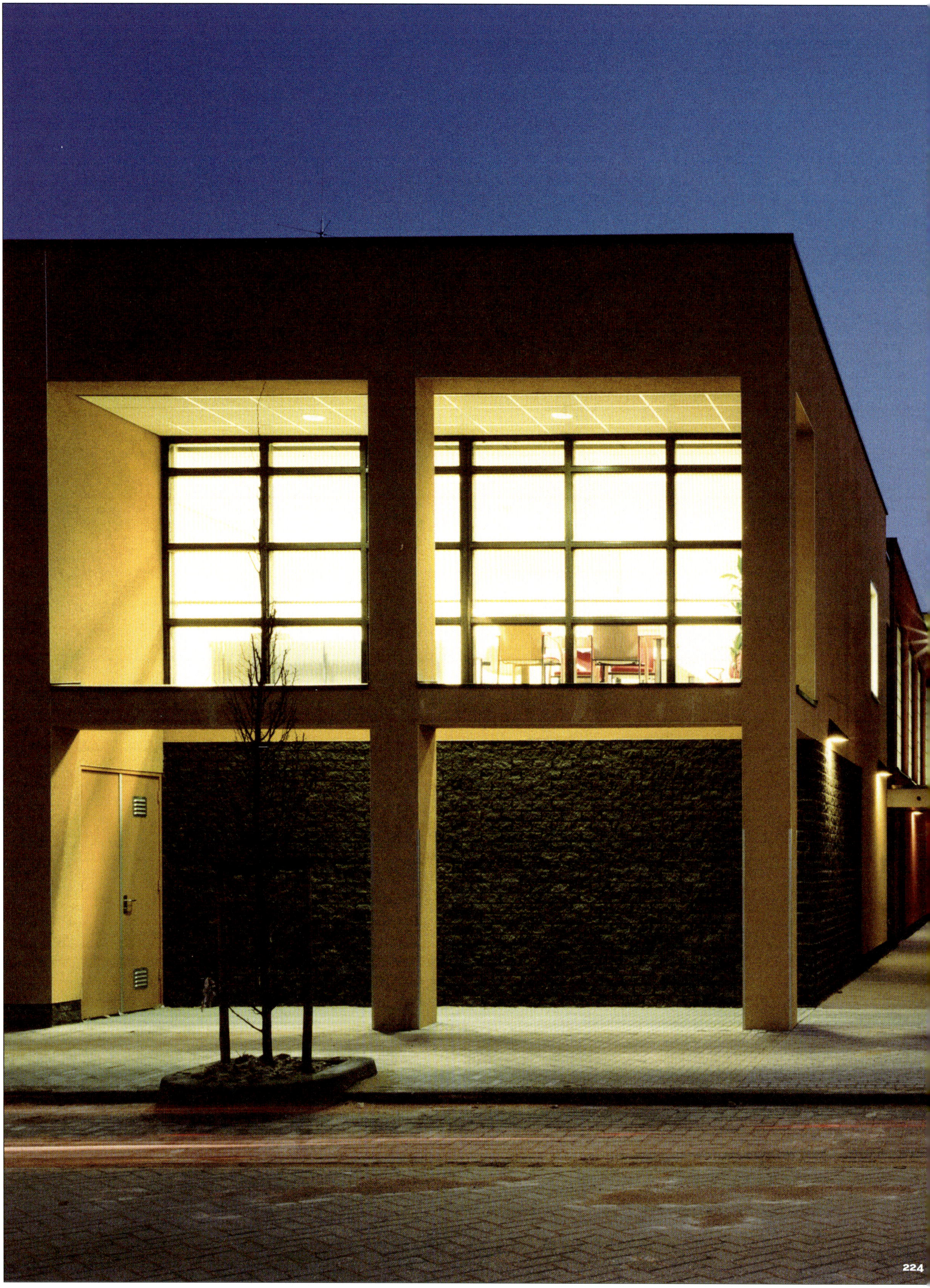

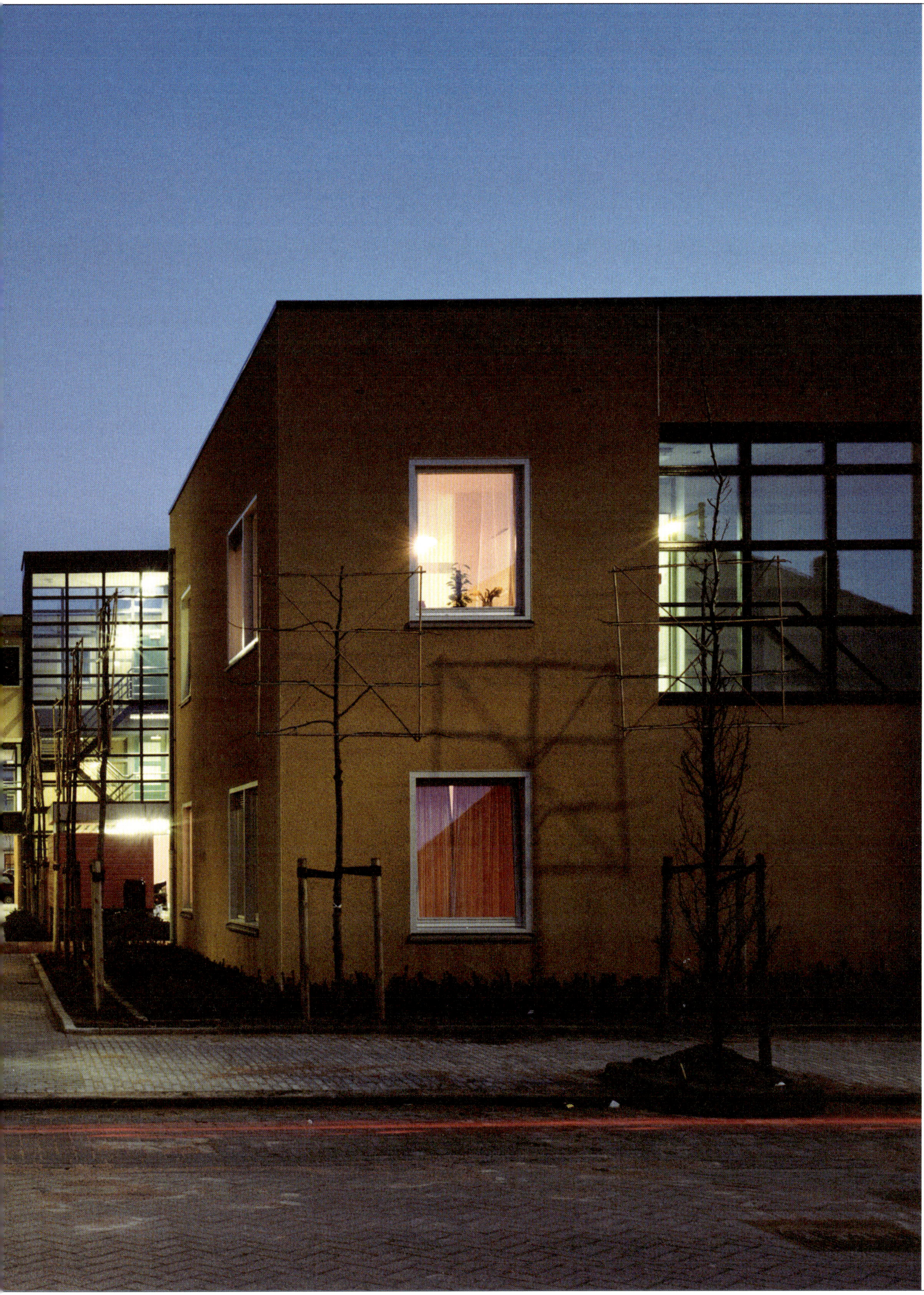

KAMSTRUKTUUR

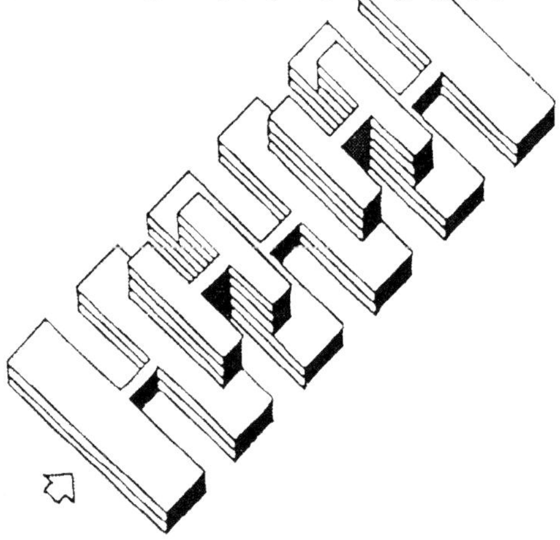

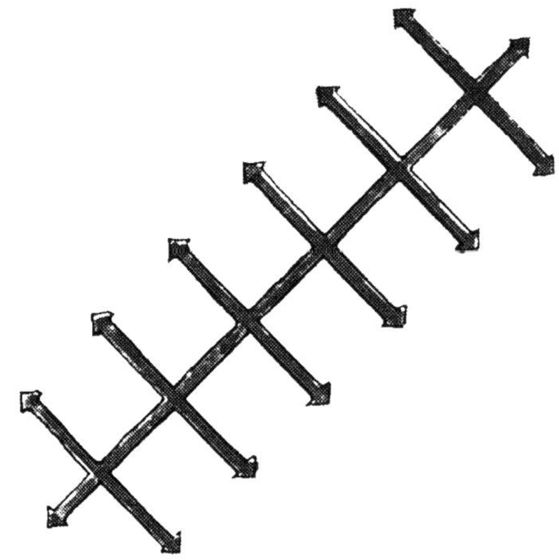

Flexibility

RIJNSTATE

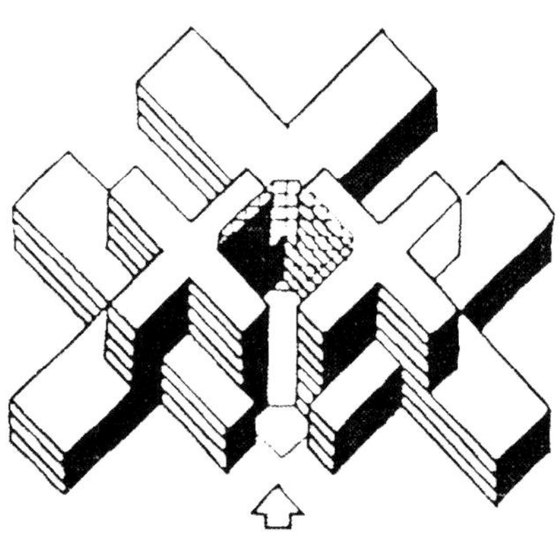

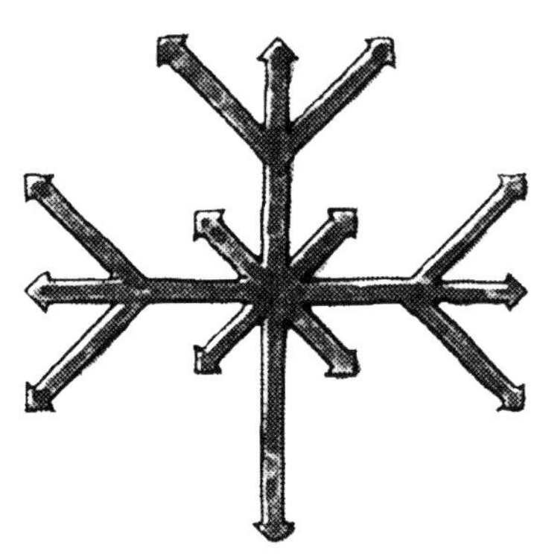

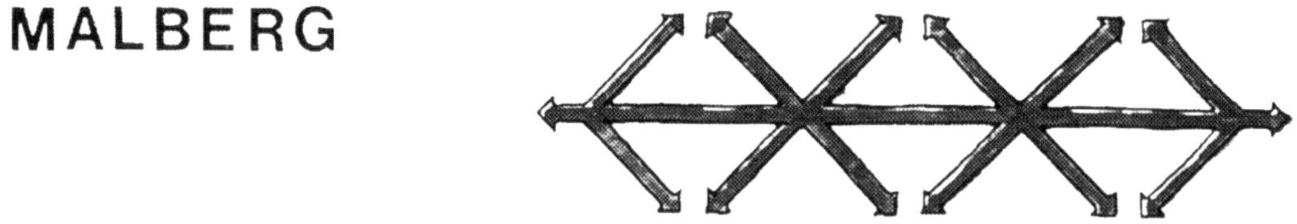

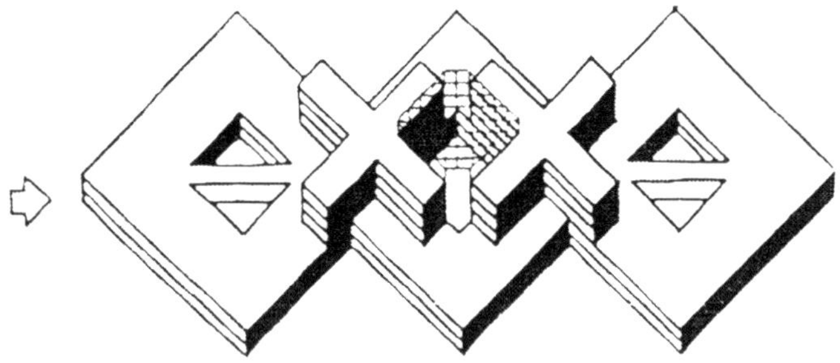

Top
Architektenburo Roelofs Nijst Lucas, structural diagrams for the new building of a hospital merger in Arnhem (Malberg – the predecessor of the Rijnstate Ziekenhuis), with possibilities for expansion

Bottom
Architektenburo Roelofs Nijst Lucas, structural diagram Rijnstate Ziekenhuis, completed in 1994

Strategic model National Hospital Institute; design for a flexible hospital

Hendriks Campman Tennekes, structure of the Streekziekenhuis Koningin Beatrix, Winterswijk, completed in 1982

Since the Second World War, hospital design has grown to become one of the most complex assignments. Besides long, opaque procedures, strict regulations and building standards, architects have to deal with a large and varied group of users. A 'principal' seventy persons strong is not unusual. A hospital is a large-scale ensemble of very diverse areas, some of which fall under the regime of a specialist. A Dutch hospital has between 1,500 and 3,000 rooms.[1] Moreover, the assignment is constantly changing during the design and construction phase. The dynamics of health care create the need for continuous renovations. A large percentage of the hospitals built in the 1960s had already been replaced by new buildings within twenty years. The Streekziekenhuis Oranjeoord in Harlingen opened in 1961; the decision to rebuild was taken in 1971.[2] Besides new building, there were renovations and extensions of the hospitals on a large scale in the 1970s. This tendency was encouraged by the Hospital Provisions Act, the imposition in 1974 of limits on the health care buildings to be built, and the ongoing specialisation. The number of specialisations in the Netherlands increased from twenty-one to thirty between 1966 and 1984.[3] The newcomers included neurology, diagnostic imaging, radiation therapy, clinical chemistry and clinic geriatrics. The uninterrupted process of renovation and extension was usually fatal to the original architectural conception. This strengthened the conviction that not building designs were required, but a strategic concept capable of accommodating the inevitable changes. The hospital had to become flexible. It must be amenable to both extension and internal contraction.

According to the National Hospital Institute (NZI), improvement of flexibility should be focused on the potential for modifications as soon as they became necessary, a minimum of interference to the normal activities of the hospital during renovation, and limitation of the expense.[4] In order to arrive at such improvements, an investigation of how modifications were effected in practice was conducted first. The renovation experiences of four hospitals made it clear that rooms were always added. Extra room could generally only be found at a distance. To avoid that, adjacent functions had to be expelled (which often had a domino effect). Twenty years later, the sum of the renovation budget amounted to half of the original investment.[5]

Flexible building, however, is a contradiction in terms. Even the infinite capacity for modification in every direction that the endlessly extendable constructional grids of the Foundation for Architects Research (SAR) had promised turned out to be difficult to achieve in practice, and the internal flexibility – the production of interchangeable infill packages independently of the supporting structure – proved to be a dead letter as well. The open-end structures with which experiments were conducted in the 1970s were similar to the SAR grids. They were expandable, but that resulted in fairly arbitrary compositions with the same drawbacks as the earlier pavilion hospitals: they occupied a lot of room and increased the distances between the different departments. Instead of these directionless, uniform grids, experiments were conducted in the 1980s with structures that had a clear centre of gravity, which often coincided with the central point in the internal traffic system. The design challenge lay in trying to find a compact form that was nevertheless flexible. This was to square the circle, in a way, because compact high-rise building was regarded as the opposite of flexible; it was not for nothing that the upper floors of the tower on a podium hospitals accommodated the wards, the least dynamic part of the hospital.

No matter how much flexibility was in the limelight, not everyone was convinced of

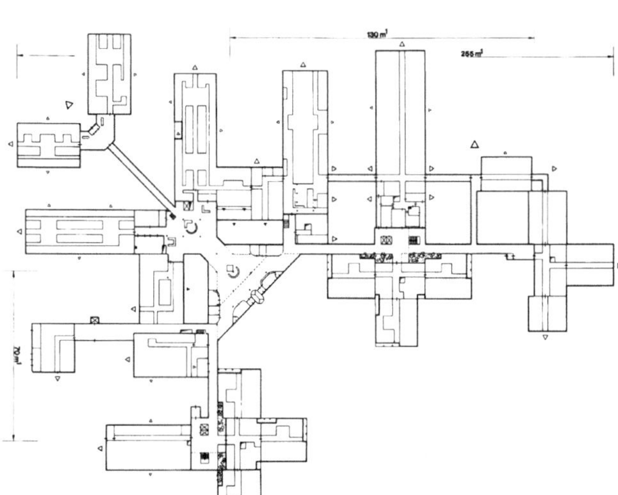

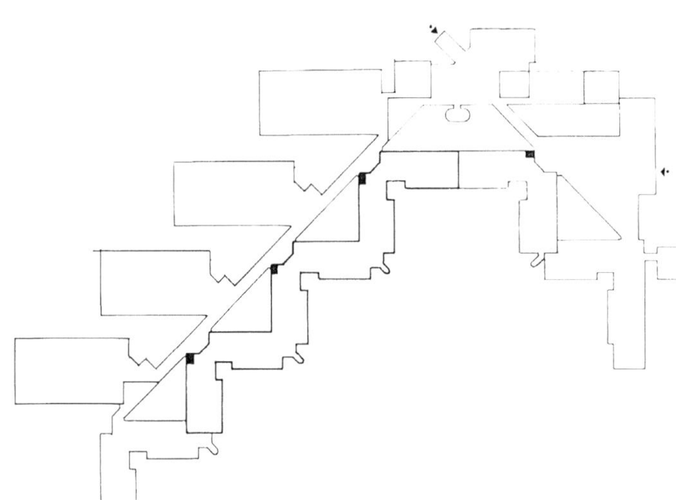

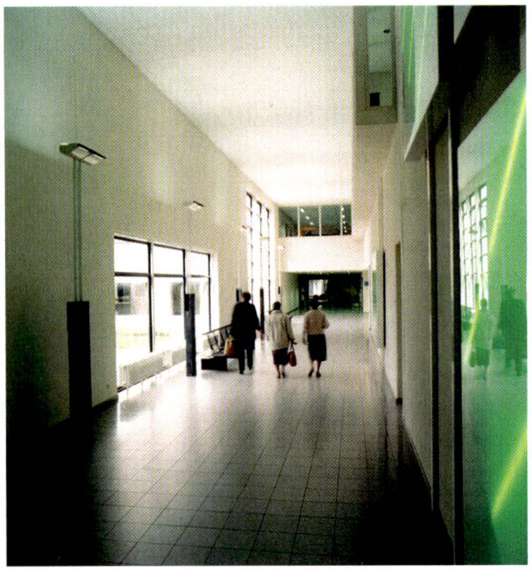

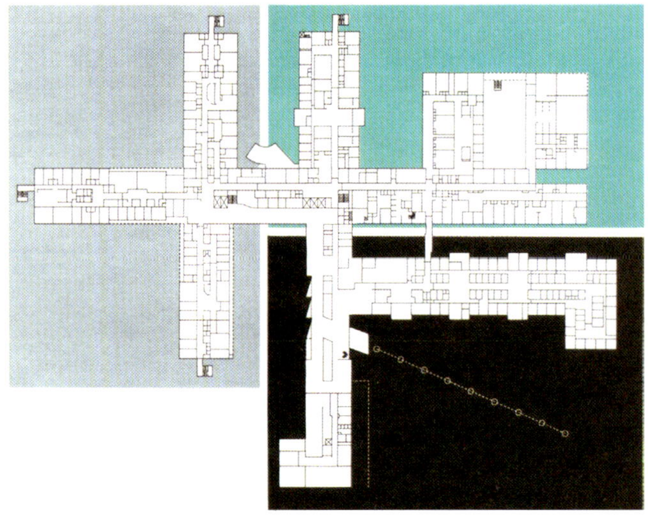

the need for it. M. le Mandat was one of the few to warn of overstatement when he claimed that the speed at which hospitals changed was usually grossly exaggerated. 'However, one should not put blind faith in the speed of obsolescence.'[6] He too emphasised the importance of easy adaptability, but believed that this was something different from the striving for flexibility. The term flexibility, he felt, was only too often a pretext to design in a sloppy way and to camouflage conceptual imperfections. It could lead to designs that were nothing but a 'feeble and imprecise response to a deliberately badly formulated problem, thereby making it possible to absorb all the future changes'.[7] These remarks by Le Mandat in fact mark the transition from a functionalism that clearly manifested itself in the exterior to a more introvert functionalism: the hospital became a traffic machine where the emphasis came to lie not on the functions but on the routing, and which was supported not only by functions clustered together, but also by those parts of the building where the function had not been pinned down for the long term.

In his study *Flexibiliteit in ziekenhuis-bouw* (Flexibility in hospital architecture), W.Q. Stolwijk of Wiegerinck Architecten referred to three types of building: the linear structure, the cruciform structure, and the square structure. These types were supposed to afford a maximal external flexibility. Most hospitals that were built in the 1980s and 1990s were examples of variations on these types. The simplest is the linear hospital, a variation on the comb type. In principle linear types can be expanded in two directions without affecting the relation with the core. In their design for the Streekziekenhuis Koningin Beatrix in Winterswijk (1979-1982), Hendriks Campman Tennekes opted for a linear structure in which the various units are at an angle of forty-five degrees to the main axis. The nursing wards are grouped in an L-shape at one end of the corridor, resulting in an unimpeded view from the rooms. In the first instance Roelofs Nijst Lucas also remained close to the comb type in their quest for the flexible hospital. In most cases they assumed a strong linear area for the main traffic, to which various units were linked that were individually expandable. An example is the design for the Rijnstate Ziekenhuis in Arnhem. The principal had ended up with Roelofs Nijst Lucas in 1984 via the Sint Elisabeth Ziekenhuis in Tilburg, which has a comb structure. The first design was similar to the hospital in Tilburg and had a linear structure. The plan changed during the design process and the various units were set at an angle of forty-five degrees to the main corridor, resulting in a structure of crosses with an atrium in the middle. At the moment when a third hospital came to take part in the merger, the whole plan was scrapped because the structure was not suitable for further expansion.[8] A new plan was drawn up in which the atrium and the angled structure were once again taken as the starting point.[9] The final design that was implemented in 1994, however, has a star-shaped structure rather than one of crosses. The ground plan still comprises a number of cross shapes, but they are no longer articulated in a straight line but are set at an angle to one another, resulting in a roofed central area in the middle. This is where the visitor enters the building and finds all kinds of provisions.

'Whoever designs a hospital designs transience', R. Nicolaï commented on the report *Flexibiliteit als bouwstrategie* (Flexibility as building strategy), which he and K. Dekker compiled for the NZI.[10] The most recent hospitals were not considered flexible enough either; the number of wings that could branch of from a central point in the cruciform and square types was taken

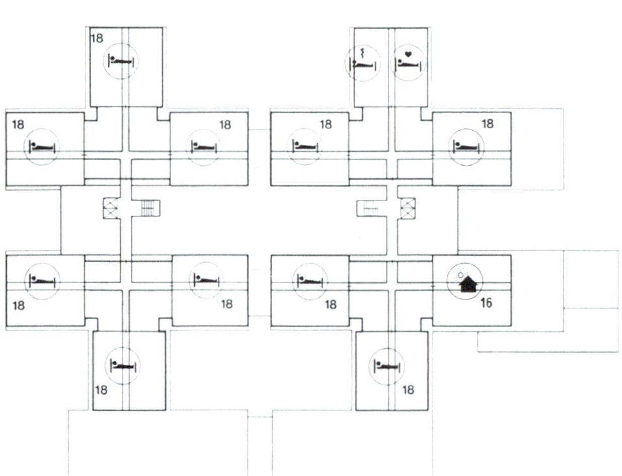

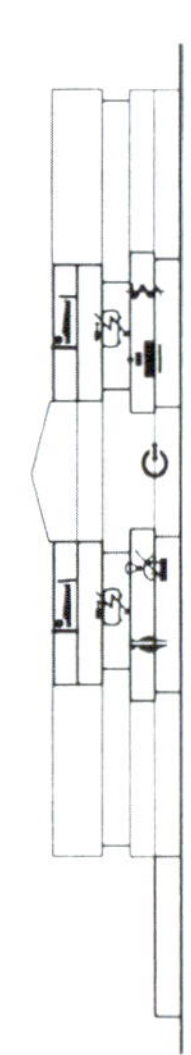

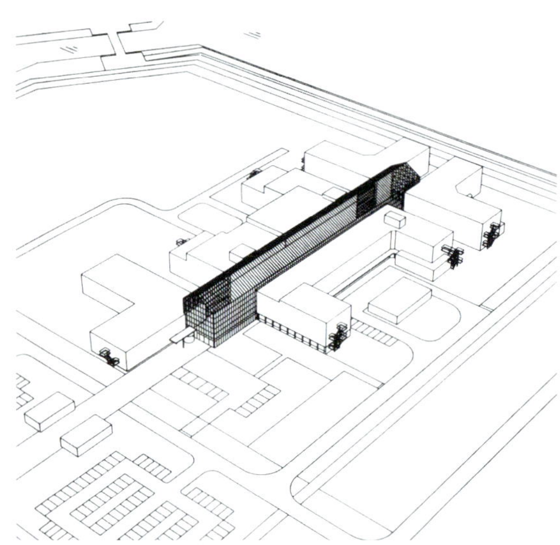

Top
Tuns + Horsting Architecten, Wilhelmina Ziekenhuis, Assen, 1990. Interior and ground plan

Wiegerinck Architecten, Antonius Ziekenhuis in Sneek, 1994. Ground plan nursing unit and scale model.

Bottom
Campman Tennekes De Jong, ground plan IJssellandziekenhuis, Capelle aan den IJssel, 1991

Campman Tennekes De Jong, Flevo Ziekenhuis, Almere, 1990. Passage model

Four-bed ward in the Antonius Ziekenhuis, Sneek, 1994

Kruisheer Hallink Arends architecten, Oosterscheldeziekenhuis, Goes, 1987. Cruciform model

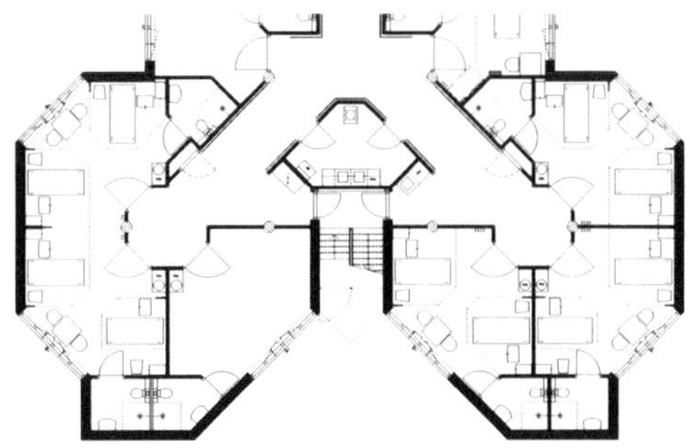

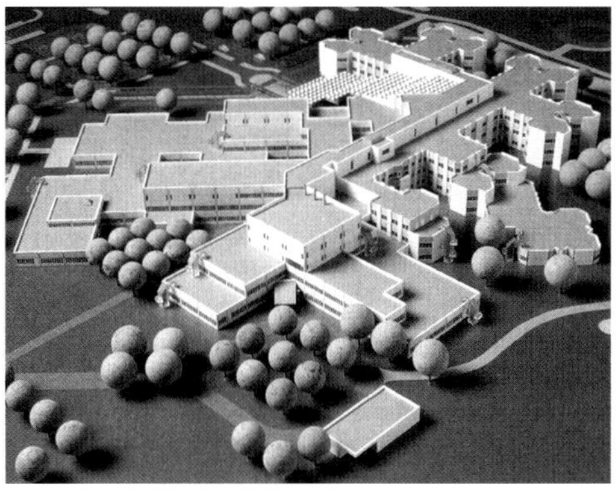

to be too small to allow sufficient possibilities for expansion. This could be improved by splitting these wings into several branches. The researchers turned a blind eye to the ragged edges that resulted, since for them a hospital was more an instrument than a building. A second innovation was the introduction of open flanks: expansion would be possible not only at the ends of the branches but also on the sides by making the areas situated there easy to extend. To prove that this strategy was both more flexible and less expensive, they compared the results with the Wilhelmina Ziekenhuis in Assen designed by A. Tuns (Tuns + Horsting Architecten) and the IJssellandziekenhuis that Campman Tennekes de Jong had built in Capelle aan den IJssel. The outcome – the NZI model would be more flexible and cheaper – was predictable, and that was the reaction of Tuns and Tennekes as well: Tuns considered it an expression of 'classic thinking' because the nursing wards determined the structure, while Tennekes questioned the claim that the project in Capelle aan den IJssel was actually more expensive than Nicolaï's alternative.[11]

The strategies that were introduced in the NZI model were reflected in the new Antonius Ziekenhuis in Sneek (1994) by Wiegerinck Architecten. F. Kolkman broke this hospital down into three parts and grouped them around a central hall. The facilities that were not directly connected with health care proper, such as the kitchen, the laboratory, the mortuary and the dispensary were taken out of the complex so that they would not stand in the way of any possible changes in the hospital. Another new element here was the structure of the rooms for patients. Each bed stands beside the window, and the rooms can be divided up into two-bed and four-bed rooms. Every room is a multiple of 15 m^2, so that outpatient functions can be accommodated there too. According to Kolkman, this was one of the most flexible hospitals that Wiegerinck Architecten had made so far. He was referring above all to the solution of the problem of internal pressure, which reduced the risk that 'hard' outpatient units (which depend on heavy equipment) might be replaced by 'soft' outpatient units (where there are hardly any installations or equipment). This enabled a hard outpatient unit to grow without any obstacle and a soft outpatient unit to be moved without many problems.[12]

These flexible hospitals have in common with the Structuralist conception of architecture of the 1960s that they are structures. What made original Structuralism so fascinating – the vision of endless, even growth, the utopia of individual freedom to organise one's own niche within the grid in accordance with individual taste and needs – has degenerated in these hospitals to become a purely technical and infrastructural basis that is subsequently fleshed out with corridors, atria and entrance halls at a number of strategic points, which usually coincide with nodes in the traffic system. The constructional support plays a subordinate role, and the most important characteristic is that of the ground plan: a corridor, a cross, a square, a combination of them, or a tree with branches. It is difficult to achieve a strong architectural design here; sometimes the ragged edges convey a sloppy, unfinished impression. This is rarely due to the incapacity of the designer: these hospitals are in principle never complete. They are buildings in progress, destined to continue to grow. They do so, of course, from the inside.

A very different way of making hospital complexes more flexible consists of detaching the non-specific parts. This 'onion rings' model, which was advocated around the turn of the century by the (no longer existing) Building Board and others, is attracting a good deal of attention. It

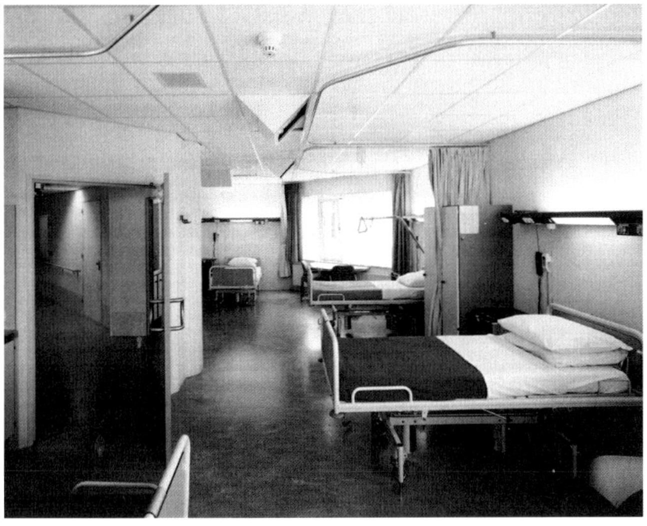

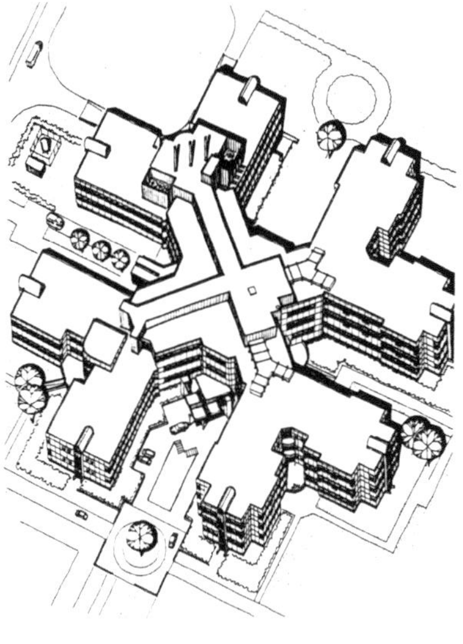

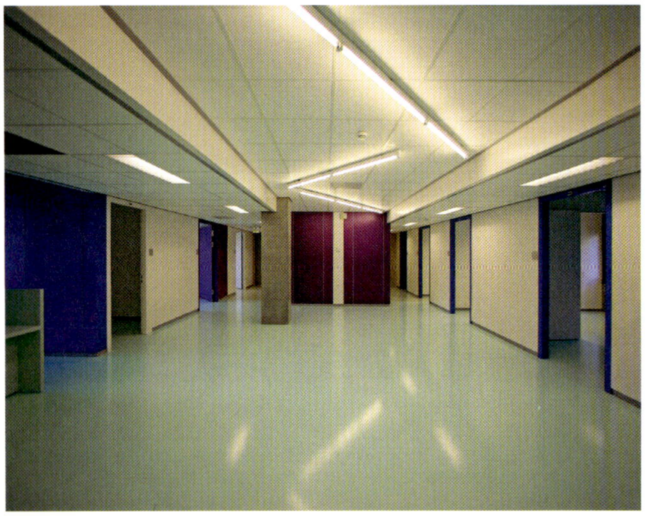

assumes that all generic functions that have no need to be located in a hospital can be accommodated better elsewhere. As a result, the hospital proper loses a lot of spatial ballast that only gets in the way when changes become necessary. Moreover, these generic parts outside the hospital are designed in such a way that they can escape from the dimensions and physical appearance of the hospital, which improves their real estate value.

It is only natural that the composition of buildings is important, and so is the fact that advantages can be drawn from distinguishing between long-term elements and an infilling that is constantly changing because changes in use demand it. A third flexibility strategy was added to these tried and tested solutions around the end of the century. The principle of Industrial Flexible and Demountable building (IFD) explores the constructional possibilities of a building package type of constructional method. In practice this targets mainly the maximal free divisibility of the spaces. Buildings with a lot of technology, and thus many cables, call for much more advanced solutions than are required in a regular building. So IFD refines the methods of the SAR, which has difficulty in guaranteeing the presupposed flexibility in a complicated technological environment. An example of a project built in accordance with IFD principles is the Martini Ziekenhuis in Groningen that opened in 2007 (Burger Grunstra architecten adviseurs). The main structure of the building is detached from the health care concept that can change in the future. It remains to be seen whether the IFD principle really is able to accommodate the presupposed changes – the axiom of the famous Modernist Ludwig Mies van der Rohe still seems to offer the best guarantee of that: make all the rooms as large as possible, that not only provides immediate ease of use but is also the best guarantee that other functions can be accommodated there too.

A very different solution can be found in a new building for the Gelre ziekenhuizen in Zutphen designed by Royal Haskoning with Wiegerinck Architectuur en Stedenbouw. As experience has shown that renovation of the 'hot floor' is not only more expensive than rebuilding but also causes considerable inconvenience, it was proposed to accommodate the 'hot floor' in a separate volume that can be demolished as soon as it no longer satisfies the requirements. Next to it there is room for a medical complex of roughly the same size that is linked with the other units in a similar way. If the existing wing becomes outdated, the new one can be placed next to it, after which the old one can be demolished. It is one of the innovative strategies of this project; another is the partial application of the 'onion rings' model: non-specific functions such as offices have been reduced to a minimum inside the hospital, and the rest have been situated elsewhere.

Flexibility of use makes it possible to assign new functions to areas without the need for drastic renovation. This means that, after being used for clinical care, a building can continue to be suitable for completely different functions such as offices or housing. As care organisations are now themselves responsible for the running costs of their real estate, this is an attractive way of building. The Parnassia Bavo Group, one of the largest institutions for mental health care, uses this method in its plans for new buildings. Extra large dimensions make the building less specific and thus more flexible. Thanks to its longer life span, the extra expenses are easily recovered, The group has commissioned a building for the so-called Triple-Ex clients (those who are addicted, in detention and unemployed) in The Hague-Loosduinen. The design is by the Inbo firm of architects. When the building is no longer suitable for this group, which requires (heavy) security

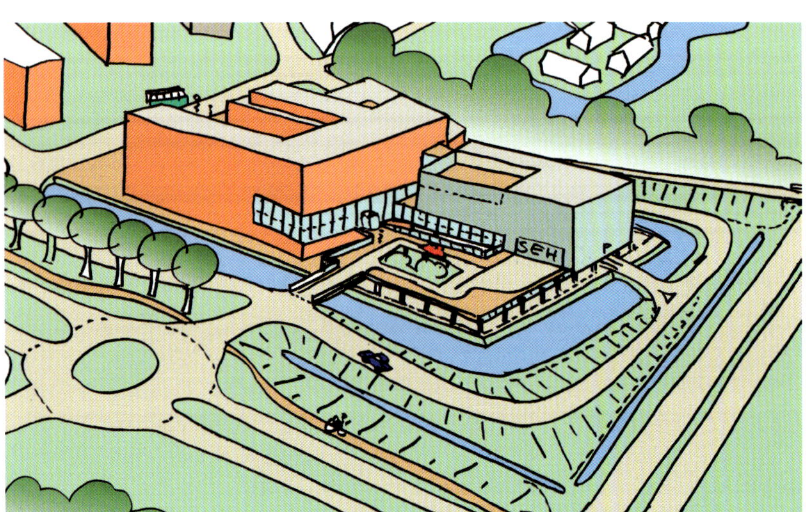

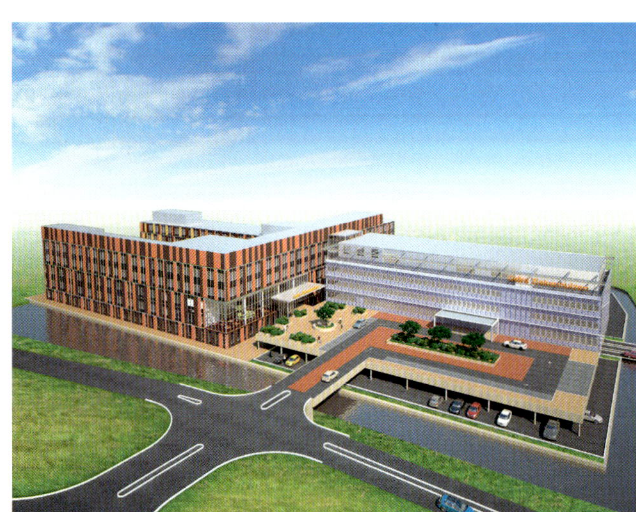

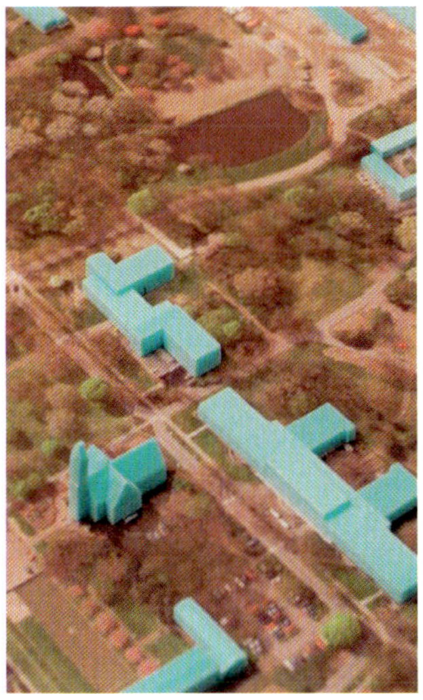

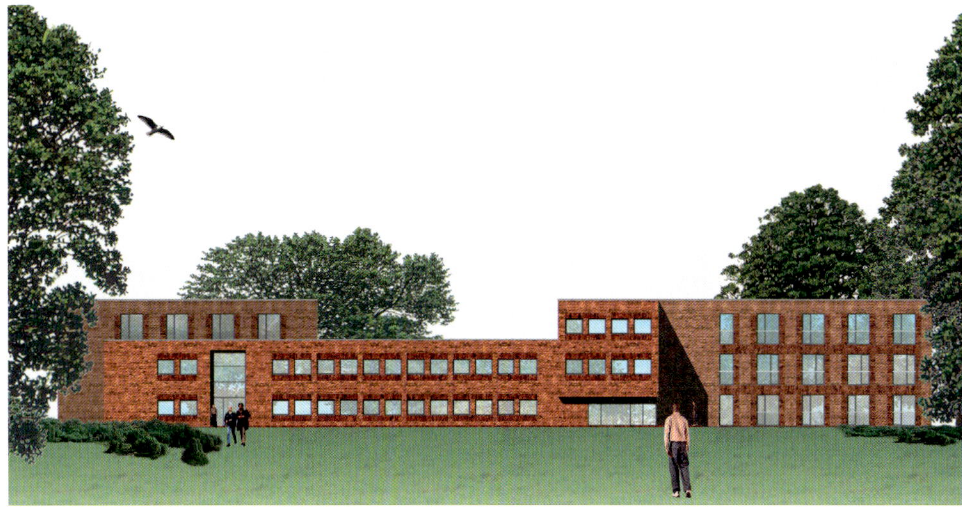

care, it can easily be made suitable for general housing.[13] The incorporation of the costs of the real estate in the product price stimulates the organisations to optimise and rationalise the use. According to Rob Scheerder and Marinus Verweij from the Building Board, it is not a question of the largest tailored suit, but of the best fitting tailored suit. 'A hospital with an excess of (inflexible) square metres can end up in a disadvantageous competitive position. The idea is to make optimal use of available capacity in combination with "shrinkage and growth" – flexibility to take fluctuations in its stride.'[14] They expect that working with clinical and care pathways will increase sharply. Serious reflection on the development of the care process is of great important for a building that faces the future. Changes in the design of the real estate can be expected above all on the borderline between first-line and second-line care. Buildings will become smaller in scale, more pluriform and more 'ordinary'.[15]

Top
Burger Grunstra architecten adviseurs, interior Martini Ziekenhuis, Groningen, 2007

Inbo, building for Triple-Ex clients, Parnassia, The Hague

Bottom
Royal Haskoning with Wiegerinck Architectuur en Stedenbouw, design for Gelre ziekenhuizen, Zutphen

Inbo, building for Triple-Ex clients, Parnassia, The Hague

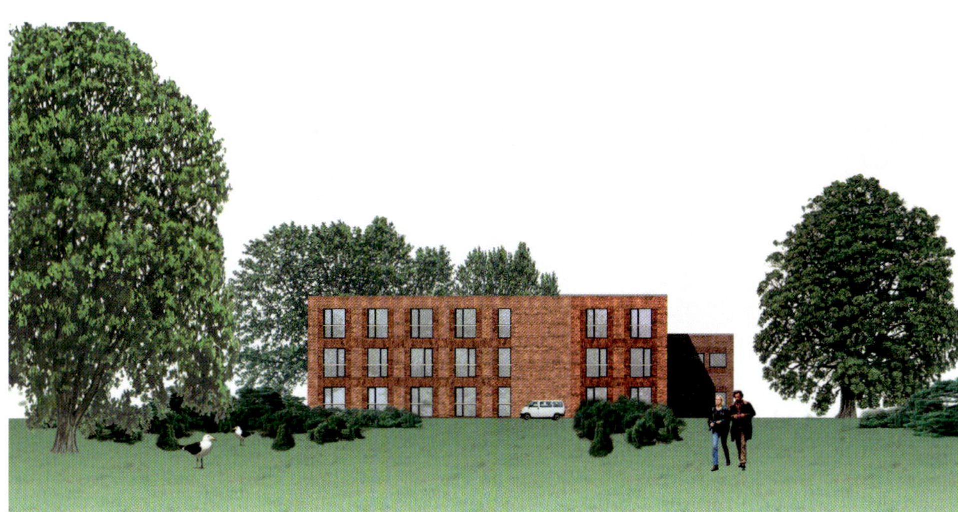

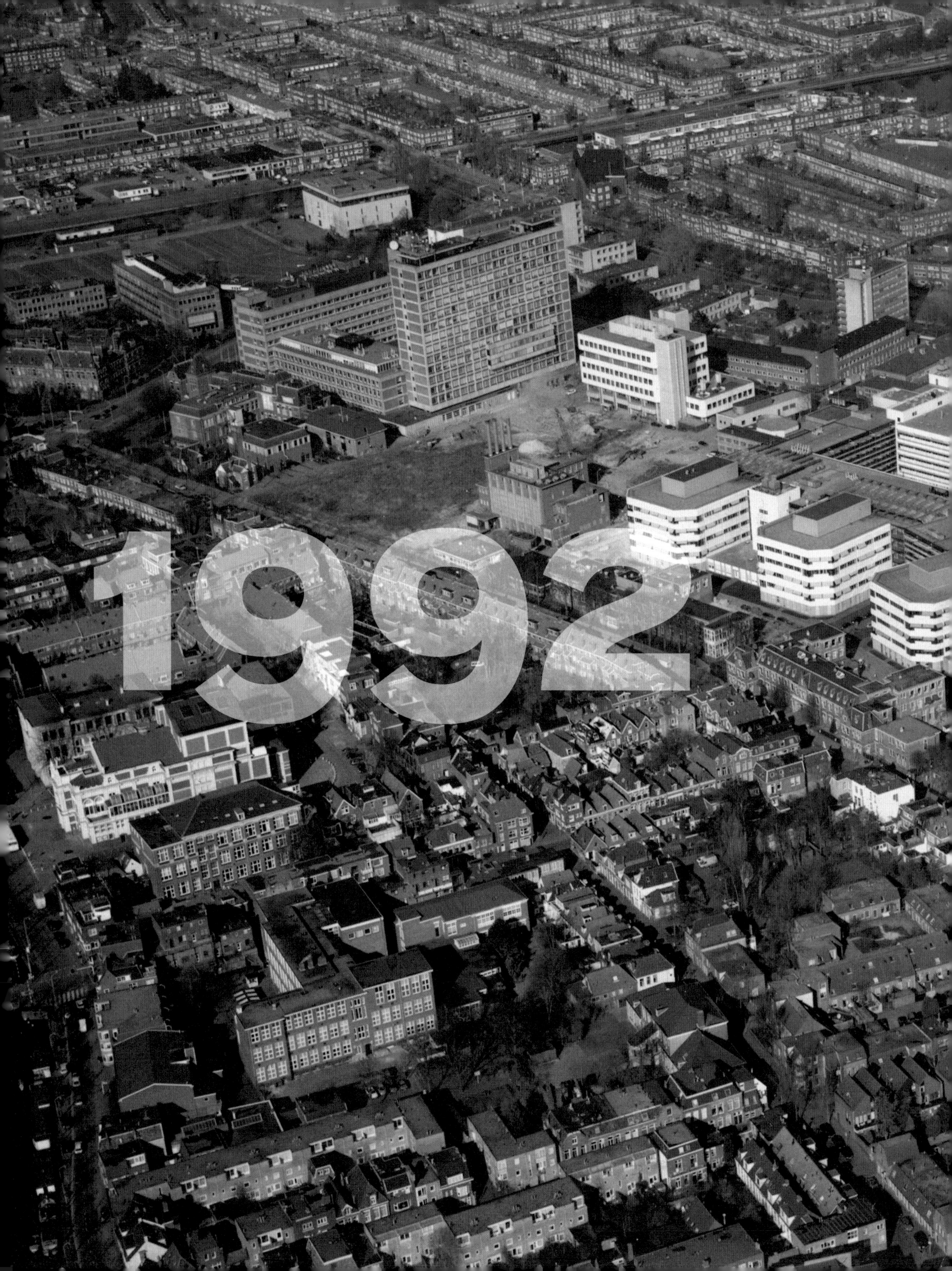
1992

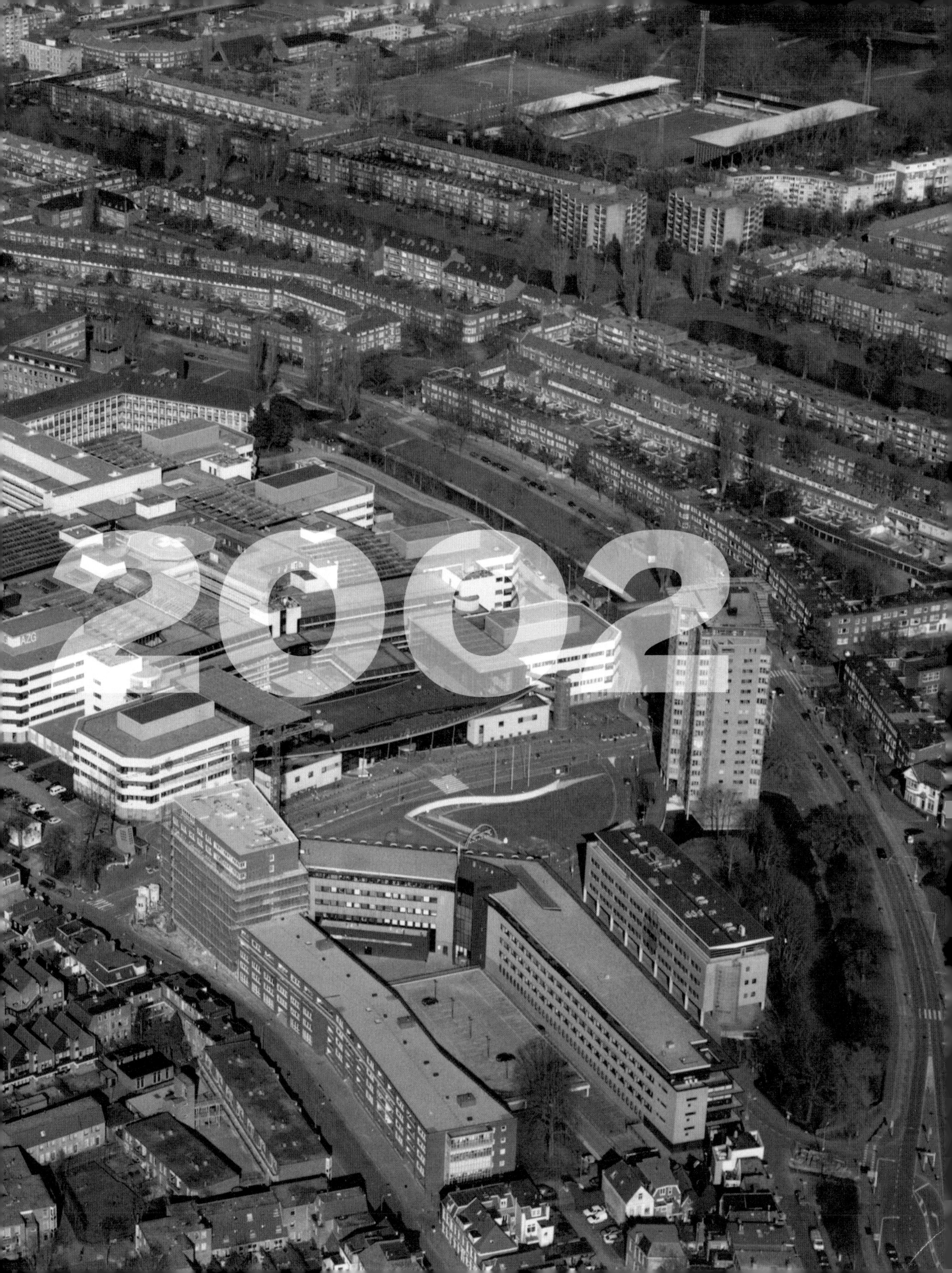
2002
AZG

Changes in the health care landscape

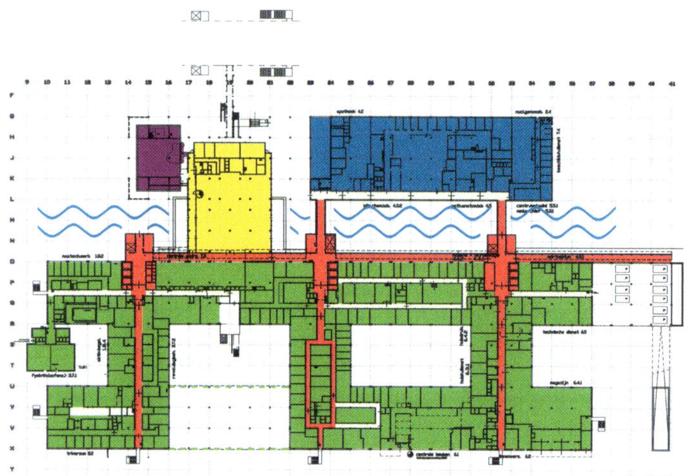

p. 232
***Kruisheer Hallink Arends architecten, Team 4 Architecten and Wytze Patijn architecten*, Academisch Ziekenhuis Groningen (AZG), Groningen, 1997**

p. 234
***Wiegerinck Architecten*, Spaarne Ziekenhuis, Hoofddorp, 1998-2004. Ground plan first floor.**

p. 235
***de Jong Gortemaker Algra architecten en ingenieurs*, extension the Netherlands Cancer Institute/Antoni van Leeuwenhoek Ziekenhuis, Amsterdam, 1998-2004**

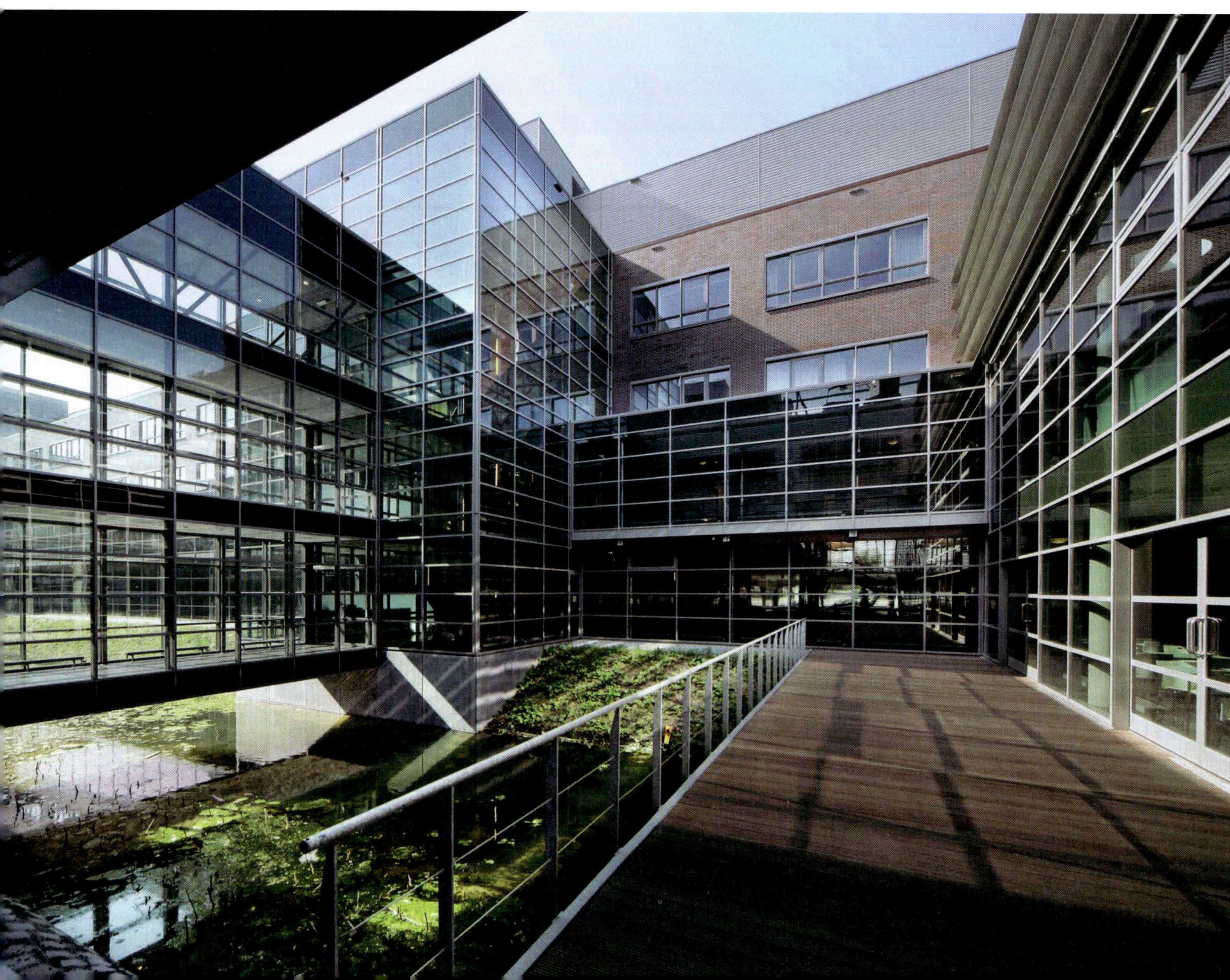

The end of the welfare state

The 1990s saw the completion of the substitution policy, by which the transition to small-scale, non-institutional provisions was largely accomplished, particularly in care for the elderly and in psychiatry. In the meantime the foundations of the welfare state, the framework within which the Dutch health system had developed after 1945, were called into question. The fall of the Berlin Wall in November 1989 marked a turning-point: the demise of Socialism was celebrated throughout the West as a victory of the free market. While the presence of a competitive system that had been legitimised by the emancipation of the lower classes had been a reason to give the welfare state a collective, planned character too, once the Socialist model had been defeated there was no longer any obstacle to the dismantling of the Western variant. It is only natural that this would have far-reaching consequences for health care: is it possible to see health care in isolation from the welfare state? In the many thought experiments that analysed the basic principles of care, this question centred on the degree to which market mechanisms were possible and desirable. Although attempts to revise the system were seen as a priority, the practical consequences remained limited for the time being.

As we have seen, the building world was marked by the completion of the tendencies that had begun earlier. It was only now that the consequences of trends that had cautiously been begun in the 1980s became fully visible. The hospitals were an exception. The conviction that here too it was impossible to avoid a change of course led to a temporary building freeze, intended as a pause for thought in order to arrive at new concepts. In psychiatry the big shift from the grounds in woods and dunes to small-scale provisions in the cities took shape, while care for the mentally disabled followed the trend towards 'normal' housing. It was care for the elderly that was marked by the most radical changes: the separation of accommodation and care. Care was only integrated with accommodation when no other solutions were conceivable – the number of categories of residents to whom this applied was reduced as far as possible. All other old people lived in regular adaptable or adapted homes and received personalised care.

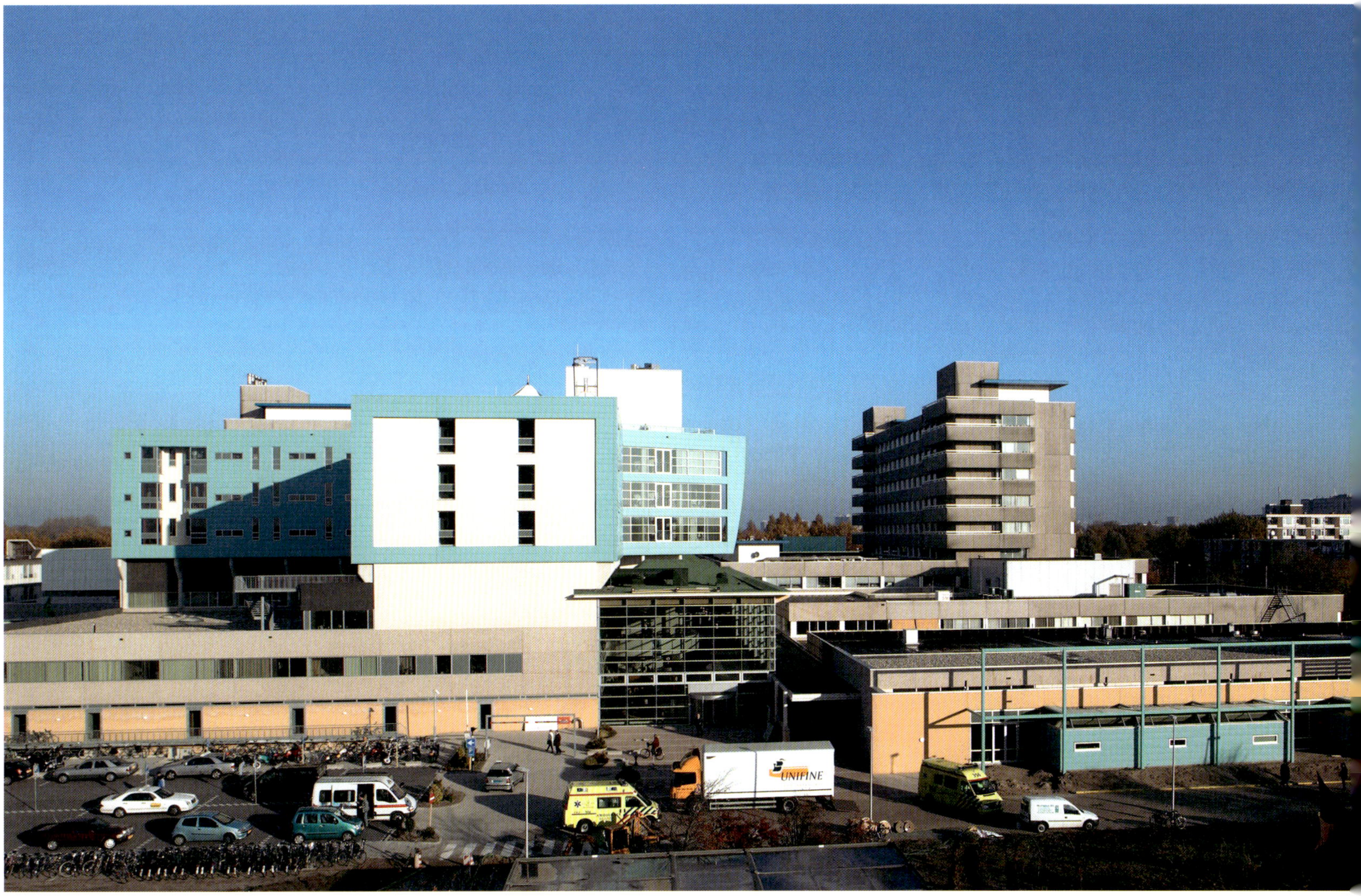

Hospitals

In the 1990s the government endeavoured to reduce the number of hospital beds from 2.8 to 2.0 per 1000 population. It still attempted to keep costs down by regulating the supply. In the light of the consideration that the scale benefit from mergers enabled working more efficiently, the lowering of the bed standard was accompanied by the building of bigger hospitals. To accommodate changes in medical technology, they had to be as flexible as possible. In that respect nothing had changed. Compared with the preceding period, however, in which mainly open-end structures had been built, a search now took place for other ways of incorporating flexibility. It was important that the architectural concept should remain intact in the long term.

According to R. Gortemaker and G. Mulkens from de Jong Gortemaker architecten en ingenieurs, most hospitals were organised in the form of a tree structure.[1] They were entered through a central hall (the trunk) that subsequently branched out to the various units (branches) and subunits (side branches). Modifications of the type often led to problems because the places where expansion was necessary were not always situated at the tips of the branches. Gortemaker and Mulkens sought their inspiration from other types of building, such as airport buildings. They often have very large halls in which smaller units are arranged. Developments in medical technology would probably mean that the physician of the future would go to see the patient with the appropriate equipment under his arm instead of receiving the patient in his room.

De Jong Gortemaker architecten en ingenieurs (now de Jong Gortemaker Algra architecten en ingenieurs) started work on designing a major extension of the Netherlands Cancer Institute/Antoni van Leeuwenhoek Ziekenhuis in Amsterdam in 1997. It was completed in 2003. The examination and consultation rooms for outpatients are on the ground floor, while above them are the work and consultation rooms of the specialists in the form of a large open office area. The firm designed a ward on the roof of this wide and elongated outpatients clinic. The result was a new type of tower on podium hospital.

In all hospitals the reduction of the bed standard inevitably led to the prospect of empty nursing wards. If they were to be used in the future, they must be capable of absorbing outpatient units, for instance. In designing the Spaarne Ziekenhuis in Hoofddorp (1990), Wiegerinck Architecten (now Wiegerinck Architectuur en Stedenbouw) opted for a structural plan to keep the hard medical and technological functions separate from the softer clinical and outpatient functions. All the same, the two building volumes are designed on a single universal grid so that the various functions are mutually interchangeable, resulting in a flexible building. The Spaarne Ziekenhuis was completed in 2004. The interchangeability of functions was also one of the main premises for the design of the Kennemer Gasthuis in Haarlem in 1999. Victor de Leeuw and Erik Fokkema (EGM architecten) called the result a network hospital. The unusual feature of their proposal is that the wards and outpatients unit are no longer conceived as separate volumes, but the whole programme is incorporated in a single rectangular block. To create the space required by the programme, the volume has been hollowed out where necessary, resulting in a building with holes. The hospital was completed between 2002 and 2006.

Hans Liscaljet from Architectengroep Duintjer (now merged with de Jong Gortemaker Algra architecten en ingenieurs) no longer conceived of the Westfries Gasthuis in Hoorn, that was completely renovated in several stages, as a hospital. He thereby hoped to escape the limitations of the classic hospital typology and to benefit from solutions for other types of building. Partly forced by the small dimensions of the site, Liscaljet proposed a long and narrow block projected on the edge of the site on the building line to make the hospital blend with the urban context. The choice of a narrow block means that the building has few indoor rooms. By separating the various units from one another by soft instead of hard architectural boundaries, the various units can be shifted in terms of one another. This use of space that is in theory multifunctional is to promote flexibility. The physical appearance of the hospital is determined to a large extent by the play of the horizontal lines and the vertical columns and disks of the supporting construction.

The trend towards the formation of clusters of specialisations with the corresponding facilities continued in both existing and newly designed hospitals. This enables a more patient-orientated form of care. An example of this is the Medisch Centrum Leeuwarden (MCL) by Architecten aan de Maas in cooperation with Bonnema Architecten.

The hospital of the twenty-first century

While an intensive search went on for alterative ways of making hospitals more flexible, it became clear that more drastic innovations were inevitable. That changes were taking place that called for a reaction was also generally recognised in the world of architects. To celebrate its twenty-fifth anniversary in 1997, the Foundation for Architects Research on Health Care Buildings (Stagg) issued a call for submissions focused on the future position of the hospital. The resulting twenty-two entries were published in *Zorg voor morgen* (Care for tomorrow).[2] The assignment was to think up a future care landscape encompassing the whole health sector (hospitals, nursing homes, specialised clinics, homes for those with a handicap, etc.). The designers were free to confine themselves to one aspect, but could also design it in combination with other aspects.

A number of experts from the field offered their views on the future of health care as the starting point. It was expected that, as a result of the developments in medical technology, a smaller, high tech core hospital would be left. After a short stay there, the patients would be transferred to other provisions. Municipal or regional treatment centres (satellites) would be set up for outpatient assistance and day treatment. The outpatient units became larger and continued to form a part of the organisation of the hospital (without necessarily forming a physical part of it), and the importance of smaller-scale care provisions that need to form either an organisational or a physical part of a hospital increased. 'Options will become available. Light forms of hospital-related care can also be delivered in care hotels (*zotels*), in sick bays or at home in cooperation with home care organisations.'[3] R.B.M.R. Bakker (physician and medical director of the Westeinde Ziekenhuis in The Hague) expected the hospital to be increasingly used as a shopping centre. The distinction between shopping street and hospital would become blurred.

A more important trend was the organisation of hospitals around medical processes rather than medical functions. Different categories of patients follow personalised courses of treatment, by which this trend results in the identification of specific groups. The medical specialisations are ideally distributed among these groups, so that the hospital becomes divided into specialised clusters. Although it was not to be

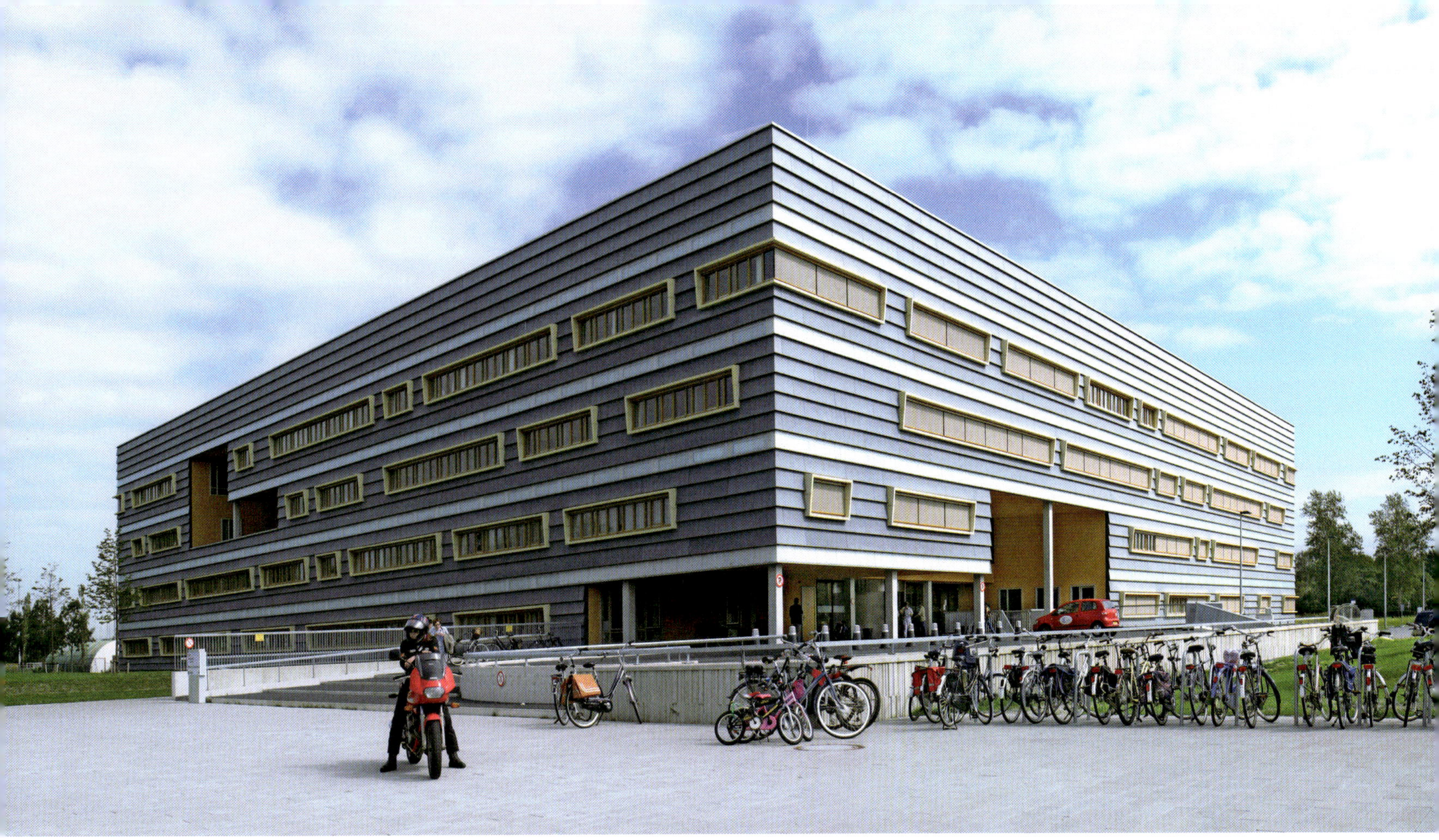

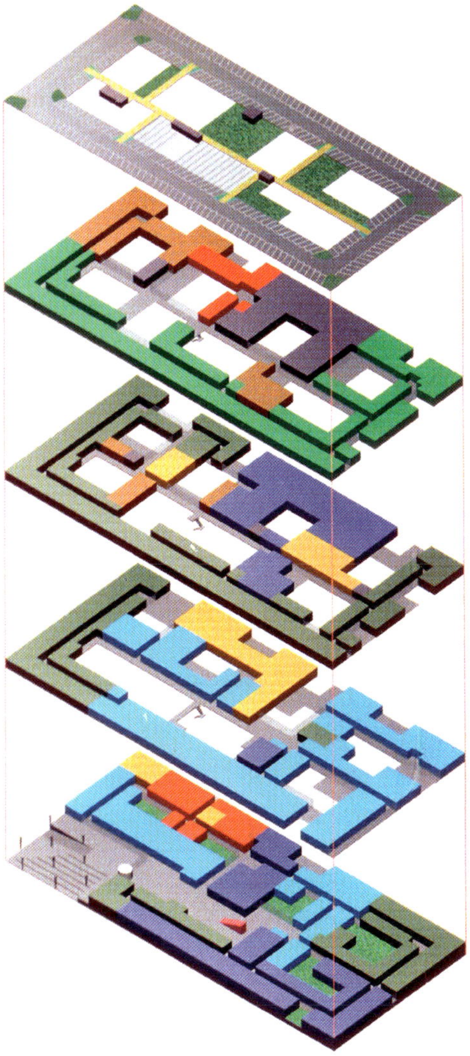

***EGM architecten*, Kennemer Gasthuis, Haarlem, 1998-2006**

***EGM architecten*, Kennemer Gasthuis, Haarlem, 1998-2006. Lay-out.**

- *patient accommodation*
- *medical care: examination*
- *medical care: treatment*
- *paramedical care*
- *management and training*
- *civil and technical service*
- *staff units*
- *technology*

***Architecten aan de Maas*, Medisch Centrum Leeuwarden (MCL), Leeuwarden, 2004**

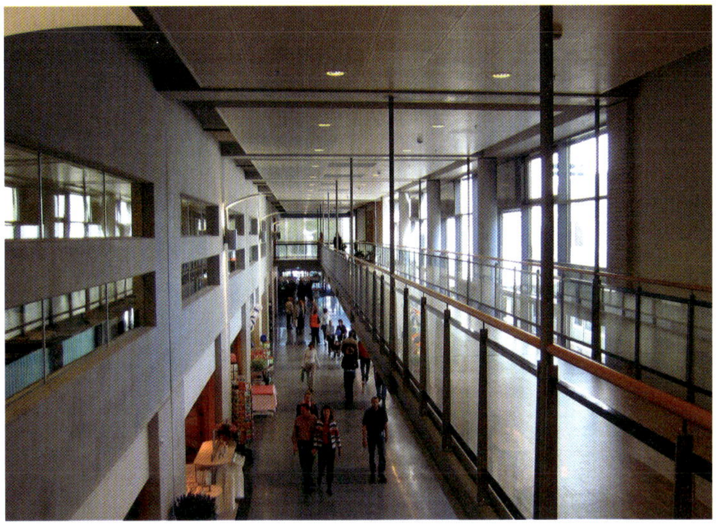

expected that the specialisations would be abandoned as an ordering principle, the clinical, outpatient and auxiliary functions would be telescoped. This should be reflected in the architecture of the hospital, for example by connecting the outpatient consultation and treatment areas with the clinical units of the same care cluster.[4]

The designers followed the future scenarios that the experts unfolded. They gave the predictions a programmatic, urban planning and architectural dimension. The term 'distribution planning' was launched for their approach: 'Which provisions are necessary, and how should they be distributed?'[5] The predictions were most explicitly visualised in 'Overstagg', the design by EGM architecten. It indicated that the care landscape would consists of three sectors by 2015: a high-care intervention centre, outpatient treatment centres, and housing provisions.

The seriousness of the predicted revolution in hospital architecture became clear from the ministerial decision to freeze a number of large-scale new building and renovation plans for hospitals until the beginning of the following century. In 1997 these hospitals received letters from the Minister of Public Health, E. Borst, stating that 'in studying the projects submitted, it is striking that they in fact elaborate on the existing and familiar concept of a hospital'.[6] She first wanted research to be conducted on whether the traditional hospital would still be able to adapt to the changes that could already be discerned in health care. 'Continuing along the well-trodden path leads to hospitals that are already out of date the minute they are completed', the minister expected.[7]

This pause for thought lasted no longer than two years. A national study tour of twenty-five hospitals with at least 250 beds revealed that the field found the regulations too rigid and too slow.[8] It was not practical to wait for the introduction of a new system, but it was also clear that the regulation of supply would not be reconcilable with the mechanisms of a freer market, and would thus have to be replaced. The first years of the twenty-first century were a period of thought experiments to comprehend the consequences for the architecture of health care.

p. 238
***EGM architecten*, design submission Stagg jubilee, 1997, motto 'Overstagg'**

p. 239
***Soeters Van Eldonk Ponec Architecten*, social-cultural centre at the Willem Arntsz Hoeve (Altrecht Foundation), Den Dolder, 2001**

***Paul van Beek*, plan of terrain lay-out for the Willem Arntsz Hoeve, Den Dolder, 1995**

***Paul van Beek*, garden plan around socio-cultural centre at the Willem Arntsz Hoeve, Den Dolder, 1995**

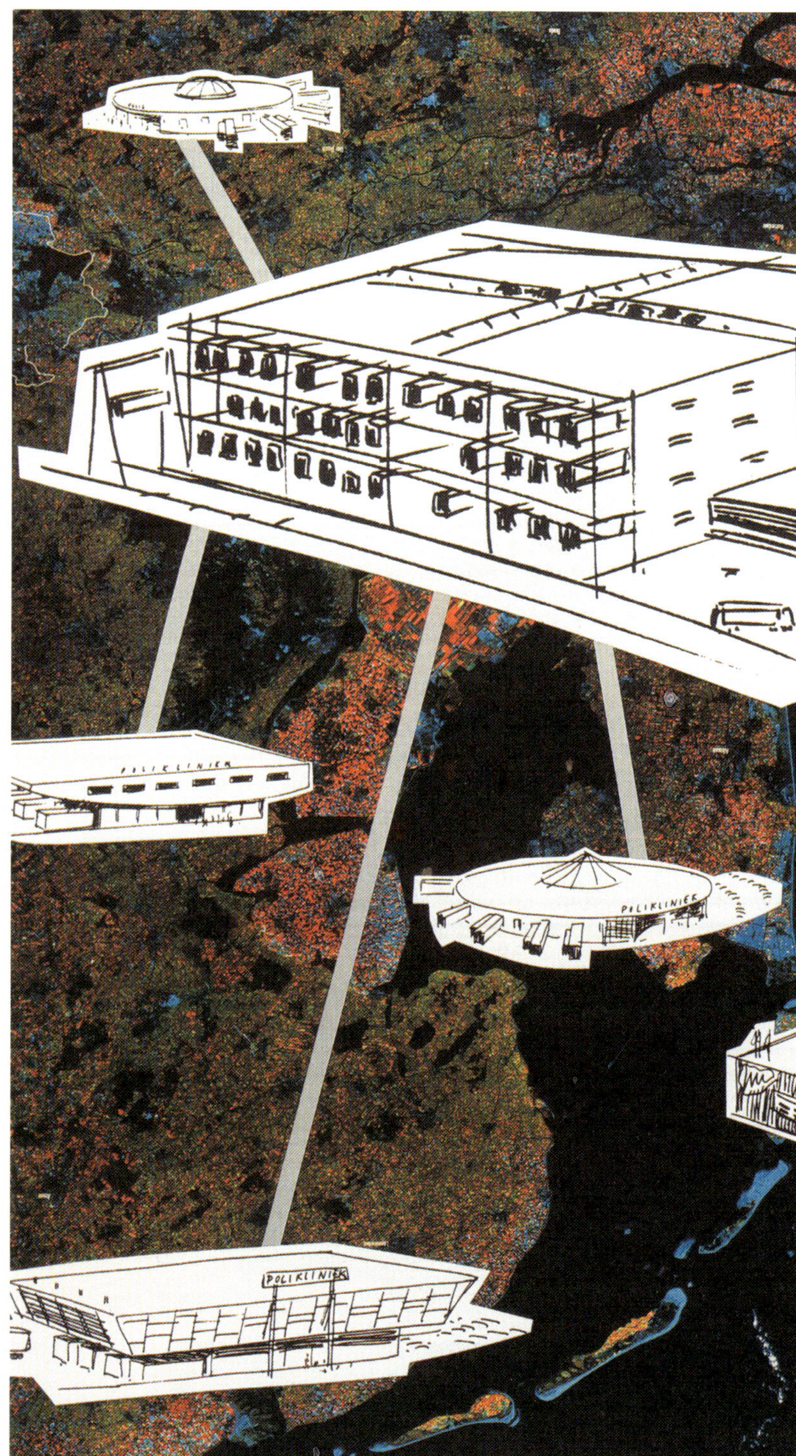

Psychiatry

In psychiatry the emphasis came to lie on ambulant and short-term care. Regionalisation became more important, as the formation of the Regional Institutes for Mental Welfare (RIAGG) and the Regional Institutions for Sheltered Forms of Housing (RIBW) in the middle of the 1980s had already underlined. While new small-scale facilities emerged in the cities, many of the classic asylums were abandoned. Nowhere were the consequences of the policy that had been implemented in the preceding years clearer than here. The 1980s were a decade of organisation, reorganisation, concentration and specialisation. Arbitrariness, chaos, lack of direction and even a certain need to settle accounts with the buildings of the past seem to have determined the appearance of many a psychiatric hospital. At the beginning of the 1990s many institutions looked like a battlefield after the battle. The main challenge in architecture and urban planning in this decade was that of reconstruction, of introducing order into the chaos.

The big cleaning up operation

The big cleaning up operation of old psychiatric hospitals got under way in the 1990s. Until the 1970s the transformations of the old institutions had been characterised by processes of densification and fragmentation, followed by the exodus. What was left were the chronic psychiatric patients who needed intensive assistance and those groups that could not be accommodated outside the institutions. If they were transferred to other institutions as well, that meant the end of the classic asylum. This was the case in Santpoort, which gradually turned into a ghost town after 1 April 1991.[9] The new clinics designed by Greiner en Van Goor, some of which had only just opened, also closed their doors. A network of small-scale institutions, in which the Valeriuskliniek and the Psychiatrisch Centrum Amsterdam formed important centres, took over their task. Almost all facilities were integrated in the residential environment, and most of them had been newly designed since the second half of the 1980s.

The Willem Arntsz Hoeve, by now a part of the Altrecht Foundation, also saw a large number of its functions transferred to small-scale institutions in the city, although a number of core activities were still located in the old grounds. This created the need for restructuring, because here too most of the original structure had gone. If the institution wanted a new, clearly visible spatial organisation, that called for a targeted injection. This was found in the building of a new socio-cultural centre with a building for psychomotoric therapy. The design was by Soeters Van Eldonk Ponec (now Soeters Van Eldonk architecten). It consists of three separate volumes for the gym rooms, activity rooms and offices respectively. The office building has two floors. Behind it are two tapering volumes, one for sports and therapy rooms, the other for creative functions such as workshops and a theatre. A light well in the office building links the three components of the design. The

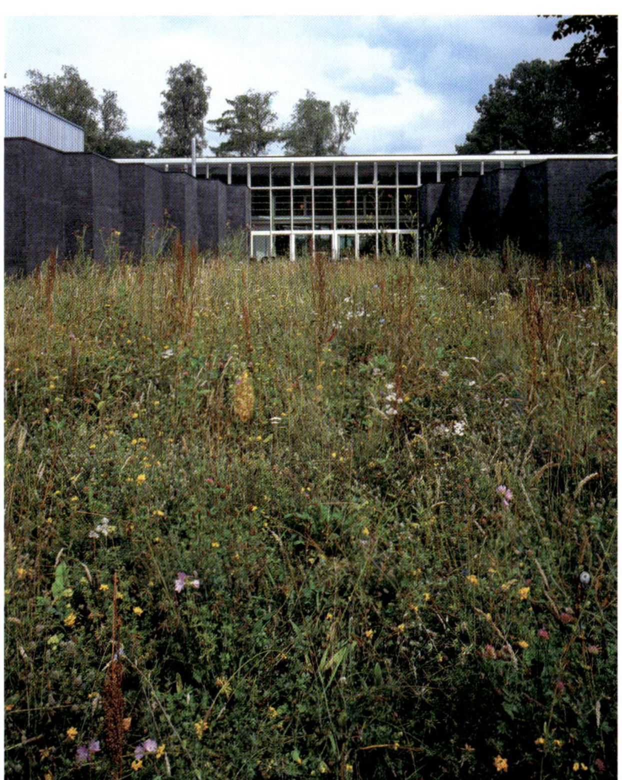

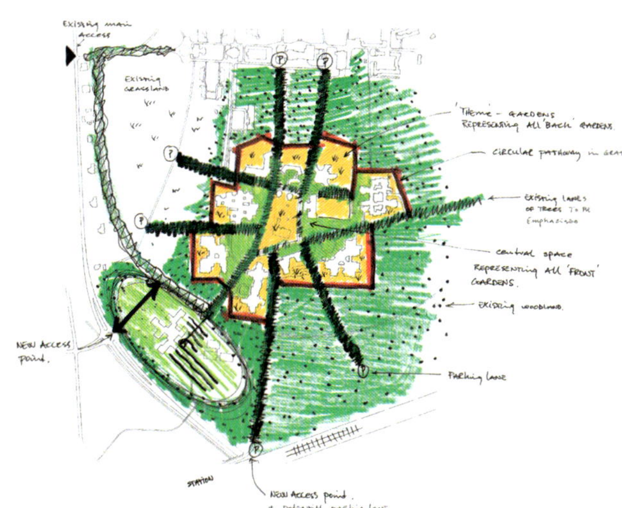

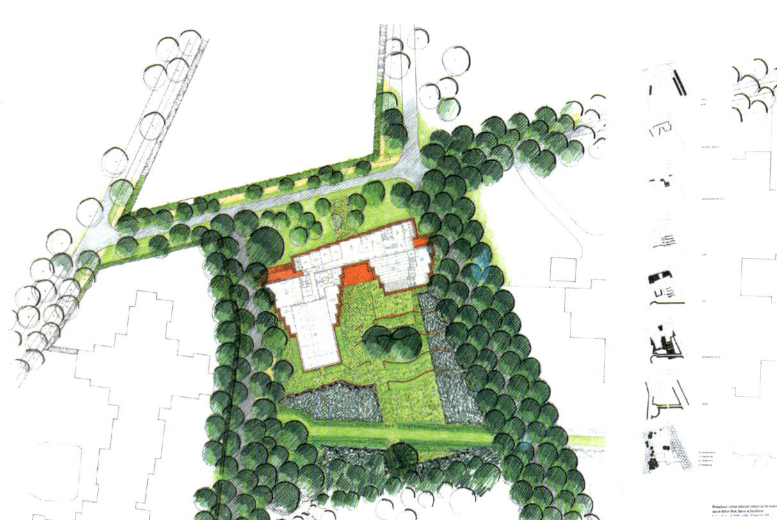

complex forms the core of a master plan for the reorganisation of the terrain drawn up by Paul van Beek.[10]

The psychiatric hospital in Goes did not escape the need for restructuring either. Here too this led to the transfer of functions connected with non-chronic patients and to a concentration on patients for whom a return to society or care in less restrictive facilities for short-term or ambulant care or in sheltered forms of accommodation were not an option. The existing buildings were not considered suitable for this group. Mecanoo was invited to submit a proposal. Their U-shaped building referred to the typology of the medieval cluster of almshouses. The more public functions (living rooms for the residential groups, kitchens) are adjacent to a corridor around an enclosed garden, while the private rooms (bedrooms) are situated on the outside.[11]

Another relatively new institution that was dismantled is the Sint Franciscushof in Raalte, which had been designed in the 1950s and had grown to become a model institution. The decision was taken in the 1990s to move from the rural idyll of the countryside of Overijssel to the city, in this case Zwolle, where the institution shared premises with the RIAGG and the RIBW in the hope that this would lead to a complete merger. When this ran aground in 1998, the institution was faced with the choice of continuing as a psychiatric hospital or changing direction and turning itself into an ambulant care institution. The latter was preferred, and since the late 1990s every effort has been devoted to that ambulant transformation.[12]

The cleaning up of the Delta psychiatric hospital in Poortugaal is also noteworthy. The old buildings and the historic planning structure were almost completely eradicated. The original idea of new buildings on the old location, which was still defended in 1988, was dropped here too. As a result of the regionalisation, the Delta had to target an area of care that was partly new: instead of serving some of the patients from the whole Rotterdam region, the care was now concentrated on the southern districts of Rotterdam and the islands of the province of South Holland. Consequently, Delta transferred a large part of its activities to locations in this region in the early 1990s. Facilities for short-term and ambulant care were set up in South Rotterdam and Hellevoetsluis, including two extramural outpatient units and two multifunctional units (MFE).[13] An ambitious reconstruction plan for the Delta psychiatric hospital in Poortugaal was begun in 1993. The institution entered a second life on the basis of an urban development plan drawn up by de Jong Gortemaker architecten en ingenieurs (now de Jong Gortemaker Algra architecten en ingenieurs) and a landscape design by Stijlgroep that won an award in 2000.

By the early 1990s there was little left of the clear structure of the Delta psychiatric hospital in Poortugaal that had been set up as Maasoord at the beginning of the twentieth century. The process of demolition and new building had completely transformed the appearance of the complex. The visible axis from the main building to the Oude Maas had practically disappeared, the main building itself had been demolished, and so had most of the original pavilions. The garden, in fact a large park, no longer had any connection with the buildings that sprang up here and there. The complex was thereby an extreme example of the process of fragmentation and disintegration. The urban development plan envisages a new axis on which the most important new buildings will be situated. The building with facilities for patients and the administration building mark both the structural plan and the landscape architecture, thereby restoring the lost unity without imitating the original layout. The new Delta looks like a very spaciously laid out suburban residential district and is barely recognisable as a psychiatric hospital.

Buildings for short-term and ambulant care

The multifunctional unit (MFE) was set up around 1990 for short-term and ambulant mental health care. The term does not have a clear definition and many institutions that share its main characteristics are nevertheless given different names: psychiatric centre, mental health care centre (*GGZ-centrum*), etc. Nowadays it is more common to speak of the Regional Mental Health Centre (RGC). In 1994 the Stagg investigated a number of the centres that had been set up and outlined three models on the basis of that investigation: a concentrated multifunctional unit in which all the functions are combined in a fairly large building; a deconcentrated variant in which various buildings are situated on different but proximate locations; and a small-scale solution that concentrates treatment and accommodation functions in a building but keeps them separate. Reference was often made to the hotel to characterise the atmosphere, which seems to have become an increasingly important source of inspiration. It was expected that the future multifunctional unit would have only single rooms. Soon after its release, the Stagg report was commented on in numerous articles, but the general purport was still the conviction that the rise of the multifunctional unit was unstoppable by now. The architectural and urban planning aspects received little comment, although the principle of the maximal integration in the urban fabric was tacitly accepted. This meant that the location helped to determine the design. 'In terms of urban design', Roelof Gortemaker remarked, 'the multifunctional unit seems to be a chameleon, a block of flats in a residential district, a hospital wing in a hospital. The multifunctional unit as such does not exist'.[14]

What they at any rate have in common is the endeavour to integrate ambulant, clinical and outpatient care, a preference for a location on the site of or in the immediate vicinity of a general hospital, and accommodation designed to look as normal as possible. For instance, the doors of the residential units in the open sections are usually in the public area, and only the closed sections are separated from them. Although the dimensions are usually modest – some forty beds – the rediscovery of architecture as the medium that adds value can nowhere be seen more clearly than in the multifunctional unit. The added value exceeds the purely aesthetic and representative aspects and is intended to contribute to the actual functioning of these institutions.

When the psychiatric centre in Oosterhout designed by Greiner en Van Goor Architecten (now Greiner Van Goor Huijten Architecten) opened its doors in 1990, the term multifunctional unit was not yet common currency; when it became a household word a few years later, the complex in Oosterhout was regarded as one of the first to comply with the basic principles of the multifunctional unit. The institution was on a relatively small scale, integration of different forms of treatment was part of the programme, and the living quarters and treatment units were both physically and organisationally separate from one another. It illustrates the attempt of existing psychiatric hospitals to decentralise. It is one of the three complexes that replaces a classic asylum, the Sint Antonius in Etten-Leur. In accordance with the principles of the Boston model, which keeps therapy and accommodation separate from one another, the treatment unit is housed in a separate volume.

The building that was completed in Schagen in 1992 is by

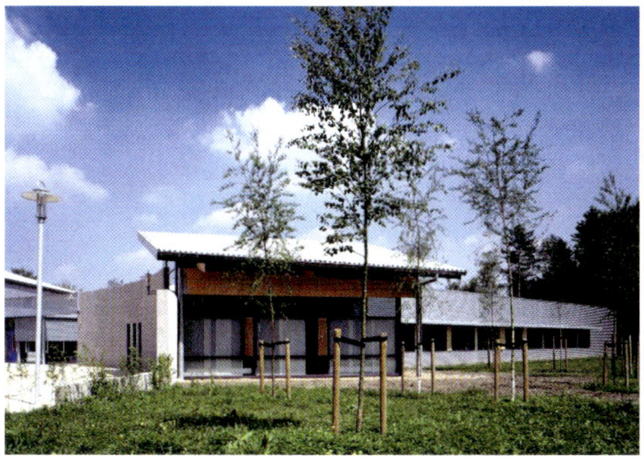

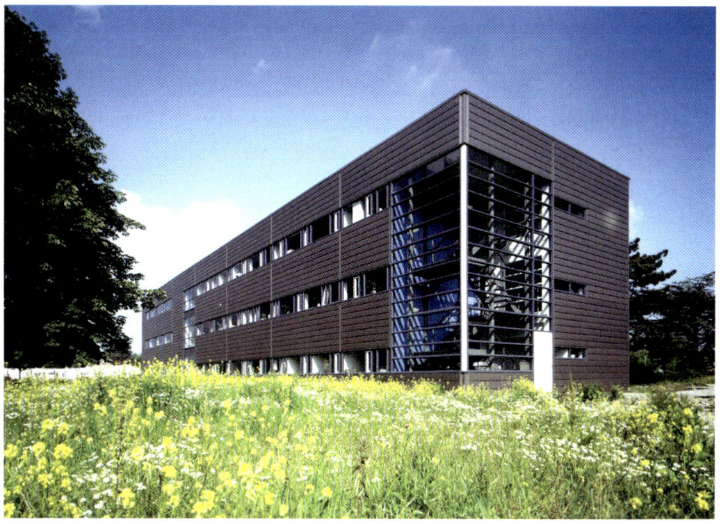

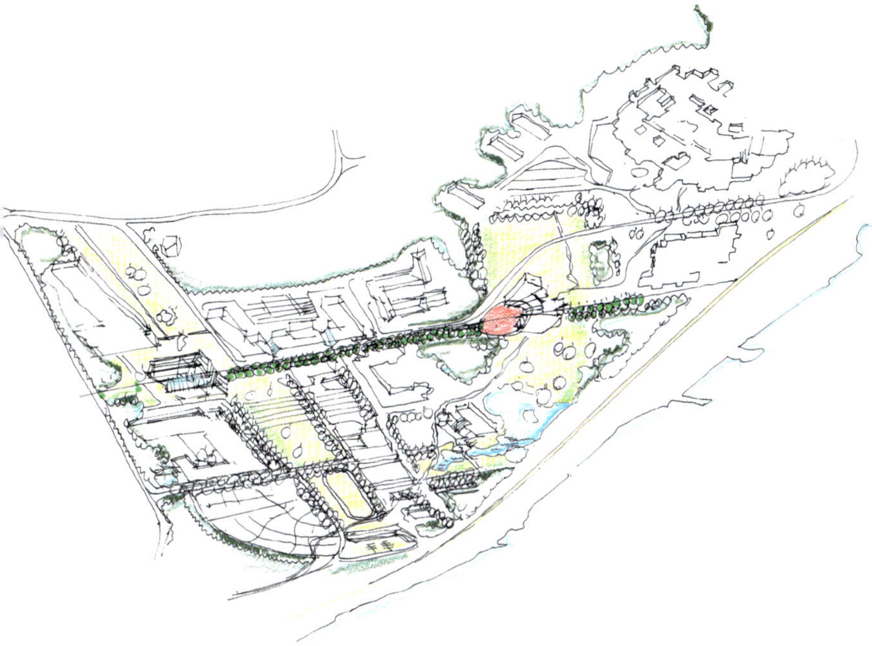

p. 241 | <
***de Jong Gortemaker architecten en ingenieurs*, social-cultural centre and structural plan Delta psychiatric hospital, Poortugaal, 1992**

p. 241 | >
***de Jong Gortemaker architecten en ingenieurs*, administration building, Delta psychiatric hospital, Poortugaal, 1999**

***Delta psychiatric hospital*, Poortugaal, with the work and activity centre (Kruisheer Elffers Architecten) beside the new visual axis**

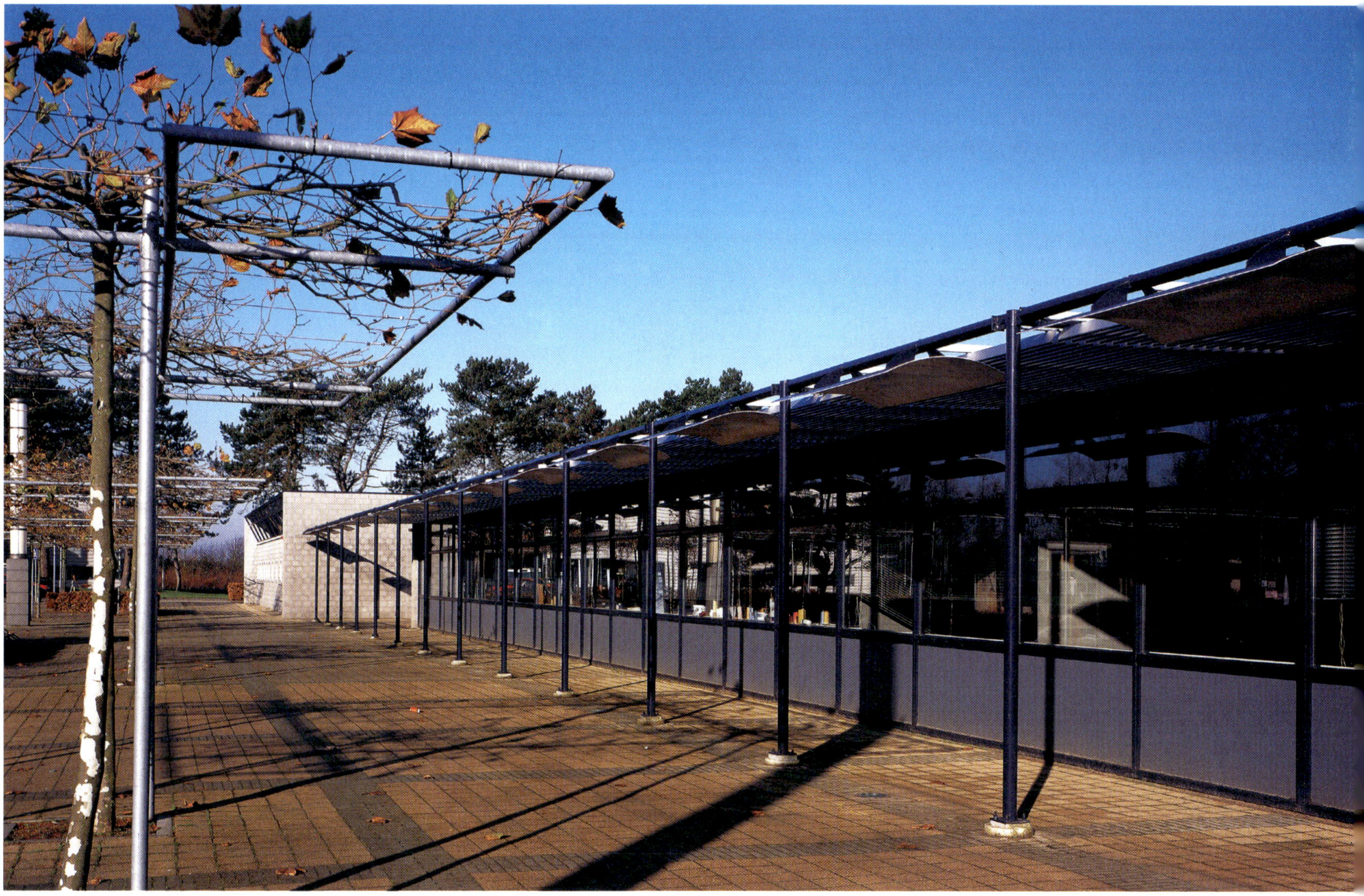

the same firm of Greiner en Van Goor. Unconventionally, it is not linked with a hospital. It consists of two buildings: a T-shaped treatment unit in front of an accommodation block around a rectangular area. The stem of the T forms the link and extends to the enclosed garden. Daylight and maximal visual transparency were important parameters in the design and resulted in an airy, friendly complex.

With the transfer of the Drentse Dennenoord to the city of Groningen, in accordance with a design by Klaas Paul de Boer and Team 4 Architecten, the enclosed terrain on which the complex is situated was transformed into a semi-public district of the city. Intimacy and openness go hand in hand, but the pressure of the city is always nearby. The grand gesture of the new hospital consists of the internal main structure that is visible everywhere: two inner streets at right angles to one another that can be recognised from inside and from outside by the two brightly coloured walls that run straight through the building and intersect. These orientation walls create a kind of street – if you follow them you always reach an exit. The murals are by the artist Pieter Bijwaard. The wall with an East-West orientation has a sky blue basic layer, the North-South wall has a yellow one.

In 1995 Hans Liscaljet from Architectengroep Duintjer (now de Jong Gortemaker Algra architecten en ingenieurs) put forward a plan for the Hoorn Mental Health Care Centre, which was connected with the new Westfries Gasthuis. Together with the psychiatric hospital Duin en Bosch and several other institutions, this hospital was responsible for the project. The three-storey treatment building has outpatient units on the ground and first floors, while treatment and administration are on the third floor. This part has the basic shape of an apostrophe; the terrain on the inside is occupied by the living quarters separated by two patios. The main entrance is located in the tail of the apostrophe. A connecting corridor provides the link with the hospital.

The multifunctional unit De Opmaat, a design by IAA Architecten, was opened in Hengelo in 1996. The psychiatric hospital Helmerzijde, the local RIAGG and RIBW, and the General Hospital Psychiatric Unit (PAAZ) of the Streekziekenhuis Midden Twente are the main partners supporting this initiative. It is therefore a typical example of the functional combining of regional institutions that is so characteristic of the formation of multifunctional units. De Opmaat has seventy-two clinical and thirty-two part-time treatment places as well as an outpatients unit and ambulant care facilities. Form followed function: the plan developed in 1993 distinguishes a treatment unit, closed accommodation, open accommodation, and various auxiliary functions. De Opmaat has rooms for six or four persons as well as single rooms. A partly covered corridor separates the living quarters from the treatment unit; the different functions are accentuated by differences in the use of colour and the shape of the roof.[15]

With its capacity of 122, De Riethorst near Ede, a design by Architectengroep Duintjer (project architect Joost Koldeweij, now Architectenbureau Koldeweij) is larger than most multifunctional units, but accommodates the same functions and is situated near a hospital, the Gelderse Vallei. The treatment unit and accommodation are separated; the shape of the curving, three-storey treatment building is repeated by the accommodation block behind it, though the latter has a sharp bend instead of a gentle curve. The hospital is connected with the treatment unit by means of an underground passageway.

Delta Spijkenisse is one of the institutions that have largely replaced the old central hospital in Poortugaal. It is a fairly large multifunctional unit in which EGM architecten clearly marked the division between living quarters and therapy building that is characteristic of the first generation of multifunctional units. The accommodation is situated on the lowest part of the grounds beside the water, while the treatment building functions as a screen to protect the complex from the bustle of the street. The 'village square' in between separates the two parts and obliges the residents

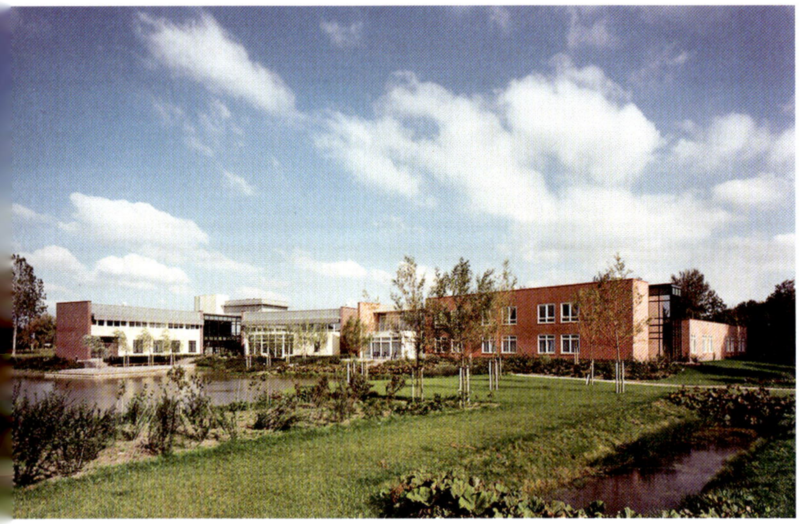

Onno Greiner en Martien van Goor Architekten, De Geestercogge mental health care centre, Schagen, 1997

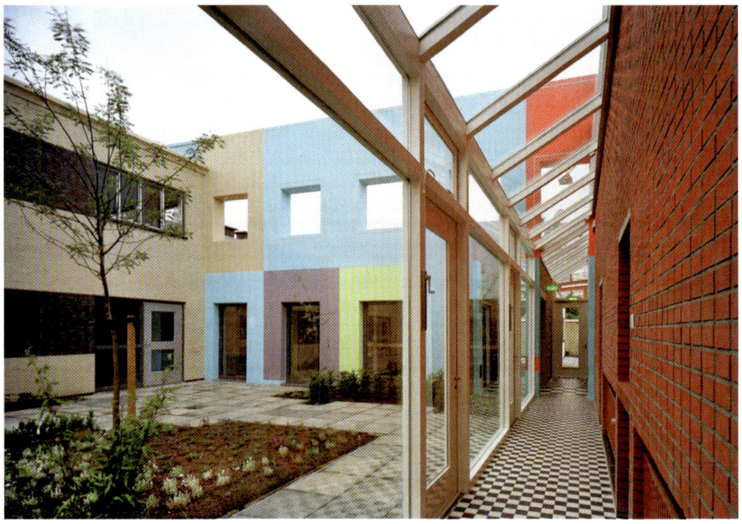

Team 4 Architecten, Dennenoord psychiatric hospital, Groningen, 1995

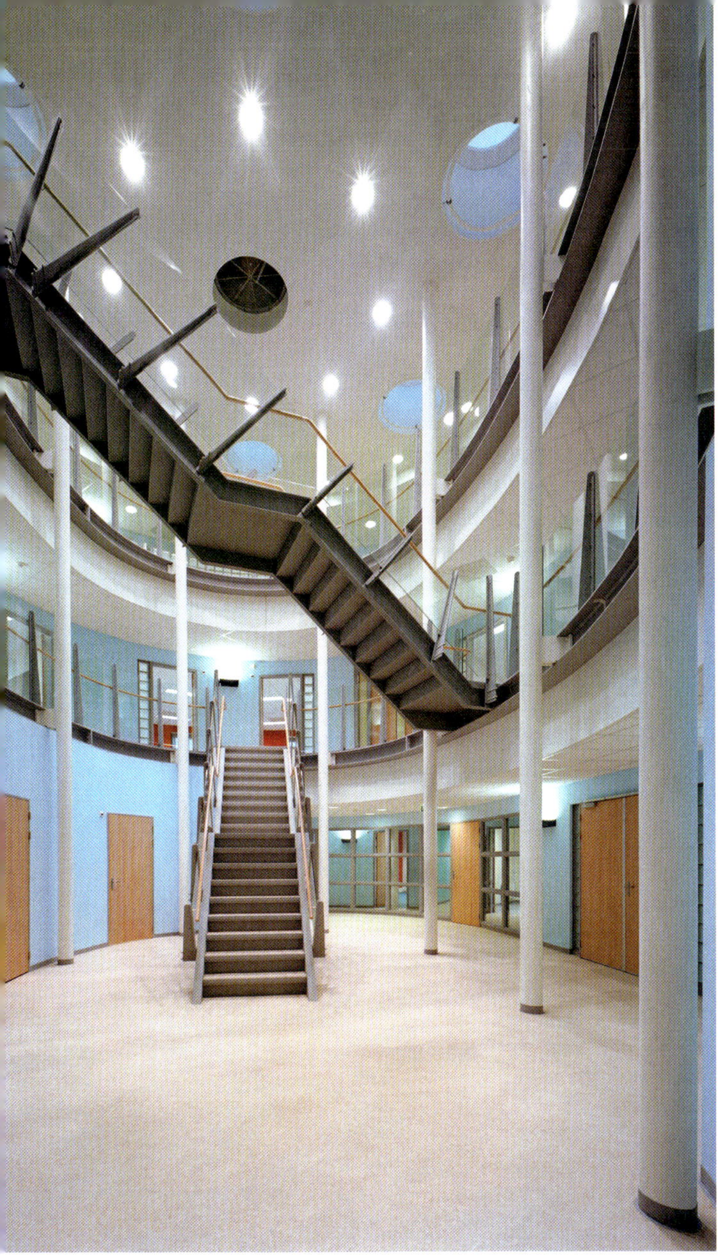

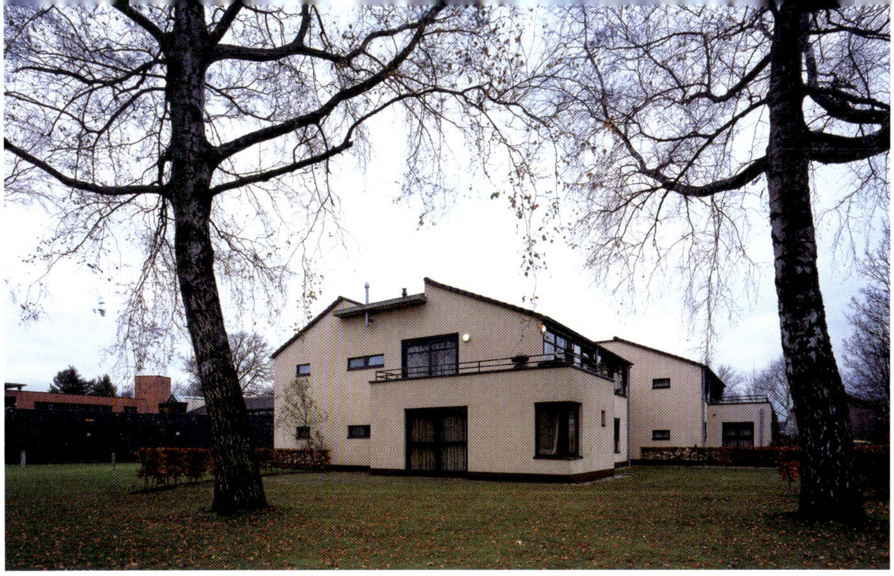

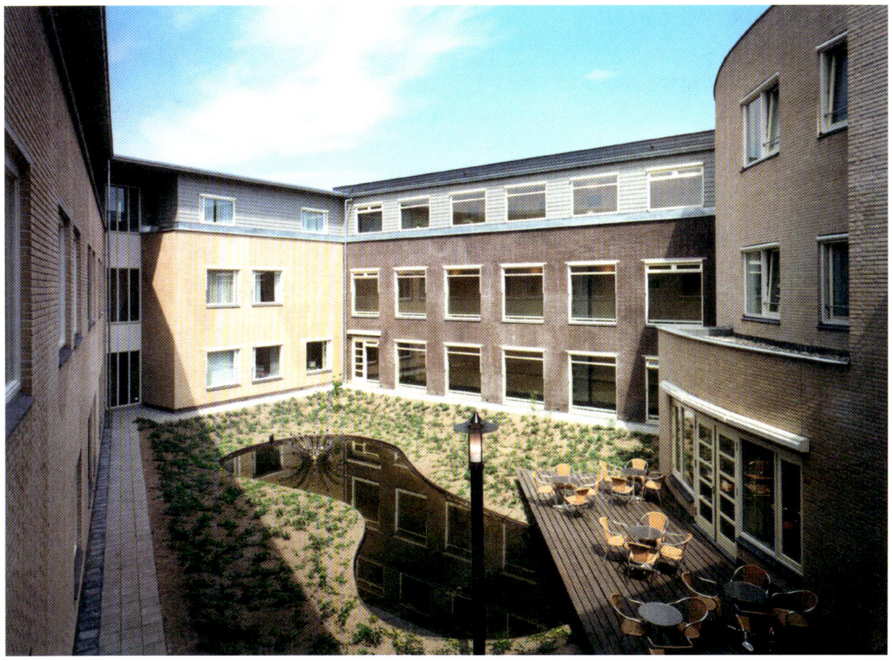

Architectengroep Duintjer, Westfriesland mental health care centre, Hoorn, 2003

IAA Architecten, De Opmaat multifunctional unit (MFE), Hengelo, 1993–1996

Architectengroep Duintjer, De Riethorst mental health care centre, Ede, 2000

EGM architecten, multi-functional unit (MFE) Delta psychiatric hospital, Spijkenisse, 2003

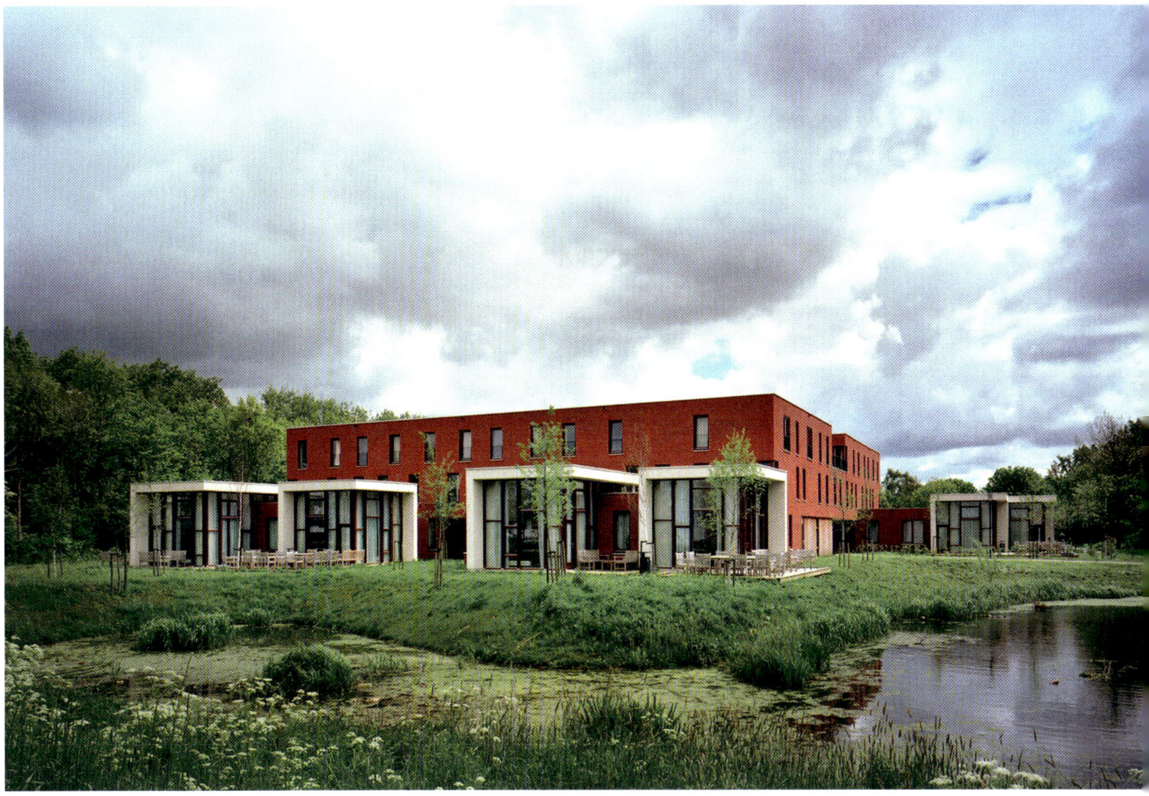

to cross a (semi-)public area whenever they want to visit the therapy rooms. Both volumes have three storeys; the accommodation building can be divided up flexibly so that the size of the group can vary between twelve and forty-eight patients.

The designs by the Alberts & Van Huut are immediately recognisable by their characteristic idiom of form. Based on an anthroposophical ideology, this firm resists the dictatorship of the right angle. 'Looser, freer, so-called "organic" forms give people a friendlier and more harmonious feeling. They determine to a large extent our intuitive development.'[16] The products of this vision include the second stage of the Hafakker in Noordwijkerhout, as well as Triversum, a centre for child and youth psychiatry in Alkmaar (awarded the Care Vision Excellence Trophy in 1996) and a multifunctional unit in Lelystad, psychiatric centre Meerzicht.

Special provisions

Besides the multifunctional units, there were always other provisions needed too. De Jong Gortemaker architecten en ingenieurs designed the general psychiatric hospital for South-East Friesland in Heerenveen which, in spite of its name, is by no means a classic institution, but has many of the features of a multifunctional unit. Unconventionally, this complex has accommodation for chronic patients and therefore has a fairly large number of beds: eighty-eight. The complex is situated on the edge of a residential district on the historic site of the former Thialf Stadium and is separated into two parts. The dayrooms and bedrooms match the architecture of the residential district in their texture and use of colour, while the treatment unit matches those of the neighbouring Tjongerschans Ziekenhuis. A characteristic feature of this complex is the separation between the parts for chronic patients and the units for acute cases. This separation is fairly hard because a wide boulevard passes in between the two parts.

De Jutter, a centre for child and youth psychiatry in The Hague, is an example of a special provision for which there is still a need besides the multifunctional units. It comprises three elongated, slightly curving volumes that enclose a triangular garden. The two residential wings were designed by Eric Wendel of EGM architecten as comb structures; the parts fanning outwards contain the bedrooms and the communal living room is adjacent to the enclosed garden. The third wing contains the treatment unit and the school. The children's hospital was erected on the location of the former Rode Kruis Ziekenhuis in The Hague and lies between the dunes and the city; the visual features of dune, beach and sea were one of the sources of inspiration for the plan, such as in the colourful storage rooms that look like beach huts.

Delta Pendrecht has a resocialisation unit for thirty-two patients to prepare them for their return to normal society. EGM architecten designed an elongated building for the residential groups and a special feature at the end in the form of a dark brick volume that houses the various services. This volume at the end of the building is next to the Slinge, a busy shopping street, and protects the residents from it. The simple complex blends imperceptibly into the layout of the Pendrecht district, which dates from the 1950s; in the meantime this district has been largely renovated, but its original features can still be recognised.

Another special provision is the forensic psychiatric clinic. These are clinics for psychiatric criminals who are sentenced by a magistrate to undergo detention and

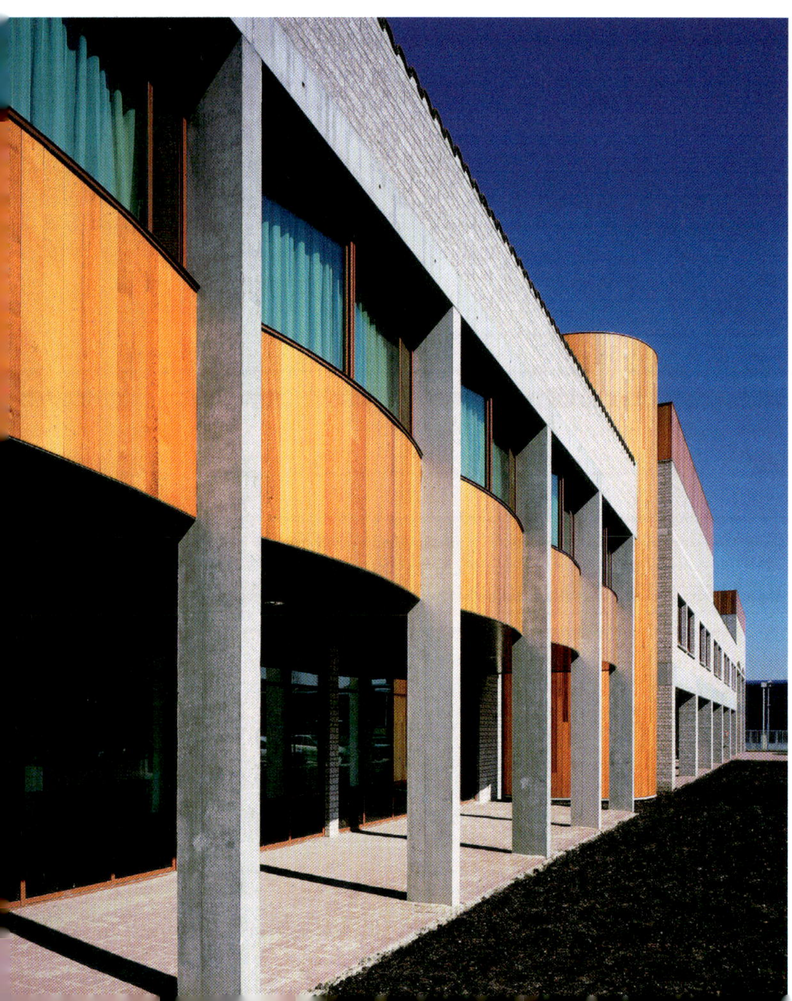

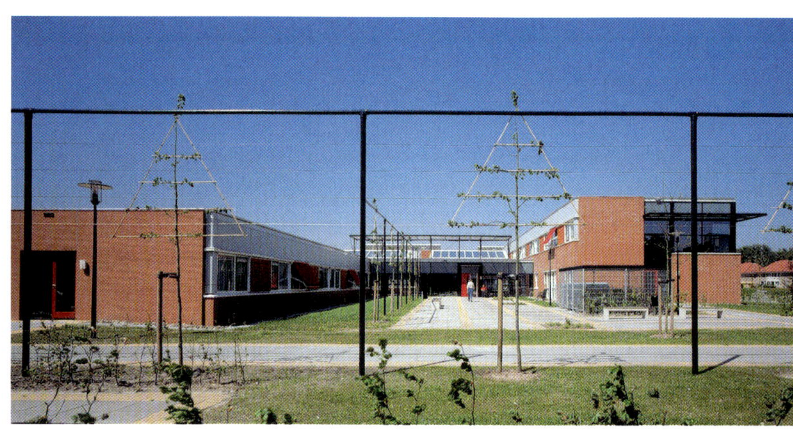

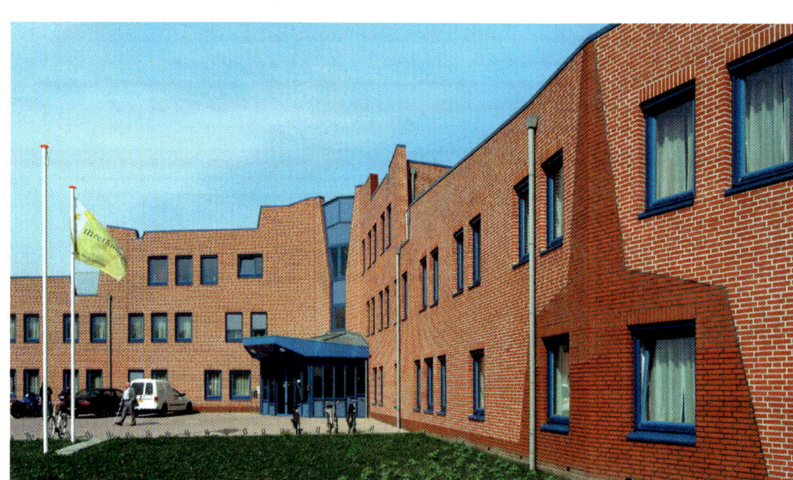

treatment. Forensic patients form a problem group. Prisons are not the place for them because they are usually severely disturbed and can make life impossible for themselves, their fellow prisoners and the staff. Moreover, prisons do not offer psychiatric treatment, while such treatment can have beneficial effects on this category. Nor are they easy to keep in psychiatric hospitals. Not only can they form a threat to their fellow inmates, but there may also be a danger of their escape, in which case they also pose a risk to the society from which they have been removed for a reason. Since the end of the 1980s there has been a building wave of new forensic psychiatric clinics. A striking example is De Meren in Amsterdam, designed by Han Westelaken from Architecten aan de Maas. The complex was built for 102 patients who were accommodated in a number of V-shaped blocks. As in every forensic institution, the motto here was that the closed units must be low in stimuli. That is why the private rooms (the bedrooms) overlook not the public highway but a canal, the Weespertrekvaart. The living rooms are next to the main volume containing the treatment units.

The architect managed to avoid prison-like fencing, for example by making the roof overhangs so big that it is impossible to climb onto the roof. His points of reference did not include prisons either. 'He had in mind the monasteries that he knew, the ruins of the Minoan palaces that he had once seen on Crete, the buildings designed by the Benedictine architect Hans van der Laan. He concluded: "The complex must be a place of reflection: the wood petrified in a building."'[17] The angle that Westelaken chose for De Meren therefore seems to underline the ambivalent character of forensic psychiatry: on the one hand the attempt to absorb the patients in the society to which they are supposed to return after treatment, on the other hand the view that they have to be kept separate, a wish that is motivated by the need to keep these patients out of regular society and by the therapeutic fact that, unlike most other mentally disturbed patients, they benefit from rest, quiet and an environment that is low in stimuli.

p. 244
***Architecten aan de Maas*, De Meren forensic psychiatric clinic, Amsterdam, 2001**

***de Jong Gortemaker architecten en ingenieurs*, general psychiatric hospital for South-East Friesland, Heerenveen, 1999**

***Alberts & Van Huut*, Meerzicht psychiatric centre, Lelystad, 2003**

p. 245
***EGM architecten*, Delta psychiatric hospital, resocialisation, Rotterdam-Pendrecht, 1998**

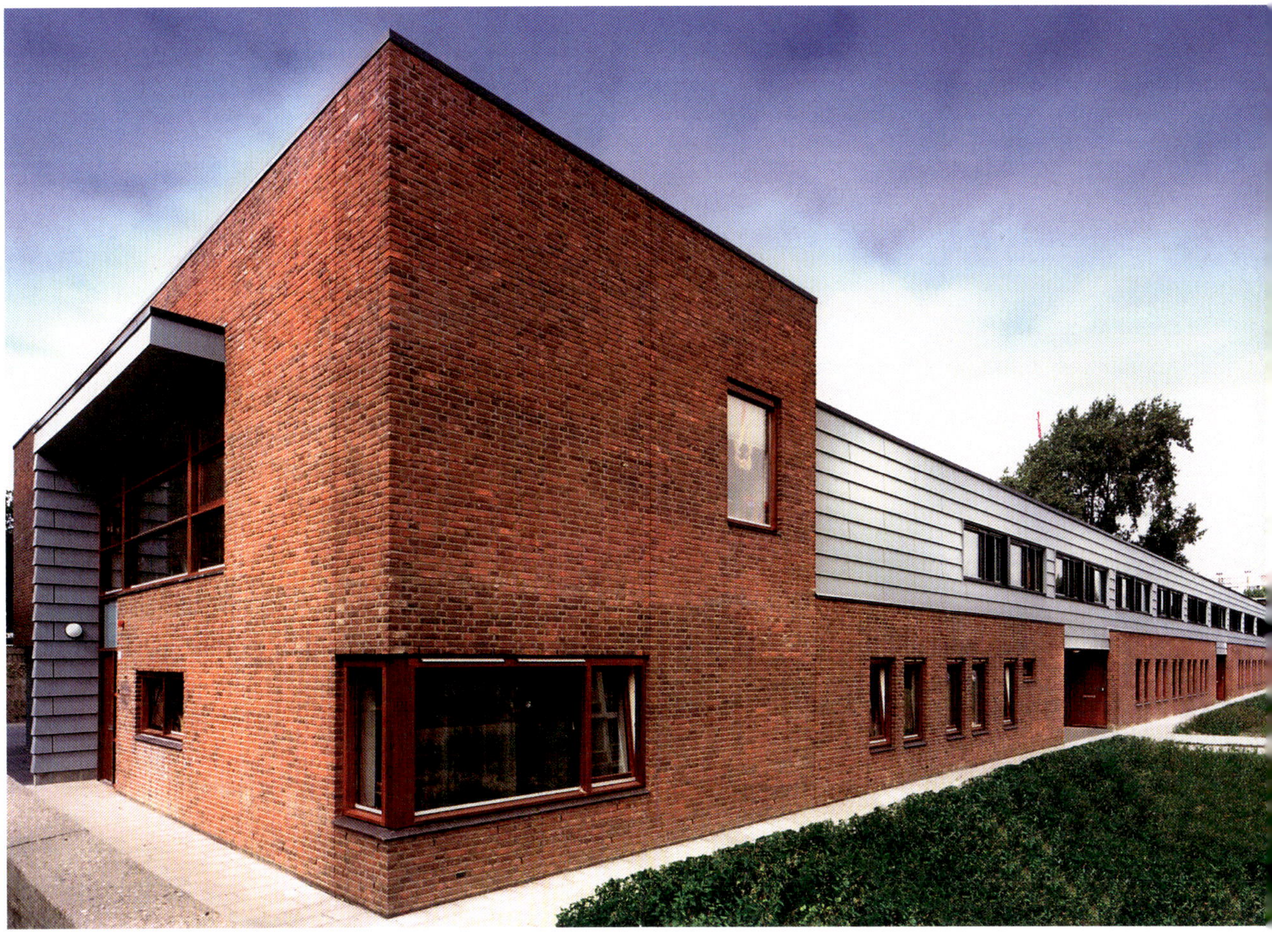

Housing and care for the elderly

Care for the elderly as it had evolved since 1945 used to have two components: domestic support and medical care. If the emphasis was on nursing, an institution was seen as a medical provision. Nursing homes therefore fell under a different ministry from the various forms of housing that offered only domestic support. The separation of care and housing presupposed a different organisation of care. The distinction between domestic and medical assistance became blurred and the entire range of care was entrusted to the Ministry of Welfare, Health and Cultural Affairs (WVC) and largely funded under the provisions of the Exceptional Medical Expenses Act (AWBZ). Housing only formed a part of this if it was impossible to separate housing from care. The report of the Care for the Elderly Modernisation Commission (Welschen Commission, 1993-1995) marked a breakthrough in the necessary reorganisation. In the light of the background of collective expenditure that was getting out of hand and would become even more insupportable because of the ageing of the population, the commission opted for the two-column model: care and housing would be separated from now on, and this would apply as far as possible to the organisation and funding as well. From now on the instance ultimately responsible for the provision and quality of the care was the health insurance company. 'The commission wants a building freeze of nursing homes to bring about a closer rapprochement between old people's home and nursing home so that the "housing component" will disappear by itself.'[18]

The Welschen Commission report triggered an even more far-reaching renewal of policy on the elderly. This operation was to be so drastic that the Dutch parliament even turned it into a major project comparable to large-scale infrastructural projects or the purchase of large quantities of military material. The major operation concluded the work that the Welschen Commission had begun. Many transitional measures and legal amendments fleshed out the principle of the separation of housing and care. The Social Support Act (WMO) transferred the responsibility for domestic assistance to the municipalities, who were assigned a key role in the new system as in other countries like Denmark. From now on care was almost entirely funded under the provisions of the AWBZ and some of the services provided outside the institutions were brought under the aegis of this regime. The implementation was decentralised in 1998 and left to regional care offices run by the health insurance companies. Finally, person-related budgets were introduced so that at least a part of the funding would no longer proceed via the institutions, but could ideally be managed directly by the 'client'. The separation of housing and care was first manifested in the so-called *wozoco* apartments for the elderly that combined housing and care in one complex. Although this type was an elaboration on the older generations of care homes, it nevertheless embodies an important step on the road towards the development of new types.

The nursing home

After having relinquished the housing component, nursing became the mainstay of care for the elderly. The classic nursing home was already making way for a more diversified range of provisions in the 1980s: small intramural provisions, small-scale residential forms with integrated nursing in which family-like situations were created, specific provisions for

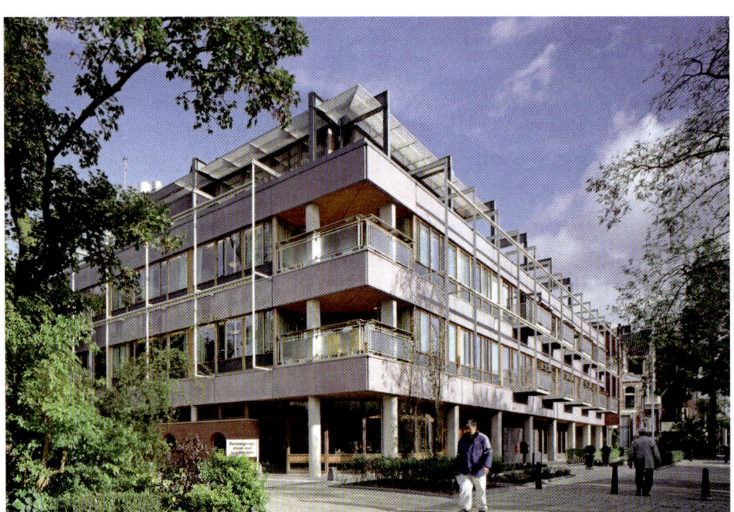

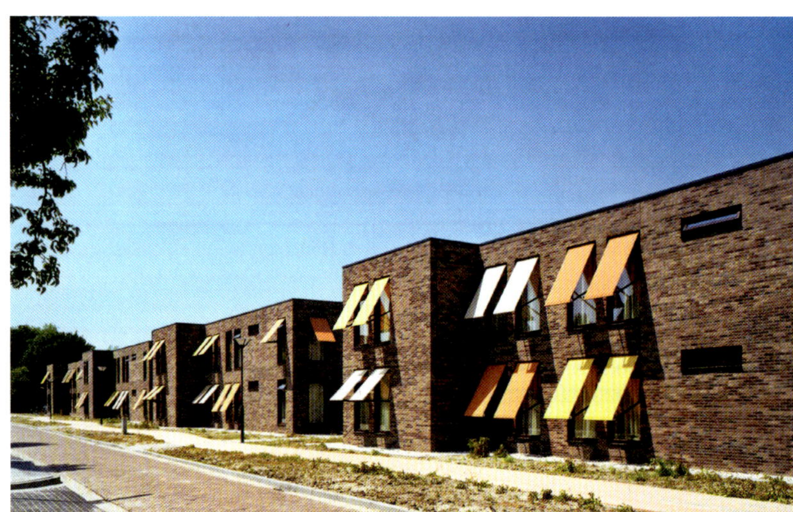

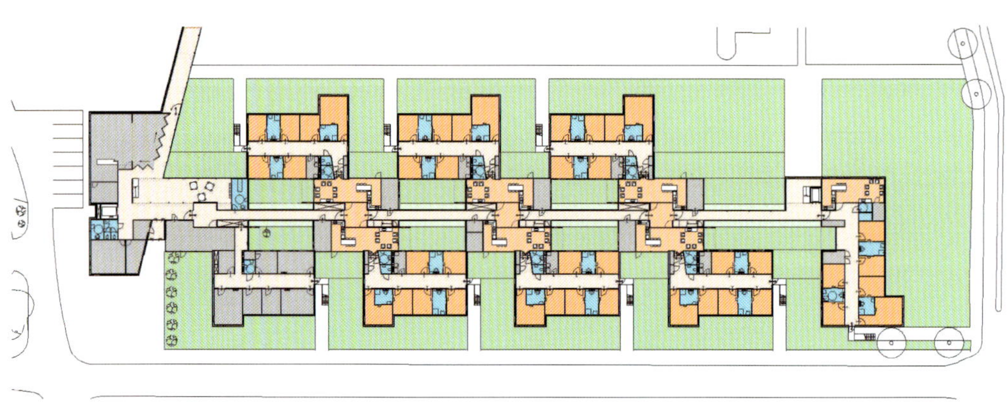

***Tjeerd Dijkstra*, nursing home for sixty somatic and sixty psycho-geriatric residents, Rotterdam-Kralingen, 1993**

***EGM architecten*, Ter Reede nursing home, Flushing, 2003**

De Nijl Architecten, Putselaan residential care complex, Rotterdam, 2000

EGM architecten, Bergweg complex, Rotterdam, 1993-1996

PBV Architecten, renovation Willem Drees-huis, The Hague, 1990

de architektengroep, Polderburen nursing home, Almere, 1995

EGM architecten, Bergweg complex, Rotterdam, 1993-1996

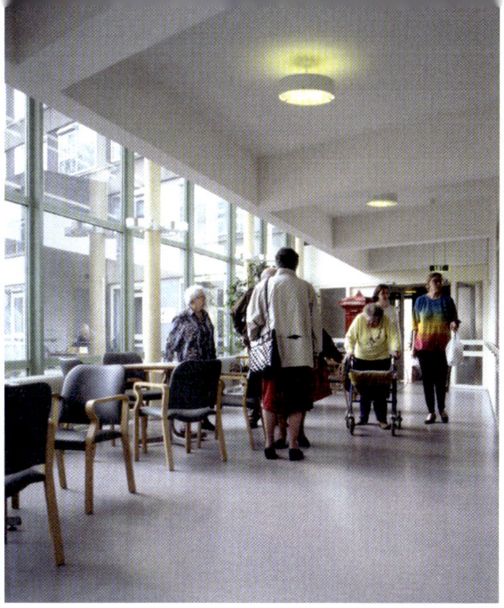

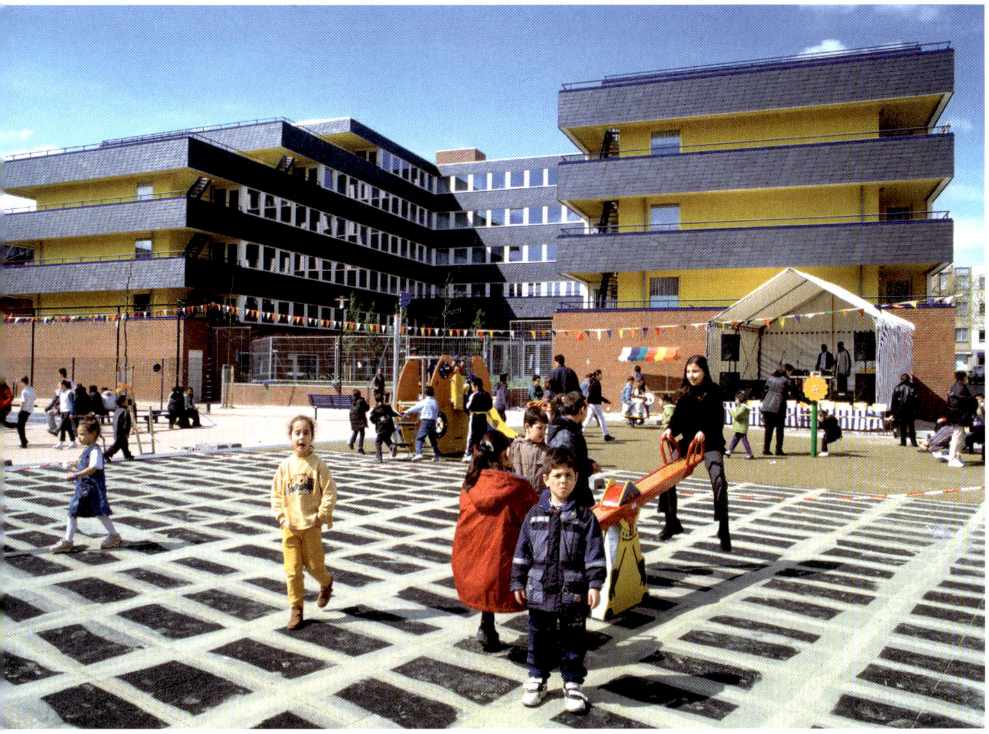

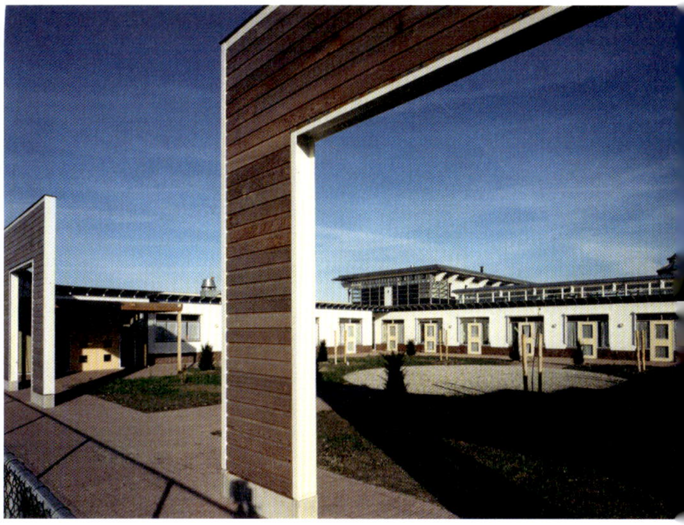

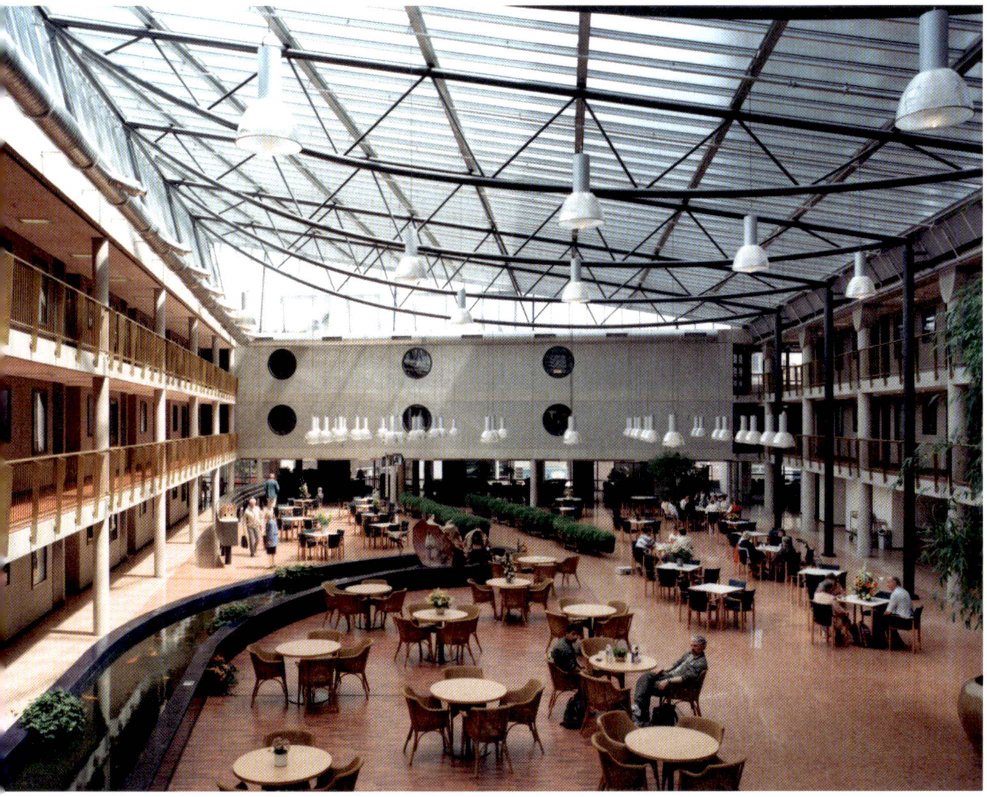

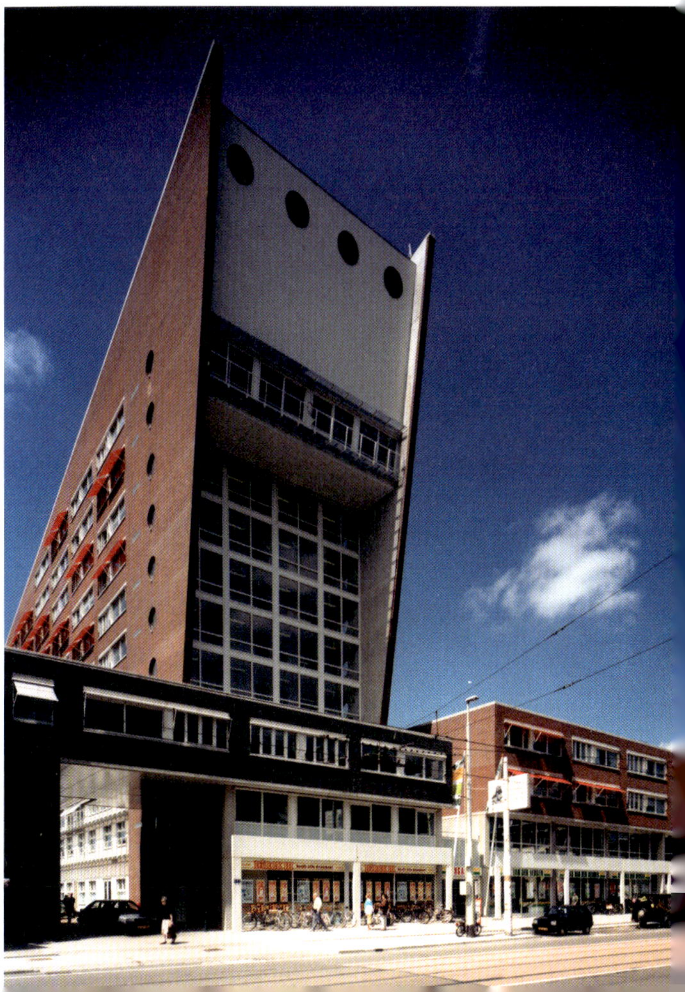

psycho-geriatric patients, separate from somatic patients.

A nursing home for sixty somatic and sixty psycho-geriatric residents was implemented in Kralingen between 1993 and 2000. Tjeerd Dijkstra designed a building consisting of two interconnected hook-shaped volumes. The one for somatic residents forms a wall on the side facing the street, with an enclosed garden at the rear for residents and locals. The other volume is intended for the psycho-geriatric residents and is more sheltered in the block. In the angle of the hook is a verandah with a route that the residents can take without encountering any obstacles. Weather permitting, this circuit can be extended to the enclosed garden around the verandah.

Polderburen in Almere, a striking extensive complex designed by de architektengroep, fills an entire block and is conceived as a spacious courtyard with residential units that are not immediately adjacent to the public space outdoors, surrounded by seven half-open inner courtyards whose open, partly screened side is in contact with the surrounding neighbourhood. These nursing homes are to a certain extent generic: they can accommodate all kinds of groups of residents and also provide accommodation for day treatment. Unlike later examples, the architecture offers few clues to distinguish the different types of residents; instead, they play an urban design game with their surroundings. Small specialist clinics for very specific target groups, for example demented old people, sprang up beside these generic nursing homes. Given the increasing importance attached to the possibility of both categories being able to live as normally as possible, the word 'patient' was replaced by 'resident'.

Ter Reede in Flushing (Zeeland), designed by EGM architecten (1999-2003), is a nursing home consisting of fifteen residential units for people with serious psycho-geriatric problems. Each unit houses six or seven elderly residents who generally have a room of their own. The residential units have a kitchen and living room of their own to offer the residents a home from home and in which they can take part in ordinary domestic activities. The units are linked to one another by means of connecting bridges and are linked to the care centre by a corridor.

Separation of housing and care: the residential care complex (*wozoco*)

Although it was the intention of the substitution policy that the institutional forms should no longer be regarded as the centre of gravity of accommodation for the elderly, many were still built. The ageing of the population made it necessary to keep expanding the stock, and besides many of the older institutions were due for replacement or renovation. Care homes remained in the first instance residential facilities, but the filtering out of residents who were able to take care of themselves increased the importance of the care component. The reverse process took place in the nursing homes, where more and more importance was attached to underlining the accommodation function. The two types thus increasingly came to resemble one another. That was the reason to experiment with a consistent separation of accommodation and care by making the accommodation independent and bringing in the care from elsewhere. Housing would fall under the responsibility of the Ministry for Housing, Spatial Planning and the Environment (VROM), while the care component became the responsible of the Ministry of Welfare, Health and Cultural Affairs. In practice it proved difficult to implement the distinction; if the residential care complex (*wozoco*) was the initiative of an institution that ran nursing homes, the ministerial involvement was different from that with an institution that usually built care homes.

The first prototypes, the Willem Dreeshuis in The Hague and the Florapark in Enschede, appeared at the end of the 1980s. A few precursors emerged in the following years, resulting in an exacerbation of the contradictions between the two ministries. The Bergweg complex in Rotterdam marked a breakthrough. At first the plan for 195 life-cycle residential units, including a substantial number for nursing home patients, stranded because the homes were not considered suitable for the latter category, or at any rate did not satisfy the standards in force at the time. All the same, the organisation behind the initiative, Humanitas, went ahead. The complex designed by Freek Prins (EGM architecten), which was opened in 1996, has a striking sloping roof. The complex separates housing and care for every category and also functions as a neighbourhood centre for care for the elderly.[19]

No less than 580 such complexes were implemented between 1987 and 1998.[20] The main differences from the care home to which they form an alternative is the size and fitting out of the apartments: they are on a par with what one would expect on the regular housing market. They are large, in principle built in accordance with the norms of the senior label. Personalised care is provided by the service centre, which often also functions as a neighbourhood support centre. The best-known example of such a complex, both in the Netherlands and internationally, is the Oklahoma complex in Amsterdam designed by MVRDV. It was commissioned by the Het Oosten housing corporation and consists of apartments for the elderly who, with the assistance of home care, should be able to continue to live on their own for as long as possible. The complex concludes a strip of provisions for the elderly, including the Leo Polak care home and a series of sheltered apartments. The architects designed a very unusual block of gallery access apartments. Eighty-seven apartments with a North-South orientation were incorporated in a long wedge. Hanging five blocks of various sizes on the outside of the wedge made it possible to add another thirteen apartments. The deep blocks protrude more than eleven metres from the wall. Access to the apartments inside and outside the wedge is via galleries on the north side of the block. The entrance with lift and staircase is at the west end of the building.

De Nijl designed a complex for Humanitas that combined housing with care in the Putselaan in South Rotterdam (1995-1999). The complex forms part of the restructuring of a residential neighbourhood from the 1930s and comprises three buildings: a central building on the site of a demolished block, and two connected buildings on the sides. The three buildings accommodate a mixed programme. The central building contains fifty-eight residential units for senior citizens, with provisions that are open to the public on the ground floor.

In many of the mixed housing and care complexes, the communal facilities are adjacent to a large atrium or winter garden. Examples of this are Hof van Orden, designed by Atelier Pro Architekten (1994-1997), and a complex of this kind on the Emerald housing estate in Delfgauw designed by KCAP (1997-2000). The atria are usually created by covering the empty areas between the blocks. In the Klooster-verzorgingshuis, a nursing home in Venlo designed by Han Westelaken (Architecten aan de Maas), a simple rectangular volume with two wings at right angles to it encloses a garden. The rectangular volume, which is adjacent to the street, contains the dining room and chapel, while the wings, which are closed off by two oval meeting areas, contain the residential units.

p. 249 | <

***Atelier Pro Architekten*, Hof van Orden residential units for the elderly, Apeldoorn, 1997**

***Wiel Arets*, housing for the elderly, Tilburg, 1995**

p. 249| >

***KCAP*, residential care complex (*wozoco*), Delfgauw, 2000**

***Vera Yanovshtchinsky*, Breeweg apartments for the elderly, Middelburg, 2001**

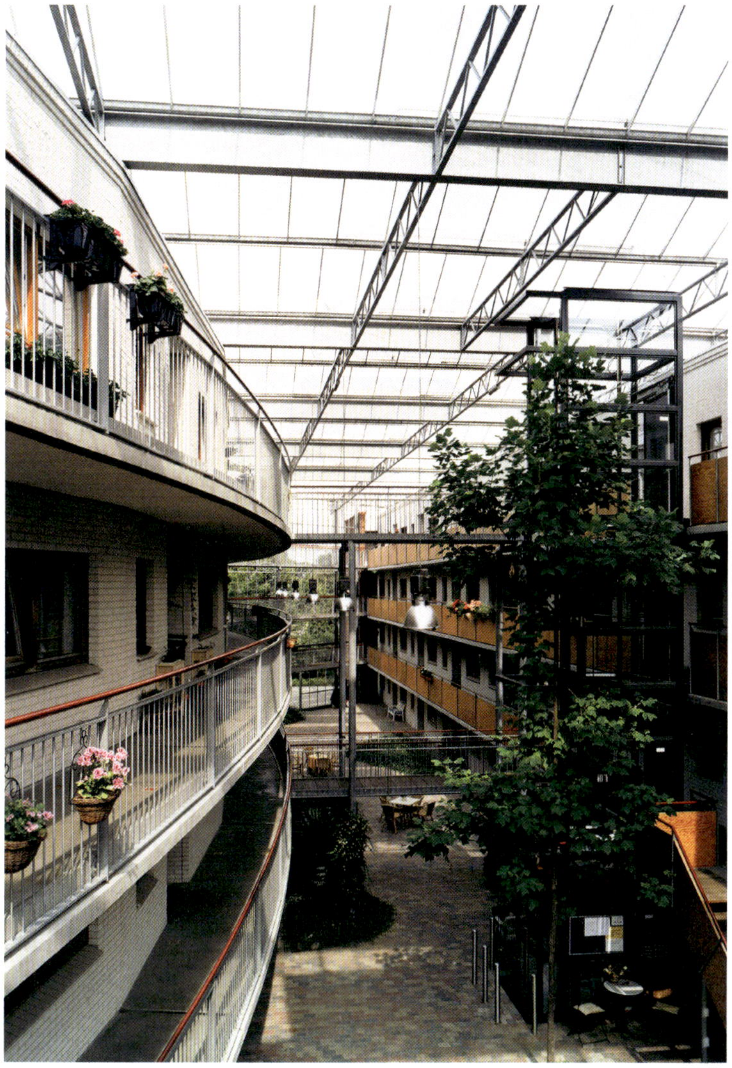

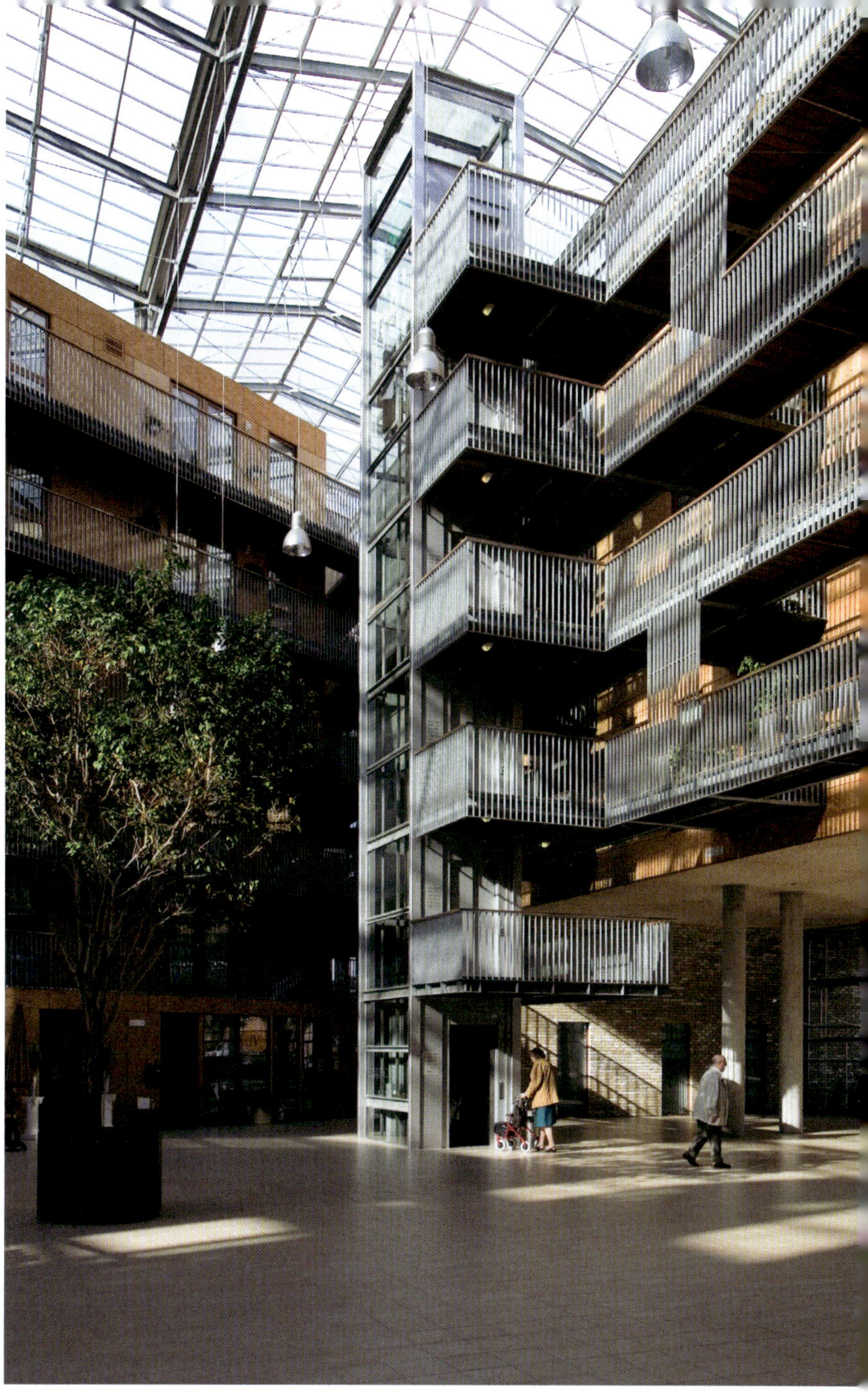

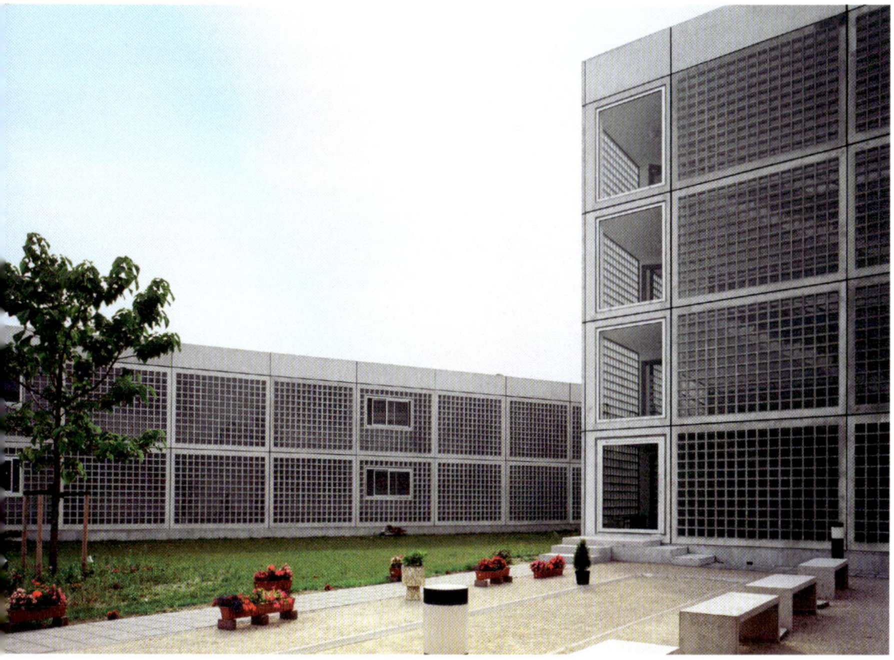

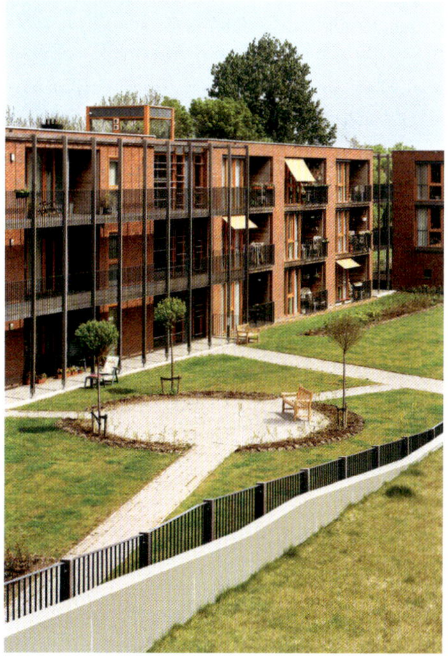

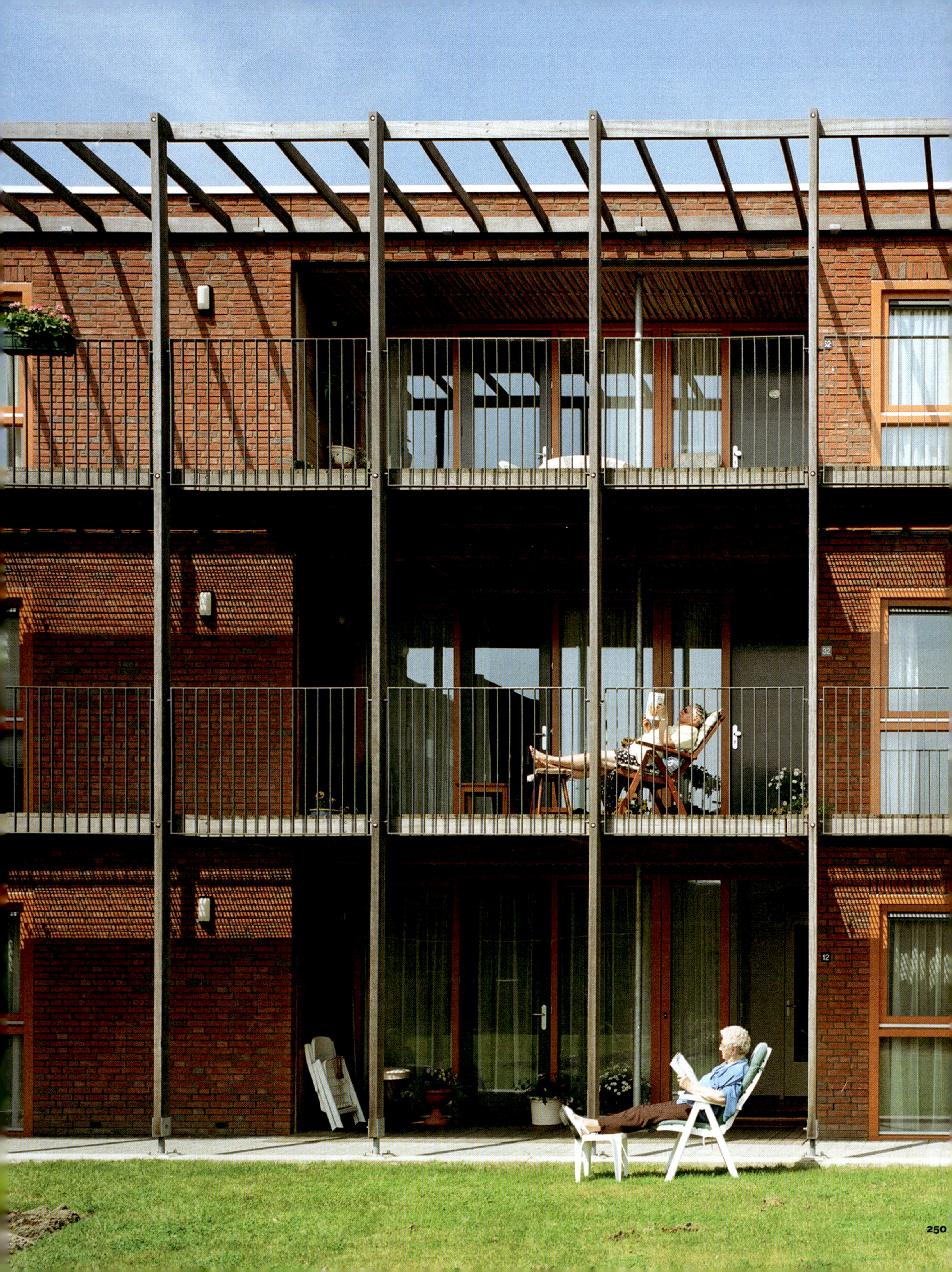

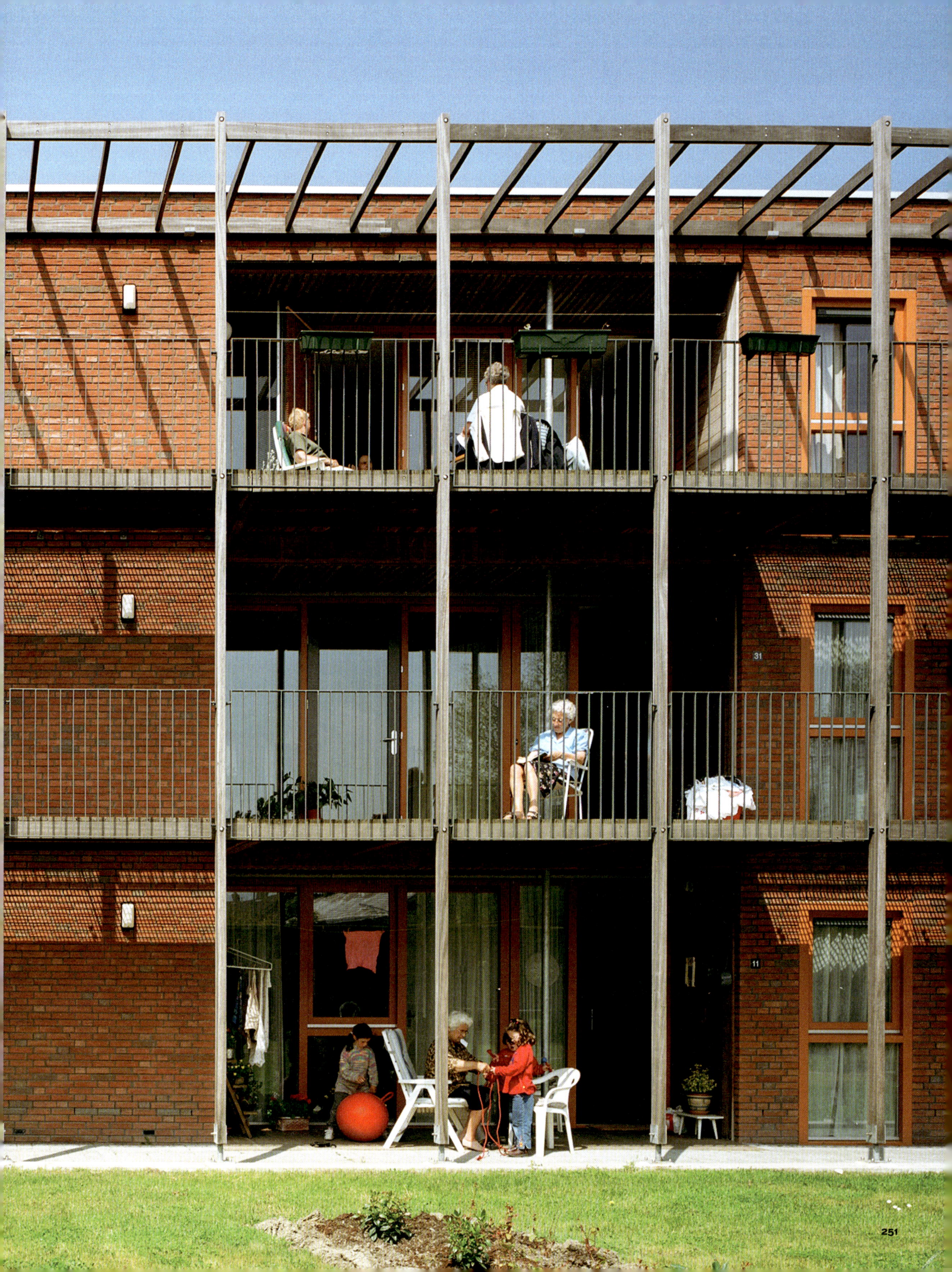
31
11

Housing for the elderly

The separation of housing and care also created an important task for housing corporations, who now started to build housing for the category of elderly people formerly accommodated in an institutional setting. The Stichting Verenigde Woningcorporaties (United Housing Corporations Foundation) (later incorporated in the WonenBreburg housing corporation) commissioned Wiel Arets to build sixty-seven apartments for the elderly in two buildings in Tilburg, which were completed in 1992. The most striking feature of one of the buildings is the entrance: a narrow shaft made of glass brick that runs all the way up the four-storey volume at a distance of more than ten metres from the outside wall. The four-storey block is one of the sides of a V-shaped building. The other side has two storeys. There are thirty apartments in this building, thirty-seven in the other. The galleries that provide access to the apartments are concealed behind outside walls of glass brick. It is fairly Minimalist architecture characterised by simplicity and the lack of decoration. The apartments are close to a care home.

The traditional cluster of almshouses proves to be an exceptionally good type for housing for the elderly.[21] The central communal courtyard offers a safe and sheltered environment. Apartments for the elderly were built on the site of a block from the 1960s in Middelburg for the Woongoed housing corporation and were completed in 2001. The architect, Vera Yanovshtchinsky, designed five different volumes that nevertheless form a unity grouped around a large communal courtyard. The residents of the thirty rented apartments and twenty-seven owner-occupied apartments can make use of the facilities of the neighbouring old people's home.

De Vonk in Nijmegen (1989-1994), designed by Erick van Egeraat (from Mecanoo at the time), was implemented on an attractive location beside a monastery garden. The complex of apartments for the elderly consists of a small volume adjacent to the street and a larger volume behind it and borders on the monastery garden and cemetery. The three-storey complex has twenty-six three-room apartments

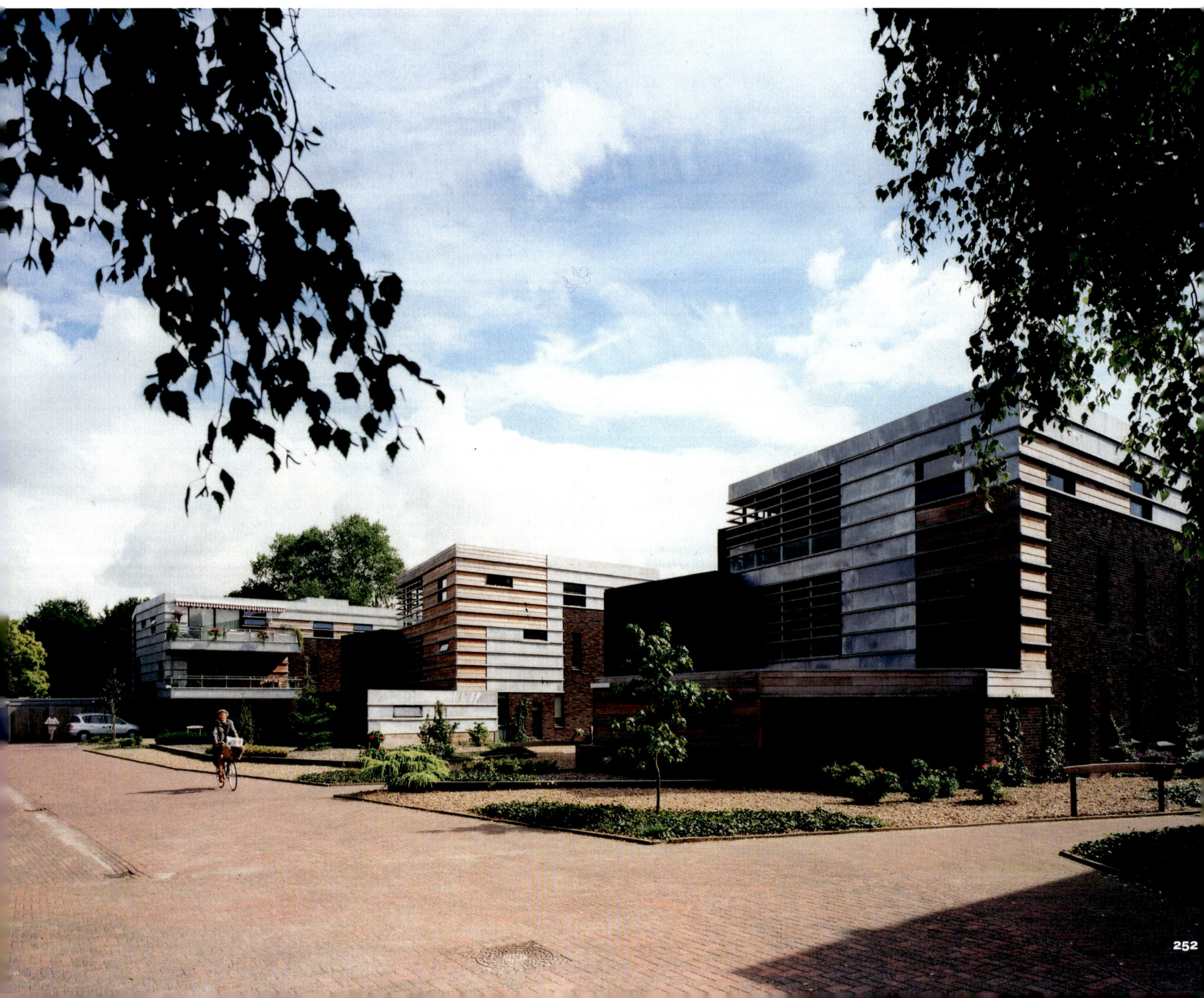

in five different standard types. A hall was projected between the two blocks. The walls facing the street have a robust and modern finish and are characterised by bare concrete. The elongated volume has galleries on the garden side that are protected from the wind and rain by heavy wooden beams and glass panels. There is a kink in this wall, and the half-open glass screen repeats it. The outside wall on the other side has a similar robust look to that of the block on the street side. The apartment next to the hall on the ground floor functions as a communal room.

Many old people who can afford it make sure that they move in good time into an apartment where they will still be able to live when they become more or less dependent on care. This group is therefore an attractive target group for project developers. Larger or smaller complexes of luxurious apartments for the elderly are springing up everywhere.

The premise of a complex of apartments for the elderly that Onix designed in Eelde (Drenthe) between 1996 and 2000 was to reinforce a series of green areas that intersect the village. Two estates, Westerbroek and Ode Marsch, form part of this green strip. Their buildings are set back behind a green front area. Onix designed a volume consisting of four clusters that are set back in a similar way. A semi-communal area is set between the articulated 'crenellations' and a communal carport. By allowing the vegetation to grow high up the brick walls, Onix wanted to tone down the distance between the building and its natural setting. The bricks that jut out at some points suggest a ruin, a classic theme in architecture that symbolises the passing of time.

p. 250
***Vera Yanovshtchinsky*, Breeweg apartments for the elderly, Middelburg, 2001**

p. 252
***Onix*, apartments for the elderly, Eelde, 1996-2000**

p. 253
***Mecanoo*, De Vonk apartments for the elderly, Nijmegen, 1989**

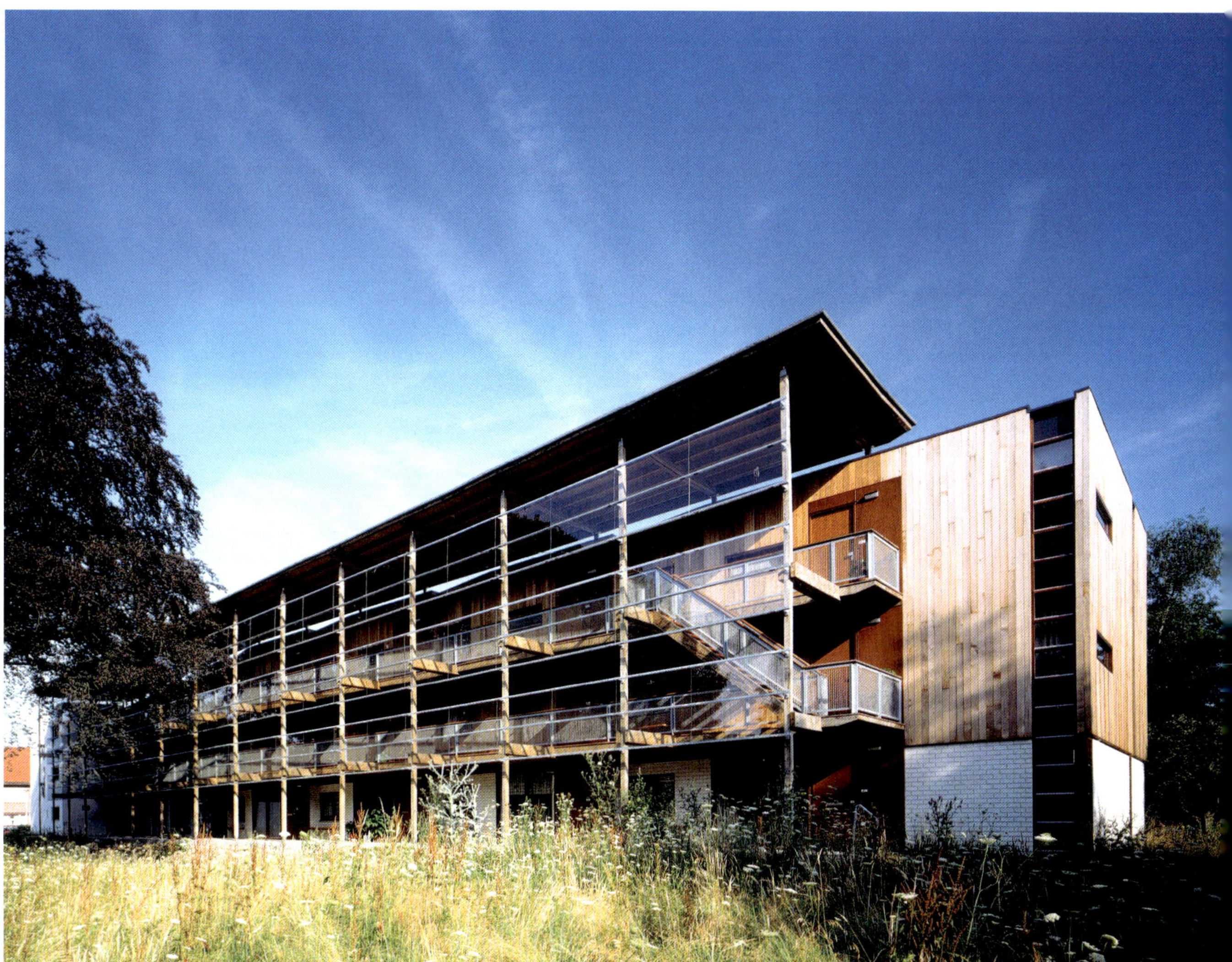

Kruisheer Hallink Arends architecten, Team 4 Architecten, Wytze Patijn architecten

Academisch Ziekenhuis Groningen (AZG)
Groningen
1975-1997

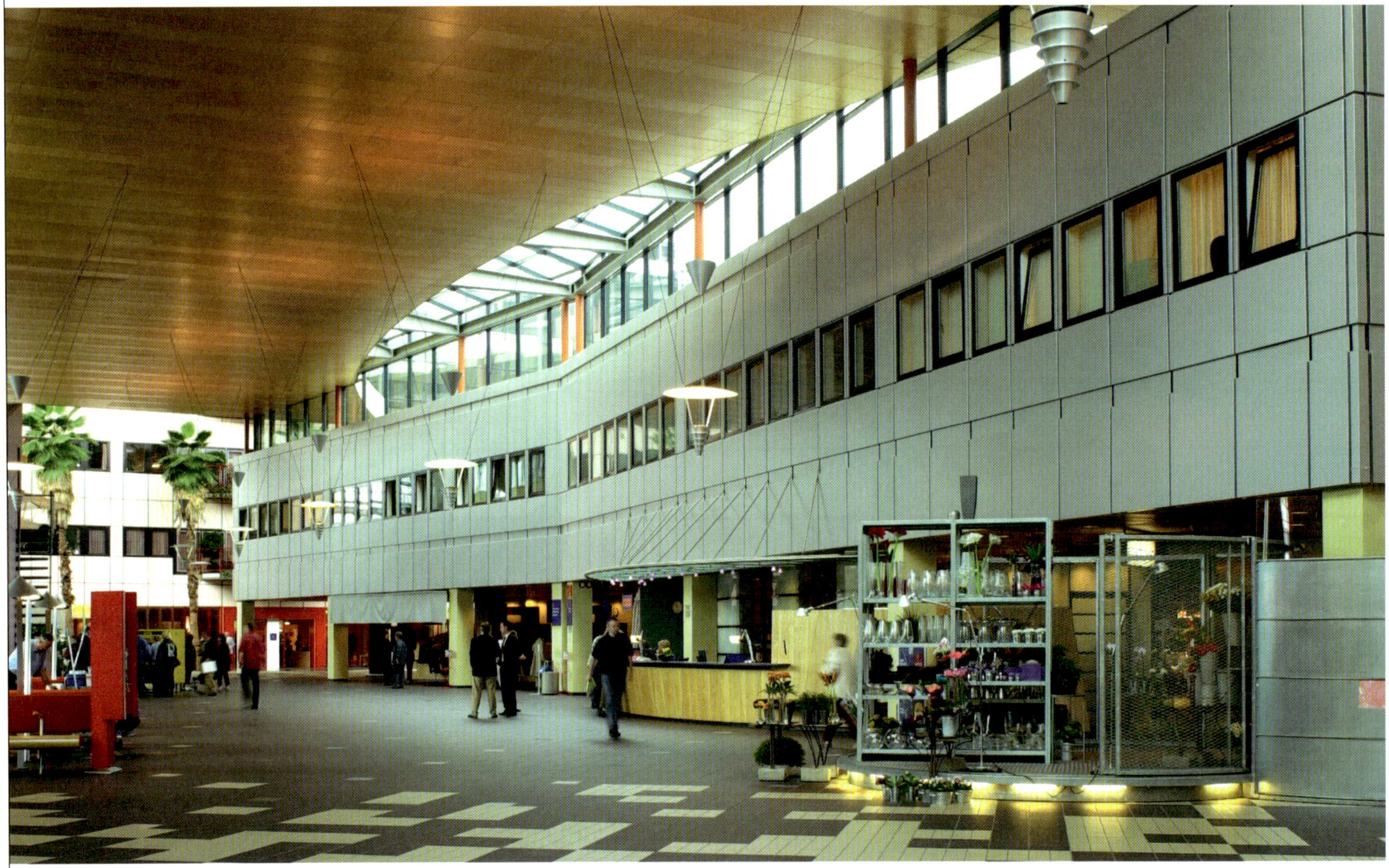

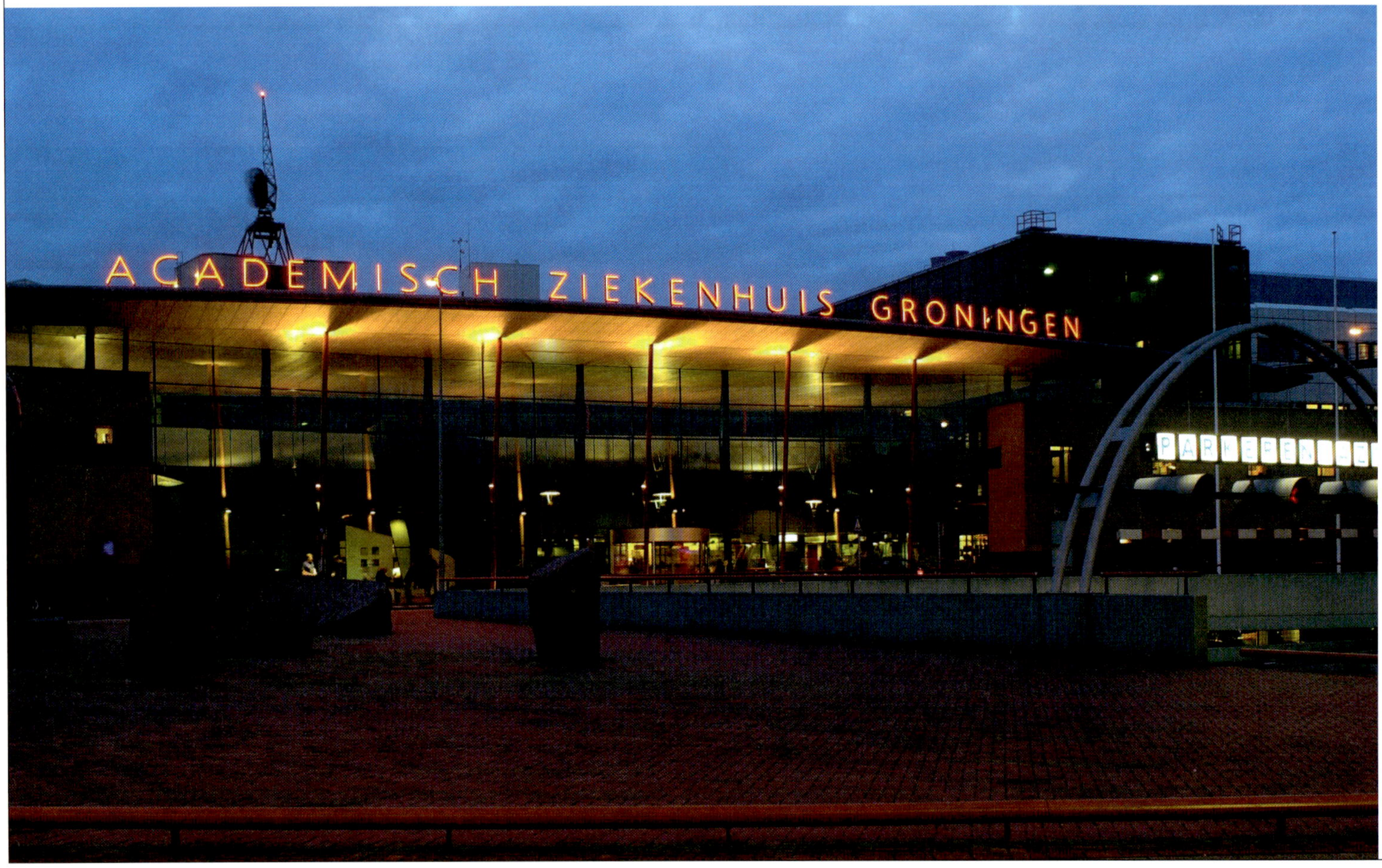

Right from the start the Ministry of Education and Science, the municipality of Groningen and the board of the AZG were resolved that the new university hospital building should be built on the location of the old pavilion hospital close to the historic city centre. J.E. Kruisheer was appointed chief architect in 1974. He presented his development plan in 1976. It was characterised by small scale, hospitality, and integration of the hospital in the urban fabric. The Central Medical Complex (CMC) was projected in the middle, with inner streets on each side that converge at the southern tip of the terrain. The underground corridors for internal service traffic follow the same pattern. Nine wards were projected beside the inner streets, each with an outpatient unit, its own underground car par and its own entrance on the ground floor.

Team 4 Architecten were brought in to design the wards. While the building was going on, the plan was more or less turned inside out in the first half of the 1980s. Decentralisation was replaced by centralisation. It was decided to place a central hall in front of the hospital to link the two inner streets with one another and to roof them. This was elaborated in a structural plan that was presented in 1987 simultaneously with the departure of Kruisheer. This about-turn was marked by the recruitment of Wytze Patijn as his successor. Patijn designed the central hall and the inner streets. He decided to introduce variety in the wards on the ground floor by inviting a different interior architect for each outpatient unit to give it a look of its own.

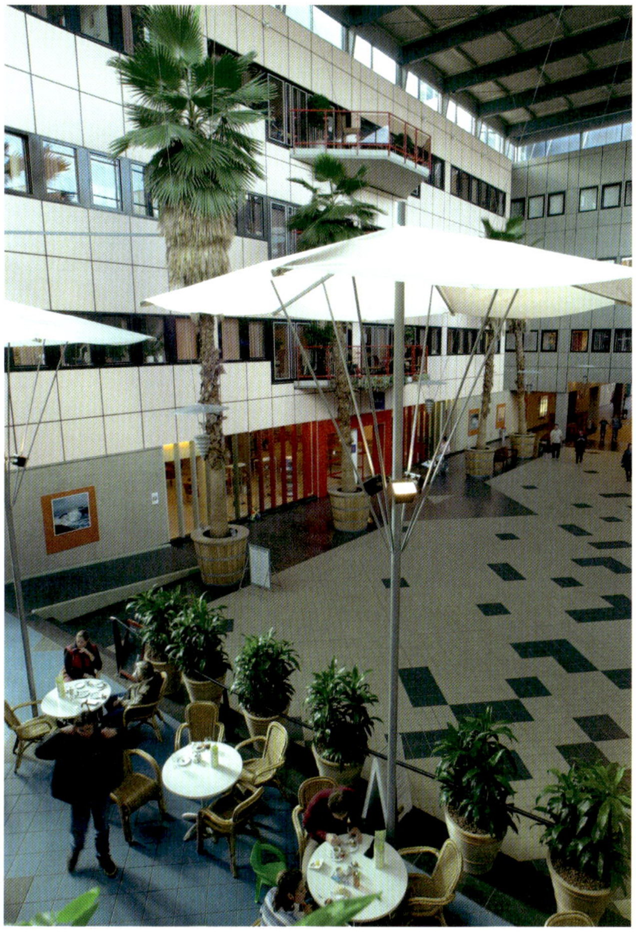

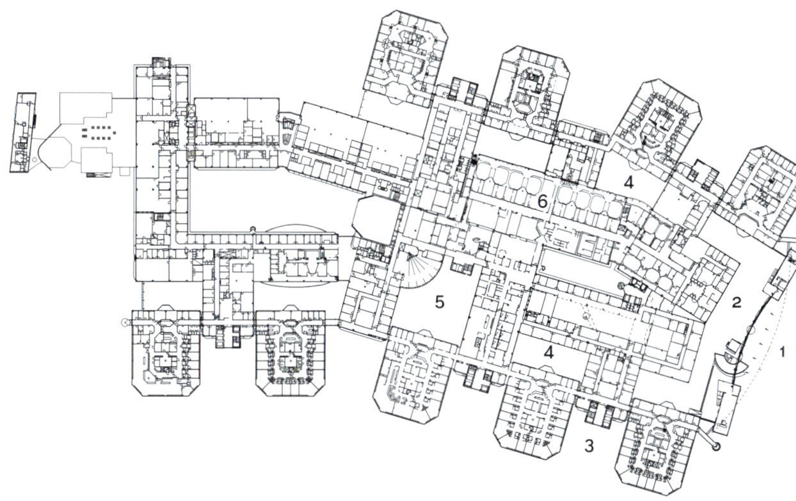

Ward on nursing floor

Ground floor
1 *entrance*
2 *entrance hall*
3 *ward with outpatients unit*
4 *inner street*
5 *atrium*
6 *Central Medical Complex*

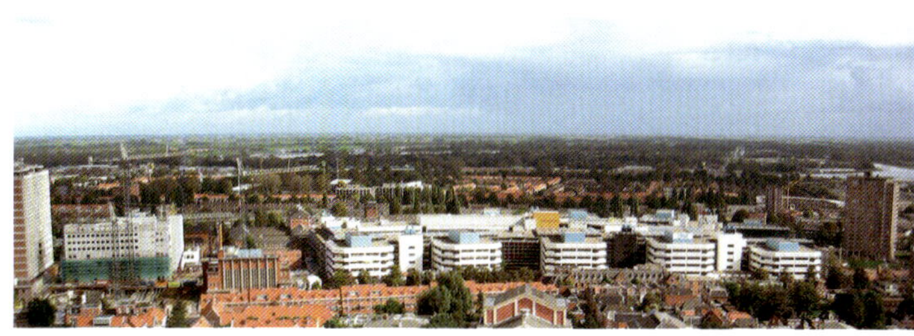

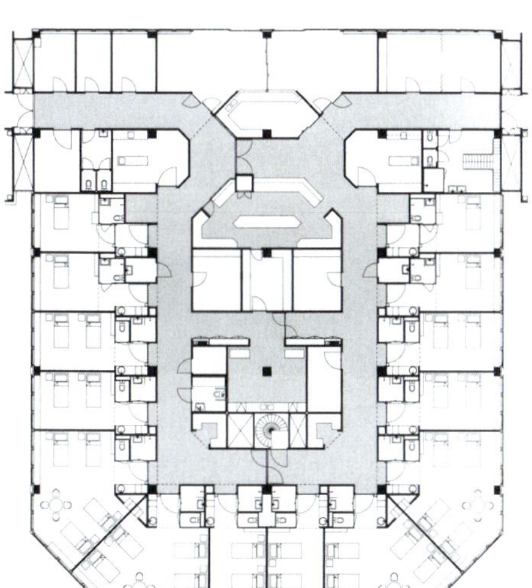

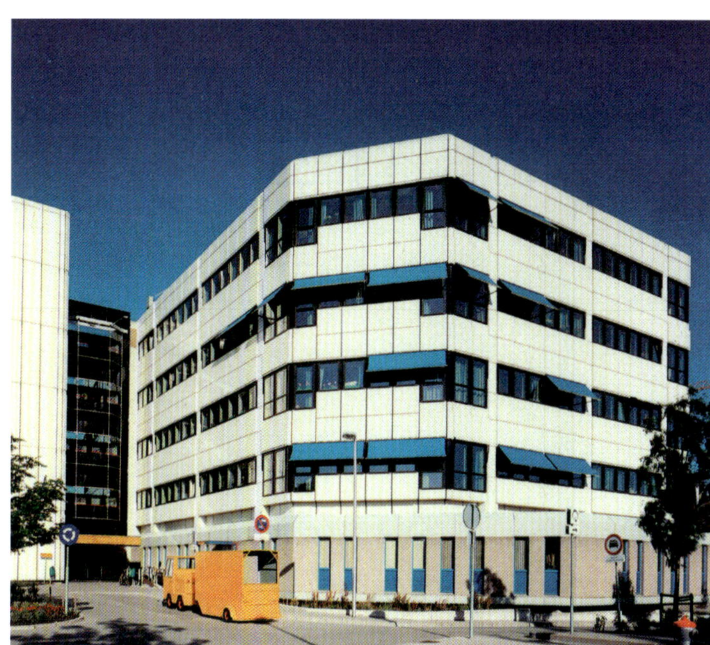

Skybox

MVRDV

Johannes de Deo residential care comlex
Amsterdam
1994-1997

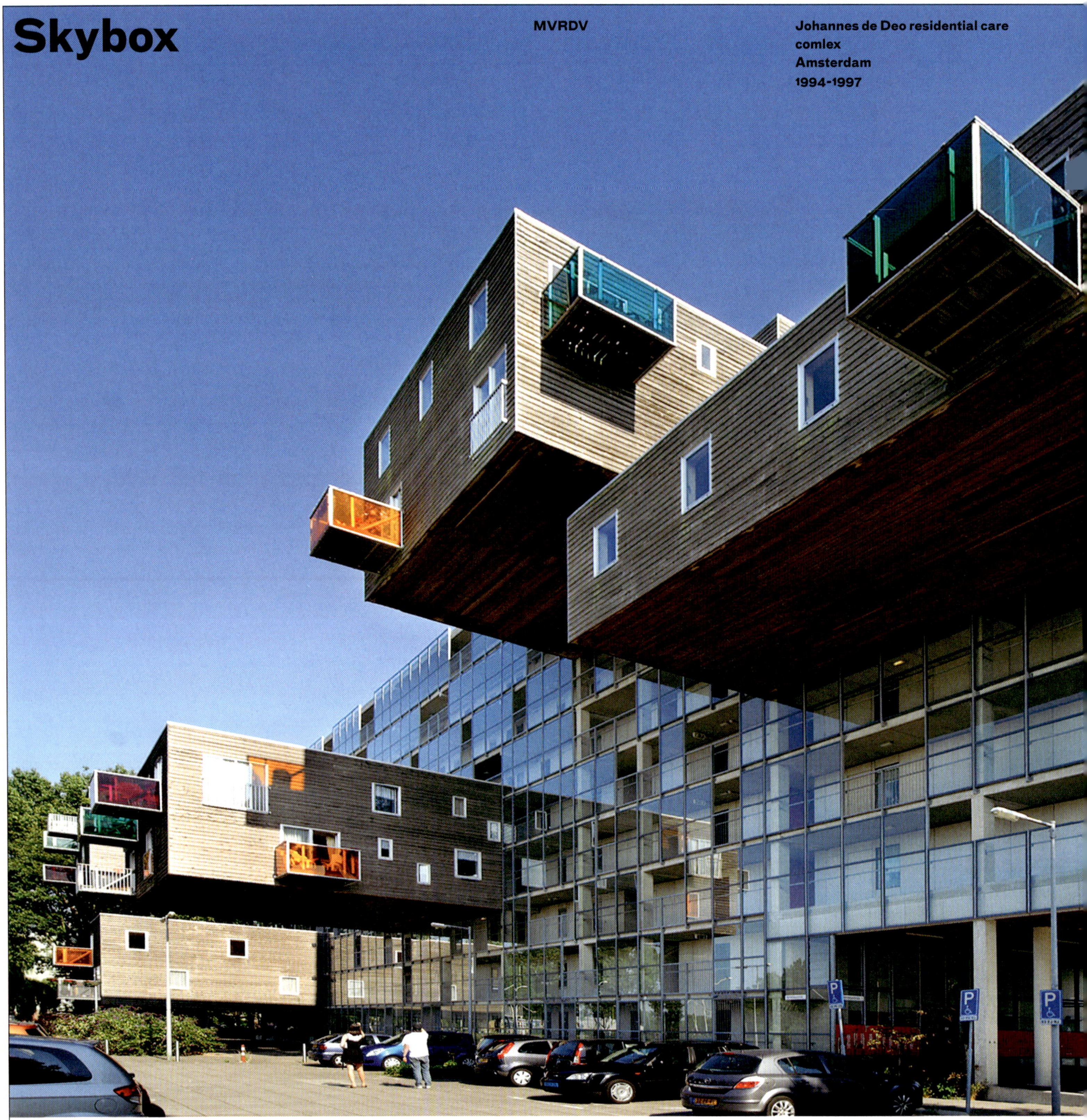

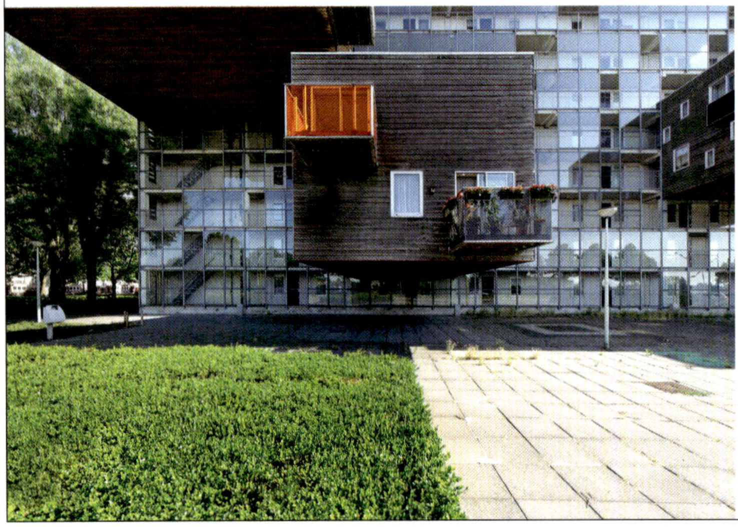

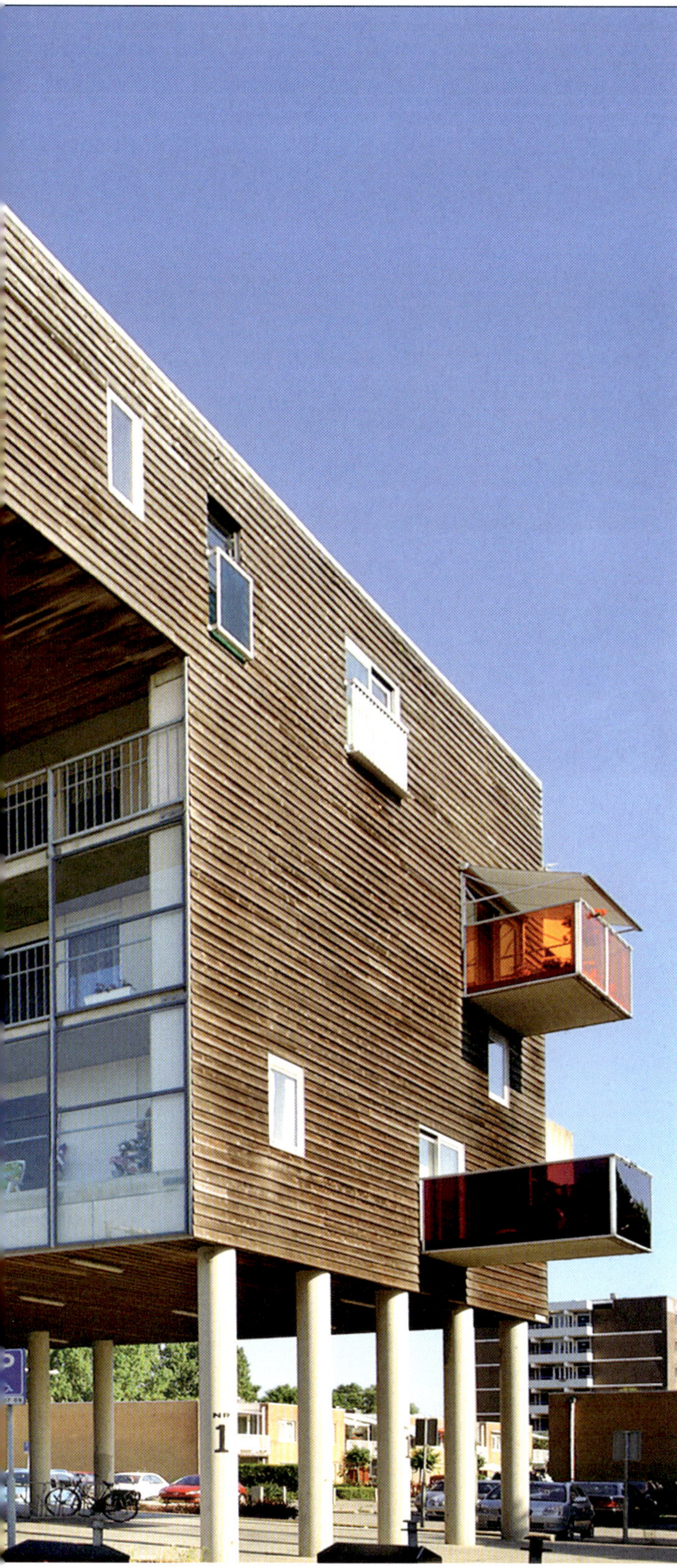

MVRDV was commissioned by the Het Oosten housing corporation in Amsterdam-Osdorp to design a residential care complex (*wozoco*) for the elderly who, with the assistance of home care, should be able to continue to live on their own for as long as possible. The complex concludes a strip of provisions for the elderly, including the Leo Polak care home and a series of sheltered apartments. The urban development plan did not leave enough space for the 100 apartments requested, as the building was not allowed to have more than nine floors on the south side and only six on the west side.

87 apartments with a north-south orientation are accommodated in a long wedge. The other 13 apartments are distributed among the five blocks that hang from the wedge. There are two deep blocks, each with two apartments side by side and two apartments one above the other, two blocks with two apartments one above the other, and one block with a singe apartment. The deep blocks extend outwards from the façade for more than eleven metres. Galleries on the north side of the block provide access to the apartments in the wedge and the blocks hanging from it. The entrance with lift and staircase is on the west side at the end of the building.

The wedge has a supporting construction of concrete poured in place. The five blocks have been kept as light as possible and hang with a steel framework construction from the walls of the block that separate the apartments. Because these are extra large in order to comply with the noise restriction criteria laid down in the Building Decree, the excess can be used to absorb the pressure and traction forces. The proportionally expensive supporting construction of the blocks was made affordable by limiting the number of inner partitions in the wedge. This gave the south façade more variation because the dimensions and position of the windows and balconies were less fixed. The finishing of the balcony fences in different colours enhances this variety.

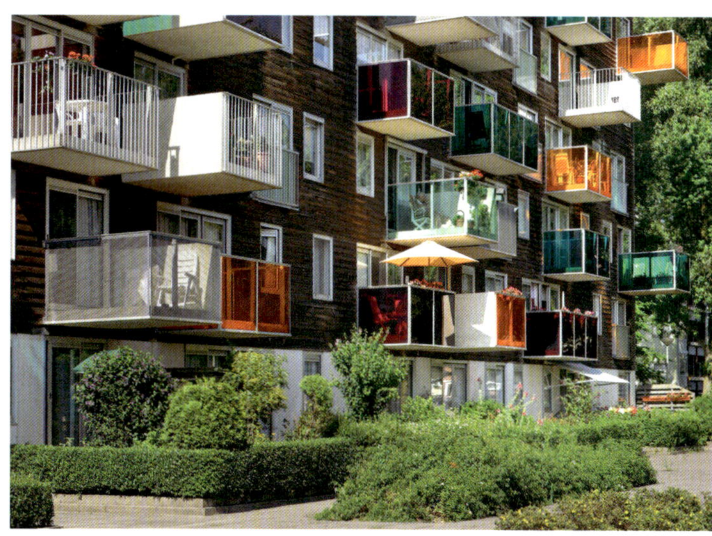

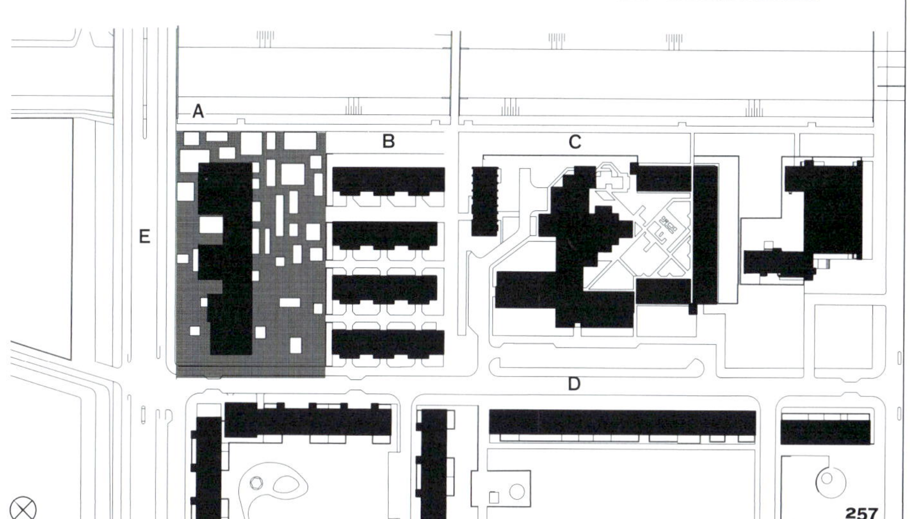

Situation
A *residential care complex*
B *sheltered homes*
C *Johannes de Deo care centre*
D *Reimerswaalstraat*
E *Ookmeerweg*

Wood

Mecanoo

Centre for mental care
Goes
1995-2001

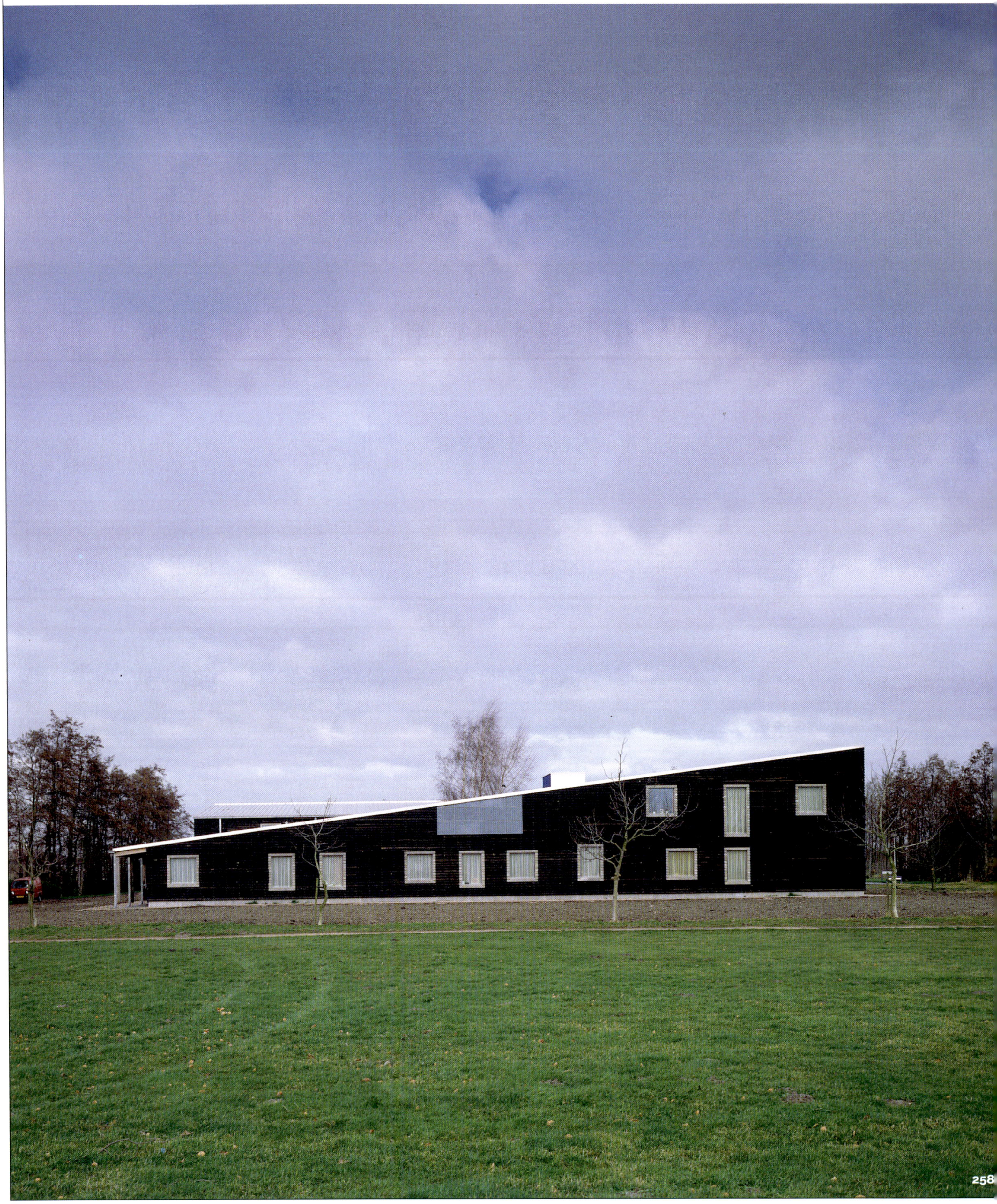

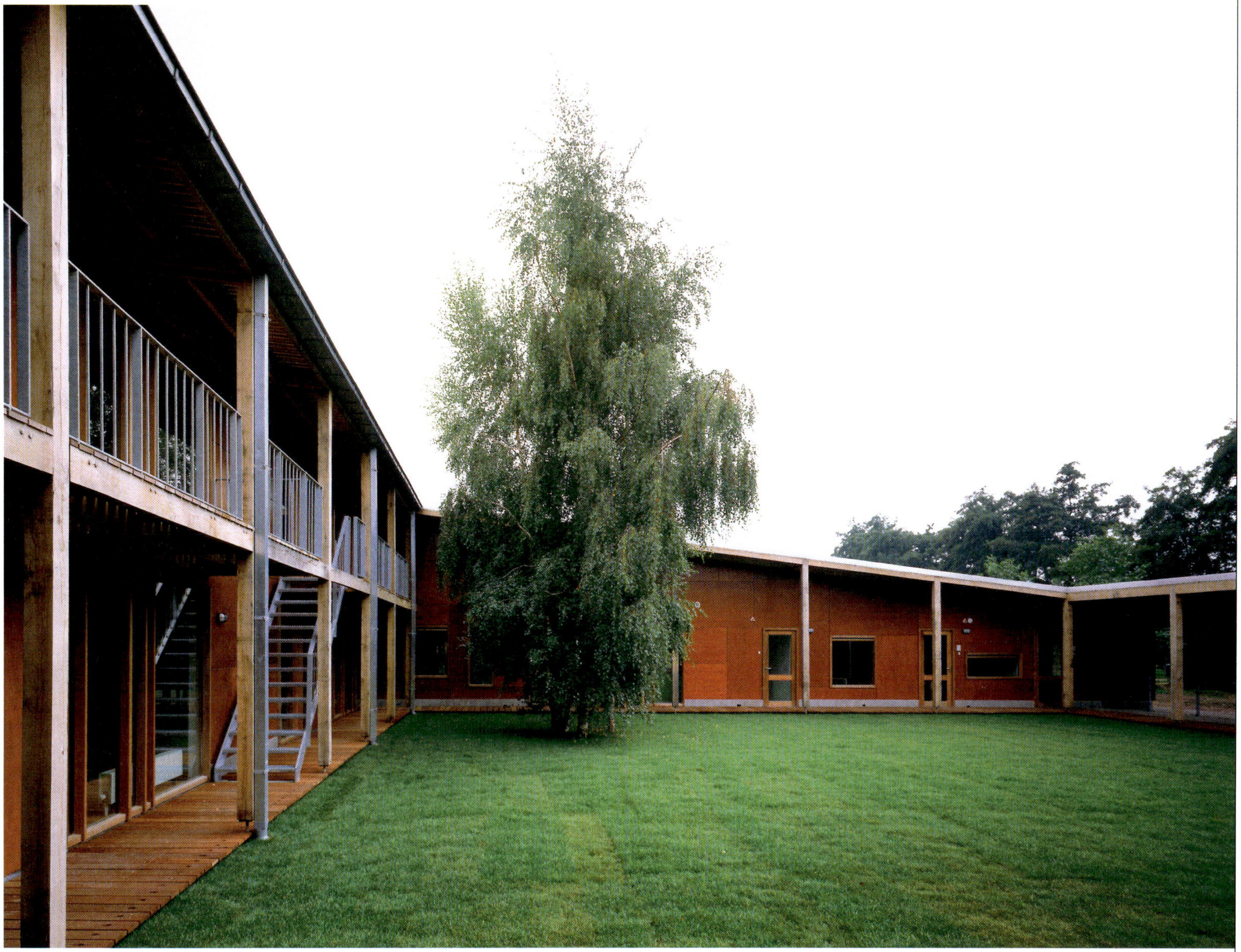

The centre for mental care designed by Mecanoo in Goes is intended for 42 long-term residential patients in need of constant care. The complex fulfils a similar role to the large institutions of the past, but reflects the preference for small-scale solutions that are integrated in their surroundings. Within this modest complex, the scale has been reduced even further by forming seven groups. The serious nature of their situation prevents them from leaving the building, so it has to satisfy all their needs. The central element is an enclosed garden, which recalls one of the two sources of inspiration of Mecanoo: the convent. A curving colonnade with wooden columns reinforces this association. The communal lounges are adjacent to this garden, while the individual living rooms and the two individual residential units are on the outside. The façades facing the enclosed garden have a warm, intimate character. One side has been left open to create a visual link between the garden and an old orchard. That represents the second source of inspiration: the landscape of the province of Zeeland. The exterior of the building continues this reference in the cladding with rough wooden panels painted black. As a result, the way the building is embedded in the landscape resembles that of rural buildings such as farmhouses and barns.

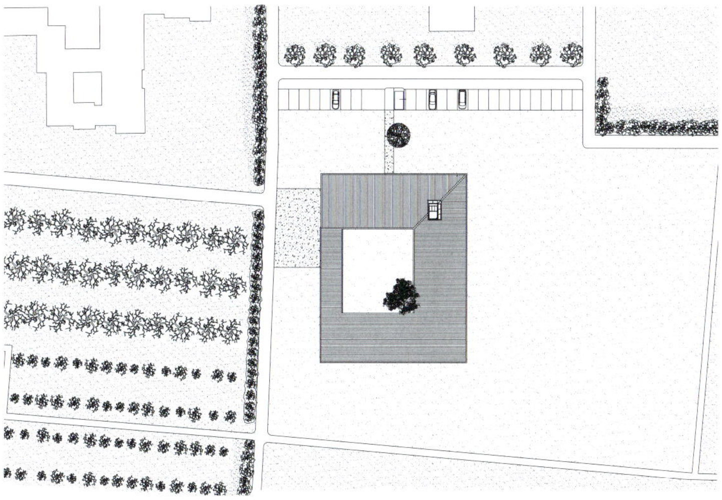

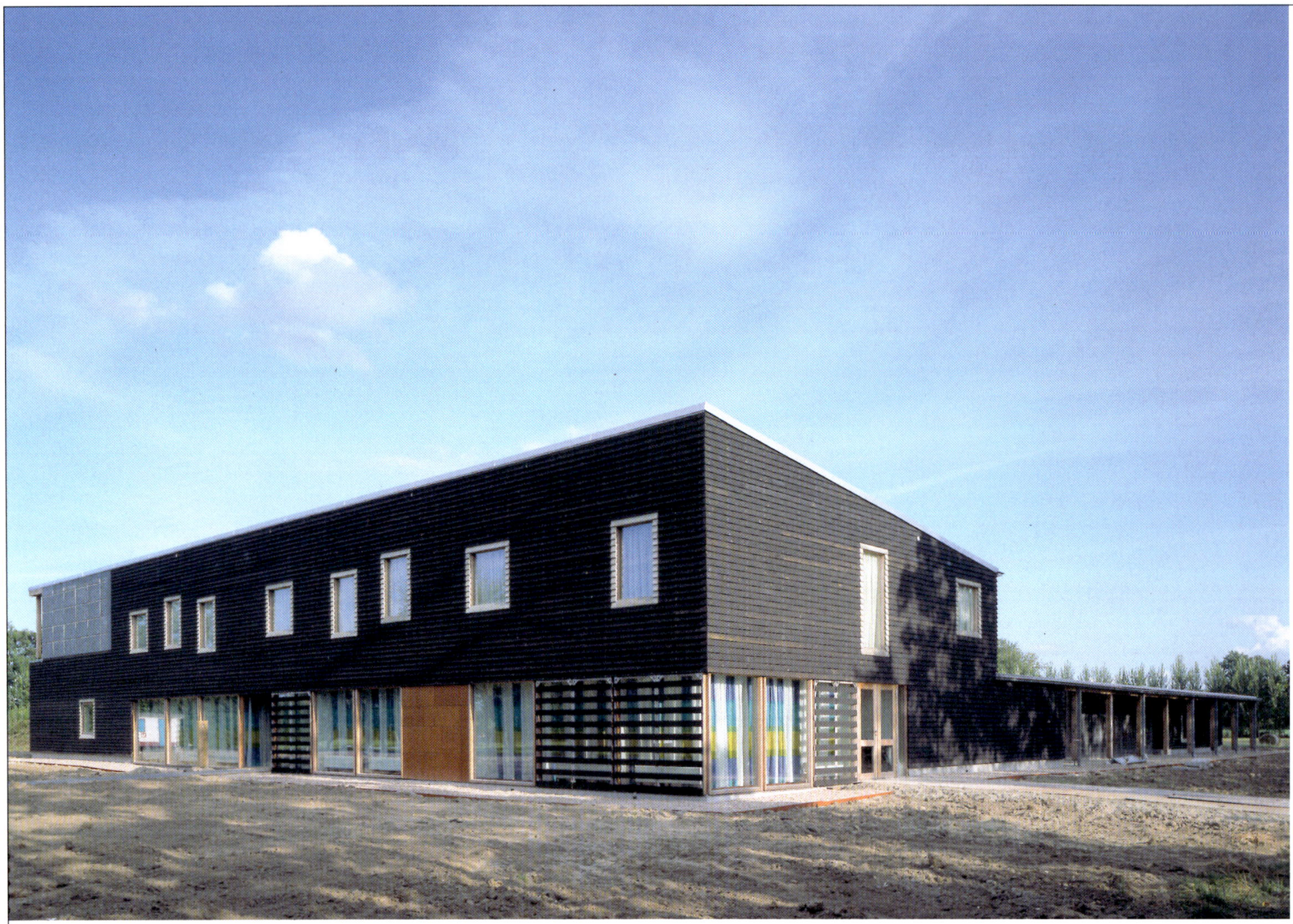

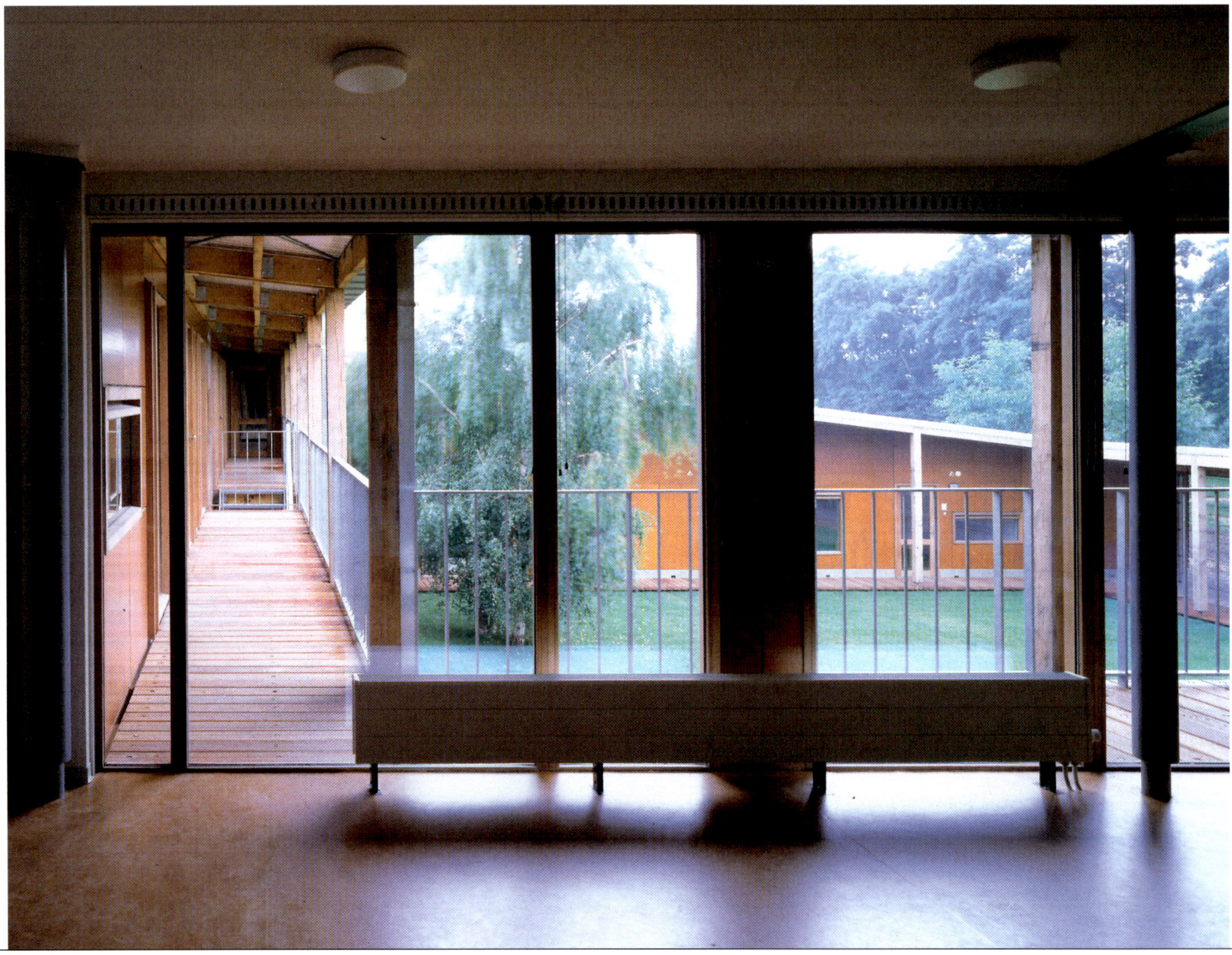

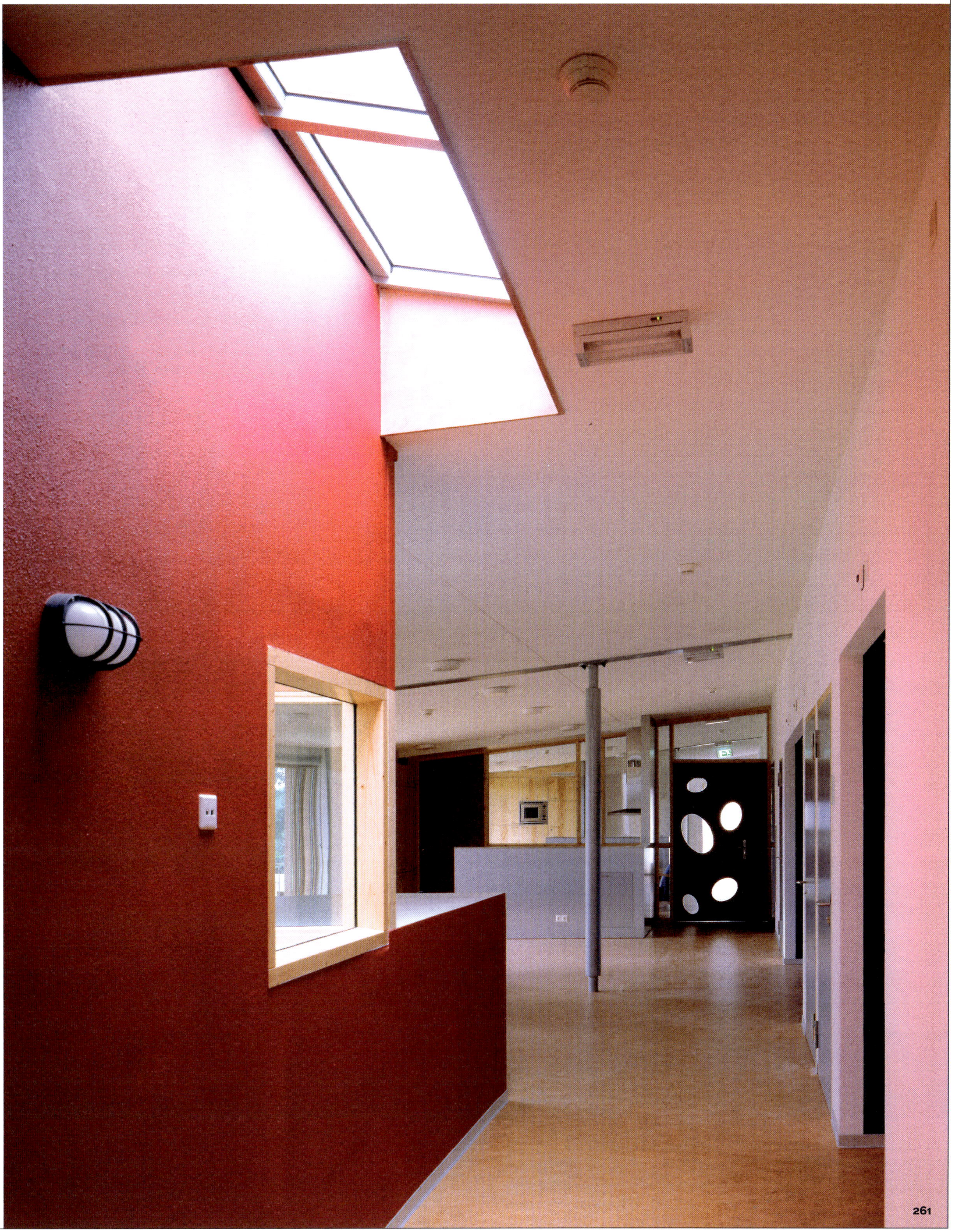

Building on the edge

Architectengroep Duintjer (now de Jong Gortemaker Algra architecten en ingenieurs)

Westfries Gasthuis (first phase)
Hoorn
2003

Hans Liscaljet built a five-storey slender and elongated volume on the edge of the terrain that accommodates the Sint-Jan Ziekenhuis in its centre. The new volume was to contribute to the formation of a closed street wall at this point. The lower three floors have a curved façade on the side facing the street. This volume is folded backwards on both sides, thereby creating a sheltered inner space. The ambulant care is accommodated in the lower floors. Above them are an intermediate level, and above that the two floors for clinical care. They are staggered and jut out at the rear, where they rest on a row of slender columns. A three-storey white box containing the day wards juts out at the front, supported on two columns. Orientation was an important motive in the choice of a slender volume. Visual contact with the outside world is possible from almost every point of the connecting corridors and waiting rooms. The mental health centre is aligned with one of the wings of the lower volume that are folded backwards. A park has been projected at the site of the existing building of the Sint-Jan Ziekenhuis. If later extensions of the Westfries Gasthuis are required, they can be located there.

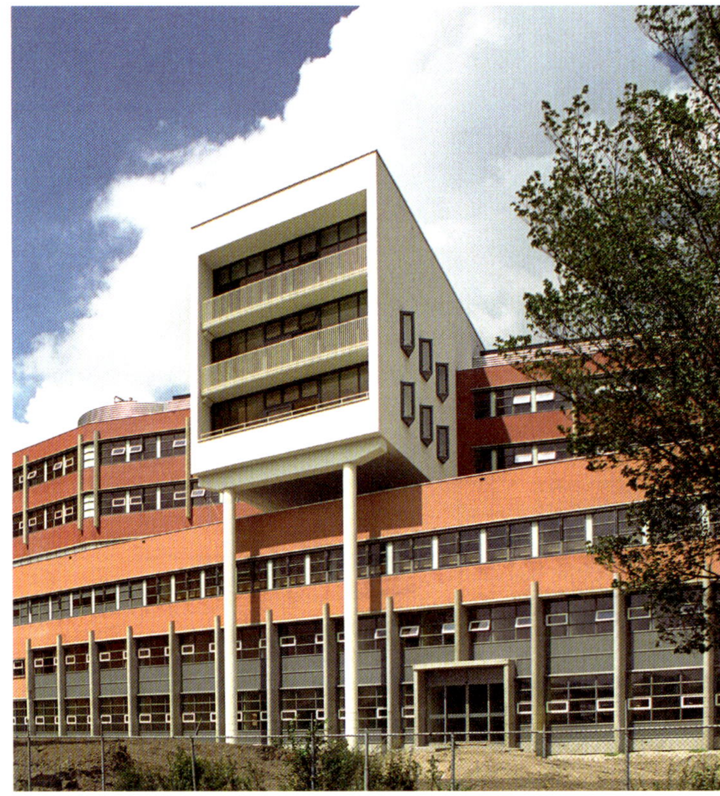

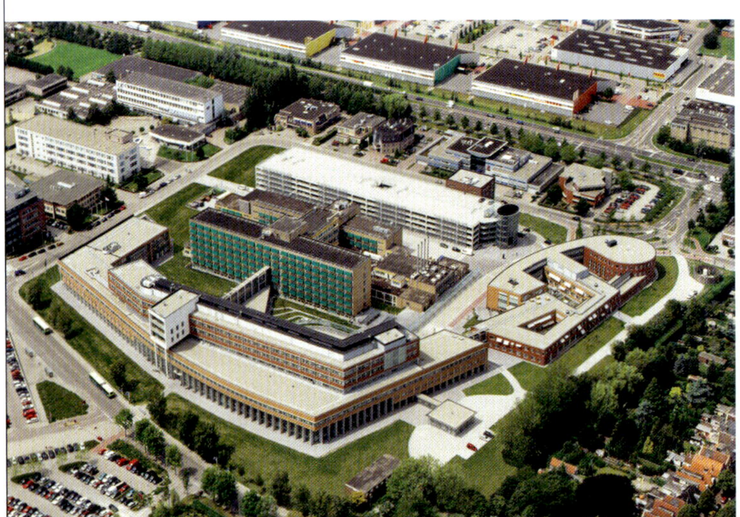

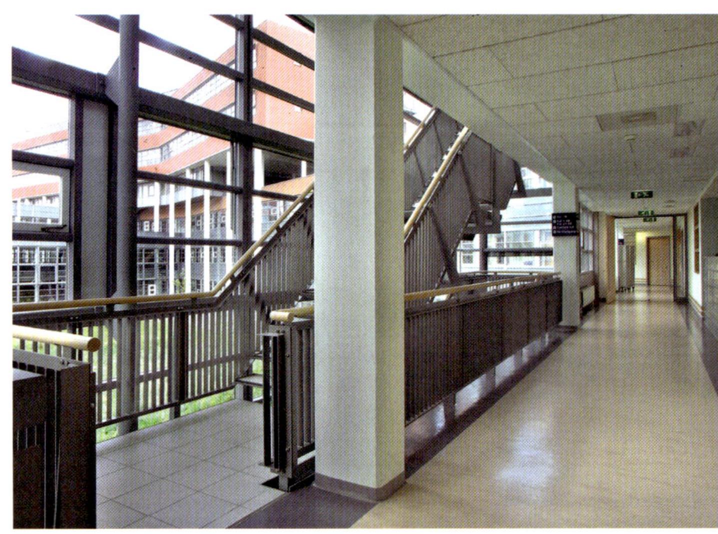

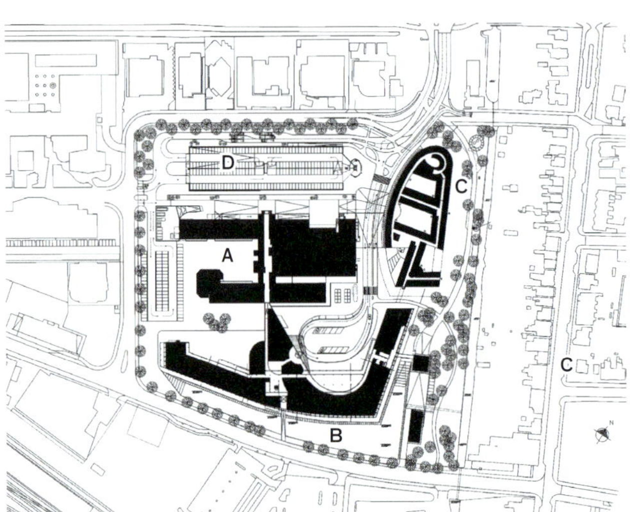

Situation
A *Old Sint-Jan Ziekenhuis*
B *new building project, first stage*
C *mental health care centre*
D *car park*

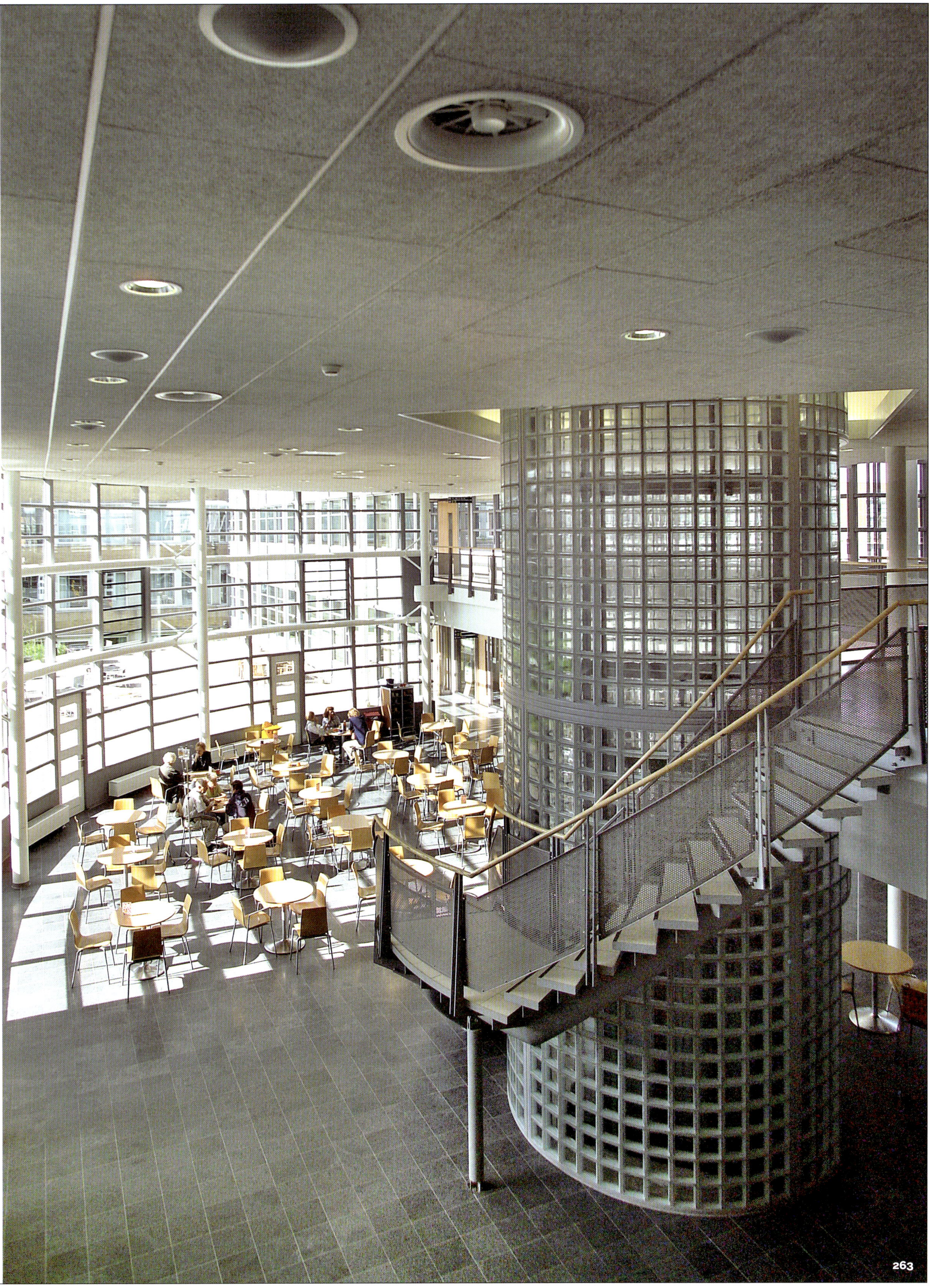

Play

EGM architecten

De Jutter centre for child and youth psychiatry
The Hague
1997-2002

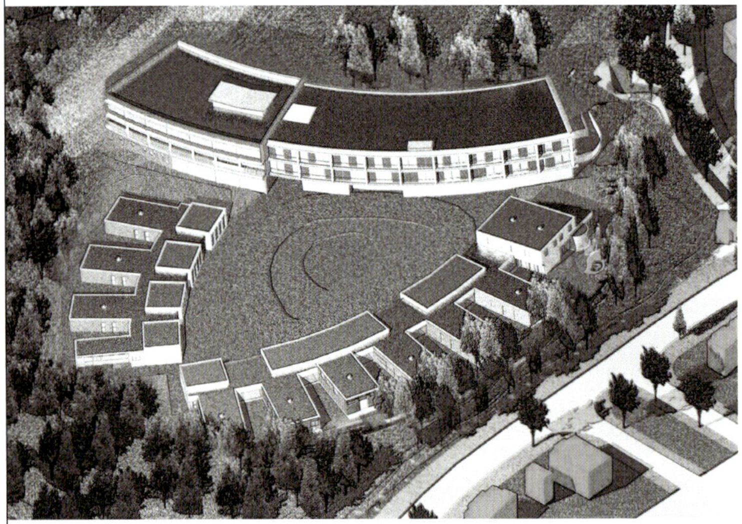

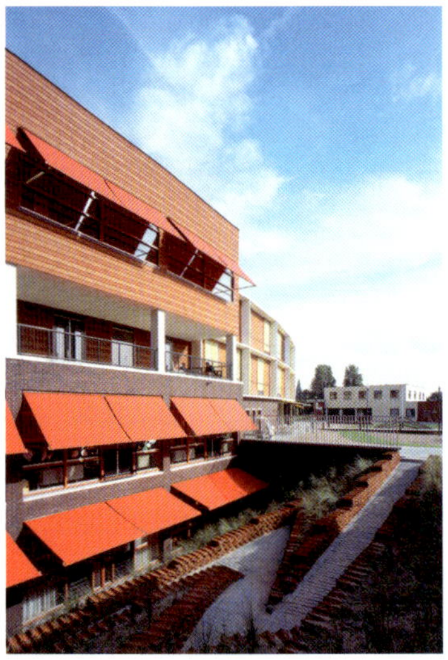

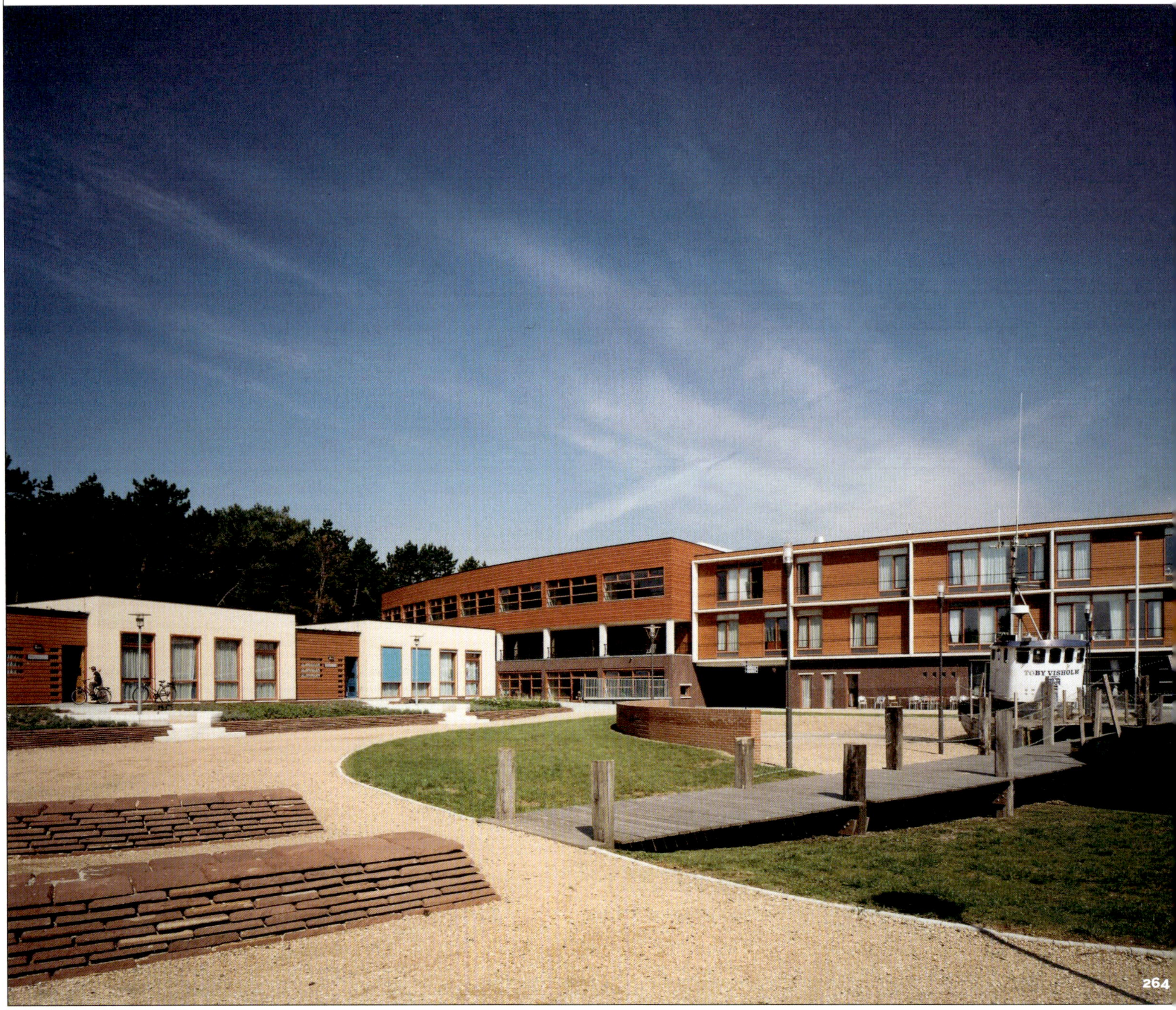

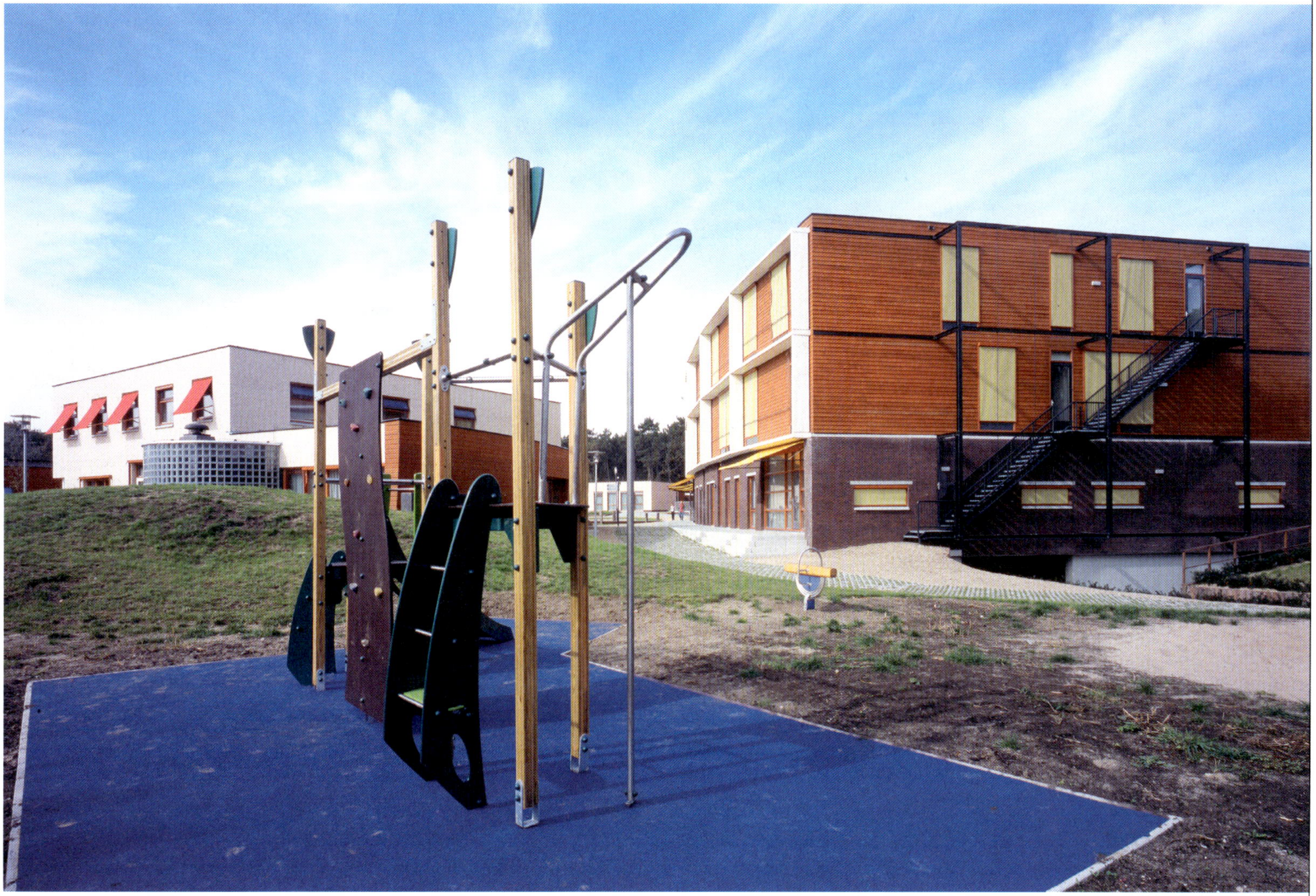

Eric Wendel (EGM) drew up a plan for the De Jutter centre for child and youth psychiatry to cater not only for the demands of the young children and adolescents but also for the emotions of their parents. A transparent structure was required to enable the staff to rapidly notice common anxieties among the children. De Jutter comprises three buildings grouped around an enclosed square: a clinic for young children, a clinic for adolescents, and a main building with the treatment rooms and the school for special education. This main building has three floors and an underground car park and houses the day treatment unit, the outpatient unit, the sports and therapy areas, the school for special education linked with De Jutter, offices and general and technical services. The treatment unit is on the left, the school on the right. The latter occupies the ground floor and the two upper floors. On the left, the treatment unit is on the ground floor, the first floor is an outpatient unit, and the second floor is occupied by offices.

The clinic consists of two buildings, one for young children and one for adolescents. The building for children is situated in the lee of the dunes. The children live in three linked residential groups of seven children per group. Each group has its own lounge and a bedroom wing with single bedrooms that poke into the dune behind like fingers. The lounges face the inner square. The building for adolescents is on the side facing the city. The bedroom wings also poke like fingers into the garden at the rear.

The placing of an old Danish ship completed De Jutter, whose name means 'beachcomber'. The ship makes it clear that play is the most normal way for children to spend their time, even when they are admitted to De Jutter.

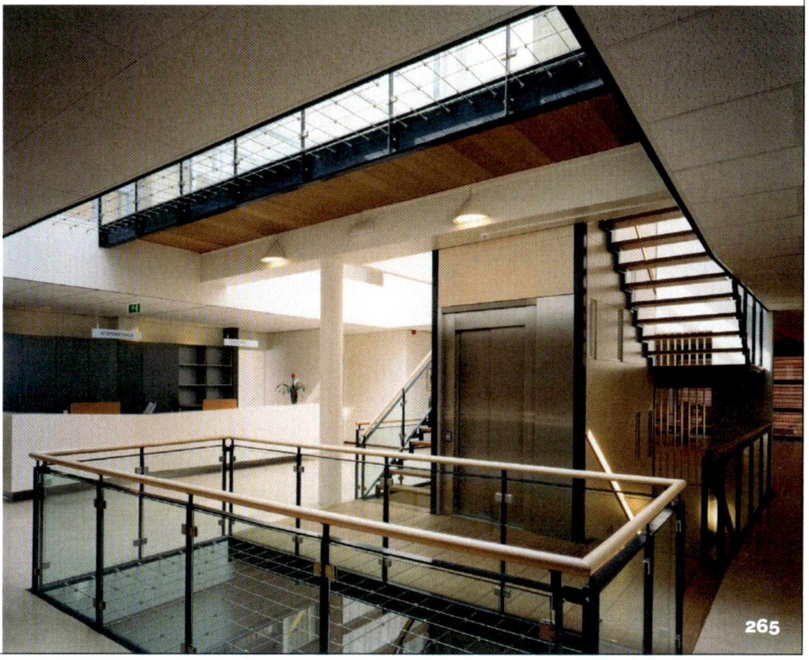

Convent

Han Westelaken
(Architecten aan de Maas)

Kloosterverzorgingshuis
Venlo (Tegelen)
1999-2002

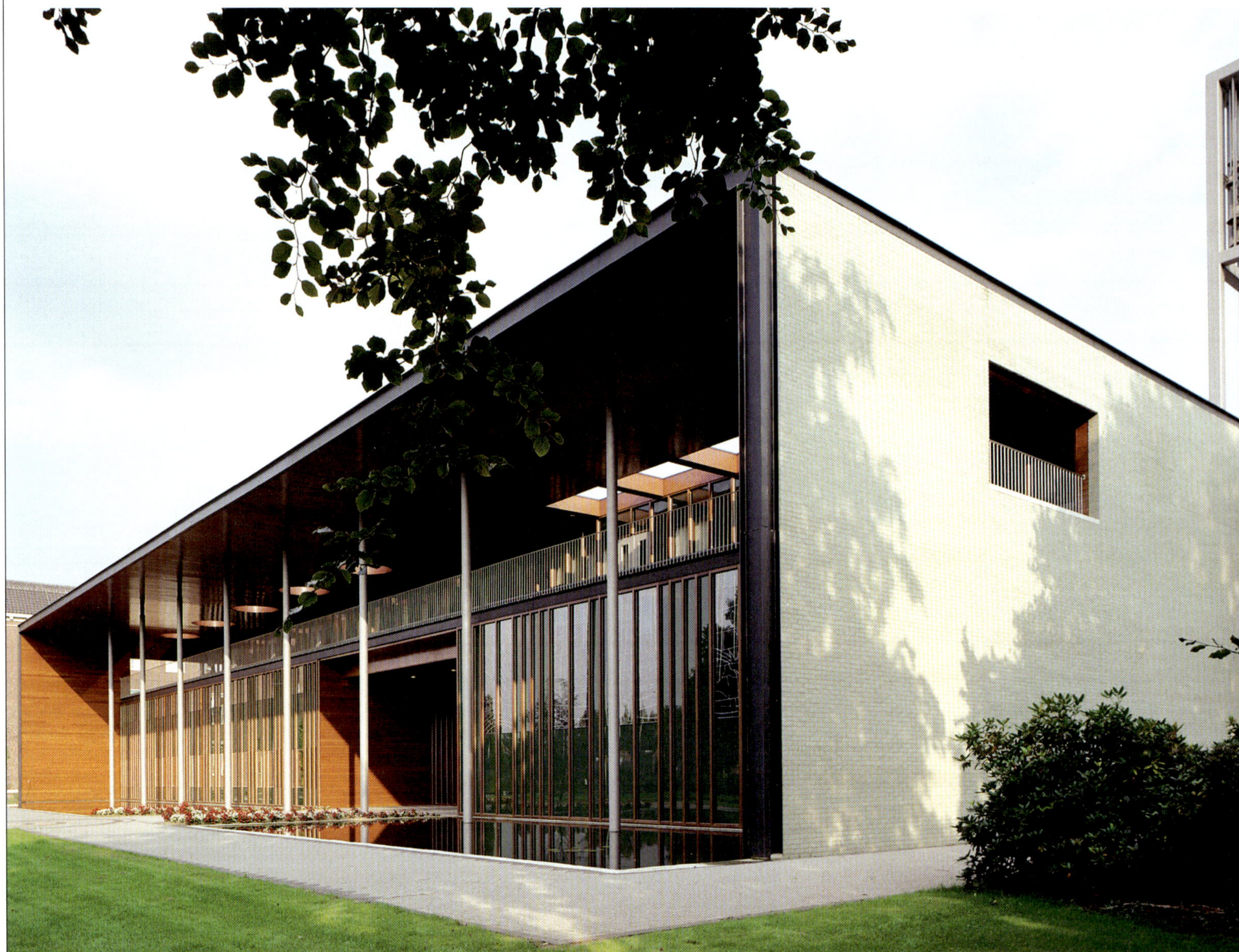

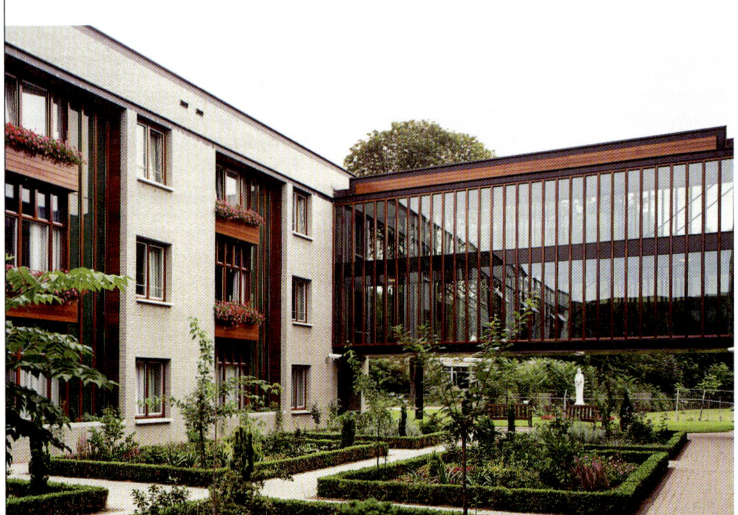

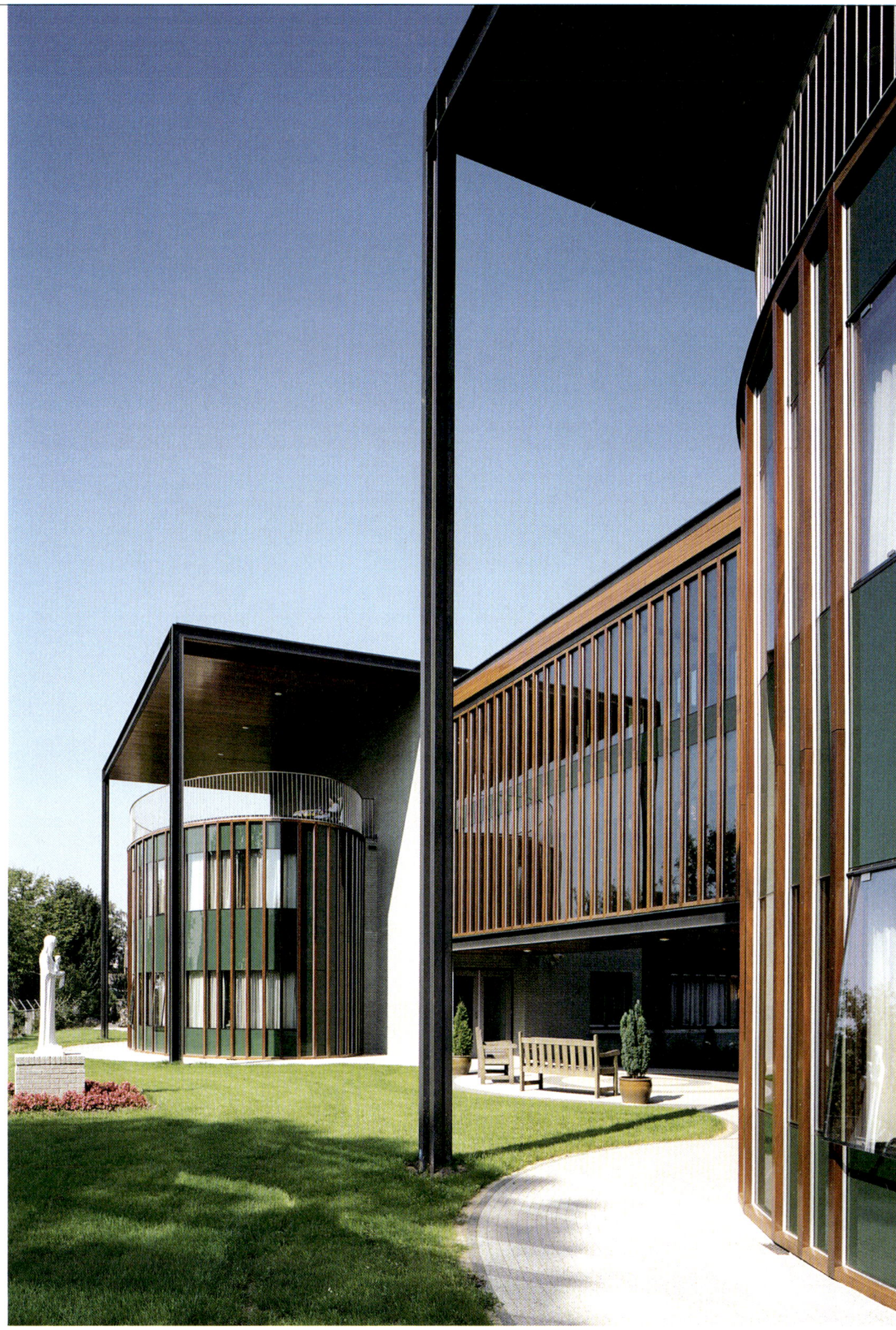

The Kloosterverzorgingshuis in Tegelen is intended for sisters of the Congregation of Our Lady there. Advancing age made nursing inevitable, and that was the reason for a new building. This complex follows the basic programme derived from the norms drawn up by the government, with the addition of a few areas specially designed for this group of residents: a chapel and a communal refectory. These characteristic functions are accommodated in a simple, rectangular volume. The overhanging roof floats above it, resting on slender columns placed in front of the refectory and the chapel. The roof merges seamlessly with that of the two wings that stand at right angles to this section. They contain the residential units. The chapel, which has an elegant spire, and the refectory are situated next to the road. The two residential wings end in two oval meeting areas. Neither these areas nor the communal areas in the volume facing the street extend over the entire three floors, so that here too the roof seems to float above the building. An intermediate section that does extend over the full height of the building connects the two façades of the residential wings.

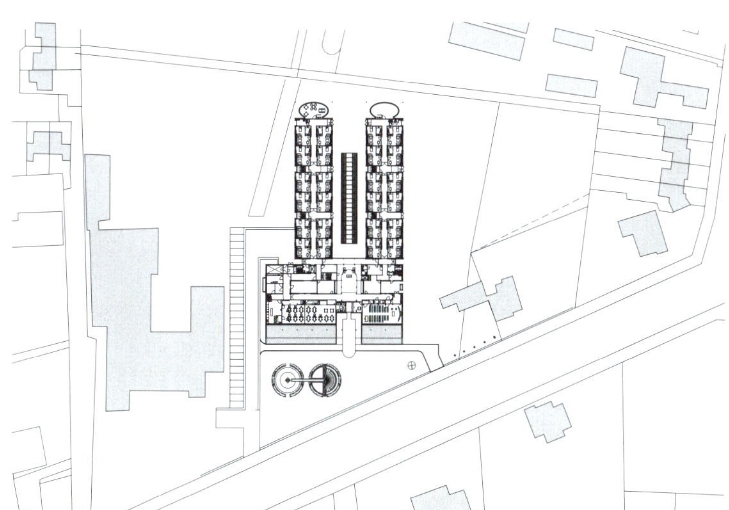

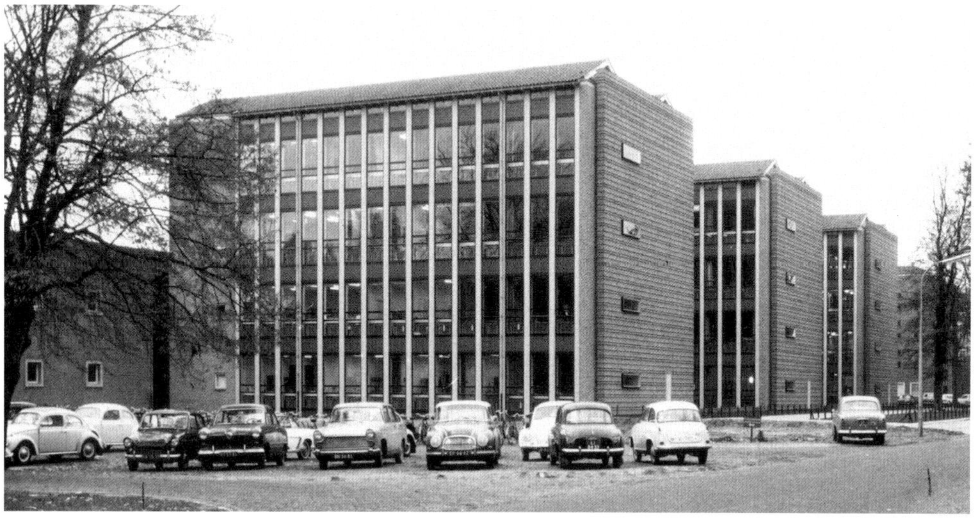

University Medical Centres

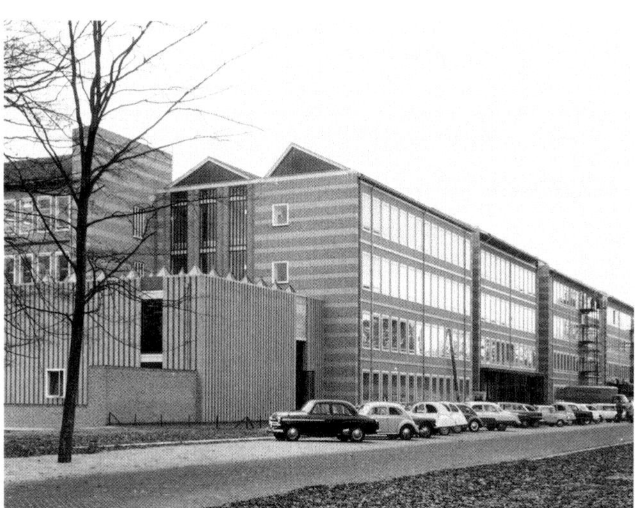

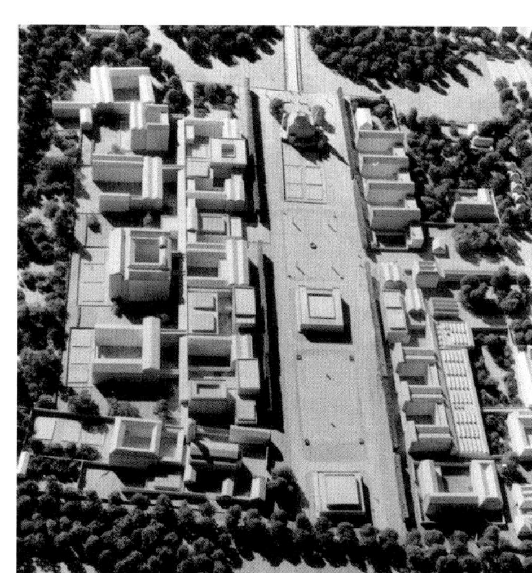

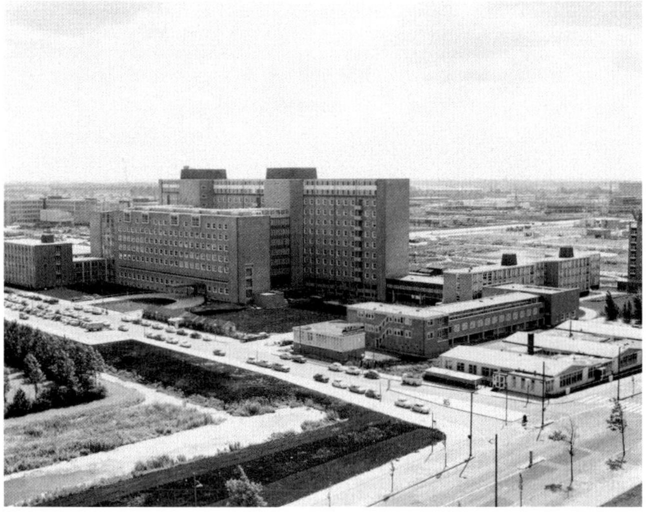

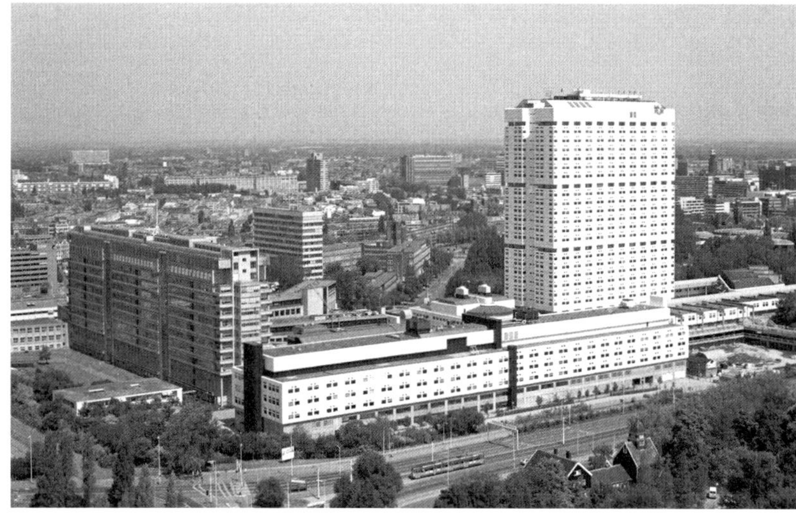

By the end of the 1950s the postwar reconstruction was practically complete. The government relaxed its tight hold, which enabled the medical world to respond to the sharp increase in demand. The demographic explosion, the development of new therapies and technological innovation resulted in a large growth in the number of medical provisions. That called for more physicians and specialists, whose training was a task of the government. The universities of Leiden, Utrecht, Groningen and Amsterdam had university hospitals at their disposal.[1]

The Catholic University in Nijmegen and the Protestant Vrije Universiteit in Amsterdam were each assigned a medical faculty in the 1950s. In 1965 the Dijkzigt Ziekenhuis in Rotterdam was also granted academic status. The core of the new university that was created in Maastricht in 1976 was the medical faculty, which brought the total of university training centres up to eight. The regulations on the building of university hospitals were different from those applying to the building of general hospitals, and the budgets were much more generous.

The first to develop plans for new buildings was the Nijmegen university hospital. J.A. van der Laan began to draw up a plan on the basis of an urban development plan that had been designed under the responsibility of M.J. Granpré Molière. Its general structure was in harmony with the park-like terrain behind Villa Heyendaal. A broad green strip separated the hospital, that lay on the north side of the green boulevard, from the faculty on the south side. The treatment units were directly adjacent to the green strip and were connected with one another and with a convent complex by a long corridor. This backbone of the hospital was also the link with the nursing wards, that were built in the park on the north side.

Work commenced on the building of the new hospital of the Vrije Universiteit in Amsterdam in 1956. The architects were A. Rothuizen and Joh. Groenewegen. The complex consists of two parallel wedges: the nursing wards with 700 beds, and the treatment unit with laboratories, operating theatres, the X-ray unit and the medical examination rooms. Two corridors link the two buildings with one another. On one side of the treatment unit are the lecture rooms and a building for pathological anatomy, on the other side are the outpatient clinics. Soon after completion the building was already too small. From 1965 on there was a particular need for more room for outpatient treatment, resulting in many renovations and extensions.

After the Minister of Education, I.A. Diepenhorst, had decided to grant the Dijkzigt Ziekenhuis in Rotterdam academic status in 1965, the building of a medical faculty was a logical step. There was no time for delay if the increasing shortage of physicians was to be met. The location of the new building was a natural choice: the former Land van Hoboken next to the hospital. One of the tasks of the OD 205 firm of architects was to integrate the new faculty with the Dijkzigt Ziekenhuis.
The programme consisted of more than 100,000 m², of which only a part was actually implemented. The new faculty was completed in 1972. Its 117-metre tower made it the highest building in the Netherlands at the time.

While the newcomers now had new, well equipped complexes at their disposal, Amsterdam, Leiden, Groningen and Utrecht were still grappling with the legacy of the past. The pavilions in which these hospitals had been housed since the beginning of the century were hardly equipped for their tasks, and the locations that lay in or close to the inner city areas became clogged up with a series of new pavilions to accommodate the latest subspecialisations and superspecialisations. G. Westerhout drew up a plan of renewal for the Groningen

Top
Van der Laan Hermans Van der Eerden with Dijkema, Radboudziekenhuis with medical faculty, Nijmegen, 1948-1965. Pre-clinical institutes

Ir. A. Rothuizen en Joh. Groenewegen, university hospital Vrije Universiteit Amsterdam, 1956

OD 205, medical faculty, Rotterdam, 1972

Bottom
Van der Laan Hermans Van der Eerden with Dijkema, Radboudziekenhuis with medical faculty, Nijmegen, 1948-1965. Clinical buildings and model of structural plan.

J. Leupen, plan for a new university hospital on the site of the Wilhelmina Gasthuis, Amsterdam, 1958

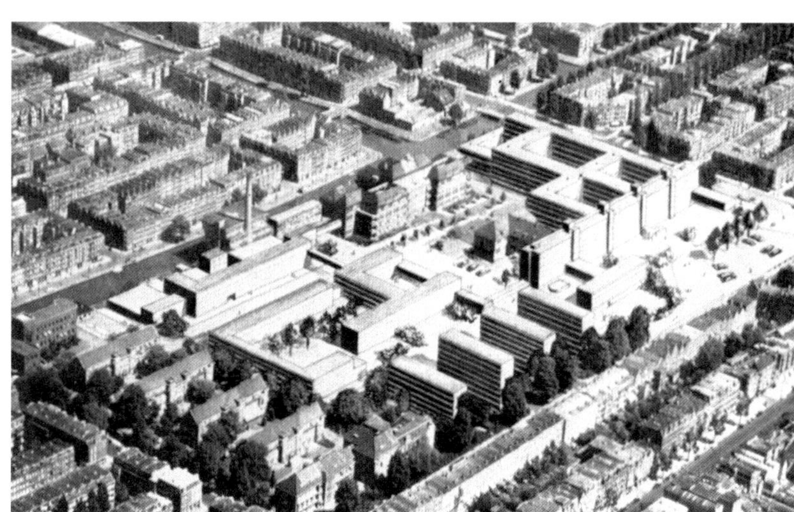

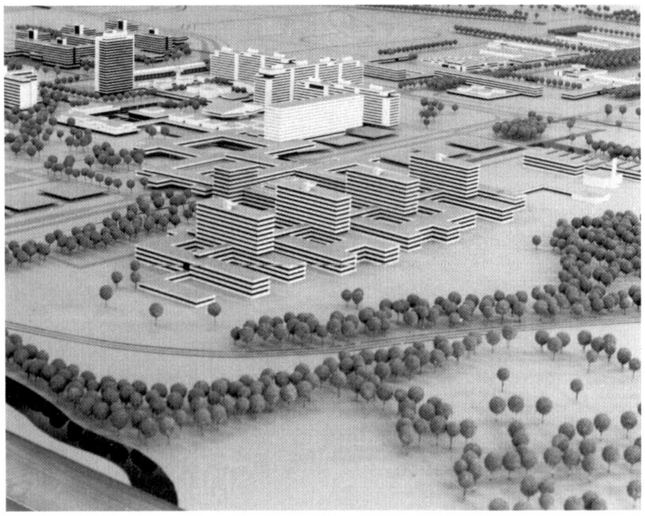

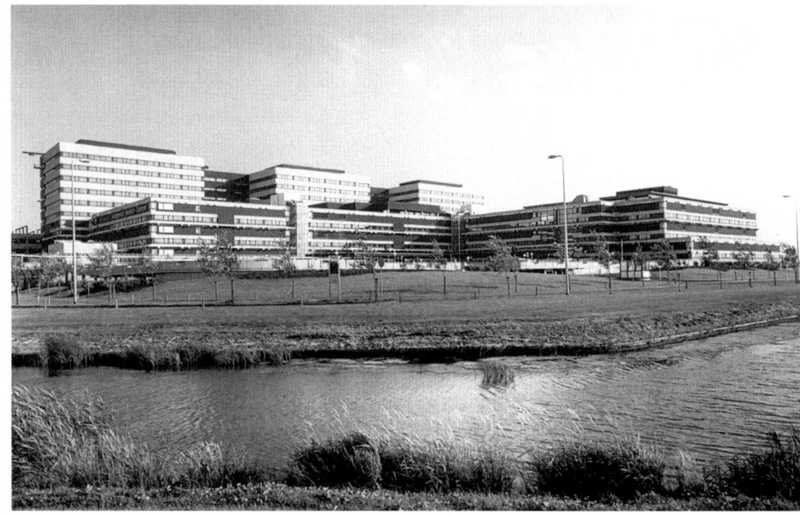

complex in 1955 that envisaged a gradual cleaning up operation by demolishing the old buildings and replacing them with new ones. The different buildings would be connected by a system of underground corridors. The Amsterdam hospital was divided between two locations, which were both at the limit of their capacity. The city architect J. Leupen designed a plan for a new university hospital on the site of the Wilhelmina Gasthuis in 1958. Its 1600 beds made it a giant: nine storeys high, articulated in two parallel volumes with lateral links and an equally massive extra building to house the outpatient clinics and laboratories.[2] The plan was highly controversial: there was hardly any room for expansion and it was difficult for the surroundings to absorb a block of that size. In 1965 the local authority offered a site on the Bijlmer housing estate, bringing the move to the periphery a lot closer.[3] The situation in Leiden and Utrecht was even worse than in Amsterdam and Groningen, where there were at any rate plans for new buildings. They too were confronted with saturated sites without any possibility of expansion. So urgent was the lack of properly functioning training institutes that the government decided on a megalomaniac project in 1966.

While Groningen continued to grapple with the new building programme in stages – which proved virtually impractical because the implementation of new pavilions rarely followed the demolition of the old ones – Amsterdam, Leiden and Utrecht were given the go ahead to draw up plans for new buildings. The government hereby launched what was to be one of the most large-scale building projects in the country. The size of the new complexes was enormous and it was decided to cluster the three assignments. That would yield major advantages: the designers did not have to reinvent the wheel each time and it facilitated standardisation of certain components. That was favourable to an industrial and thus less expensive building method. The cooperation was so intensive that the three firms selected for the task – Du Pon en Van Mourik for Amsterdam, Brouwer en Deurvorst for Leiden, and Duintjer en Istha for Utrecht – set up a joint office in Haarlem.

The structural plans drawn up in 1966 were typical: they were variants of the 'tower on a podium' type. Duintjer and Istha sketched a comb-shaped treatment unit with four high ward units on the 'teeth' for the Utrecht university hospital (AZU). The outpatient clinics were an extension of the teeth; the laboratories and teaching areas were on the other side of the passage that connected them. The height of the complex ran up against criticism. Changes in the urban framework subsequently made revision inevitable. There were objections to the choice of the location in Leiden, and all that was known in Amsterdam was that the hospital could not remain on the site of the Wilhelmina Gasthuis.

In 1967 J. Wester was commissioned to develop a standard programme of requirements for the new university hospitals. Ten years later this Wester programme contained more than eighty parts, in a certain sense *the* monument to the belief in a (medical) society that can be designed. A characteristic of the hospitals that followed these standards is the formation of functional units by specialisation. Wards, outpatient units and treatment units were integrated per specialisation and connected with a 'hot floor'. The latter was called the Central Medical Complex at the time and contained high tech provisions such as the operating theatres.

The building of the Academisch Medisch Centrum (AMC) in Amsterdam began in 1974. It was completed in stages between 1981 and 1984. It was built before the Wester programme was ready and therefore required a high degree of flexibility. C.A. Doets, the building coordinator of the university

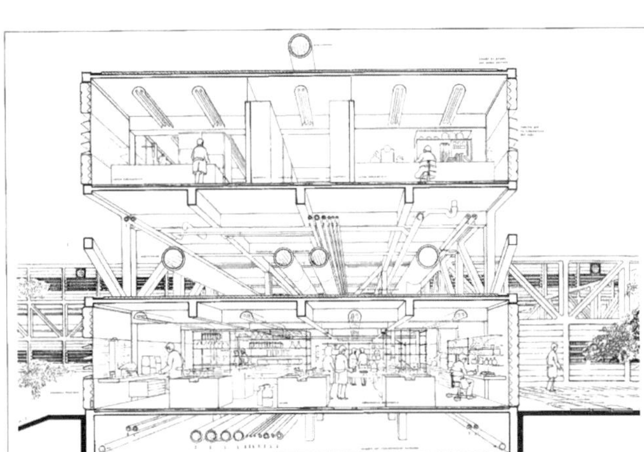

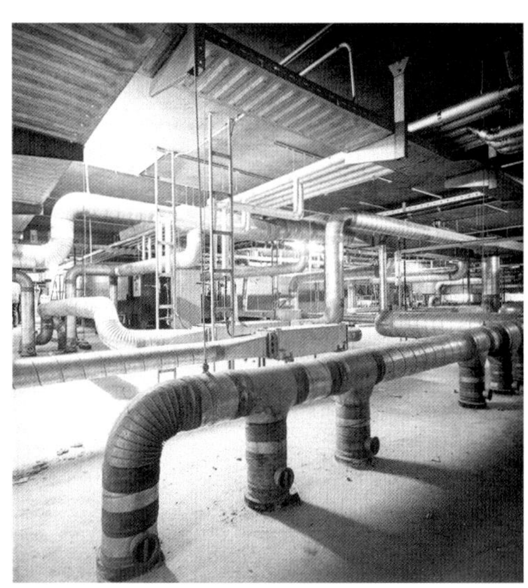

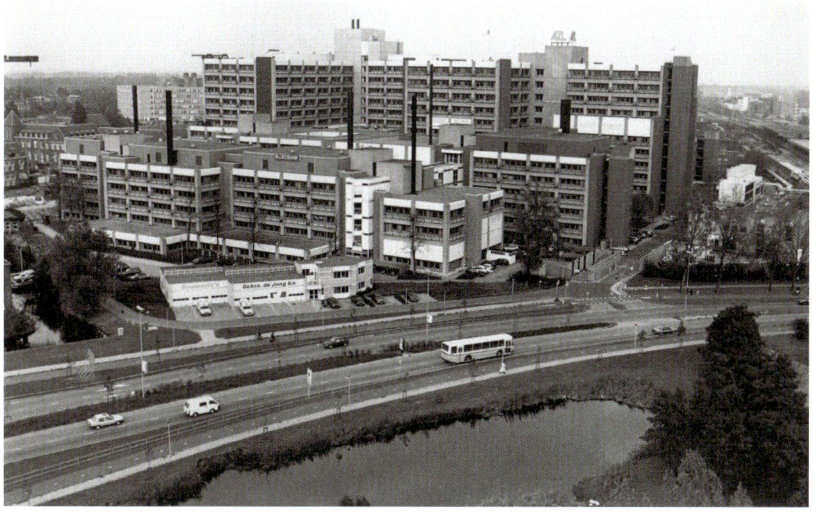

Top
Duintjer en Istha, plan for university hospital, Utrecht, 1966

Duintjer Istha Kramer Van Willegen with D. van Mourik architecten en ingenieurs, Academisch Medisch Centrum (AMC), Amsterdam, 1966-1981/1985

B&D Architecten, Academisch Ziekenhuis Leiden (AZL), Leiden, 1985/1994

Bottom
Mc Master University Health Sciences Center, Hamilton, Canada. Cross-section technical intermediate floor

Technical intermediate floor in the AMC

EGM architecten, Academisch Ziekenhuis Utrecht (AZU), Utrecht, 1989

hospitals, stated: 'The supporting construction was built and the infill of rooms and installations could be determined at a later stage to meet the latest requirements. Progress in medical science is so fast that before you know it you are opening a building that is already outdated'.[4] When the decision was taken during the building operations to reduce the number of beds and related provisions from 1040 to 950, the advantage was immediately obvious. There was no difficulty in redistributing the space that had become vacant and giving it new functions.[5]

The model for the university hospitals was the McMaster University Health Sciences Center in Hamilton, Canada. This institute was famous all over the world for the revolutionary teaching model that had been developed there, based on the concept of learning by practice. That made it only natural to combine teaching with hospital departments. Not only was this model subsequently exported, but the pioneering new building based on the concept, which was completed in 1971, provoked considerable interest as well. The designers, Craig, Zeidler and Strong, designed a megastructure with a large degree of flexibility which made it possible to combine and exchange functions. 'This constructional mechanical structure is to be understood as a therapy for the malady of the hospital called flexibility', is how the *Deutsche Bauzeitung* praised the solution adopted, which included service subfloors (interstitial spaces).[6] This meant that if a hospital was expanded or modified, there would be no need to break open the always extremely large networks of pipes and cables running through the whole complex. The McMaster Health Sciences Center was in fact less of a building than a moment in an ongoing process of transformation.[7] The industrial building technique with prefab façade elements, the application of service subfloors and the hard appearance were highly appreciated by Doets and the three firms of architects (joined by a fourth later) who built the Dutch university hospitals.[8]

The solution for the concentration of similar functions and the promotion of optimal contact between these functions was found by creating three parallel zones. As in the general hospitals, these linear strips could easily be enlarged simply by extending them. The difference was that they had a specific function: one strip with wards, one with treatment units, and one with outpatient clinics. The teaching units were located partly in the treatment zone, and partly on a separate location outside the three zones.

With its shops and restaurants, the Academisch Medisch Centrum (AMC) in Amsterdam has the appearance of a safe city closed off from the outside world. This look was so successful that the integration of shops, supermarkets, travel agencies and similar urban functions has become one of the fixed elements of hospital architecture since the 1980s. Far from the real city, a pseudo-city was created in the AMC which, entirely in line with the philosophy of the 1960s, bore hardly any relation to its surroundings.[9]

The university hospital in Utrecht (Academisch Ziekenhuis Utrecht, AZU) also exchanged the old location in the city for a peripheral one. That decision was already taken in 1960, when the parachuting of hospitals in the periphery was still regarded as ideal.[10] When the original structural plan of Duintjer and Istha for the AZU proved not to be feasible, their successors, Eijkelenboom Gerritse Middelhoek (EGM), removed the wards from the treatment zone to arrive at the characteristic division into three zones here too. The first pile was driven in 1981 and the hospital opened eight years later. Covered streets and squares determine how the complex presents itself to the visitor in Utrecht too.

The third and last hospital to be built on

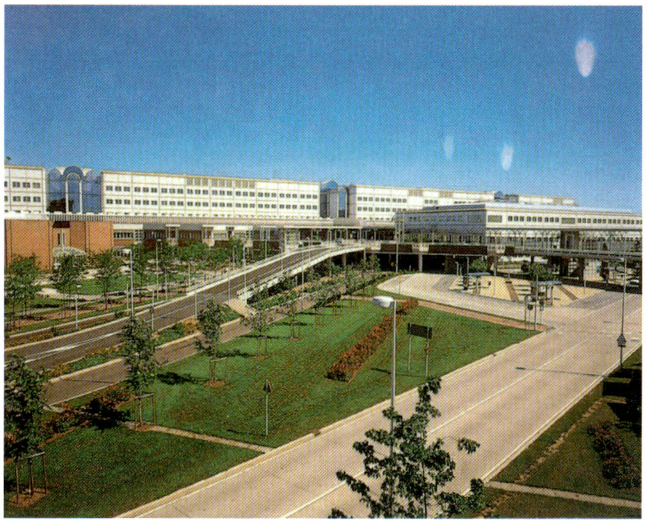

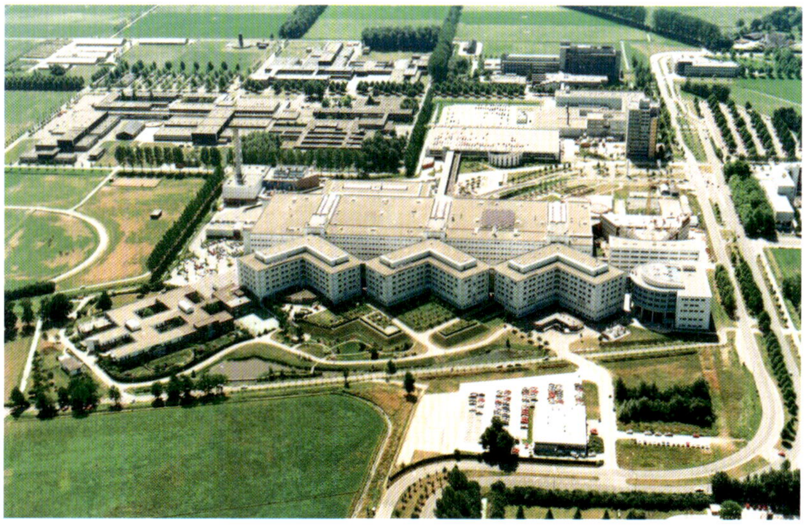

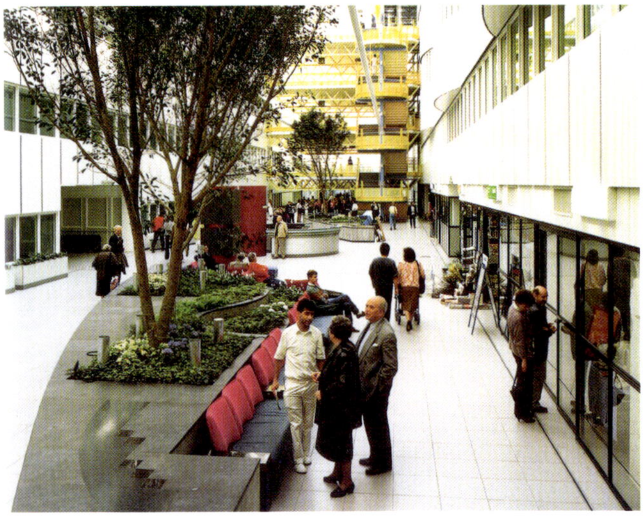

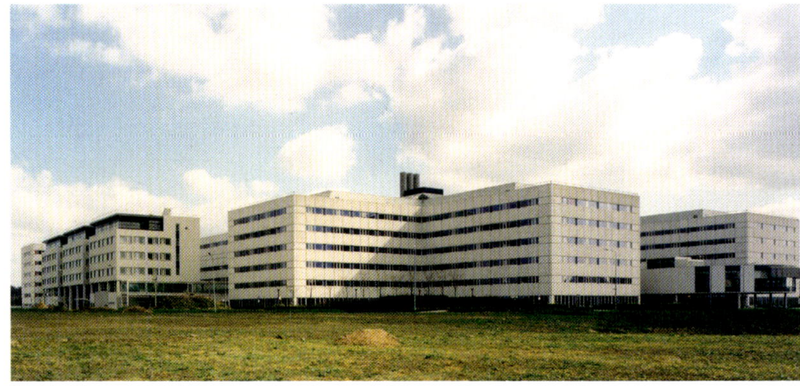

the basis of this standard design is the Leiden university hospital (Academisch Ziekenhuis Leiden, AZL). Unlike its counterparts in Amsterdam and Utrecht, after years of debates on the most suitable location the Leiden university hospital was allowed to remain in the city, just behind the station and only separated from the inner city by the railway track. Work on building began in 1981 and it was carried out in stages. The relatively small plot of land available forced the designers, Brouwer en Deurvorst (later B&D Architekten), to partly telescope the zones and to create a tower on a podium hospital with a broad podium, but also an exceptionally high tower (five storeys). In spite of the necessary compactness, covered streets and patios also play a prominent role in this design.[11] This is where the three megastructures try to harmonise their introverted medical technological culture with the more pleasant aspects of everyday life. The most characteristic and imitated feature is 'the undisguised recreational flirt in the lighting rows and atria where not only the catering establishments with all their trimmings twinkle, but also an unprecedented concentration of art purchased from the building budget fills the empty space of these parts of the building. Nowhere is the membrane between suffering and entertainment so thin.'[12] Leiden was the last of the three hospitals that together formed an almost megalomaniac project.

The university hospital in Maastricht (Academisch Ziekenhuis Maastricht, AZM) was initially housed in the outdated Sint Annadal, but it was already clear that new premises were essential. The Maastricht firm Swinkels/Passchier/Bonneur/Westelaken architekten & ingenieurs was responsible for the design. It was still based on the 84-part Wester programme, but because that programme had not been geared to the specific situation of Maastricht, a 'Memorandum of divergence' was added.[13] Unlike the other university hospitals, the AZM in Maastricht has the classic tripartition into a treatment unit, nursing wards, and outpatient clinics. It was built between 1984 and 1991 on a location on the periphery. The complex has a symmetrical plan. The main entrance is situated on the central axis, and from there the traffic system branches out in a completely logical way in the form of a ladder. According to the designers, this displays characteristics of what is called the 'public domain' in the city. The way in which large buildings are divided up must possess all the characteristics that make a public domain legible and pleasant for the users. Streets and squares perform that function in the city. The architects of the AZM fleshed it out in a similar way: 'Walking through the ladder offers surprising views of the interior of this complex, but at the same time it provides the insight and general picture that are needed to find one's way and to feel at home, just like in the city'.[14]

The university hospital in Groningen (Academisch Ziekenhuis Groningen, AZG) opened in 1997.[15] Work had been going on to the building for more than twenty years, starting with the structural plan by Kruisheer + Hallink from the 1970s. The hospital had to be built on the site of the old building. It consisted of separate buildings with the nursing and outpatient units organised around a Central Medical Complex with operating theatres, X-ray unit and laboratories. Team 4 Architecten was invited to design the nursing wards, each of which was to have an entrance of its own according to the Kruisheer + Hallink structural plan. Insights changed during the design and construction process. It was decided to roof the streets between the different buildings to form one large whole. The two main streets between the wards and the medical core were connected with one another on the south by a large entrance

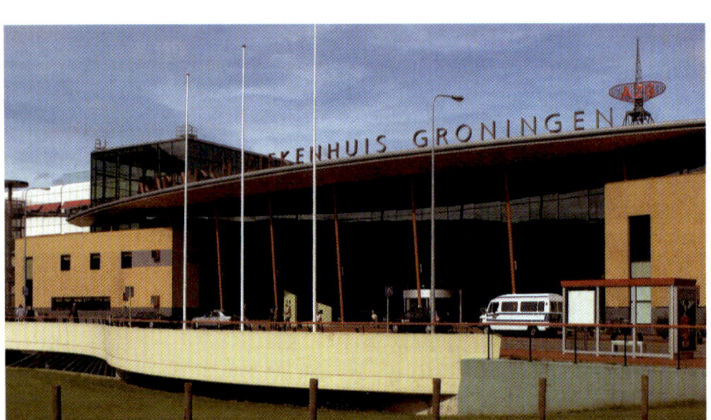

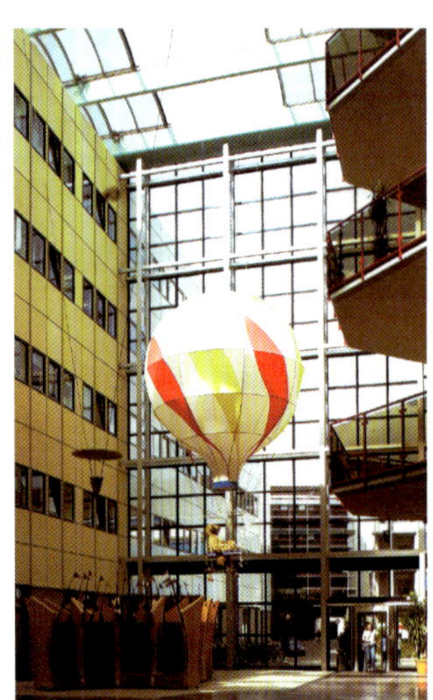

Top
Swinkels/Passchier/Bonneur/Westelaken architekten & ingenieurs, Academisch Ziekenhuis Maastricht, 1990

Sponge Architects & Rupali Gupta with IOU Architecture, Ronald McDonald VU Kinderstad, Amsterdam, 2008

EGM architecten, plan for Erasmus MC, Rotterdam, 2004. Work in progress.

Bottom
Wytze Patijn, Academisch Ziekenhuis Groningen (AZG), Groningen, 1997. Entrance hall and inner street.

EGM architecten, Teaching building, UMC St Radboud, Nijmegen, 1999. Part of the restructuring.

Kuiper Compagnons, V. Yanovshtchinsky, plan for extension of the UMCG, Groningen, 2009

View of the UMCG, Groningen with teaching building by Thomas Rau and laboratory by UN Studio

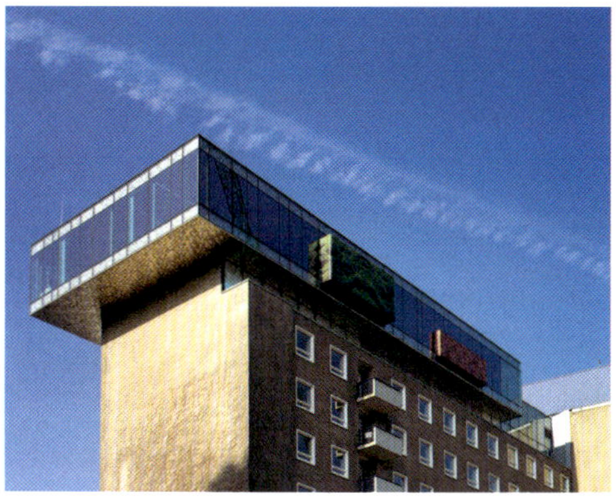

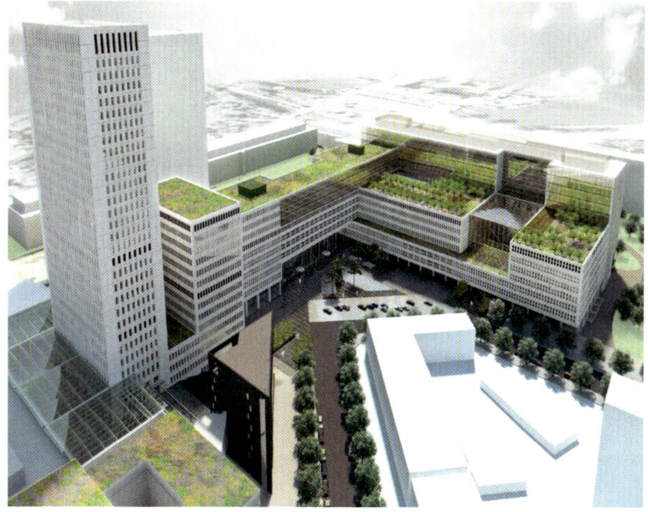

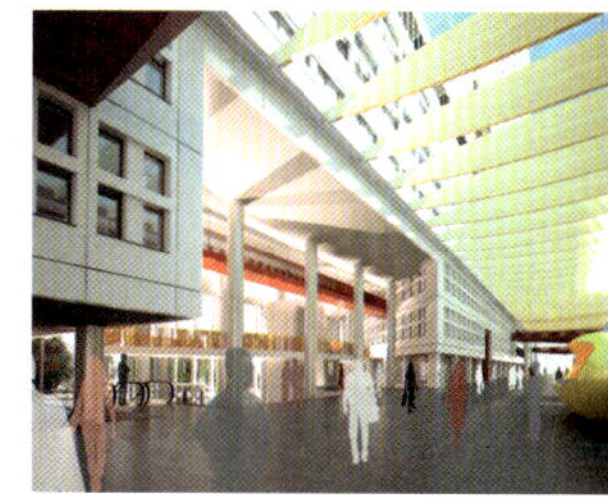

hall and on the north by a side street. Wytze Patijn designed several features including the entrance hall, under which a car park was built. Beneath the rest of the complex is a tunnel structure, a remnant from Westerhout's 1955 plan. After the opening of the connecting building, the Bridge, between the hospital and the medical faculty in 2005, another teaching building designed by Thomas Rau, as well as the Research Laboratory designed by Ben van Berkel (UN Studio), were built between 2005 and 2007. By now there are also plans to expand with medically related functions and housing on the north side of the site in the course of the next twenty years.

Work has continued on a long-term accommodation plan for the Vrije Universiteit (VU) since the 1980s. It entails renovation of the old building and the implementation of a series of new buildings. The Ronald McDonald VU Children's City, placed on top of the existing building, was opened in 2008. It was designed by Sponge Architects & Rupali Gupta in cooperation with IOU Architecture.

After fifty years, the Nijmegen university hospital (UMC St Radboud since 2004) is ripe for renewal. It has been further expanded with new buildings and functions in the course of time. A large-scale restructuring, renovation and new building programme was approved in 1992. It is being implemented in two stages after a design by the EGM architecten.

The Erasmus Medisch Centrum (Rotterdam) is being largely replaced by new buildings too. Once again a design by EGM architecten is being implemented in two stages. The first entails the construction of three patient themes: Oncology, Immunity, metabolism and ageing, Acute care and the locomotive apparatus, and most of the auxiliary functions. These sections are due to be completed in 2014. Afterwards the old Dijkzigt Ziekenhuis, which was built in the aftermath of the Second World War, will be demolished and the second stage will get under way. It comprises the themes Brains and senses, Circulation, and Reproduction, growth and development. When the Erasmus Medisch Centrum will be completed, all eight university teaching hospitals will have up-to-date facilities at their disposal – but as the continuous addition and reconstruction processes of even the newer complexes demonstrate, it is unlikely that work on these complexes, which represent the top level of what Dutch medicine has to offer, will ever end...

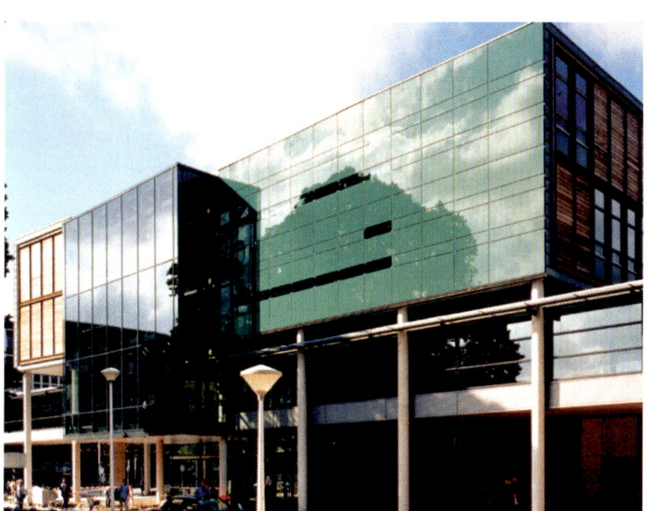

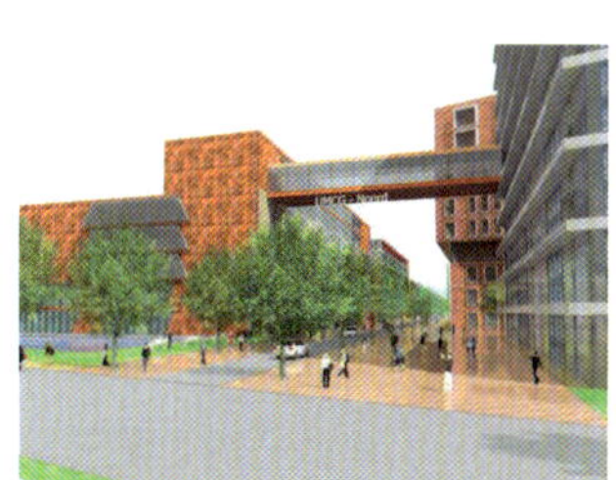

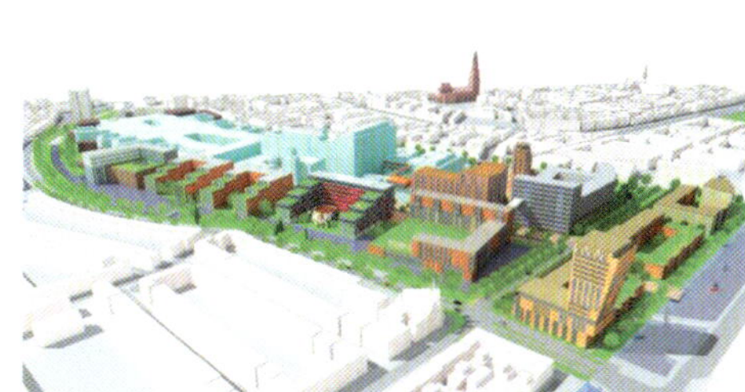

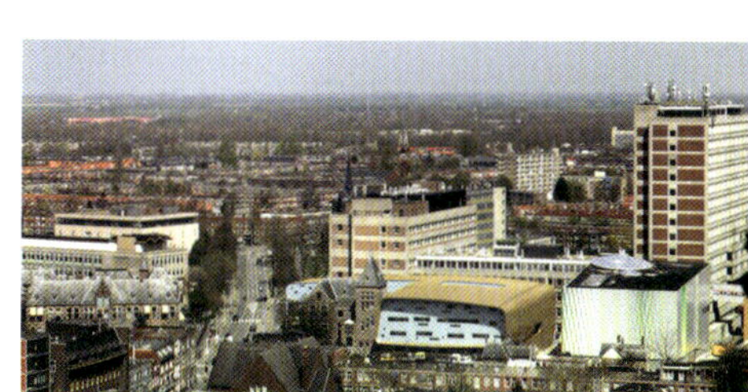

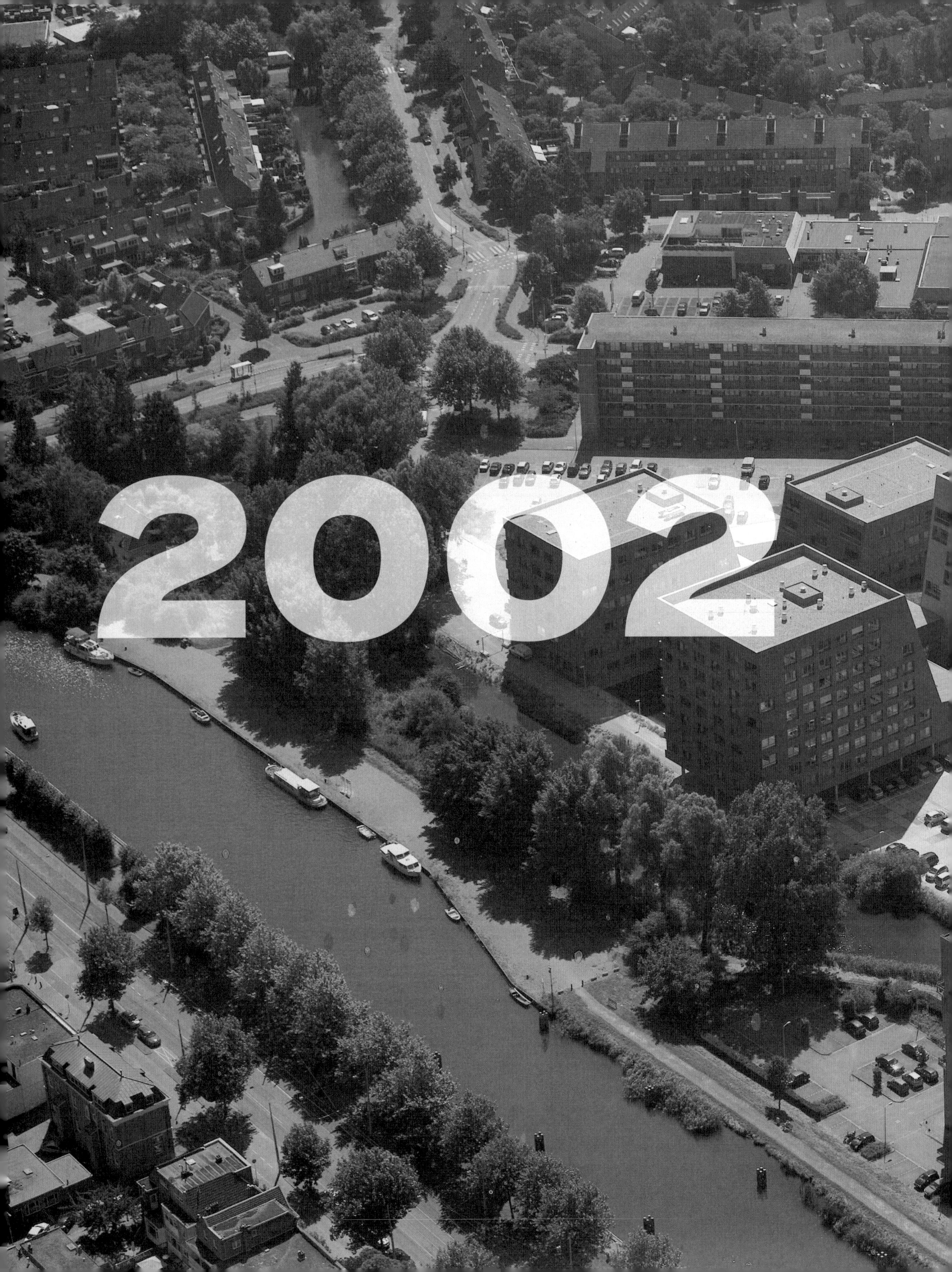

2002

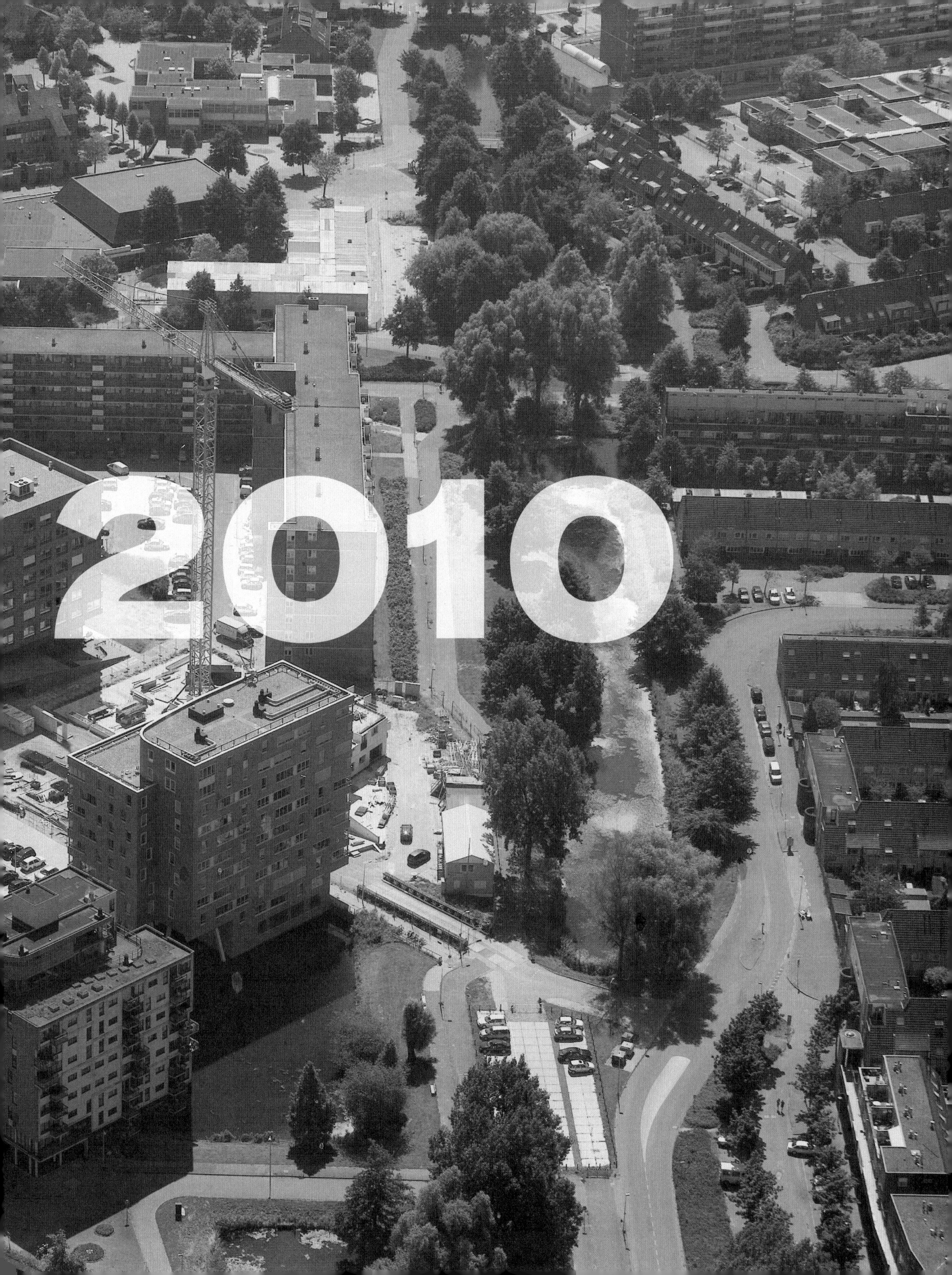
2010

Beyond health care architecture: the way to the future

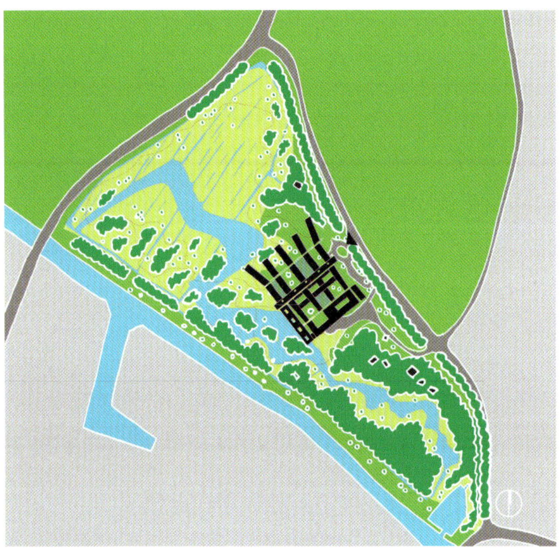

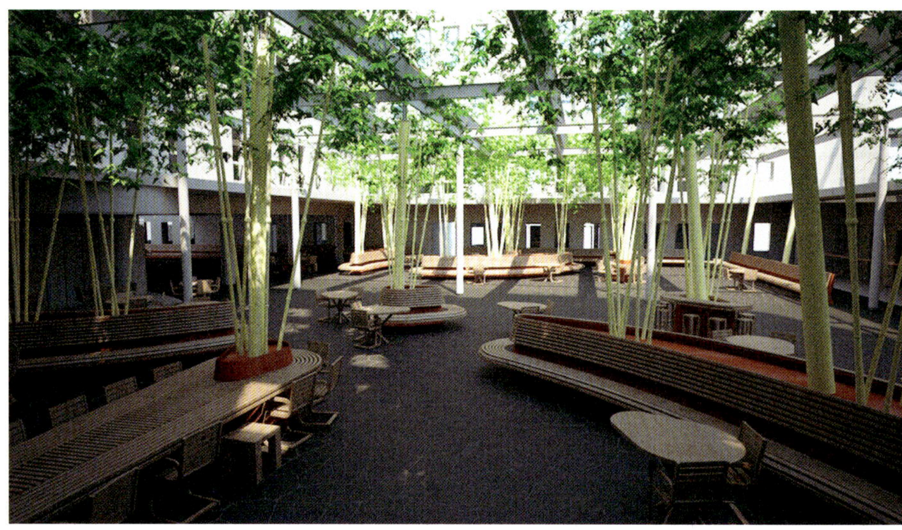

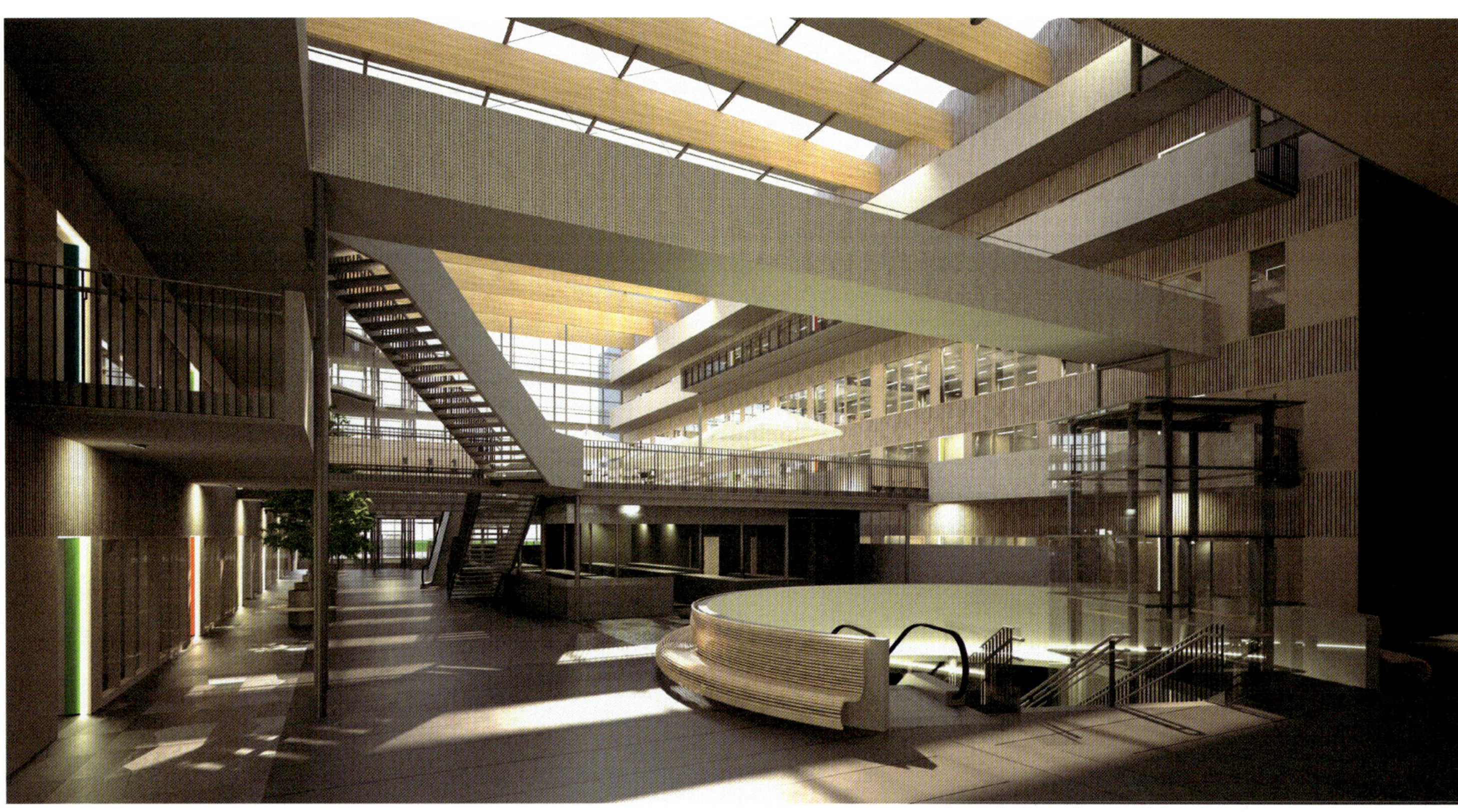

Architecture and health care buildings

Health care buildings are among the most fascinating architectural assignments. Their evolution began when hospitals and psychiatric institutions deliberately began to distinguish themselves some 250 years ago by the way in which they were determined by their purpose. Their function was to contribute to the recovery of the patients who were admitted to them, and the architecture was deployed as an instrument to make that possible. Even if these buildings already had to be designed to accommodate medical processes and nursing, more importance was attached to the surroundings that they offered their users. A natural, healthy environment was believed to make an essential contribution to their wellbeing and to promote their recovery. This resulted in specific types of building – the first in the history of architecture. The further evolution of this type was determined by medical, technological and social developments. This book documents the changes inspired by them. No matter how drastic they were, until the 1990s health care buildings were still clearly distinguished as special types, and hospitals in fact still are. However, developments have been taking place in the last ten years that seem to herald the end of the typological series. The determinant factor seems to be the gradual transition to a health care system in which market mechanisms are given a prominent role. The magical formula that is constantly repeated is the replacement of supply by demand regulation. In a liberalised market, the demand – in this case for health care – determines the supply. Expenses are not cut by limiting supply, but by competition, and that competition will only increase as the market acquires an increasingly open character.

The regulation of supply was characterised by an extensive system of permits, restrictions on the possibility of running a care institution, and exemptions from them. The new system gradually does away with most restrictions. Institutions themselves become responsible for their real estate and have to pass the building and running costs on to the price of the care. While in the past it was a fine art to obtain permission from the government to build as many square metres as possible – the costs were covered by the state – it is now a question of building flexible and above all sellable buildings that function optimally without wasting space. Although there are as many definitions of optimal functioning as there are different parties and perspectives, there is a consensus on the desirability of reducing the number of parts of the building specifically designed for their function to a minimum.[1]

All institutions in the health care sector are forced to think about the usefulness and necessity of their buildings – and thus of architecture. Two extreme positions can be discerned. On the one hand there is the view of architecture as a necessary evil whose costs must be kept as low as possible. On the other hand is the view that architecture is a business instrument that directly influences the business results. Two aspects play a major role here: logistics and the way a building is perceived and experienced by its users. Frustration of the logistical processes leads to high costs, while innovative concepts can involve considerable savings. In the most radical visions, the hospital is seen as a differentiated network of small-scale specialised clinics in which the potential of the multimedia and the internet are utilised to the full for mutual communications and for the relation with the patients. The way in which architecture is experienced by the users is also at the focus of attention. In the last resort it is the user who passes judgement, and in a genuinely liberalised market it is the user who represents the demand which the supply should be targeting.

p. 274
***Dick van Gameren architecten*, Berkenstede care centre, Diemen, 2006**

p. 276
***Atelier Pro*, the projected new Meander Medisch Centrum, Amersfoort, 2010, situation and artist impressions**

p. 277
***Rothuizen Van Doorn 't Hooft architecten en stedenbouwkundigen*, Rijnland Ziekenhuis, care boulevard, Alphen aan den Rijn, 2008**

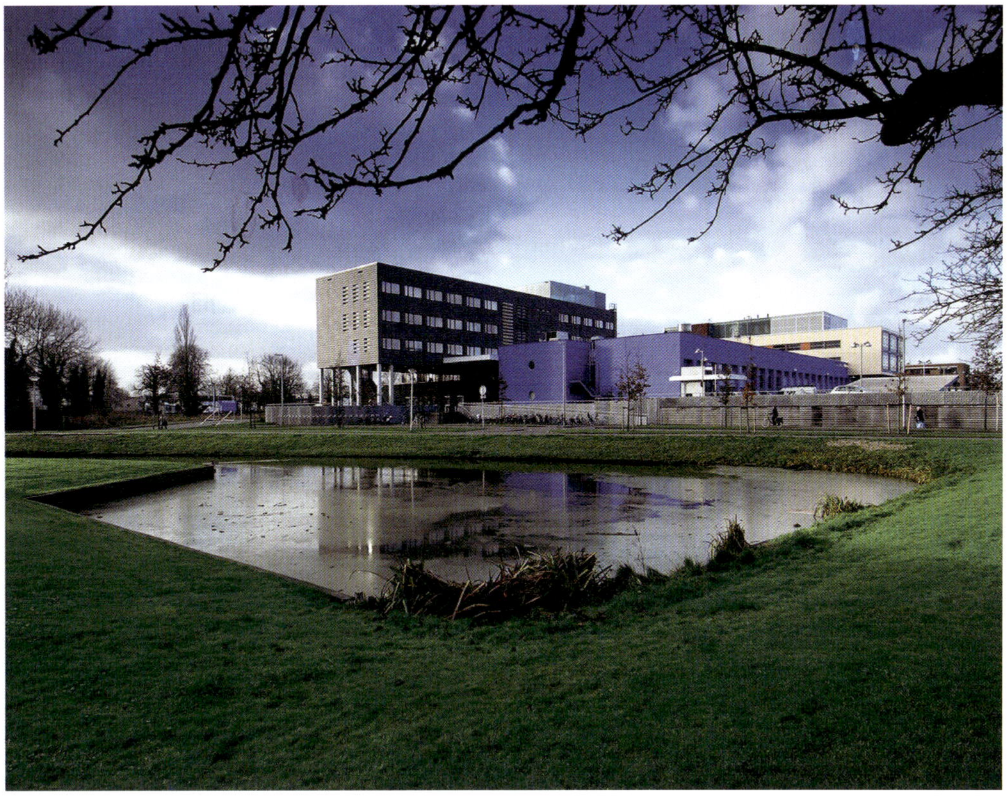

Hospitals

A notable difference can be seen in the architecture of hospitals between the development of new concepts and the implementation of the last dinosaurs for the time being. Conferences like 'The Architecture of Hospitals' organised in the Universitair Medisch Centrum Groningen (UMCG) in 2005 illustrate that there is an urgent need for reorientation.[2] Research specifically geared to the situation in the Netherlands yields points of anchorage for drastic and sometimes controversial new models, but in practice it proves difficult to implement them because of the organisational consequences, the uncertainty of funding, and the persistence of set ways of thinking. No doubt an even greater obstacle is the inadequate awareness of the potential of architecture, which is still often seen as a necessary evil instead of a powerful instrument to achieve better performance. Still, that situation seems to be changing too, witness the growing interest in the concepts of the Healing Environment and Evidence-Based Design. Publications such as *Au! Bouwen aan de architectuur van de zorg* (Ow! Building care architecture), master classes in the Berlage Institute in Rotterdam, the UMCG and elsewhere, various initiatives of the Netherlands Architecture Fund, increasing interest within the university world, the creation of the Hedy d'Ancona Award for excellent care architecture and the work of the atelier Rijksbouwmeester (Chief Government Architect studio) – all these developments indicate that hard work is being done on the rediscovery of the significance of architecture in health care in general, and in hospitals in particular.[3]

From medical bulwark to secure enclave

In the last few years the complexes have been completed that were developed from the mid-1990s as the hospitals of the twenty-first century. The pause for thought that was introduced when the ministry announced a temporary building freeze has borne fruit. In spite of the often vast scale and the large concentration of the most diverse medical functions, the designers do their very best to avoid giving these buildings the character of medical bulwarks while still

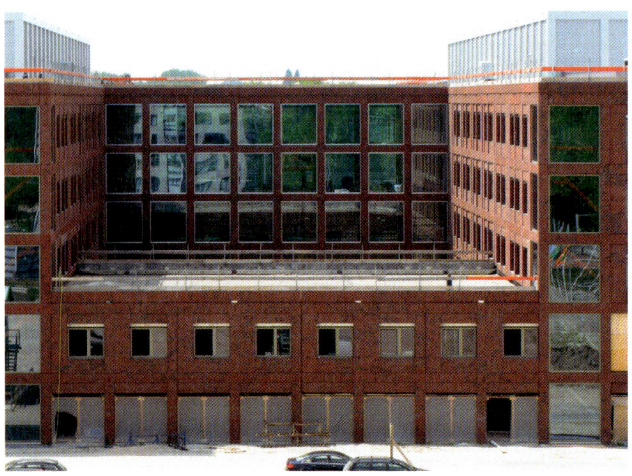

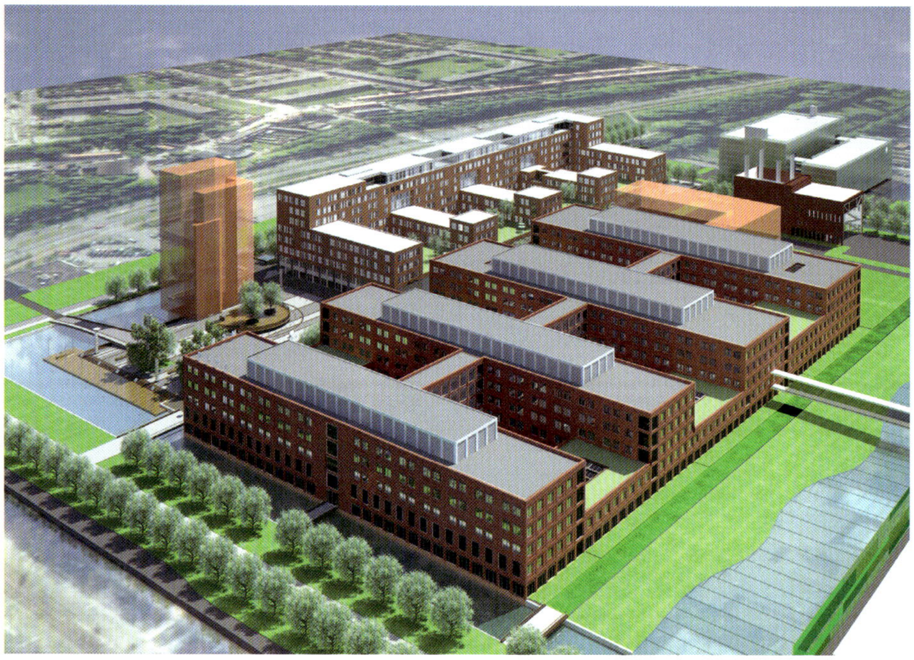

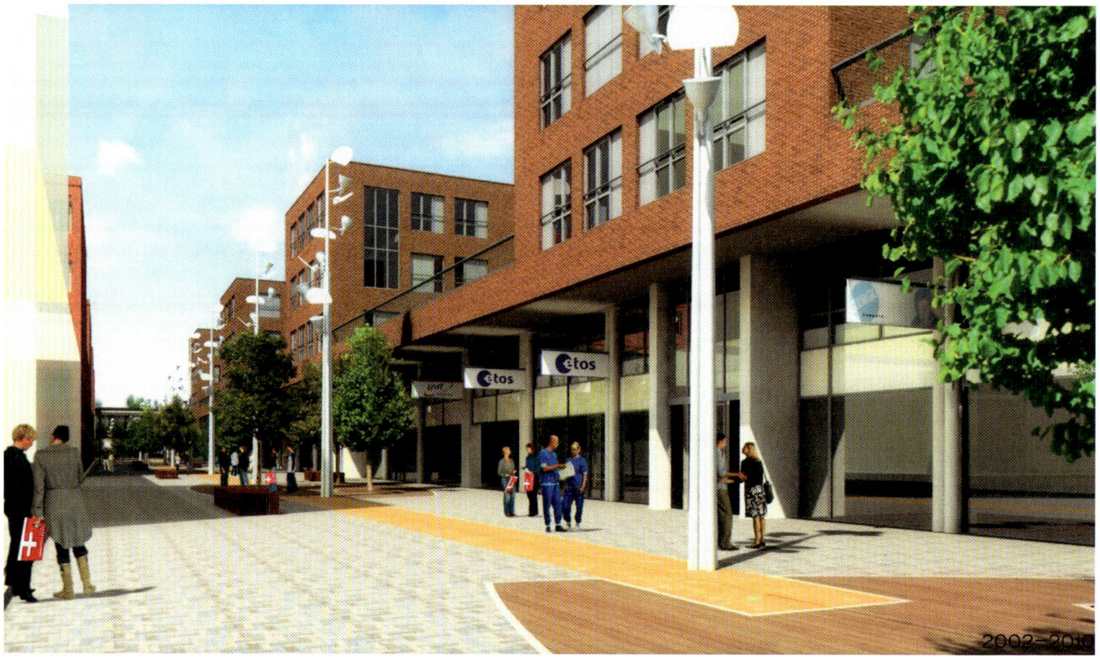

p. 278
***Wiegerinck Architectuur en Stedenbouw*, Maasstad Ziekenhuis, Rotterdam, 2001–2010**

Impression of care boulevard Rotterdam and the Maasstad Ziekenhuis (Wiegerinck Architectuur en Stedenbouw) and the medimall (EGM architecten)

***EGM architecten*, impression of care boulevard Rotterdam**

p. 279
***Burger Grunstra architecten adviseurs*, Martini Ziekenhuis, Groningen, 2007**

allowing them to profile themselves as special provisions. An example of this is the Maasland Ziekenhuis in Sittard, but there are other recent projects too. All the attempts to drastically modernise the classic all-under-one-roof hospital culminate in the Maasland Ziekenhuis in Sittard designed by Bonnema Architecten. The architecture is luxurious and transparent, the materials – a lot of wood – are robust and elegant, the details are extremely refined. More important is that only single rooms have been applied, and the idea of four clusters of consultation rooms that are used by different specialists – the era of a consultation room of one's own is past – is truly pioneering. The individual study has gone too; it has been replaced by four centres of expertise. The main principle is the rigorous separation of the different groups of users. The medical staff have their own lift and staircase in the middle of the building, at the point where the atrium leads to the wing with high tech medical provisions, including the operating theatres.

The main theme of the Deventer Ziekenhuis (de Jong Gortemaker Algra architecten en ingenieurs), completed in 2008, is the distinction between different categories of patients: those who come for intensive planned care use a different zone from visitors to the outpatients clinics or who need acute care. The building is situated in the landscape like a boomerang. The outpatient zone provides access to the complex; this zone consists of a hall with patios containing separate 'boxes' for the various outpatient units.

The design of the Isalakliniek in Zwolle by Alberts & Van Huut in collaboration with a/d amstel architecten stands out for the idiosyncratic architectural idiom, which is referred to as organic.[4] The building avoids a technical or clinical appearance. It consists of four 'butterflies', each of which has its own function. The internal division is based on target groups and types of complaints.

The Martini Ziekenhuis in Groningen (2007) designed by Arnold Burger (Burger Grunstra architecten adviseurs) consists of two elongated volumes. One has a flowing serpentine shape, the other a zigzag. The two volumes are connected at two points. A striking feature is the glass façade on the side of the access road: this double façade gives the complex many of its salient characteristics. The hospital is a model project for industrial, flexible and

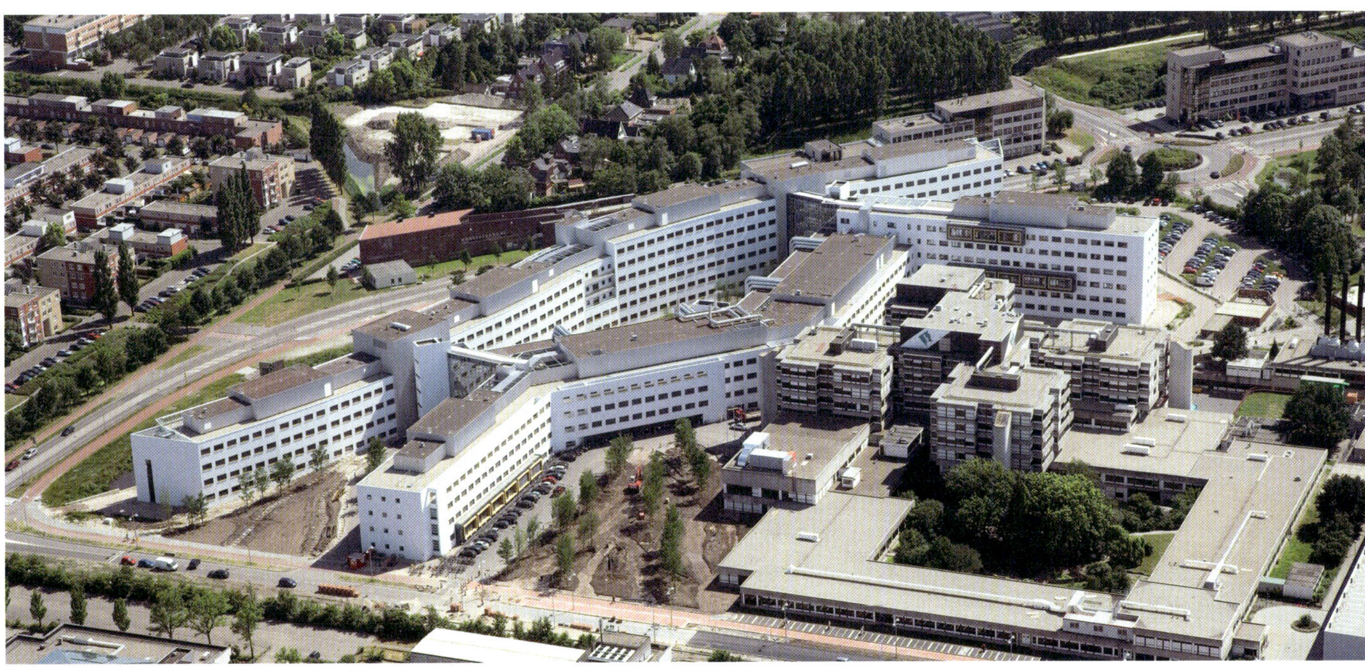

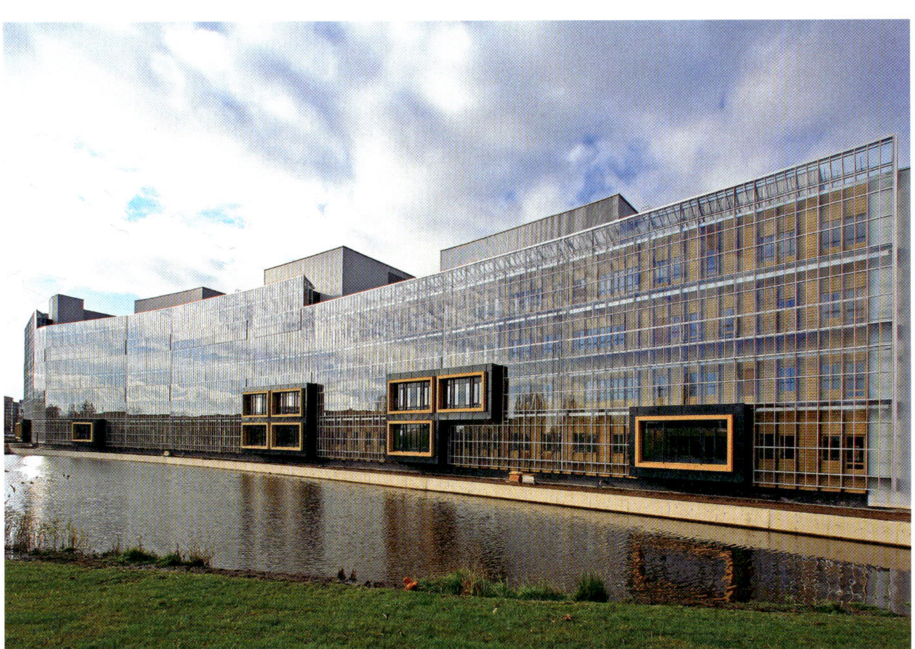

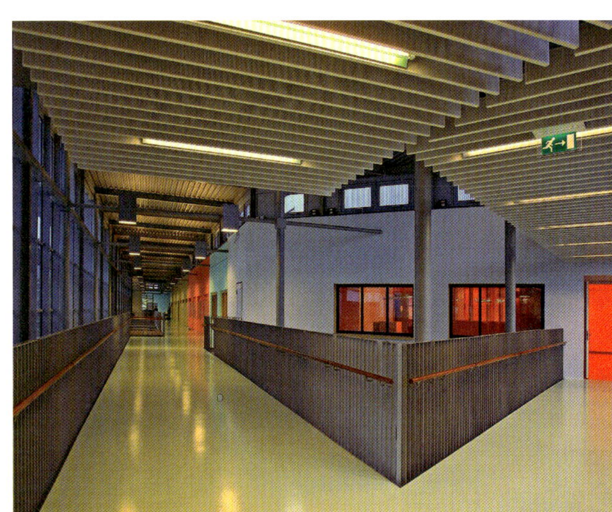

demountable architecture. This is manifested here in a system of partitions that are easy to move in spite of the mass of cables and other technical elements. The interior design is by Bart Vos (Vos Interieur) with a range of colours by the artist Peter Struycken.

Flexibility was also a priority for the Vlietland Ziekenhuis in Schiedam (EGM architecten). It consists of a linear string with a bend in the middle. The section of the building is the same everywhere so that functions can be moved. Each floor has one or more nursing units that can be replaced by other functions in the future if necessary.

The creation of links with the green, parkland surroundings is one of the guiding principles of the design of the Meander Medisch Centrum in Amersfoort. Like the Isalakliniek in Zwolle, it is one of the first examples of a hospital that has not been designed by a specialist in hospital architecture. The design by Hans van Beek (Atelier Pro Architecten) envisages three main zones. The 'hot floor' contains the key medical functions. The ambulance entrance is on the side, the goods entrance is beneath this zone. The hotel is located parallel to this strip. The complex consists of four volumes, of which the central two with seven storeys are the tallest, giving the hospital the character of a landmark. The third zone accommodates the outpatient units and the offices. Three fingers have been designed in line with three of the four hotel wings and bent slightly outwards to open the building towards the landscape on this side. A car park for patients and visitors is projected beneath the hotel and some of the outpatient units. It is surrounded by a logistical corridor that connects with the goods entrance. The idea is that the entire logistical process takes place out of everyone's view.

The Maasstad Ziekenhuis in Rotterdam, designed by Wiegerinck Architectuur en Stedenbouw, is an urban building according to an almost Rossi-like pattern. With its clear articulation it could easily drop units or put them to another use, and thereby anticipates the possibility of shrinkage – a prospect that has present-day hospital building in its grip too.

Care boulevards

Although the nursing units of hospitals are increasingly regarded as hotel facilities, and thus as temporary residential units, hospitals can never offer an everyday living environment. Patients do not behave like residents – they are often too ill or too frightened for that. Whereas in psychiatry and care for the elderly normal everyday surroundings formed the bridge to a link with society, this link is absent from hospitals. If there is any question of normalisation in their case, it proceeds along other paths. The concept of the care boulevard is popular. This consists of attracting medical and commercial activities close to the hospital so that it hides behind a complex of businesses that look most like a shopping centre. The concept of the care boulevard can therefore be regarded as the medical equivalent of the turning of the whole of social life into a shopping experience. It is mainly applied in general hospitals. Although the size of the recently completed buildings is sufficient to absorb extra facilities internally, as in the big university hospitals that have followed the lead of the Amsterdam and Groningen university medical centres, these facilities are grouped on a separate location near the main entrance, where a public area emerges with medical, paramedical and supplementary non-medical functions, often in separate buildings. The term 'boulevard' is somewhat misleading: the combination of functions that is characteristic of the classic boulevard is there, but the physical form is completely different. Most of them are based on the shopping mall or medical mini mall and often consist of an ensemble of separate buildings – there are rarely any streets or squares. What is the reason behind this concept? Its commercial look seems to be attuned to the transition to a customer-orientated form of provision of services; in that sense the care boulevard represents the increasing influence of market thinking. Pragmatic considerations are of greater importance: mainly thanks to the outpatient units, hospitals attract a constant flow of clients, which is attractive for the businesses on the boulevard. The boulevard in turn provides extra revenue for the hospital, especially when the hospital itself exploits the facilities or manages to conclude favourable contracts with the private parties who exploit them. These are so interested in this model that they also adopt initiatives in this direction themselves, and that too is in line with the breaking open of what was once the hermetically sealed world of health care.

Moreover, a care boulevard forms a seamless transition to normal forms of urban services, and that can help to make the hospital manifest itself less as an isolated bulwark. On the other hand, the concept stands or falls with a high degree of concentration. It is a supplement to the classic central hospital, which swells even more thanks to this addition. The one-stop medical centre implies that the whole range of provisions, from non-medical to top-medical, are clustered together. The popularity of the care boulevard and the fact that it brings about drastic changes in the previously stable care landscape prompted the Stagg to set up a design study.[5]

Rothuizen van Doorn 't Hooft Architecten Stedenbouwkundigen was one of the firms that took part in the Stagg study of care boulevards. The firm investigated how existing care institutions with limited potential for expansion can be supplemented with commercial facilities, using the Rijnland Ziekenhuis in Alphen aan den Rijn as the study model. The new premises of this centre comprise three volumes with care functions beside an inner street. The project was implemented between 2005 and 2009. The concept of the care boulevard was also deployed for the renewal plans for the Elisabeth Ziekenhuis in Tilburg. Completed in 2001, it was the first care boulevard in the Netherlands. The design is by Nijst Idema Architecten (now a/d amstel architecten), the successive firm of the architect of the hospital.

The concept of the Maasstad Ziekenhuis in Rotterdam includes a care boulevard (designed by EGM architecten), due to be completed in 2011. Besides a psychiatric centre, a care supplier for nursing home and home care, a 'medimall' with care-related provisions, a care hotel, a maternity hotel and a central general practitioners' centre also belong to the care boulevard, making it the largest in the Netherlands. In this way it becomes a location for health, care and wellbeing and is more than a care boulevard in the original sense. A similar development has taken place in Dordrecht, although there it is called a health park. Care is linked with sports, recreation and commercial facilities. The master plan is by Döll – atelier voor bouwkunst. The area comprising the Albert Schweitzerziekenhuis (the former Merwedeziekenhuis) and a sports park has been divided into five zones. The first consists of the existing hospital and the fifth of the sports park. In between them are three zones of hospital extensions with parking facilities, the care-related functions, and a location for large-scale events and offices on the side of the sports park.

Top
***Döll – atelier voor bouwkunst*, master plan health park with the different zones and elevations of the zone with the care-related functions, Dordrecht, 2002-2006**

Middle
***Ton Venhoeven CS Architecten with Itten + Brechbühl*, competition entry College Bouw, motto 'Core Hospital', 2004. The plan was projected on the Binnenrotteplein in Rotterdam.**

Bottom
***C. Weeber and L. Kaper*, competition entry College Bouw, motto 'Big Bang', 2007**

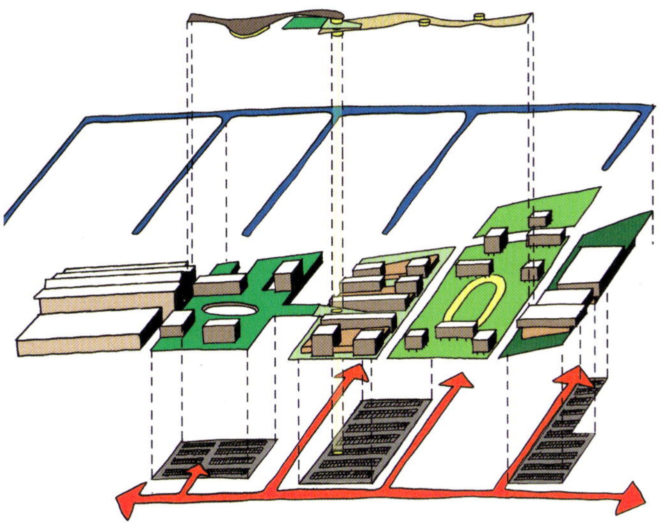

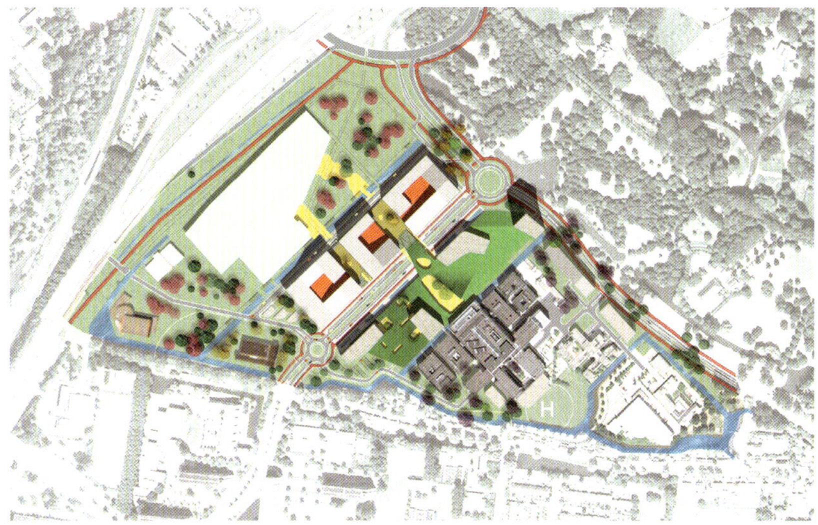

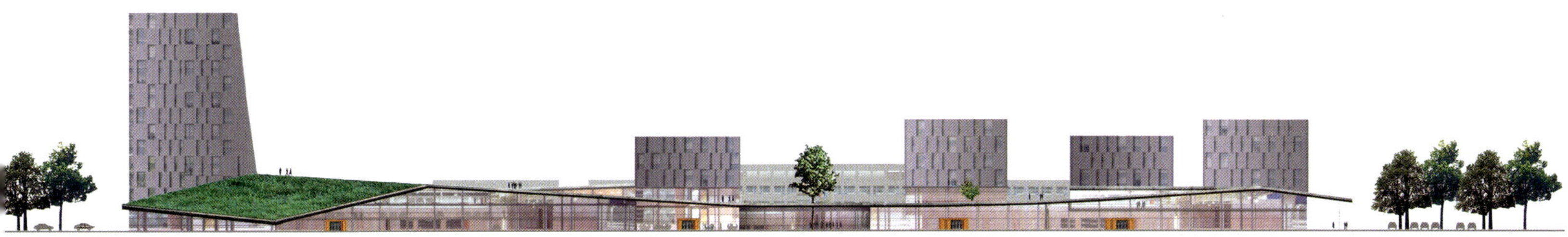

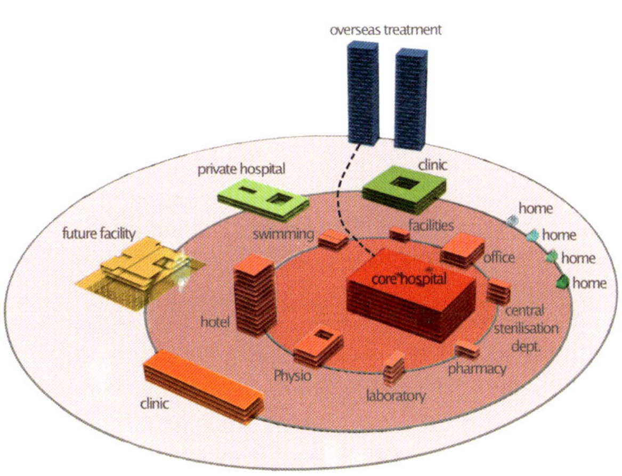

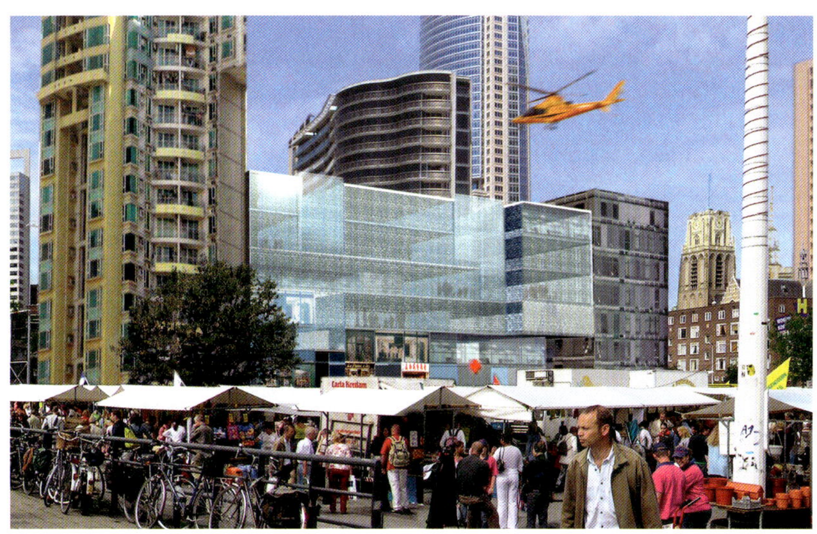

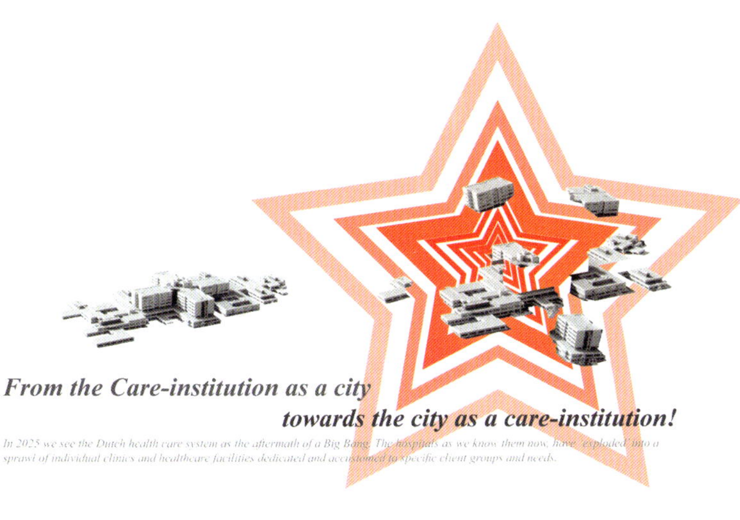

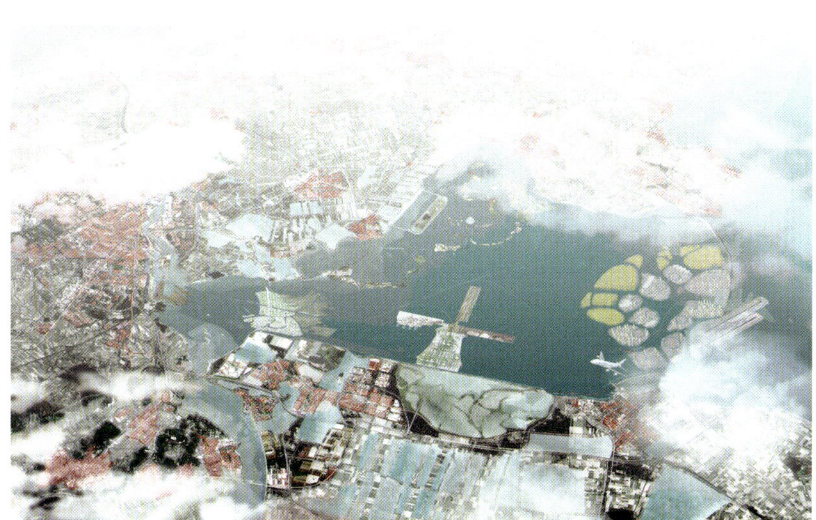

Decentralisation

While the previous decades were marked by an increase in scale, partly because it was the only way to get the most out of the never ending stream of mergers, now the tide slowly turns. Of course, there are many medical functions that can only be properly accommodated in large hospitals. That is the only place for complicated and hazardous interventions. If multidisciplinary work is required, that implies the availability of a concentration of different specialisations. Smaller institutions are also less suitable for training and research, so there will always still be a considerable number of large complexes. All the same, the conviction that a large scale is always better has been shaken. The search for ways of decentralising large hospitals is triggered by several motives. Fist of all there are the consequences of the new building legislation, which sharpens the differences between the 'hot floor', offices and hotel functions and thereby encourages the fragmentation of the building into separate parts.[6]

Second, there is the awareness that the classic all-under-one-roof hospital entails major problems of logistics, is not flexible, generates a mass of traffic, and combines things that have no functional relation with one another – all within an inevitable institutional setting. These criticisms have found their way to many reports, of which the report by the TPG postal company *Sneller Beter* (Faster better) is the best-known.[7]

Third, the revolution in the multimedia increasingly often makes the bridging of physical distances redundant. Information can be exchanged at lightning speed, not only between the departments within hospitals, psychiatric institutions and nursing homes, but also between these institutions and their ambulant patients. The use of the internet by Jan Kremer, a specialist in the field of artificial insemination, is exemplary in this area.[8] It opens up the possibility of transferring part of the front office of hospitals to smaller institutions. Moreover, there are many stages in the most complex treatment routines in which the interaction between medical staff and patient is limited to the taking of a simple blood sample: why should that not take place as close to home as possible? Finally, the idea is gaining ground that small-scale clinics are closer to the 'client', can play an important role in the field of information and prevention, and are not hindered by the massive scale and coldness of the large hospital when it comes to approaching patients.

At the same time, however, these small-scale clinics can only take over a small part of the range offered by larger hospitals: specialisation is inevitable. That presupposes the existence of networks of care clusters, extramural outpatient units and medical neighbourhood and community centres. It was already supposed in the 1990s that the classic central hospital would be reduced to a small high tech clinic. While the organisation of a large hospital remains intact and may even be expanded with provisions from other sectors, the accommodation is spread over a large number of locations which are in intensive contact with one another thanks to the internet. The internet ideally enables patients to exercise optimal control over the processes to which they are subjected, thereby reversing the relation between customer and provider of services – a reversal that has already taken place in sectors of society such as banking and travel agencies. In return for the responsibilities and work that are transferred to the customers, the latter gain more influence, especially when they can choose from several providers on different locations. Having a wide choice at their disposal is a condition for the empowerment of the patients.

p. 282
***De Nijl Architecten*, the decentralised hospital as catalyst of urban renewal, Rotterdam, 2008. Locations of the various components.**

***De Nijl Architecten*, design for a clinic for women and children and a centre for youth and the family as part of the decentralised hospital, Rotterdam, 2008**

p. 283
***DP6 architectuurstudio*, Het Noorderdok health centre, Almere, 2009**

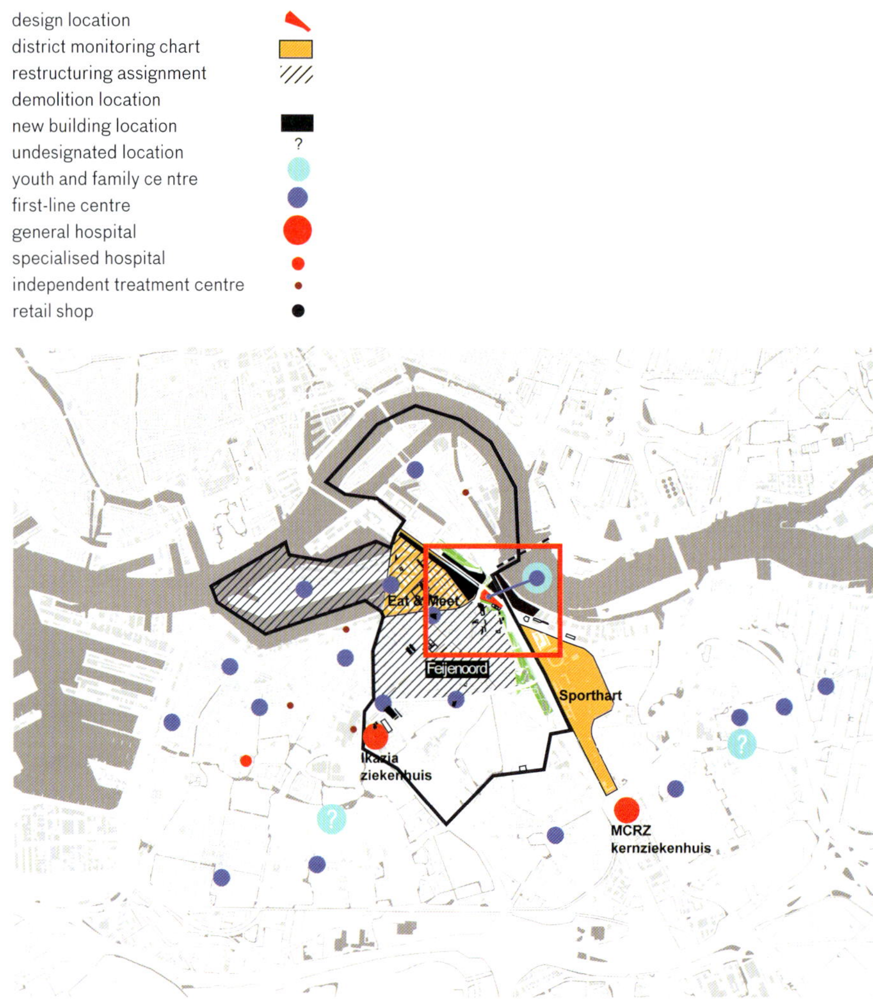

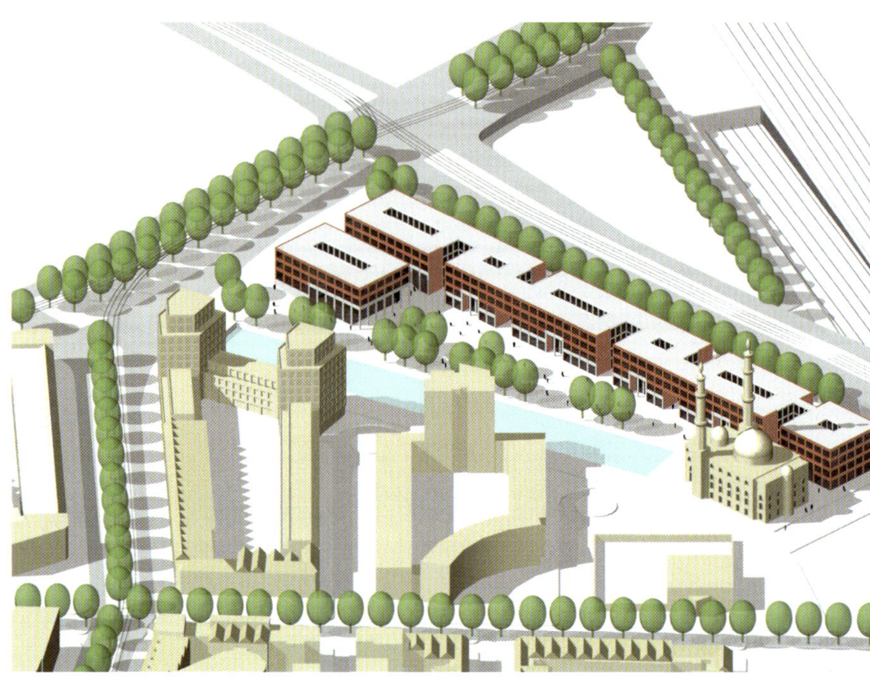

Ton Venhoeven and the Swiss firm Itten + Brechbühl (Thomas Guthknecht) presented a convincing concept for a fragmented hospital. Their Core Hospital won the first prize in the competition organised by the Building Board in 2004. Carel Weeber and Laura Kaper went a step further with their Big Bang entry for a competition organised by the same board in 2007. Their (winning) proposal assumes that the traditional large hospitals will explode by 2025 as a result of market mechanisms and become a scattered swarm of small-scale specialist clinics and care provisions. This underlines how attractive the concept of the decentralised hospital is. A Stagg study of the future of the outpatients unit explored the possibilities of transferring most ambulant health care to separate, small-scale institutions that link a certain degree of specialised care with community functions.[9] The business model was borrowed from that of airports and filling stations: although they have no raison d'être either without their core business, they earn the most money with all kinds of retail functions. The view of these separate outpatient units as 'normal' forms of services pre-eminently suitable for thinking in terms of shop formulae (not every supermarket is the same, even though the products are very similar) was rather controversial. In connection with a series of projects in the field of design research initiated by the Netherlands Architecture Fund, De Nijl Architecten, the Delft University of Technology and Colette Niemeijer from CEANconsulting designed a decentralised hospital that combines youth and family facilities with those for mothers with children. The result indicated that a relatively small hospital can still represent a considerable volume. However, that was no obstacle to the planned integration of this project in a district undergoing a process of urban renewal – part of the concept was that it should boost this process.[10]

While these concepts are based on an unravelling of the classic large-scale hospital, in practice the decentralisation of hospital care can also turn out to be a bottom-up operation. While existing hospitals seem to be remarkably resistant to the apparently growing demand for fundamental changes, health centres with general practitioners, physiotherapists and psychologists are springing up all over the place. DaF-architecten designed De Pionier (completed in 2008) in Nieuw-Vennep; the former Sint Jozef Ziekenhuis in Deventer was transformed into a health centre designed by One Architecture in 2009; and Het Noorderdok health centre designed by DP6 architectuurstudio in Almere shows similar tendencies. These centres have the potential to secure an increasingly prominent position and to take over many front office functions of hospitals and psychiatric institutions, especially if the empowerment of the patient turns out to be more than a dead letter.

Whether the decentralisation of the hospital is initiated from below or is the result of a reduction of the traditional all-under-one-roof hospital, that this concept is on the way up is clear from recent research too – paradoxically enough, even from the counterarguments that are sometimes advanced.[11] If the supply is brought too close to the users, it is argued, that might needlessly increase the demand for care, and there might be a tendency to offer forms of treatment that belong in a hospital and not in institutions that are too small and not specialised enough. Practice seems to refute these arguments, and the possibilities of decentralisation have by no means been exhausted yet.

Architectural quality

Many recently built hospitals are characterised by the striving for high quality. This is in line with the rediscovery of the potential of architecture referred to earlier and is also encouraged by the revision of the system that obliges the institutions to develop strategies for the optimal deployment of their buildings. Similar trends can be seen in psychiatric institutions and housing for the elderly, where the same motives play a role. That quality can confer added value, both in use and – literally – in terms of accountancy is no recent discovery; what is new is the discovery that optimal profit can be derived from health care architecture.

As always, it all depends on the role of the principal. Koen van Velsen was already invited at an early stage by the directors of the Groot Klimmendaal convalescent centre in Arnhem to think about a new building. The result is a building that is already regarded as pioneering. It forms part of a rolling up strategy by which most of the idyllically located terrain is evacuated. Van Velsen's building is lower

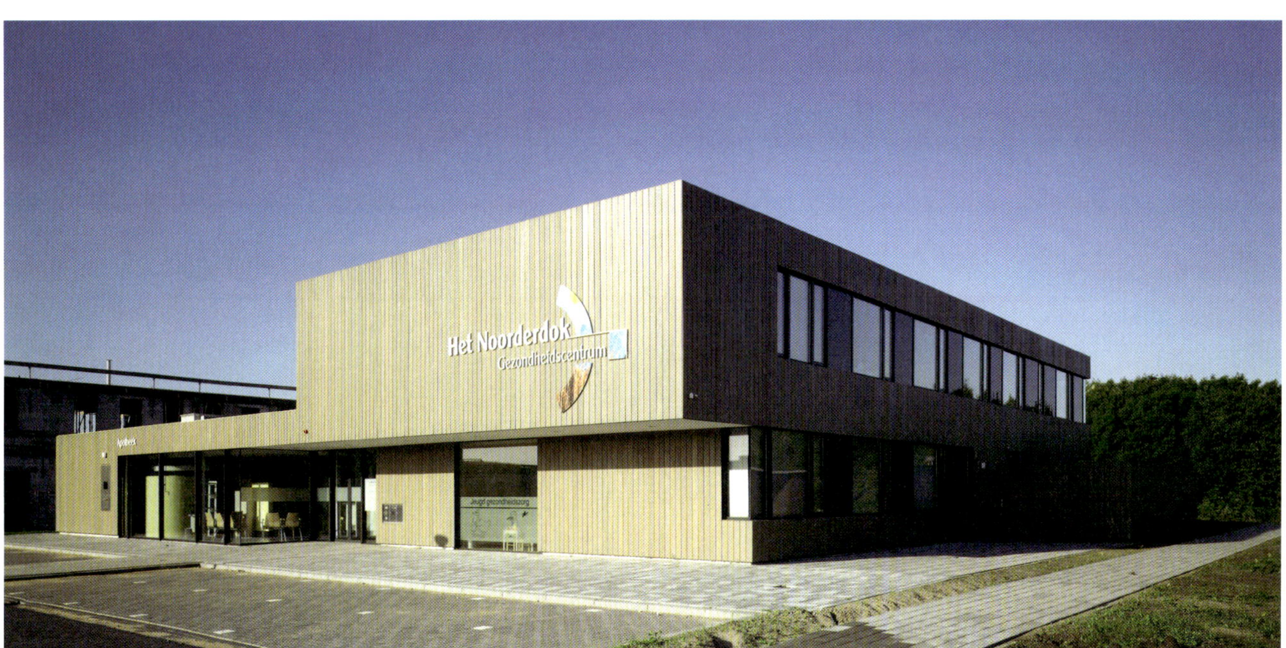

than the treetops, has a dark colour, adds relief with the aluminium façade cladding to prevent the complex from becoming a cold and smooth box, and thereby provides the ideal dialogue with its setting. By opening some of the functions to the public – the 'health spa' aspects of a convalescent centre are ideal for that – and avoiding everything that recalls the atmosphere of an old-fashioned hospital, Van Velsen has shown that health care architecture can have a place in the vanguard.[12]

The striving for quality also characterises the two buildings that Thomas Rau and UN Studio added to the Universitair Medisch Centrum in Groningen. The first is based on the One Planet Architecture principle that translates sustainability into a change of behaviour stimulated by the spatial environment. People must be made aware that everything they do can affect our environment and habitat. Rau's teaching and research building includes a lecture hall for 450 students and the cycle shed that no Dutch student city can afford to miss with room for no less than 1,350 bicycles. The design of the building contrasts with the historic premises next door. A gold-coloured shell envelops the building, resulting in a flowing blob-like volume that seems to have been cut open on one side, affording passers-by a view of the interior.

In view of its function, the laboratory designed by UN Studio could have no such transparency, but here too the unusual appearance of the building is entirely due to the unusual façade. The remarkable layout of the interior remains hidden from sight. From the outside it is impossible to see that it contains two conical shapes.

In all these examples, a logistically clear solution is combined with a design that both supports and represents use. That makes them interesting examples in a series that is growing by now and points to a renaissance of health care architecture.

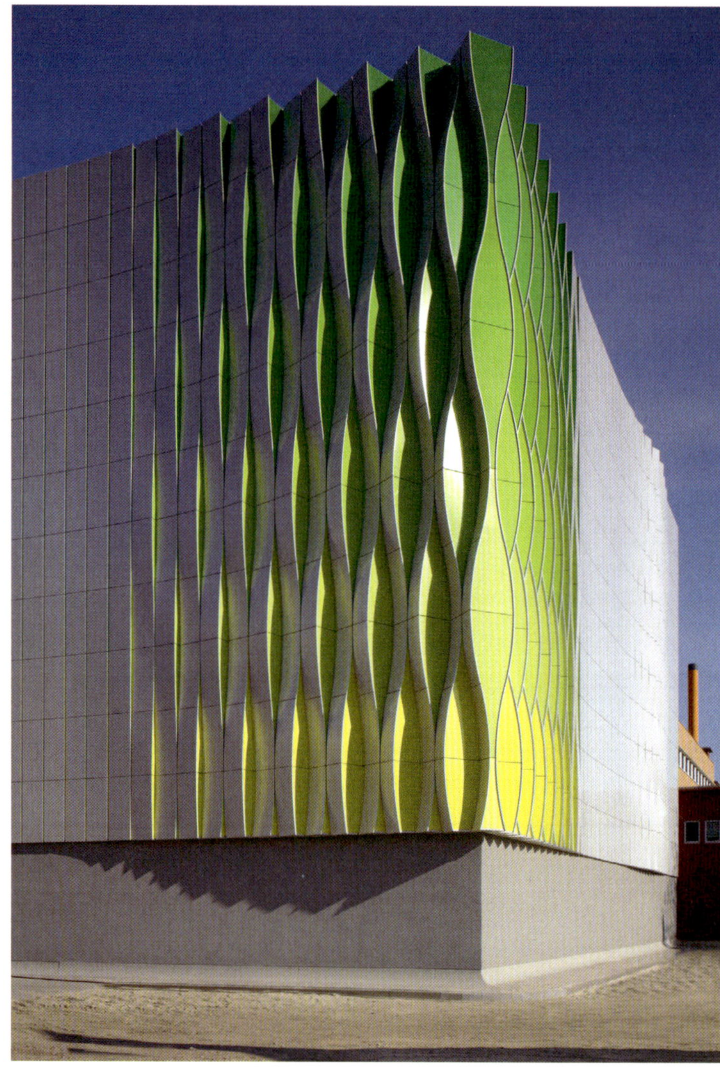

p. 284
***UN Studio*, laboratory Universitair Medisch Centrum Groningen, 2008**

***RAU*, Faculty of Orthopaedics and Kinesiology, Universitair Medisch Centrum Groningen, 2007**

p. 159
***Architectenbureau Koen van Velsen*, Groot Klimmendaal rehabilitation centre, Arnhem, 2009**

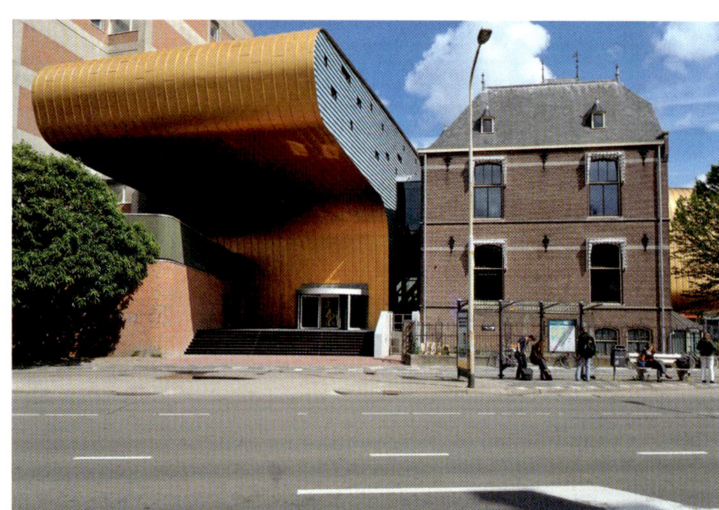

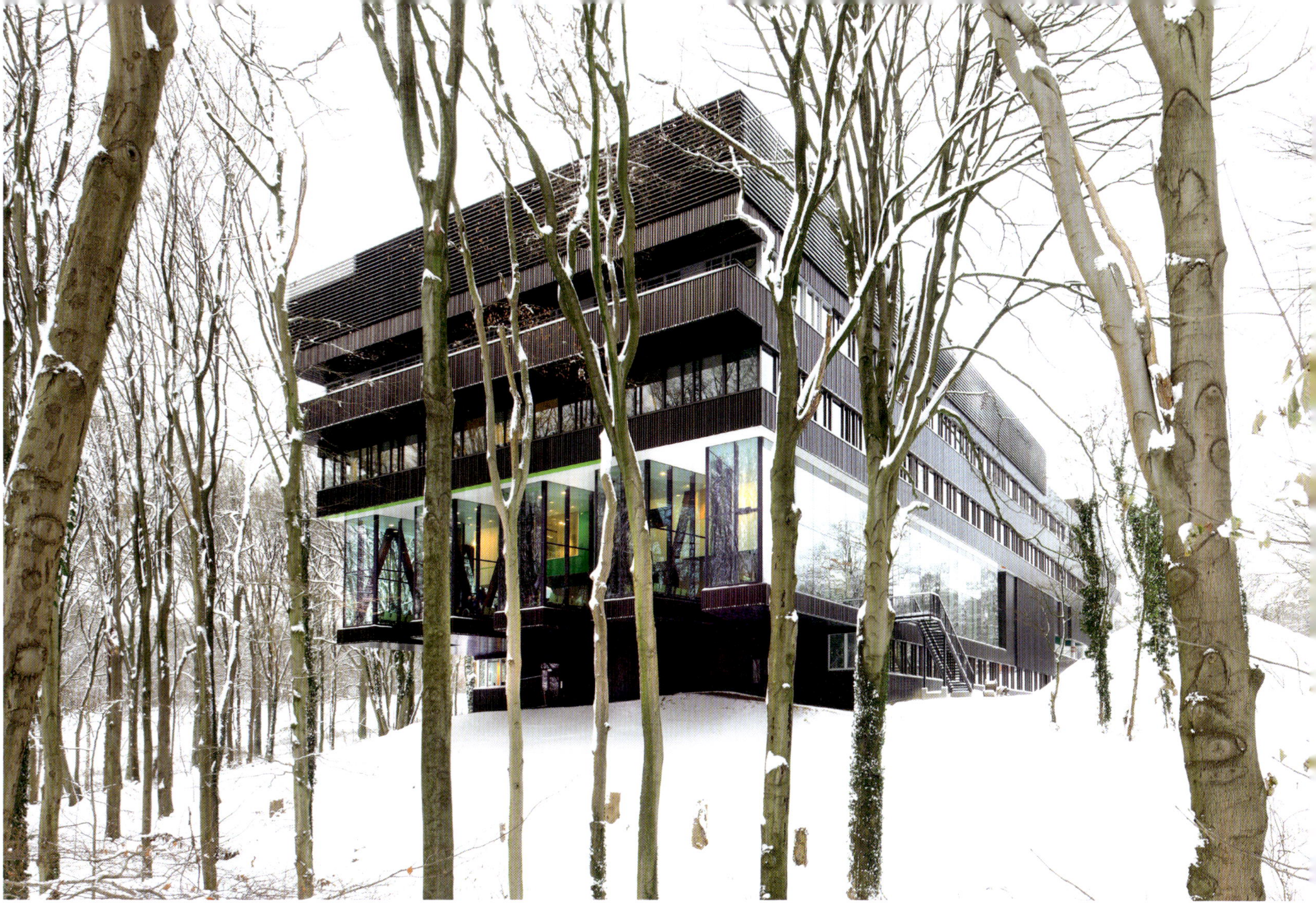

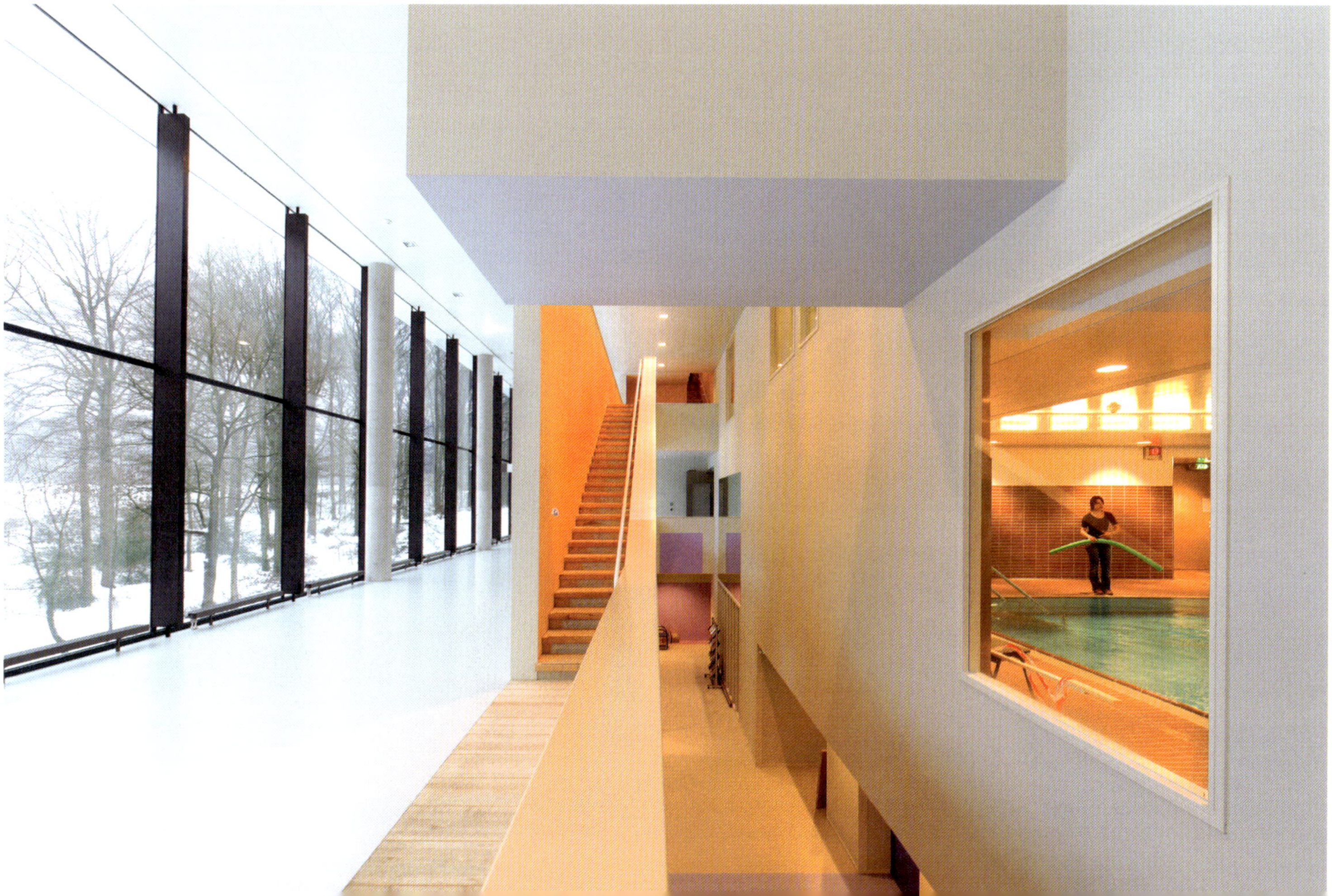

Psychiatry

Compared with the world of the hospitals, the developments in psychiatry have taken place at lightning speed. The transition to small-scale, multifunctional units was already largely complete by the end of the 1990s. In the meantime a remarkable reappraisal of the terrains that were left empty as a result is taking place.

Reverse integration

The big cleaning up operation that heralded the end of many classic institutions in the woods has been more or less completed. Some of them, including the most famous ones such as Meerenberg in Santpoort, have lost their function. Others have been transformed and to a certain extent have taken on the guise of the de-institutionalised, small-scale provisions that now determine the landscape of mental health care. Yet others have been turned into residential colonies for patients who are in need of constant specialised care. Small buildings for specific groups are being implemented on various sites. VXM Architects designed the Eikenboom pavilion, a facility for psychosomatic patients, in the grounds of the sanatorium in Zeist. While the present appearance of the old psychiatric hospitals is often the result of an exodus except for a certain residual category, in the meantime these sites have been discovered as rich in potential. Certain groups of patients benefit from living in green surroundings. For some it is the only option, but there are also patients who prefer a rural to an urban setting. Research by UR architects has shown that institutions can benefit financially from the redevelopment of these locations. Moreover, they often have a cultural historical value that can make them all the more attractive. Now that institutions are themselves responsible for their own real estate, the possession of these sites is a major asset, all the more so if it is possible to designate parts of them for healthy people. Besides the financial motives, there are also others that make this trend attractive. For instance, the mixing of healthy residents and patients could have a therapeutic value.[13] For the time being this trend is the latest stage in the development of the traditional institutions. In Venray Sint Anna has been closed down and Sint Servatius retained. New buildings are going up to provide 371 clinical places to replace the loss, and existing buildings are being renovated for treatment, day patients and auxiliary services. Bureau B+B urban design and landscape architecture drew up an urban development plan for the restructuring. Greiner Van Goor Huijten Architecten designed the buildings. The site includes facilities for long-term care, forensic psychiatry and Korsakoff's syndrome. Housing for the free market sector is going up on the edge of the terrain, resulting in reverse integration. Urban villas, apartments and residences designed by Klunder Architecten and KOW are being built.

The Medical Health Centre for North Holland North is building a mixture of care homes and regular rented property on the edge of the Sint Willibrordus terrain in Heiloo, next to a new housing estate. This enables long-term patients who depend on care, shelter and counselling to live as independently as possible. The homes were designed by Architectenbureau Zijlstra Schipper.

The small-scale urban clinics seem to be developing in the meantime to become more or less autonomous units. When the proximity of a regular hospital is not a necessity, they may pop up elsewhere in the neighbourhood too and form clusters with other small-scale medical provisions. As a result, what is to a certain extent a separate circuit emerges for psychiatric patients who are not a danger to themselves nor to society. This circuit offers sheltered forms of housing, outpatient treatment and short-term admission to day treatment centres. Every association with the traditional psychiatric hospital is avoided. Of course, these provisions too belong to the domain of mental health care and although normality is the ideal in every respect, designing it is a highly specialised, particular task. Still, they are not asylums. The classic asylum was initially an architectural instrument to promote healing processes and later a functional translation of therapeutic demands for the same purpose. In both cases it offered an environment that was not to be found in 'normal' society. The multifunctional units and small-scale mental health centres, on the other hand, are fully integrated in

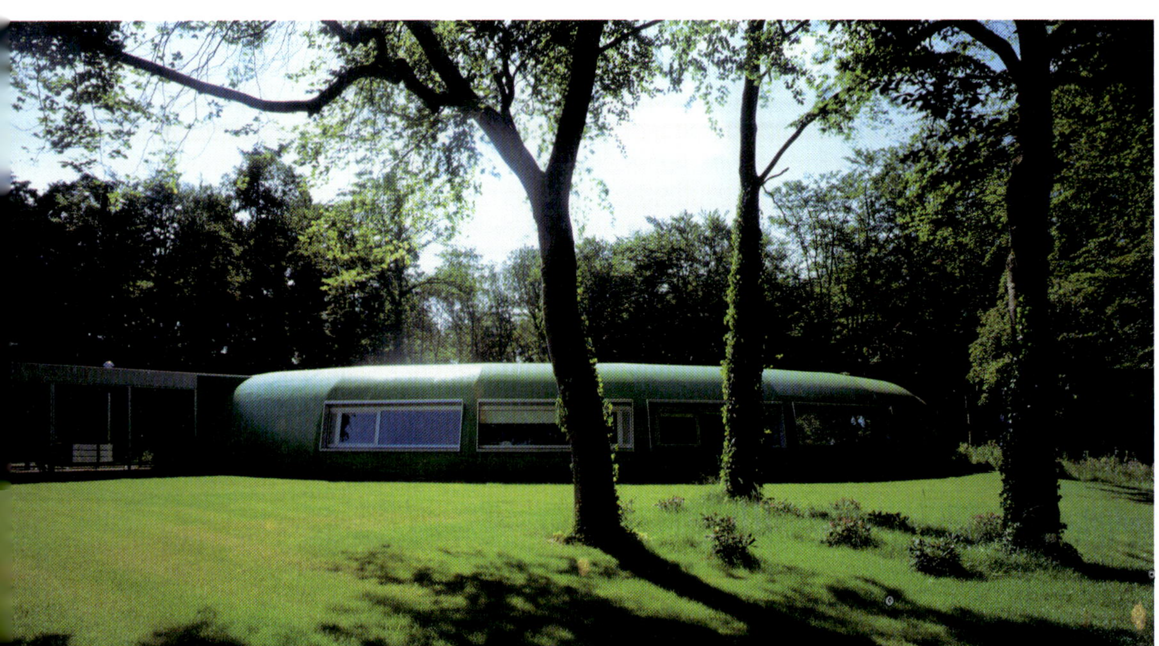

p. 286
***VMX Architects*, Eikenboom pavilion, a unit for psychosomatic patients, Zeist, 2003**

p. 287
***Greiner Van Goor Huijten Architecten*, Sint Servatius, building for intensive residential care, Venray, 2008**

***Greiner Van Goor Huijten Architecten*, Sint Servatius, housing on the edge of the terrain, Venray, 2009**

***Bureau B+B*, development plan for the restructuring Sint Servatius, Venray**

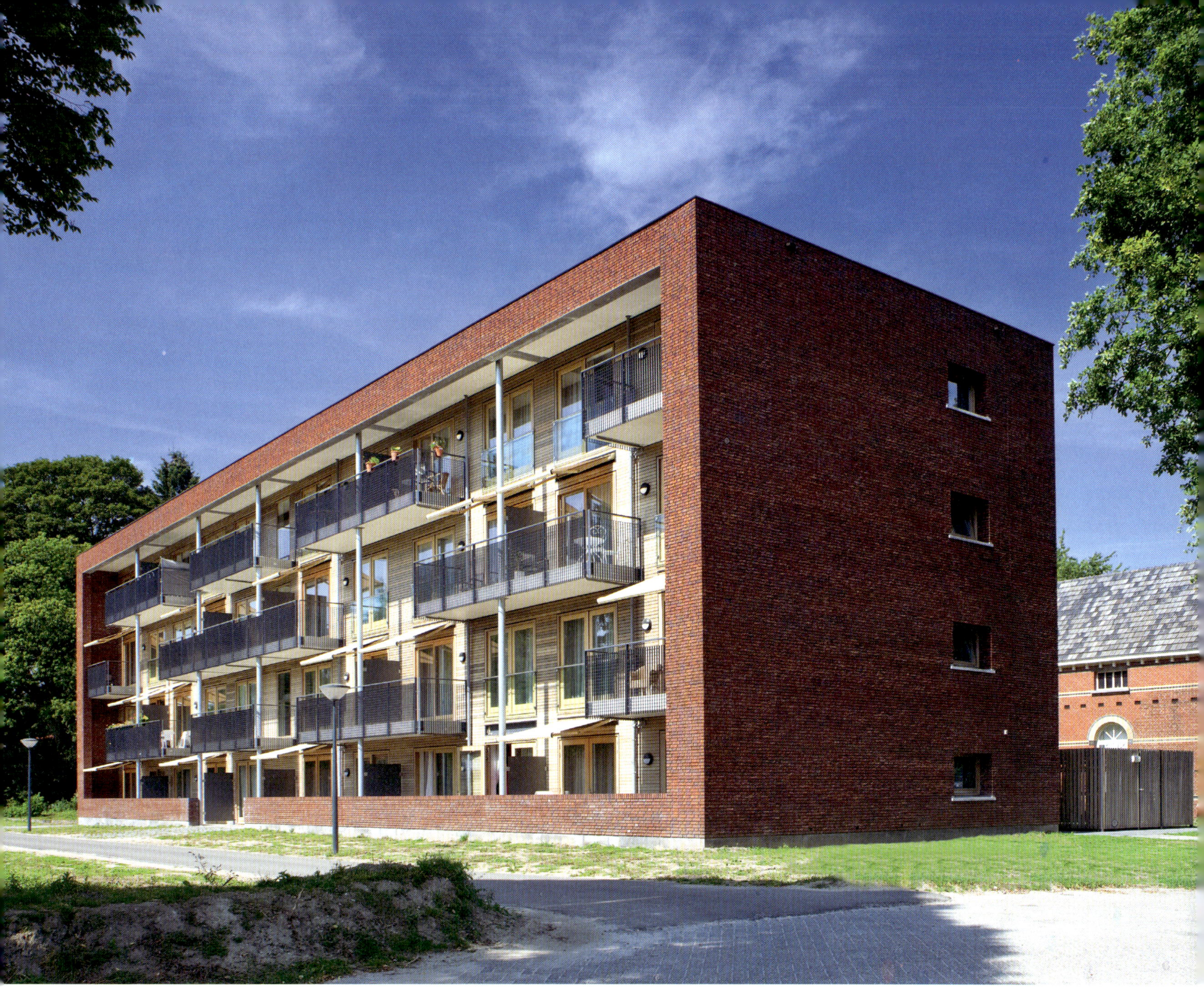

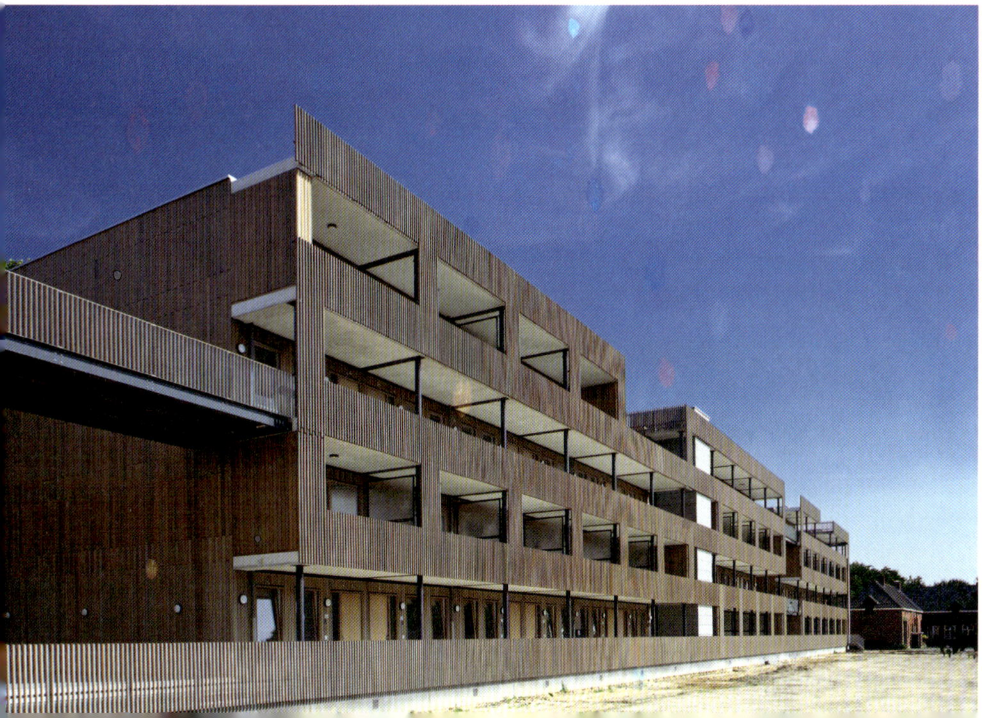

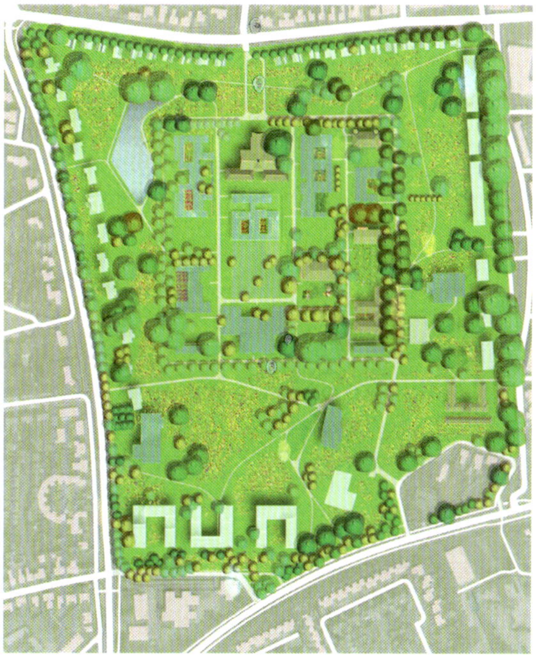

'normal' society and in their architecture they strive to offer the patients an environment that is hardly distinguishable from what is normally found in cities or new urban districts.

An example is the new building of a combined residential and treatment facility for short-term treatment in Amsterdam, commissioned by the mental health institution Mentrum. The design is by Van Panhuys & Bais in collaboration with de Jong Gortemaker Algra architecten en ingenieurs. The building is situated in a busy traffic street with a high building density and matches the scale of the other buildings. A particular inner city project is the new building of the historic Willem Arntsz Huis in the inner city of Utrecht. This famous institution that played such a prominent role in the renewal of psychiatric institutions in the nineteenth century decided on new buildings and renovation on the historic location. The result is a psychiatric hospital integrated in the urban fabric that tries to establish contact with its surroundings. VMX Architects achieved this by making a cruciform design that defines four urban gardens. On the front is a representative forecourt with the main entrance. Opposite is the local square and playground. The therapy garden and the enclosed garden have a more closed character, but are also open to passers-by.[14]

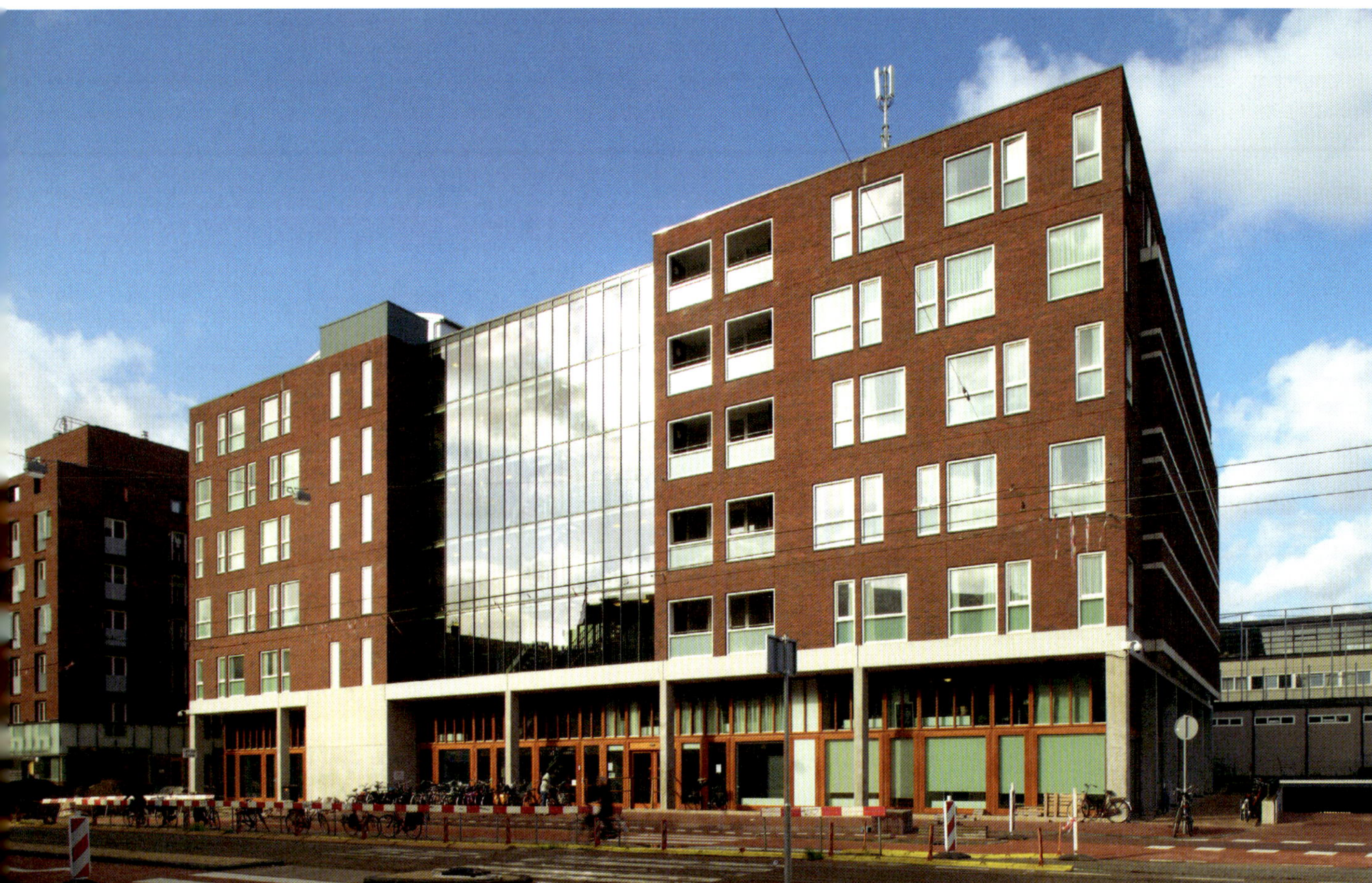

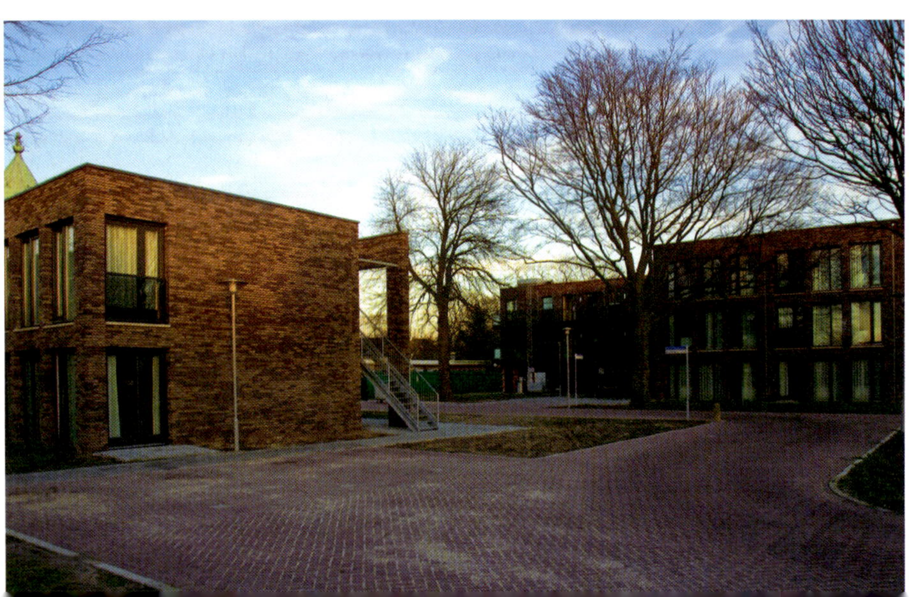

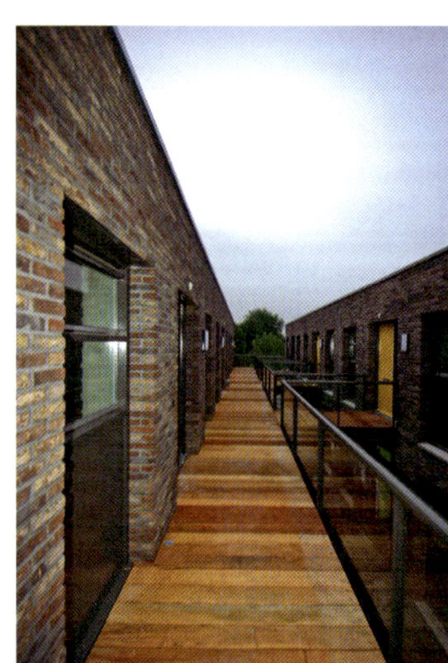

Housing and care for the elderly

Combined with the need to find less expensive accommodation than the traditional institutional facilities, the practically unrecognisably changed position of old people has culminated in a complete overhaul of the system that evolved after 1945. Of course the roots of this change sometimes go back a few decades, but it is only now that it is crystallising. While accommodation in old people's homes is a thing of the past, more is being built for this generation than ever before. The share of specific care provisions, however, has dropped dramatically; in proportion, the types that combine care and housing in particular have been cut back sharply. What seems difficult in other fields is feasible in that of care for the elderly: the shift from the regulation of supply to the regulation by demand. This shift is reflected in architecture in the abandonment of functionally distinct building types. They have been replaced by what M. Boekholdt calls domains. He distinguishes three types: complex care with a home of one's own, sheltered housing, and (intramural) residential housing.[15] While in the past care had three standardised layers – home care, domestic help and medical support – it now works with personalised care arrangements. This is possible within the institutional parameters of a residential home that combines individual and communal facilities – it is likely that this form will continue to exist and even expand – but care can also be brought to the home provided it is close to the care providers or forms a part of the urban fabric and can be serviced from community support points. The position of the care providers is completely new as well. Until recently they operated within the framework of a policy orientated towards regulation of

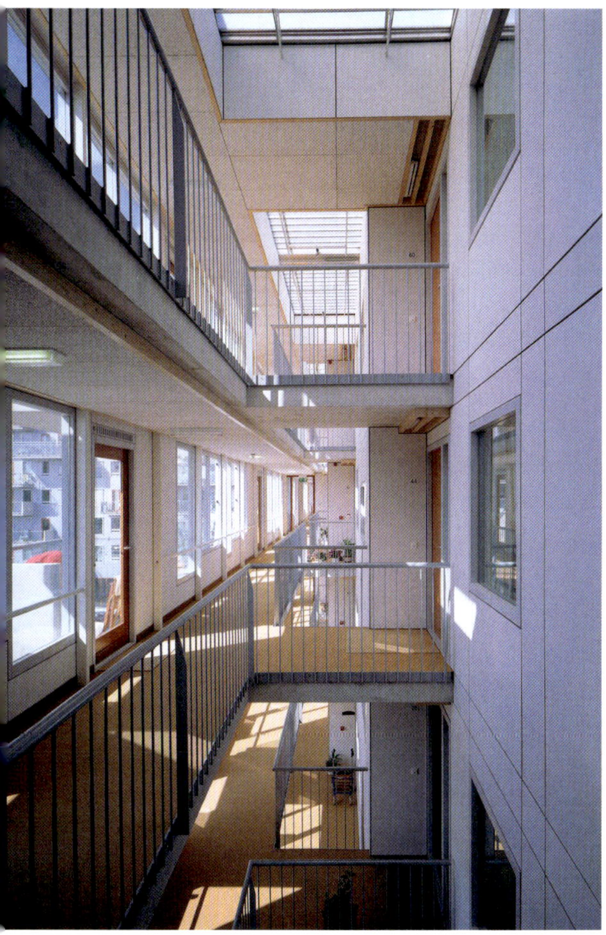

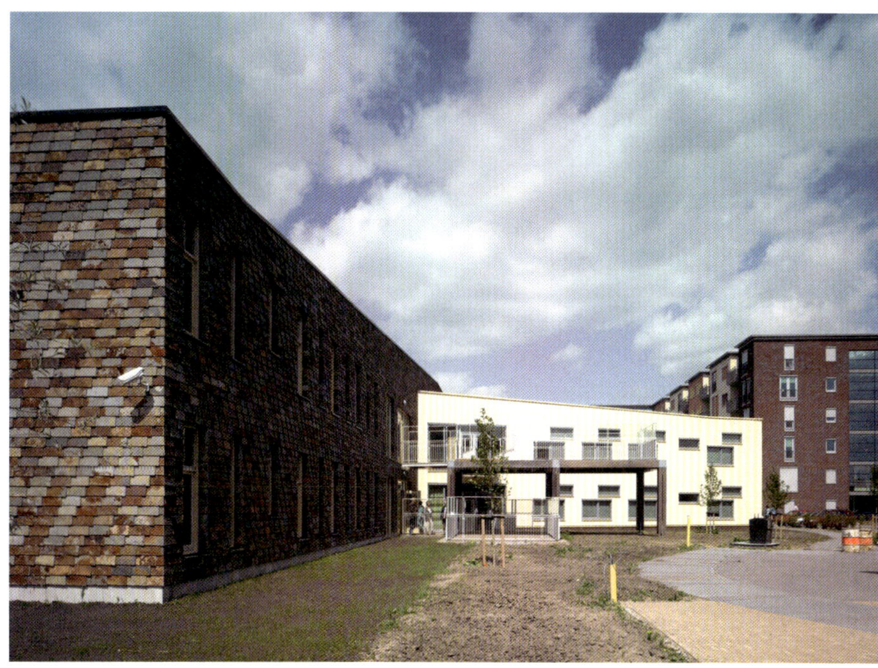

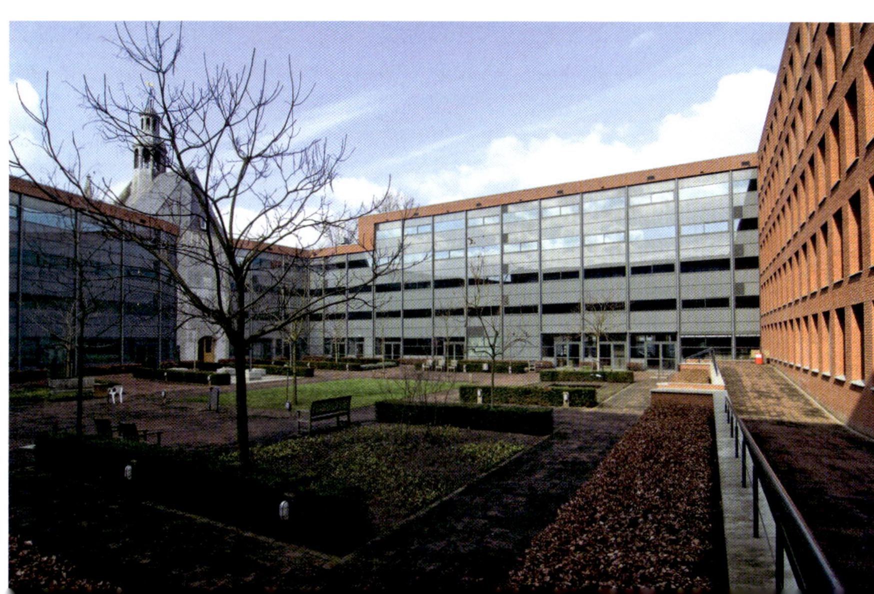

p. 288
***Van Panhuys & Bais with de Jong Gortemaker Algra architecten en ingenieurs*, combined residential and treatment facility for short-term patients, Amsterdam, 2003-2007**

***Zijlstra Schipper Architectenbureau*, housing for chronic psychotic patients on the edge of the terrain of Sint Willibrordus, Heiloo, 2007-2009. The homes form part of a mixture of care homes and ordinary rented homes.**

p. 289
***Döll – atelier voor bouwkunst*, Nieuw Bleyenburg, Utrecht, 2007**

***RAU*, Het Zonnehuis nursing and reactivation centre, Zwolle, 2007**

***KOW with Molenaar en Koeman architecten*, Nieuw Antoniegaarde, 's-Hertogenbosch, 2003**

supply, which reduced their room for manoeuvre to such an extent that their role was mainly that of policy executive organs. Now they are social entrepreneurs. Other players have appeared on the field that they service too. Housing corporations in particular play a much larger role than in the past.

What are the consequences for building? The most essential consequence of the primacy of the demand side is the emergence of integration frameworks that are not dominated by the institutions, even though they play a large role in their organisation. The new frameworks are geographical, not sectoral, and the municipalities are assigned a major role in their coordination. Whole urban districts are gradually being transformed into residential care or service zones (*wozozo*), although these terms are by no means always used. The programmes of some of the new large-scale housing estates also include care along the lines of the residential service zones.

Nursing and care homes

As a result of the substitution policy, nursing and care homes have gradually converged. What initially complicated the telescoping of the two categories was the different organisation and financial structure, but in the course of the 1990s not even that obstacle was able to prevent the creation of an essentially new division of the categories of care for the elderly. By coupling accommodation to care for only particular groups of the elderly, a highly diversified range of care facilities was created, as well as a range of extramural or day care independent of the form of accommodation. What are the consequences for the existing institutions? More emphasis is being put on the residential aspect in nursing homes. All the same, there were still fifteen with bedrooms for five or six persons in 2002. At that moment there were 1,340 nursing homes with more than 100,000 intramural residents[16] – a large number, most of which also offered extramural and day care. They therefore have to make strategic choices, which are generally characterised by getting rid of a large part of their intramural capacity. An exploration of the future conducted by Arcares offers several options.[17] The prospects are often not very bright. Two-thirds of the places in care homes (and half of those in nursing homes) failed to satisfy the basic quality criteria in 2006.[18] A large-scale renovation programme was inevitable, and that provided the impulse to replace some of these homes by the newer hybrid types discussed below, or to go completely extramural.[19] Whichever option was chosen, the further normalisation of the nursing home was facilitated by the emergence of a new care concept, the commune (*leefgemeenschap*) model.[20] The category of nursing home residents who are accommodated in such communes have little or nothing against the idea, since normal functioning in society outside the institutions is usually not an option for them. The commune model usually entails individual bedrooms with communal living rooms. Members of one of these communes play a role in supporting one another and have a certain responsibility for the domestic tasks that the group as a whole can manage on the basis of a mutual division of labour. To a certain extent nursing thus becomes a kind of assisted living at home. This development shows how much the accent is shifting from the accommodation of nursing as a function linked in the first instance with the medical profession to an emphasis on the quality of human life in its final stage. This shift coincides with the choice of the experience of the nursing home resident as the main criterion – an approach that was to leave its mark on the architecture too.

When most institutions decide to join a network of small-scale provisions, the phenomenon of ageing and the often desolate state of the old building stock often make the building of new institutions unavoidable too. There is very little of the classic nursing home about them. To a certain extent they are generic, representative, public buildings, often with a restaurant that is open to local residents. Priority is given to ease of use, comfort, and the avoidance of reminiscences of what used to be the customary institutional character of these facilities in the past. The number of specific facilities is growing gradually – while their share may drop in relative terms, the phenomenon of ageing makes expansion and new building inevitable. The trends that began earlier are continued in most projects.

In many cases the homes accommodate all categories of patients who are eligible for admission, and sometimes even groups who do not yet need assistance. In that case it is natural to cooperate with housing corporations, who exploit the part that cannot be considered a hospital provision. A great advantage of the bringing together of different categories of residents, even if in separate wings, is that it prevents the degeneration of the institutional old people's homes into 'dumping grounds for really hopeless cases'.[21]

Recent examples of such combinations of different categories of residents within a single building are Berkenstede in Diemen, designed by Dick van Gameren (2007), the nursing and reactivation centre Het Zonnehuis in Zwolle by RAU & Partners (2007), Nieuw Antoniegaarde in 's-Hertogenbosch (KOW in collaboration with Molenaar en Koeman architecten, 2003), and Laurens de Elf Ranken in Barendrecht by EGM architecten (2003). The Leo Polakhuis in Amsterdam was renovated and expanded by Claus en Kaan in 2006, resulting in a similar hybrid complex. Henk Döll designed the large-scale Nieuw Bleyenburg complex for the elderly in Utrecht (2007).

The difficulty in implementing such hybrid buildings is partly due to the number of parties involved: care providers, housing corporations, local government bodies at provincial and municipal level, developers, national government, the care office, the Health Insurance Board, the Building Board, the Health Care Rates Board, and external stakeholders.[22] The role of the housing corporations is noteworthy: they often show themselves prepared to invest in complexes of this kind, even though the rents for the sections that are paid for under the Exceptional Medical Expenses Act (AWBZ) do not cover the costs. This is compensated by the increased attractiveness of the rented apartments in the other sections and the neighbourhood around such a centre.

Reduction of scale is also a key term in the larger institutions. Reduction of scale (residential groups of a maximum of six or seven persons) and increase of scale complement one another; the latest trend contributes to strengthening the basis of support for the desired facilities. The mixing of different categories of residents and the emphasis on a small scale signify a once and for all victory over the classic old people's home.[23] An example is Bruggerbosch, designed by Jorissen Simonetti architecten. It houses two hundred residents in the top category of psycho-geriatric care, as well as having seventy places for day treatment where people with a dementia syndrome can be helped to live by themselves for as long as possible. The residents live in groups of six with regular counsellors and in a recognisable house. The building comprises six apartment blocks in which the groups are accommodated and a central building with the auxiliary functions. A corridor connects the buildings with one another. Bruggerbosch is 'the last institution in the Netherlands to have evaded the obligatory decentralisation

p. 291 | <
***Jorissen Simonetti architecten*, Bruggerbosch, Enschede, 2006**

***EGM architecten*, Laurens de Elf Ranken care centre, Barendrecht, 2003**

p. 291 | >
***AWG Architecten*, Bijdorp housing, welfare and care complex, Zoetermeer, 2007**

***Claus en Kaan*, Leo Polakhuis, Amsterdam, 2006**

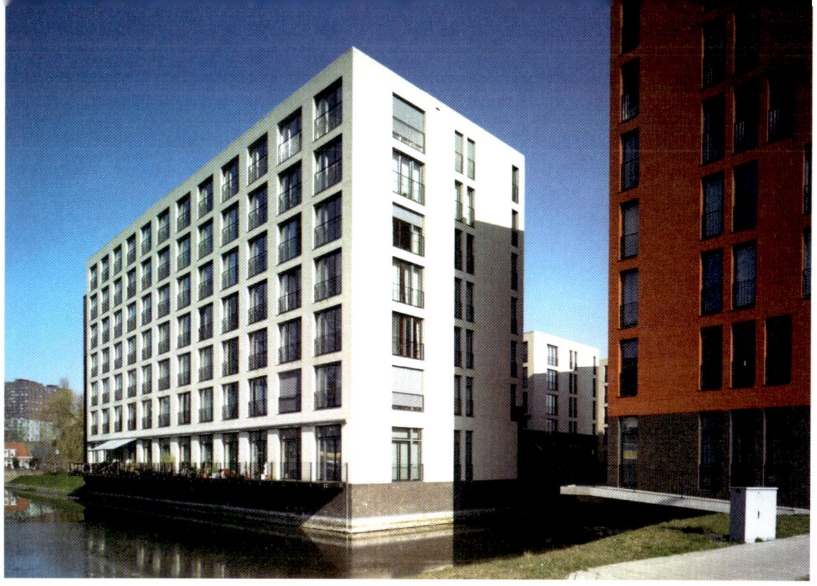

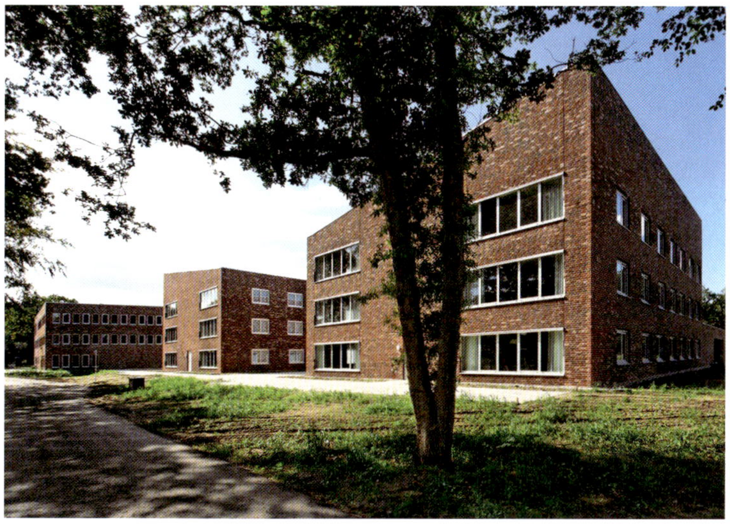

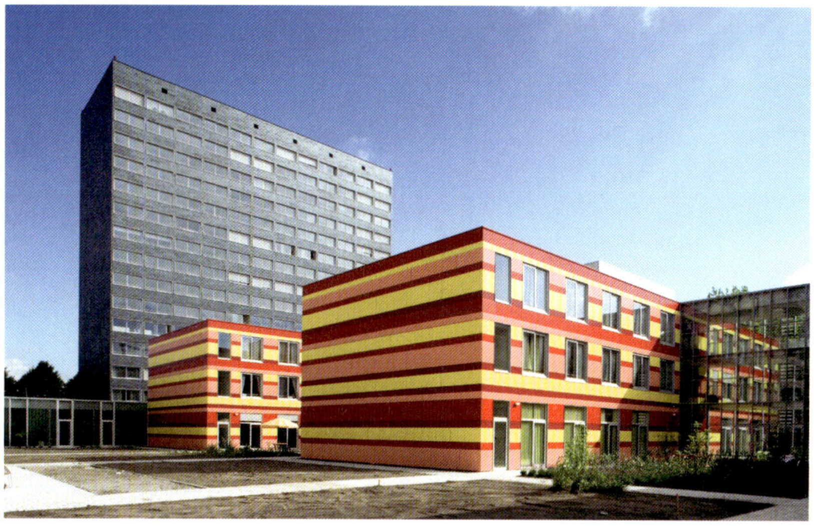

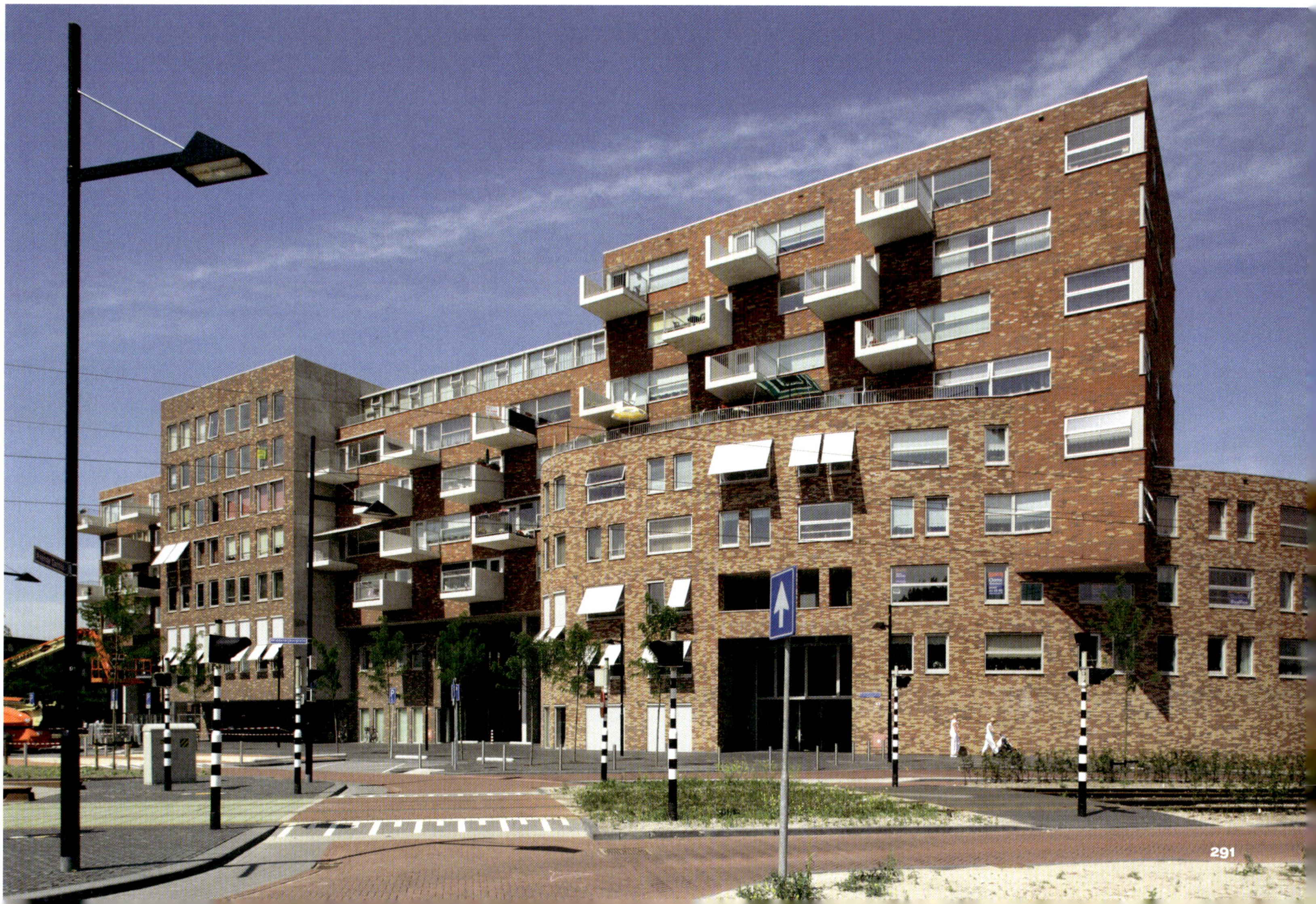

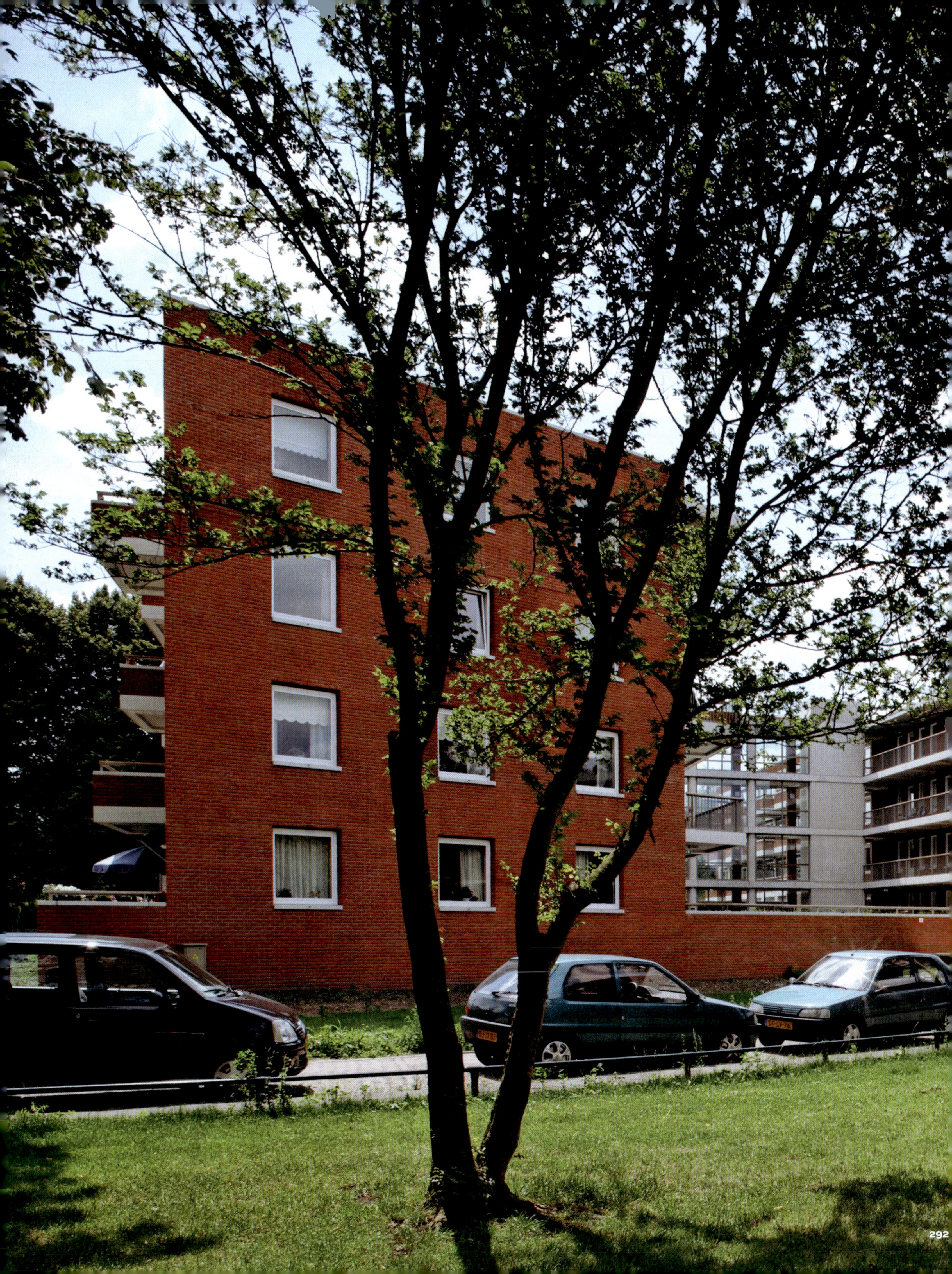

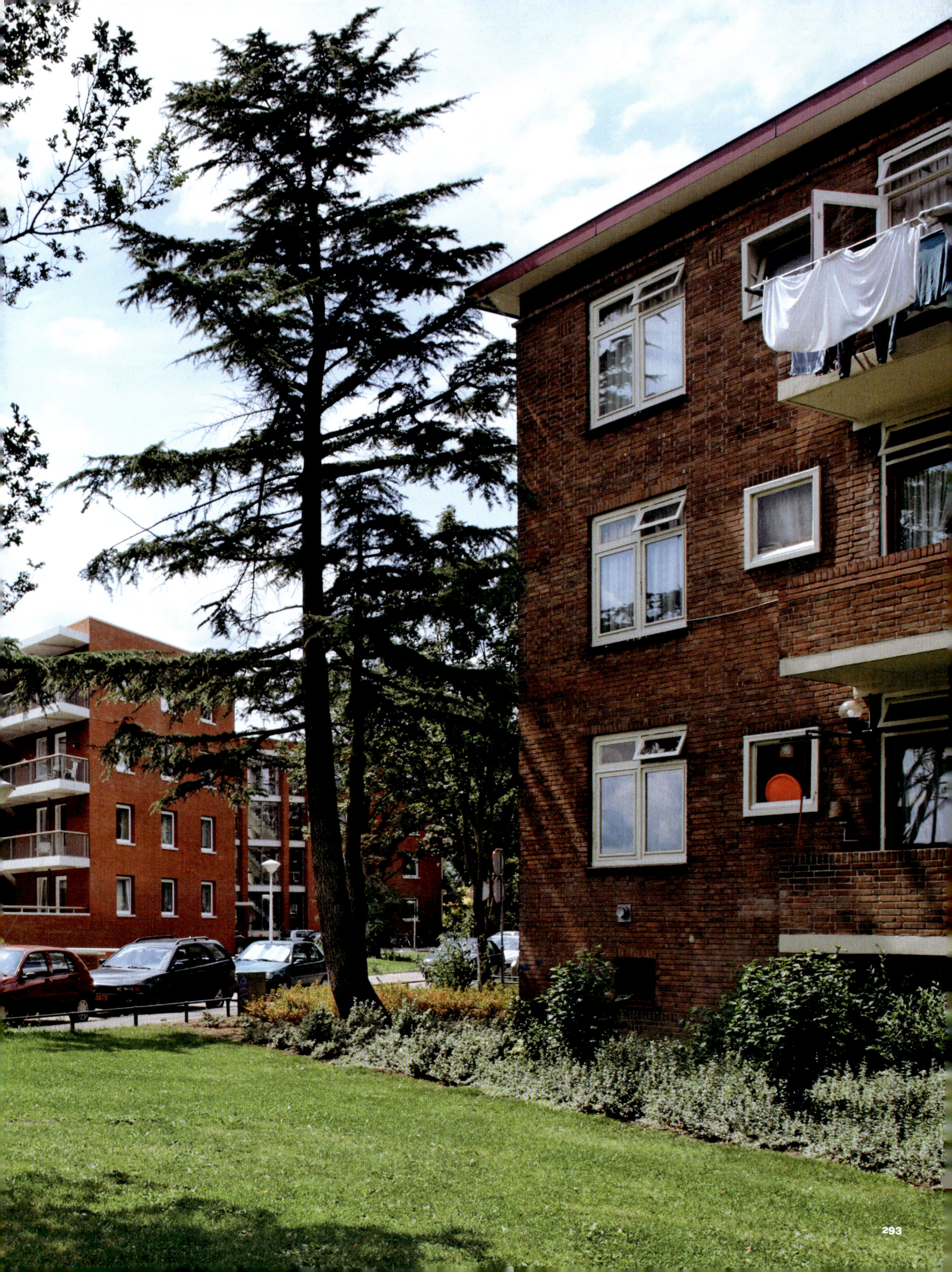

of care'. The target groups would not benefit from a location in the city, hence the choice of a number of more or less closed environments in clearly separated volumes.[24]

Another complex that combines increase and reduction of scale at the same time is the Bijdorp housing, welfare and care complex in Zoetermeer, commissioned by Vidomes and designed by AWG Architecten. These are life-cycle rented and owner-occupied apartments in which old people can continue to live on their own for as long as possible. The complex consists of seven different buildings with three to seven floors. Three buildings linked by a gallery are grouped around a central square. These three buildings contain apartments, including a psycho-geriatric unit with five group residential units and commercial units. Besides intramural assistance, Bijdorp also offers extramural care (home care). Another component is a health centre including three general practices, a dispensing chemist, and a physiotherapy and remedial therapy practice. The architect wanted to achieve a small scale by locating the functions in separate buildings.

The building of more or less luxurious apartment blocks next to existing nursing and care homes may be the finishing touch to the attempt to cluster the largest number of categories of residents together. A condition of its success is its clear identity as a separate facility – these apartments want to clearly distinguish themselves from the care buildings, even though their immediate proximity is a decisive factor for many buyers. Examples are Berkendaal in Diemen, designed by the Döll – atelier voor bouwkunst, De Plussenburgh, a project of Arons en Gelauff in Rotterdam (2006), and De Rokade by the same designers in Groningen. The residents of these tower blocks can make use of the provisions of the care institutions next door without literally having to live in a care institution. In complexes of this kind, a corridor connects the apartment section with the care or nursing home. It is impossible to tell from the apartments that they are a part of a care complex. De Nijl Architecten designed a building in Dieze-Oost, Zwolle, that houses both starters on the housing market and old people. It consists of three parts that follow the direction of the classic strip building, and are connected with a narrow volume the whole length of the building.

It is noteworthy that the successor to the traditional old people's home, the residential care complex (*wozoco*), which was previously the link between the nursing home and 'ordinary' housing, has become outdated by now. They are still being built, but according to Jeroen Singelenberg their heyday was over long ago. In the jubilee issue of Aedes Arcares, he calls this model a 'coproduct of the rented social sector and the intramural care sector and as such connected with the typically Dutch postwar system'.[25] There is apparently no longer any demand for a provision of this kind now that the nursing home has been split into a large number of small-scale complexes and larger hybrid buildings. The extramural and day care that they offer is a good match for the regular, modified or modifiable housing stock. The framework in which supply and demand have to strike a balance is the neighbourhood. The residential care or service zone seems more popular than ever.

Residential care or service zones (*wozozo*)

Care for the elderly may have rid itself of housing to a large extent, but housing is still the framework within which care provisions are harmonised with one another in the concept of the residential care or service zone. By now this goes much further than just amenities for the elderly. Psychiatry has been decentralised too and thereby made suitable to function

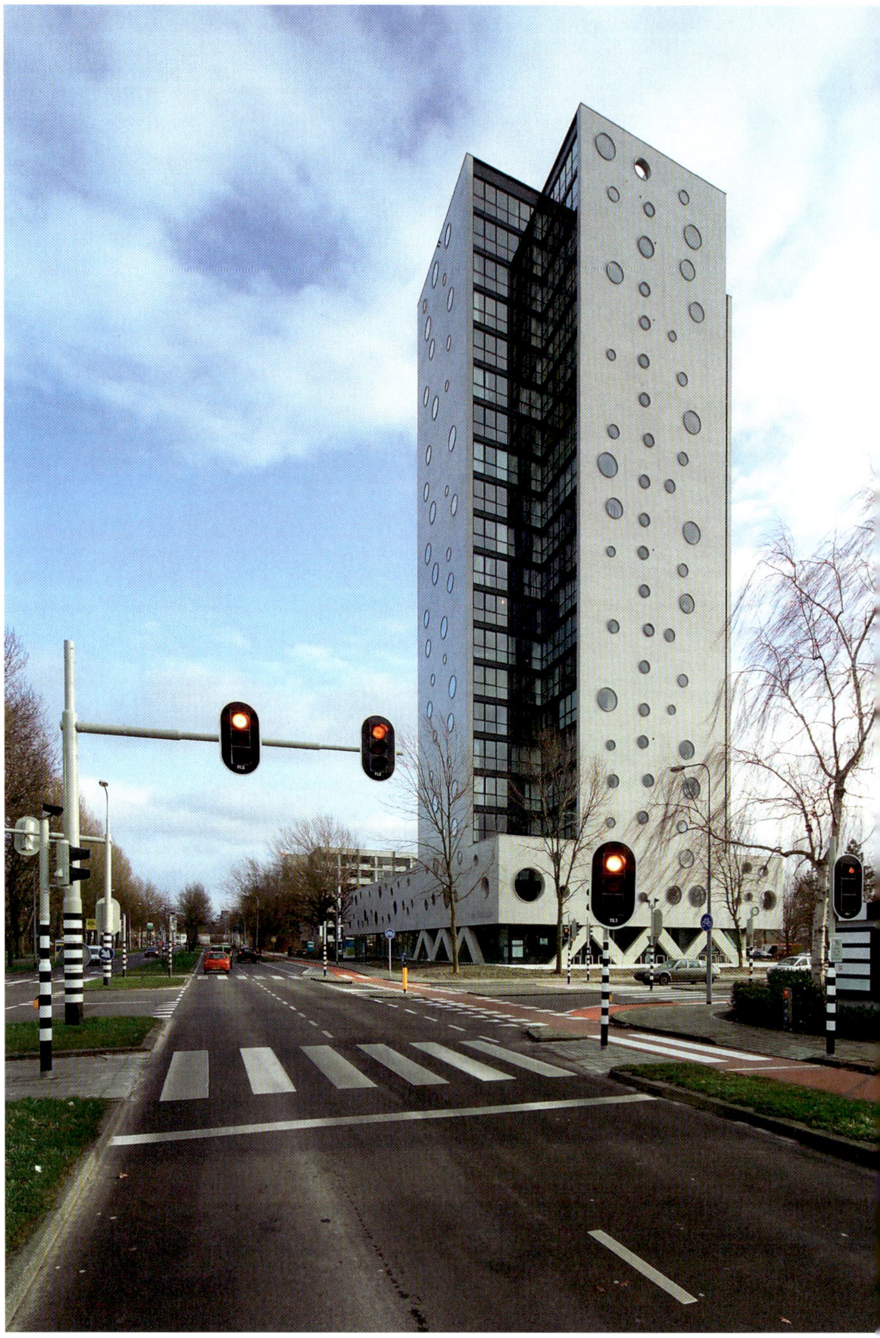

p. 292
***De Nijl Architecten*, residential building Hobbemastraat (homes for the elderly and starters on the housing market), Zwolle, 2008**

p. 294
***Arons en Gelauff*, De Rokade, Groningen, 2007**

***Meyer en Van Schooten*, De Kristal residential care centre, Rotterdam Nesselande, 2008**

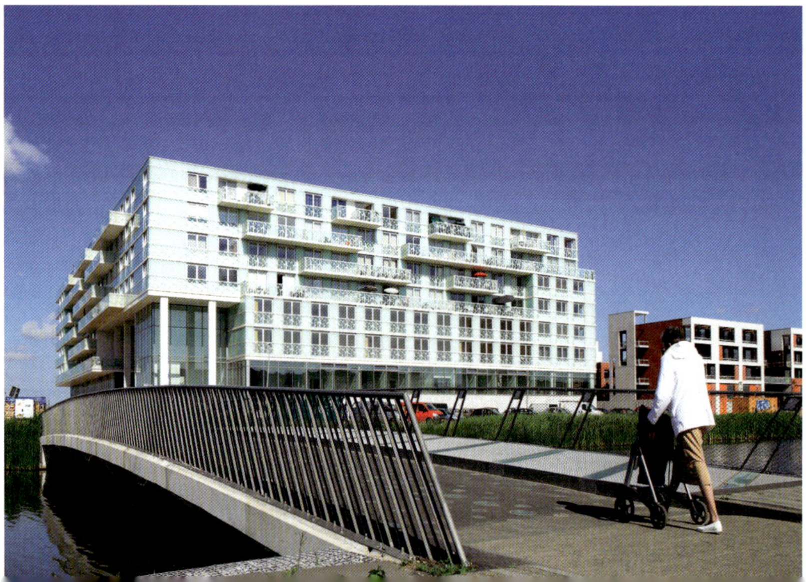

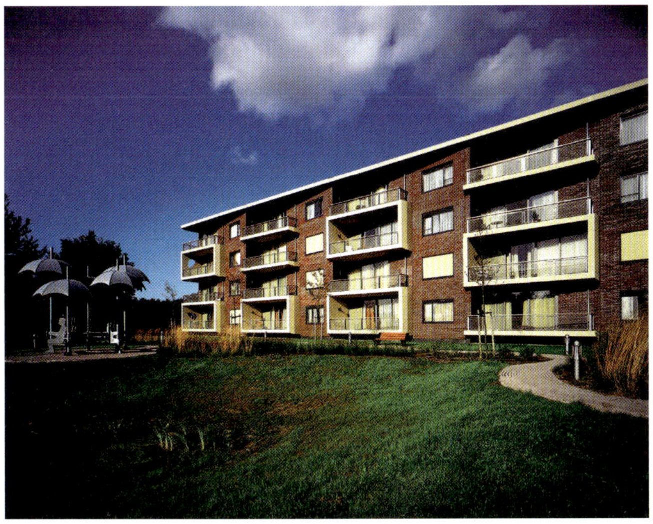

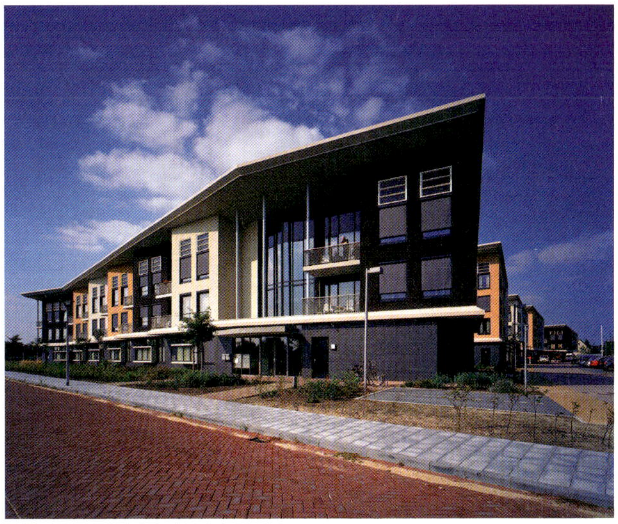

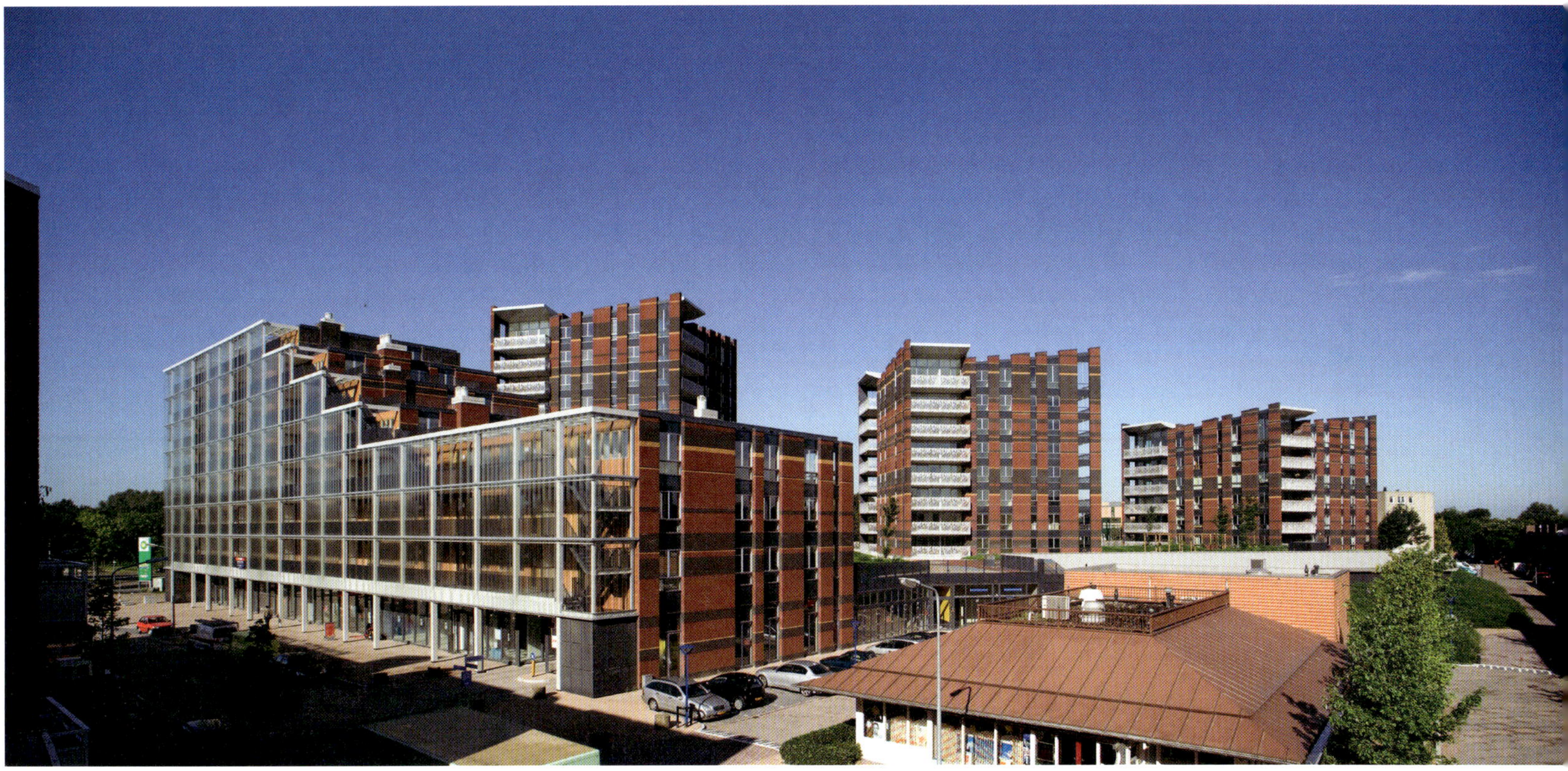

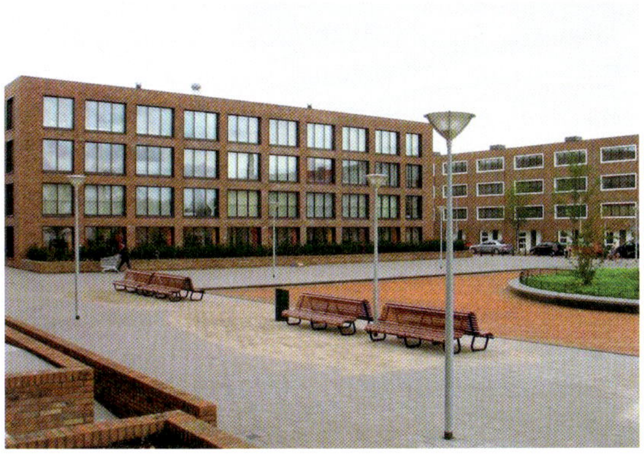

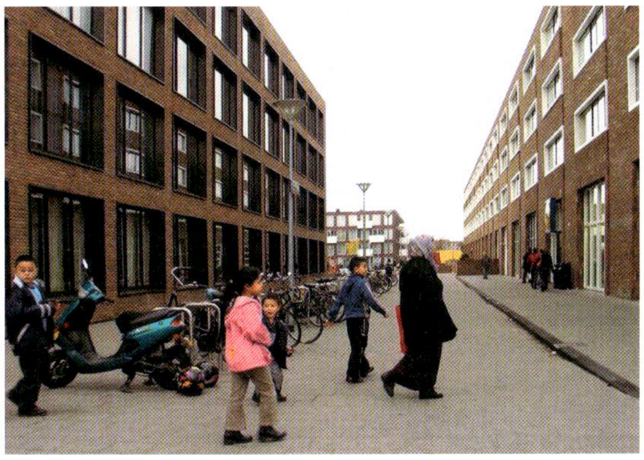

Top
***RDH architecten en stedenbouwkundigen*, Blankershof residential care centre, Oud-Gastel, 2005**

***RDH architecten en stedenbouwkundigen*, Kroonestede residential care complex, Hoeven, 2007**

Middle
***de Architekten Cie.*, De Regentesse, Huizen, 2008**

Bottom left
***Marlies Rohmer*, Transvaal district, residential care complex, The Hague, 2005**

Bottom right
***Jef Reintjes Architecten*, Onder-de-Pannen, Amsterdam, 2006**

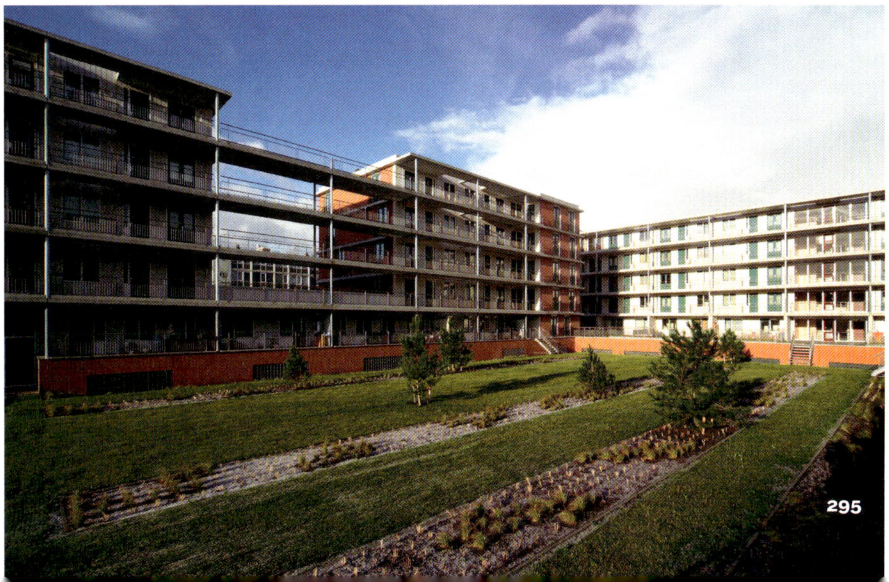

as a community service. Health centres complete the diverse range of services. The community support points were the renaissance of the service centre. Now they were usually created via forms of cooperation involving care institutions, childcare centres, libraries, health centres, general practitioners or schools: they combined their extramural and day services with existing or ar least regular facilities and were able to form the distinctive element in the residential care zones – in fact the concept of the residential care zone coincided with that of the elderly-friendly or life-cycle community, which led the Building Board and others to encourage the development.[26] If a full support point was to be practicable, a catchment neighbourhood or village of 10,000 residents was the minimal requirement. A full-time equivalent (FTE) of 8.7 would be required to guarantee round-the-clock care.[27] Health centres can assume the role of community support point. They can be organised in a general practitioners' centre (for example a so-called HOED: General Practitioners Under One Roof), or on a location in a centre that may not be permanently manned as part of a public building, such as a school, or part of a residential complex.

A remarkable project in every way is the renovation of the Garden Towns to the west of Amsterdam. Sixty per cent of the 54,000 homes here are due to be demolished and replaced between 2011 and 2015. Part of the programme is the supply of six hundred housing units with care (partly in the stock that is not demolished), twenty-five service centres and many care support points. This care component is part of what is called the social foundation. Including the implementation of four per cent adapted homes, the budget for this is around 270 million euro (the budget for the total project is 8 billion). The project is fleshed out by the cooperation of different clusters of institutions. The local government organs (urban district councils, municipal councils) combine to form a Park City Bureau, while the institutions for nursing and care, physical and mental handicaps, mental health care (GGZ) and social work are combined in a group called CareWest. Characteristic, but certainly not without its complications, is the fact that almost everything in the social foundation is connected with the social sector and is thus financed from collective funds. Moreover, the limit of the decentralisation concept seems to be approaching. The dispersal of what used to be called self-sufficient homes is supposed to lead to loneliness and isolation, and thus to work counterproductively. (This dilemma is apparently less frequent in the case of decentralised housing where care is available.) Part of the project is a complex of rented and owner-occupied apartments developed by the Algemene Woningbouwvereniging in cooperation with CareWest. The architect Jef Reintjes designed the Onder-de-Pannen (Roof-over-our-Head) complex on the basis of the Design for All principle. Tenants, owner occupiers, those with a physical or multiple handicap and old people live together there in spacious, adaptable homes.

A large restructuring project is also under way for the Transvaal district in The Hague. It is supposed to be transformed from a problem district into a showcase district within the next ten years, and the offer of care facilities plays a large role in this process. Marlies Rohmer has implemented various projects, including the Stellenbosch housing complex, that comprises a large diversity of types of rented or owner-occupied homes in different categories, including a housing-cum-care complex for the elderly and the handicapped.

Soon after the emergence of the first massive new housing estates built as part of the Vinex programme in the 1990s, it was concluded that they were not very suitable for old people. 'The conclusions (...) regarding the possibility of meeting the demands of the (future) older generation by means of new buildings on the large-scale housing estate appear to give little reason for optimism', the Ministry for Housing, Spatial Planning and the Environment (VROM) concluded in 1997.[28] Facilities were often implemented after the houses had been built, and the prices were too high. An attempt was made to learn from past mistakes in the setting up of IJburg, the large-scale new housing estate on artificial islands in the IJsselmeer. Sixty per cent of the homes in the first building stage were built to be adaptable, and five per cent were already adapted. They were dispersed, clustered and even built in the form of clusters of almshouses. In addition, packages of basic medical care and domestic support were developed to bridge the separation between housing and care.[29] Meyer en Van Schooten implemented De Kristal, a combination of housing, services and community amenities on the large-scale Nesselande housing estate in Rotterdam. The homes are all life-cycle homes. As one would expect, the residential care zone is fleshed out particularly in urban regions, where catchment numbers are sufficient for a differentiated supply of small-scale provisions. Their success or failure depends on good accessibility, which presupposes short distances. This is often not the case in the countryside, which is why central provisions persist there. All the same, a decentralisation trend can be perceived in rural areas too, in which ideally each village is assigned its own provisions. This is the case in the province of Brabant, for example. Whereas in the past old people in need of assistance from Oud-Gastel, Hoeven and Oudenbosch were accommodated in the Halderberge district in the Zellebergen in Oudenbosch, since 2006 each of the three village centres has had its own residential care centre. This enables old people to continue to live in their own surroundings for as long as possible. The centres consist of several apartment buildings in which homes with a surface area of 90 m^2 are incorporated. General provisions such as a restaurant, a cosy bar, a fitness centre, hairdresser, launderette and care areas form the links between the buildings.

Practically synonymous with the residential care zone is the residential service zone, the first of which was opened in 2000. This concept targets not only the distribution of care provisions but also housing and welfare. The Escamp district in The Hague is regarded as a textbook example; in 2007 the Aedes-Actiz knowledge centre acclaimed this district as the most innovative integrated neighbourhood project. It targets all 110,000 residents. The initiative to consider the whole of Breda as an ensemble of integrated neighbourhood services is also intended for all residents irrespective of age of demand for care.

Ordinary housing

The creation of residential care zones, and in general the transfer of care services to buildings without housing facilities, is only possible if the regular housing stock is suitable for the elderly. Vice versa, that only makes sense if it meets certain architectural demands and is located in an environment that is suitable for the elderly – and that in turn presupposes in the first place the presence of sufficient care facilities. As soon as the contours of a broad category of well-to-do elderly became visible, private developers saw a gap in the market. It is only natural for them to do their utmost to create the impression that the buildings and complexes they offer exactly match the demands of the target tenants or owner-occupiers. Although the presence of care facilities is often praised as one of the unique selling points, the priority lies elsewhere:

in the attempt to address specific lifestyles. Age in itself is no longer a distinctive criterion, it has been replaced by a wide range of separate categories that have been demarcated as neatly as possible by all kinds of research agencies. Motivaction is probably the best-known research agency to target lifestyles, but it is certainly not the only one. For instance, the IVA Institute distinguishes three main types: cosmopolitan, critical and committed, conservative. These can be found in each of the five senior segments that the agency described as lively, lively in the future, able to cope on their own, able to cope with cognitive limitations, and dependent on assistance.[30]

The cabinet supports the building of homes that are suitable for the elderly in the project 'Beter (t)huis in de buurt' (Better (at) home in the neighbourhood), which envisages 406,000 new housing units and the modification of a part of the existing stock.[31] It was expected that eight per cent of the 150,000 housing units that the housing corporations provided until 2010 would be suitable for old people. Private building was promoted too, for example by encouraging the elderly to implement joint projects themselves. The diversity is the largest in the higher rented and owner-occupied segment. Developers like the Stichting Initiatieven Realisatie 55+ (SIR-55) discovered a gap in the market. The target group is described as 'mediors', the group from middle aged to senior[32], and provided with service flats. As in the latest generation of care complexes, a certain diversity is sometimes sought without marring the chic appearance. The complex De Regentesse designed by de Architekten Cie. in Huizen comprises three tower blocks and a fairly low apartment building. Besides fifty-three owner-occupied apartments, there are ninety-four rented ones. Care and comfort facilities are located on the ground floor of the apartment building. Detached villas are also popular as homes for the elderly. If the concept does not include access to care facilities in the purchase contract, a location near a community support point or a nursing and care home proves to be preferred.

Besides these products of senior-orientated marketing, the campaigns for modifiable renovation, building and life-cycle homes continued. The only specific feature of these homes is that they are suitable for the elderly. They are not distinguished by attempts to address the lifestyles of (well-to-do) seniors.

As has been noted before, neither the concept of the residential care zone nor the range of provisions that form the hybrid care landscape at the moment can perform their role properly if the supply of homes on the regular owner-occupied and rented property market does not enable old people to live at home for as long as possible. Not a type of housing, but an increasingly everyday component of more and more homes (for the elderly) is home automation or domotics. This usually includes a number of standard applications in the communal areas: burglar alarms, fire and smoke alarms, gas and water leak alarms, devices to report breakdowns and to give an alarm signal for lifts, and entrance warning systems that come into operation if the entrance is left open too long. Inside the apartments themselves there are controls for the central heating as well as burglar, fire and smoke alarms. What the combination of modifiable building and domotics could achieve was demonstrated in a mobile model home.[33] Home automation is making rapid progress, especially with regard to user friendliness. All the same, this technology turns out to be too complicated to operate for, for instance, victims of dementia. Recent innovations seem to have overcome that obstacle: they react independently and are set and operated if necessary by the personnel.[34]

Ordinary housing that is inconspicuously absorbed among the buildings of streets and neighbourhoods where the whole range of age categories live side by side proves not to be ideal for all old people. Fairly homogeneous residential groups because they consist exclusively of old people seem to satisfy a need for certain lifestyle groups. Market research has shown that they like to live together. Living together in a much smaller community is characteristic of the commune. This form continues to attract interest. Its architectural elaboration, however, is extremely diverse, and that is also true of the social backgrounds of the different groups and, related to that, their economic status.

While these complexes are usually situated in an ordinary neighbourhood in a city, town or village, the villages designed specifically for the elderly present a very different picture. The famous Sun City is always cited as the prime model. Inbo, BAM and TNC Property Project took the lead in setting up the Senior City Initiative Group in 2004. Although this concept had been considered impossible in the Netherlands for a long time, it suddenly seemed to achieve a good chance of success. Five locations were selected, including a 'walhalla' for the elderly in the Noordoostpolder.[35] Villages of this kind have not been implemented yet, but their precursor has: the small-scale concentrations inside urban contexts that are advertised as 'golden years'.[36]

Shelter

Greiner Van Goor Huijten Architecten

Sinai Centrum
Amstelveen
2007

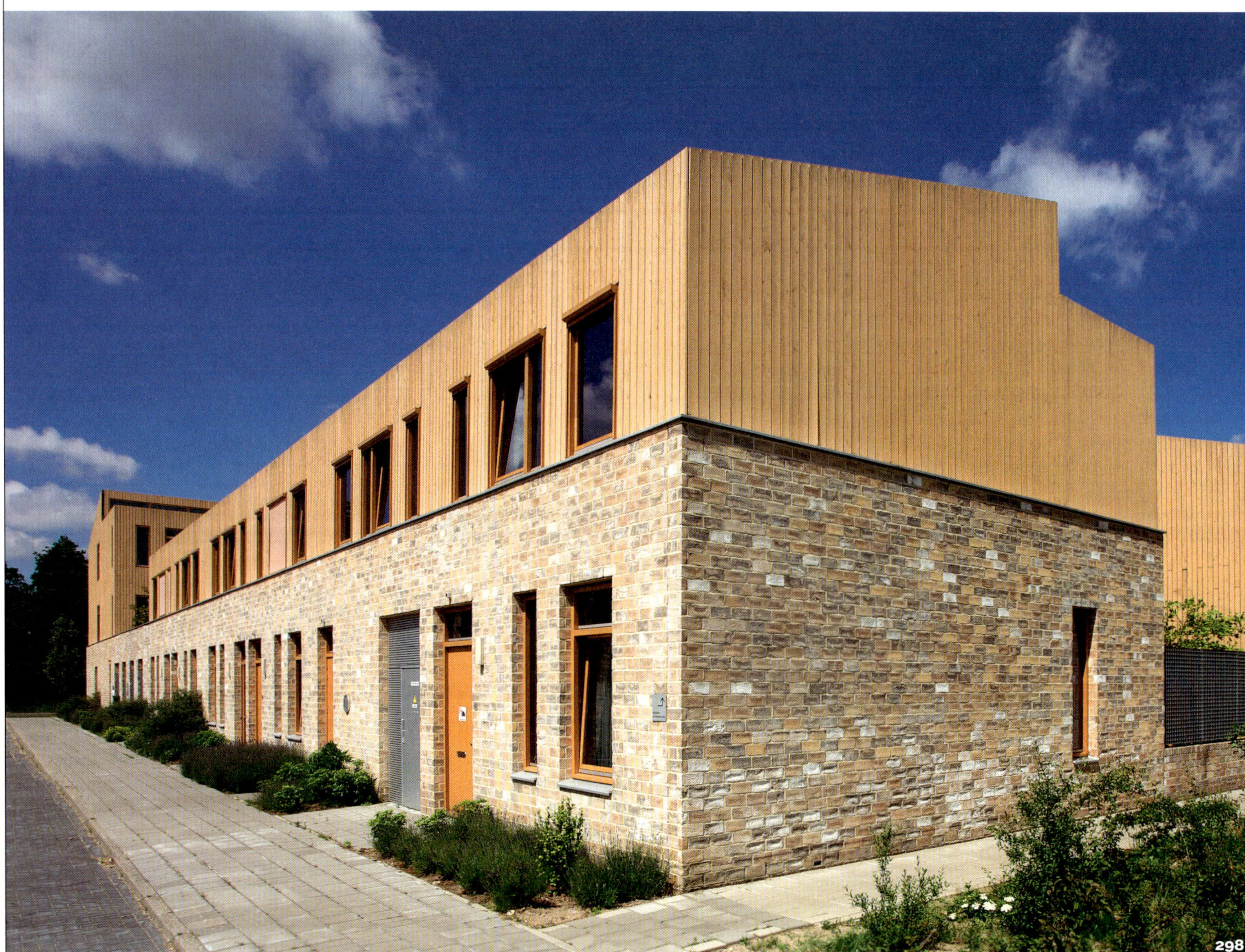

The Sinai Centrum in Amstelveen is for Jewish residents with a psychiatric or mental handicap. The new facility has been built on two locations in Amstelveen (Bankras and Langerhuize). The Bankras location consists of an apartment block built around an inner garden with front doors on the street side and on the gallery on the first and second floors. There is a clear distinction between the residential units and a learning and work centre. The internal connection of the units means that residential groups can be made larger or smaller to suit their requirements.

The Langerhuize location gives the impression of being on a small scale thanks to the articulation of the volumes and by giving the different sections small gardens of their own. A distinction has also been made between treatment and residential areas. Flexibility is guaranteed by the continuous series of sections grouped around an inner garden, which makes it simple to alter their size. Bedrooms and work rooms are also interchangeable. The supporting structure would allow a completely different internal division.

The architects used a variegated sand-coloured stone to evoke associations with the sandstone blocks to be seen in Jerusalem. Besides this cultural reference, attention has also been paid to the atmosphere and the potentially positive effect of the materials. Bricks stands for shelter, wood for a warm, natural look, and the light wooden panels in the interior are intended to promote the wellbeing of the residents. The interiors are simple and cosy and designed to make the residents feel at ease. These complexes are not the place for exaggerated spectacle; a clear articulation of the façade, which is determined above all by the use of materials, highlights the distinction between residential and work areas.

The garden designs for both locations are by Copijn: two enclosed gardens, two patios and a roof garden. Jewish identity and Jewish customs play an important role in the designs of both gardens.

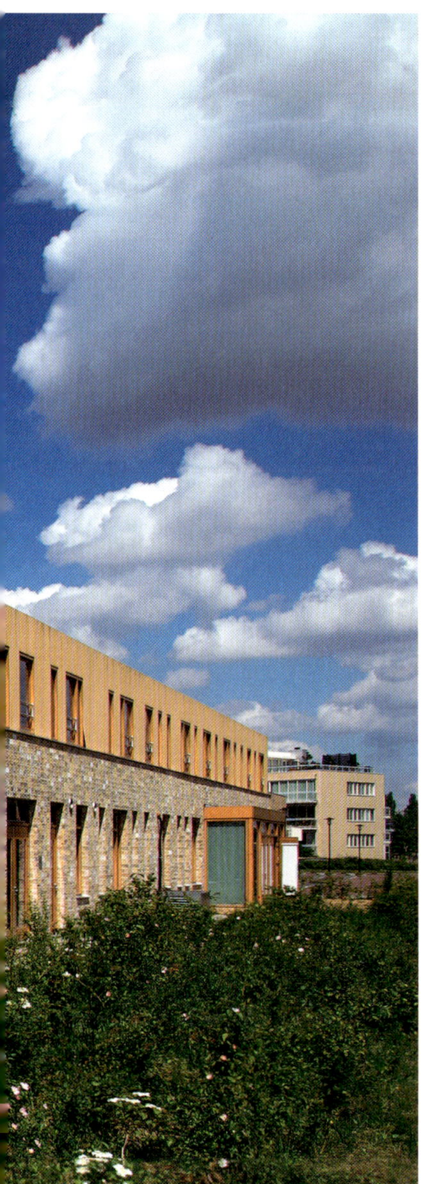

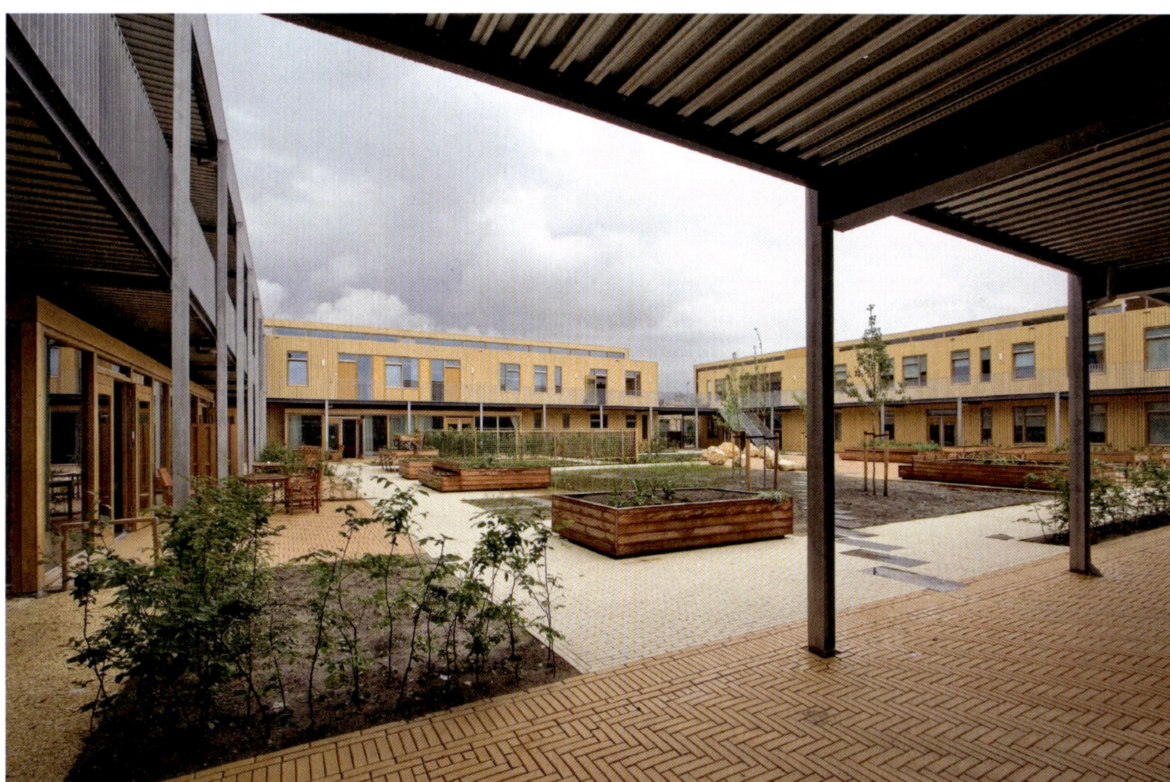

Situation Bankras location

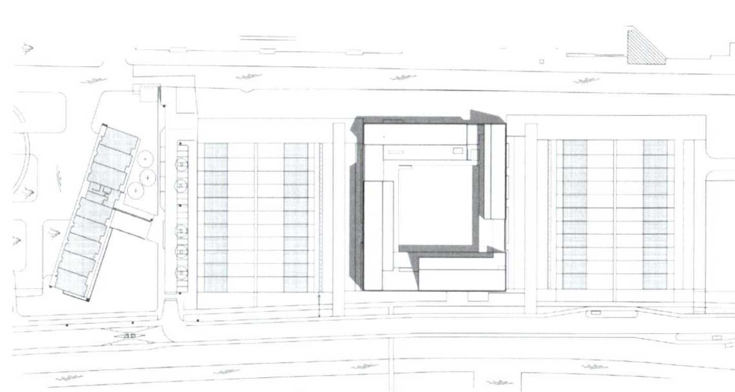

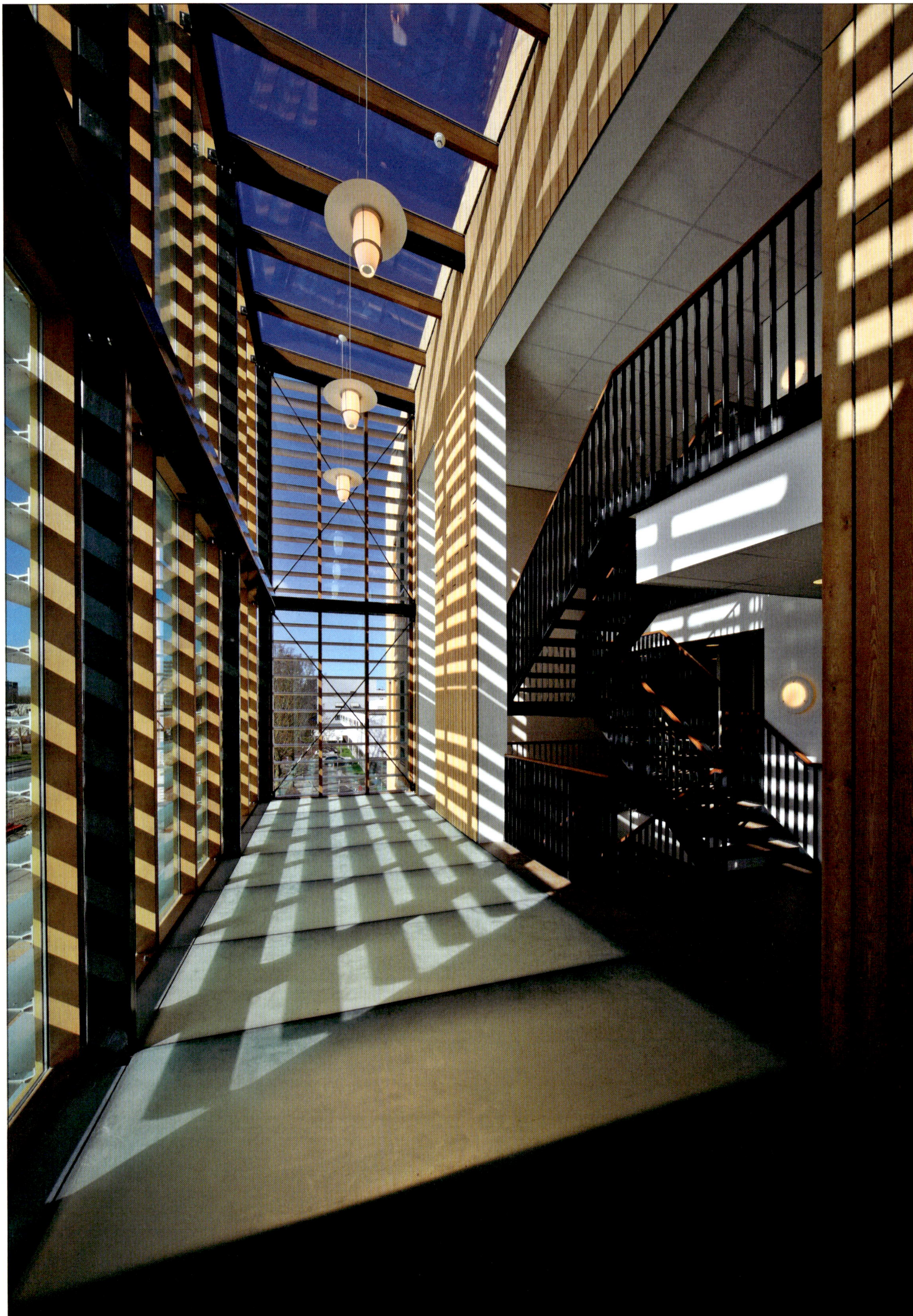

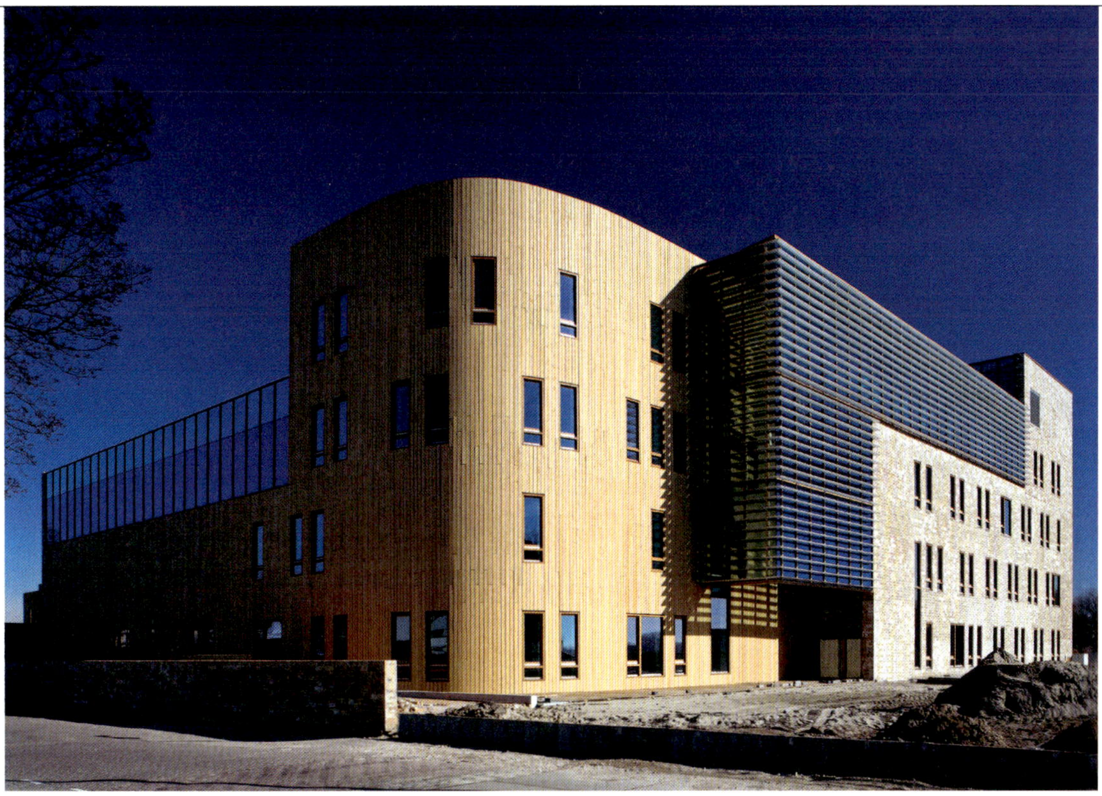

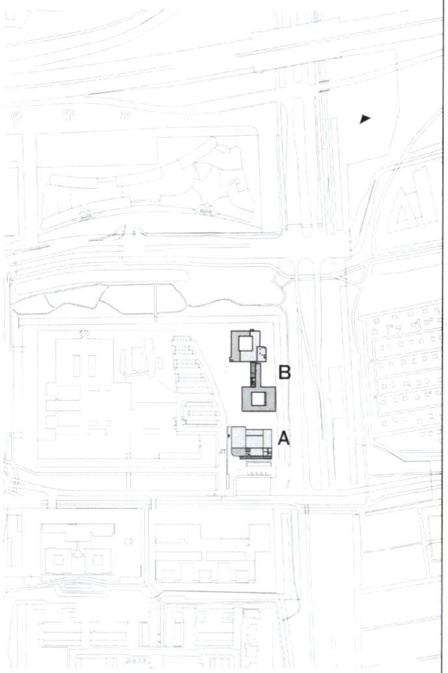

Situation Langerhuize location
1 *treatment building*
2 *clinics*

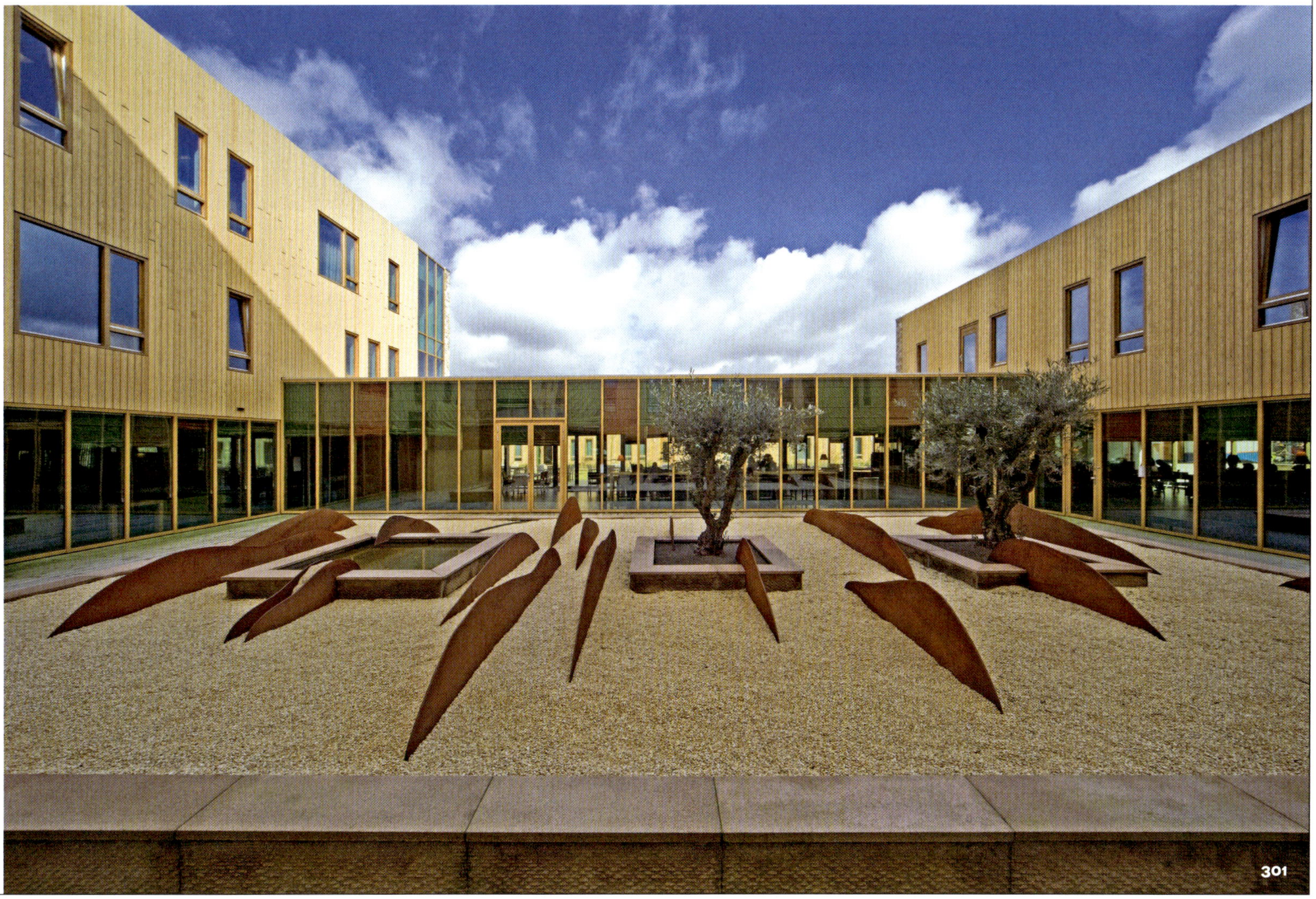

Residential blocks

Dick van Gameren architecten

Berkenstede care centre
Diemen
1999-2006

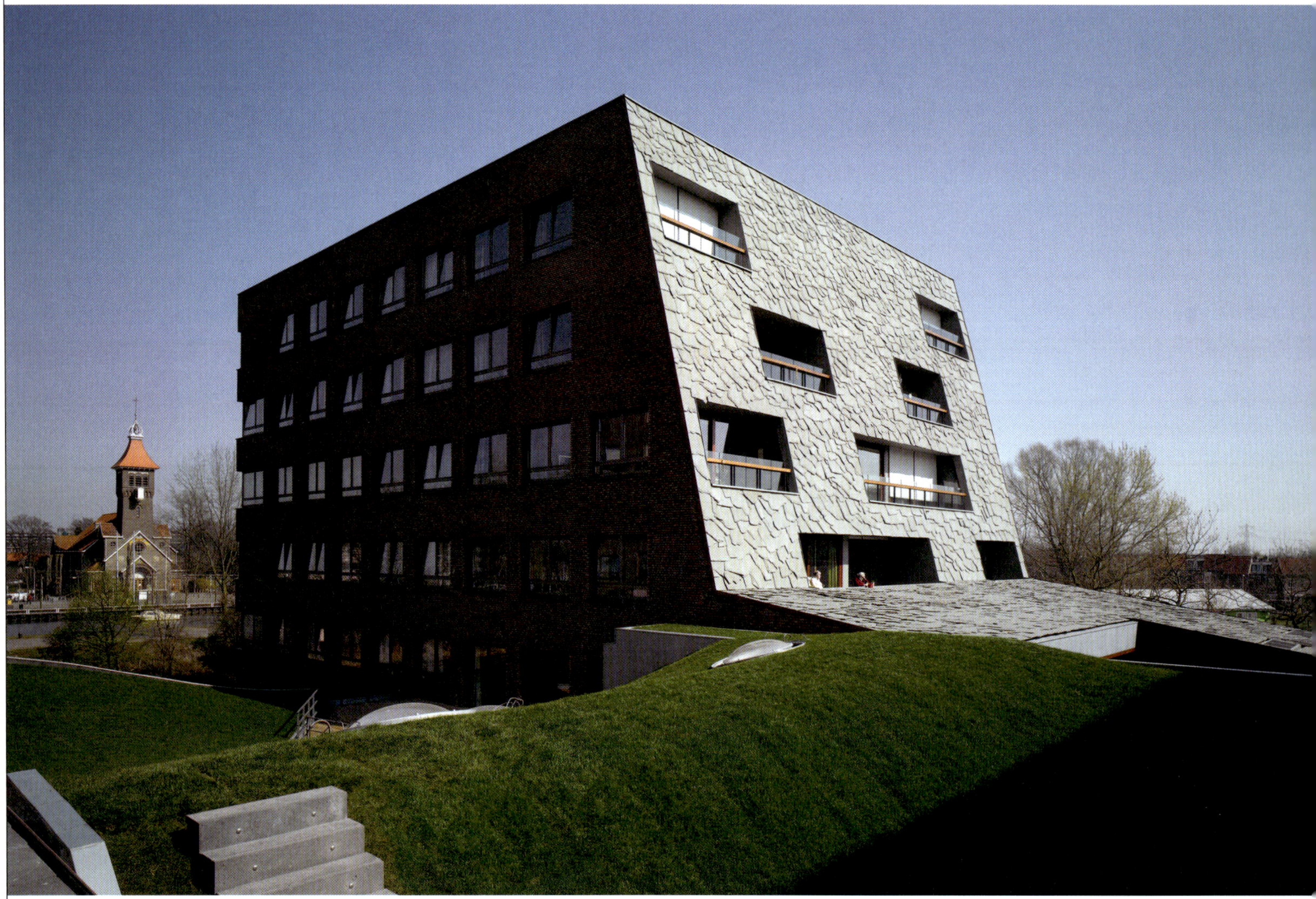

The Berkenstede residential care centre replaced the Oude Vrouwenhuis Amstelhof in Amsterdam and a 1970s block of flats for the elderly in Diemen. The new building was implemented in the nearby village of Diemen. The urban development plan prescribed a unity in the choice of materials. Moreover, the Berkenstede residential care centre, which is situated in the heart of the neighbourhood, had to consist of four separate volumes from the second floor up. The architect deliberately refrained from resorting to the flat box with towers on top. The complex comprises four tower blocks of different heights, each with a sloping façade. The ground floor blocks are connected with one another by an inner street, where the general amenities are situated which the locals are also free to use, such as a restaurant, a grand café, a relaxation area, a physiotherapist, paramedical facilities and a hairdresser. On the first floor is a service corridor that connects the residential with the nursing areas. Between the buildings are gardens, terraces, patios and slopes. The outdoor design is by the landscape architect Lodewijk Baljon.

The building accommodates different target groups per tower block. The first block (the tree tower) has 85 residential units for intramural care of approximately 50 m². The second block (the fruit tower) contains 46 independent service flats with a larger surface area that varies from 60 to 80 m². The third block (the flower tower) has rooms for temporary stay and revalidation. The fourth block (the fauna tower) contains ten group residential units for patients suffering from advancing dementia.

The rooms are on the large side to be able to cater for future changes in care and to keep the building up to date for a longer period. The roof and sloping walls of each block are clad in a different (natural) material: metal, stone, grass, and wood.

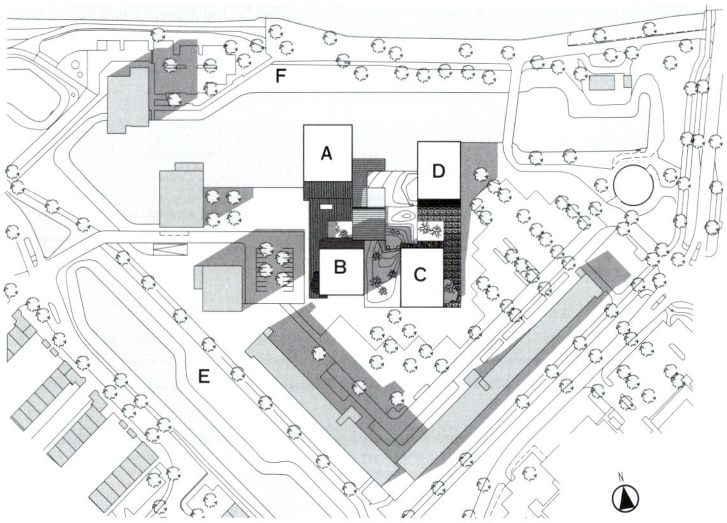

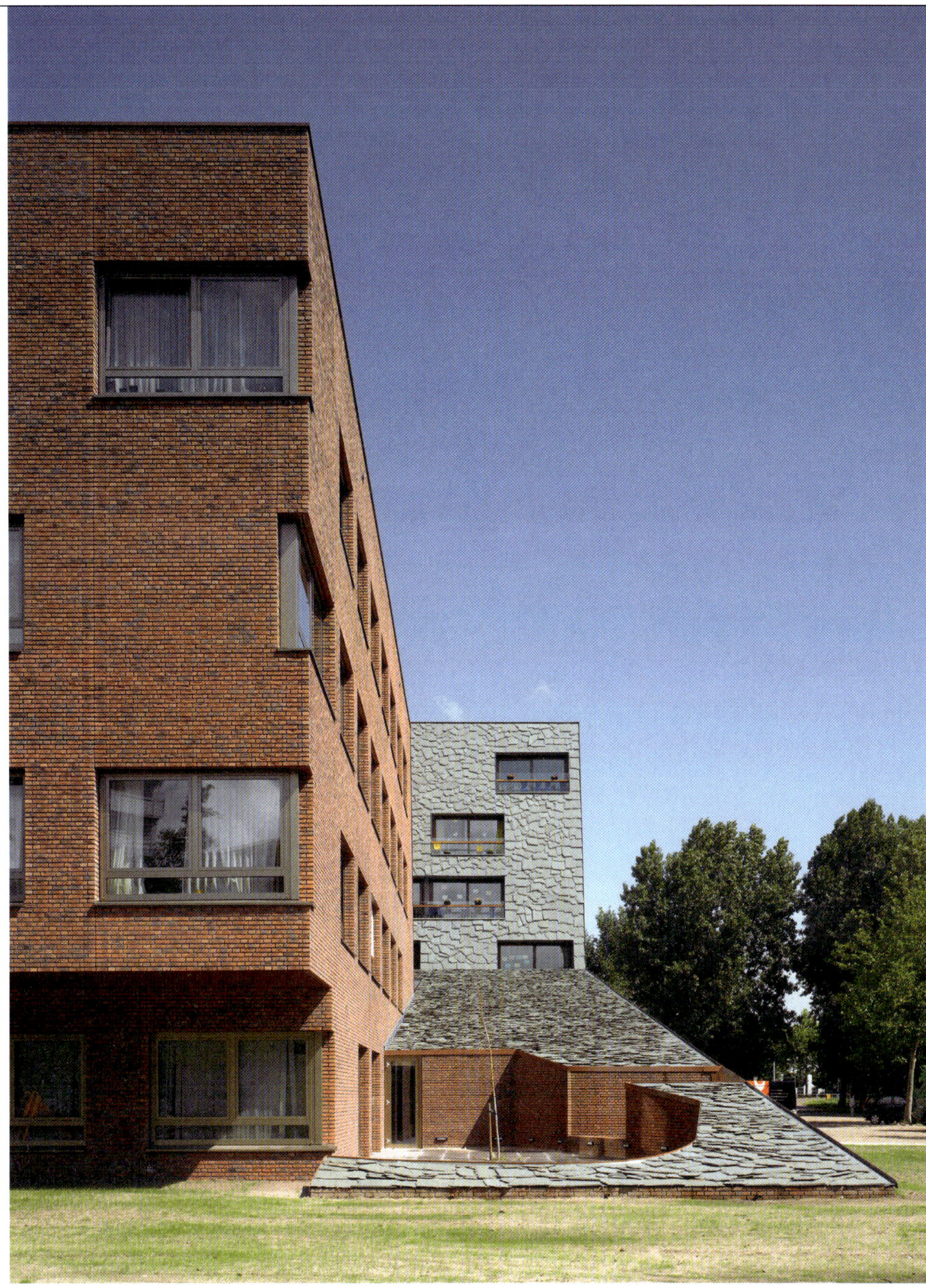

Situation

A *housing for the elderly*

B *housing for invalids and regular housing*

C *rehabilitation*

D *psycho-geriatrics*

E *Berkenstede*

F *Venserkade*

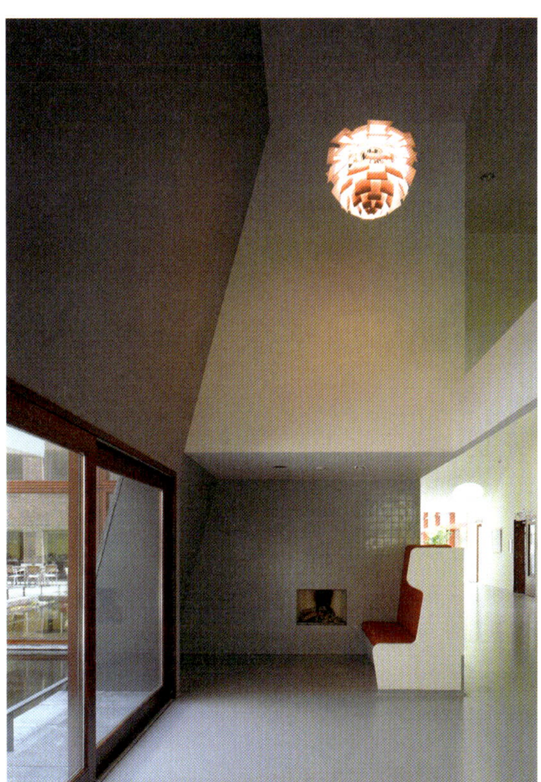

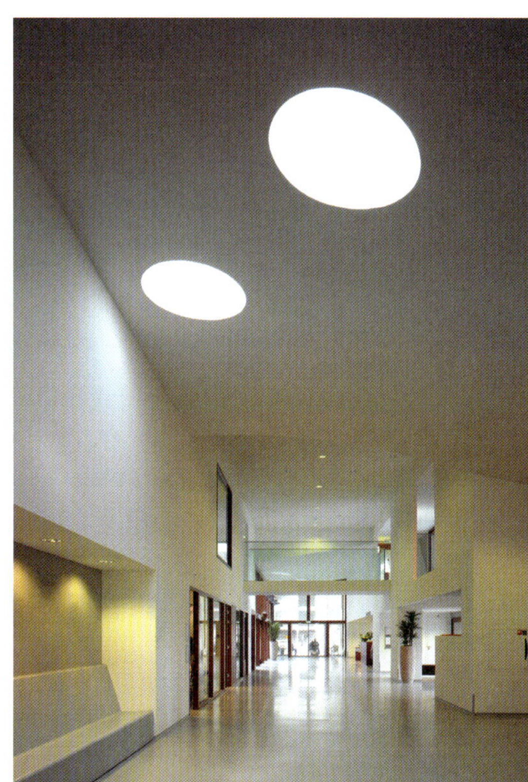

Hip

Arons en Gelauff Architecten

De Plussenburgh
Rotterdam
2001-2006

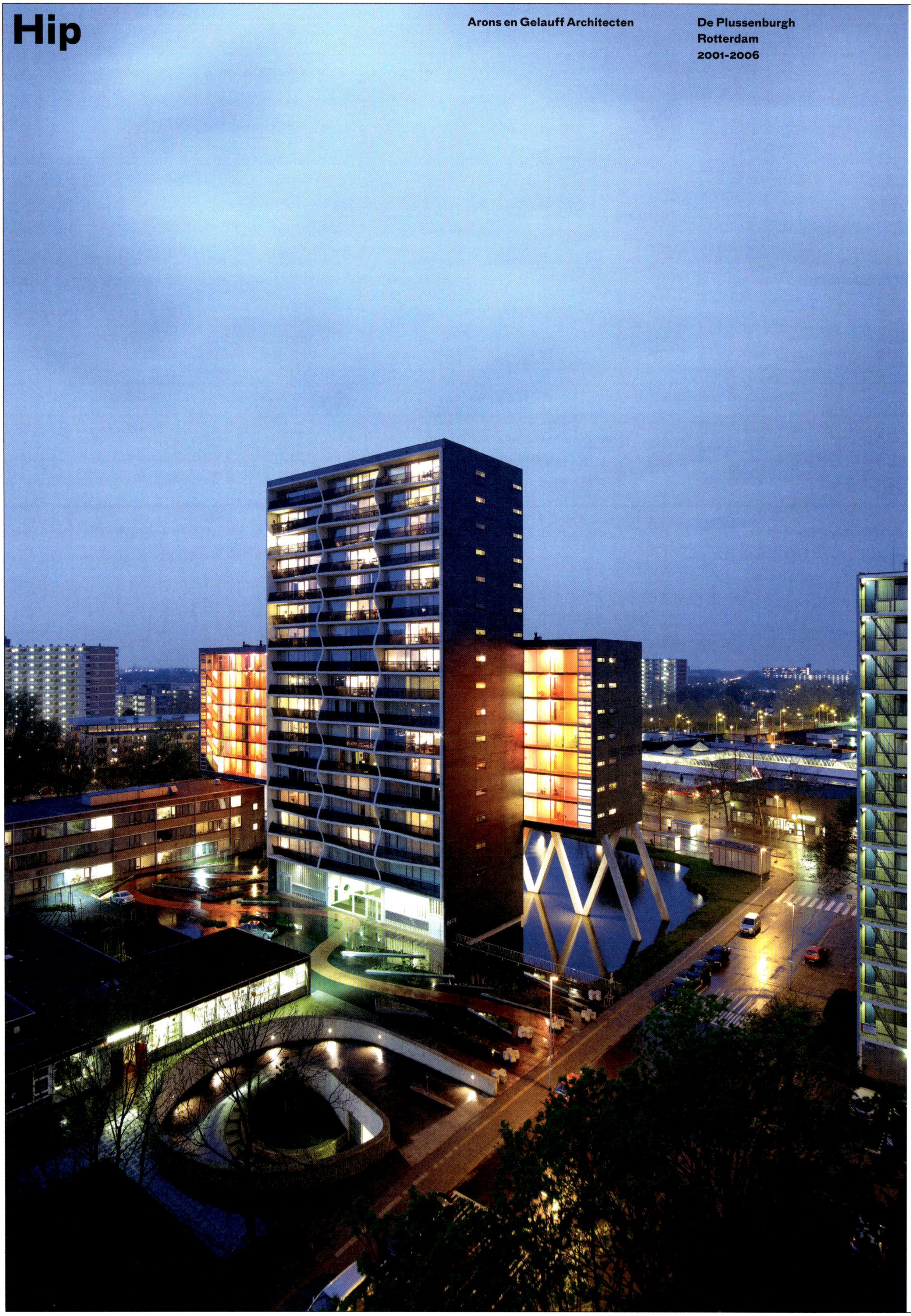

De Plussenburgh combines two topical architectural and urban development assignments: urban renewal in a postwar district, and the implementation of housing for the elderly close to facilities and public transport. The urban development plan for the revitalisation of IJsselmonde is by Rein Geurtsen, the further elaboration by Kees Rijnboutt. It envisages a renovation of the Keizerswaard shopping centre and the construction of a market square with a tower apartment block, the district office, catering amenities and a library. De Plussenburgh is the first step in this plan for the centre. It consists of a seventeen-storey tower block with 48 rented apartments and, at right angles to it, a lower seven-storey volume with 56 rented apartments. The latter rests on angular struts ten metres above ground level. Beneath it is an artificial lake.

A square consisting of different triangles with reed vegetation designed by Inside Outside landscape architects links the new block to the existing residential care centre. There is a communal meeting area beside the lake. The design is based on the fact that those aged 55 or more today formed the hippie generation in the 1960s. That explains the strikingly hip building with panels to which two hundred different colours have been applied. The most eye-catching feature, however, is the wavy shape of the balconies. The widest part affords full opportunity to spend time out of doors, while the narrowest part still satisfies the minimal norms for a balcony from which the windows can be washed to avoid expensive cleaning equipment. Twisted steel balustrades accentuate the rhythm, which is further emphasised by alternating wide and narrow parts per floor. Parking facilities are below ground level. The apartments are more than 80 m² in size and relatively flexible thanks to the generous wall-to-wall dimensions of 9.8 metres. The corridors are wide enough for two people in wheelchairs to pass one another without any difficulty.

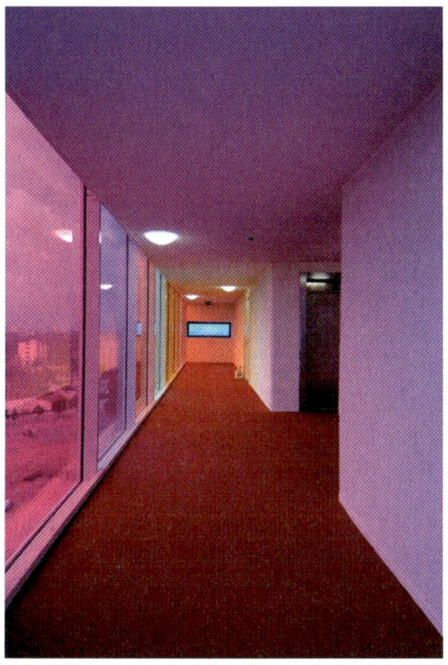

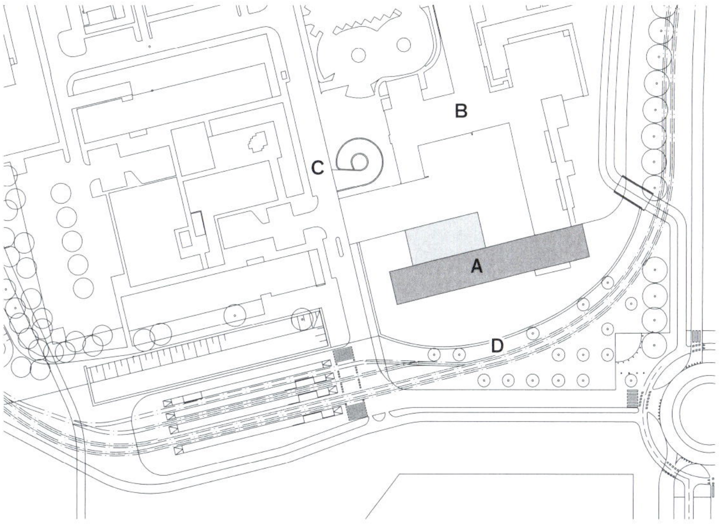

Situation
A *De Plussenburgh*
B *adjacent care centre*
C *Grote Hagen*
D *Herenwaard*

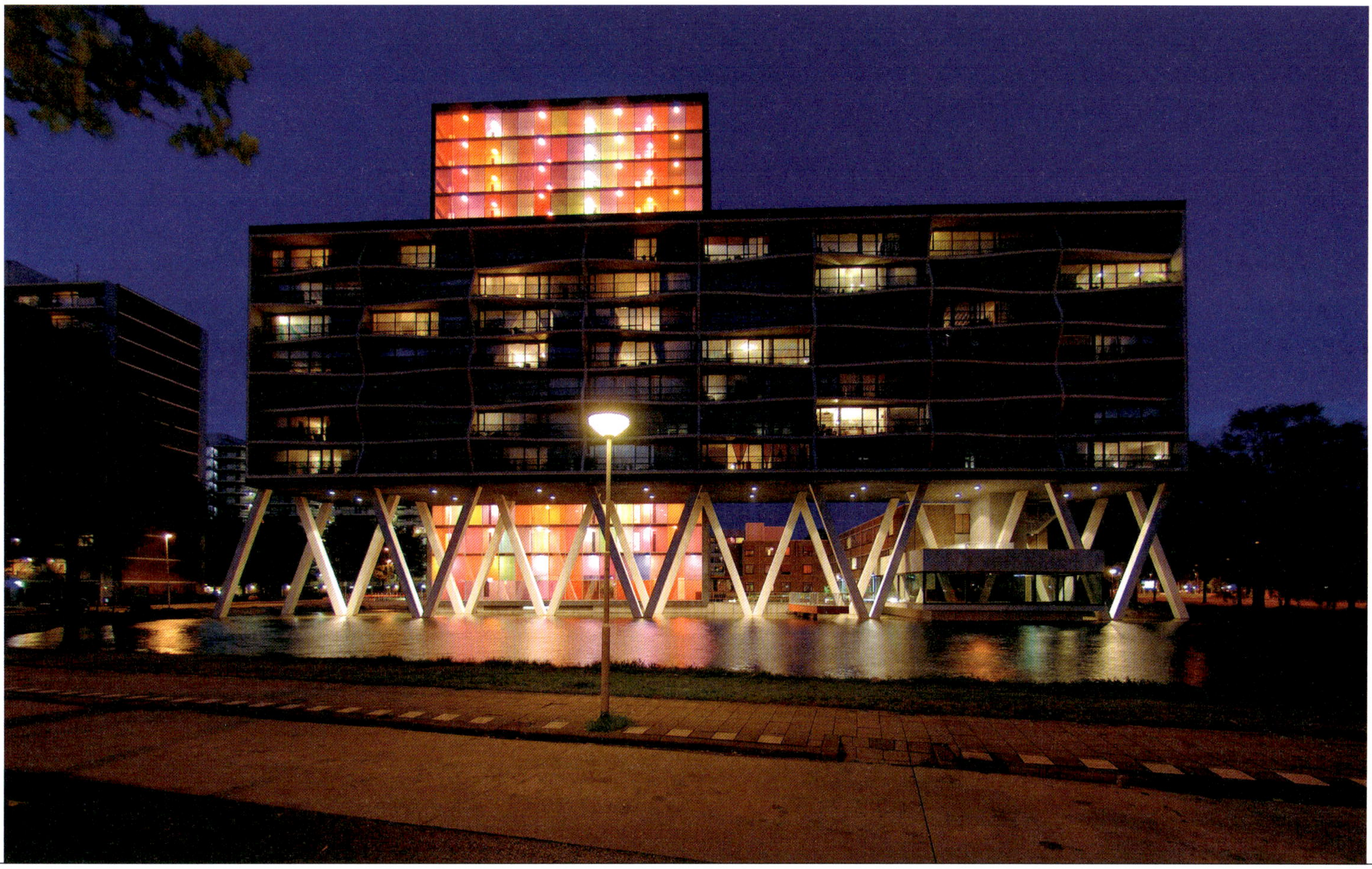

VMX Architects

Willem Arntsz Huis
Utrecht
2003-2007

Situation
A *Lange Nieuwstraat*
B *Agnietenstraat*
C *closed courtyard*
D *public courtyard*

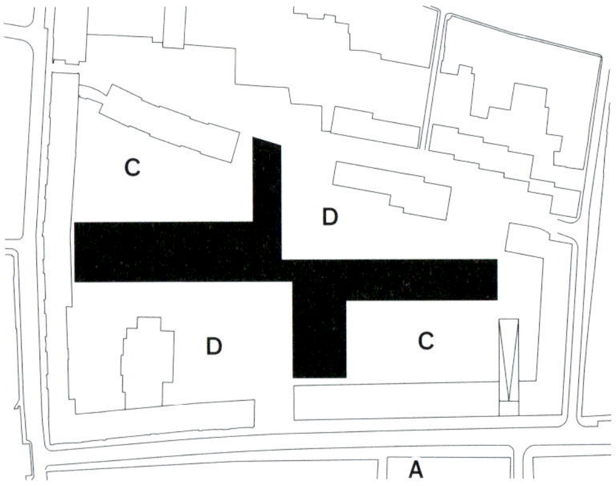

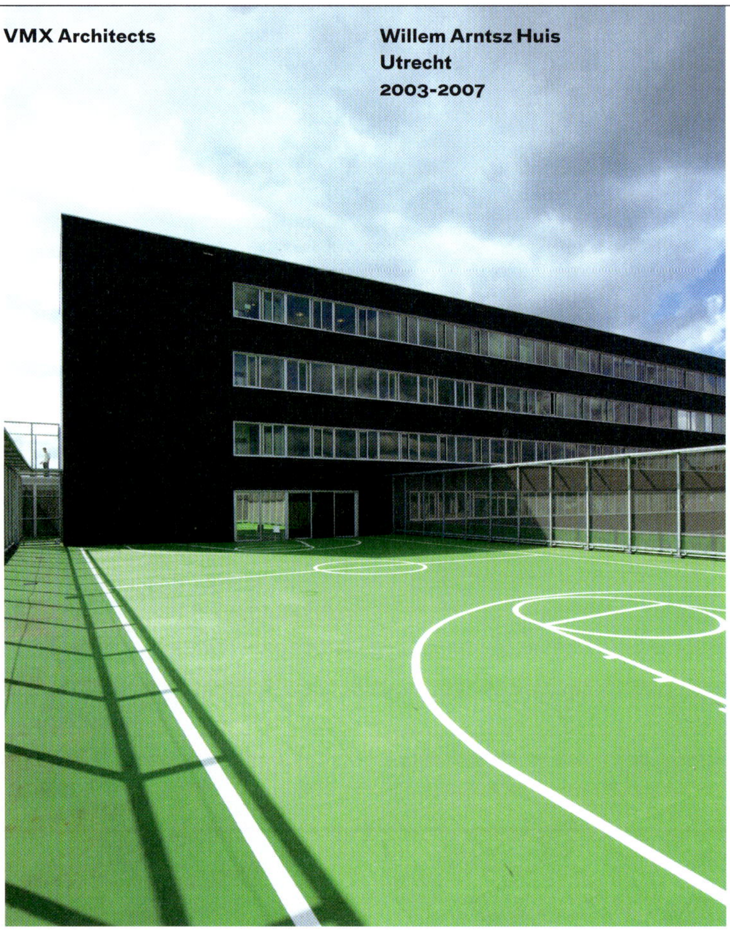

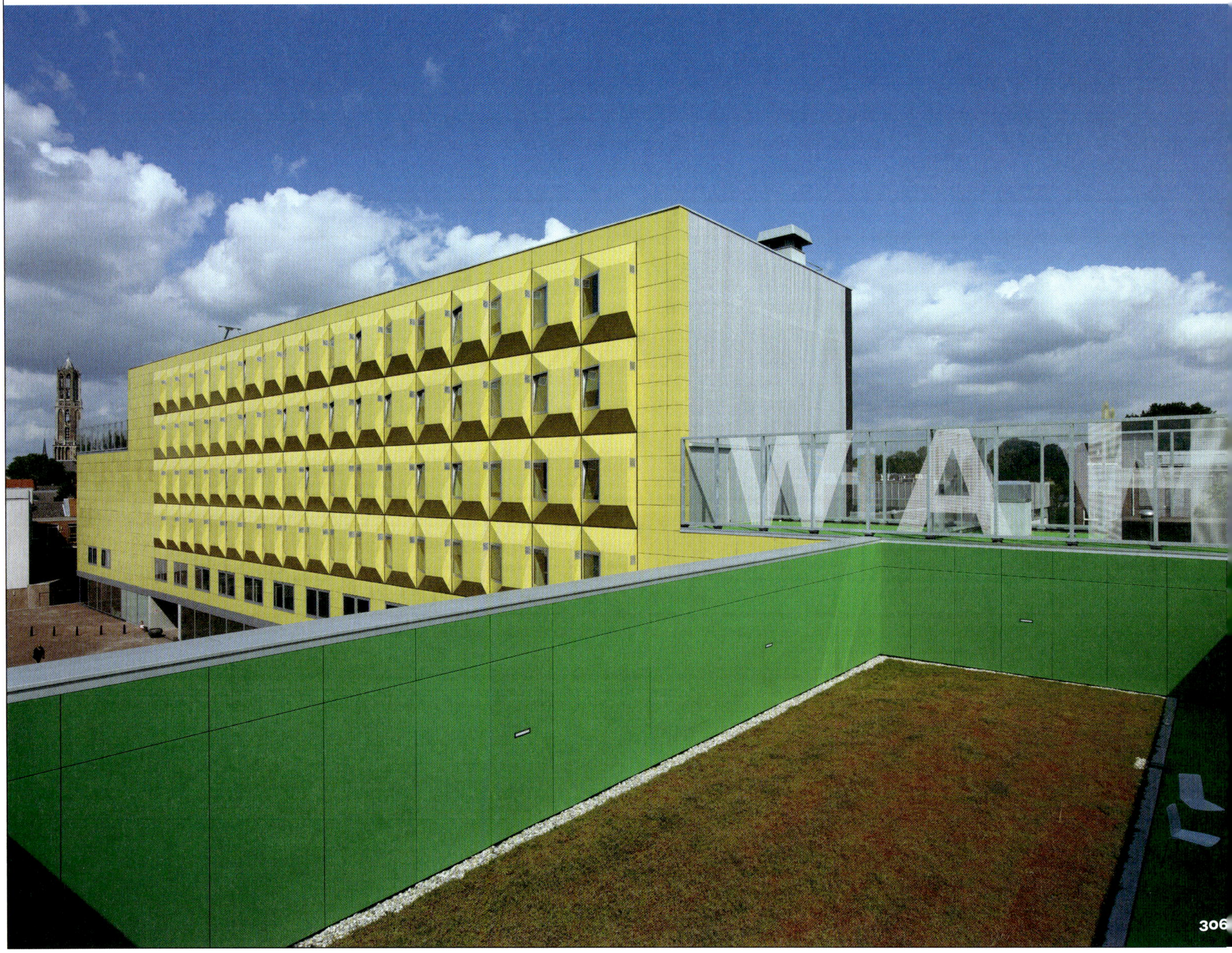

Stichting Altrecht and the Centrum Maliebaan commissioned VMX Architects to implement a substitute new building in the historic museum quarter of Utrecht. All that is left of a grey concrete monster from the 1970s is the underground car park. Integration with the surroundings was an important criterion for the new design. Homes and social functions are situated on the edge of the terrain, while the psychiatric functions are accommodated on the terrain enclosed by them. The new building has a cruciform design and delimits four gardens, two of which are open to the public. The different kinds of façade cladding give each of these gardens a character of its own. Most of the complex is for short-term patients; there are also a few areas for long-term care. The buildings combine treatment and residential units. The latter are based on the hotel concept. Most of the public functions such as reception, therapy and the crisis service, which must be easy to reach, are on the ground floor. The treatment areas are on the first and second floors, and the wards are on the top four floors with a residential unit on each floor. The new Willem Arntsz Huis owes its character above all to the application of coloured polyester panels, which have been shaped to form bays in one of the walls. The roofs are of a green synthetic material. There is a basketball field on top of the east wing. The complex is due to be expanded in the future, partly over existing buildings.

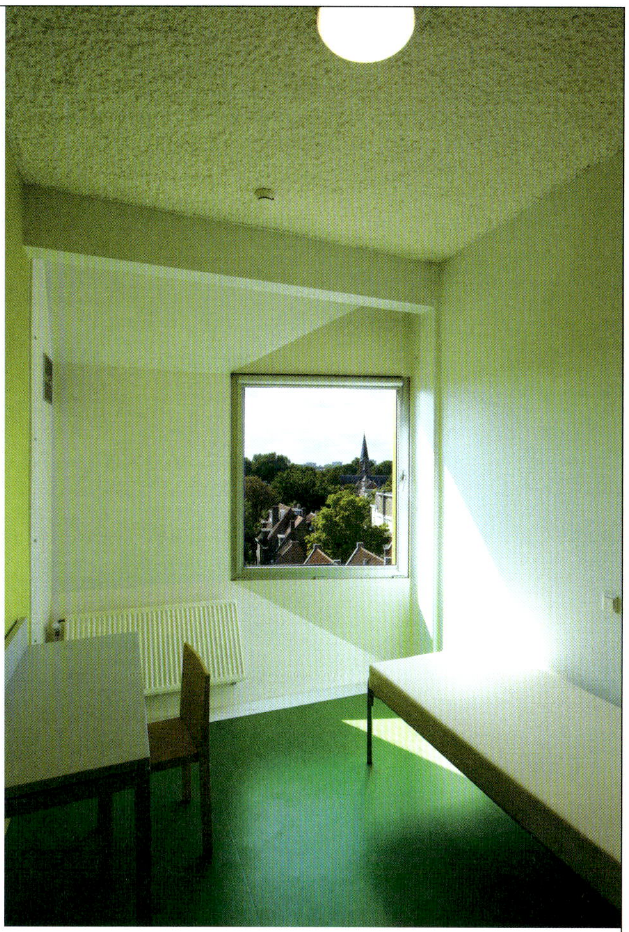

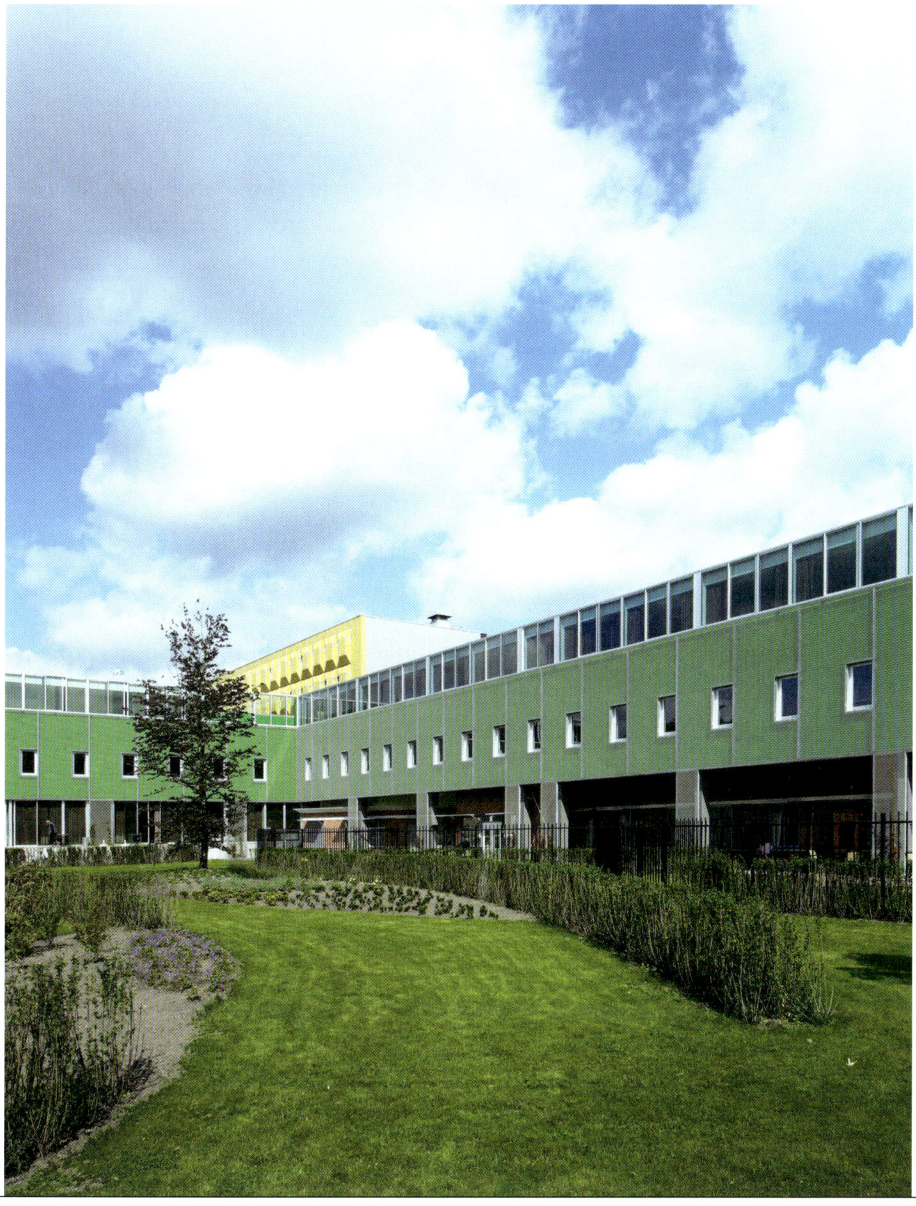

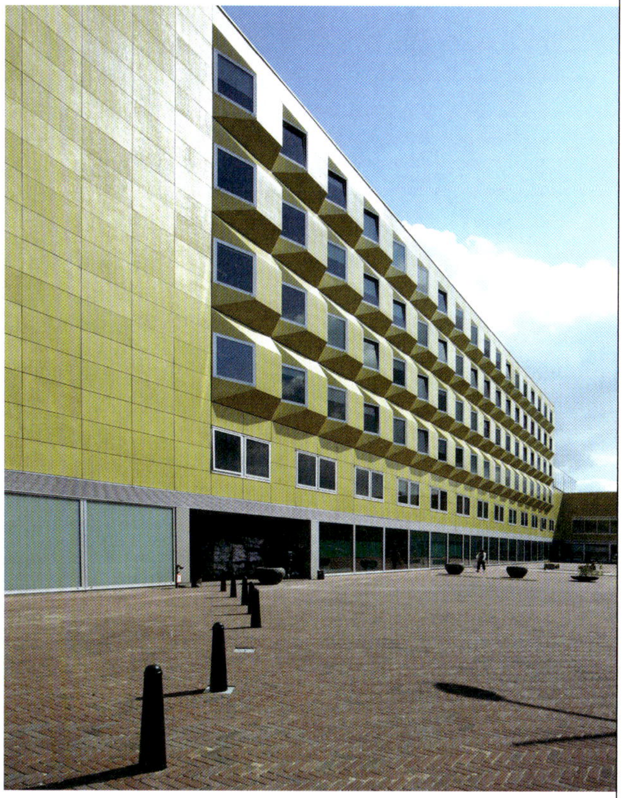

Teeth

Architecten aan de Maas

La Valence nursing home
Maastricht
2007

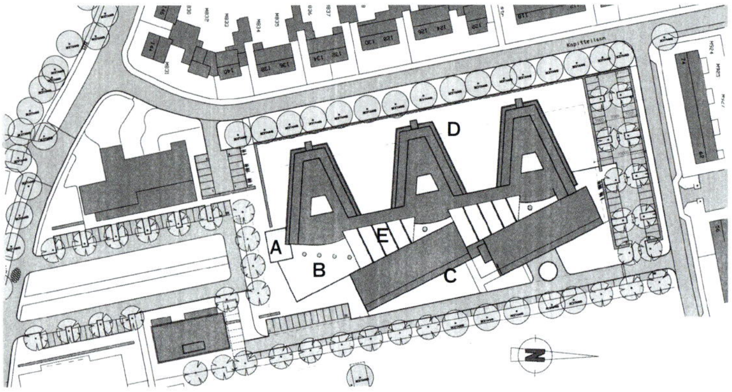

Situation
A *main entrance*
B *restaurant, recreation*
C *care homes, general provisions*
D *residential groups*
E *atrium*

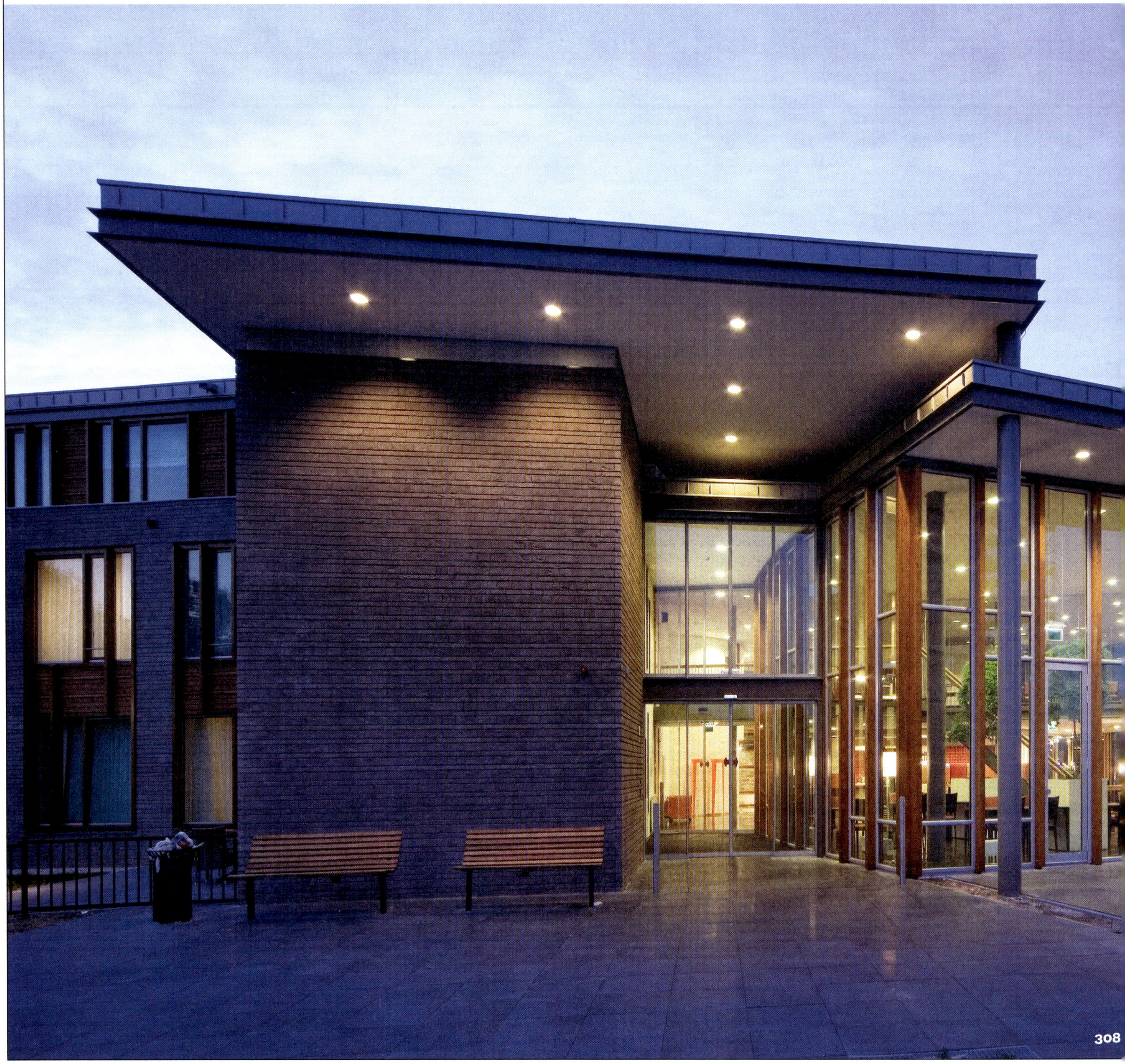

La Valence is a nursing home for 130 somatic and psycho-geriatric patients, who are divided into groups of eight to twelve persons. The complex includes 24 sheltered homes for couples one of whom is entitled to nursing care, and a further 18 sheltered homes in a detached volume at the front of the terrain. The floor plan of La Valence shows a sequence of three rectangular volumes like a row of teeth, and three teeth opposite them with eight rooms on each side on the ground floor and second floor that together form a group. The middle section of each of the three teeth contains communal facilities and a small patio. The entrance to the complex is in the first of the three rectangular volumes, which is also the shortest. The restaurant, reception and an audiovisual lounge are here too. Three triangular gardens are demarcated between the two other rectangular blocks and the three teeth. In one of them the central library can be found, the last one accommodates a meditation room with fitness and health amenities above it. The ground floor further accommodates a hair-dresser's and various activity areas. The individual residents have a single room of their own with its own front door, name plate and letter box. The greenery, the natural materials and the reticent colours give La Valence a warm, welcoming atmosphere that marks a break with the hospital-like character of the older institutions.

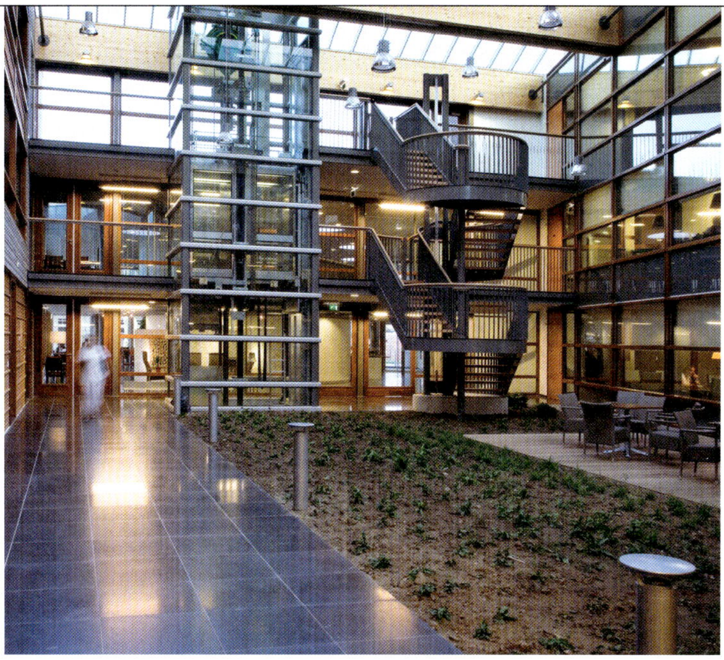

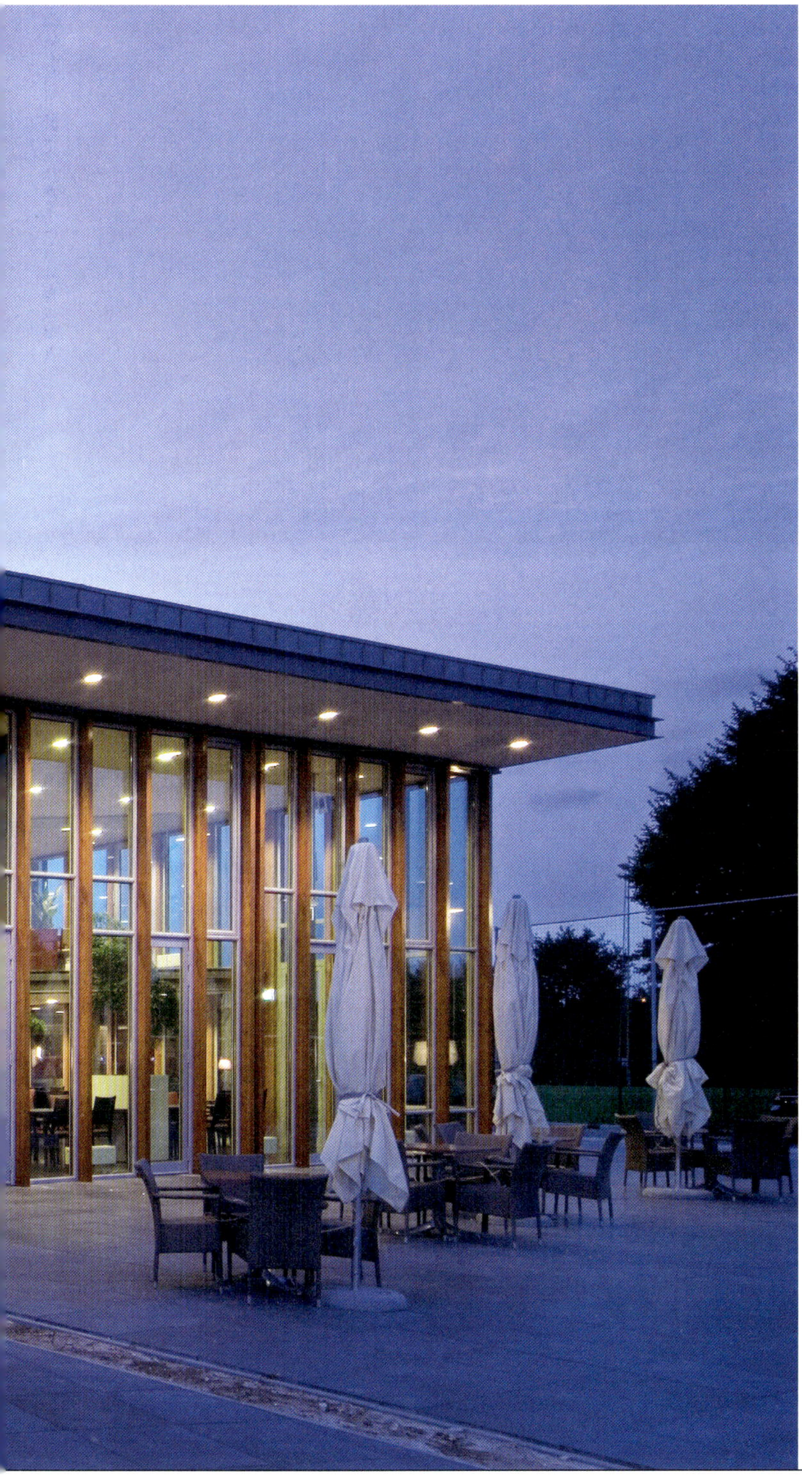

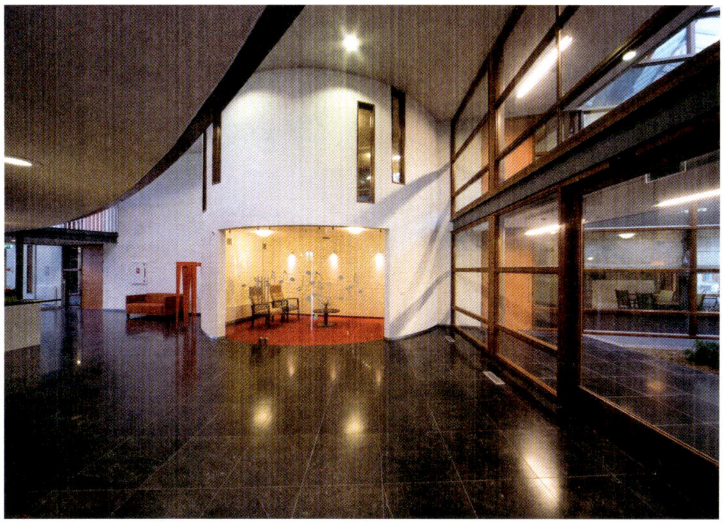

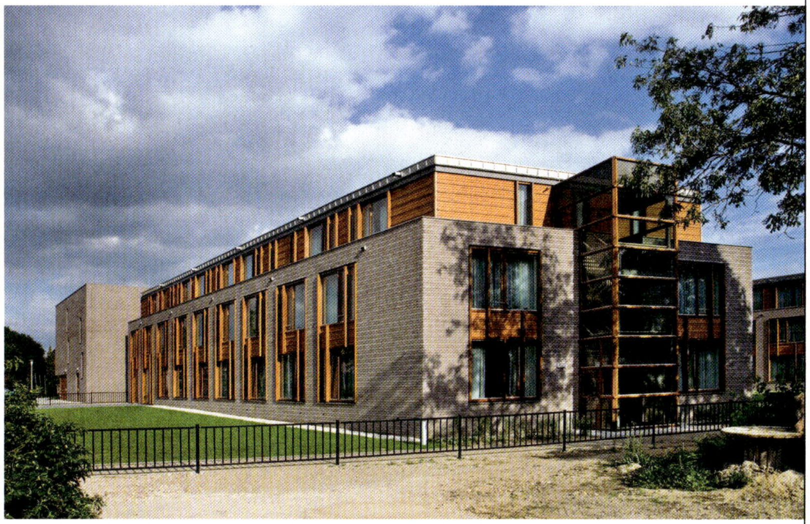

Airport

de Jong Gortemaker Algra
architecten en ingenieurs

Deventer Ziekenhuis
Deventer
2007

Deventer Ziekenhuis is situated on a natural mound in the historical landscape formed by the River IJssel to the east of the city. This mound connects the open cultivated landscape with the wooded Brinkgreve estate in the west. The hospital articulates the various elements in this historical landscape, which accommodates a sports field complex on the south side of the building. The design reflects this natural situation. It leaves the low-lying cultivated landscape intact by allowing a number of fingers raised on stilts to float above it. A curbed 'back' connects these fingers with one another. The medical 'hot floor' and other facilities are housed here and are connected with the outpatient clinics on the other side. The outpatient area offers a large degree of flexibility in contrast to the robust architecture of the back and fingers. It is designed as a continuous high roof with apertures below which the patios are situated. The standardised consultation and treatment rooms and the entrance are located beneath this roof. This makes the hall with the entrance and outpatient clinics the busiest part of the complex. It looks rather like an airport. The thread running through this design is the distinction between acute, urgent, scheduled and chronic patients. The division of the building reflects this distinction and reinforces the landscape articulation. Patients and visitors do not go further into the hospital than is required by their specific case. With the support of a clear routing system, the four flows of patients are more or less automatically kept apart. The façade on the entrance side consists of panels that can easily be dismantled and replaced. The building is regarded as a European model for sustainable decision-making.

Third floor, second floor, first floor, ground floor, basement
1 *laboratories*
2 *dispensary*
3 *nursing units*
4 *operating theatre complex*
5 *staff/offices*
6 *day care*
7 *intensive care*
8 *children's nursing unit*
9 *maternity clinic*
10 *outpatients*
11 *urgent care*
12 *imaging techniques*
13 *dialysis*
14 *hall with restaurant for visitors and general services*
15 *technical service*
16 *kitchen*
17 *car park*
18 *multifunctional unit*

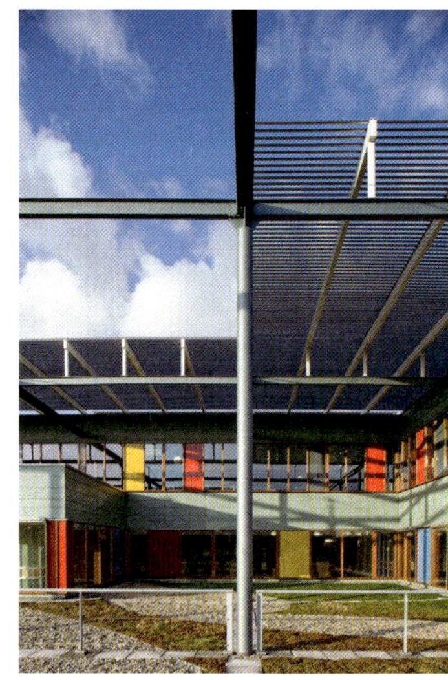

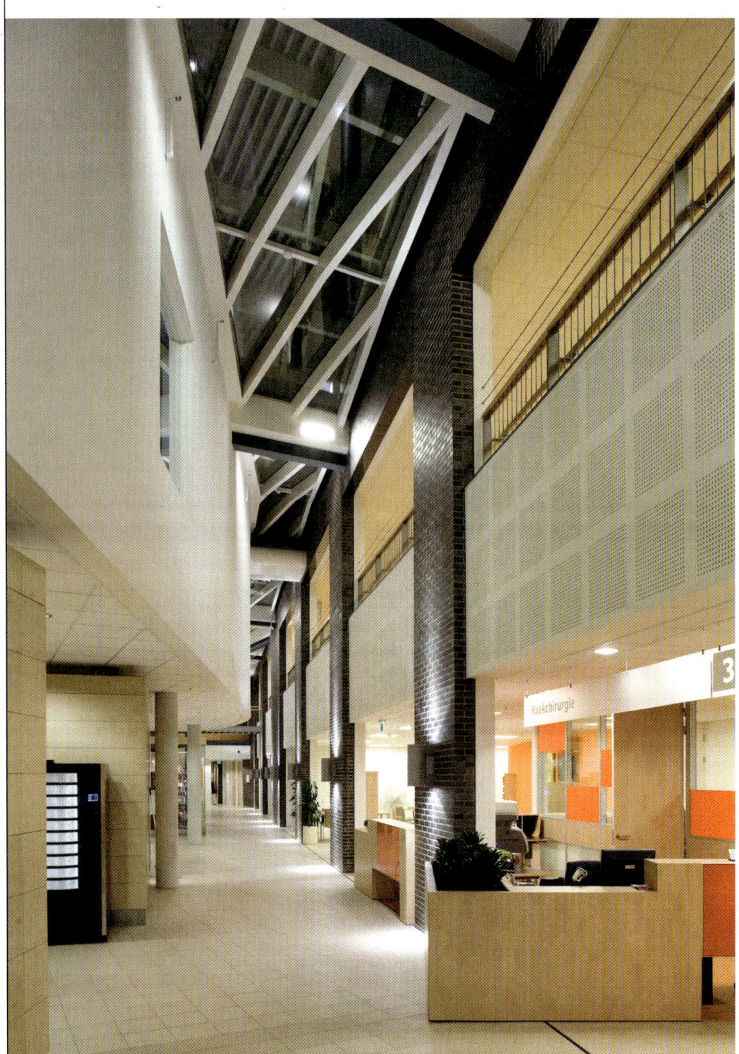

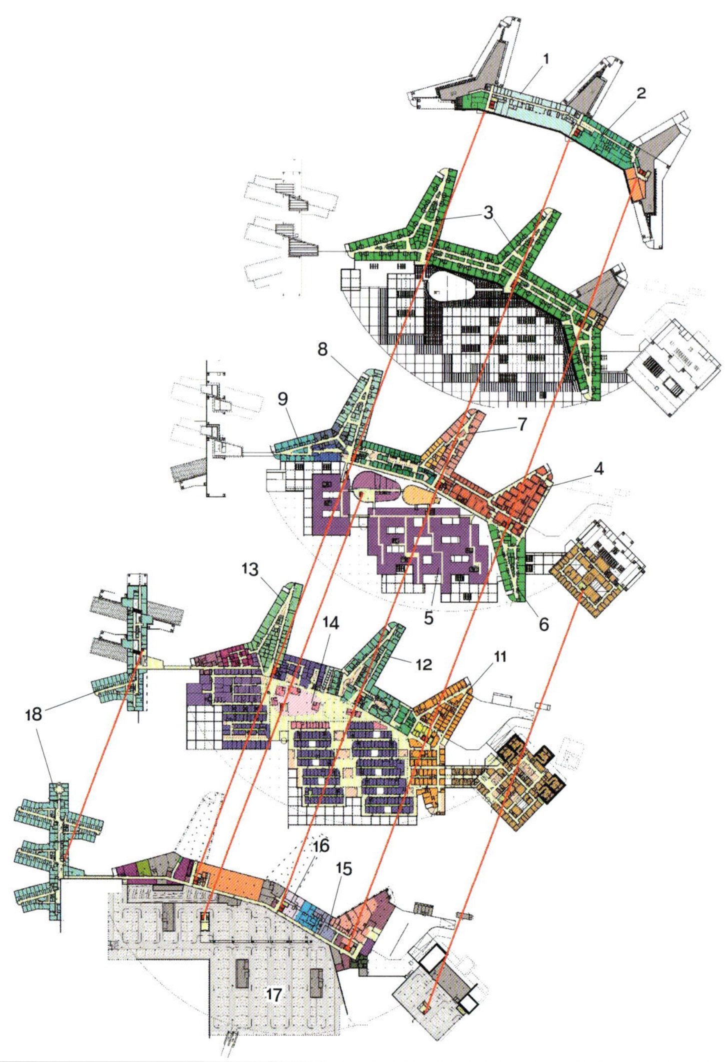

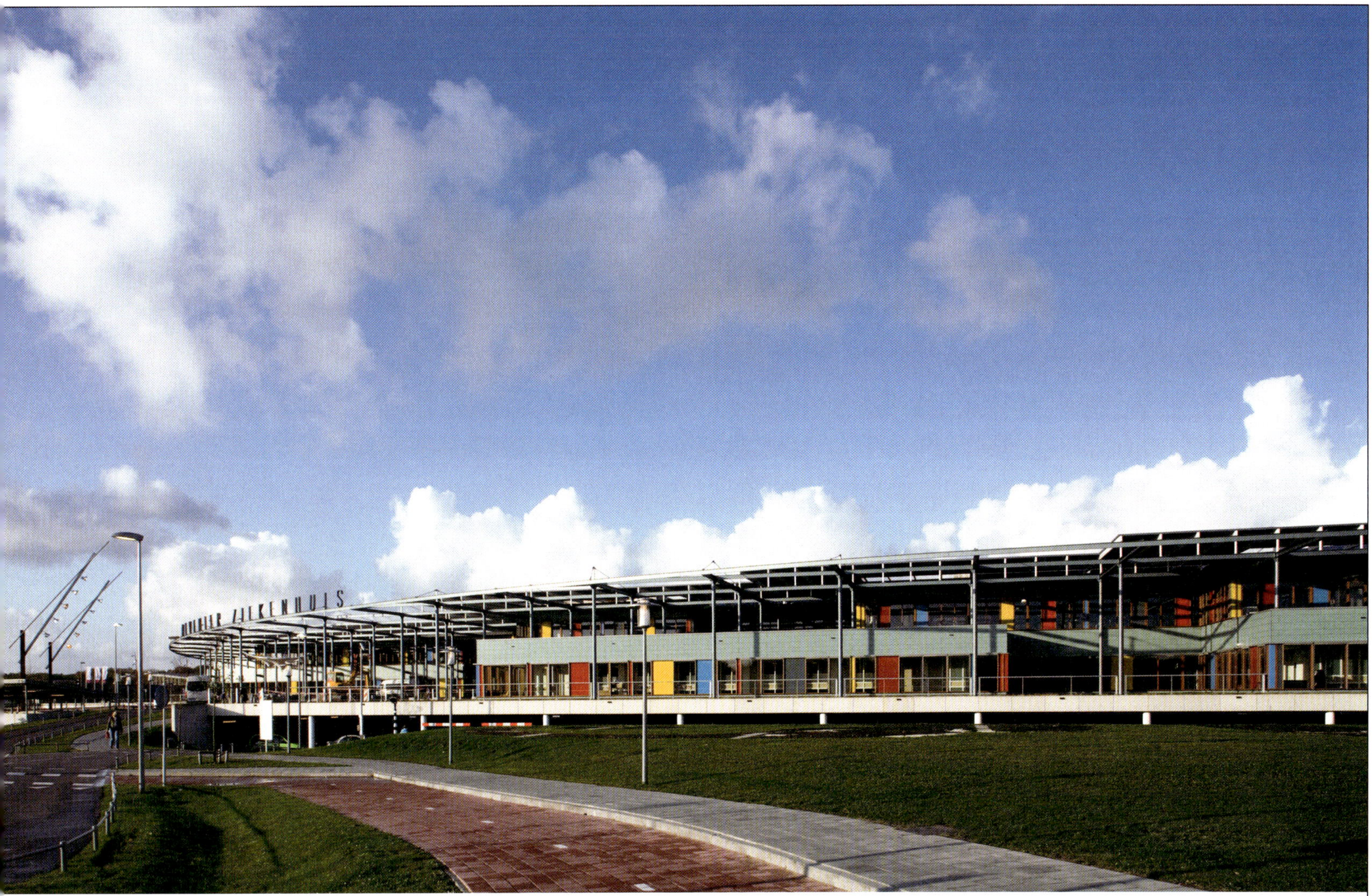

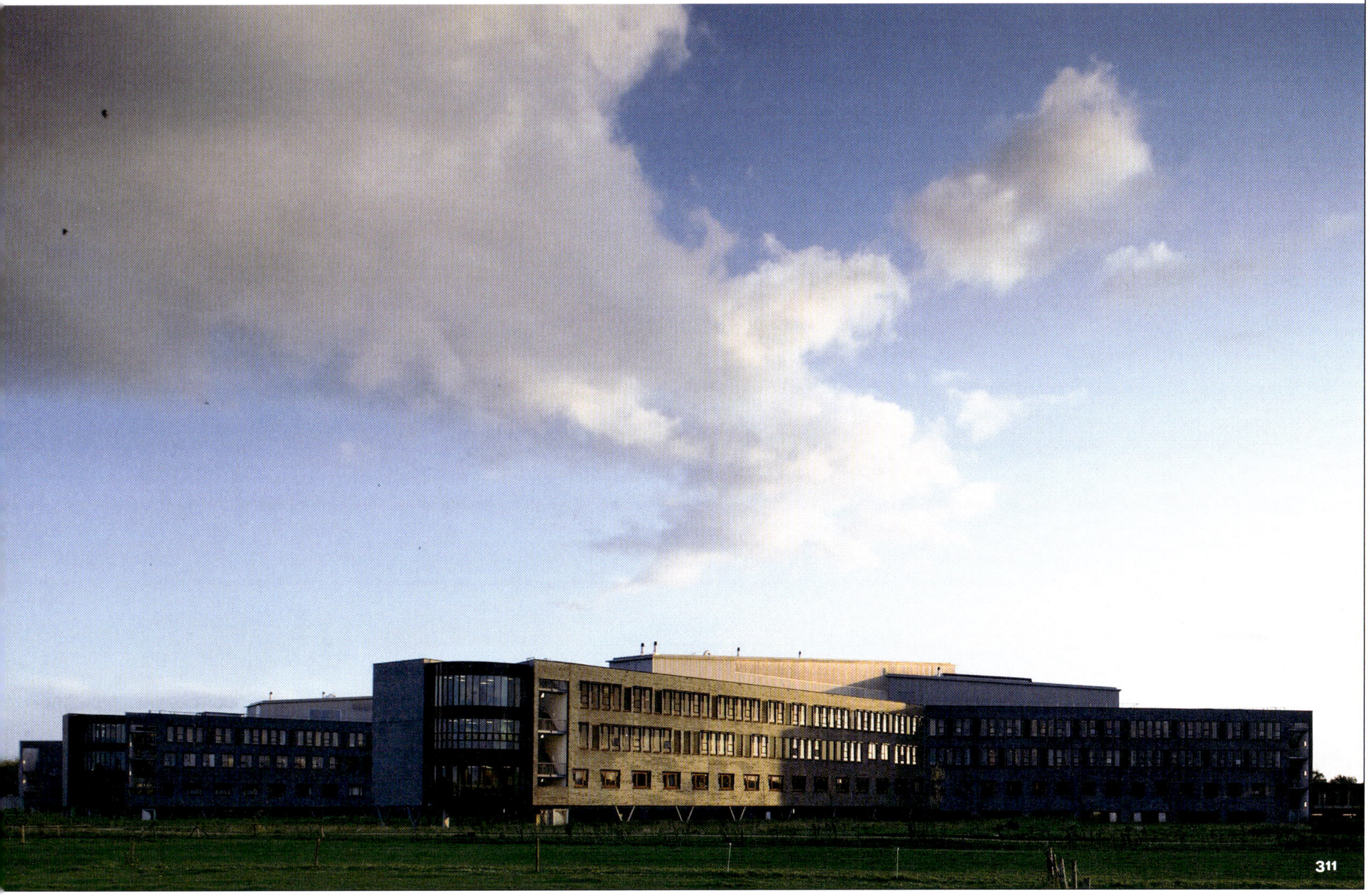

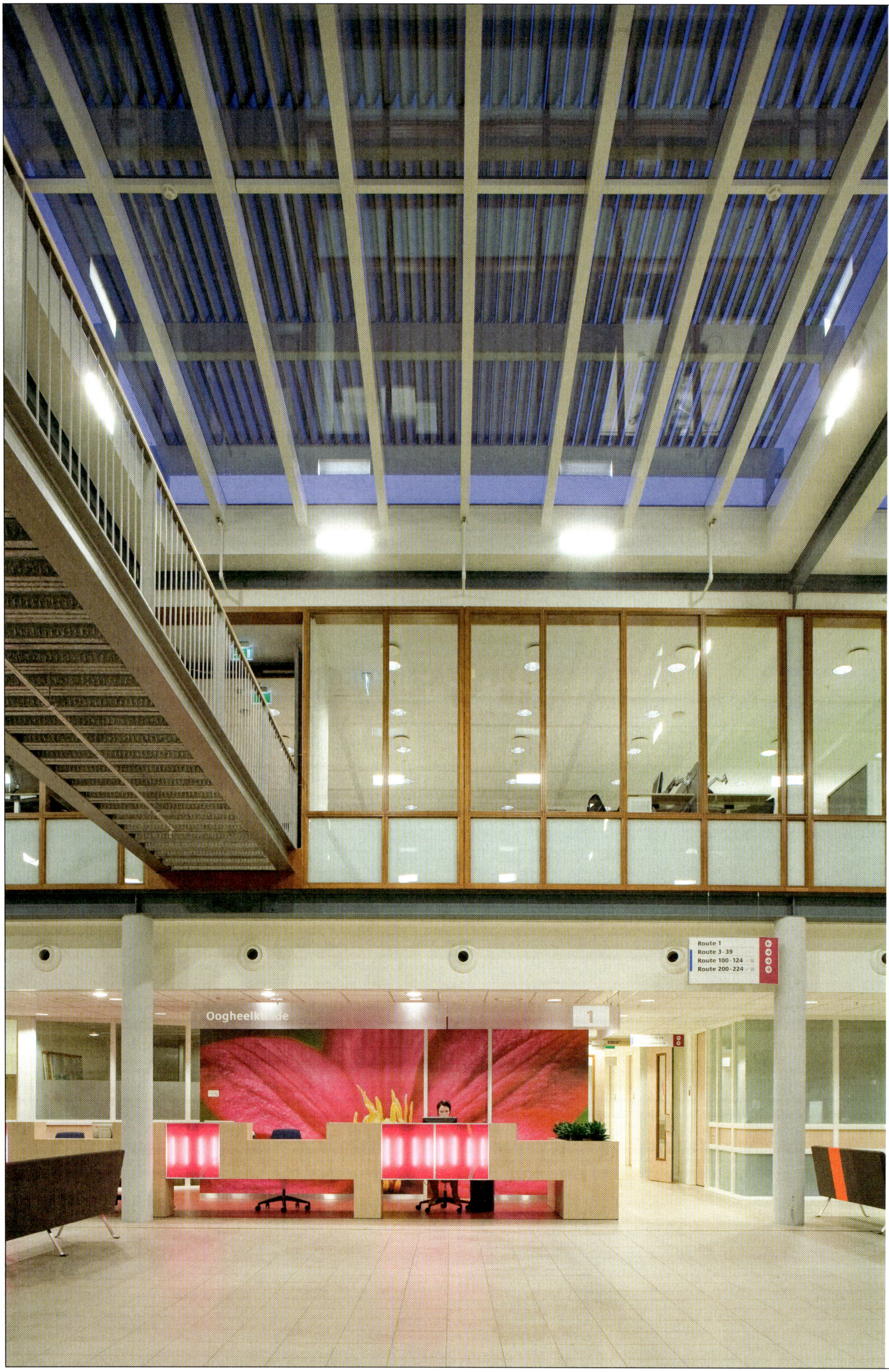
Route 1
Route 3 - 39
Route 100 - 124
Route 200 - 224
1

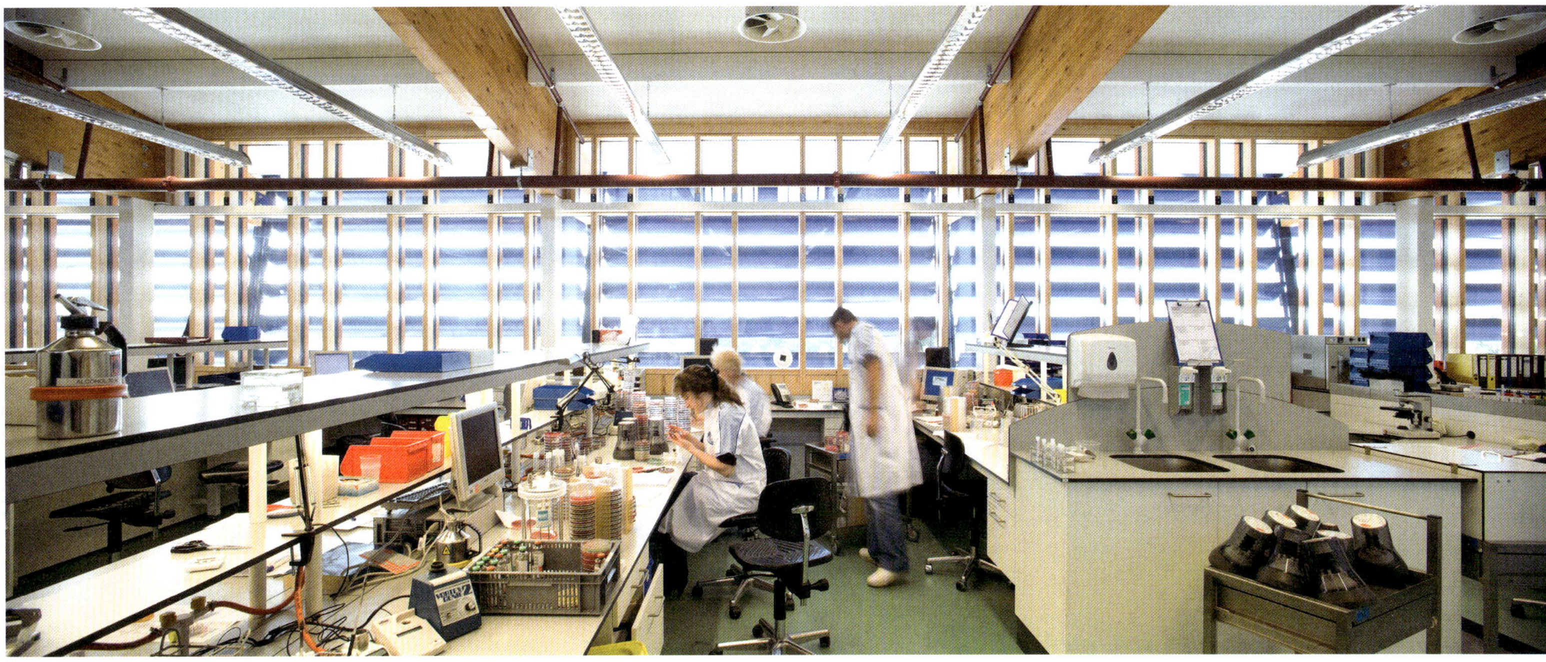

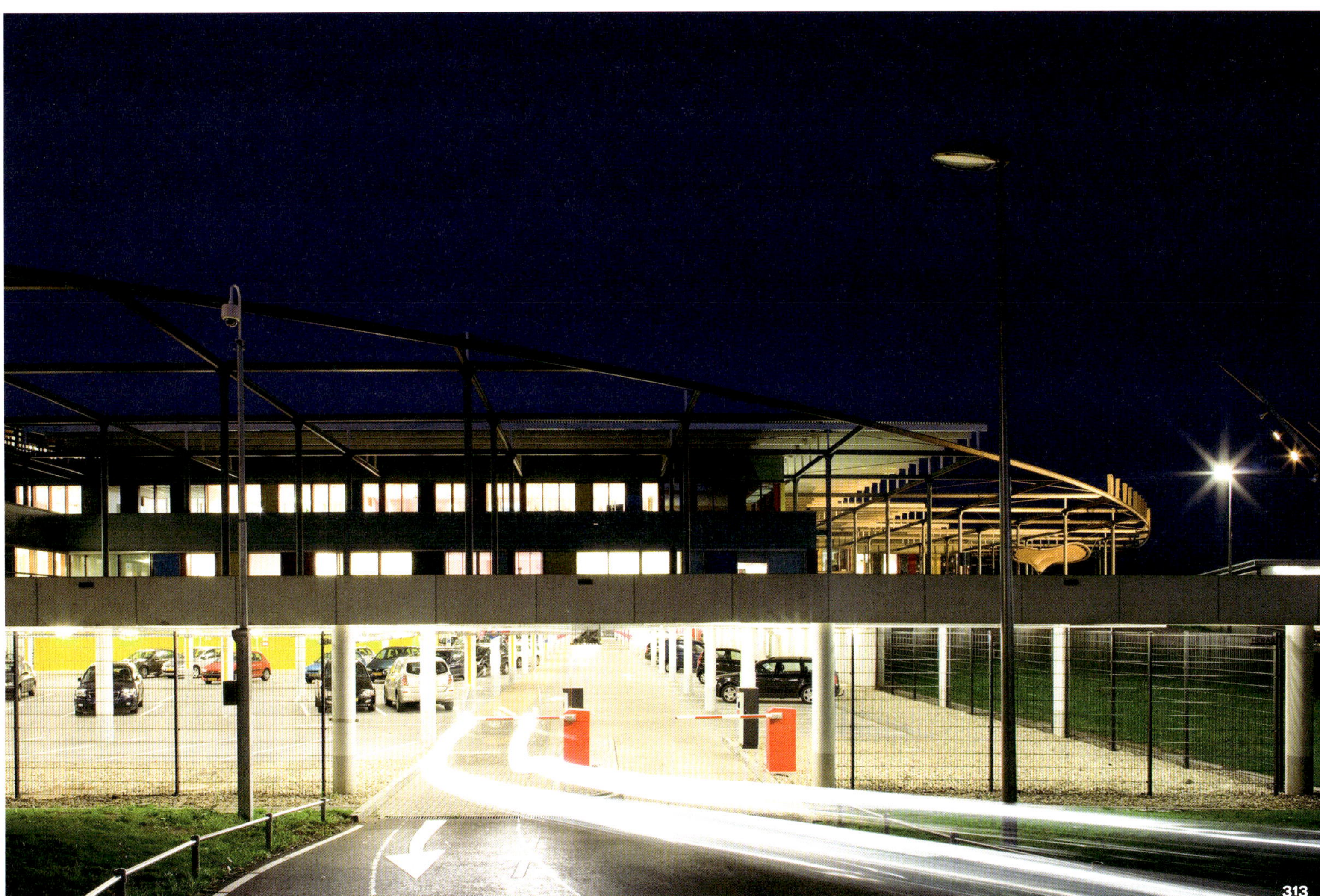

Zigzag

EGM architecten

Vlietland Ziekenhuis
Schiedam
1999-2008

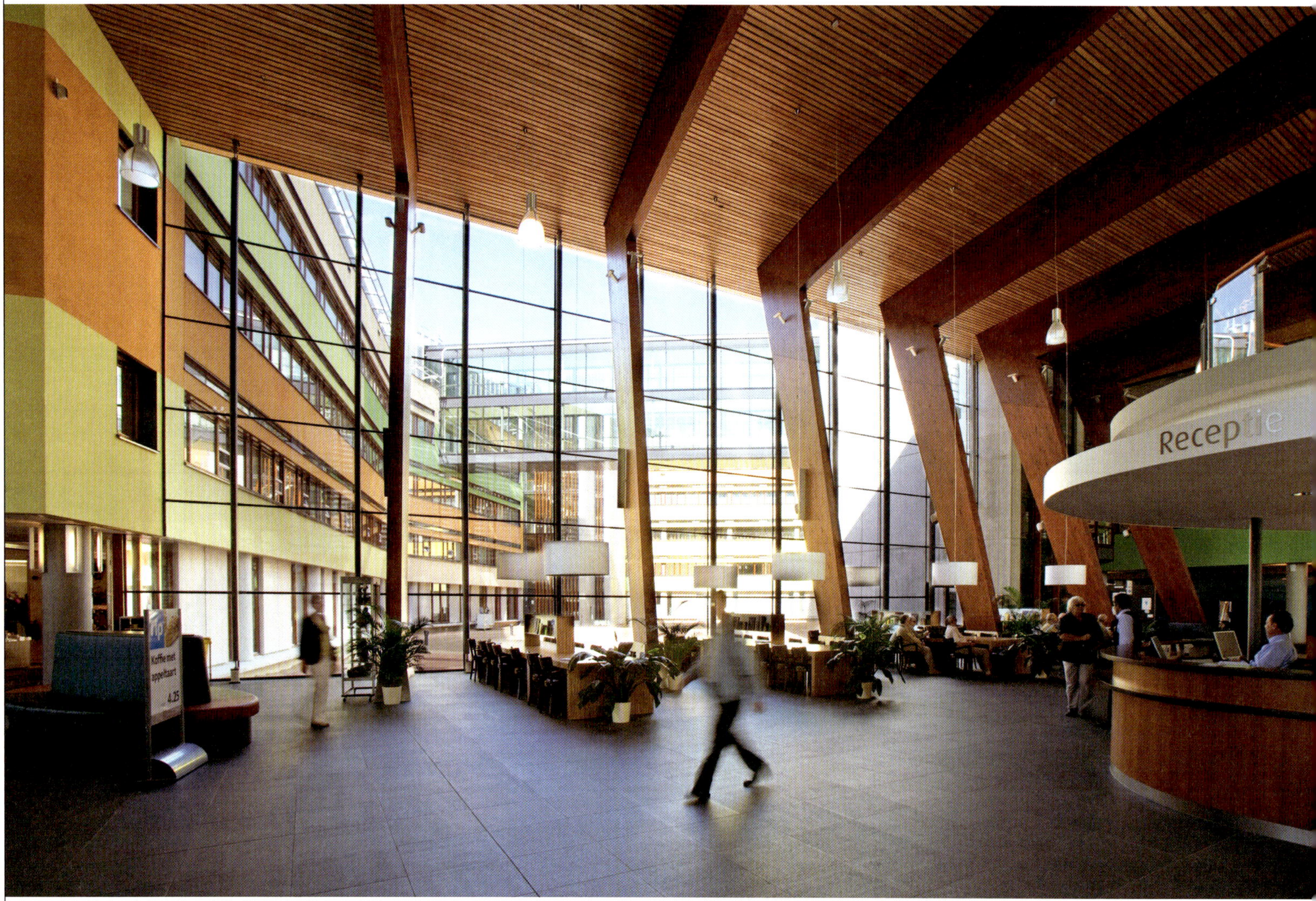

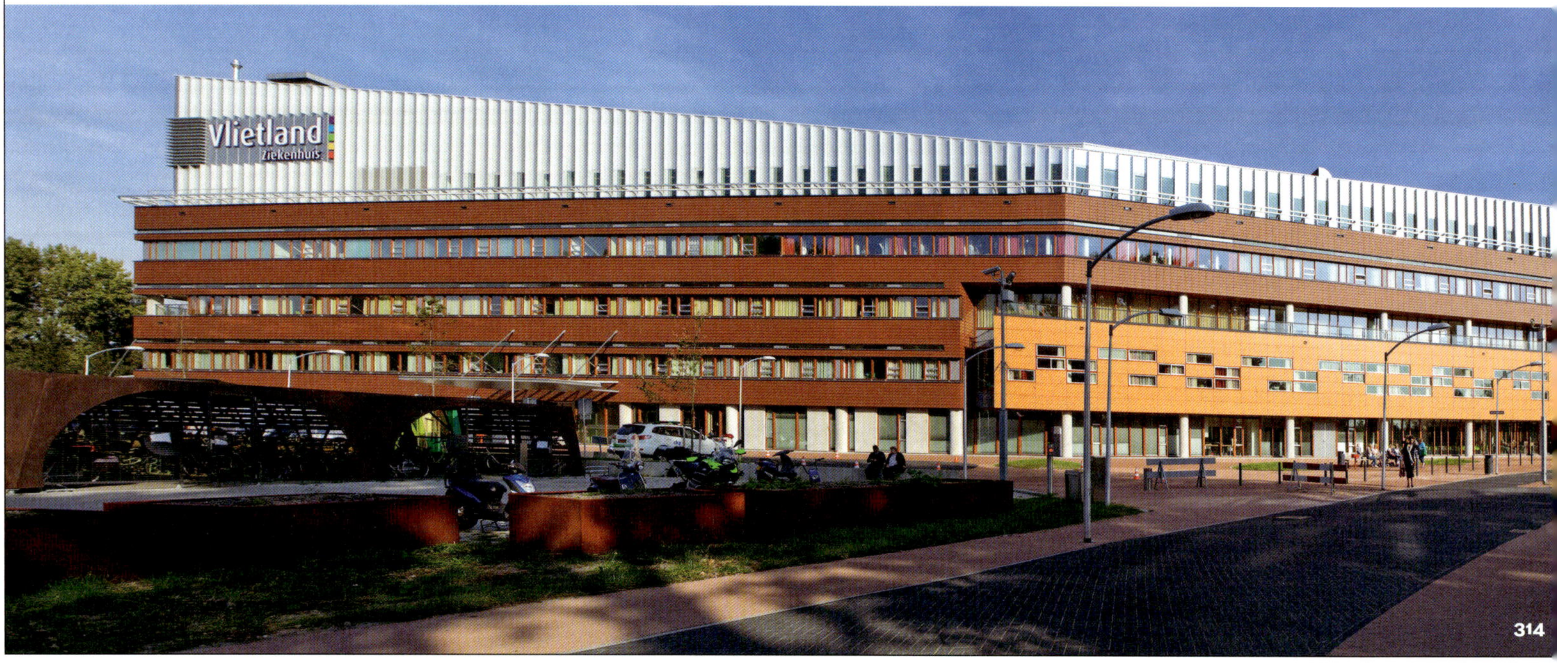

Stichting Samenwerkende Schiedamse en Vlaardingse Ziekenhuizen decided to build a new hospital on the northern outskirts of Schiedam beside a tram line towards Vlaardingen. The hospital forms a link between the urban environment and the countryside and is designed to offer the patients a setting that will promote their wellbeing while being extremely flexible at the same time. The designers linked these two demands by building a strip with the same cross-section at all points. In principle any function can be accommodated at any point in this strip. In that sense the elongated building has been designed as generically as possible: if an area is to be given a different function, the dimensions will not be an obstacle. However, the strip is too long for the parcel of land so it has been bent. The result is the characteristic double-folding ruler that encloses a garden. Glass galleries connect the various parts of the ruler. On the inside the façades have long window strips on top of a completely glass plinth. The outside is clad with dark ceramic tiles and broken with irregularly placed windows in an aluminium frame.

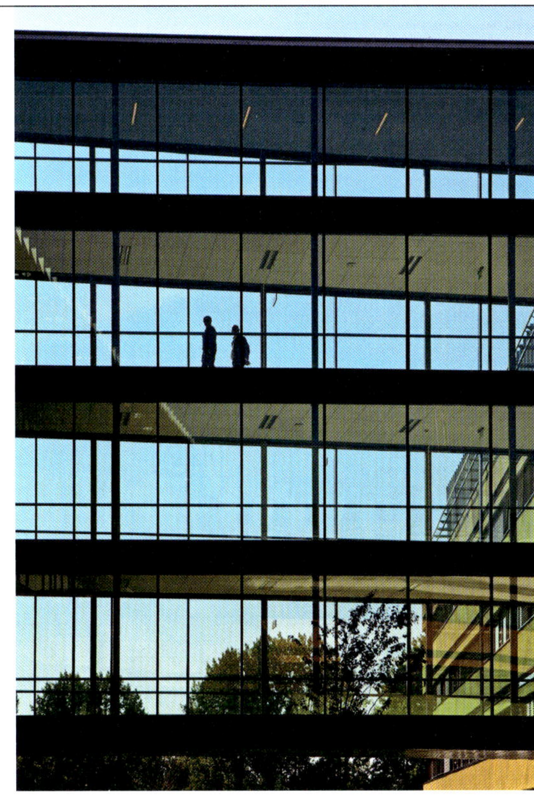

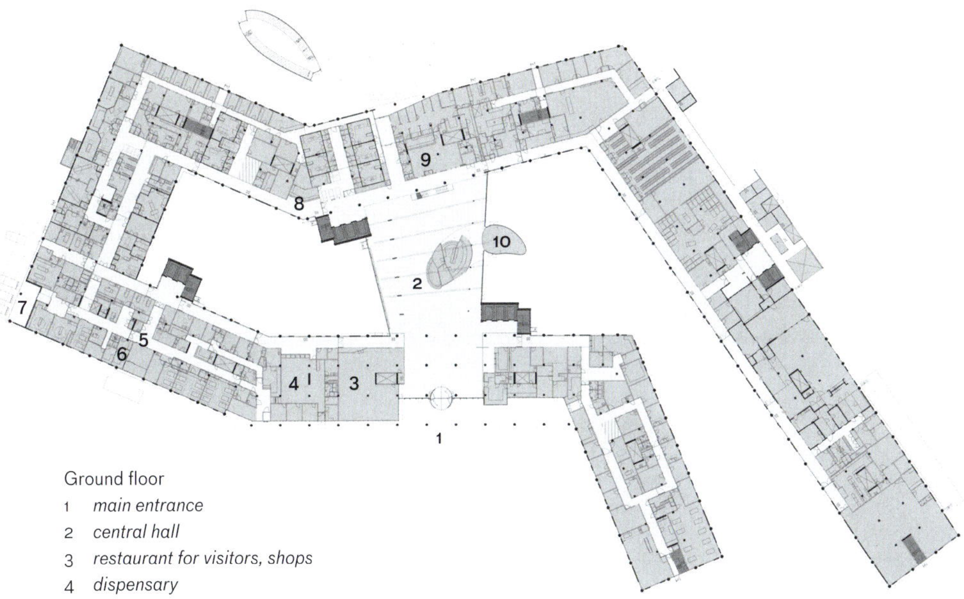

Ground floor
1 *main entrance*
2 *central hall*
3 *restaurant for visitors, shops*
4 *dispensary*
5 *emergency*
6 *general practitioners*
7 *entrance for ambulances*
8 *radiology*
9 *blood transfusion / laboratory*
10 *meditation centre*

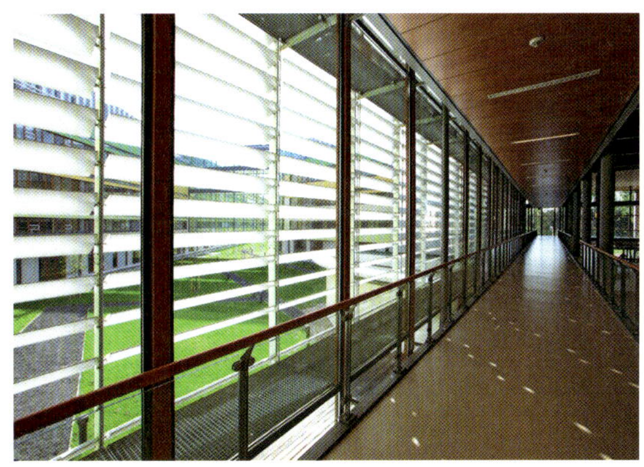

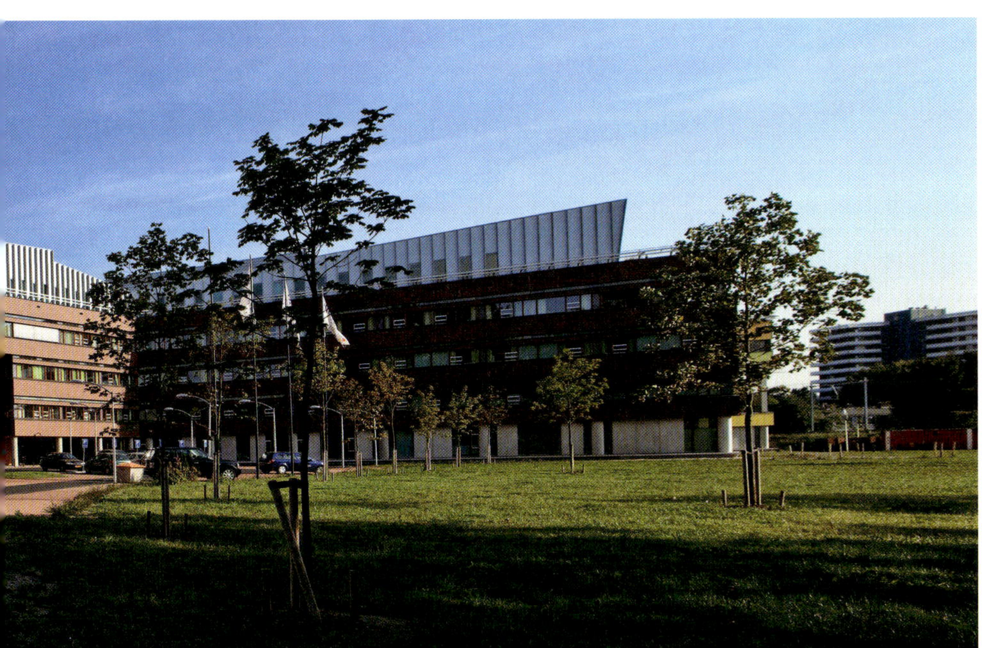

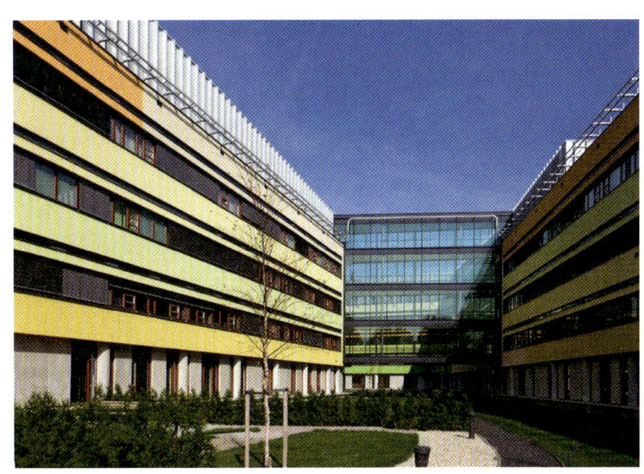

Bonnema Architecten

Maasland Ziekenhuis
Sittard
2001-2008

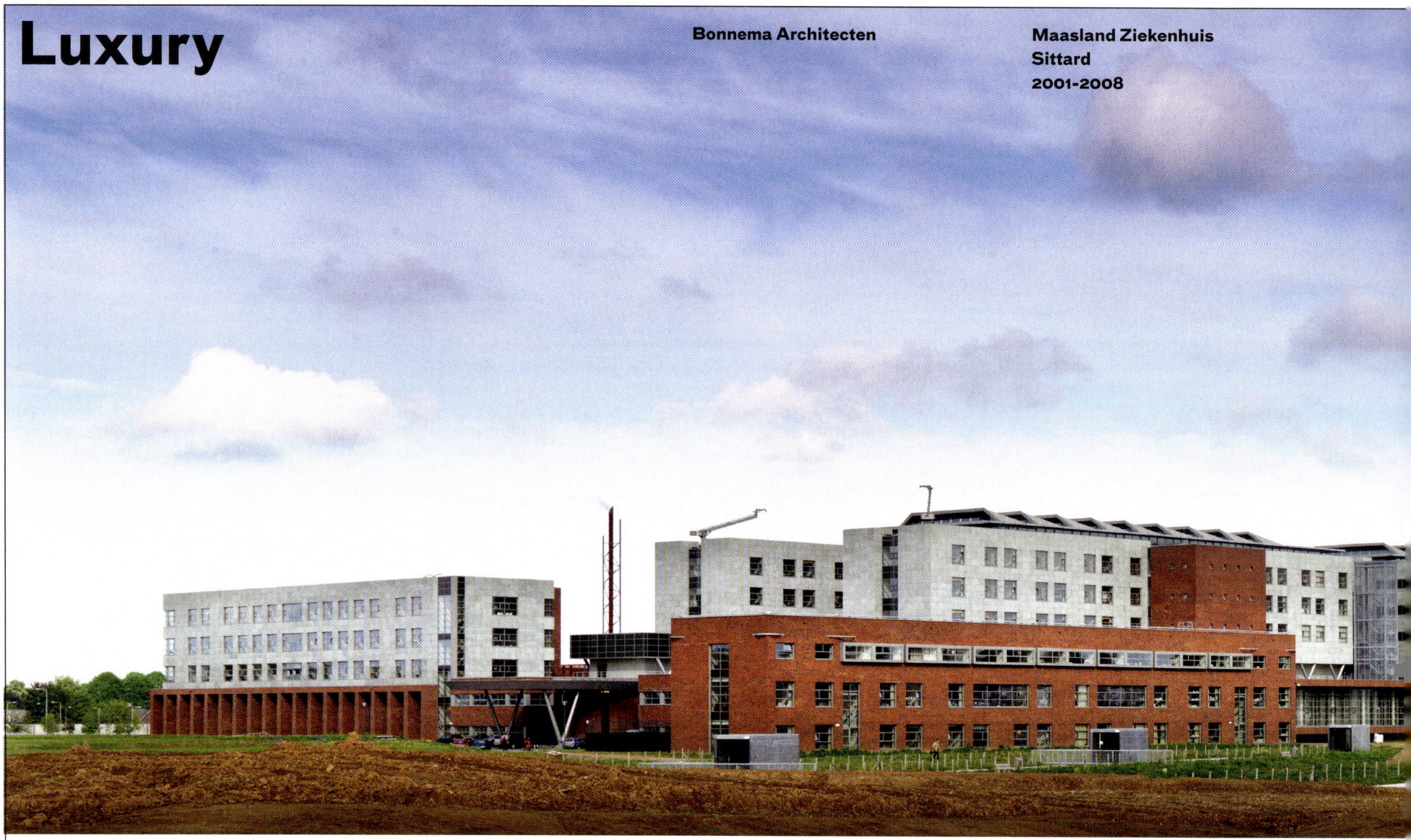

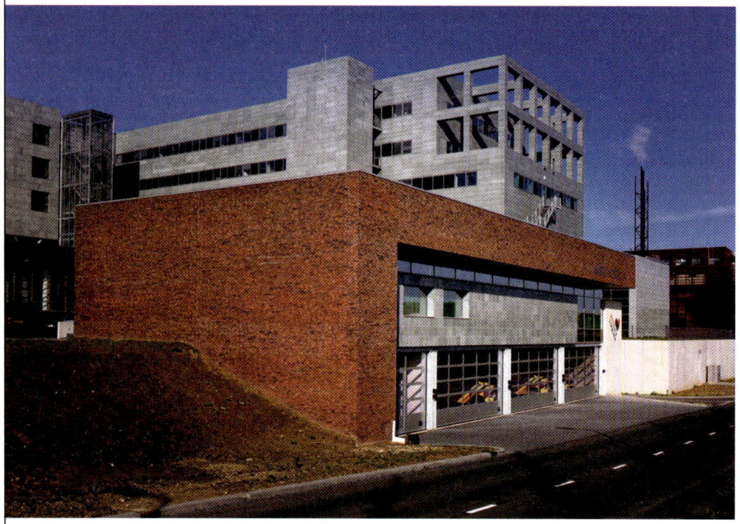

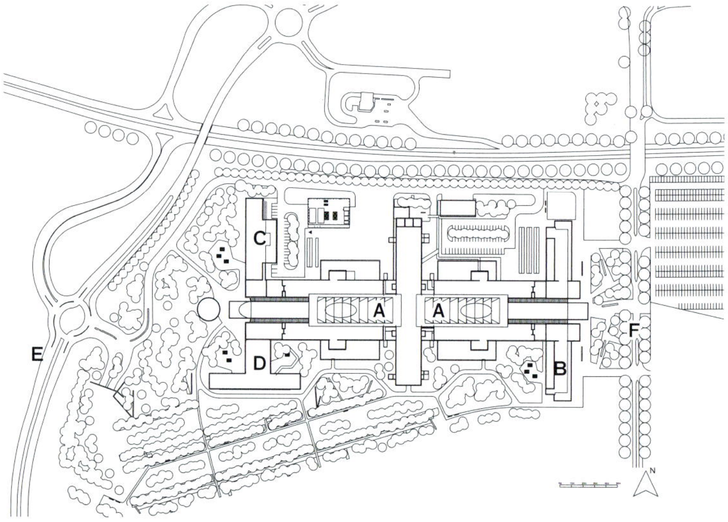

The most striking feature of the Maasland Ziekenhuis is the elongated roofed hall that forms the backbone of the spatial composition. The wooden panels in the ceiling, the dark grey of the window frames and the balustrades, the glass of the consultation rooms on the upper floors with its print decorations, and the shops on the ground floor, combined with the spaciousness of the hall, all produce a decidedly chic effect. The hall is also the logistical core of the building. Visitors use it as the central waiting room. It is flanked on either side by four series of consultation rooms above ground level that are used by different doctors – the time when the specialists had a domain of their own has gone. The consultation rooms physically separate the front office from the back office; the latter is fleshed out in the form of four centres of expertise. Specialists can be by themselves there, but the rooms invite mutual consultation and multi-disciplinary cooperation. The distinction between front and back office reflects the main theme of the design: the separation of traffic flows. This can already be seen in the hall: the middle one of the three colossal towers for staircases and lifts that have been placed here is for the exclusive use of the staff and for supplying and removing medical material. This tower gives access to a volume at right angles to the hall where the so-called hot floor is located. Goods transport is automated: electric carts that find their way by themselves pass to and from with containers and make use of the same lift as the staff. The logistical centre from which all this is directed is located beneath the building. The Maasland Ziekenhuis has a psychiatric centre linked to one of the extremities next to the hall. There are many works of art in the meditation centre and in the rest of the building.

Situation
A *atrium*
B *care boulevard*
C *convalescence*
D *mental health care*
E *Westelijke Randweg*
F *Rijksweg Noord*

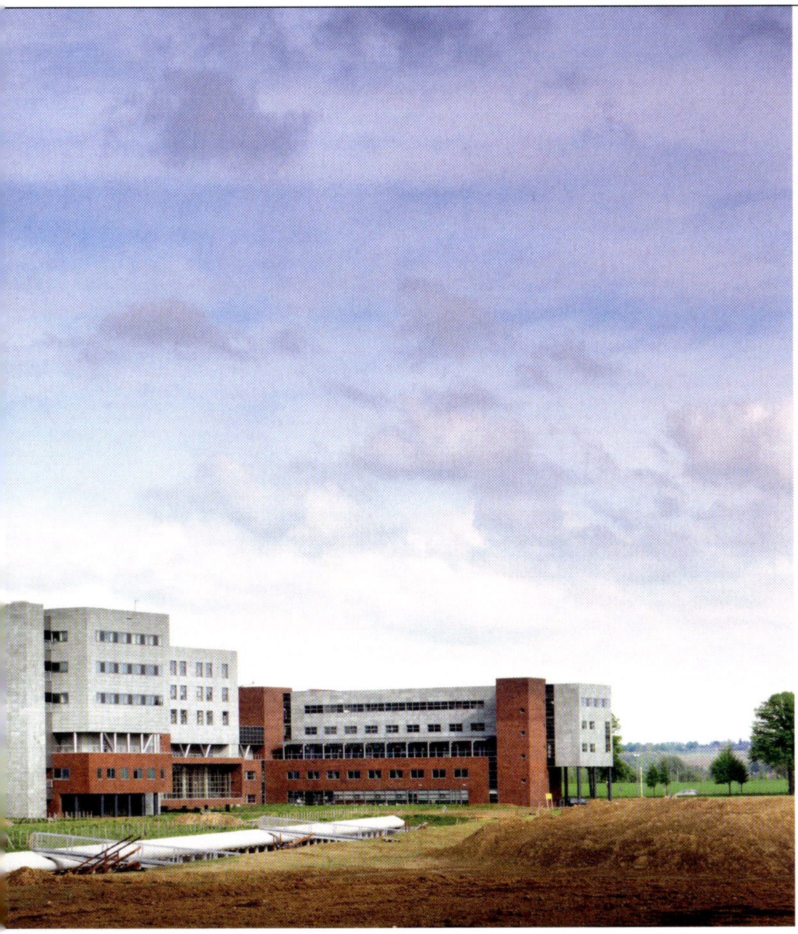
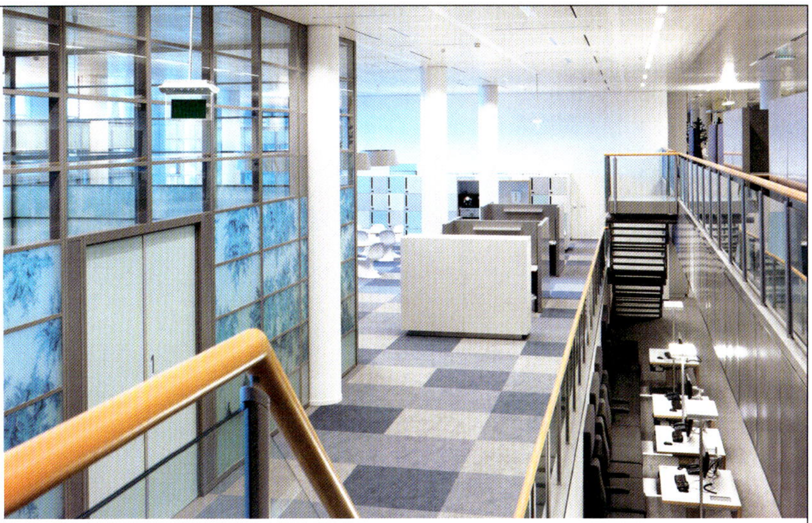
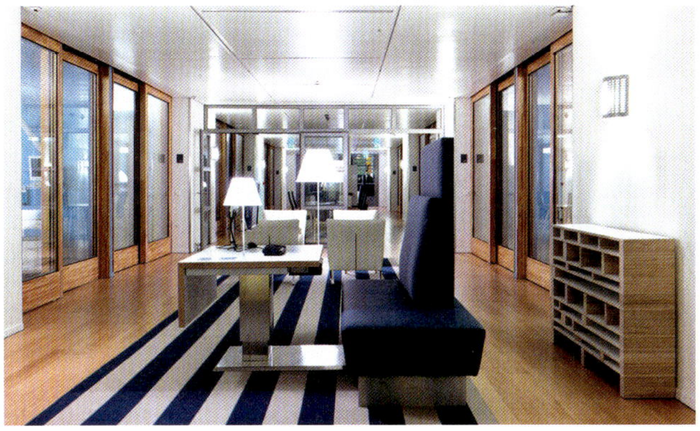
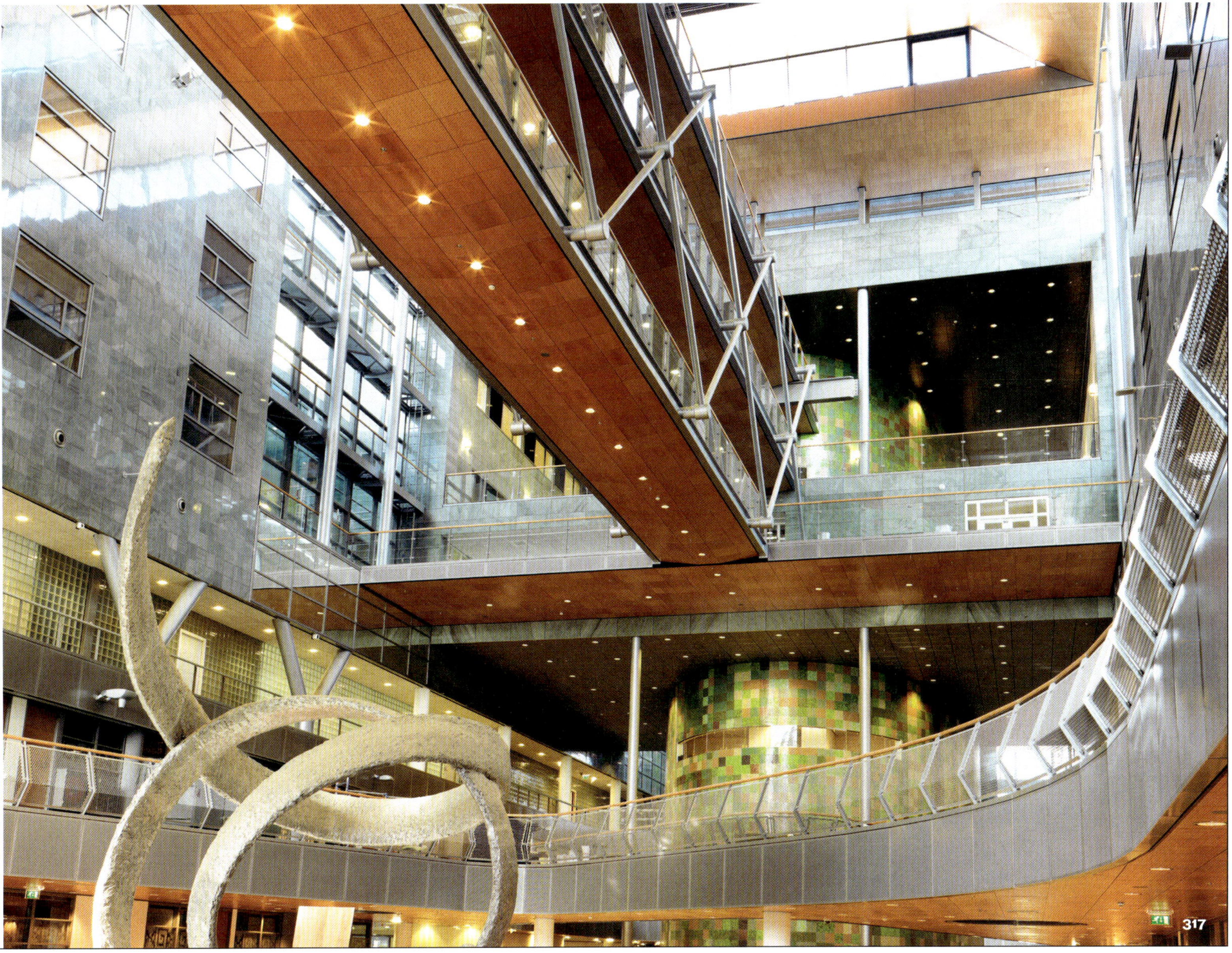

DaF-architecten

De Pionier medical centre
Nieuw-Vennep
2008

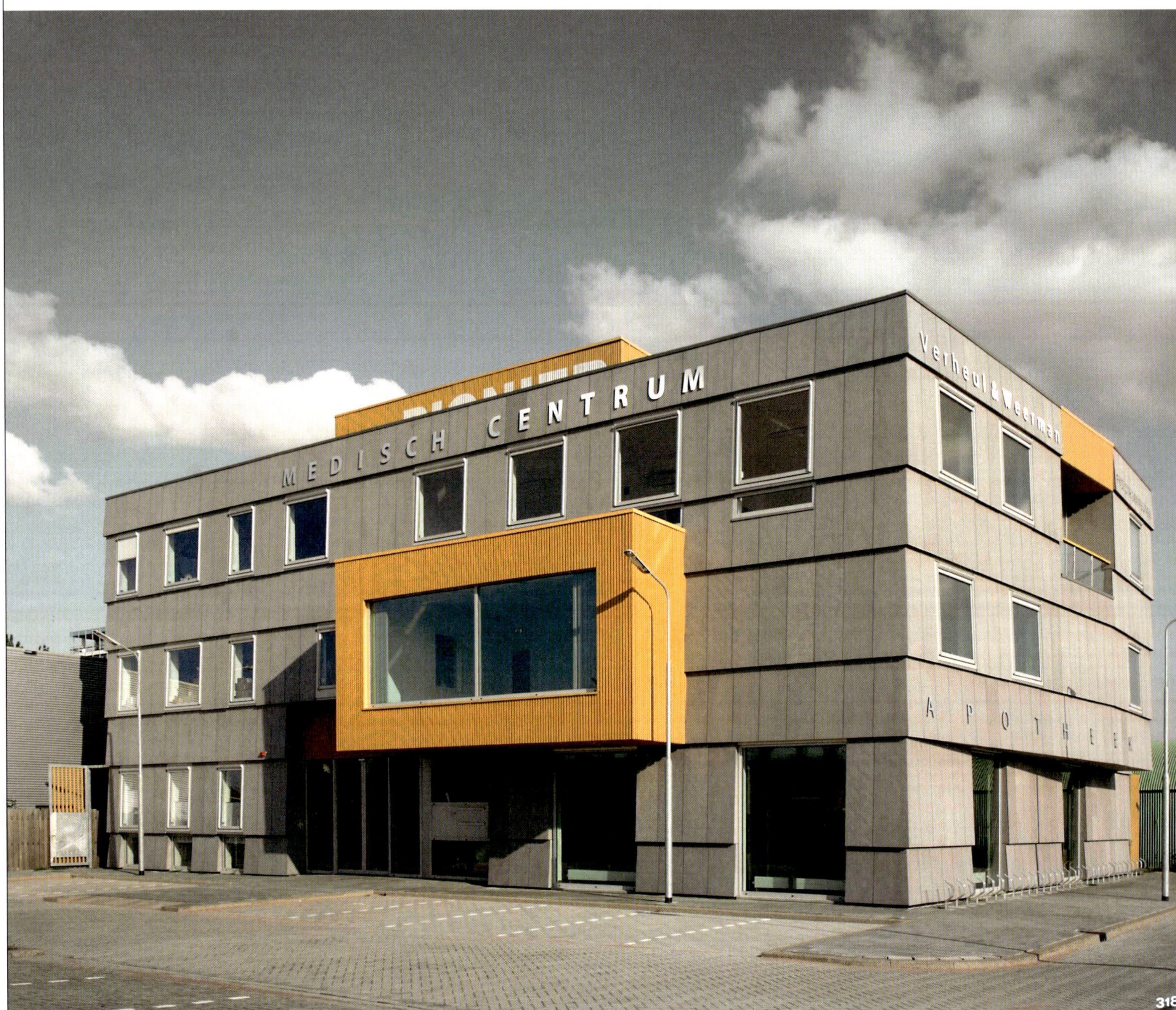

Nieuw-Vennep in the Haarlemmermeer has realised the new housing district Getse Woud and thereby expanded towards an existing industrial estate. The urban development department wants to transform this industrial estate into a service zone for the new housing estate and to alter the street pattern for that purpose. This medical centre is the first project to flesh out that ambition. It occupies a strategic position in the new pattern of roads and its design anticipates that pattern. It houses a joint general practice, a practice for physiotherapy, midwives, psychotherapy and a dispensing chemist. It therefore concentrates the low-threshold facilities within a complex that anticipates the possibility of far-reaching decentralisation of a part of health care. De Pionier has three floors linked to one another by a striking hall with a central staircase and large light wells. This hall determines the character of the building, which remains intact when the users themselves design their own part of the complex. The building has a strong sculptural quality. This is achieved by the articulation: the entrance is set back, the waiting room on the first floor hangs like a box from the outside wall, the hall has a bright skylight in the roof, and the side wall that overhangs the pavement anticipates the new road pattern. The outside walls are clad with bevel sided Eternit sheets.

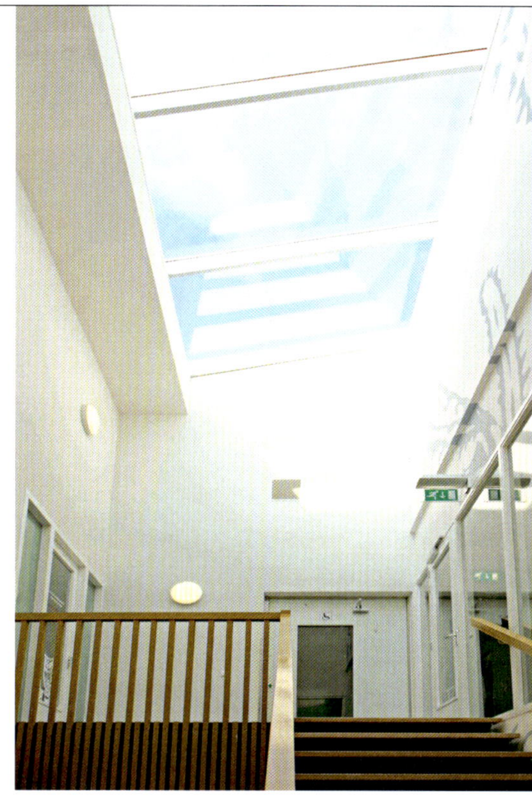

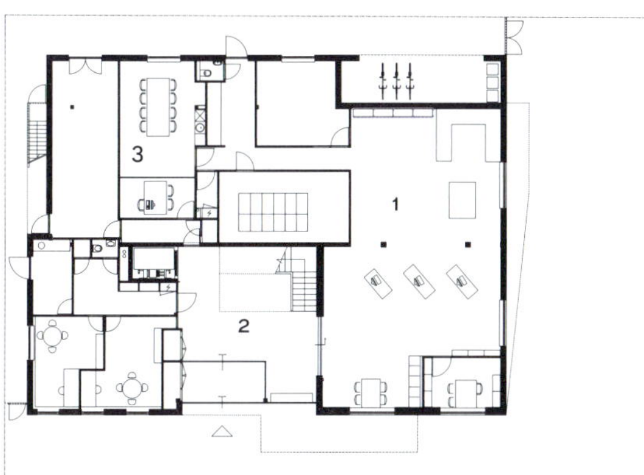

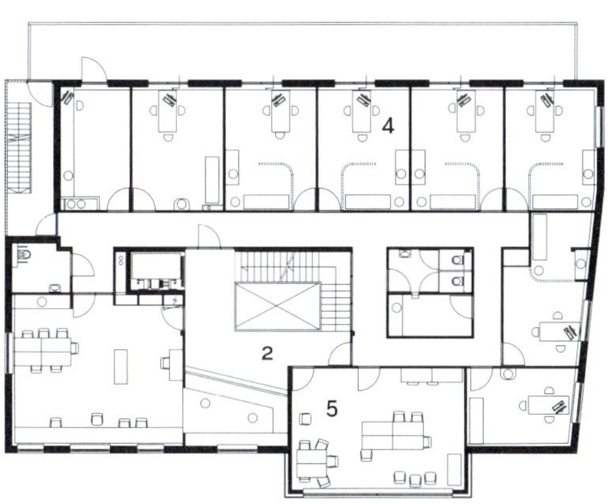

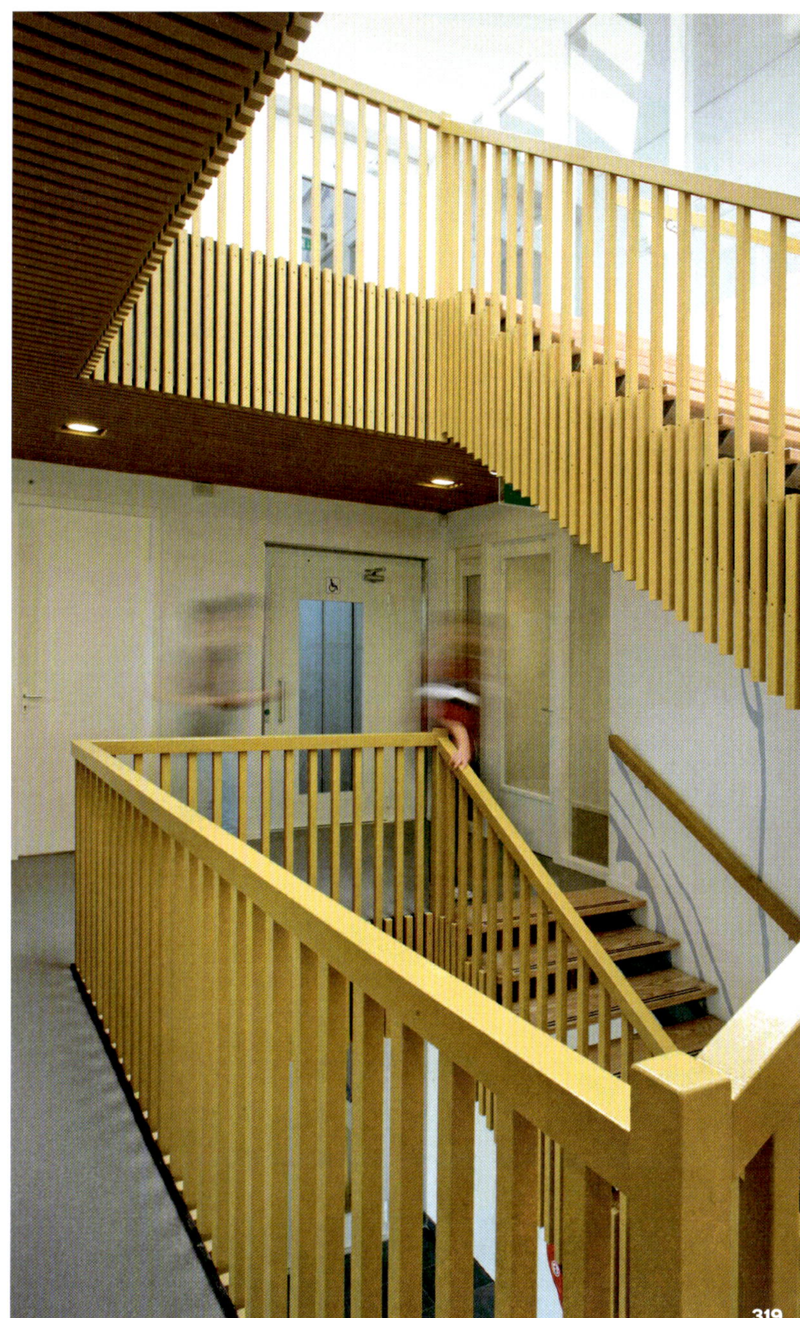

Ground floor and first floor
1 *dispensary*
2 *staircase*
3 *conference room*
4 *consultation room*
5 *waiting room*

Second life

One Architecture

Gezondheidscentrum St. Jozef
Deventer
2009

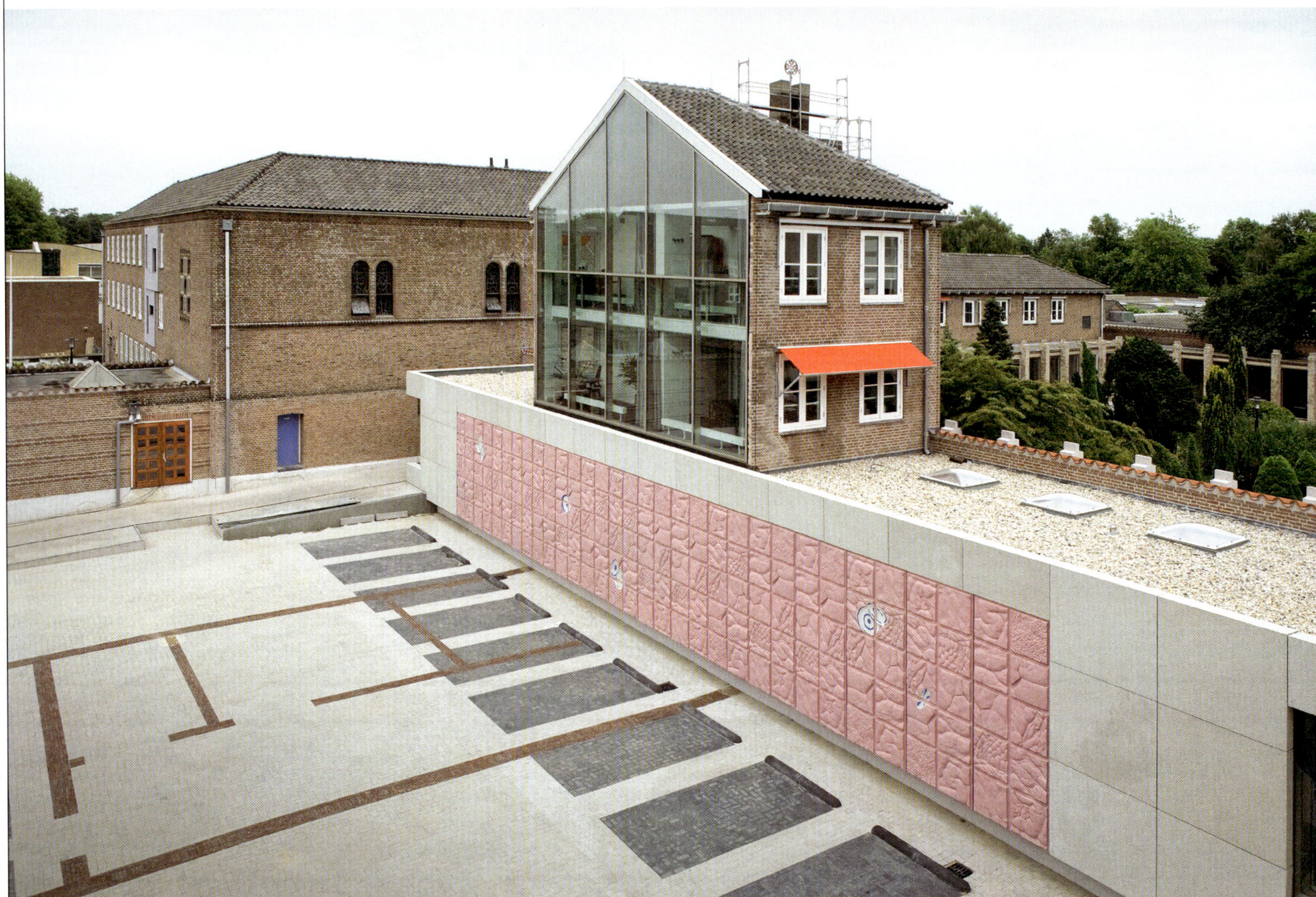

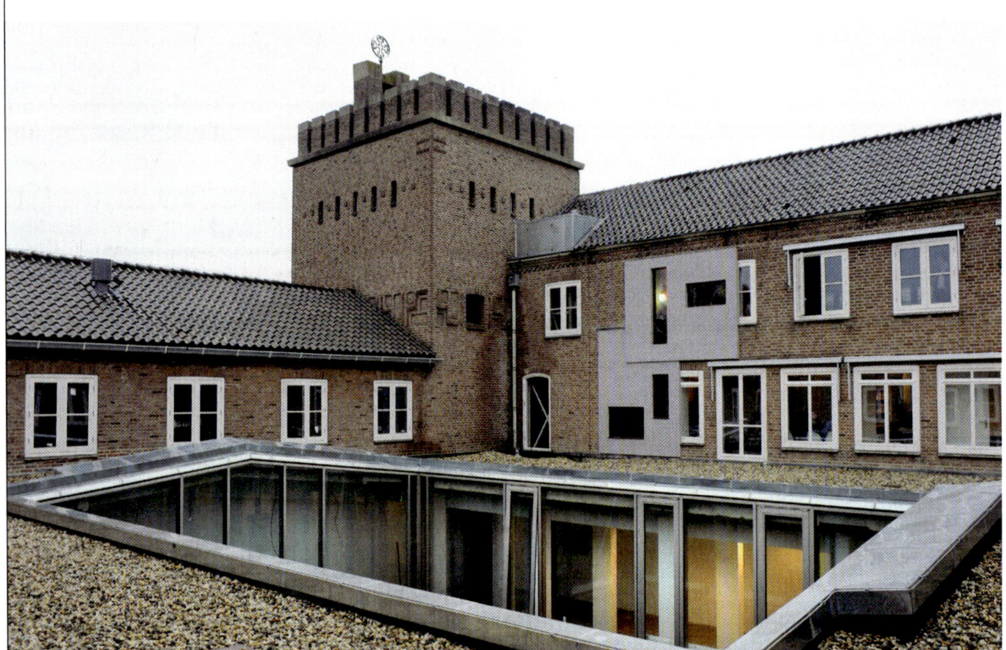

The original St. Jozef monastery and hospital designed by Jan van der Laan was completed in 1952. It was one of the first hospitals to be built after the war. Van der Laan combined a modern concrete construction with the traditional features of the monastery, of which two enclosed gardens were important elements. When a new hospital building was erected, it was decided to give St. Jozef a different function as a health centre. The programme includes a general practice, midwives, physiotherapists, speech therapists, psychologists, dentists and a laser clinic. One Architecture decided to revise the logistics completely in order to accommodate this extensive programme. The main entrance next to the car park leads to the tower, which forms the easily recognisable central point. A wooden wall fences off a part of the adjacent chapel, where a striking white staircase has been placed. The rest of the chapel remains in its original state and houses the dispensary. One Architecture mounted eye-catching concrete panels with designs in stained glass by the artist Berend Strik outside the waiting rooms. Strik is also responsible for the other works of art including the elongated closed wall next to the car park, behind which the blood bank is situated. Part of the former nurse's home had to be demolished to make room for this car park. This wing has been literally cut open and the interior exposed behind a glass wall. The garden design by Inside Outside replaces the traditional rectangular geometry with a radial design that fans outwards, with a fountain in the monastery garden as its centre. The radial lines that extend from here recur in the other three gardens. The building was placed on the list of 100 young national monuments in 2007 during the planning stage.

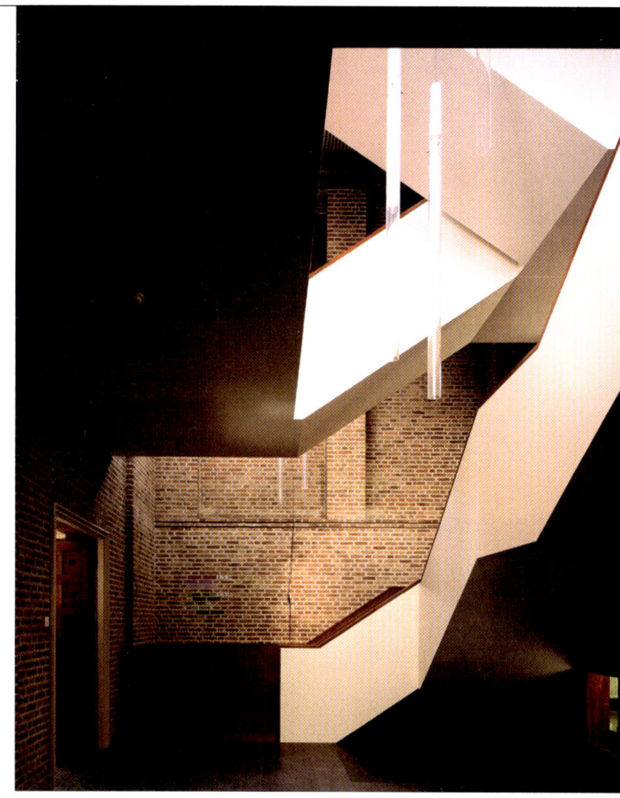

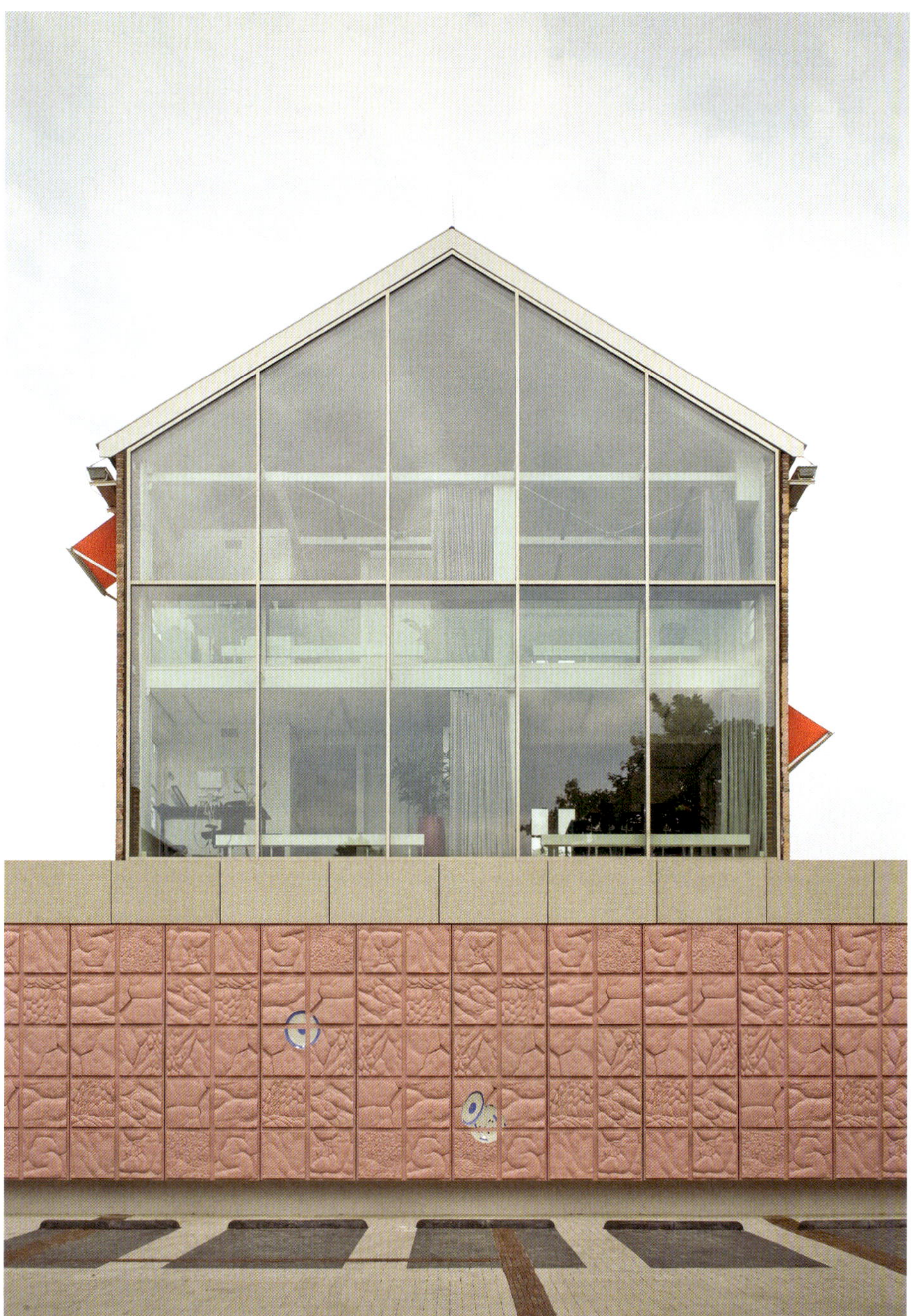

Ground floor

1 *enclosed garden*
2 *gallery*
3 *tower*
4 *reception*
5 *chapel*
6 *mortuary*
7 *blood bank*
8 *car park*
9 *physiotherapy*
10 *former kitchen*
11 *general practitioners*

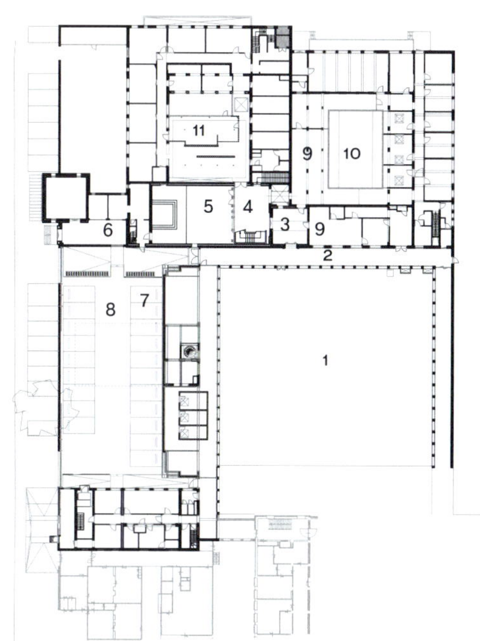

Lifestyles

Molenaar&Bol&Van Dillen Architects

De Hogeweyk
Weesp
2008

De Hogeweyk replaces an older high-rise nursing home which looked like a classical hospital by a residential district that at first sight resembles any other contemporary new building. All the same, it is a geriatric nursing home with 23 units for old people in an advancing state of dementia. It has been designed, not as a building, but as an urban district with streets, squares, courtyards and parks. Different lifestyles have been designed for the residents. 'Gooi' is rather formal, politeness is appreciated, and the home takes pride of place. A larger dining kitchen is important in 'Indonesia', while the kitchen marks the entrance to the home in 'Brabant'. In this way the seven different lifestyles introduce variation into the architecture and the communal areas, including the outdoor areas and a roofed square. Every home has contact with the outside world, but the streets and squares are only genuinely public to a certain extent. The district has a high level of amenities. These include a café and restaurant, theatre, information centre, hairdresser's, and a beauty salon. Niek Roozen landscape architects drew up a vegetation plan with plenty of diversity that gives the district a well tended character. Although facilities for professional (medical) care have been included too, they have been inconspicuously absorbed by the district. This underlines the ambition of making the nursing home as normal as possible.

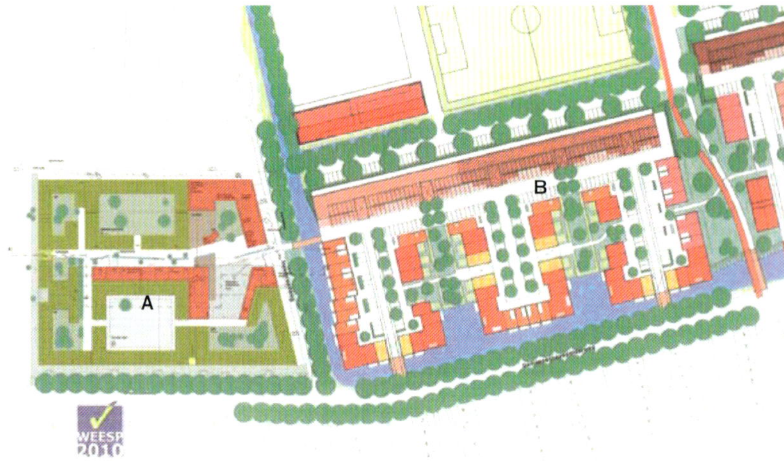

Situation
A *De Hogeweyk*
B *Papenlaan apartment block*

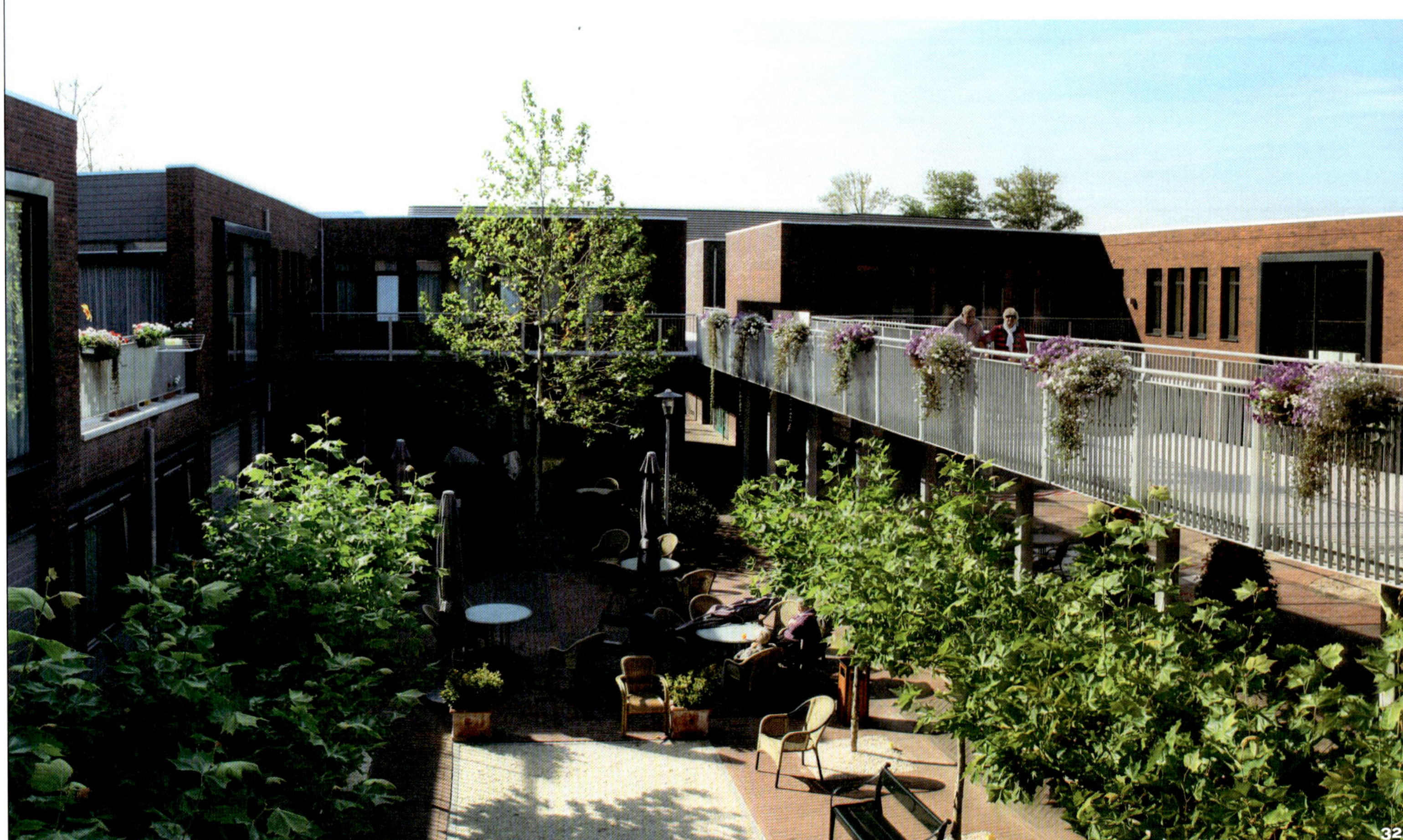

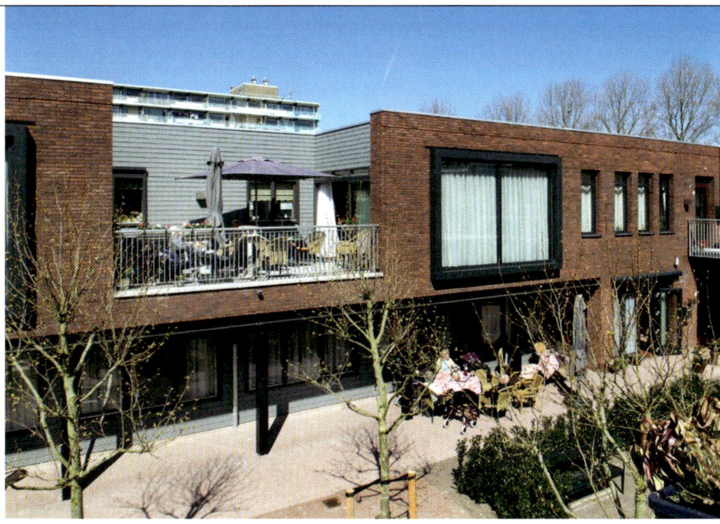

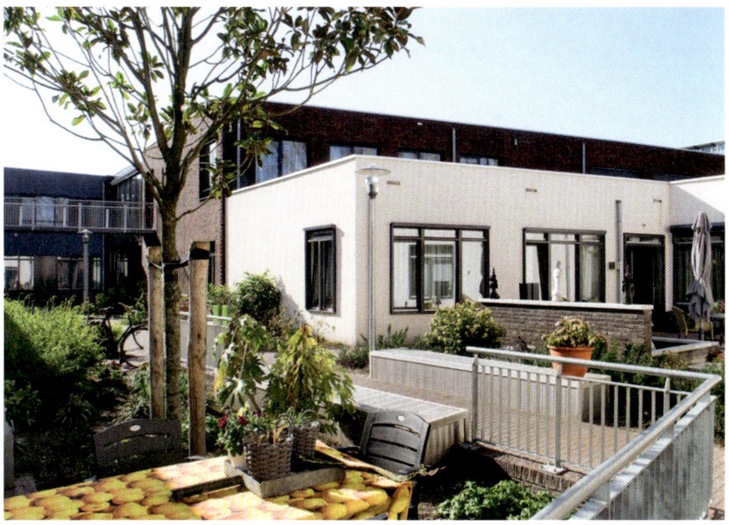

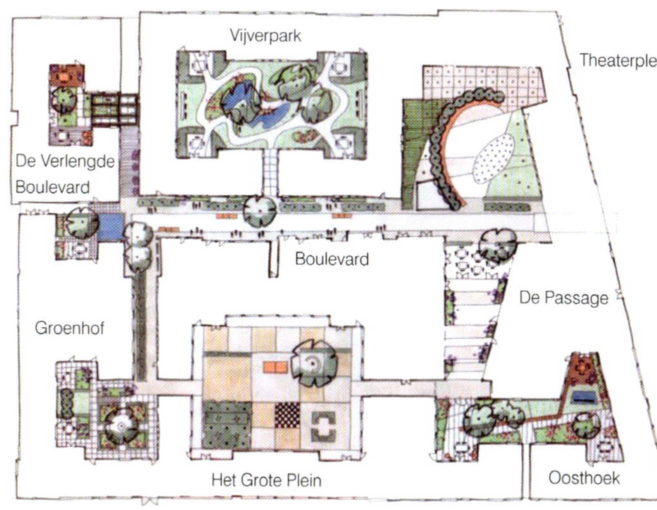
Vijverpark
Theaterplein
De Verlengde
Boulevard
Boulevard
De Passage
Groenhof
Het Grote Plein
Oosthoek

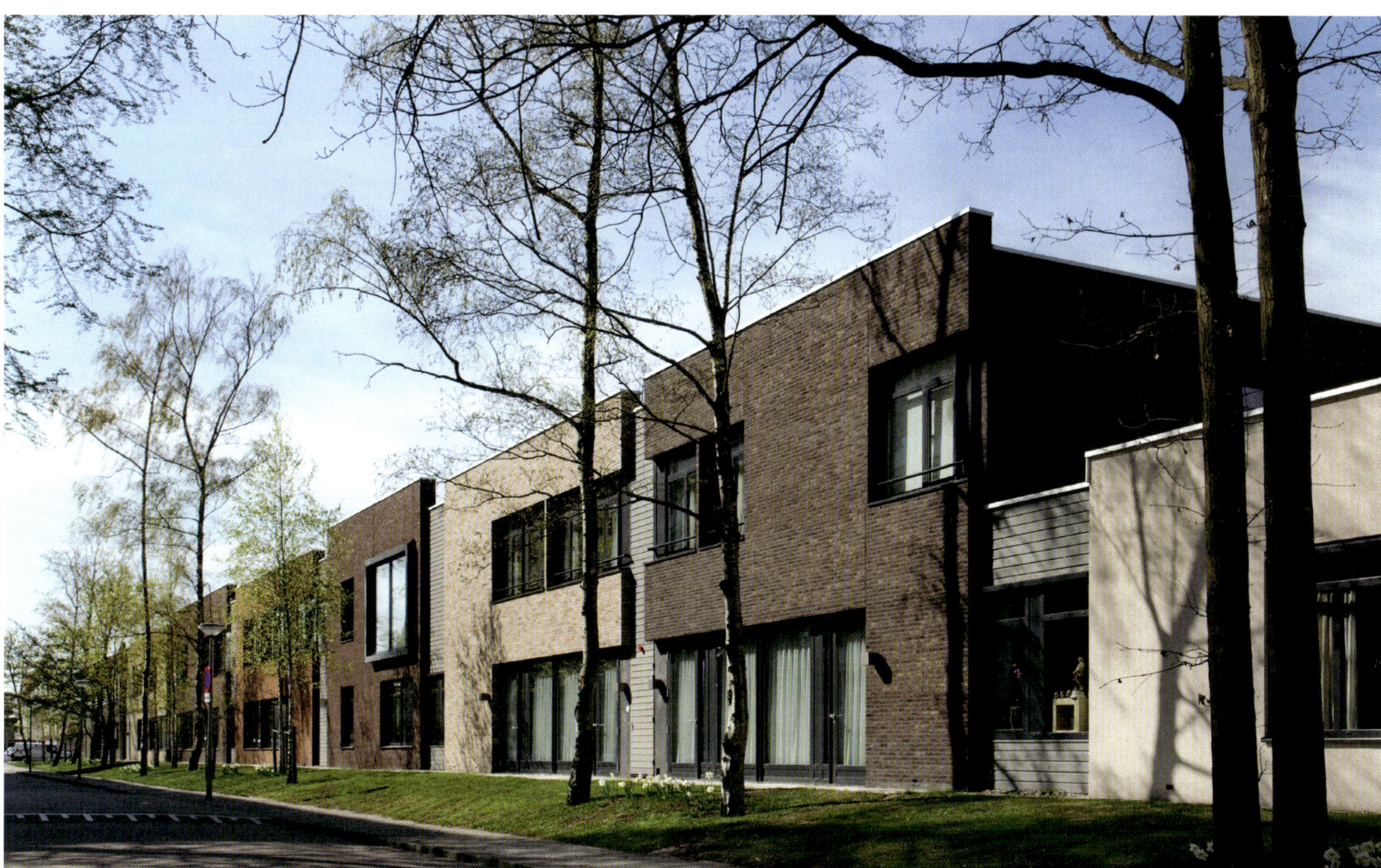

Industrial

Marlies Rohmer

Dobbelmanterrein residential care centre
Nijmegen
2009

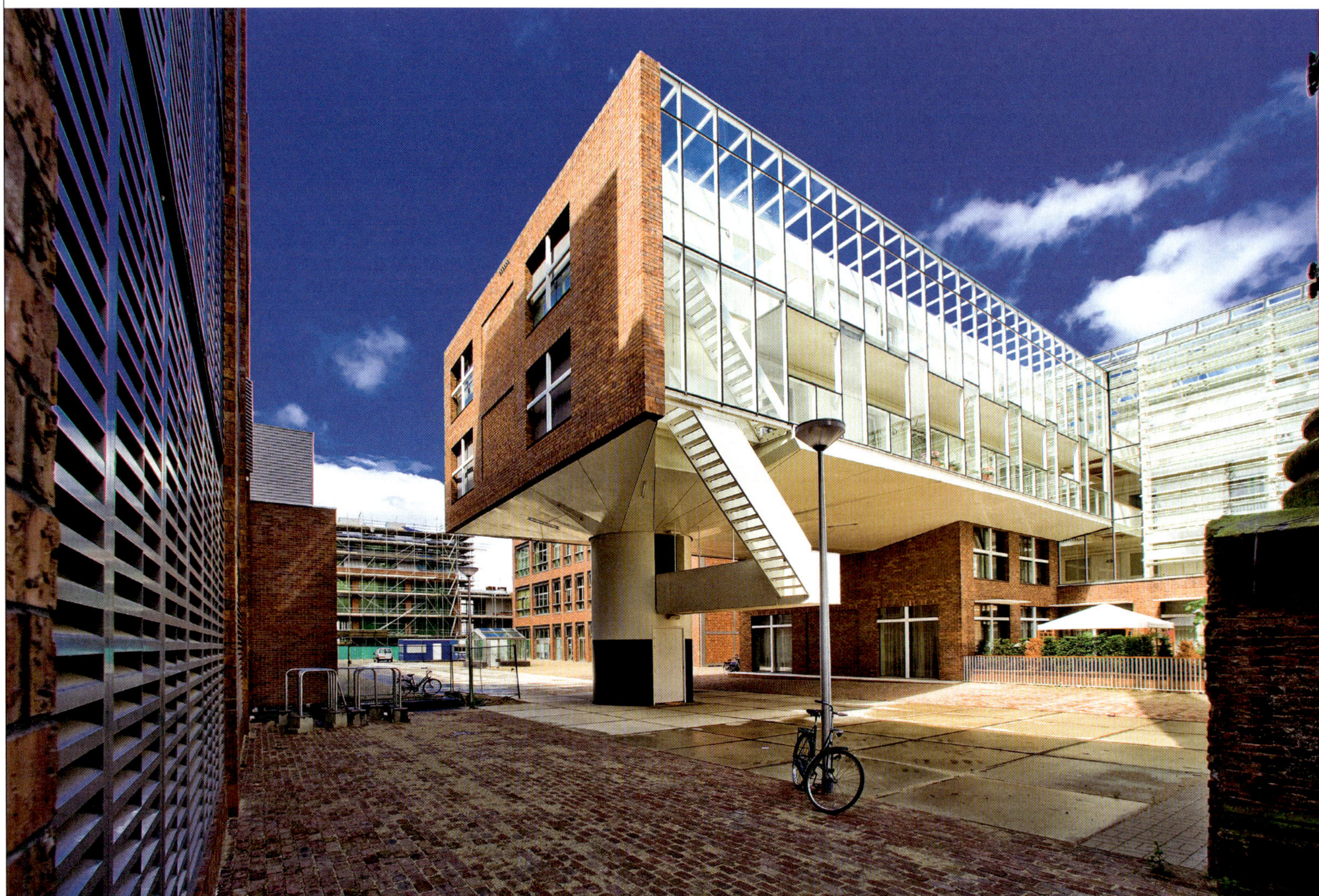

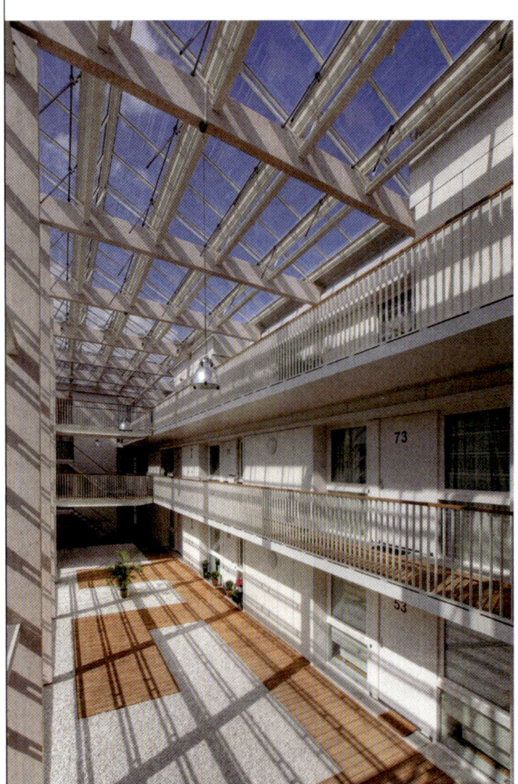

Situation
A *residential care complex*
B *studio and apartment complexes*
C *Graafseweg*
D *Graafsedwarsstraat*
E *De Ruyterstraat*

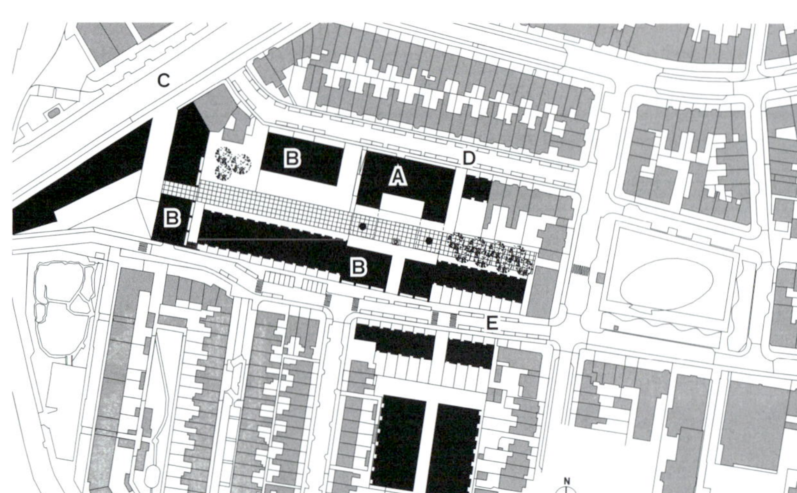

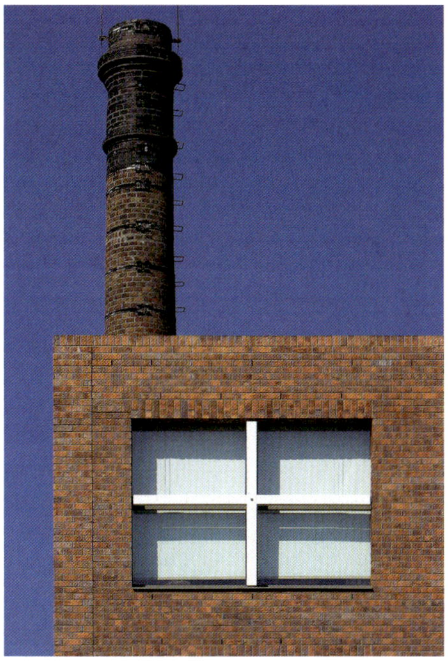

Like many other cities, Nijmegen is obliged to breathe new life into abandoned industrial estates, which often lie close to the city centre. After the departure of the Dobbelman soap factory, several parties worked together on redeveloping the area. Marlies Rohmer provided the master plan and also designed the residential care complex, an initiative of Talis Woondiensten. It contains three group homes for psycho-geriatric patients, twenty residential units for old people of non-Dutch origin, and six homes each for the mentally or the physically handicapped. This combination is characteristic of the bringing together of different categories of users who were kept separate in the past because they corresponded to different sectors in the health care organisation. The possibility of giving priority to housing and supplying personalised care favours this combination. Marlies Rohmer has given the building an industrial look in keeping with the robust character of the recycled and extended factory architecture. A striking feature is formed by the large columns beneath the building where it boxes in the communal courtyard. The four floors of the complex give the residents access to shared public areas – winter gardens on the upper storeys, and the communal courtyard on the ground floor. These communal areas are intended to promote contact between the residents and to prevent the complex from turning its back on its surroundings.

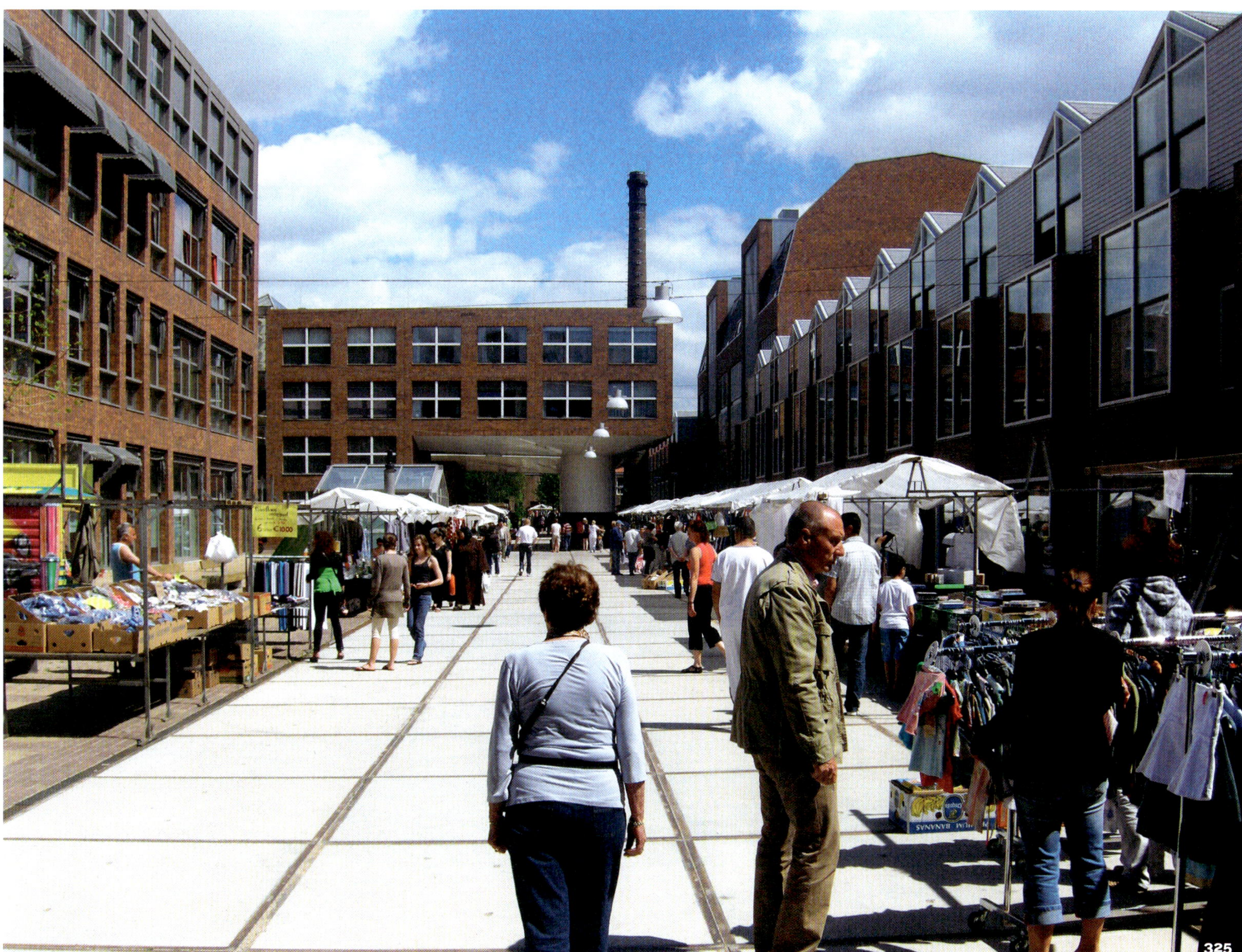

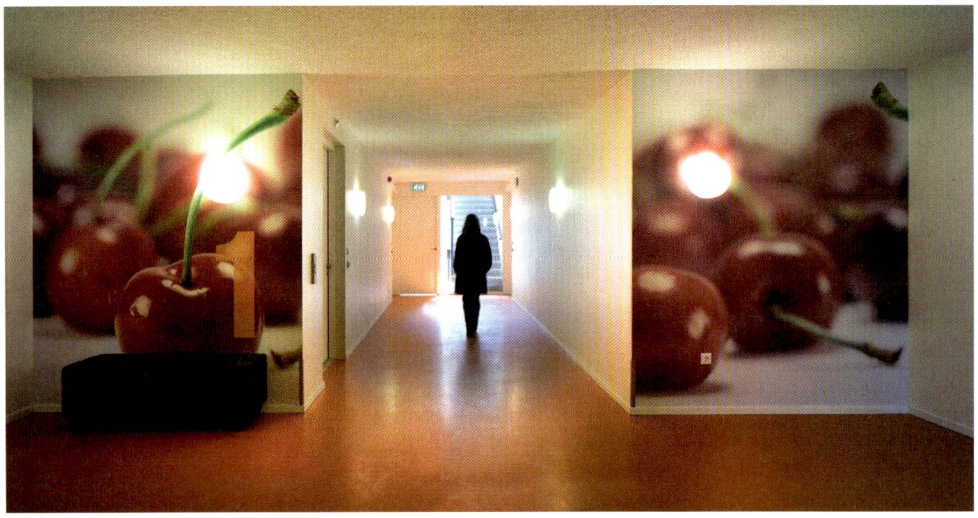

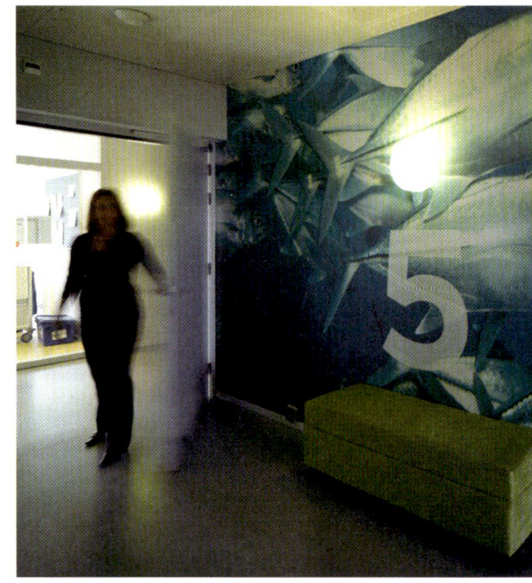

Healing environment

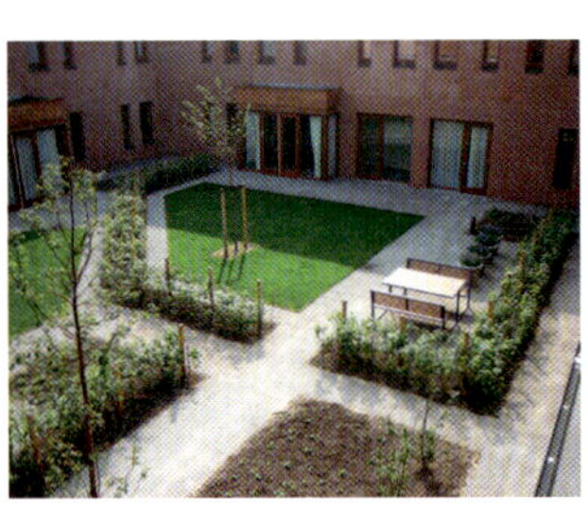

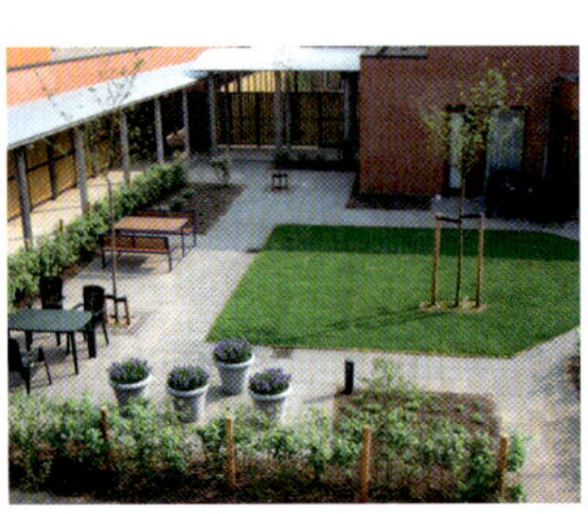

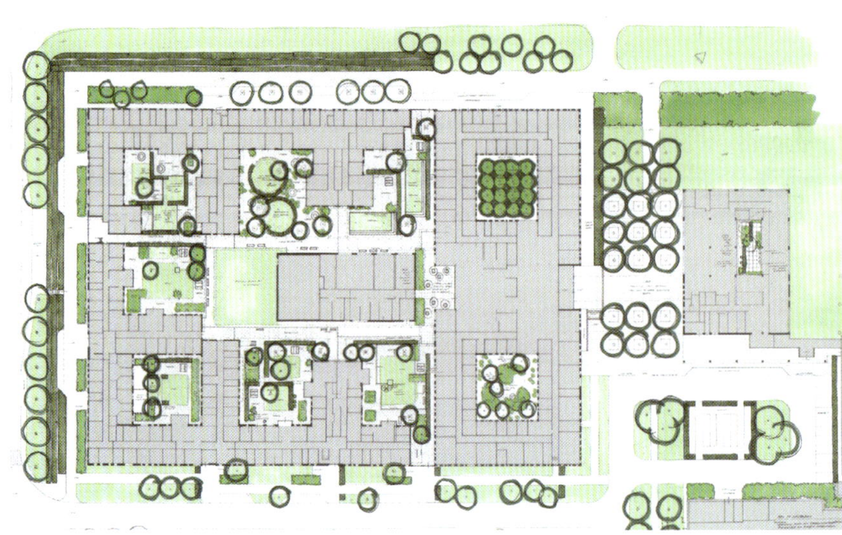

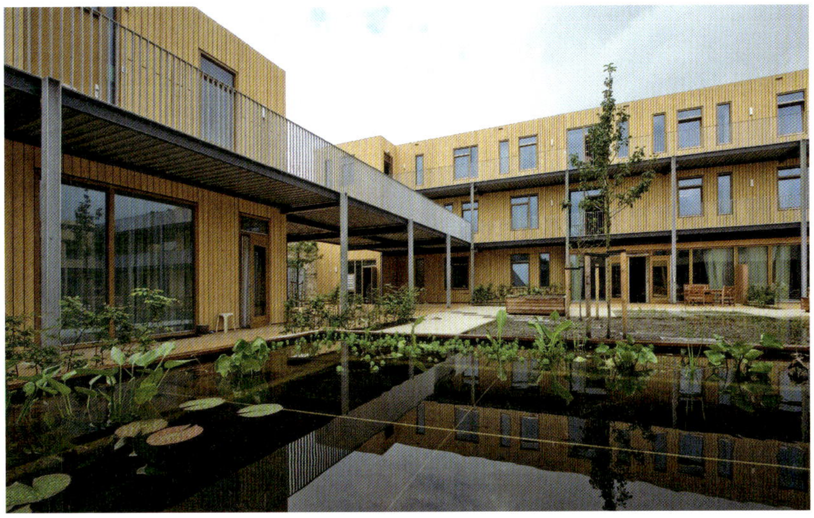

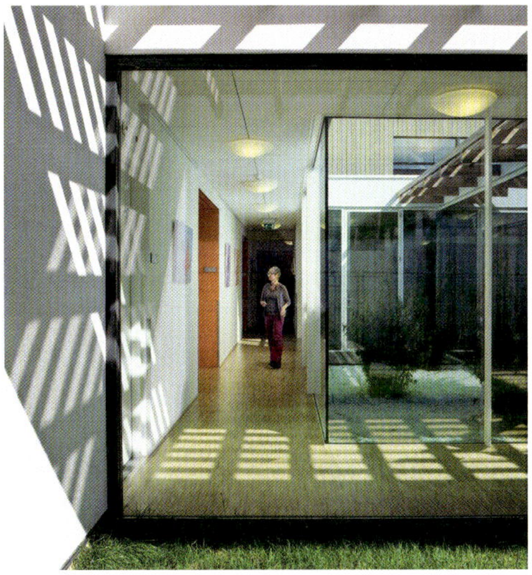

The idea that the environment in which people live and work influences their health is not new. Statistics were already made available in the eighteenth century that showed that life expectancy in the city was considerably less than in the countryside. At the time this was blamed on the polluted water and the stench that was often insufferable as a result. Those who could afford to do so bought a home in the country with a garden, far from the bustle of the city. A large part of the nineteenth century was characterised by making the city healthy, which was to a major extent a civil engineering operation. Sewers were constructed to counter the worst pollution, and the water supply brought purified drinking water into the home. Attention then shifted to social housing – down to the end of the nineteenth century, watertight, draught-free working-class homes with at least one room that could be reasonably heated were the exception rather than the rule. Extensive statistics, often provided by municipal services specially created for this purpose, charted the effects of these measures on public health. The results were often striking. The manipulation of the environment was undoubtedly one of the most effective ways of improving health standards in the city.

The situation changed at the beginning of the twentieth century when a much more powerful instrument appeared on the scene: the increasing possibility of combating illnesses where they occurred – in the patient. Improved diagnosis (partly thanks to the invention of X-ray photography), new medicines, better operating techniques, and above all the rapid progress in medical science all clouded the awareness that environmental factors had lost none of their importance. It was not until the 1960s that the downside of technological progress came into view – in particular, the effects of industrial pollution on the air and water – and the importance of the environment was rediscovered. It is characteristic of the political climate of the time that this was linked with Marxist theories of social critique, which acquired a strong psychological component under the influence of New Left philosophers and theoreticians such as Herbert Marcuse. The damaging effects of modern mass housing as the cause of much psychological suffering – loneliness, boredom, stress – had already been discovered in the 1950s.[1] From the 1970s on, these developments formed the framework within which psychology evolved as the discipline that specialised in the study of the effects of the environment on human behaviour and welfare. It seems but a small step from the study of these effects by environmental psychologists to the devising of interventions in the environment to achieve certain effects – the work of architects, landscape architects and urban developers. This laid the foundation for the concept of the healing environment, and its more scientifically orientated pendant, Evidence Based Design (EBD). Hospitals are a spearhead, for it was precisely there that the emphasis on medical processes had pushed attention for environmental factors into the background. Now research on the interaction between building, patient and staff brought them back to the centre of attention. Psychological effects, especially the aim of reducing stress, play a prominent role.

Roger Ulrich's research on the effect of the view from the patients' room on the healing process is still regarded as a breakthrough. 'Patients who were exposed to pictures of nature in the hospital suffered fewer signs of stress; patients who could look through a window at trees rather than at a brick wall were able to leave the hospital faster and suffered fewer complications.'[2] Perhaps the main importance of this finding is the direct relation between a spatial given – in fact primarily a visual one – and its

Top
Dick van Gameren architecten, Berkenstede care centre, Diemen, 2006

Greiner Van Goor Huijten Architecten, Sinai Centrum, Amstelveen (Langerhuize location), 2004

DP6 architectuurstudio, Het Noorderdok health centre, Almere, 2009

Bottom
Buro Mien Ruys, enclosed gardens, AMC psychiatric centre, Amsterdam, 2007

Patio and atrium AZG (now UMCG), Groningen, 1997

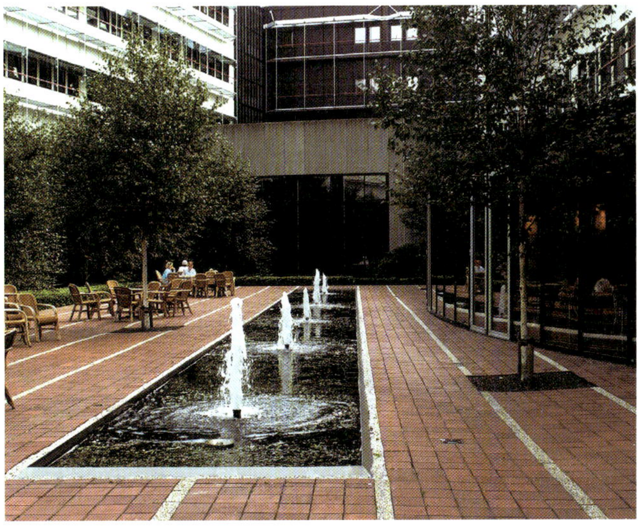

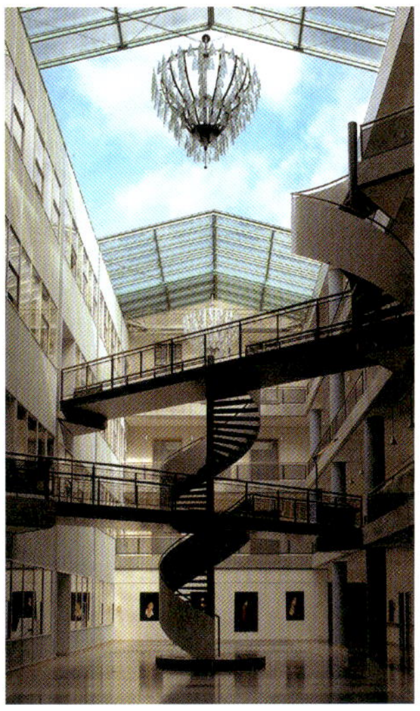

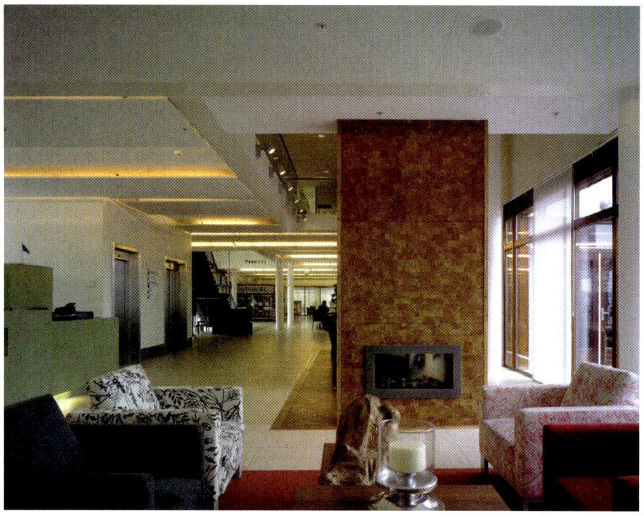

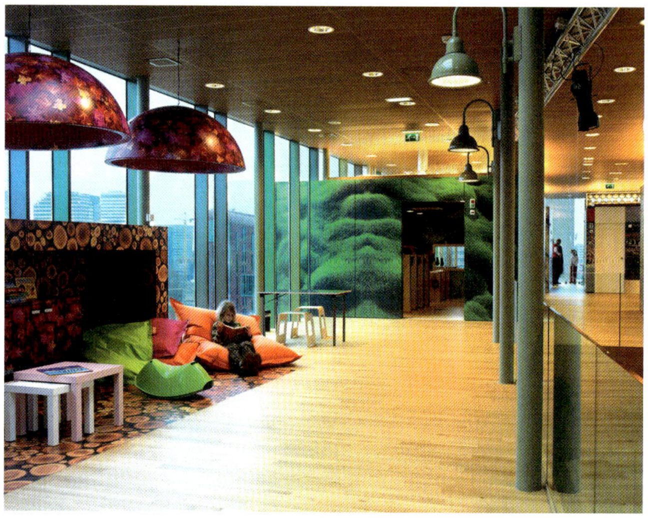

measurable effects. Elaborating on this type of research, the theoreticians of the healing environment and the EBD have considerably widened the scope of these concepts. The essence of the healing environment is that a well designed building contributes to the healing of the patient, an aim that recalls the old Enlightenment ideal of transforming the hospital through design into a healing machine. E. Zeidler, whose McMaster University Health Sciences Center in Hamilton, Canada, created a major stir in the 1970s, claimed that thirty per cent of the drop in the use of certain medicines in the Walter C. Mackenzie Health Sciences Center in Edmonton, Canada, which he had also designed, was due to the design.[3]

How does a hospital earn the title of a healing environment? It is not difficult to draw up a long list of elements that are considered to contribute to that. The natural surroundings are the primary factor: the view of nature alone has a positive effect. Green patios, whether roofed or not, and a large number of plants can give the whole hospital a far more natural appearance. It is of great importance to remove the somewhat alarming, mechanical and clinical character of the building. A large hospital with many patients and visitors and a large staff is something like the public space in a city, where a cross-section of the entire population is also to be found. The Academisch Medisch Centrum (AMC) in Amsterdam is the first hospital to provide a pleasant and secure urban space with streets and squares that are protected from the weather. The most exuberant urban atmosphere is to be found in the Universitair Medisch Centrum Groningen (UMCG). The pendant of the urban is the domestic: the areas where patients are alone or only accompanied by a few people should resemble an ordinary domestic setting in the use of colour and material (even if they have little in common with 'ordinary' homes). A number of basic qualities can also be drawn up for the areas that it is impossible to render 'normal'. Privacy is of great importance, and starts at the entrance where the patient registers for the first time. Single rooms are to be preferred, although it is advisable to offer the patient a choice from several options. Patient empowerment is also important, and vice versa care should be taken to ensure that the patient does not have the feeling of losing control – that is the case, for instance, when the routing in the building is inadequate. Finally, a number of other factors that increase stress have been identified that can often be avoided at little expense. Special acoustic ceiling tiles, for instance, can reduce noise.

Some categories of patients call for specific solutions, such as demented old people. Therapy orientated towards healing does not generally make much sense in their case. In the case of these patients, treatment and accommodation belong together. That is why a special role can be played by the architecture of clinics for this category: intervening in the environment, Van der Voordt and Terpstra claim, cannot stop their decline, but it can slow it down.[4] The colour and use of materials play a role, but so does the presence of stimuli to the senses. Various strategies have been developed in which the environment plays a larger or more prominent role. Many come from the United States, such as reality orientation training, which is intended to offer residents anchor points to enable them to function better in their present situation. It thus targets the here and now. An opposite tendency is the notion of validation, which assumes that many patients prefer to live in the past. This notion is reflected in the Netherlands in the Humanitas 'memory museum' in a nursing home in Rotterdam (part of Humanitas-Akropolis). Whether these qualities really do have an effect is not a question of conviction but of

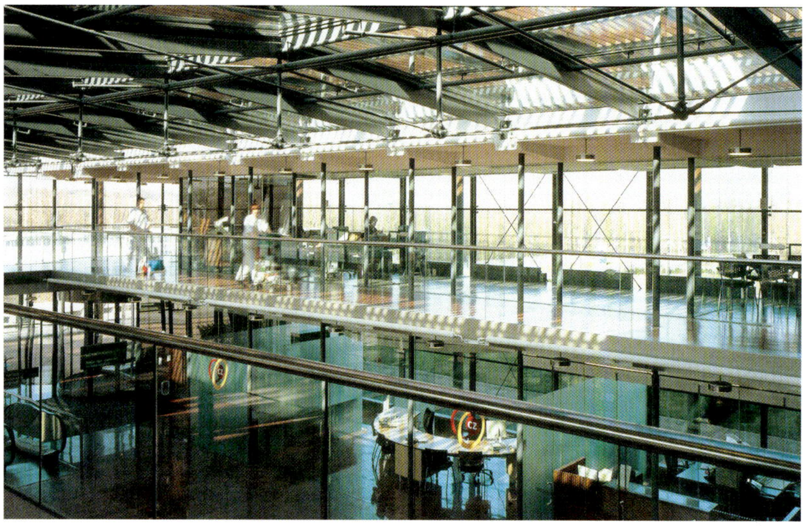

Top
RAU, Het Zonnehuis, Zwolle, 2007

Sponge Architects & Rupali Gupta with IOU Architecture, Ronald McDonald VU Kinderstad, Amsterdam, 2008

De Jong Gortemaker Algra architecten en ingenieurs, the Netherlands Cancer Institute/Antoni van Leeuwenhoek Ziekenhuis, 2004

Wiegerinck Architecten, Spaarne-ziekenhuis, Hoofddorp, 2004

Bottom
Han Westelaken, Atrium Medisch Centrum, Heerlen, 2003. Entrance building

Architecten aan de Maas, La Valence nursing home, Maastricht, 2007

De Jong Gortemaker Algra architecten en ingenieurs, operating theatre, Ziekenhuis De Lievensberg, Bergen op Zoom, 2005

Bonnema Architecten, Maasland-ziekenhuis, Sittard, 2008

Architectenbureau Koen van Velsen, Groot Klimmendaal rehabilitation centre, Arnhem, 2009

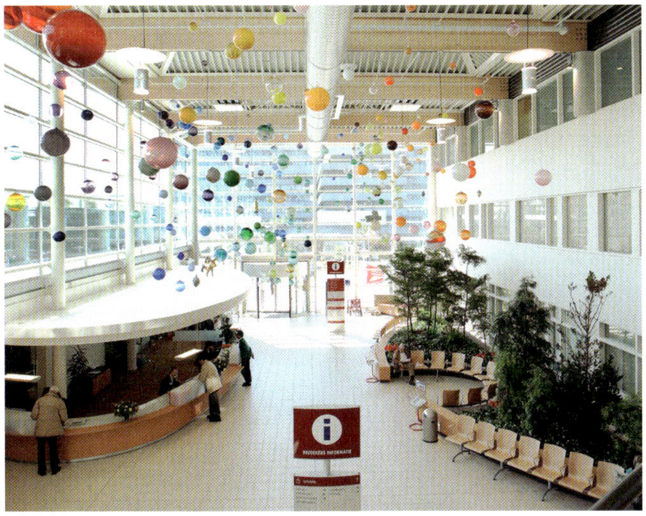

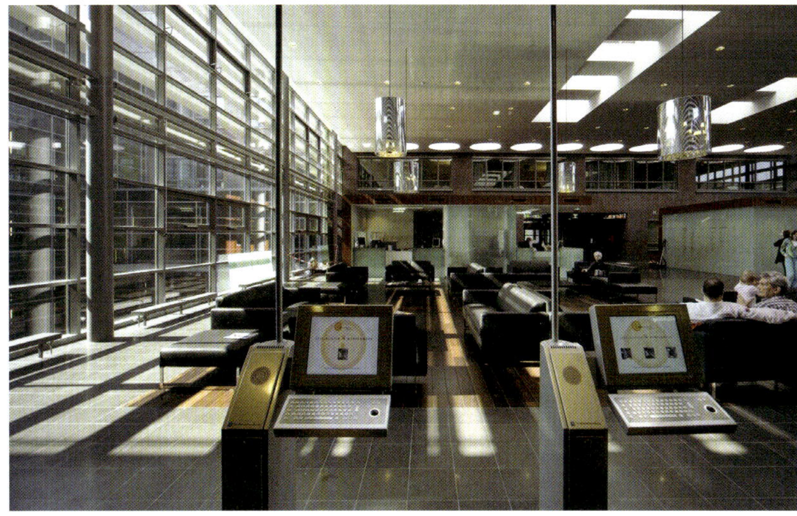

measuring for the advocates of EBD. An ideal measuring moment is when an institution moves into new premises, even if the patient population is floating. The pebbles project that documents the distribution of EBD (like the ripples around a pebble thrown into the water) likes to make use of this method, but it is not unknown in the Netherlands either. When a new nursing home opened in Maastricht, the patients in the new building turned out to behave more independently and actively than they had done in the Klevarie, one of the large-scale predecessors.[5]

It is perhaps not surprising that the concepts of the healing environment and EBD initially met with scepticism in the world of architects – although they emphasise the scope and importance of architecture, they come mainly from the world of environmental psychologists, which prompted fear of extra external regulations and guidelines. In the meantime, a slow but sure change of attitude seems to be taking place. The fear of curbs on design freedom does indeed seem to be unfounded. When high-quality architecture proves able to make use of the findings of EBD, this appears to be to everyone's benefit.

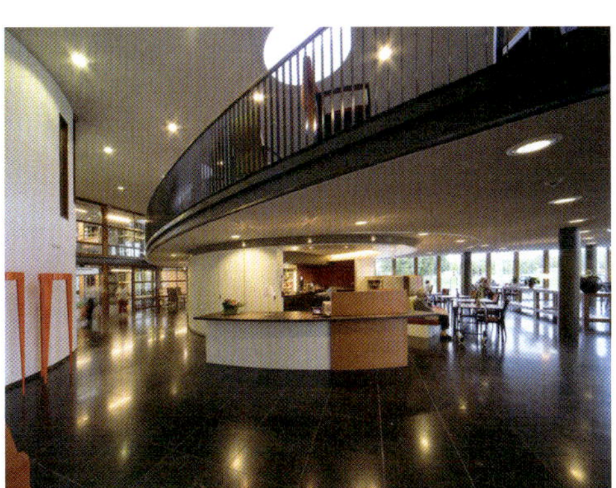

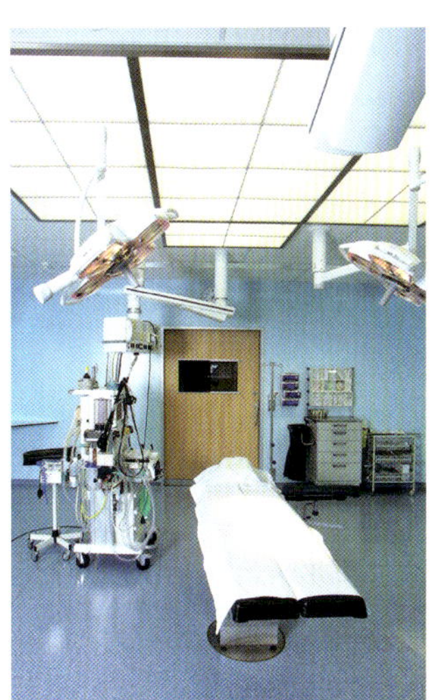

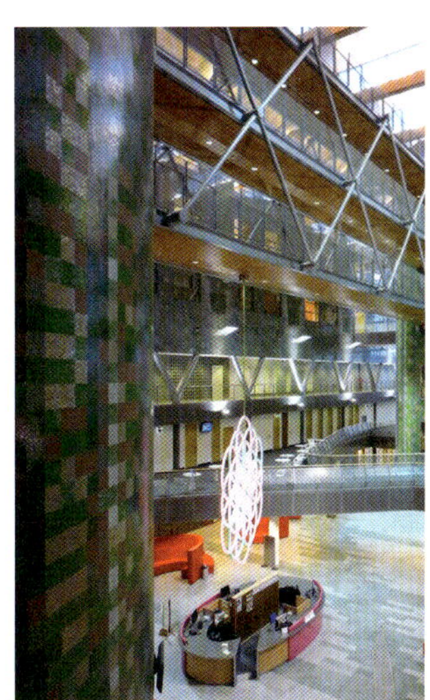

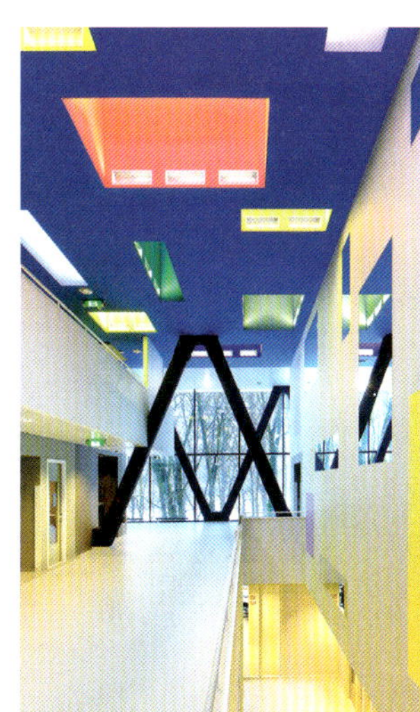

Conclusion

Architecture plays a much larger and more fundamental role in health care that is usually recognised. There are two sides to this role, as we stated in the introduction: the way a complex is designed has direct consequences for the running of it. It can seriously frustrate the running, which is hardest to avoid in the classic all-under-one-roof hospital. It can also order those processes in such a way that loss of time due to excessive internal traffic via illogical and impractical routes is avoided. Moreover, architecture has a direct relation to the real estate value. Buildings that do not require modification before they can be used for other purposes are preferable. This presupposes a standardisation of the rooms with dimensions that make them usable for other purposes too, flexibility of the parts that do not belong to the constructional core, a well conceived system of dimensions, and above all surplus space. This effect of architecture is important enough, but in health care the way design influences how the building is experienced is crucial. Research on such concepts as the healing environment and evidence-based design has shown that this effect is directly connected with what in the last analysis is the core business of health care buildings: to improve the wellbeing of the patients (which ideally includes contributing to their cure), and to create an environment in which it is pleasant for the staff to work. The aim of this publication is to provide insight into how these premises have been elaborated in health care architecture in the Netherlands. Their importance – and also the importance of driving home the need for a proper understanding of the architecture – turns out to go beyond the domain of health care and to apply to architecture in general.

Ten years into the new millennium, is there still such a thing as specific health care architecture? The substitution policy that was launched in the 1970s, the gradual abolition of the regulation of supply, and the emergence of small-scale, bottom-up institutions heralded the end of buildings that are immediately recognisable as a hospital, psychiatric institution, care home or nursing home. The classic health care building, that usually consisted of several clearly identifiable functional components but still formed a clear unity, is under pressure. In fact, there seems to be a consensus on the need to abandon buildings whose structure and appearance are completely tailored to their specific function. The most important consideration is the negative effect on their real estate value: what is completely designed for a single function has a much lower market value than a building that can be used for several different purposes. So it looks as though the phenomenon of building typology, which was introduced some 250 years ago by the development of rationally conceived hospital designs, is coming to an end. After all, the essence of these buildings is that they are pre-eminently specific. Of course, the advantages of generic architecture are important for every type of building, but an additional factor in health care architecture is that the abandonment of the typology coincides with a victory over the intensely regretted institutional character of hospitals, psychiatric clinics and nursing homes.

Does the end of thinking in typologies mean that health care buildings will no longer be different from any other type of building on the same scale? That does not appear to be the case at all. The specificity of the type has been replaced by the specificity of the transformation strategy, which still proceeds within different frameworks for each sector. Even if a hospital consists for eighty per cent of generic volumes, their evolution is specific of developments that are characteristic of hospitals, and the same goes for the other sectors too. In every case the result is the distinction between generic and specific building components, and the recruitment of provisions that, related or not, are of a different kind. In the first trend as many components as possible are so designed that they can be let or sold to third parties if that should prove necessary or desirable (most new hospitals follow this strategy). Another possibility is to accommodate these generic parts in separate buildings (which leads to a variant of the pavilion system) or to rent or newly develop buildings outside the main location. The recruitment of other functions besides the core business immediately makes buildings multifunctional. A contemporary phenomenon is that of the so-called 'window hospitals': often complexes of a relatively modest size that, like 'window schools', offer all kinds of extra functions in the building.[1]

Although the various sectors evolve within their own frameworks, there are striking similarities. Normalisation is the trend everywhere. In psychiatry and above all in care for the elderly, this leads to an emphasis on ordinary housing, and in all sectors to the attempt to create a less institutional impression. Efforts are being made everywhere to strengthen the role of the user (patient or resident). Apart from the top clinical and academic segment, the potential of decentralisation is being given serious thought even in the hospital world. Where large-scale complexes are unavoidable, that decentralisation is sought in the principle of small scale in large scale, which is often applied in care for the elderly and psychiatry.

An interesting question is how hospital functions will relate to the phenomenon of the residential care zone, the final station in the evolution of the health care landscape in the Netherlands for the time being. Small-scale institutions with extramural and day functions are replacing the vast majority of traditional care institutions. Residential facilities with internally organised care have been reduced to the level where separation is simply impossible: acute somatic nursing, dementia, or temporary admission to a psychiatric clinic. Outside the residential care zone, there seem to be only a number of residual categories left who have been left untouched by the processes of substitution under the regulation of supply regime and the transition to a demand-side provision of health care. It is gradually becoming clear that a part of the large-scale residential care complexes will probably remain in use for longer than was supposed only a short while ago. Perhaps they offer the best solution for the group of old people who lack the resources to pay for a reasonable old age health provision themselves and whose relatively poor health makes a certain centrally administered care attractive.

Moreover, this standardised, no-frills care in institutions of this kind is believed to be less expensive than in the small-scale solutions in the residential care zones. A concentration of long-term care provisions of this kind is taking place in psychiatry; the partly evacuated sites outside the urban zones are the ideal location for this. Concentration, deconcentration, integration but also isolation again for some categories of patients, which are then sometimes tempered by attracting other functions (the reverse integration in psychiatry, for example), specialisation or being at home in every market – the evolution of health care architecture continues without flagging. The future will show how it will develop further, but one thing is certain: the unprecedented possibilities of health care architecture that have been at the centre of attention for some time now designate this field as one of the most vital and challenging for the years to come.

Notes
Bibliography
Index

Notes

Preface

1 N. Mens, A. Tijhuis, *De architectuur van het ziekenhuis. Transformaties in de naoorlogse ziekenhuisbouw in Nederland*, Rotterdam 1999; N. Mens, *De Architectuur van het psychiatrisch ziekenhuis*, Wormer 2003; C. Wagenaar (ed.), *The Architecture of Hospitals*, Rotterdam 2006; *Au. Bouwen aan de Architectuur van de Zorg*, Utrecht 2007; N. Mens, C. Wagenaar, *De architectuur van de ouderenhuisvesting. Bouwen voor wonen en zorg*, Rotterdam 2009.

1750–1914
The origin of health care buildings

1 M. Le Mandat, *Prévoir l'espace hospitalier*, Paris 1989, p. 72.
2 Idem, p. 59.
3 A.H. Murken, *Vom Armenhospital zum Großklinikum. Die Geschichte des Krankenhauses vom 18. Jahrhundert bis zur Gegenwart*, Cologne 1988, p. 25.
4 Idem, p. 21.
5 Idem, p. 37.
6 M. Foucault et al., *Les Machines à guérir (aux origines de l'hôpital moderne)*, Brussels 1979, p. 80.
7 A. Vidler, *Writing of the Walls. Architectural Theory in the Late Enlightenment*, Princeton 1987, p. 60.
8 J.B. Leroy, *Précis d'un ouvrage sur les hôpitaux dans lequel on expose les principes, résultats des observations de physique et de médecine qu'on doit avoir en vue dans la construction des édifices, avec un projet d'hôpital disposé d'après ces principes*, Paris 1787.
9 A. Vidler, *Writing of the walls. Architectural theory in the late enlightenment*, Princeton 1987, p. 60.
10 A. Husson, *Étude sur les hopitaux considérés sous la rapport de leur construction, de la distribution de leurs batiments, de l'ameublement, de l'hygiène & du service des salles de malades*, Paris 1862, p. 8.
11 R. Middleton, 'Sickness, madness and crime as the grounds of form', *AA files*, (1993) 25, p. 26.
12 J.-L. Binet, *Les architectes de la médecine*, Besançon 1996.
13 H. Burgerhout, 'Plan en functie bij ziekenhuizen', in: *Handboek voor het ziekenhuiswezen*, s.l. 1939.
14 M.J. van Lieburg, *Het Coolsingelziekenhuis te Rotterdam (1839–1900)*, Amsterdam 1986, p. 188.
15 Idem, pp. 25-26.
16 D. Schiffczyk, *Die intellektuelle Revolution im europäischen Krankenhausbau um 1800. Zur systematischen Entwicklung neuzeitlicher Bauformen vor dem Hintergrund des mittelalterlichen Hospitaltypus*, Frankfurt am Main 1985, p. 223.
17 M.J. van Lieburg, *Het Coolsingelziekenhuis te Rotterdam (1839–1900)*, Amsterdam 1986, p. 31.
18 R. van der Woude, W. van der Schuit, *Oude tradities, nieuw ambities. 200 jaar Academisch Ziekenhuis Groningen*, Groningen 1998, p. 44.
19 J. Vijselaar, 'Van kleine en grote gestichten. Een overzicht van de institutionalisering van de krankzinnigenzorg vanaf 1400', in: H. Marens et al., *Voor gek gehouden. Geschiedenis van de krankzinnigenzorg in Nederland*, Gouda/Haarlem 1982, p. 42.
20 L. van den Berg, *Rijp voor paviljoen III. Krankzinnig in Amsterdam vanaf 1565*, Amsterdam 1989, pp. 38-40.
21 Verslag betreffende eenige Krankzinnigengestichten in Duitsland. Historisch Documentatiecentrum voor het Nederlands Protestantisme, Vrije Universiteit Amsterdam, Archief Vereniging tot Christelijke Verzorging van Geestes- en Zenuwzieken, 1884-1987 (archive no. 501), inv. no. 52.
22 K. Roosjen, 'Werken aan genezing. Het therapeutische klimaat in Brinkgreven tussen 1892 en 1940', in: J. Vijselaar (ed.), *Over de IJssel, over de schreef. De geschiedenis van de geestelijke gezondheidszorg in Overijsel en van het Psychiatrisch Ziekenhuis Brinkgreven in het bijzonder*, Utrecht 1993.
23 H.G.M. Rooijmans, *Negenennegentig jaar tussen wal en schip. Geschiedenis van de Leidse Universitaire Psychiatrie*, Houten/Diegem 1998, p. 6.
24 A. Kerkhoven, J. Vijselaar, 'De zorg voor zenuwlijders rond 1900', in: G. Hutschemaker, C. Hrachovec (ed.), *Heer en Heelmeester. Negentig jaar zorg voor zenuwlijders in het christelijk sanatorium te Zeist*, Nijmegen 1993, p. 29.
25 H.G.M. Rooijmans, *Negenennegentig jaar tussen wal en schip. Geschiedenis van de Leidse Universitaire Psychiatrie*, Houten/Diegem 1998, p. 19.
26 A. Kerkhoven, J. Vijselaar, 'De zorg voor zenuwlijders rond 1900', in: G. Hutschemaker, C. Hrachovec (ed.), *Heer en Heelmeester. Negentig jaar zorg voor zenuwlijders in het christelijk sanatorium te Zeist*, Nijmegen 1993, pp. 29-30.
27 A. Kerkhoven, *Beeld van de psychiatrie 1800–1970*, Zwolle 1996, p. 98.
28 Verslag van een bezoek aan eenige zenuwinrichtingen. Historisch Documentatiecentrum voor het Nederlands Protestantisme, Vrije Universiteit Amsterdam, Archief Vereniging tot Christelijke Verzorging van Geestes- en Zenuwzieken, 1884-1987 (archive no. 501), inv. no. 52.
29 N.Y. Schuyt-Lucassen, G.J.F. Leene, P.P.J. Houben, *Hofjes in perspectief. Een onderzoek naar de identiteit en actualiteit van de Hofjes Codde en Van Beresteyn in het licht van de modernisering van de ouderenhuisvesting*, Amsterdam 1995; N.Y. Schuijt-Lucassen, G.J.F. Leene, P.P.J. Houben, *Hofjes met perspectief. Al eeuwen een moderne woonvorm voor ouderen*, Bussum 1997.

Sanatoria for tuberculosis patients

1 M.A. van Nieukerken, *Sanatoria voor tuberculose patiënten*, Deventer 1909.
2 Idem, p. 19.
3 *Zonnegloren. Soestduinen. Provincie Utrecht*, [Utrecht 1921].

1914–1940
Light, air and space

1 J. Abram, 'The Filter of Reason: Experimental Projects, 1920-1939', in: J. Abram, T. Riley, *The Filter of Reason*, New York 1990, pp. 52-62.
2 A. Querido, *Godshuizen en gasthuizen*, Amsterdam 1960, pp. 50-51.
3 J.W. Wicherink, 'Het nieuw Academisch Ziekenhuis te Leiden', *Het Ziekenhuis*, 14 (1923), pp. 87-99.
4 B.J.K. Cramer, 'Eenige beschouwingen over ziekenhuisbouw in hoogbouw', in: *Handboek voor het Ziekenhuiswezen*, s.l. 1939.
5 E.M. Dolné, 'Katholieke ziekenzorg in Nijmegen', in: D. Nicolaisen (ed.), *Een veelkleurig habijt. Kloosters in Nijmegen in de negentiende en twintigste eeuw*, Nijmegen 1989, pp. 79-91.
6 Ed. Cuypers, 'Het nieuwe Gast- of Ziekenhuis te Dordrecht', *Het Ziekenhuis*, 13 (1922), pp. 37-52.
7 Brief van de Commissie voor de Gemeentewerken aan de wethouder van Gemeentewerken, 16 November 1931. GAR, Plaatselijke Werken Archive, file 1931/16129, inv. no. 2576.
8 J. de Jonge, *Handelingen van de Gemeenteraad* 1931, meeting 15 January, p. 11.
9 W.M. van der Scheer, *Nieuwere inzichten in de behandeling van geesteszieken*, Groningen, The Hague/Batavia 1933, p. 77.
10 Ibid.
11 J.A.J. Barnhoorn, *De Moderne Psychiatrische Inrichting en de Nieuwere Behandelmethode van Geesteszieken*, offprint from *Ons Ziekenhuis*, p. 3.
12 Geciteerd in R. Blijdenstein, *Zeist, groei en bouw. Den Dolder en Bosch en Duin. Een inventarisatie van waardevolle gebouwen en gebieden*, Zeist 1984, p. 169.
13 G.A. Lindeboom, M.J. van Lieburg (ed.), *Gedenkboek van de Vereniging tot Christelijke Verzorging van Geestes- en Zenuwzieken, 1884-1984*, Kampen 1984, p. 196.
14 C.B. Posthumus Meyjes, 'Het sanatorium "Koningsheide" te Arnhem', *Bouwkundig Weekblad Architectura*, 57 (1936) 48, p. 489.
15 J.H. Furnée, J.H.G. Jonkman, *Het Noorder Sanatorium te Zuidlaren. Geschiedenis en architectuur van een psychiatrisch monument*, Zuidlaren 1994, pp. 8, 41.

16 M. Casciato, *De Amsterdamse School*, Rotterdam 1991, p. 191.
17 W. Swart, *Van sinaasappelkistje tot kangoeroe woning. Het Amsterdam-Noord van Arie Keppler*, Amsterdam 1992, p. 47.
18 'Nieuw gebouw voor de Remonstrantsche Stichting voor ouden van dagen e.d.', *Bouwkundig Weekblad Architectura*, 59 (1937) 50, pp. 474-475.
19 T. Idsinga, J. Schilt, *Architect W. van Tijen, 1894-1974. 'Ik ben een rationalist, maar er is meer op de wereld...'* , The Hague 1987, 28-30, pp. 241-244.
20 Letter from N.V. Volkswoningbouw Rotterdam to Mayor and Aldermen, 13 November 1929. GAR, Plaatselijke Werken Archive, file 1929/6521, inv. no. 2470.
21 Letter from the director of the Building Commission and the Housing Department to the Alderman of Social Affairs, 3 June 1930. GAR, Plaatselijke Werken Archive, file 1929/6523, inv. no. 2470.
22 'Jury-rapport over de openbare prijsvraag voor een woongebouw voor oude mannen en vrouwen te Alkmaar (Karenhuizen)', *Bouwkundig Weekblad*, 38 (1917) 31, p. 176.
23 A. van der Woud, *Waarheid en karakter. Het debat over de bouwkunst 1840-1900*, Rotterdam 1997.
24 'Jury-rapport over de openbare prijsvraag voor een woongebouw voor oude mannen en vrouwen te Alkmaar (Karenhuizen)', *Bouwkundig Weekblad*, 38 (1917) 31, p. 178.
25 *Rapport van de Studiecommissie voor de verzorging en huisvesting van Ouden van Dagen*, s.l. 1950.
26 W. Bruin, 'De Rusthoeve, tehuis voor ouden van dagen te Purmerend', *Bouwkundig Weekblad Architectura*, 60 (1938) 35, p. 289.
27 J.H. Groenewegen, 'Een nieuw rusthuis te Driebergen. Ontwerp Ir J.B. van Loghem, Rotterdam', *De 8 en Opbouw*, 3 (1932) 10, p. 97.

Utility and aesthetics

1 J. Hudnut, 'Architecture and the art of medicine', *Journal of The American Institute of Architects*, Vol. VIII, October 1947, nr. 4, p. 147.
2 J.L.C. Wortman, 'De bouw van kleine ziekenhuizen', *Het Ziekenhuis*, 2 (1910), pp. 35-40; J.L.C. Wortman, 'Enige wenken over de bouw en organisatie van ziekenhuizen', *Het Ziekenhuis*, 3 (1911), pp. 87-97.
3 S. Kroonenberg (ed.), *Handboek voor het ziekenhuiswezen*, s.l. 1939.
4 J.B. van Loghem, 'Theorie en Praktijk', *De 8 en Opbouw*, 3 (1932) 20, p. 198.
5 J.B. van Loghem, 'Vergrooting van het Sophiaziekenhuis te Zwolle', *De 8 en Opbouw*, 6 (1935) 20, p. 212.
6 J.B. van Loghem, 'Uitbreiding van de Diaconesseninrichting te Rotterdam', *De 8 en Opbouw*, 10 (1939) 26, p. 281.

1940–1960
The Reconstruction

1 K. Schuyt, E. Taverne, *1950. Welvaart in zwart-wit*, The Hague 2000.
2 The interest in Switzerland is revealed by book and periodical publications, for example, P.C. Cleyndert, 'Indrukken over het Zwitsersche ziekenhuiswezen', in: *Handboek voor het Ziekenhuiswezen*, s.l. 1939.
3 M.J. Groot Wesseldijk, 'Ziekenhuisbouw in den vreemde', *Het Ziekenhuiswezen*, 19 (1946), pp. 187-191.
4 K. Bosma, C. Wagenaar, 'Het Regeringscommissariaat zoekt een stelsel', in: K. Bosma, C. Wagenaar (ed.), *Een geruisloze doorbraak. De geschiedenis van architectuur en stedebouw tijdens de bezetting en de wederopbouw van Nederland*, Rotterdam 1995, pp. 215-216.
5 L.J. Zielstra, 'Samenwerking tussen de Stichting "Het Nederlandse Ziekenhuiswezen" en het "Bouwcentrum"', *Het Ziekenhuiswezen*, 22 (1949), p. 32.
6 P.C. Cleyndert, 'Bouwcentrum-Rotterdam (II)', *Het Ziekenhuiswezen*, 22 (1949), p. 41.
7 P.C. Cleyndert, 'De Verpleegeenheid', *Het Ziekenhuiswezen*, 24 (1951), pp. 108-125.
8 C. Zervos, 'Introduction', in: P. Nelson, *Cité hospitalière de Lille*, Paris 1933, xiii. Van den Broek adopted this line too after the war: he referred to a synthesis of the individual elements that would form the core of the architectural conception. 'The analysed elements form the building bricks with which the designer puts together the whole.' J.H. van den Broek, 'De architectonische conceptie van het ziekenhuis', *Het Ziekenhuiswezen*, 23 (1950), special issue on buildings, p. 69.
9 P.C. Cleyndert, 'De verpleegeenheid', *Het Ziekenhuiswezen*, 21 (1948), pp. 356-357; P.C. Cleyndert, 'Isometrische afbeeldingen van ziekenhuisafdelingen', *Het Ziekenhuiswezen*, 22 (1949), p. 201 and seperate annex.
10 P.C. Cleyndert, 'De medische en verpleegtechnische organisatie van het ziekenhuis en zijn afdelingen', *Het Ziekenhuiswezen*, 23 (1950), special issue on buildings, p. 24.
11 J.H. van den Broek, 'De architectonische conceptie van het ziekenhuis', *Het Ziekenhuiswezen*, 23 (1950), special issue on buildings, p. 73.
12 A. Viergever, 'Recente buitenlandse inzichten en ervaringen', *Het Ziekenhuiswezen*, 23 (1950), special issue on buildings, p. 60.
13 H.A.F. Königs, C. de Kievit, 'Studie commissie voor poliklinieken, röntgen-afdelingen enz. Rapport inzake poliklinieken', *Het Ziekenhuiswezen*, 21 (1948), p. 361.
14 Ibid.
15 A. Viergever, 'Recente buitenlandse inzichten en ervaringen', *Het Ziekenhuiswezen*, 23 (1950), special issue on buildings, p. 52.
16 P.C. Cleyndert, 'De medische en verpleegtechnische organisatie van het ziekenhuis en zijn afdelingen', *Het Ziekenhuiswezen*, 23 (1950), special issue on buildings, p. 22.
17 H. Hoekstra, 'De bouwkundige Organisatie van het ziekenhuis en zijn afdelingen', *Het Ziekenhuiswezen*, 23 (1950), special issue on buildings, p. 31.
18 R. Nicolaï, *Inleiding tot het bouwen voor de gezondheidszorg*, Utrecht 1983, p. 116.
19 H. Hoekstra, 'De bouwkundige Organisatie van het ziekenhuis en zijn afdelingen', *Het Ziekenhuiswezen*, 23 (1950), special issue on buildings, p. 35.
20 A. Viergever, 'Recente buitenlandse inzichten en ervaringen', *Het Ziekenhuiswezen*, 23 (1950), special issue on buildings, p. 51.
21 Interviews with J.P. Kloos, 18 December 1996 en 10 November 1997.
22 'Woningbouw in IJmuiden (Oost)', *Bouwkundig Weekblad*, 68 (1950) 38, p. 577.
23 H.G. van Beusekom, 'Mogelijkheden voor de Huisvesting van Bejaarden, *Tijdschrift voor Maatschappelijk werk*, 2 (1948) 13, p. 200.
24 B. Colenbrander (ed.), *Stijl. Norm en handschrift in de Nederlandse architectuur*, Rotterdam 1993, p. 258.
25 A. Evers, G.J.M. Sarlemijn, 'Tehuis voor bejaarden te Breda', *Bouwkundig Weekblad*, 70 (1952) 19/20, p. 145.
26 *Bouwstenen in het Damspel. Opstellen over de bouw van ziekenhuisvoorzieningen*, Utrecht 1983, p. 84.
27 H. van Bergeijk, *Jan Wils. De Stijl en verder*, Rotterdam 2007, pp. 56-59.

Compartmentalisation

1 C.A. Drogendijk, *Het protestants-christelijke ziekenhuis in Nederland*, p. 44.
2 Idem, p. 52.
3 W. Bruin, 'De Rusthoeve, tehuis voor ouden van dagen te Purmerend', *Bouwkundig Weekblad Architectura*, 60 (1938) 35, p. 289.

1960–1970
Building boom

1 J.J.P. Oud, 'Randstad dreigt kuststad te worden', *Bouw*, 21 (1966) 13, p. 471.
2 C. Lijnzaad, 'Het bejaardenvraagstuk – een maatschappijprobleem', *Forum*, 13 (1958) 5, p. 147.
3 M.J. van Lieburg, 'Overheid, medisch beroep in instellingswezen. De contouren van de overheidsbemoeienis met de infrastructuur van de Nederlandse gezondheidszorg in deze eeuw', in: R.B.M. Rigter (ed.), *Overheid en gezondheidszorg in de twintigste eeuw*, Rotterdam 1993, p. 66.
4 M. Roemer, 'Bed supply and utilization: a natural experiment', *Hospitals, Journal of the American Hospital Association*, (1961), 33, pp. 35-42. Quoted in: A. van der Zee, 'Vraag en Aanbod in de Gezondheidszorg', in: *Het ziekenhuis in de eenentwintigste eeuw. Een achtergrondstudie. Basisanalyse 1945–1988 en overzicht van toekomstonderzoek*, s.l. 1989, p. 235.
5 A. Ankoné, 'Greve's visie op planning en bouw. Over twintig jaar is één van de drie ziekenhuizen weg', *Het Ziekenhuiswezen*, 41 (1968), p. 744.
6 P. Muntendam, 'Gezondheidszorg in ontwikkeling', in: G. Schrijvers, J.M. Boot (ed.), *Een halve eeuw gezondheidszorg: 1950–2000*, Lochem [etc.] 1983, pp. 37-38.
7 F.J. van der Velde, 'Integratie en ziekenhuiszorg', in: *Het ziekenhuis in de eenentwintigste eeuw. Een achtergrondstudie. Basisanalyse 1945-1988 en overzicht van toekomstonderzoek*, p. 377, s.l. 1989.
8 B.T.G. de Jong, 'Zorgen over ziekenhuisplanning', in: *Nederlands Symposium Ziekenhuisbouw Amsterdam*, Amsterdam 1964, p. 56.
9 M. Plooij, 'Openingsrede', in *Nederlands Symposium Ziekenhuisbouw Amsterdam*, Amsterdam 1964, p. 51.
10 P.A. Heeres, 'Enkele gedachten over ziekenhuisbouw in deze tijd', *Bouwkundig Weekblad*, 76 (1958), p. 449.
11 W. Eijkelenboom, 'De architectuur. Holy-ziekenhuis in Vlaardingen', *Bouw*, 21 (1966) 40, p. 1526.
12 T. Noakes, P. James, *Hospital Architecture*, Harlow 1994, p. 14; A. Tengbom, 'Recent Developments in the Design of Hospitals in Scandinavia', *World Hospitals: l'Hôpital dans le Monde*, 2 (1966) 1, p. 3; G. Guez, 'Image ouverte de l'hôpital', *L'Architecture d'Aujourd'hui*, (1970) 120, p. 8.
13 'Ontwerp voor een gemeenteziekenhuis en gemeenteapotheek te Den Haag', *Polytechnisch Tijdschrift*, 20 (1965), p. 541B.
14 'Psychiatrisch ziekenhuis St. Franciscushof te Raalte', *Bouw*, 23 (1968) 8, pp. 301, 303.
15 'Architect Hendriks: Ontwerpers moeten de gemeenschapsidee "inbouwen"', *Baksteen*, 14 (1972) 4, p. 3.
16 'Onno Greiner: "Ik heb me aangepast aan de omliggende natuur..."', *Baksteen*, 14 (1972) 3, pp. 14-16.
17 M.A. Reinalda, 'Gebouwen voor bejaardenzorg', *Bouw*, 11 (1956) 4, p. 84.
18 C. Lijnzaad, 'Het bejaardenvraagstuk – een maatschappijprobleem', *Forum*, 13 (1958) 5, p. 146.
19 R. Nicolaï, *Typologie van Gebouwen. Handleiding bij het ontwerpen van verpleeghuizen voor somatisch zieken*, s.l. 1982, p. 17.
20 P.J. van Leeuwen, H. Schreuders, 'Ontwikkeling van de verpleeghuizen', in: *Bouwstenen in het Damspel*, Utrecht 1983, p. 85.
21 G. ten Cate, *EGM architecten*, Rotterdam 2003, p. 95.
22 'Bejaardencentrum Crabbehoff te Dordrecht', *Bouw*, 22 (1967) 9, pp. 335-336.
23 R.H. Fledderus, 'Het Zonnehuis te Vlaardingen', *Bouw*, 22 (1967) 12, p. 440.
24 Ibid.
25 *Voorschriften en wenken voor het ontwerpen van verzorgingstehuizen voor bejaarden (1965)*, The Hague 1966, p. 6.
26 'Voorschriften bouw bejaardenhuizen', *Bouw*, 21 (1966) 13, p. 471.

Standardisation

1 C.A. Vietsch, *Anamnese, diagnose, therapie: een onderzoek naar de bouwvoorbereiding van algemene ziekenhuizen*, Eindhoven 1987, p. 16.
2 Idem, p. 21.
3 F.W. van Gulick, *Aspecten van het ziekenhuis van de toekomst*, Utrecht 1969.
4 N. Mens, A. Tijhuis, *De architectuur van het ziekenhuis. Transformaties in de naoorlogse ziekenhuisbouw in Nederland*, Rotterdam 1999, p. 127.
5 I.C. Stofberg, 'Bejaardentehuizen in een productie-

stroom', *Bouw*, 23 (1968) 21, p. 832.

6 College bouw ziekenhuisvoorzieningen, *Signaleringsrapport inzake IFD-Bouwen. Uitbreidingen verpleeghuizen en verzorgingshuizen*, Utrecht 2001.

1970–1980
The critical Seventies

1 W. van Gorp, J.C.M. Hattinga Verschure, J.L.M. Zuidberg (ed.), *Heel het Ziekenhuis*, Lochem 1980, p. 256.

2 E. Bernatzik, 'Zivilisationsschäden bei Naturvölkern', in: E. Kühn, P. Vogler (hrsg.), *Medizin und Städtebau. Ein Handbuch für gesundheitlichen Städtebau*, München/Berlin/Vienna 1957, pp. 1-25. Bernatzik applied the following definition of 'primitive' peoples: 'Wir verstehen darunter jene kulturarmen Völker farbiger Rasse, deren Lebensbedingungen noch weitgehend von der Natur abhängig sind. Idem, p. 1. For a survey of the relation between urban planning and health see: M. Rodenstein, *'Mehr Licht, mehr Luft'. Gesundheitskonzepte im Städtebau seit 1750*, Frankfurt/Main/New York 1988.

3 'Het ziekenhuis van de toekomst', *Het Ziekenhuiswezen*, 33 (1960), p. 428.

4 L. Söderberg, 'Trends in Swedisch Hospital Design', *World Hospitals = l'Hôpital dans le Monde*, 2 (1965), p. 217.

5 Hassenpflug, prijsvraagontwerp voor een Academisch Ziekenhuis in München, 1955; K. Gutschow, 'Gedanken aus der Planungspraxis', *Architektur Wettbewerbe. Schriftenreihe für richtungweisendes bauen*, 28 (1960), p. 5.

6 'Hvidovre general hospital', *World Hospitals = l'Hôpital dans le Monde*, 3 (1966), p. 62.

7 *Le Corbusier. Oeuvre complète 1957–1965*, Zürich 1965, pp. 140-151.

8 W. Fuchs, R. Wischer, *H VEN LC. Le Corbusiers Krankenhausprojekt für Venedig*, Berlin 1985, p. 68.

9 H.P. Lenke, 'Under dem Einfluß des Strukturalismus. Das Krankenhausprojekt im Gesamtwerk', in: W. Fuchs, R. Wischer, *H VEN LC. Le Corbusiers Krankenhausprojekt für Venedig*, Berlin 1985, p. 58.

10 A. Tengbom, 'Recent Developments in the Design of Hospitals in Scandinavia', *World Hospitals = l'Hôpital dans le Monde*, 3 (1966), p. 3.

11 I. Rosenfield, geciteerd in J. Delrue, 'Van zieken-huis naar huis-om-te-genezen', *Plan*, (1977) 8, p. 8.

12 The following hospitals were visited: Diaconessenhuis in Leiden (1963), VU Ziekenhuis (1957-1966), Andreas Ziekenhuis (1969) and Sint Lucas Ziekenhuis (1968) in Amsterdam, Nicolaas Tulp Ziekenhuis in Amstelveen (1968), De Lichtenberg (1957) and Sint Elisabeth Ziekenhuis in Amersfoort (1969), Diaconessenhuis in Eindhoven (1966), Mariaziekenhuis in Tilburg (1966), Sint Hippolytusziekenhuis in Delft (1970), Sint Clara Ziekenhuis and Ikazia Ziekenhuis (1966) in Rotterdam, Sint Franciscusziekenhuis (1968) in Roosendaal, Centraal Ziekenhuis in Alkmaar, Sint Joseph Ziekenhuis in Heemskerk (1964), Juliana Ziekenhuis, Zaandam (1961), Diaconessen Ziekenhuis in Voorburg (1966), Ziekenhuis Oudenrijn in Utrecht (1968), Ziekenhuis De Weezenlanden in Zwolle (1967), Sint Radboudziekenhuis in Nijmegen (1956-1965), De Wever Ziekenhuis in Heerlen (1968), Algemeen Ziekenhuis in Schiedam (1969) and Diaconessen Ziekenhuis in Breda (1960).

13 J.B. Stolte, 'IHF Study Tour of Hospitals in the Netherlands', *World Hospitals = l'Hôpital dans le Monde*, 7 (1971), p. 27.

14 Zie *Het Ziekenhuis*, (1974), p. 99; rapport van de Centrale Raad voor de Volksgezondheid, 'Benadering van de ontwikkeling van de kosten van de Nederlandse gezondheidszorg in de periode 1950-1980', 1974.

15 R. Nicolaï, 'De stijging van de kosten van ziekenhuisbouw', in: *Het ziekenhuis in onze samenleving*, Amersfoort 1974.

16 *Jaarverslag College voor Ziekenhuisvoorzieningen en Ziekenhuiscommissie 1975*, p. 80. Utrecht.

17 *Jaarverslag College voor Ziekenhuisvoorzieningen en Ziekenhuiscommissie 1979*, pp. 126-127.

18 Idem, p. 113, Utrecht.

19 A.J.H. Thiadens (ed.), *Ziekenhuis menselijk en modern. De patiënt als kritische consument van intramurale gezondheidszorg*, Deventer 1972 [supplements 1973 and 1975], p. xvii.

20 Idem, pp. 7.6-11.

21 Idem, pp. 7.6-03.

22 Idem, pp. 7.6-29.

23 N. Mens, A. Tijhuis, *De architectuur van het ziekenhuis. Transformaties in de naoorlogse ziekenhuisbouw in Nederland*, Rotterdam 1999, p. 151.

24 'Ziekenhuis te Dordrecht', *Bouw*, 28 (1973) 43, p. 1280.

25 Ibid.

26 J. van den Noort, *Blokken op de bres. Geschiedenis van planning en bouw van het nieuwe Academisch Ziekenhuis Groningen*, Groningen 1999, p. 102.

27 S. Schmid, *Vrijheid is de beste medicijn. Over de democratische psychiatrie in Italië*, Amsterdam 1979.

28 E. Tellegen, *Waar was de dood nog meer*, Bilthoven 1971; C.A. van Eijk, *Laat ze het maar voelen... Een verhaal over psychiatrische inrichtingen*, Amsterdam 1981.

29 A.J. Heerma van Voss, 'De geschiedenis van de gekkenbeweging', in: *Voor de gek gehouden. Geschiedenis van de krankzinnigenzorg in Nederland*, Haarlem/Gouda 1982, p. 74.

30 *Basisfilosofie PC Jan Wier*, geciteerd in J. Huizenga, *Memorabele mensen en memorabele momenten uit de geschiedenis van de intramurale gezondheidszorg*, Lochem 1991, pp. 247-248.

31 C. van Winkel, *Modern leegte. Over kunst en openbaarheid*, Nijmegen 1999, p. 39.

32 G. Blok, J. Vijselaar (ed.), *De weg van Welterhof. 25 jaar psychiatrie in Oostelijk Zuid-Limburg*, Utrecht 1999, p. 49, 33.

33 'Nota bejaardenbeleid 1970', *Bouw*, 25 (1970) 41, p. 1571.

34 'Huisvesting van bejaarden', *Bouw*, 8 (1953) 17, p. 318.

35 *College voor Ziekenhuisvoorzieningen. Jaarverslag 1981*, Utrecht, p. 107.

36 Idem, p. 102.

37 J.A.J. Meijer, 'De bejaarde als mens', *Bouw*, 11 (1956) 4, pp. 84, 85.

38 'L. van der Meer, 'Verzorgingstehuizen voor bejaarden. Onderdeel van een sociaal-structureel bejaardenbeleid', *Bouw*, 25 (1970) 9, p. 336.

39 B.B. Westerveld, 'Bejaardentehuizen en -woningen', *Forum*, 13 (1958) 4, p. 115; '"Geef bejaardentehuis meer contact met de buitenwereld"', *Bouw*, 14 (1959) 17, p. 471.

40 'Spiegel van de week', *Bouw*, 25 (1970) 19, p. 813.

41 R.J. van Zonneveld, 'Medische aspecten van de huisvesting van bejaarden', *Forum*, 13 (1958) 4, p. 132.

42 'Bejaardencomplex voor Cappelle aan den IJssel', *Bouw*, 25 (1970) 20, p. 887.

43 'Bejaardenhuis "De Esdoorn" te Zwolle', *Bouw*, 29 (1974) 5, p. 115-117; 'Bejaardenwoningen te Zoetermeer', *Bouw*, 27 (1972) 7, p. 249.

44 'Bejaardenwoningen te Zoetermeer, *Bouw*, 32 (1977) 11, pp. 291-294.

45 G.J.V. Hotze, 'Openbaar verkeer in en om een bejaardencentrum', *Bouw*, 28 (1973) 1, pp. 11-12.

46 N. Mens, *De architectuur van het psychiatrisch ziekenhuis*, Wormer 2003, p. 269.

47 'Verzorgingscomplex voor bejaarden te Amsterdam', *Bouw*, 31 (1976) 12, p. 207.

48 N. de Vreeze, *Woningbouw, inspiratie & ambitie. Kwalitatieve grondslagen van de sociale woningbouw in Nederland*, Almere 1993.

49 L. de Klerk, *Particuliere plannen. Denkbeelden en initiatieven van de stedelijke elite inzake de volkswoningbouw en de stedebouw in Rotterdam, 1860-1950*, Rotterdam 1998.

50 'Bejaardencomplex Zonnetrap te Rotterdam-Lombardijen', *Bouw*, 35 (1980) 18, p. 64.

Housing for the mentally handicapped

1 *Bouwstenen in het damspel. Opstellen over de bouw van ziekenhuisvoorzieningen*, Utrecht 1983, p. 152.

2 Stagg/bbi, *Rapportage doeleinden-analyse zwakzinnigenzorg*, Amsterdam, Utrecht 1977.

3 '"De Merwebolder" te Sliedrecht', *Bouw*, 28 (1973) 6, p. 829.

4 P.R. Siebesma, 'Kleinschalig wonen. Van gezinsvervangend tehuis naar begeleid zelfstandig wonen', in: G.H. van Gemert, R.B. Minderaa (ed.), *Zorg voor mensen met een verstandelijke handicap*, Assen 1997, p. 229.

5 W.H. van der Sluijs, M.A. Maaskant, 'Huizen of luchtkastelen? Wonen door mensen met een verstandelijke handicap', in: O. Koekebakker (ed.), *Zorg voor morgen. Ontwerpen voor de gezondheidszorg'*, Rotterdam 1997, pp. 27-28.

6 J.N. Broeders, 'De inrichting', in: G.H. van Gemert, R.B. Minderaa (ed.), *Zorg voor mensen met een verstandelijke handicap*, Assen 1997, p. 240.

1980–1990
Flexibility and urbanity

1 N.A.A. Baakman, 'De veranderde legitimaties van het Nederlandse Ziekenhuisbouwbeleid 1945-1980', *Mens en Maatschappij*, (1987) 4, p. 351.

2 *Jaarverslag College voor Ziekenhuisvoorzieningen 1982*, Utrecht 1983, p. 13.

3 P. Mulder, 'Met de WZV in de hand, sluit de minister ziekenhuizen in het hele land. Overleg over beddenreductie is mogelijk, maar uitkomsten staan nu vast', *Het Ziekenhuis*, (1982), p. 759. This article includes the list of the hospitals due for closure.

4 P. Mulder, 'Met de WZV in de hand, sluit de minister ziekenhuizen in het hele land. Overleg over beddenreductie is mogelijk, maar uitkomsten staan nu vast', *Het Ziekenhuis*, (1982), p. 759.

5 J. Rentes de Carvalho, 'Door het oog van de gebruiker', in: G. Staal, H. Wolters (ed.), *Holland in vorm. Vormgeving in Nederland 1945-1987*, The Hague 1987.

6 A. Tuns, 'Flexibiliteit. NZi beknot vrijheid in constructie', *Architectuur/Bouwen*, (1991) 6/7, p. 28.

7 L. Veldhoen, 'Nieuw psychiatrisch oord in Nijmegen: "geïsoleerd gekkengetto in de bossen"', *NRC Handelsblad*, 18 January 1983.

8 J. Huizenga, *Memorabele mensen en memorabele momenten uit de geschiedenis van de intramurale gezondheidszorg*, Lochem 1991, p. 241.

9 H. van de Beek, J.W. van Zuthem, *Thuis in de samenleving. Samenwerken aan maatschappelijke ondersteuning vanuit beschermd en begeleid wonen in de geestelijke gezondheidszorg*, Utrecht 2002, p. 14.

10 N. Mens, A. Tijhuis, *De architectuur van het ziekenhuis. Transformaties in de naoorlogse ziekenhuisbouw in Nederland*, Rotterdam 1999, p. 63.

11 L. Perquin, *'Het Boston model', een alternatief voor 24-uurs psychiatrische opname?*, Amsterdam 1985.

12 J. Huizenga, *Memorabele mensen en memorabele momenten uit de geschiedenis van de intramurale gezondheidszorg*, Lochem 1991, p. 228.

13 J. Cannegieter, 'Psychiatrisch ziekenhuis Helmerzijde. Een therapeutische woonwijk in Enschede', *Architectuur/Bouwen* 1 (1985)10, pp. 33-38.

14 L.J.A. Straathof, *Uittreksel basisplannen Psychiatrisch Ziekenhuis Zeeland*, Goes 1977, p. 22.

15 J. Molenaar, 'Architectuur achter de zintuigen van de waarnemer. ESTEC en Padua, twee nieuwe werken van Aldo en Hannie van Eyck', *Archis* (1990) 1, p. 32.

16 E. Koster, 'Alternatief functionalisme in low-tech en barok. Twee projecten van Aldo en Hannie van Eyck', *de Architect* 20 (1989), 12, p. 54.

17 *Deconcentratie. Een nieuw APZ in de gezondheidsregio Dordrecht*, Bennekom 1983, p. 6.

18 J. Vijselaar, (ed.), *Gesticht in de duinen. De geschiedenis van de provinciale psychiatrische ziekenhuizen van Noord-Holland van 1849-1994*, Hilversum 1997, p. 222.

19 T. Vroon: in M. Spanjer, *Dynamiek in Steen. Jubileumuitgave College voor Ziekenhuisvoorzieningen, 1972-1997*, Delft 1997, p. 78.

20 B. Biemold, M. Noordmans, 'Woningbedrijf: van flats serviceflats maken', *Bouw*, 42 (1987) 17, pp. 34-35.

21 *Advies inzake het experiment aanpasbaar bouwen*, Rotterdam 1991, p. 3.

22 I. Folgerts, E. Kalle (ed.), *Seniorenlabel. Consumenten-*

keurmerk voor Ouderenhuisvesting. Versie experimenteerfase 1993/1994, Rotterdam 1993, p. 8.
23 *Senioren thuis test*, s.l., s.a.
24 J.H. van der Veek, F. van Holland, M.J.J. van Leent, *Bestaande woningen aanpassen voor ouderen. Ontwerpanalyse van acht praktijkprojecten*, The Hague 1994; *Aanpasbaar bouwen en verbouwen. Doelbewust de toekomst tegemoet*, s.l., s.a..
25 L. Donk, B. Fris, J. Lamers, *Vrijheid, Zelfstandigheid & Vriendschap. Groepswonen van ouderen*, Amsterdam 1989.
26 'Woongemeenschappen van ouderen', *Woonkwaliteit*, 2 (1990) 9, p. 11.
27 J. Peters, C. Woldringh, *Groepswonen voor ouderen*, Nijmegen 1989, p. 80.
28 P. Sep, *Tot in lengte van dagen. Zelfstandige ouderenhuisvesting en architectuur*, Amsterdam 1993.
29 A. Lambert, 'De huisvesting van ouderen. Zelfstandig wonen in een zorgzame samenleving', *Architectuur/Bouwen*, 4 (1988) 1, p. 13.
30 P. Sep, *Tot in lengte van dagen. Zelfstandige ouderenhuisvesting en architectuur*, Amsterdam 1993, p. 30.
31 R. Meijer, 'Woongebouw Kreilerburcht', in: A. Devolder, H. Damen (ed.), *Architectuur Rotterdam 1970-1995. 75 gebouwen gedocumenteerd*, Rotterdam 1995.
32 J.C.M. Hattinga Verschure, *Het verschijnsel zorg*, Lochem 1977, p. 114.
33 J.C.M. Hattinga Verschure, *Zelfredzame ouderen*, Lochem/Ghent, 1987, p. 12.
34 Idem, p. 104.
35 *Ouderen en hun woonbehoeften*, Delft 1981, p. 53.

Flexibility

1 W. Algra, '"Ziekenhuizen zijn de meest gecompliceerde gebouwen"', *Het Ziekenhuis*, 24 (1994) 3, p. 116.
2 R. Nicolaï, K.H. Dekker, *Flexibiliteit als bouwstrategie voor een veranderende gezondheidszorg. Band I handleiding*, Utrecht [1991], p. 3.
3 W.Q. Stolwijk, *Flexibiliteit in ziekenhuisbouw*, Arnhem 1987, p. 123.
4 R. Nicolaï, K.H. Dekker, *Flexibiliteit als bouwstrategie voor en veranderende gezondheidszorg. Band I handleiding*, Utrecht [1991], XVI, 11. The study was commissioned and published by the NZI.
5 R. Nicolaï, K.H. Dekker, *Flexibiliteit als bouwstrategie voor en veranderende gezondheidszorg. Band I handleiding*, Utrecht [1991], XVII, pp. 15-22. The four hospitals investigated were: Julianaziekenhuis in Zaandam, Bethesda Ziekenhuis in Hoogeveen, Sint Clara Ziekenhuis in Rotterdam en Sint Elisabeth Ziekenhuis in Amersfoort. For the research see: Vol. II supplementary information.
6 M. Le Mandat, *Prévoir l'espace hospitalier*, Paris 1989, p. 3.
7 Idem, p. 13.
8 ' Arnhem: Ziekenhuis Rijnstate nadert zijn voltooiing', *Stedenbouw*, (1994) 512, p. 63.
9 N. Mens, A. Tijhuis, *De architectuur van het ziekenhuis. Transformaties in de naoorlogse ziekenhuisbouw in Nederland*, Rotterdam 1999, p. 171.
10 R. Nicolaï, 'NZi-rapport niets zo veranderlijk als een ziekenhuis', *Architectuur en Bouwen*, (1991) 6/7, p. 25.
11 A. Tuns, 'NZi beknot vrijheid in constructie', *Architectuur en Bouwen*, (1991) 6/7, p. 28; H.J. Tennekes, 'Duur NZi-model kan goedkoper', *Architectuur en Bouwen*, (1991) 6/7, p. 31.
12 N. Mens, A. Tijhuis, *De architectuur van het ziekenhuis. Transformaties in de naoorlogse ziekenhuisbouw in Nederland*, Rotterdam 1999, p. 172.
13 T. Zoethout, 'Bestemmingsvrije zorgbouw', *Stedebouw & Architectuur*, 26 (2009) 9, p. 20-21.
14 R. Scheerder, M. Verweij, 'Flexibel bouwen. Vastgoed in de cure op een kruispunt van wegen', *Medisch Contact*, 60 (2005) 5, p. 190.
15 Idem, p. 191.

1992–2002
Changes in the health care landscape

1 R. Gortemaker, G. Mulkens, 'Luchthavengebouw is vertrekpunt voor nieuw ziekenhuis', *ZorgVisie*, (1996) 15, pp. 30-32.
2 O. Koekebakker (ed.), *Zorg voor morgen. Ontwerpen voor de gezondheidszorg*, Rotterdam 1997; N. Mens, A. Tijhuis, 'Het ziekenhuis van de toekomst', *Archis*, (1998) 1, pp. 78-79.
3 Letter from minister E. Borst-Eilers to W.B. Meijer, General secretary of the Hospital Provisions Board, 23 July 1997.
4 O. Koekebakker (ed.), *Zorg voor morgen. Ontwerpen voor de gezondheidszorg*, Rotterdam 1997, pp. 14-15.
5 Idem, p. 39.
6 Letter dr. E. Borst-Eilers, minister of Health, Welfare and Sport to the Hospital Provisions Board, 23 June 1997.
7 *de Volkskrant*, 27 June 1997.
8 Minister VWS E. Borst, letter and report 'Big Hospitals Study Tour', 31 March 2000.
9 G. Blok, 'Enkele reis op z'n retour', in: J. Vijselaar (ed.), *Gesticht in de duinen. De geschiedenis van de provinciale psychiatrische ziekenhuizen van Noord-Holland van 1849 tot 1994*, Hilversum 1997, p. 238.
10 N. Mens, 'De bouwgeschiedenis van de Willem Arntsz Hoeve', *Open*, 1 (2002) 2, p. 73-77.
11 K. Havik, 'Mecanoo gebruikt kloostertypologie voor zorginstelling', *de Architect Interieur*, (2002) 7, pp. 60-63.
12 G. Huiskes, R. van der Kroeg, *Van Rooms tot Rome, 1952-2002. Van Sint Franciscushof naar Zwolse Poort*, Zwolle 2002, p. 92.
13 C.Th. Bakker, G. Blok, J. Vijselaar, *Delta. Negentig jaar psychiatrie aan de Oude Maas*, Utrecht 1999, p. 168.
14 Geciteerd in R. Katz, 'Behandelfilosofie is de belangrijkste bouwsteen', *Het Ziekenhuis*, 25 (1995) 2, p. 23.
15 *De Opmaat. Wat vooraf ging aan de bouw van de MFE Midden Twente*, [s.p., s.a.].
16 *Bureau Presentatie Gezondheidszorg*, [Amsterdam] 2002.
17 H. de Haan, 'Nieuwe kliniek lijkt op een paleis', *de Volkskrant*, 9 June 2001.
18 *Ouderenzorg met toekomst. Advies van de Commissie modernisering ouderenzorg aan de minister van Welzijn, Volksgezondheid en Cultuur*, The Hague 1994, p. 12.
19 F. Hazewinkel, *Van 'slaapzaal' naar 'levensloopbestendige woning'. Van 'handen uit de mouwen' naar 'handen op de rug'. Veertig jaar Stichting Humanitas Rotterdam 1959-1999*, Rotterdam 1999, p. 94-102; E. Bassa, G. van Nifterik, 'Op de grens van wonen en zorg. Levensloopbestendige woningen in Bergwegcomplex Rotterdam', *Architectuur/Bouwen*, (1996) 10, p. 12-15.
20 R. Schippers, *Het subsidie-instrument kritisch bekeken. Evaluatie van de tijdelijke woonzorgstimuleringsregeling*, [The Hague 2004; master's thesis].
21 N.Y. Schuyt-Lucassen, G.J.F. Leene, P.P.J. Houben, *Hofjes in perspectief. Een onderzoek naar de identiteit en actualiteit van de Hofjes Codde en Van Beresteyn in het licht van de modernisering van de ouderenhuisvesting*, Amsterdam 1995; N.Y. Schuijt-Lucassen, G.J.F. Leene, P.P.J. Houben, *Hofjes in perspectief. Al eeuwen een moderne woonvorm voor ouderen*, Bussum 1997.

University Medical Centres

1 The term 'academic hospital' has in most cases been replaced by the term 'university medical centre' (UMC). The UMC is a merger of the university hospital and the medical faculty. At first these training institutes fell under the Ministry of Education, later the hospital sector fell under the aegis of the ministry responsible for health, and since the middle of the 1990s this ministry has been responsible for everything connected with the University Medical Centres – that even turned out to be one of their raisons d'être. (The Ministry of Education still pays one-quarter of the expenses of these centres.)
2 J. Leupen, 'De plannen van het nieuwe Academisch Ziekenhuis te Amsterdam', *Het Ziekenhuiswezen*, 31 (1958), pp. 247-255.
3 M. Jonker, D. Schuiling, 'Godshuis, gasthuis, ziekenhuis, medisch centrum, cité medicale', *Wonen-TA/BK*, 24 (1974), p. 27.
4 'Interview met ir. C.A. Doets te Baarn', *Architectuur/Bouwen*, 2 (1986) 2, p. 29.
5 D.H. Cox, 'Het Academisch Medisch Centrum. De eerste uit een reeks van academische ziekenhuizen', *Architectuur/Bouwen*, 2 (1986) 11, p. 19.
6 'Health Sciences Centre McMaster University, Kanada', *Deutsche Bauzeitung*, 1969, p. 717.
7 'Questo ospedale è particolarmente interessante per l'approccio al processo costruttivo considerato non come un atto temporalmente definito, ma come un "continuum" che persiste anche dopo il completamento della costruzione.' F.R. Prodi, A. Stocchetti, *L'architettura dell'ospedale*, Florence 1990, p. 84.
8 'Health Sciences Centre McMaster University', *World Hospitals*, 1970, pp. 34-38; 'McMaster University Health Sciences Centre Hamilton Ontario (Canada)', *Werk/Oeuvre*, 1974, pp. 157-162; N.J. Meyer, 'De relatie tussen leefbaarheid, programma's van eisen en bouwplannen bij een academisch ziekenhuis (II)', *Het Ziekenhuis*, 7 (1977), pp. 290-294.
9 J.G. Constant, *AMC gebouwd*, Wormer 1984.
10 C. Zwinkels, 'Een gebouw als een woonwijk. Academisch Ziekenhuis Utrecht van EGM', *de Architect*, (1989) 11, pp. 121-129.
11 P. van Dam, *Academisch Ziekenhuis Leiden. Uit de steigers*, Leiden 1985; P. van Dam, *Academisch Ziekenhuis Leiden*, Leiden [1990].
12 K. Bosma, 'Tussen leed en vermaak: vijf academische ziekenhuizen', in: R. Brouwers (red.), *Architectuur in Nederland. Jaarboek 1989-1990*, Deventer 1990, p. 32.
13 G. Passchier, *Academisch Ziekenhuis Maastricht. AZM*, Maastricht 1991, p. 8.
14 Idem, p. 12.
15 J. van den Noort, *Blokken op de Bres. Geschiedenis van planning en bouw van het nieuwe Academisch Ziekenhuis Groningen (1967-1997)*, Groningen 1999.

2002–2010
Beyond health care architecture: the way to the future

1 M. Verweij, F. Bisschop, 'Ingrijpende systeemwijziging voor financiering zorgvastgoed', *ZM*, (2006) 1, pp. 7-10.
2 The following was published in connection with the conference/congress: C. Wagenaar (ed.), *The Architecture of Hospitals*, Rotterdam 2006.
3 *Au! Bouwen aan de architectuur van de zorg*, Utrecht [etc.] 2007.
4 The Isala partnership of architects (AMI) was specially created for this hospital consisting of Alberts & Van Huut, a/d amstel architecten and Alberts, Van Huut & Partners.
5 N. Mens, *Zorgboulevards. Verkenningen in het zorglandschap van morgen*, Bussum 2005.
6 M. Verweij, F. Bisschop, 'Ingrijpende systeemwijziging voor financiering zorgvastgoed', *ZM*, (2006) 1, pp. 7-10.
7 There was room for improvement in logistical processes in health care. The TPG postal service, where logistics is all-important, was asked to conduct an investigation. TPG, *Het kan écht: betere zorg voor minder geld. Sneller beter. De logistiek in de zorg*, Amsterdam 2004.
8 N. Mens, C. Wagenaar, *Anders bouwen voor betere zorg. De toekomst van de polikliniek*, Amsterdam 2007, pp. 86-87.
9 N. Mens, C. Wagenaar, *Anders bouwen voor betere zorg. De toekomst van de polikliniek*, Amsterdam 2007.
10 'Het decentrale ziekenhuis, Katalysator van de stedelijke vernieuwing', *Lay-out*, no. 6; 'Urban Hospitality. Kleinschalige zorg in de stedelijke omgeving', *Lay-out*, no. 7.
11 M. Hinkema, J. Nauta, 'De chirurg in de buurt. Het

relatieve succes van decentrale ziekenhuisvoorzieningen', *Medisch Contact* 64 (2009) 33/34, pp. 1392-1395.
12 Kirsten Hannema, 'Revalideren als in een luxe hotel', *de Volkskrant*, 4 March 2010.
13 UR architects, *De psychiatrische instelling ontmanteld*, October 2009.
14 H. Tilman, 'Bejaardenhuis gepasseerd station. Grotere rol voor architectuur in de zorg', *de Architect*, 37 (2006) 10, pp. 53-54.
15 M.G. Boekholdt, 'Verpleeg- en verzorgingshuis voorbij', in: P. van Beek, H. Hoes (ed.), *Zorg en Architectuur. Verslag Jubileumcongres Bouwkunde*, Utrecht 2002, p. 22.
16 J.M.D. Boot, *Organisatie van de Gezondheidszorg*, Assen 2007, p. 58.
17 *De toekomst van het verzorgingshuis*, s.l. 2004.
18 Letter from the Netherlands Board for Healthcare Institutions to the state secretary for Health, Welfare and Sport, 16 October 2006.
19 T. Mandemaker, L. Christ, *De volledige extramuralisering van het verzorgingshuis*, Utrecht 2005.
20 D.J.M. van der Voordt, D. Terpstra, *Verpleeghuizen: varianten en alternatieven*, Delft 1995, p. 44.
21 M. Spanjer, interview with Gerrit I. Almekinders, Federation of nursing institutions, in: *Dynamiek in Steen. Jubileumuitgave College voor Ziekenhuisvoorzieningen 1972-1997*, Delft 1997, p. 85.
22 H. Nouws, *Het transformatieproces van verzorgingshuizen: vier recente cases. "Gundaphorus' Paleis"*, Utrecht 2004, p. 4.
23 H. Tilman, 'Bejaardenhuis gepasseerd station. Grotere rol voor architectuur in de zorg', *de Architect*, 37 (2006) 10, p. 49.
24 J.E. Abrahamse, 'De buitenwereld binnen. Verpleeghuis Bruggerbosch in Enschede door Jorissen Simonetti architecten', *de Architect*, 37 (2006) 10, p. 82.
25 Jeroen Singelenberg, 'Welke innovaties hebben echt het aangezicht van woonzorgland veranderd?', in: *Innovatieve kracht in wonen en zorg*, Utrecht 2008, p. 8.
26 *Multifunctioneel bouwen in de ouderenzorg*, Utrecht 2004.
27 *Verzorgd wonen: een concept met toekomst!*, Enschede 2005, p. 38.
28 *Huisvesting van ouderen op het breukvlak van twee eeuwen*, The Hague 1997.
29 M.H. Boon, 'Voorbeeld Vinex-project: IJburg, wijk zonder scheidslijnen', in: H. Priemus, E. Philipsen (ed.), *Levensloopbestendig in Europees perspectief*, Delft 2000, p. 58.
30 K.G. Luijkx, D. Brinkhof, 'Behoeften wonen, welzijn en zorg in beeld', *ZM Magazine*, 22 (2006) 6, pp. 2-5.
31 VROM, VWS, *Beter (t)huis in de buurt. Actieplan Samenwerken aan welzijn en zorg, 2007-2011*, The Hague 2007.
32 P. Bekkering, 'Ontwikkelen voor Medioren', *Stedebouw & Architectuur*, 25 (2008) 9, pp. 10-13.
33 A. van Berlo, *Veilig en comfortabel wonen*, Knegsel 1994.
34 P. Bekkering, 'Domotica aan vooravond van doorbraak', *Stedebouw & Architectuur*, 25 (2008) 9, pp. 26-29.
35 R. Hartgers, 'Amerikaanse praktijken? Seniorensteden in Nederland', *Stedebouw & Ruimtelijke Ordening*, 88 (2007) 1, pp. 33-35.
36 R. Hartgers, 'Zelfstandig wonen', *Stedebouw & Ruimtelijke Ordening*, 88 (2007) 1, p. 36.

Healing environment

1 P. Vogler, E. Kühn (hrsg.), *Medizin und Städtebau. Ein Handbuch für gesundheitlichen Städtebau*, Munich 1957.
2 V.K. Dorris, 'Health Trends', *Architecture*, 82 (1993) 3, p. 93.
3 'Boston Symposium Addresses Healing Designs', *Architecture*, January 1992, p. 75.
4 D.J.M. van der Voordt, D. Terpstra, *Verpleeghuizen: varianten en alternatieven*, Delft 1995, p. 52.
5 'Vraaggestuurde zorg in verpleeghuis. Interview met Wilma van den Groenendaal', in: N. Mens, C. Wagenaar, *Healing Environment. Anders bouwen voor betere zorg*, Bussum 2009, p. 109.

Conclusion

1 The term 'window hospital' was introduced by Frans Jaspers, member of Executive Board University Medical Center Groningen (UMCG).

Bibliography

40 jaar bouwen voor ouderen, 1950-1990, Amsterdam 1991

Aanpak van de Woonomgeving, The Hague 1994
Aanpassing van de woningvoorraad, The Hague 1994
Abrahamse, J.E., 'De buitenwereld binnen. Verpleeghuis Bruggerbosch in Enschede door Jorissen Simonetti architecten', *de Architect*, 37 (2006) 10, pp. 82-85
Abram, J., T. Riley, *The Filter of Reason*, New York 1990
De Academische ziekenhuizen in Nederland, Utrecht 1993
Advies inzake het experiment aanpasbaar bouwen, Rotterdam 1991
Advies inzake het experimententhema serviceplus bij huurwoningen (als onderdeel van het experimentenprogramma Ouderenhuisvesting/Diensten aan Huis), Rotterdam [1994]
Algra, W., '"Ziekenhuizen zijn de meest gecompliceerde gebouwen"', *Het Ziekenhuis*, 24 (1994) 3, p. 116
Algra, W., 'De lange weg van het APZ Zuidoost-Friesland. Bedden hadden we zo mogen bouwen', *Zorgvisie*, 26 (1996) 14, pp. 14-18
Alle ontwerpers gebruiken onderzoek. Evidence-Based Design in de praktijk, Utrecht 2009
Allen, R.W., I. von Karolyi, *Hospital Planning Handbook*, New York 1976
Amersfoort, J.M.M. van, 'De huisvesting van bejaarden', *Bouw*, 20 (1965) 41, pp. 1508-1509
d'Ancona, H., 'Woonstijl – en niet leeftijd – moet bindend buurtelement worden', *Bouw*, 31 (1976) 20, pp. 349-351
Ankoné, A., 'Greve's visie op planning en bouw. Over twintig jaar is één van de drie ziekenhuizen weg', *Het Ziekenhuiswezen*, 41 (1968), p. 744
'Architect Hendriks: Ontwerpers moeten de gemeenschapsidee "inbouwen"', *Baksteen*, 14 (1972) 4, pp. 1-8
'Architektenburo Campman – Tennekes: Complexe, grootschalige gebouwen herkenbaar en vooral leefbaar ontwerpen', *Progres Projekten*, December 1984, pp. 16-19
Architektengroep Duintjer bv, Amsterdam 1985
'Arnhem: Ziekenhuis Rijnstate nadert zijn voltooiing', *Stedenbouw*, 46 (1994) 512, pp. 63-64
Au. Bouwen aan de Architectuur van de Zorg, Utrecht, Groningen 2007
Aurousseau, P., R. Cheverry, *L'Hôpital de Demain*, Paris 1964
Axeisson, S., D. Lindberg, 'Trends in hospital care', *Hospital Management International*, 1991, pp. 223-225
AZG ontwikkelingsplan 76, Rotterdam [s.a.]

Baakman, N., *Kritiek van het openbare bestuur. Besluitvorming over de bouw van ziekenhuizen in Nederland tussen 1960 en 1985*, Nijmegen 1990
Baakman, N.A.A., 'De veranderende legitimaties van het Nederlandse ziekenhuisbouwbeleid', *Mens en Maatschappij*, 1987, no. 62, pp. 340-357
Bak, J. (et al., ed.), *J. Duiker bouwkundig ingenieur*, Rotterdam 1982
Bakker, C.Th., G. Blok, J. Vijselaar, *Delta, negentig jaar psychiatrie aan de Oude Maas*, Utrecht 1999
Balen, H.J. van, 'Achtergronden en problemen bij ziekenhuisbouw', *Katholiek Bouwblad*, 34 (1967), pp. 540-562
Ban, W. van den, 'De betekenis van historisch bezit. Ziekenhuisarchitectuur goede indicatie voor visie op de gezondheidszorg', *Het Ziekenhuis*, 16 (1986) 8, pp. 269-272
Banning, C., *Bouwplannen van verpleeg- en behandelingsinrichtingen*, *Bouw* 3 (1948) 5, p. IV
Barnhoorn, J.A.J., *De Moderne Psychiatrische Inrichting en de Nieuwere Behandelmethode van Geesteszieken* [offprint from *Ons Ziekenhuis*] s.a. s.p.
Barnhoorn, J.A.J., L.A.M. Pennock, J.P. de Smet, *Gedenkschrift St. Willibrordusstichting 1929-1954*, s.p. 1954
Bassa, E., G. van Nifterik, 'Op de grens van wonen en zorg. Levensloopbestendige woningen in Bergwegcomplex Rotterdam', *Architectuur/Bouwen*, 12 (1996) 10, pp. 12-15
Becker, H.A. (ed.), *Het ziekenhuis in de eenentwintigste eeuw. Een achtergrondstudie. Basisanalyse 1945-1988 en overzicht van toekomstonderzoek*, Utrecht 1989
Becker, H.M., *Verboden af te blijven. Het herinneringsmuseum, spiegel van Humanitas' zorgfilosofie*, Delft 2008
Beek, P. van, H. Hoes (ed.), *Zorg en architectuur. Verslag Jubileumcongres Bouwcollege*, Utrecht 2002
Beek, W.J.A., *De toepassing van systeembouw bij ziekenhuizen*, IJsselstein 1970
'Behoefte aan bedden in verpleeghuizen groeit', *Bouw*, 32 (1977) 19, p. VI
'Bejaardencentrum Crabbehoff te Dordrecht', *Bouw*, 22 (1967) 9, pp. 335-336
'Bejaardencomplex voor Capelle aan den IJssel', *Bouw*, 25 (1970) 20, p. 887
'Bejaardencomplex Zonnetrap te Rotterdam-Lombardijen', *Bouw*, 35 (1980) 18, pp. 63-67
'Bejaardenhuis "De Esdoorn" te Zwolle', *Bouw*, 29 (1974) 5, pp. 115-117
'De bejaardenhuisvesting in internationaal verband', *Bouw*, 20 (1965) 49, pp. 1891-1895
'Bejaardenwoningen te Zoetermeer', *Bouw*, 27 (1972) 7, p. 249
'Bejaardenwoningen te Zoetermeer', *Bouw*, 32 (1977) 11, pp. 291-294
Bekkering, P., 'Domotica aan vooravond van doorbraak', *Stedebouw & Architectuur*, 25 (2008) 9, pp. 26-29
Bekkering, P., 'Ontwikkelen voor Medioren', *Stedebouw & Architectuur*, 25 (2008) 9, pp. 10-13
Bennekom advies, *Multifunctionele eenheid geen droom maar werkelijkheid. Bouwprojectdocumentatie*, Bennekom 1993
Berg, L. van den, 'Rijp voor paviljoen 3. Een eeuw psychiatrische zorg', *Ons Amsterdam*, 41 (1989) 11, pp. 266-273
Berg, L. van den, *Rijp voor paviljoen III. Krankzinnig in Amsterdam vanaf 1565*, Amsterdam 1989
Berg, M. van den (ed.), *Bouwkundige uitgangspunten van woonzorgprojecten*, Rotterdam 1992
Bergeijk, H. van, *Jan Wils. De Stijl en verder*, Rotterdam 2007
Bergvelt, D. (ed.), *'Dan heb je alles in de buurt'. Ideeën over een voor ouderen geschikte woonomgeving*, Rotterdam 1991
Bergvelt, D. (ed.), *Woningcorporaties en ouderenbeleid. Van aanleunwoning tot zorggarantie*, Rotterdam 1992
Bergvelt, D. (ed.), *Wonen met zorg. Gebouw en financiering van vijf lichte projecten*, Rotterdam 1993
Bergvelt, D., A. Janzen, J. Singelenberg (ed.), *Zorg dat je thuis blijft wonen. Alternatieven voor het verzorgings- of verpleeghuis*, Rotterdam 1992
Bergvelt, D., J. Leijen, H. Nouws, *Kleinschalig wonen voor dementerenden. Een waaier aan ervaringen*, Amersfoort 2000
Bergvelt, D., H. van Rossum, *Een tweede jeugd. Ouderenhuisvesting in ontwikkeling*, Amsterdam 2004
Bergvelt, D., H. van Rossum, J. Oosterbaan, *Het beste van drie werelden. De architectuur van wonen en zorg*, Amsterdam 2002
Bergvelt, D., R. Scherpenisse, J. Singelenberg, 'Zelfstandig wonen met zorg aan huis', in: *Praktijkhandboek bouw en beheer. Wonen met zorg voor ouderen*, Houten/Diegem 1998
Berkemeier, B.L., G.C. Kaper, J.R.S.K. Vleesblok (ed.), *Ziekenhuisplanning als schouwtoneel. Opstellen over de planning van de intramurale gezondheidszorg en de Wet ziekenhuisvoorzieningen*, Leidschendam 1982
Berlo, A. van, *Veilig en comfortabel wonen*, Knegsel 1994
Berlo, A. van, P. Vermijs, *Domotica opent deuren*, Knegsel 1993
Berns, A.W.C., *De Gasthuizen van Amsterdam van de 14de eeuw tot heden*, Amsterdam 1883, p. 55
Besamusca-Ekelschot, A., P. de Natris, 'Debat Toekomst van het APZ (II). Ziekenhuis en samenleving zijn uitersten van een continuüm', *Het Ziekenhuis*, 24 (1994) 9, pp. 400-402
Beusekom, H.G. van, *Woningbouw. Problemen en perspectieven*, Amsterdam 1944
Beusekom, H.G. van, *Woningvoorziening in een nieuwen tijd*, Alphen aan den Rijn 1946
Beusekom, H.G. van, 'Mogelijkheden voor de Huisvesting van Bejaarden', *Tijdschrift voor maatschappelijk werk*, 26 (1948) 13, pp. 200-202
Beusekom, H.G. van, 'Een kwart eeuw bejaardenhuisvesting', *Bouw*, 25 (1970) 1, p. 10
Biemold, B., M. Noordmans, 'Woningbedrijf: van flats serviceflats maken', *Bouw*, 42 (1987) 17, pp. 34-35
Binet, J.-L., *Les architectes de la médecine*, Besançon 1996

Binneveld, H., *Filantropie, repressie en medische zorg. Geschiedenis van de inrichtingspsychiatrie*, Deventer 1985
Binneveld, J., 'Om de plaats van de psychiatrische inrichting', in: J. van Genabeek (ed.), *Balans en perspectief van de Nederlandse cultuurgeschiedenis. Het wonen*, Amsterdam 1990, pp. 64-82
Binneveld, J.M.W., 'De organisatie van de geestelijke gezondheidszorg in de 19e eeuw. Het ontstaan van het krankzinnigengesticht', *Groniek*, 15 (1981) 71, pp. 37-40
Binneveld, J.M.W. (et al.), *Een psychiatrisch verleden. Uit de geschiedenis van de psychiatrie*, Baarn 1982
Binneveld, J.M.W., M.J. van Lieburg, *Psychiatric Reform in the Netherlands in the 19th Century*, Rotterdam 1979
Birch-Lindgren, G., 'American Hospitals Through Swedish Eyes', *Journal of the American Institute of Architects*, 1947, 5, pp. 208-215
Birch-Lindgren, G., *Modern Hospital Planning in Sweden and other Countries*, Stockholm 1951
Bisschop, F., J.G.M. Hendriks, 'Bouwbeleid in de jaren negentig', *ZM Magazine*, 6 (1990) 1, pp. 13-16
Blijdenstein, R., *Zeist, groei en bouw. Den Dolder en Bosch en Duin. Een inventarisatie van waardevolle gebouwen en gebieden*, Zeist 1984
Bloemendaal, G., M. Duijnstee, J.C.M. Hattinga Verschure, *Thuis in het verpleeghuis. Werken-wonen-bezoeken*, Nijkerk 1985
Blok, G., J. Vijselaar, *Terug naar Endegeest. Patiënten en hun behandeling in het psychiatrisch ziekenhuis Endegeest 1897-1997*, Nijmegen 1998
Blok, G., J. Vijselaar (ed.), *De Weg van Welterhof. 25 jaar psychiatrie in Oostelijk Zuid-Limburg*, Utrecht 1999
Blom, R., J. Schuyt, B. Wouters (ed.), *Vergrijzen en verzilveren. Experimenten voor oudere eigenaar-bewoners*, Rotterdam 1992
Bock, M., K. Somer, *Architect J.P. Kloos (1905). De ethiek van de constructie*, Amsterdam 1986
Boekholdt, M.G., 'Maatschappelijk ondernemen in zorg: mythe en werkelijkheid', inaugural lecture Vrije Universiteit Amsterdam 29 March 2007
Boekholdt, M.G., 'Verpleeg- en verzorgingshuis voorbij', in: P. van Beek, H. Hoes (ed.), *Zorg en Architectuur. Verslag Jubileumcongres Bouwkunde*, Utrecht 2002
Boer, F. de, 'Architectuur en krankzinnigen. De typologie van krankzinnigengestichten in de negentiende eeuw in Nederland', *Akt*, 7 (1983) 1, pp. 48-60
Boer, F. de, 'Bouwen voor gekken. De typologie van het psychiatries ziekenhuis in histories perspektief', *Psychologie en Maatschappij*, 9 (1985) 1, pp. 47-63
Boer, J., P. Sijtsma (ed.), *Ouderenhuisvesting: tijd voor een nieuw beleid*, Groningen 1990
Boom, H. van der, *De geschiedenis van het ziekenhuis-wezen in Nederland 1900-1940. Het ontstaan van het moderne ziekenhuis vanuit sociaal constructivistisch perspectief*, Maastricht 1997 (thesis)
Boomen, T. den, 'Het Steen. Grootheidswaanzin', *Psy*, 6 (2002) 2, pp. 28-29
Boot, J.M.D., *Organisatie van de Gezondheidszorg*, Assen 2007
Borgesius, E., W. Brunenberg, 'Nieuwe zorg van het Psychiatrisch Ziekenhuis. Een inventarisatie van zorgvernieuwingsprojecten', *Maandblad Geestelijke Volksgezondheid*, 51 (1996) 12, pp. 1267-1281
Borselen, J.W. van, 'Dienstencentra voor bejaarden', *Bouw*, 24 (1969) 25, p. 1068
Borst-Eilers, J.E., G.M. van Etten, D.M. Sluimers (ed.), *Continuïteit en verandering. De zorgagenda voor de jaren '90*, [Rijswijk] 1991
Bosma, K., 'Tussen leed en vermaak: vijf academische ziekenhuizen', in: R. Brouwers (ed.), *Architectuur in Nederland. Jaarboek 1989/1990*, Rotterdam 1990, pp. 25-32
Bosma, K., D. van Hoogstraten, M. Vos, *Housing for the Millions. John Habraken and the SAR (1960-2000)*, Rotterdam 2000
Bosma, K., C. Wagenaar (ed.), *Een geruisloze doorbraak. De geschiedenis van architectuur en stedebouw tijdens de bezetting en de wederopbouw van Nederland*, Rotterdam 1995
Bosma, K. (et al. ed.), *Bouwen in Nederland 600-2000*, Zwolle 2007
'Boston Symposium Addresses Healing Designs', *Architecture*, January 1992, p. 75
'De bouw van een mammoet ziekenhuis. Interview met ir. C.A. Doets c.i. te Baarn', *Architectuur/Bouwen*, 2 (1986) 11, pp. 27-29
'Bouwen in de gezondheidszorg', *Baksteen*, 22 (1980) 1/2, pp. 10-16
'Bouwen in de gezondheidszorg: je moet er wat voor in huis hebben', *Stedenbouw*, 40 (1988), 453 (special), p. 2
Bouwen voor bejaarden, s.l. [1972]
'Bouwen voor gezondheidszorg: integratie', *Plan*, 8 (1977) 7, p. 3
Bouwen voor ouderen, Amsterdam 1981
Bouwmaatstaven voor een Regionaal GGZ-centrum (RGC), Utrecht 2001
Bouwstenen in het Damspel. Opstellen over de bouw van ziekenhuisvoorzieningen, Utrecht 1983
Braaksma, S.B., 'Marktwerking in de gezondheidszorg', *ZM Magazine*, 13 (1997) 5, pp. 13-15
Bresler, J., *Deutsche Heil- und Pflegeanstalten für Psychischkranke in Wort und Bild*, Halle 1910
Bresler, J., *Heil- und Pflegeanstalten für Psychischkranke in Wort und Bild* (Band 1), Halle 1914
Brinke, A. ten, L. Eikelboom, *Een leven lang wonen. Huisvesting en zorg*, Amsterdam 1999
Broek, J.H. van den, 'De architectonische conceptie van het ziekenhuis', *Het Ziekenhuiswezen*, 23 (1950), special on building, pp. 65-116
Brouwers, R., 'Prof. Jacques Choisy: "in de stad bouwen is goed als er maar geen barrières uit voortkomen"', *TA/BK Tijdschrift voor Architektuur en Beeldende Kunsten*, (1972), pp. 470-471
Brouwers, R., 'Precaire contacten over zorg voor gezondheid en medisch onderwijs', *Wonen-TA/BK*, 2 (1974) 24, p. 14
Brouwers, R., 'Zieke bouw en ziekenhuisbouw', *Wonen-TA/BK*, 2 (1974) 2, pp. 1-2
Brouwers, R., C. Weeber, 'De hoogopwaaiende slip van de witte jas van de dokter. Mediese fakulteit Rotterdam – een tempel der wetenschap die geen barrière mag worden', *TA/BK Tijdschrift voor Architektuur en Beeldende Kunsten*, (1972), pp. 453-460
Bruegmann, R., 'Les Machines à Guerir', *Journal of the Society of Architectural Historians*, 1979, pp. 210-211
Bruin, R. de, M. Heurneman, F. van der Veeke, *Van aalmoes tot AOW: zes eeuwen ouderenzorg in een Nederlandse stad*, Utrecht 1996
Bruin, W., 'De Rusthoeve, tehuis voor ouden van dagen te Purmerend', *Bouwkundig Weekblad Architectura*, 60 (1938) 35, pp. 289-295
Buchanan, P., L. Lefaivre, A. Tzonis, *Aldo en Hannie van Eyck. Recent werk – Recent work*, Amsterdam 1989
Burdett, C., *Hospitals and Asylums of the World*, London 1892-1893
Butler, C., A. Erdman, *Hospital Planning*, New York 1946

Casciato, M., *De Amsterdamse School*, Rotterdam 1991
Cate, G. ten, *EGM architecten*, Rotterdam 2003
Cederström, H., 'Hospital in Stockholm', *Architectural Review*, 1946, nr. 99, pp. 135-140
Cederström, H., *Södersjukhuset Stockholm*, Stockholm 1946
Centralisatie of decentralisatie in de gezondheidszorg, Lochem 1978
'Charenton', *Revue général de l'architecture et des travaux publics*, 1852, pp. 384-359
Choisy, J.L.C., 'Toelichting op de mediese fakulteit Rotterdam', *TA/BK Tijdschrift voor Architektuur en Beeldende Kunsten*, 1972, pp. 461-469
Claassen, J., *Van Buitenplaats tot Bijlmerflat. De ontwikkeling in de architectuur van psychiatrische ziekenhuizen in Nederland vanaf de eerste geneeskundige gestichten, gebouwd na de eerste Krankzinnigenwet uit 1841, tot heden* [thesis RU Leiden 1999]
Cleyndert, P.C., 'De verpleegeenheid', *Het Ziekenhuis-wezen*, 21 (1948), pp. 356-357
Cleyndert, P.C., 'Isometrische afbeeldingen van ziekenhuisafdelingen', *Het Ziekenhuiswezen*, 22 (1949), p. 201 and separate annex
Cleyndert, P.C., 'Bouwcentrum-Rotterdam (II)', *Het Ziekenhuiswezen*, 22 (1949), p. 41.
Cleyndert, P.C., 'De medische en verpleegtechnische organisatie van het ziekenhuis en zijn afdelingen', *Het Ziekenhuiswezen*, 23 (1950), special on building, pp. 18-28
Cleyndert, P.C., 'De Verpleegeenheid', *Het Ziekenhuis-wezen*, 24 (1951), pp. 108-125
Cleyndert, P.C., 'Een halve eeuw later. I. Het ziekenhuis: medische en sociale vooruitgang', *Bouw*, 12 (1957) 13, pp. 282-285
Cohen, D., H.E. Sanders, 'De transformatie van een klassieke psychiatrische opname-afdeling. College bouw ziekenhuisvoorzieningen', *Bouwmaatstaven voor Langdurige zorg GGZ* [report no. 0.99], Utrecht 2002
Colenbrander, B. (ed.), *Stijl. Norm en handschrift in de Nederlandse architectuur*, Rotterdam 1993
College bouw ziekenhuisvoorzieningen, *Referentiekader bestaande voorzieningen voor Langdurige Zorg (GGZ)* [report no. 0.99a], Utrecht 2002
College bouw ziekenhuisvoorzieningen, *Signalerings-rapport inzake IFD-Bouwen. Uitbreidingen verpleeghuizen en verzorgingshuizen*, Utrecht 2001
College voor Ziekenhuisvoorzieningen, *Inventarisatie 1978 psychiatrische inrichtingen in Nederland*, Utrecht 1979
Constant, J.G., *AMC gebouwd*, Wormer 1984
'Constructions hospitalières', *L'Architecture d'Aujourd'hui*, 1938, 5, pp. 2-102
Cox, A., Ph. Groves, *Design for Health Care*, London [etc.] 1981
Cox, A., Ph. Groves, *Hospitals and Health-care Facilities. A Design and Development Guide*, London 1990
Cox, D.H., *AMC: Academisch Medisch Centrum bij de Universiteit van Amsterdam*, Amsterdam 1984
Cox, D.H., 'Het Academisch Medisch Centrum. De eerste uit een reeks van academische ziekenhuizen', *Architectuur/Bouwen*, 2 (1986) 11, pp. 11-23
Cramer, B.J.K., *Technische bouwkundige onderwerpen*, 1936
Cusdin, S.E.T., J. Murray Easton, 'Recent Trends in Hospital Design', *RIBA Journal*, July 1947, p. 456
Cüsters, J., 'Programma in gevaar. Ziekenhuisbouw speelbal van zeer trage procedures', *Bouw*, 46 (1991) 1, pp. 9-12
Cüsters, J. (ed.), *Een derde levensfase voor flatcomplexen*, Rotterdam 1997
Cüsters, J., *Wonen op leeftijd*, Amsterdam/Utrecht 1998
Cuypers, Ed., 'Het nieuwe Gast- of Ziekenhuis te Dordrecht', *Het Ziekenhuis*, 13 (1922), pp. 37-52

Dankers, J.J., A.A.M. van der Linden, *Om het geluk van de zwakzinnige. De geschiedenis van Dennendal 1969-1994*, Den Dolder 1994
Dankers, J., J. van der Linden, *Van regenten en patiënten. De geschiedenis van de Willem Arntsz Stichting. Huis en Hoeve Van der Hoeven Kliniek en Dennendal*, Amsterdam/Meppel 1996
Darton, E., 'The Evolution of the Hospital', *Metropolis*, October 1996, pp. 66-68
Das Bürgerspital Basel 1260-1946, Basel 1946
De Opmaat. Wat vooraf ging aan de bouw van de MFE Midden Twente, s.l. s.a.
Deben, L., 'Het betrekkelijk belang voor zieken van ziekenhuizen in onze welvaartstaat', *Wonen-TA/BK*, 2 (1974) 24, pp. 15-19
Debets, C., 'Omgekeerde wereld. Mini-psychiatrisch centrum dichtbij de mensen', *Bouwwereld*, 93 (1997) 20, pp. 18-20
Deconcentratie. Een nieuw APZ in de gezondheidsregio Dordrecht, Bennekom 1983
Degess, L., *Der Bau der Krankenhäuser*, Munich 1862
Dekker, J.J.M., *Het Amsterdamse Sociaal Psychiatrisch Diensten Centrum. Een vergelijkend onderzoek naar een multi-functionele eenheid en de reguliere 24-uurs zorg* [dissertation Universiteit van Amsterdam], Amsterdam 1996
Dekker, J.J.M., 'De multifunctionele eenheid in opmars', *Medisch Contact*, 52 (1997) 15, pp. 465-466
Delft, S. van, 'Wie is er bang voor het Bouwcollege', *Zorgvisie*, 30 (2000) 10, pp. 16-21
Delrue, J., 'Van zieken-huis naar huis-om-te-genezen', *Plan*, 8 (1977) 8, pp. 5-15
Diederich, J., 'Enkele sociologische aspecten van het vraagstuk der bejaarden', *Tijdschrift voor maatschappelijk werk*, 26 (1948) 13, pp. 45-46
'Dienstencentra voor bejaarden', *Bouw*, 23 (1968) 11, p. 422

'Dienstencentra voor bejaarden', *Bouw*, 24 (1969) 44, p. 1761
Dijkema, P., 'Menselijk en modern', *Plan*, 8 (1977) 7, pp. 27-28
Dijkman, F.J.M., W. Eijkelenboom, 'Het ziekenhuis als weefsel', *Plan*, 8 (1977) 8, pp. 39-46
Dijkstra, T., 'Nieuwe ontwikkelingen in het bouwen voor geestelijk gehandicapten', *Plan*, 8 (1977) 7, pp. 18-28
Dijl, P.W. van, 'Bouwsystemen voor gezondheidszorg', *Bouw*, 25 (1970) 45, pp. 1713-1717
Dirichlet, G.L., F. Labryga, P. Poelzig, G. Schlenzig, *Krankenhausbau. Maßkoordination. Entwurfsstrategie. Anwendungsbeispiele*, Berlin 1980
Dolné, E.M., 'Katholieke ziekenzorg in Nijmegen', in: D. Nicolaisen (ed.), *Een veelkleurig habijt. Kloosters in Nijmegen in de negentiende en twintigste eeuw*, Nijmegen 1989, pp. 79-91
Donk, B. van de, J. Singelenberg (ed.), *Eindevaluatie Seniorenlabel*, Rotterdam 1998
Donk, L., B. Fris, J. Lamers, *Vrijheid, Zelfstandigheid & Vriendschap. Groepswonen van ouderen*, Amsterdam 1989
Dooghe, G., L. van den Boer (ed.), *Sheltered accommodation for elderly people in an international perspective*, Amsterdam/Lisse/Berwyn 1993
Dorris, V.K., 'Health Trends', *Architecture*, 82 (1993), 3, p. 93
Draaisma, A., 'Plaats van de basisfilosofie bij het ziekenhuisontwerp', *Bouw*, 30 (1975) 3, pp. 45-48
Driest, P.F., 'Zorg en huisvesting aan elkaar klinken', *Stedebouw & Architectuur*, 21 (2005) 10, pp. 4-5
Drogendijk, C.A., *Het protestants-christelijke ziekenhuis in Nederland*, Utrecht 1975
Duurkoop, P., 'Van traditioneel APZ naar nieuwe woonmogelijkheden in de stad', *Passage*, 8 (1999) 4, pp. 238-246
Duurkoop, W.R.A., J.W. van Zuthem, 'Tussen Algemeen Psychiatrisch Ziekenhuis en Beschermde Woonvorm (3)', *Maandblad Geestelijke Volksgezondheid*, 51 (1996) 11, pp. 1181-1183

Eck, R. van, *Innovatie in de ouderenhuisvesting*, Delft 1992
Eck, R. van, T. Weggemans, *Wooncentrum voor ouderen: aspiraties en praktijk. Een analyse van gewenste en mogelijke kwaliteiten van een grootschalige woonconcept voor ouderen*, The Hague 1990
Eefsting, J., 'Inconsistente maatschappelijke eisen in de dementiezorg', *ZM Magazine*, 23 (2007) 5, pp. 14-15
Een eeuw krankzinnigenverpleging 1849-1949. Gedenkboek ter gelegenheid van het honderdjarig bestaan van het Provinciaal Ziekenhuis nabij Santpoort (voorheen Meerenberg), Santpoort 1949
Eijk, C.A. van, *Laat ze het maar voelen... Een verhaal over psychiatrische inrichtingen*, Amsterdam 1981
Eijkelenboom, W., 'De architectuur. Holy-ziekenhuis in Vlaardingen', *Bouw*, 21 (1966) 40, pp. 1526-1531
Engel, H.J.J., P.W.G. van der Broek, G. Wesseling, J.C. Tukker, 'Medische Faculteit Rotterdam', *Polytechnisch Tijdschrift*, 26 (1971) 25, pp. 989-1001
Esch, P. van der, *Jacobus Ludovicus Conradus Schroeder van der Kolk, 1797-1862, leven en werken*, 1954 s.p. [dissertation Universiteit van Amsterdam]
Esch, P. van der, *Geschiedenis van het Staatstoezicht op Krankzinnigen. Deel I*, Leidschendam s.a. [1975-1980]
Esch, P. van der, *Geschiedenis van het Staatstoezicht op Krankzinnigen. Deel II*, Leidschendam s.a. [1975-1980]
Esch, P. van der, *Geschiedenis van het Staatstoezicht op Krankzinnigen. Deel III*, Leidschendam s.a. [1975-1980]
Evans, R., 'The Rights of Retreat and the Rites of Exclusion. Notes towards the Definition of Wall', *Architectural Design*, 41 (1971) 6, pp. 335-339
Evers, A., G.J.M. Sarlemijn, 'Tehuis voor bejaarden te Breda', *Bouwkundig Weekblad*, 70 (1952) 19/20, pp. 145-151
Everts, J., 'De huisvesting en verzorging van bejaarden', *Economisch-statistische berichten. Algemeen weekblad voor handel, nijverheid, financiën en verkeer*, 9 February 1944, pp. 77-80
Eyck van Heslinga, C. van, 'Verzorgingstehuizen voor bejaarden', *Bouw*, 25 (1970) 37, pp. 1395-1396
Eyk, C.A. van, *Laat ze maar voelen... Een verhaal over psychiatrische inrichtingen*, Amsterdam 1981
Eynde, I.E.I.M., 'Enkele nieuwe woonvormen voor psychiatrische patiënten', *Tijdschrift voor psychiatrie*, 20 (1978), pp. 79-94
Eysselsteijn, G. van, *Het Algemeen Provinciaal-, Stads- en Academisch- Ziekenhuis te Groningen*, Groningen [s.a.]

Fedderson, E., I. Lüdtke, *Living for the Elderly. A Design Manual*, Bazel 2009
Fiset, M., 'Architecture and the Art of Healing', *The Canadian Architect*, 35 (1990) 3, pp. 25-26
Fledderus, R.H., 'Bejaardencentra', *Bouwkundig Weekblad*, 74 (1956) 46, pp. 497-500
Fledderus, R.H., 'Het Zonnehuis te Vlaardingen', *Bouw*, 22 (1967) 12, pp. 440-446
Folgerts, I., E. Kalle (ed.), *Seniorenlabel. Consumentenkeurmerk voor Ouderenhuisvesting. Versie experimenteerfase 1993/1994*, Rotterdam 1993
Forty, A., 'The modern hospital in England and France: the social and medical uses of architecture', in: A.D. King (ed.), *Buildings and society. Essays on the Social Development of the Built Environment*, London/Boston/Henley 1980
Foucault, M., *Naissance de la clinique. Une archéologie du regard médical*, Paris 1963
Foucault, M., *Discipline, Toezicht en Straf. De geboorte van de gevangenis*, Groningen 1989
Foucault, M., et al., *Les machines à guérir. Aux origines de l'hôpital moderne*, Brussels/Liège 1979
Foudraine, J., *Wie is van hout... Een gang door de psychiatrie*, Bilthoven 1971
Fowler, Ch., 'On the arrangement of lunatic asylums', *The Builder*, 4 (1846) 25, pp. 349-352
Fuchs, W., R. Wischer, *H VEN LC. Le Corbusiers Krankenhausprojekt für Venedig*, Berlin 1985
Fuente Saez, V.P de la, *De S.A.R. en het ziekenhuis*, Eindhoven [s.a.]
Fuks-Mansfeld, R., A. Sunier, *Wie in tranen zaait... Geschiedenis van de Joodse Geestelijke Gezondheidszorg in Nederland*, Assen 1997
Funk, A., *Gebäude für Heil- und sonstige Wohlfahrtanstalten. Handbuch der Architektur Vierter Teil 5. Halb-Band 2. Heft*, Darmstadt 1891
Furnée, J.H., J.H.G. Jonkman, *Het Noorder Sanatorium te Zuidlaren. Geschiedenis en architectuur van een psychiatrisch monument*, Zuidlaren 1994

'"Geef bejaardentehuis meer contact met buitenwereld"', *Bouw*, 14 (1959) 17, p. 471
'"Geef bejaardentehuis meer contact met buitenwereld"', *Bouw*, 14 (1959) 24, p. 681
Gelder, H.E. van, 'De "intellectueel" en het Bejaarden-Centrum', *Bouwkundig Weekblad*, 77 (1959) 49/50, pp. 607-608
Gemeren, P. van, 'Naar een nieuwe huisvesting voor alle groepen ouderen (1)', *Bouw*, 32 (1977) 2, pp. 29-31
Gemeren, P. van, 'Naar een nieuwe huisvesting voor alle groepen ouderen (2)', *Bouw*, 32 (1977) 3, pp. 57-59
Gemert, G.H. van, R.B. Minderaa (ed.), *Zorg voor mensen met een verstandelijke handicap*, Assen 1997
Gerlach, B., *Ed. Cuypers Architect*, Amsterdam 1979
Giedion, S., 'Een ziekenhuiscomplex voor de stad Rijssel', *De 8 en Opbouw*, 5 (1934) 1, pp. 1-8
'Giganten in opmars. Academische centra', *Wonen-TA/BK*, 2 (1974) 24, p. 5
Gijswijt-Hofstra, M., H. Oosterhuis, 'Leeswijzer voor het psychiatrisch verleden', *Maandblad Geestelijke volksgezondheid*, 56 (2001) 7/8, pp. 627-643
Gijswijt-Hofstra, M., H. Oosterhuis, 'Psychiatrische geschiedenissen', *BMGN*, 116 (2001) 2, pp. 162-197
Goedmakers, H., 'Bejaardenzorg, een vraagstuk van de hedendaagse samenleving', *Bouwkundig Weekblad*, 77 (1959) 49/50, pp. 585-586
Goei, L. de, *De psychohygiënisten. Psychiatrie, cultuurkritiek en beweging voor geestelijke volksgezondheid in Nederland, 1924-1970*, Nijmegen 2001
Goor, M. van, 'De inrichting ontmanteld. Nieuw psychiatrisch ziekenhuis als onderdeel van de stad', *Architectuur/Bouwen*, 3 (1987) 6/7, pp. 17-21
Gorp, W. van, J.C.M. Hattinga Verschure, J.L.M. Zuidberg (ed.), *Heel het ziekenhuis*, Lochem 1980
Gortemaker, R., G. Mulkens, 'Luchthavengebouw is vertrekpunt voor nieuw ziekenhuis', *ZorgVisie*, 26 (1996) 15, pp. 30-32
Grevelt, E.R.E., *Geestelijke gezondheidszorg in deconcentratie. Een APZ in wording. Nota over de totstandkoming van een algemeen psychiatrisch ziekenhuis in de gezondheidsregio Dordrecht*, Amsterdam 1990
Groenewegen, J.H., 'Een nieuw rusthuis te Driebergen. Ontwerp Ir J.B. van Loghem, Rotterdam', *De 8 en Opbouw*, 3 (1932) 10, pp. 96-99
Groot, A. de, *Veldwijk in verleden tijd. De eerste 50 jaar van Psychiatrisch Ziekenhuis Veldwijk te Ermelo*, Harderwijk 1976
Groot Wesseldijk, M.J., 'Ziekenhuisbouw in den vreemde', *Het Ziekenhuiswezen*, 19 (1946), pp. 187-191
Guez, G., 'Image ouverte de l'hôpital', *L'Architecture d'Aujourd'hui*, 40 (1970) 120, pp. 5-11
Guislain, J., *Traité sur l'aliénation et sur les hospices des aliénés*, Amsterdam 1826 (two parts)
Guislain, J., *Leçons orales sur les phrénopathies, ou traité théorique et pratique des maladies mentales. Cours donné a la clinique des établissements d'aliénés a Gand*, Ghent 1852
Guislain, J., P.J. Triest, *Reglement voor de krankzinnigengestichten der stad Gent*, Ghent 1829
Gulick, F.W. van, *Aspecten van het ziekenhuis van de toekomst*, Utrecht 1969
Gutschow, K., 'Gedanken aus der Planungspraxis', *Architektur Wettbewerbe. Schriftenreihe für richtungweisendes bauen*, 28 (1960), p. 5

Haan, H. de, 'Nieuwe kliniek lijkt op een paleis', *de Volkskrant*, 9 June 2001
Haneveld, G.T., *Oude medische gebouwen van Nederland*, Amsterdam 1976
Hannema, K., 'Revalideren als in een luxe hotel', *de Volkskrant*, 4 March 2010
Hartgers, R., 'Amerikaanse praktijken? Seniorensteden in Nederland', *Stedebouw & Ruimtelijke Ordening*, 88 (2007) 1, pp. 33-35
Hartgers, R., 'Zelfstandig wonen', *Stedebouw & Ruimtelijke Ordening* 88 (2007) 1, pp. 36-37
Harwood, E., 'Hospital and Asylum Architecture in England 1840-1914. Building for Health Care', *AA Files*, (1992) 23, pp. 105-106
Hattinga Verschure, J.C.M., *Patiënt, Ziekenhuis, Gezondheidszorg op weg naar 2000*, Amsterdam 1971
Hattinga Verschure, J.C.M., 'Kostenontwikkeling in de ziekenhuisbouw', *Bouw*, 27 (1972) 39, pp. 1229-1230
Hattinga Verschure, J.C.M., *Het verschijnsel zorg*, Lochem 1977
Hattinga Verschure, J.C.M., *Nieuwbouw en variabiliteit. Vijf herfstvoordrachten*, Utrecht 1978
Hattinga Verschure, J.C.M., 'Trends in de ziekenhuisbouw', *De Ingenieur*, 91 (1979), pp. 731-732
Hattinga Verschure, J.C.M., *Zelfredzame ouderen*, Lochem/Ghent, 1987
Hattinga Verschure, J.C.M., 'Ziekenhuisbouw caleidoscoop', *ZM Magazine*, 15 (1999) 6, pp. 28-30
Have, H. ten H, *Het verpleeghuis: veld van onderzoek*, Deventer 1979
Havik, K., 'Mecanoo gebruikt kloostertypologie voorzorg-instelling', *de Architect Interieur*, (2002) 7, pp. 60-63
Hazewinkel, F., *Van 'slaapzaal' naar 'levensloop-bestendige woning'. Van 'handen uit de mouwen' naar 'handen op de rug'. Veertig jaar Stichting Humanitas Rotterdam 1959-1999*, Rotterdam 1999
'Health Sciences Centre McMaster University, Kanada', *Deutsche Bauzeitung*, 103 (1969), 10 pp. 717-723
'Health Sciences Centre McMaster University', *World Hospitals*, 1970, pp. 34-38
Heeres, P.A., 'Enkele gedachten over ziekenhuisbouw in deze tijd', *Bouwkundig Weekblad*, 76 (1958) 38, pp. 449-462
Heerma van Voss, A.J., 'De geschiedenis van de gekkenbeweging', in: *Voor de gek gehouden. Geschiedenis van de krankzinnigenzorg in Nederland*, Haarlem/Gouda 1982
Hermans, J.B., 'Hoe komen gebouwen voor gezondheidszorg tot stand?', *Bouw*, 29 (1974) 10, pp. 227-228

Heuvel, W.J. van, *Structuralisme in de Nederlandse architectuur*, Rotterdam 1992
Heuvel, W.J., van 'Een "Cité Médicale" aan de rand van de Bijlmer. Het AMC tussen andere academische ziekenhuizen', *Architectuur/Bouwen*, 2 (1986) 11, pp. 37-47
Heuvel, W.J.A. van den, 'Sociale en ruimtelijke omgeving van de verpleeghuispatiënt', *Bouw*, 29 (1974), 5, pp. 119-121
Heuvelink, J.J.W., *Verblijven of wonen; zorg voor eenieder*, Amsterdam 2000
Heyden, J.T.M. van der, *Het ziekenhuis door de eeuwen. Over geld, macht en mensen*, Rotterdam 1994
Hillen, M., 'Over het modelleren van het totale ding. Zwolle, Dieze-Oost, Hobbemastraat', *Stadscahiers 2008/2009. Buitenwereld – binnenwereld. Ontwerpen aan opdrachtgeverschap*, Amsterdam 2008, pp. 86-93
Hinkema, M., J. Nauta, 'De chirurg in de buurt. Het relatieve succes van decentrale ziekenhuisvoorzieningen', *Medisch Contact* 64 (2009) 33/34, pp. 1392-1395
Hoekstra, E., I. van Liemd, *Ruimte – Vragen. Bouwen aan zorginstellingen vanuit cliëntenperspectief*, s.l. s.a.
Hoekstra, E.K., H.M.J.A. van Liempd, *Bouwen aan MFE's. Stagg-studie naar de huisvesting van multifunctionele eenheden in de psychiatrie*, Amsterdam 1994
Hoekstra, E., I. van Liempd, 'Bouwen aan MFE's. Een onderzoek naar de huisvesting van multifunctionele eenheden', *Maandblad Geestelijke Volksgezondheid*, 50 (1995) 7/8, pp. 781-790
Hoekstra, H., 'De bouwkundige Organisatie van het ziekenhuis en zijn afdelingen', *Het Ziekenhuiswezen*, 23 (1950), special on building, pp. 29-46
Hoekstra, H., 'De bouwkundige organisatie van het ziekenhuis en zijn afdelingen', *Bouwkundig Weekblad*, 68 (1950) 25, pp. 385-391
Hornstra, J.J., 'Het ontwerpen van een bejaarden-tehuis', *Bouwkundig Weekblad*, 77 (1959) 49/50, pp. 599-600
Hospital Care in the United States, New York 1947
Hospital Handbook for Architects and Engineers, New York 1949
Hotze, G.J.V., 'Openbaar verkeer in en om een bejaardencentrum', *Bouw*, 28 (1973) 1, pp. 11-12
Houben, P.P.J., A. Mulder, *Ouderenhuisvesting in Europees perspectief*, Delft 1999
Houben, P.P.J., F. Wind, H. Moeskops, *Herstructurering van voorzieningen voor ouderen op wijkniveau*, Delft 1984
Houben, P.P.J., F. Wind, H. Moeskops, *Ouderen op de bres voor huisvesting in hun wijk*, Delft 1984
Housing for the Elderly in the Netherlands, The Hague s.a.
Houwaart, E.S., *De hygiënisten. Artsen, staat & volksgezondheid in Nederland 1840-1890*, Groningen 1991
Houwaart, E.S., 'Medische statistiek', in: *Techniek in Nederland. De wording van een moderne samenleving 1800-1890*, Zutphen 1993, pp. 19-45
Houwaart, E.S., 'Het ziekenhuis; de ontwikkeling van het ziekenhuis in de moderne tijd', in: *Techniek als cultuurverschijnsel*, Amsterdam 1997
Huddleston Slater, W.B., *Nederlandsche sanatoria en herstellingsoorden, gids*, The Hague [1933]
Hudnut, J., 'Architecture and the art of medicine', *Journal of The American Institute of Architects*, 8 (1947) 4, pp. 147-156
Huffmeijer, G.J., 'De toekomst van de ziekenhuisbouw: bouw jij of bouw ik?', *ZM Magazine*, 11 (1995) 6, pp. 2-3, 29
Huijsman, R., 'Het Nederlandse ouderenzorgbeleid: verleden, heden en toekomst', in: *Morele problemen in de ouderenzorg*, Rotterdam 1999
Huijsman, R., *Model van voorzieningen voor ouderen*, Zeist 1990
Huijsman, R., *Ouderenzorgbeleid in Nederland*, Rotterdam 1999
Huijsman, R., F.F.H. Rutten (ed.), *De economie van de ouderenzorg. Visies vanuit wetenschap en beleid*, Assen, Maastricht 1989
Huiskes, G., R. van der Kroef, *Van Rooms tot Rome. Van Sint Franciscushof naar Zwolse Poort 1952-2002*, Groningen 2002
'Huisvesting bejaarden "nieuwe stijl"', *Bouw*, 29 (1974) 15, p. VI
Huisvesting van bejaarden, s.l. [1949]
Huisvesting van bejaarden, Rotterdam 1959
'Huisvesting van bejaarden. Studiegroep, waarin Bouwcentrum-deskundigen en andere specialisten samenwerken', *Bouw*, 7 (1952) 17, p. 318
'Huisvesting van bejaarden', *Bouw*, 8 (1953) 17, pp. 301-320
De huisvesting van bejaarden in Nederland, The Hague 1970
Huisvesting van ouderen, Almere 1991
Huisvesting van ouderen op het breukvlak van twee eeuwen, The Hague 1997
Huizenga, J., *Memorabele mensen en memorabele momenten uit de geschiedenis van de intramurale gezondheidszorg*, Lochem 1991
Huizenga, J., *Memorabele mensen en momenten uit de geschiedenis van de intramurale gezondheidszorg*, Lochem 1991
Hulst, W. van, '"Humanitas runt meer restaurants dan MacDonalds"', *Zorgvisie*, 36 (2006), p. 4
Hunt, W.A. (ed.), *Hospitals, Clinics and Health Centers. An Architectural Record Book*, New York 1960
Husson, A., *Etude sur les hopitaux considérés sous le rapport de leur construction de la distrubution de leurs batiments de l'ameublement, de l'hygiène & du service des salles de malades*, Paris 1862
Hutschemaekers, G., Chr. Hrachovec (ed.), *Heer en heelmeesters. Negentig jaar zorg voor zenuwlijders in het Christelijk Sanatorium te Zeist*, Nijmegen 1993
Hutter, A., 'Klinieken voor zenuwzieken', *Het Ziekenhuiswezen*, 9 (1936) 12, pp. 629-631
'Hvidovre general hospital', *World Hospitals = l'Hôpital dans le Monde*, 2 (1966) 1, pp. 62-63

Idsinga, T., J. Schilt, *Architect W. van Tijen 1894-1974. 'Ik ben een rationalist, maar er is meer op de wereld'*, The Hague 1987
In dienst der zieken. Het St. Joseph-ziekenhuis te Heerlen 1904-1954, Bussum 1954
Inspection reports: Feith, C.J., J.L.C. Schroeder van der Kolk, *Geschiedkundig overzigt der verbetering (...) in de verpleging van krankzinnigen etc.* (The Hague 1848); *Verslag over den staat der gestichten voor krankzinnigen, in den jaren 1849-1884; Verslag van het Staatstoezicht op krankzinnigen en krankzinnigengestichten (...) in de jaren 1885-1936*

Jager, I., *Willem Kromhout Czn. 1864-1940*, Rotterdam 1992
James, T., P. Noakes, *Hospital Architecture*, Harlow 1994
James, W.P., W. Tatton-Brown, *Hospitals, Design and Development*, London 1986
Janssen, A.M.A.J., 'Integrale benadering van de bejaardenzorg', *Bouw*, 23 (1968) 21, pp. 830-831
Janssen, A.M.A.J., 'Vrije vestiging voor bejaarden', *Bouw*, 29 (1974) 12, pp. 275-276
Janssen, M., 'De Multifunctionele Eenheid als kleine inrichting', *Maandblad Geestelijke Volksgezondheid*, 50 (1995) 7/8, pp. 766-780
Janssen, M., *Wel en wee van de MFE. Een eerste evaluatie van Multifunctionele Eenheden in Nederland*, Utrecht 1995
Jaspers, Fr.C.A., G.J. Vermaeten, 'Waartoe bestaat het ziekenhuis?', *ZM Magazine*, 11 (1995), 1, pp. 18-23
Jelgersma, G., 'De inrichting der psychiatrische kliniek', *Psychiatrische en Neurologische Bladen*, 24 (1920), pp. 396-410
Jetter, D., *Geschichte des Hospitals*, Wiesbaden 1966
Jetter, D., *Grundzüge der Krankenhausgeschichte (1800-1900)*, Darmstadt 1977
Jetter, D., *Grundzüge der Geschichte des Irrenhauses*, Darmstadt 1981
Jetter, D., *Das Europäische Hospital*, Cologne 1986
Joedicke, J., 'Krankenhaus auf neuen Wegen?', *Bauen + Wohnen*, 29 (1974) 3, pp. 93-107
Jonker, M., D. Schuiling, 'Godshuis, gasthuis, ziekenhuis, medisch centrum, cité medicale', *Wonen-TA/BK*, 2 (1974) 24, pp. 22-28
'Jury-rapport over de openbare prijsvraag voor een woongebouw voor oude mannen en vrouwen te Alkmaar (Karenhuizen)', *Bouwkundig Weekblad*, 38 (1917) 31, pp. 176-178

Kaath, G. te, L. van de Cappelle (ed.), *Bouwen op Woonzorg Nederland*, s.l. 2006
Kamminga, I.F., *Van hervormde zorg naar zorghervorming. Verhalen over het Psychiatrisch Centrum Licht en Kracht te Assen*, Assen 1995
Kappelhof, A.C.M., *Reinier van Arkel 1442-1992. De geschiedenis van het oudste psychiatrische ziekenhuis van Nederland*, 's-Hertogenbosch 1992
Katz, R., 'Behandelfilosofie is de belangrijkste bouwsteen', *Het Ziekenhuis*, 25 (1995) 2, pp. 22-25
Keijsers, G., 'De tijd van ziekenhuisarchitecten is voorbij', *BNABlad*, (2008) 5, pp. 20-21
Kerkhof, M.P.N. van, 'Interview. Paul Schnabel: "We laten mensen leven in een sociale isoleercel"', *Psy*, 6 (2002) 12, p. 7
Kerkhoven, A., *Beeld van de psychiatrie 1800-1970. Historisch bezit van de psychiatrische ziekenhuizen in Nederland*, Zwolle 1996
Kersloot, J.M., *Woongedrag van draagkrachtige senioren*, Delft 1993
Klaver, A.M.J., *Bouwen voor een vergrijzende samenleving*, Amsterdam 2004
Klazinga, A.F., N.S. Casparie, 'Het ziekenhuis van de toekomst', *Medisch Contact*, 53 (1998), 51/52 pp. 1630-1634
Kleinschalig wonen, grote verschillen. Bouwkundige verschijningsvormen van kleinschalig wonen in de ouderenzorg, Utrecht 2007
Klerk, L. de, *Particuliere plannen. Denkbeelden en initiatieven van de stedelijke elite inzake de volkswoningbouw en de stedebouw in Rotterdam, 1860-1950*, Rotterdam 1998
Kleuren in de ziekenkamer: onderzoek en aanbevelingen, s.l. 1993
Kloos, J.P., 'Ziekenhuisbouw', *Bouwkundig Weekblad*, 76 (1958) 38, pp. 458-461
Kloos, J.P., *Architectuur, een gewetenszaak*, The Hague 1985
Kloos, J.P., N. Mens, 'Het functionele ziekenhuis. Complexiteit wordt soms overschat', *ZM Magazine*, 15 (1999) 6, pp. 14-17
Knol, C.F.A., 'Optimale planning in de ziekenhuisbouw', *Bouw*, 28 (1973) 12, pp. 385-386
Koekebakker, O. (ed.), *Zorg voor morgen. Ontwerpen voor de gezondheidszorg*, Rotterdam 1997
Kohnstamm, P.P., L.J. Regterschot, *De manager als bouwheer. De rol van de bestuurder bij de realisatie van nieuwe huisvesting*, The Hague 1994
Kok, J.B., *The elderly and urban planning in Amsterdam*, Amsterdam 1986
Kolkman, F., 'Integratie van de gezondheidszorg. Het model van een wijksteunpunt, *Architectuur/Bouwen*, 3 (1987) 6/7, pp. 25-26
Kolkman, F.A.J., 'Veranderende zorgvoorzieningen', *ZM Magazine*, 6 (1990) 1, pp. 23-27
Königs, H.A.F., C. de Kievit, 'Studie commissie voor poliklinieken, röntgen-afdelingen enz. Rapport inzake poliklinieken', *Het Ziekenhuiswezen*, 21 (1948), p. 361
Koster, E., 'Alternatief functionalisme in low-tech en barok. Twee projecten van Aldo en Hannie van Eyck', *de Architect* 20 (1989), 12, pp. 42-54
Kothe, F.H.A., *Het Academisch ziekenhuis van de Vrije Universiteit te Amsterdam. Introductieboek uitgegeven ter gelegenheid van de officiële ingebruikneming van het ziekenhuis*, Amsterdam 1966
Kramer, F., 'De geneeskundige behandeling en de verpleging van geesteszieken van de middeleeuwen tot heden', *Groniek*, 15 (1981) 71, pp. 29-36
Krankenhäuser in Berlin. Bauten und Projekte der 80er Jahre, Berlin 1989
Krijger, E., *Receptuur voor kleinschaligheid. Een onderzoek naar de stand van zaken, kansen en knelpunten van acht kleinschalige initiatieven in de zorg voor mensen met dementie*, Utrecht/Rotterdam 2002
Krol, B., J.W. Groothoff, *Kleinschalige woonvoorzieningen voor ouderen: de ervaring gemeten, de behoefte gepeild*, Groningen 2000
Krol, D.A., M.K.J.J. ter Kuile, 'Is heroriëntering bij de huisvesting van bejaarden geboden?', *Bouw*, 24 (1969) 21, pp. 866-869
Kroonenberg, S. (ed.), *Handboek voor het ziekenhuiswezen*, s.l. 1939
Kruisheer, J.E., *AZG ontwikkelingsplan 76*, Rotterdam 1976
Kruisheer, J.E., 'Vormgeving ziekenhuis in relatie tot omgeving', *Plan*, 8 (1977) 8, pp. 16-27
Kruisheer, J., 'Zonder inspraak geen schoonheid', *Plan*, 9 (1978) 3, p. 20
Kruisheer, J., 'Integratie', *Plan*, 10 (1979) 4, p. 5

Kruisheer, J., 'Het stadsziekenhuis in de toekomst. Emancipatie van de gezondheidszorg vraagt om spreiding', *Architectuur/Bouwen*, 3 (1987) 6/7, pp. 13-16
Kruisheer, J.E., 'Het Regionaal Model Gezondheidszorg', *ZM Magazine*, 6 (1990) 1, pp. 17-22
Kruisheer, J.E., *Van appeltje tot gemberstok. Herinneringen van een ziekenhuisarchitect*, Oberägeri 1997 [manuscript]
Kühn, E., P. Vogler (ed.), *Medizin und Städtebau. Ein Handbuch für gesundheitlichen Städtebau*, Munich/Berlin/Vienna 1957
Kuhn, F.O., *Entwerfen, Anlage und Einrichtung der Gebäude. Des Handbuches der Architektur vierter Theil. 5. Halb-Band: Gebäude für Heil- und sonstige Wohlfahrts-Anstalten. 1. Heft: Krankenhäuser*, Stuttgart 1897
Kuhn, F.O., *Krankenhäuser. Handbuch der Architektur Vierter Teil 5. Halb-Band 1. Heft*, Stuttgart 1903
Kuiper, I., *VPR-Stimuleringsprijs 2005. 'Het beste woonzorginitiatief voor ouderen'. 20 creatieve voorbeelden die navolging verdienen*, s.l. 2005
Kullberg, J., *Ouderen van nu en van de toekomst. Hun financiële spankracht, zorgbehoefte en woonwensen,* The Hague 2005
Kwee, L., J. Hacquebord (ed.), *Preventief wonen. Ouder worden zonder zorg*, s.l. 2005
Kwee, L., J. Hacquebord, *Preventief wonen. De dynamiek van de derde levensfase*, s.l. 2007

'Laagbouw voordeliger voor ziekenhuizen', *Bouw*, 29 (1974) 6, p. IV
Labryga, F., *Moderne Gesundheitsbauten*, Munich 1970
Laddé, E., H.Th. Hopman, 'Ouderenhuisvesting', special of *RIW-cahier*, Delft 1991
Lambert, A., 'De huisvesting van ouderen. Zelfstandig wonen in een zorgzame samenleving', *Architectuur/Bouwen*, 4 (1988) 1, pp. 11-15
Le Corbusier. Oeuvre complète 1957-1965, Zürich 1965
Leene, F., Chr. Hermsen, J. Stelwagen, 'De Multi-functionele Eenheid als Paard van Troje?' *Maandblad Geestelijke Volksgezondheid*, 50 (1995) 1, pp. 15-27
Leeuw, J.J. van der, *Domotica voor zelfstandige huisvesting*, Rotterdam 2000
Leijen, J., *Woonzorg Nederland in beeld*, Amsterdam s.a.
Leistikow, D., *Hospitalbauten in Europa aus zehn Jahrhunderten. Ein Beitrag zur Geschichte des Krankenhausbaues*, Ingelheim am Rhein 1967
Leroy, J.B., *Précis d'un ouvrage sur les hôpitaux dans lequel on expose les principes, résultats des observations de physique et de médecine qu'on doit avoir en vue dans la construction des édifices, avec un projet d'hôpital disposé d'après ces principes*, Paris 1787
Leupen, J., 'De plannen van het nieuwe Academisch Ziekenhuis te Amsterdam', *Het Ziekenhuiswezen*, 31 (1958), pp. 247-255
Lichtenberg, J., 'Ziekenhuizen bij oplevering al verouderd', *Bouw IQ*, 13 (2008) 7, pp. 28-29
Lieburg, M.J. van, *Het Coolsingelziekenhuis te Rotterdam (1839-1900). De ontwikkeling van een stedelijk ziekenhuis in de 19e eeuw*, Amsterdam 1986
Lieburg, M.J. van, W.W. Mijnhardt (ed.), *Geneeskunde en gezondheidszorg in Nederland 1940-1945*, Amsterdam 1992
Lieshout, P. van, 'Veertig jaar geestelijke volksgezondheid', *Tijdschrift Geestelijke Volksgezondheid*, 40 (1985) 12, pp. 1243-1274
Ligtelijn, V., *Aldo van Eyck. Werken*, Bussum 1999
Lijnzaad, C., 'Het bejaardenvraagstuk – een maatschappijprobleem', *Forum*, 13 (1958) 5, pp. 146-147
Lindeboom, G.A., M.J. van Lieburg (ed.), *Gedenkboek van de Vereniging tot Christelijke Verzorging van Geestes- en Zenuwzieken, 1884-1984*, Kampen 1984
Loghem, J.B. van, 'Theorie en Praktijk', *De 8 en Opbouw*, 3 (1932) 20, pp. 195-199
Loghem, J.B. van, 'Vergrooting van het Sophiaziekenhuis te Zwolle', *De 8 en Opbouw*, 6 (1935) 20, pp. 210-214
Loghem, J.B. van, 'Uitbreiding van de Diaconessen-inrichting te Rotterdam', *De 8 en Opbouw*, 10 (1939) 26, pp. 279-284
Luijkx, K.G., D. Brinkhof, 'Behoeften wonen, welzijn en zorg in beeld', *ZM Magazine*, 22 (2006) 6, pp. 2-5
Luthmann, M.J., 'Ziekenhuisbouw', *Bouw*, 4 (1949) 11, pp. 161-171
Maas, T., 'Omgaan met de machteloosheid. Nieuwe types huisvesting psychiatrische patiënten', *Architectuur/Bouwen*, 3 (1987) 6/7, pp. 22-24
Maas, T., 'Maak van een ziekenhuis een stad', *Architectuur/Bouwen*, 7 (1991) 6/7, pp. 33-34
Malkin, J., *Hospital Interior Architecture*, New York 1992
Mandat, M. le, *Prévoir l'espace hospitalier*, Paris 1989
Mandemaker, T., L. Christ, *De volledige extramuralisering van het verzorgingshuis*, Utrecht 2005
Manen, N.F. van, *De medische specialist in het algemene ziekenhuis*, Deventer 1976
Marberry, S.O. (ed.), *Journal of Healthcare Design. Proceedings from the Fourth Symposium on Healthcare Design*, [s.l.] 1992
Marberry, S.O. (ed.), *Innovations in Healthcare Design: Selected Presentations from the First Five Symposia on Healthcare Design*, New York 1995
Marens, H., et al., *Voor gek gehouden. Geschiedenis van de krankzinnigenzorg in Nederland*, Gouda/Haarlem 1982
Marlet, J.J.C. (ed.), *Een halve eeuw, ter herdenking van het vijftig-jarig bestaan van het psychiatrisch ziekenhuis St. Anna Venray*, Venray 1961
Martin, M., *Abe Bonnema Architect*, Rotterdam 1998
'McMaster University Health Sciences Centre Hamilton Ontario (Canada)', *Werk/Oeuvre*, 1974, pp. 157-162
Medische faculteit Rotterdam en Academisch Ziekenhuis Dijkzigt: Visie 1965-1970, Rotterdam 1971
Meer, L. van der, 'Verzorgingstehuizen voor bejaarden. Onderdeel van een sociaal-structureel bejaardenbeleid', *Bouw*, 25 (1970) 9, pp. 336-338
Meer dan oud alleen. De huisvesting van ouderen in een breder perspectief, [Amsterdam 1993]
Meijer, J.A.J., 'De bejaarde als mens', *Bouw*, 11 (1956) 4, pp. 84-85
Mens, N., 'Academisch Ziekenhuis Groningen; spiegel van de stad', *de Architect*, 28 (1997) 6, pp. 14-15
Mens, N., 'De metamorfose van het ziekenhuis', *Medisch Contact*, 53 (1998) 51/52, pp. 1636-1641
Mens, N., 'Neue Konzepte in den Niederlanden', *Bauwelt*, 89 (1998), pp. 2230-2231
Mens, N., 'De architectuur van het ziekenhuis', *ZM Magazine*, 15 (1999) 6, pp. 4-12
Mens, N., 'De bouwgeschiedenis van de Willem Arntsz Hoeve', *Open*, 1 (2002) 2, pp. 73-77
Mens, N., *De Architectuur van het psychiatrisch ziekenhuis*, Wormer 2003
Mens, N., *Zorgboulevards. Verkenningen in het zorg landschap van morgen*, Bussum 2005
Mens, N., 'De toekomst van de senioren', *Suncity Eindhoven. De zilveren kracht*, Eindhoven 2007
Mens, N., A. Tijhuis, 'Het Ziekenhuis van de toekomst= The hospital of the future', *Archis*, (1998) 1, pp. 78-79
Mens, N., A. Tijhuis, *De architectuur van het ziekenhuis. Transformaties in de naoorlogse ziekenhuisbouw in Nederland*, Rotterdam 1999
Mens, N., C. Wagenaar, *De toekomst van de polikliniek. Anders bouwen voor betere zorg*, Amsterdam 2007
Mens, N., C. Wagenaar, *Healing Environment. Anders bouwen voor betere zorg*, Bussum 2009
Mens, N., C. Wagenaar, *De architectuur van de ouderen-huisvesting. Bouwen voor wonen en zorg*, Rotterdam 2009
Mens, N., C. Wagenaar (ed.), *De toekomst van de polikliniek. Anders bouwen voor betere zorg*, Amsterdam 2009
'"De Merwebolder" te Sliedrecht', *Bouw*, 28 (1973) 6, pp. 829-831
Meurs, R. van, 'Breng de maatschappij binnen Dennendal, zegt architect Van Klingeren', *Trouw*, 21 juni 1971
Meuser, Ph., C. Schirmer, Neue Krankenhausbauten in Deutschland, Berlin 2006
Meyer, N.J., 'De relatie tussen leefbaarheid, programma's van eisen en bouw plannen bij een academisch ziekenhuis (II)', *Het Ziekenhuis*, 7 (1977), pp. 290-294
Middleton, R., 'Sickness, madness and crime as the grounds of form', *AA Files*, (1992) 24, pp. 16-30; (1993) 25, pp. 14-29
Mignot, C., *Architecture of the 19th Century*, Freiburg 1983
Miller, R.L., E.S. Swensson, *New Directions in Hospital and Healthcare Facility Design*, New York 1995
'Mini-ziekenhuis in wijk', *Health Management Forum*, (1997), pp. 4, 24-25
'Minister Suurhoff opende het Ziekenhuiscentrum', *Bouw*, 12 (1957) 44, pp. 1112-1116
Ministerie van VWS, *Nota Ouderenbeleid in het perspectief van de vergrijzing*, The Hague 2005
Molen, F. van der, *Ouderenhuisvesting. Belangrijkste ontwikkelingen en trends*, s.l. 1998
Molenaar, B., 'Architectuur en/of ziekenhuizen in 80/90/00. Ruimte voor vernieuwend bouwen gezondheidszorg neemt toe', *ZM Magazine*, 15 (1999) 6, pp. 26-27
Molenaar, J., 'Architectuur achter de zintuigen van de waarnemer. ESTEC en Padua, twee nieuwe werken van Aldo en Hannie van Eyck', *Archis* (1990) 1, pp. 32-41
Mouton, R., 'Het binnenstebuitengekeerde APZ', *Maandblad Geestelijke Volksgezondheid*, 52 (1997) 11, pp. 1153-1160
Mulder, P., 'Bejaardenhuizen en architectuur', *Bouw*, 24 (1969) 52, pp. 2090-2091
Mulder, P., 'Met de WZV in de hand, sluit de minister ziekenhuizen in het hele land. Overleg over beddenreductie is mogelijk, maar uitkomsten staan nu vast', *Het Ziekenhuis*, 12 (1982), p. 759
Mulders, H., 'Debat Toekomst van het APZ (IV). Werkwijze moet veranderen', *Het Ziekenhuis*, 24 (1994) 12, pp. 525-527
Multifunctioneel bouwen in de ouderenzorg, Utrecht 2004
Murken, A., *Die bauliche Entwicklung des deutschen allgemeinen Krankenhauses im 19. Jahrhundert*, Göttingen 1979
Murken, A.H., *Vom Armenhospital zum Großklinikum. Die Geschichte des Krankenhauses vom 18. Jahrhundert bis zur Gegenwart*, Cologne 1988
Murken, A.H., 'The Church hospital and the municipal hospital in Germany from the Biedermeier period to the Weimar Republic', *Planning Perspectives*, 9 (1994) 2, pp. 181-203

Naafs, J., *Met zorg wonen*, Houten/Diegem 1997
Nationaal Ziekenhuisinstituut, *Hoog- of laagbouw voor een algemeen ziekenhuis*, Utrecht 1973
Nationaal Ziekenhuisinstituut, *Prijsvraag ziekenhuisbouw 1975. Documentatie van inzendingen*, Utrecht 1975
Nationaal Ziekenhuisinstituut, *Bouwplan-documentatie woonareaal psychiatrische ziekenhuizen*, [s.l.] 1976
Nationale raad voor de volksgezondheid, College voor ziekenhuisvoorzieningen, *Rapport multifunctionele eenheden 1984-1990. Stand van zaken*, Zoetermeer 1991
Nauta, J., 'Architectuur van zorggebouwen', *ZM Magazine*, 23 (2007) 10, pp. 2-4
Nederlands Symposium Ziekenhuisbouw Amsterdam, Amsterdam 1964
Neergaard, C.F., 'New Standards in Hospital Design', *Architectural Record*, July 1937, pp. 117-120
Nelissen, H. (ed.) *Wonen met Zorg*, Amsterdam 1991
Nelissen, L.L.M.F., *Huisvestingsvormen voor psychiatrische patiënten (een typologische beschrijving)*, [scriptie 1982]
Nelson, P., *Cité hospitalière de Lille*, Paris 1933
Nickl-Weller, C., H. Nickl (ed.), *Hospital Architecture*, Berlin 2007
Nicolaï, R., 'Architectuur voor de gezondheidszorg een contradictio in terminis?', *de Architect*, 12 (1981), 2, pp. 31-33
Nicolaï, R., 'Het "panta Rhei", uitdaging van de ziekenhuisbouw', *Bouw*, 30 (1975) 15, pp. 299-301
Nicolaï, R., 'De aanpak van het bouwproces in de gezondheidszorg', *Bouw*, 31 (1976) 2, pp. 33-36
Nicolaï, R., 'Prijsvraag ziekenhuisbouw 1975', *Plan*, 8 (1977) 7, pp. 29-45
Nicolaï, R., *Typologie van Gebouwen. Handleiding bij het ontwerpen van verpleeghuizen voor somatisch zieken*, s.l. 1982
Nicolaï, R., *Inleiding tot het bouwen voor de gezondheidszorg*, Utrecht 1983
Nicolaï, R., 'NZi-rapport niets zo veranderlijk als een ziekenhuis', *Architectuur/Bouwen*, 7 (1991) 6/7, pp. 25-27
Nicolaï, R., K.H. Dekker, *Flexibiliteit als bouwstrategie. Band I handleiding*, Utrecht [1991]
Nicolaï, R., K.H. Dekker, *Flexibiliteit als bouwstrategie. Band II aanvullende informatie*, Utrecht [1991]
Nierstrasz, F.H.J., 'Het grote verzorgingstehuis voor bejaarden', *Bouw*, 21 (1966) 45, pp. 1779-1782

Niet van later zorg, The Hague 2007
Nieukerken, M.A. van, *Sanatoria voor tuberculose patiënten*, Deventer 1909
'Nieuw gebouw voor de Remonstrantsche Stichting voor ouden van dagen e.d.', *Bouwkundig Weekblad Architectura*, 59 (1937) 50, pp. 474-475
Nieuwe woonzorgvoorzieningen voor ouderen. Documentatie en beknopte evaluatie van zeven (semi-) intramurale projecten, Delft 1992
Nijenhuis, R.G.A., *Ziekenhuisbouw. Een programmeringsstudie naar het voorbereidingsproces van algemene ziekenhuizen*, Delft 1991
Noakes, T., P. James, *Hospital Architecture*, Harlow 1994
'Nodig: 982 bejaardentehuizen', *Bouw*, 16 (1961) 26, p. 822
Noort, J. van den, *Blokken op de bres. Geschiedenis van planning en bouw van het nieuwe Academische Ziekenhuis Groningen (1967-1997)*, Groningen 1999
'Nota bejaardenbeleid 1970', *Bouw*, 25 (1970) 41, p. 1571
Nouws, H., *Het transformatieproces van verzorgingshuizen: vier recente cases. 'Gundaphorus' Paleis'*, Utrecht 2004
Nuffield Studies in the functions and design of hospitals, London/New York, Toronto 1955
Nuyens, Y., 'Ziekenhuisbouw: experimenteren met integratie', *Plan*, 8 (1977) 8, pp. 34-38

'Onno Greiner: "Ik heb me aangepast aan de omliggende natuur..."', *Baksteen*, 14 (1972) 3, pp. 14-16
'Ontwerp voor een gemeenteziekenhuis en gemeente-apotheek te Den Haag', *Polytechnisch Tijdschrift*, 20 (1965), pp. 541-551
Ontwerpmethode voor standaardziekenhuizen, s.l. 1973
Oosterhuis, J.P., 'Tien jaar bejaardenhuisvesting', *Bouw*, 21 (1966) 27, pp. 1037-1041
Opwaarderen. Maatregelen voor het langer zelfstandig wonen van ouderen in de bestaande woningvoorraad, Utrecht 2003
Oude bomen? Oude bomen moet je niet verplanten. Advies over ouderenbeleid en wonen, The Hague 2005
De oudeliedenzorg, Haarlem 1950
Ouder worden in uw eigen huis, s.l. s.a.
Ouderen en hun woonbehoeften, Delft 1981
Ouderen wonen met toekomst. Overzichtspublikatie ouderenhuisvesting, The Hague 1994
Ouderenbeleid en onderzoek in perspectief. 20 jaar Nederlands overheidsbeleid, s.l., 1993
Ouderenhuisvesting op regionaal niveau. Samenvatting, The Hague 1989
Ouderenzorg met toekomst. Advies van de Commissie modernisering ouderenzorg aan de minister van Welzijn, Volksgezondheid en Cultuur, The Hague 1994
Overbeek, R. van, A. Schippers (ed.), *Vergrijzing in Nederland. Naar een toekomstgericht ouderenbeleid*, Utrecht 2005

Paris d'hospitalité, Paris 1990
Pasch, T. van de, 'Vergrijzing in een ander daglicht', interview with Martin Boekholdt, *Tijdschrift voor Verpleegkundigen*, 26 (2007) 4, pp. 20-22
Passchier, G., *Academisch Ziekenhuis Maastricht. AZM*, Maastricht 1991
Peeters, J., C. Woldringh, *Groepswonen van ouderen*, Nijmegen 1989
Pelicaan, J.C., 'Voorschriften en wenken voor bejaardentehuizen', *Bouw*, 22 (1967) 5, pp. 161-162
Perquin, L., *'Het Boston model', een alternatief voor 24-uurs psychiatrische opname?*, Amsterdam 1985
Peters, J., C. Woldringh, *Groepswonen voor ouderen*, Nijmegen 1989
Petersen, C., W. Bokkes, *Inkomen, vermogen en het eigen woningbezit van ouderen. Gebruik van de woningvoorraad*, The Hague 1991
Pevsner, N., *A History of Building Types*, London 1976
Pinon, P., *L'Hospice de Charenton. The Charenton Hospital*, Liège/Brussels 1989
Pistor, R., A. Lambert, 'Geestelijke gezondheidszorg 2. De heerschappij van het medisch model', *B-nieuws*, 8 (1975) 32, pp. 552-553
Pluym, Y. van der, 'Het ziekenhuis van klooster tot kamstructuur. De geschiedenis van de ziekenhuisbouw', *Architectuur/Bouwen*, 2 (1986) 11, pp. 51-57
Poel, D.C. van der, 'Het pensiontehuis op de helling', *Bouw*, 16 (1961) 21, pp. 652-654
Poel, D.C. van der, 'De bejaarden en hun huisvesting', *Bouw*, 17 (1962) 17, pp. 588-590
Poel, E. van der, M. Romme, K. Trimbos, H. van der Wilk, *Het psychiatrisch ziekenhuis in diskussie. Verslag van de actie Moratorium Nieuwbouw APZ'en*, Amsterdam 1985
Post, H.E., *Bouwen in de gezondheidszorg*, Amsterdam 1992
Posthumus Meyjes, C.B, 'Het sanatorium "Koningsheide" te Arnhem', *Bouwkundig Weekblad Architectura*, 57 (1936) 48, p. 489
Povel, H., 'Hoe maak ik een flexibel ziekenhuis? Ziekenhuizen Assen en Almere eerste stap in door NZi onderzochte trend', *Architectuur/Bouwen*, 7 (1991) 6/7, pp. 14-15
Praktijkhandboek bouw en beheer. Wonen met zorg voor ouderen, Houten/Diegem 1998
Priemus, H., E. Sjoer (ed.), *Ouderenhuisvesting: modernisering van wonen en zorg*, Delft 1997
Prins, H., 'Kleinschaligheid in de psychiatrie', *Reformatorisch Dagblad*, 12 July 1985
Prodi, F.R., A. Stocchetti, *l'Architettura dell'ospedale*, Florence 1990
'Psychiatrie en Hoogbouw', *Bouw*, 13 (1958) 32, pp. 822-823
'Psychiatrisch ziekenhuis St. Franciscushof te Raalte', *Bouw*, 23 (1968) 8, pp. 300-309
Pütsep, E., *Planning of Surgical Centres. Basic Studies*, London 1969
Pütsep, E., *Modern Hospital. International Planning Practices*, London 1979

Querido, A., *Godshuizen en gasthuizen*, Amsterdam 1960
Querido, A., 'Prijsvraagontwerpen getoetst aan structuur van de gezondheidszorg', *Plan*, 8 (1977) 7, pp. 46-47

Ramaer, J.N., 'De ontwikkeling van het krankzinnigengesticht in deze eeuw', *Weekblad van het Nederlandsch Tijdschrift voor Geneeskunde*, 22 (1886) 15, pp. 365-389
Rapport van de Studiecommissie voor de verzorging en huisvesting van Ouden van Dagen, s.l. 1950
Ravelli, D.P., A.J.P. Schrijvers, 'Eindtijd van de Nederlandse APZ-en', *Maandblad Geestelijke Volksgezondheid*, 54 (1999) 5, pp. 490-504
Redstone L.G., (ed.), *Hospitals and Health Care Facilities; an Architectural Record Book*, New York/ Washington D.C. 1978
Reinalda, M.A., 'Gebouwen voor bejaardenzorg', *Bouw*, 11 (1956) 4, pp. 84-86
Rentes de Carvalho, J., 'Door het oog van de gebruiker', in: G. Staal, H. Wolters (ed.), *Holland in vorm. Vormgeving in Nederland 1945-1987*, The Hague 1987, pp. 7-17
Reyers, J.G., 'Huisvesting van bejaarden. Een sociaal vraagstuk voor de geheele bevolking', *Bouw* 1 (1946) 15, pp. 372-379
Rigter, R.B.M. (ed.), *Overheid en gezondheidszorg in de twintigste eeuw*, Rotterdam 1993
Rodenstein, M., *'Mehr Licht, mehr Luft'. Gesundheitskonzepte im Städtebau seit 1750*, Frankfurt/ Main/New York 1988
Rodermond, J., 'Architectonische innovatie gevraagd. Kwaliteitsslag noodzakelijk in verpleeg- en verzorgingstehuizen', *de Architect*, 37 (2006) 10, pp. 56-61
Rodermond, J.G., H. Weyde, *Huisvesting van ouderen. Een terreinverkennende studie naar de mogelijkheden van ouderenhuisvesting binnen de algemene volkhuisvestingsregelgeving*, Leiden 1992
Rombouts, A.L.G.M., 'Voorbereiding van ziekenhuisprojecten. De noodzaak van een weldoordacht programma van eisen', *Bouw*, 12 (1957) 41, pp. 1027-1029
Rombouts, A.L.G.M., 'Voorbereiding van ziekenhuisprojecten', *Katholiek Bouwblad*, 25 (1958), 397-398
Rondagh, F., 'Psychiatrisch centrum wordt anders met gewone huizen', *de Volkskrant*, 19 juli 1975
Rongen, M.J.Th., J.C.M. de Heij, *Huisvesting en huisvestingswensen van oudere huishoudens*, The Hague 1993
Rooijmans, H.G.M., *Negenennegentig jaar tussen wal en schip. Geschiedenis van de Leidse Universitaire Psychiatrie*, Houten/Diegem 1998
Rosenau, H., 'Antoine Petit und sein Zentralplan für das Hôtel-Dieu in Paris. Ein Beitrag zur Architektur-Typologie', *Zeitschrift für Kunstgeschichte*, (1964) 3/4, pp. 228-237
Rosenau, H., 'The Functional and the Ideal in late eighteenth-century French Architecture', *Architectural Review*, October 1966, pp. 253-258
Rosenfield, I., *Hospitals. Integrated Design*, New York 1947
Rosenfield, I., *Hospital Architecture and Beyond*, New York [etc.] 1969
Rosenfield, I., *Hospital Architecture. Integrated Components*, New York 1971
Rubbens-Franken, E., 'Moderne bejaardentehuizen', *Linoleumnieuws*, 20 (1963) 1, pp. 2-31
Rütte, J.L.A.G.A. le, 'Inrichting van separeervertrekken voor geesteszieken', *Het Ziekenhuis*, 3 (1912) 6, pp. 59-62
Rütte, J.L.A.G.A. le, 'Een nieuwe richting in de wijze van interneering en verpleging der krankzinnigen', *Het Ziekenhuis*, 7 (1916) 2, pp. 9-13

Sannen, H., L. de Ree, Th. Royers, *Hoe wij senioren willen leven en wonen. Huisvesting van ouderen in de stad= Housing for the elderly in the city*, Amsterdam 1987
Schachner, R., H. Schmieden, *Krankenhausbau*, Berlin 1930
Schade, H.J.M., 'Geschiedkundige ontwikkeling van het krankzinnigenwezen in Nederland', *Het Ziekenhuiswezen*, 9 (1936) 9, pp. 481-485
Scheer, W.M. van der, 'Vooruitgang in de krankzinnigenverpleging 1850-1925', *Het Ziekenhuiswezen*, 1 (1928), pp. 188-196
Scheer, W.M. van der, *Nieuwere inzichten in de behandeling van geesteszieken,* Groningen/The Hague/Batavia 1933
Scheerder, R., M. Verweij, 'Flexibel bouwen. Vastgoed in de cure op een kruispunt van wegen', *Medisch Contact*, 60 (2005) 5, pp. 189-191
Scheerens, R. (ed.), *Scandinavië als voorbeeld voor Nederland? Deense, Noorse en Zweedse experimenten in ouderenhuisvesting en -zorg*, Rotterdam 1992
Scherpenisse, R. van, J. Singelenberg, B. van de Donk (ed.), *Seniorenscore en Opplussen. Opsporen en aanpassen van bestaande woningen*, Rotterdam 1995
Scherpenisse, R. van, J. Singelenberg, *Voortgangsverslag opplussen*, Rotterdam 1996
Schiffczyk, D., *Die intellektuelle Revolution im europäischen Krankenhausbau um 1800. Zur systematischen Entwicklung neuzeitlicher Bauformen vor dem Hintergrund des mittelalterlichen Hospitaltypus*, Frankfurt am Main 1985
Schippers, R., *Het subsidie-instrument kritisch bekeken. Evaluatie van de tijdelijke woonzorgstimuleringsregeling*, [The Hague 2004; thesis]
Schmid, S., *Vrijheid is de beste medicijn. Over de democratische psychiatrie in Italië*, Amsterdam 1979
Schmidt, F.J.M., *Die Entwicklung der Irrenpflege in den Niederlanden. Vom Tollhaus bis zur gesetzlich anerkannten Irrenanstalt*, Herzogenrath 1985 [dissertation Aken]
Schnabel, P., 'Over fanfares, feesten en fusies', *Maandblad Geestelijke Volksgezondheid*, 52 (1997) 5, p. 466
Schrijvers, G., J.M. Boot (ed.), *Een halve eeuw gezondheidszorg: 1950-2000*, Lochem [etc.] 1983
Schuurmans Stekhoven, J.H., *Ontwikkeling van het krankzinnigenwezen in Nederland, 1813-1914. Verzameling van archiefstukken, statistische tabellen, platen, kaarten, grafische voorstellingen, bouwkundige teekeningen, enz.*, The Hague 1922
Schuyt-Lucassen, N.Y., G.J.F. Leene, P.P.J. Houben, *Hofjes in perspectief. Een onderzoek naar de identiteit en actualiteit van de Hofjes Codde en Van Beresteyn in het licht van de modernisering van de ouderenhuisvesting*, Amsterdam 1995
Schuijt-Lucassen, N.Y, G.J.F. Leene, P.P.J. Houben, *Hofjes met perspectief. Al eeuwen een moderne woonvorm voor ouderen*, Bussum 1997
Schuyt, K., E. Taverne, *1950. Welvaart in zwart-wit*, The Hague 2000
Senioren thuis test, s.l. s.a.
Seniorenlabel. Geschikt voor alle Leeftijden. Consumentenkeurmerk, Rotterdam 1995
Seniorenstad een eigenzinnig dorp, s.l. 2006
Sep, P., *Tot in lengte van dagen. Zelfstandige ouderenhuisvesting en architectuur*, Amsterdam 1993

Singelenberg, J. (ed.), *Tussen wonen en zorg. Experimenteren met woonzorgprojecten voor ouderen*, Rotterdam 1993
Singelenberg, J., *Levensloop van een vinex-wijk. Bouwen met het oog op ouderen en gehandicapten, nu en in de toekomst*, Rotterdam 1996
Singelenberg, J., *Eindrapport nationale Survey Woonzorgcomplexen*, Rotterdam 1999
Singelenberg, J., 'Welke innovaties hebben echt het aangezicht van woonzorgland veranderd?', in: *Innovatieve kracht in wonen en zorg*, Utrecht 2008
Singelenberg, J., D. Bergvelt, *Woon- en Zorgservice voor verspreid wonende ouderen*, Rotterdam 1994
Söderberg, L., 'Trends in Swedisch Hospital Design', *World Hospitals = l'Hôpital dans le Monde*, 2 (1965), p. 217
Spanjer, M., *Dynamiek in Steen. Jubileumuitgave College voor Ziekenhuisvoorzieningen 1972-1997*, Delft 1997
'Spiegel van de week', *Bouw*, 25 (1970) 19, p. 813
Stagg/bbi, *Rapportage doeleinden-analyse zwakzinnigenzorg*, Amsterdam, Utrecht 1977
Stam, M., 'Ziekenhuizen', *De 8 en Opbouw*, 6 (1935), pp. 245-249
Stichting Architektenonderzoek Gebouwen Gezondheidszorg (Stagg), *Programmeringsmethodiek ziekenhuizen*, Amsterdam 1974
Stichting Architektenonderzoek Gebouwen Gezondheidszorg (Stagg), *Goedkeuringsprocedure*, Amsterdam 1974
Stichting Architektenonderzoek Gebouwen Gezondheidszorg (Stagg), *Kostenbegeleiding vanaf de elementenbegroting*, Amsterdam 1976
Stichting Architektenonderzoek Gebouwen Gezondheidszorg (Stagg), *Proces bouwvoorbereiding*, Amsterdam 1978
Stichting Architektenonderzoek Gebouwen Gezondheidszorg (Stagg), *Regionaal Model gezondheidszorg: een architektenbijdrage over integratie en schaal in de zorg*, Amsterdam 1982
Stichting Architektenonderzoek Gebouwen Gezondheidszorg (Stagg), *Supplement op het rapport proces bouwvoorbereiding*, Amsterdam 1983
Stichting Architektenonderzoek Gebouwen Gezondheidszorg (Stagg), *Wijksteunpunt 'Ontkokering van de zorg' haalbaar of niet haalbaar?*, Amsterdam 1986
Stichting Architektenonderzoek Gebouwen Gezondheidszorg (Stagg), *Planning in de gezondheidszorg. Voorstel tot bijstelling van de toestemmingsprocedure*, Amsterdam 1986
Stichting Architektenonderzoek Gebouwen Gezondheidszorg (Stagg), *Veranderende zorgvoorzieningen*, Amsterdam 1992
Stockman, R. (et al.), *Geen rede mee te rijmen. Geschiedenis van de psychiatrie*, Ghent 1989
Stockman, R. (et al.), *Met Recht en Rede. Waanzin tussen Wet en Kabinet*, Ghent 1997
Stockman, R., 'Prof. Dr. Joseph Guislain: zijn leven en zijn werken', *Psychiatrie en verpleging*, 73 (1997) 3, pp. 214-226
Stofberg, I.C., 'Bejaardentehuizen in een produktiestroom', *Bouw*, 23 (1968) 21, pp. 832-834
Stolte, J.B., 'IHF Study Tour of Hospitals in the Netherlands', *World Hospitals = l'Hôpital dans le Monde*, 6 (1971) 1, p. 27
Stolwijk, W.Q., 'Van het programma van eisen naar het ontwerp', *De Ingenieur*, 91 (1979), pp. 734-735
Stolwijk, W.Q., *Flexibiliteit in Ziekenhuisbouw: een onderzoek naar de bouwkundige ontwikkeling van algemene ziekenhuizen in relatie tot in- en externe factoren om te komen tot aanbevelingen voor een optimaal gebruik van ziekenhuiscomplexen*, Delft 1987
Stone, P.J., 'Elements of the Hospital: 1300–1900', *Architectural Review*, June 1965, pp. 413-416
Straathof, L.J.A., *Uittreksel basisplannen Psychiatrisch Ziekenhuis Zeeland*, Goes 1977
Strauven, F., *Aldo van Eyck. Relativiteit en verbeelding*, Amsterdam 1994
Structuurnota Gezondheidszorg, The Hague 1974
Swinkels, T., 'Leven en wonen van psychiatrische patiënten, gewoon of buitengewoon', in: L.H. Kroeks (et al.), *Voordrachten en discussies van het symposion ter gelegenheid van de St. Joseph-stichting op 24 en 25 november 1975*, Apeldoorn 1977, pp. 35-50
Swinkels, T., 'Tussen mens en methode. De architectuur van het ziekenhuis 1970-1980, *ZM Magazine*, 15 (1999) 6, pp. 18-21
Tanke, G., 'Nieuwe Zorgarchitectuur. Solidariteit in een individualistische samenleving', *Zorgvisie*, 36 (2006) 5
Taylor, J., *Hospital and Asylum Architecture in England 1840-1914. Building for Health Care*, London 1991
Taylor, J., *The Architect and the Pavillon Hospital. Dialogue and Design Creativity in England 1850-1914*, London/New York 1997
Tellegen, E., *Waar was de dood nog meer*, Bilthoven 1971
Tengbom, A., 'Recent Developments in the Design of Hospitals in Scandinavia', *World Hospitals = l'Hôpital dans le Monde*, 2 (1966) 1, pp. 1-4
Tennekes, H.J., 'Ontwikkeling van een ziekenhuisarchitectuur. Ontwerp streekziekenhuis Waterland in Purmerend', *Architectuur/Bouwen*, 3 (1987) 6/7, pp. 9-12
Tennekes, H.J., 'Duur NZi-model kan goedkoper', *Architectuur/Bouwen*, 7 (1991) 6/7, pp. 31-32
Tennekes, H.J., 'De arrogantie van de macht. Jaren tachtig; bouwen voor een snel veranderende samenleving', *ZM Magazine*, 15 (1999) 6, pp. 22-25
Tenon, J.R., *Mémoires sur les hôpitaux de Paris*, Paris 1788
Term, J. van, *Twee faculteiten onder één dak*, Maastricht 1992
'The architect and the hospital', *Architectural Record*, August 1946, pp. 69-75
Thiadens, A.J.H. (ed.), *Ziekenhuis menselijk en modern. De patiënt als kritische consument van intramurale gezondheidszorg*, Deventer 1972 [supplements 1973 and 1975]
Thompson, J.D., G. Goldin, *The Hospital. A Social and Architectural History*, London 1975
Tilanus, J.W.R. *De vernieuwing der stedelijk ziekenhuizen te Amsterdam in de negentiende eeuw*, Amsterdam 1907
Tilman, H., 'Bejaardenhuis gepasseerd station. Grotere rol voor architectuur in de zorg', *de Architect*, 37 (2006) 10, pp. 44-55
De toekomst van het verzorgingshuis, s.l. 2004
Tollet, C., *De l'Assistance publique et des hôpitaux jusqu'au XIXe siècle*, Paris 1889
Tollet, C., *Les édifices hospitaliers depuis leur origine jusqu'à nos jours*, Paris 1892
Tollet, C., *Les hôpitaux modernes au XIXe siècle*, Paris 1894
Top, W., *Woongemeenschappen van ouderen: licht en tegenlicht*, Utrecht s.a.
TPG, *Het kan écht: betere zorg voor minder geld. Sneller beter. De logistiek in de zorg*, Amsterdam 2004
Trimbos, C.J., 'Moratorium voor psychiatrie-bouw nodig', *NRC Handelsblad*, 6 October 1982
Trimbos, K., *Antipsychiatrie. Een overzicht*, Deventer 1975
Troost-Filipovic, B. (ed.), *Zorgzame architectuur. Zorg voor wonen, wonen met zorg. Verslag van een prijsvraag*, Utrecht 2003
Tuns, A., 'Flexibiliteit. NZi beknot vrijheid in constructie', *Architectuur/Bouwen*, 7 (1991) 6/7, pp. 28-30

UR architects, *De psychiatrische instelling ontmanteld*, s.p., October 2009

Valentijn, D. (ed.), *Van buitenplaats tot zorgcentrum*, The Hague 1995
Veek, J.H. van der, F. van Holland, M.J.J. van Leent, *Bestaande woningen aanpassen voor ouderen. Ontwerpanalyse van acht praktijkprojecten*, The Hague 1994
Veen, W.J. van der, *Oudelieden in gestichten. Bewoners van 19de-eeuwse bejaardenhuizen: een schets van de situatie in Den Haag*, The Hague 1992
Veldhoen, L., 'Nieuw psychiatrisch oord in Nijmegen: "geïsoleerd gekkengetto in de bossen"', *NRC Handelsblad*, 18 januari 1983
'Veldwijk. Het paviljoen-stelsel', in: *Het Eerste Jaarverslag der Vereeniging voor Christelijke Verzorging van krankzinnigen en zenuwlijders in Nederland*, 17 april 1884-15 april 1885
Verblijven of wonen; zorg voor ouderen. Varianten van wonen met zorg voor ouderen, Amsterdam 1995
Verderber, S., D. Fine, *Healthcare Architecture in an Era of Radical Transformation*, London 2000
Vermeulen, M., 'Den Haag. Woonwijk geïntegreerd met psychiatrisch centrum', *Stedenbouw*, 49 (1997) 540, pp. 42-43
'Vermaatschappelijking van ziekenhuizen', *Stedebouw & Architectuur*, 21 (2005) 10, pp. 10-11
Verpleeghuizen. Onderzoek naar de konsekwenties van verschillen in maatafspraak en aantal bouwlagen bij vijftien ontwerpen voor verpleeghuizen. Een studie uitgevoerd in opdracht van het ministerie van volksgezondheid en milieuhygiëne, Amsterdam 1976
Versteegen, M., *Wonen zonder zorgen?*, [Rotterdam 2003]
Verweij, M., F. Bisschop, 'Ingrijpende systeemwijziging voor financiering zorgvastgoed', *ZM Magazine*, 22 (2006) 1, pp. 7-10
'Verzorgingscomplex voor bejaarden te Amsterdam', *Bouw*, 31 (1976) 12, pp. 207-212
Verzorgingstehuizen voor bejaarden, Rotterdam 1970
Verzorgingstehuizen voor bejaarden', *Bouw*, 24 (1969) 42, pp. 1667
Vidler, A., *Writing of the Walls. Architectural Theory in the Late Enlightenment*, Princeton 1987
Viergever, A., 'Ziekenhuisbouw in Amerika', *Polytechnisch Tijdschrift*, 2 (1949), pp. 190-192, 222-226, 252-255
Viergever, A., 'Recente buitenlandse inzichten en ervaringen', *Het Ziekenhuiswezen*, 23 (1950), special on building, pp. 47-64
Vietsch, C.A., *Anamnese, Diagnose, Therapie. Een onderzoek naar de bouwvoorbereiding van algemene ziekenhuizen*, Eindhoven 1987
Vijselaar, J., 'Bronnen voor de geschiedenis van de psychiatrie in Nederland. Een duistere poel', *Groniek*, 15 (1981) 71, pp. 11-15
Vijselaar, J., *Krankzinnigen gesticht. Psychiatrische inrichtingen in Nederland 1880-1910*, Haarlem 1982
Vijselaar, J., 'Schroeder van der Kolk en de Krankzinnigenwet van 1841. Oude wetgeving in een nieuw licht', *Maandblad Geestelijke Volksgezondheid*, 40 (1985) 3, pp. 271-285
Vijselaar, J. (ed.), *Over de IJssel, over de schreef. De geschiedenis van de geestelijke gezondheidszorg in Overijsel en van het Psychiatrisch Ziekenhuis Brinkgreven in het bijzonder*, Utrecht 1993
Vijselaar, J. (ed.), *Dolhuizen – madhouses. Chapters from the history of madhouses in Europe 1400-1800*, Utrecht 1995
Vijselaar, J. (ed.), *Gesticht in de duinen. De geschiedenis van de provinciale psychiatrische ziekenhuizen van Noord-Holland van 1849-1994*, Hilversum 1997
Vletter, M. de, *De kritiese jaren zeventig. Architectuur en stedenbouw in Nederland 1968-1982*, Rotterdam 2004
Vogler, P., E. Kühn (ed.), *Medizin und Städtebau. Ein Handbuch für gesundheitlichen Städtebau*, Munich 1957
Vogler, P., G. Hassenpflug, *Handbuch für den neuen Krankenhausbau*, Munich 1951
Vogler, P., G. Hassenpflug (ed.), *Handbuch für den neuen Krankenhausbau*, Munich, Berlin 1962
Voor gek gehouden. Geschiedenis van de krankzinnigenzorg in Nederland, Haarlem, Gouda 1982
Voordt, D.J.M. van der, D. Terpstra, *Verpleeghuizen: varianten en alternatieven*, Delft 1995
'Voorschriften bouw bejaardenhuizen', *Bouw*, 21 (1966) 13, p. 471
Voorschriften en wenken voor het ontwerpen van verzorgingstehuizen voor bejaarden (1965), The Hague 1966
Vreeze, N. de, *Woningbouw, inspiratie & ambities. Kwalitatieve grondslagen van de sociale woningbouw in Nederland*, Almere 1993
Vries, M. de, 'Woonzorgzones', *Stedebouw & Architectuur*, 25 (2008) 9, pp. 16-18
VROM, VWS, *Beter (t)huis in de buurt. Actieplan Samenwerken aan welzijn en zorg, 2007-2011*, The Hague 2007
VRR-Stimuleringsprijs 2006. 'Het beste woonzorginitiatief voor ouderen'. 10 creatieve voorbeeldprojecten die navolging verdienen, s.l. 2006
Vuister, F., 'Boston in Brabant. Het gedecentraliseerde Psychiatrisch Centrum Oosterhout', *Maandblad Geestelijke Volksgezondheid*, 45 (1990) 10, pp. 1050-1063
Vuister, F., 'Boston in Brabant (2). Vijf jaar Psychiatrisch Centrum Oosterhout', *Maandblad Geestelijke Volksgezondheid*, 49 (1994) 10, pp. 1097-1110

Wagenaar, C. (ed.), *The Architecture of Hospitals*, Rotterdam 2006
Walker, A., G. Naegele, *The Politics of Old Age in Europe*, Buckingham, PA 1999

Walsem, G.C. van, 'Iets over den aanleg van afdeelingstuinen in krankzinnigengestichten', *Het Ziekenhuis*, 1 (1910) 7, pp. 69-72
Ward, K., *The Design and Equipment of Hospitals*, London 1949
Weeber, C., 'Academisch Medisch Centrum: een der grootste gebouwen ter wereld', *Wonen-TA/BK*, 2 (1974) 24, pp. 6-13
Wennink, H.J., 'Armoede en verschraling van zorg in het APZ', *Maandblad Geestelijke Volksgezondheid*, 54 (1999) 9, pp. 916-926
Wennink, H.J., G.W.M.M. de Wilde, J. van Weeghel, H. Kroon, 'De metamorfose van de GGZ. Kanttekeningen bij de vermaatschappelijking', *Maandblad Geestelijke Volksgezondheid*, 56 (2001) 10, pp. 917-937
Werkgroep bouwen-wonen van Nieuw-Dennendal, *Een goede buurt. Filosofie van de verdunning op Dennendal* [*nieuwSchrift* 1974, nr. 5]
Wessels, L., 'Sober en doelmatig. Bouwmaatstaven hebben geen eeuwigheidswaarde', *ZM Magazine*, 15 (1999) 6, pp. 35-36
Westerveld, B.B., 'Bejaardentehuizen en -woningen', *Forum*, 13 (1958) 4, p. 115
Wet van den 27. April 1884 (Stbl. No. 96) betreffende het Staatstoezicht op Krankzinnigen en Krankzinnigengestichten, The Hague 1884
Wiarda Beckman Stichting, *Ziekenhuisbouw in Nederland*, Amsterdam 1961
Wicherink, J.W., 'Het nieuw Academisch Ziekenhuis te Leiden', *Het Ziekenhuis*, 14 (1923), pp. 87-99
Wiercx, R., 'Multifunctionele eenheden. De onstuitbare opmars', *Gazet* (1994) 1, pp. 11-15
Wildt, A. de, W. van der Ham, *Tijd van Laven. Ouder worden in Nederland vroeger en nu*, [publication at the exhibition by the same name at the Amsterdams Historisch Museum, 1993]
Winkel, C. van, *Modern leegte. Over kunst en openbaarheid*, Nijmegen 1999
Wischer, R., H.-U. Rietmüller, *Zukunftoffenes Krankenhaus. Fakten, Leitlinien, Bausteine*, Vienna 2007
Wislocki, P., 'The Architecture of the feel-good factor', *World Architecture*, no. 47, June 1996, pp. 124-145
Wit, J.P. de, 'Provinciale gestichten: mislukt beleid in de 19e eeuw', *Maandblad Geestelijke Volksgezondheid*, 45 (1990) 4, pp. 405-412
Wit, R. de, 'Project Beschut Wonen. Een eigen leven in het APZ', *Psy*, 1 (1997) 11, pp. 17-19
Wonen en zorg voor ouderen. Met een blik over de landsgrens, Almere 1994
Wonen met Zorg. Advies over de samenhang van wonen met zorg- en dienstverlening, Rijswijk 1991
Wonen, zorg en welzijn van ouderen, The Hague 2003
'Woningbouw in IJmuiden (Oost)', *Bouwkundig Weekblad*, 68 (1950) 38, pp. 577-584
'Woongemeenschappen van ouderen', *Woonkwaliteit*, 2 (1990) 9, p. 11
'Woonvriendelijke zones voor ouderen. Aanzet tot een integrale benadering van huisvesting, zorg en voorzieningen in geselecteerde gebieden', special of *Signalen*, Amsterdam 1989
Woonzorg, Amsterdam 1991
Wortman, J.L.C., 'De bouw van kleine ziekenhuizen', *Het Ziekenhuis*, 2 (1910), pp. 35-40
Woud, A. van der, *Waarheid en karakter. Het debat over de bouwkunst 1840-1900*, Rotterdam 1997
Woude, R. van der, W. van der Schuit, *Oude tradities, nieuwe ambities. 200 jaar Academisch Ziekenhuis Groningen*, Groningen 1998

Zaal, K., M. Kastelein, R.J.M. Perenboom, *Vernieuwingen in ouderenhuisvesting en ouderenzorg: voorbeelden van experimenten en onderzoek*, Leiden 1993
Zeeuw, F. de, 'Dé senior bestaat niet!', *Suncity Eindhoven. De zilveren kracht*, Eindhoven 2007
'Ziek zijn, beter worden', *de Architect*, 10 (1979) 5, pp. 107-112
'Het ziekenhuis in de stad', *Plan*, 8 (1977) 8, p. 4
'Ziekenhuis te Dordrecht', *Bouw*, 28 (1973) 43, pp. 1280
'Het ziekenhuis van de toekomst', *Het Ziekenhuiswezen*, 33 (1960), p. 428
Ziekenhuizen. Hospitals, Rotterdam 1961
Zielstra, L.J., 'Samenwerking tussen de Stichting "Het Nederlandse Ziekenhuiswezen" en het "Bouwcentrum"', *Het Ziekenhuiswezen*, 22 (1949), p. 32
Zoethout, T., 'Bestemmingsvrije zorgbouw', *Stedebouw & Architectuur*, 26 (2009) 9, pp. 20-21
Zonnegloren. Soestduinen. Provincie Utrecht, [Utrecht 1921]
Zonneveld, R.J. van, 'Medische aspecten van de huisvesting van bejaarden', *Forum*, 13 (1958) 4, pp. 130-134
Zorg voor ouderen in het jaar 2010, Rijswijk 1990
'Zorginstellingen, poets je tafelzilver', *Zorgvisie*, 30 November 2009
Zorgvernieuwingsprojecten nader bezien. Een inventarisatie in het licht van de woonzorgdiscussie, Leiden 1997
Zwinkels, C., 'Een gebouw als een woonwijk. Academisch Ziekenhuis Utrecht van EGM', *de Architect*, 20 (1989) 11, pp. 121-129

Index

Persons and firms

Locations

Picture credits

a/d amstel architecten 62b, 63, 64, 65, 116bl
a/d amstel architecten/photo Sybolt Voeten 186, 187
Alvar Aalto Museum, Helsinki 43bl, 46t
Aerophoto Eelde 279t
Aerophoto Schiphol 262ml
Alberts & Van Huut 244br
Roos Aldershoff 243tl, 302t, 326t
Altrecht, Den Dolder 24bl, 36, 37, 54
Archief Eemland 67tr, 98, 116tr,
Architecten aan de Maas 120, 121l, 123, 150t, 171t/m, 188tr, 237b, 328b
Architecten aan de Maas/Wiek Ernst luchtfotografie 150b
Architecten aan de Maas/photo F. Keuzenkamp 272t
Architecten aan de Maas/photo F. Lahaye 117br, 151
Architecten aan de Maas/photo Norbert van Onna 308, 309, 329bl
Architecten aan de Maas/photo Martin Thomas 244bl
L'Architecture d'Aujourd'hui, 1938 47t, 128
Architectuurstudio Herman Hertzberger 183b, 208b
Architectuurstudio Herman Hertzberger/photo Martin Charles 208t, 209
Architectuurstudio Herman Hertzberger/photo Walter de Maar 158-159
de Architekten Cie. 281b
Architektur DK, 1975, no. 8 161
Articapress, Sint Lucas Andreas Ziekenhuis Archives, Amsterdam 117bl
Atelier Pro Architekten 276
Aviodrome, Lelystad 10-11, 49mr, 52, 55t, 56, 73bl, 89, 122, 191tl, 193t
AWG architecten/photo Niels Donckers 291tr
J. Bedaux Archives 97t
Bibliothèque nationale de France, Paris 16
Hélène Binet 321t
Bonnema Architecten/photo De Beer en Zwarts Visuele Vertalers 316t/ml, 317
Bonnema Architecten/photo Jan Versnel 137
Brabants Historisch Informatie Centrum, 's-Hertogenbosch 59bl
Stijn Brakkee 299t, 327tl
Eric Brinkhorst 320b
Joost Brouwers 207t/b, 221b, 247tr/mr, 249tr, 291b
Bureau B+B 287br
Burger Grunstra architecten adviseurs/photo Jan Buwalda 157bl
Burger Grunstra architecten adviseurs/photo Rob Hoekstra 230t, 279b
Burger Grunstra architecten adviseurs/photo Derk Jan de Vries 157br
CODA, Apeldoorn 41bl
College Bouw, Utrecht 91b, 172, 173, 201, 203
Das Bürgerspital Basel 1260–1946, Basel 1946 82t
de Jong Gortemaker Algra 117tr, 168, 196, 198, 199, 210, 212, 213, 214, 215, 241t, 243mr, 244mr, 270tr/br, 310br
de Jong Gortemaker Algra/photo P.H. Goede 117tr
de Jong Gortemaker Algra/photo Piet Mobach 129br, 176l
De Nijl Architecten 282
Marco de Nood 202r
De Nudehof, Wageningen 144, 145
René de Wit 291ml
Willem Diepraam 183t
Döll – atelier voor bouwkunst 281t
Philip Driessen 310t/bl, 311, 312, 313
EGM architecten 124, 167b, 216, 217, 237bl, 238, 273tr
EGM architecten/photo Roos Aldershoff 243b
EGM architecten/photo Coks Prins 133b
EGM architecten/photo Evert van Reijswoud 237t, 246r, 314, 315
EGM architecten/Zorgboulevard Rotterdam 278r
Fotoarchief voormalige gemeente Zuidlaren, Historische Vereniging Gemeente Zuidlaren 72t
Fotocollectie gemeentearchief Veenendaal 174
A. Funk, *Gebäude für Heil- und sonstige Wohlfahrtanstalten. Handbuch der Architektur Vierter Teil 5. Halb-Band 2. Heft*, Darmstadt 1891 24br
Gelderland in Beeld, Bibliotheek Arnhem 40br, 41mr, 191tr
Gelders Archief, Arnhem 41t, 60b
Gemeentearchief Bergen op Zoom (Het Markiezenhof) 53tr
Gemeentearchief Goes 194-195
Gemeentearchief Leidschendam 135bl
Gemeentearchief Rotterdam 17br, 24ml, 29mr, 49t/ml, 87mr/br, 156b, 185b, 269tr
Gemeentearchief Rotterdam/photo Wim K. Steffen 91tr
Gemeentearchief Soest 42b
Ggz Drenthe, Assen 51b
Ggz Noord-Holland-Noord, Heiloo 51t/m
Greiner Van Goor Huijten Architecten/photo Frank Greiner 222, 224-225
Greiner Van Goor Huijten Architecten/photo Jac ten Bbrek 130, 152, 153
Dr. Guislain Museum, Paris 21tr
Haags Gemeentearchief, The Hague 29tl, 77bl, 115tl, 190t
Martijn Heil 262mr, 263, 329mbl
Het Eerste Jaarverslag der Vereeniging voor Christelijke Verzorging van krankzinnigen en zenuwlijders in Nederland, 17 april 1884–15 april 1885 23ml
Het Huis Oud en Nieuw, 1918–1919, p. 276 62t
Het Huis Oud en Nieuw, 1928 pp. 35-36 48, 49b
Het Zonnehuis, Beekbergen 61
Het Zonnehuis, Vlaardingen 133t
Historisch Archief Almelo 83b, 167t
Historisch Centrum Limburg, Maastricht 99
Historisch Centrum Overijssel, Zwolle 87t
Historisch Documentatiecentrum Vrije Universiteit, Amsterdam 57br
Kees Hummel 273tl, 328tr
A. Husson, *Etude sur les hopitaux considérés (...)*, Paris 1862 12t/bl, 17tl
IAA Architecten 207m
Hvidovre Hospital, Copenhagen 160
H. Ibelings (ed.), *Van den Broek en Bakema 1948–1988. Architectuur en Stedenbouw. De functie van de vorm*, Rotterdam 2000 192br
Inbo 231
Institut für Geschichte der Medizin und des Krankenhauswesens, Aachen 15l
KOW/photo Ronald Schludt 289b
Luuk Kramer 291mr, 295m
L.H. Kroeks (et al.), *Voordrachten en discussies van het symposion ter gelegenheid van de St. Joseph-stichting op 24 en 25 november 1975*, Apeldoorn, 1977 188tl
Photo Tom Kroeze/photo Johan Aarssen 235, 288t, 329tl
Kruisheer Elffers Architecten 155b
Kruisheer + Hallink architecten/adviseurs, Academisch Ziekenhuis Groningen development plan, 1976 164t
F.O. Kuhn, *Krankenhäuser. Handbuch der Architektur Vierter Teil 5. Halb-Band 1. Heft*, Stuttgart 1903 12br, 14b, 17tr/m
Kuipercompagnons 220, 221t, 254, 255tl, 272b, 273bm/mr, 327
Le Corbusier, *Oeuvre complète*, vol. 7: 1957–1965, Zurich 1965 162, 163
Jannes Linders 189, 200, 218, 223, 239l, 241b, 243tr, 247tl, 264tr, 265t, 292-293
London Metropolitan Archives, City of London 13, 14t
Manten en Lugthart architecten 118-119, 142, 143
John Lewis Marshall 287t/bl, 298, 300, 301
MAS architectuur/photo P&G Morisson 197, 228tl
Meerenberg Collection, Santpoort 20tr, 23t, 24tl, 25, 30
Meerkanten, Ermelo 26, 32, 57t/mr, 114tr
N. Mens, A. Tijhuis, *De architectuur van het ziekenhuis. Transformaties in de naoorlogse ziekenhuisbouw in Nederland*, Rotterdam 1999 78t, 79t
Moderne Bouwkunst in Nederland, dl 17. Community and club-buildings, Rotterdam 1934 68b, 69t/b, 78b, 79b
Molenaar&Bol&Van Dillen architecten 322t, 323mr
Marijke Mooy 324bl, 325t
Jeroen Musch 286, 304, 305ml/b, 306, 307
Nationaal Archief, The Hague 21l
Netherlands Architecture Institute, Rotterdam 17bl, 34br, 35, 38, 39, 53br, 59t/mr/b, 70, 71, 74, 75mr/br, 77br, 83t, 85tl/b, 90m, 91m, 93, 100, 101t, 102, 103, 104, 105, 115tr, 116tl, 125, 126-127, 129mr, 135t/br, 138, 139, 146, 147br, 148-149, 154t, 177t/br, 180, 181, 184, 191br, 192bl
The New York Public Library 46b
Harry Noback 249tl
Noord-Hollands Archief, Haarlem 27, 40bl, 55b, 129ml
Pharma Bio-Research, Zuidlaren 73t/br
Prent & Landman Architekten/photo Van Ojen 108, 109, 110, 111
RAU/photo Bjorn Utpott 284b
RDH Architecten Stedenbouwkundigen/photo Ruden Riemens 277, 295t
Regionaal Archief Leiden 90b, 140, 141r, 271t
Regionaal Archief Nijmegen 41br, 88, 116mr, 191bl, 268t/bl
Regionaal Archief West-Brabant, Oudenbosch 132
Revue général de l'architecture et des travaux publics, 1852 20tl
RHC Eindhoven 117tl, 154b
RHC Groninger Archieven, Prentbriefkaart collectie 96m, 190bl
Christian Richters 253, 258, 259t, 260, 261, 273br, 283, 284t, 289t, 303, 328tl
Rijksarchief Tilburg 29br, 60t, 77t, 115br
C.F.W. Roller, *Grundsätze für Errichtung neuer Irrenanstalten: insbesondere der Heil- und Pflegeanstalt bei Achern im Großherzogthum Baden*, Karlsruhe 1838 20br
Rondom Dennendal, Odijk 1974 170
RoVorm 274-275
Royal Haskoning 230b
Buro Mien Ruys Tuin- en Landschapsarchitecten 326b
Isaac Salomons 182
Saph 252
Madeleine Sars Photography 322b, 323t/b
Daria Scagliola & Stijn Brakkee 193bl, 327tr
J.H. Schuurmans Stekhoven, *Ontwikkeling van het krankzinnigenwezen in Nederland, 1813–1914*, 's-Gravenhage 1922 23mr/br
Sinai Centrum, Amersfoort 80-81, 112, 113
Smook Architecten 202l
John Sondeyker 266, 267t
Spaarnestad Photo, Haarlem 40tr, 44-45, 47b
Spatie, Apeldoorn 188b
Stadsarchief Amsterdam 18mr/b, 28, 29tr/ml, 94-95, 96t, 116br, 133m, 156tl, 157t, 269tl
Stadsarchief Breda 43br, 96b, 114tl
Stadsarchief en Athenaeumbibliotheek, Deventer 85tr, 117ml
Stadsarchief 's-Hertogenbosch 20bl, 76t
Symfora Groep, Amersfoort 57ml/bl, 66, 67br
Rob 't Hart 256, 257t, 285, 329br
Team 4 Architecten 255mr/br
A.J.H. Thiadens (ed.), *Ziekenhuis menselijk en modern. De patiënt als kritische consument van intramurale gezondheidszorg*, Deventer 1972 164b, 165
Van Tilburg Ibelings von Behr Architecten 179
Tresoar 42t, 97b
Tuns + Horsting Architecten/photo J. v.d. Plas 129bl
Universiteitsmuseum Groningen, Historische Collectie UMCG department 34t/bl, 232-233
Het Utrechts Archief 20bm, 21br, 43t, 76b, 115bl, 270tl, 271b
VBW architecten/photo Wim K. Steffen 131
Paul van Beek Landschappen 239r
Van den Berg architecten 193br
Marcel van der Burg 318, 319r, 320t, 321bl
Allard van der Hoek 294t, 295br
Ger van der Vlugt 246l, 249bl
Aldo & Hannie van Eyck Architecten 219
Frans van Harlingen 262t
Marcel van Kerckhoven 245, 247b, 264b, 265b, 273bl
Michael van Oosten 324t, 325b
Harry van Reeken 295bl
Venhoeven CS 281m
Verslag van het Staatstoezicht op krankzinnigen en krankzinnigengestichten, 1888 t/m 1890 33r
Verslag van het Staatstoezicht op krankzinnigen en krankzinnigengestichten, 1903 t/m 1908 24tr
Arnoud Verhey 294b
Jan Versnel/MAI 106b, 107
Vincent van Gogh Instituut, Venray 23bl, 90t, 114bl
Sybolt Voeten 242
P. Vogler, G. Hassenpflug, *Handbuch für den neuen Krankenhausbau*, Munich/Berlin 1962 47tm, 128l
Wageningen UR Library, Special Collections 72b, 91tl
Wiegerinck Architectuur en Stedenbouw 155t, 169, 229tr/bl, 234, 278l, 329tr
Vera Yanovshtchinsky/photo Sjaak Henslemans 249br, 250-251
Het Ziekenhuiswezen, 1950 83mr, 87bl
Zijlstra Schipper Architectenbureau 288b
Zorgcomplex Zwolle 176r

abbreviations
b = below
bl = below left
bm = below middle
br = below right
l = left
m = middle
ml = middle left
mr = middle right
r = right
t = top
tl = top left
tm = top middle
tr = top right

The authors

Noor Mens (1962) studied art history at the Vrije Universiteit (VU) in Amsterdam with the history of architecture as her specialisation. She has been a freelance historian of architecture based in Rotterdam since 1993. She publishes on Dutch architecture and urban planning in the twentieth century, with special emphasis on the postwar period. *De architectuur van het ziekenhuis. Transformaties in de naoorlogse ziekenhuisbouw in Nederland* (co-authored with Annet Tijhuis) was published in 1999, *De architectuur van het psychiatrisch ziekenhuis* in 2003, en *W.G. Witteveen en Rotterdam* in 2007 in the series of monographs on Dutch urban planners. She wrote *Zorgboulevards. Verkenningen in het zorglandschap van morgen* (2005) and (with Cor Wagenaar) *De toekomst van de polikliniek.* (2007) and *Healing Environment* (2009) for the Foundation for Architects Research on Public Health Buildings (Stagg).

Cor Wagenaar (1960) studied history at the University of Groningen, where he wrote a dissertation on the postwar reconstruction of Rotterdam. He has worked for the Netherlands Organization for Scientific Research (NWO) on Dutch urban planning in a European context and for the Royal Netherlands Academy of Sciences (KNAW) on research on J.J.P. Oud. He was responsible for the publication *Happy. Cities and Public Happiness in Post-War Europe*. With Fr.C.A. Jaspers he organised an international conference on *The Architecture of Hospitals* for the University Medical Centre Groningen (UMCG) and edited the book with the same title. In 2004 he was an advisor to the Netherlands Foundation for Fine Arts, Design and Architecture on the setting up of a study trip to Central and Eastern Europe, which resulted in the publication *Ideal in Concrete. Exploring Central and Eastern Europe*. He is an associate professor at the Institute of History of Art, Architecture and Urbanism (IHAAU) of Delft University of Technology. He was a member of the editorial team of the *Yearbook Architecture in the Netherlands* from 2006 to 2008. He is a founding member and editor of the journal *Positions.*

Scientific Committee

M.G. Boekholdt, PhD, former CEO Zonnehuisgroep and professor Vrije Universiteit Amsterdam
Fr.C.A. Jaspers, Msc., M.D., chairman of scientific committee, member executive board University Medical Centre Groningen; chairman Thomassen à Thuessink Foundation, Groningen
E.R.M. Taverne, PhD, emeritus professor of the History of Architecture, University of Groningen
Teun Swinkels, Msc., architect, Maastricht
A.P.J. Höppener, Msc., M.D., management consultant, member Care Innovation Platform (ZIP), former CEO Altrecht Group Utrecht

Colophon

This publication is an initiative of the University Medical Centre Groningen (Thomassen à Thuessink Foundation).

This book was produced with the assistance of Ms C.J. Klijnsma, University Medical Centre Groningen.

Research, texts: Noor Mens, Cor Wagenaar
Image research and photo editing: Noor Mens, Ingrid Oosterheerd
Copy editing: Els Brinkman
Translation: Peter Mason
Design: Joseph Plateau Grafisch Ontwerpers
Printing: Drukkerij Die Keure, Bruges
Coordination Editing: Marianne Lahr
Production: Caroline Gautier, Alma Timmer
Publisher: Eelco van Welie (NAi Publishers)

This publication has received generous financial support from:
PRC
Royal Haskoning
Siemens Nederland B.V.
University Medical Centre Groningen (Thomassen à Thuessink Foundation)
Woonzorg Nederland

NAi Publishers is an internationally orientated publisher specialized in developing, producing and distributing books on architecture, visual arts and related disciplines.
www.naipublishers.nl
info@naipublishers.nl

Available in North, South and Central America through D.A.P./Distributed Art Publishers Inc, 155 Sixth Avenue 2nd Floor, New York, NY 10013-1507, tel +1 212 627 1999, fax +1 212 627 9484, dap@dapinc.com

Available in the United Kingdom and Ireland through Art Data, 12 Bell Industrial Estate, 50 Cunnington Street, London W4 5HB, tel +44 208 747 1061, fax +44 208 742 2319, orders@artdata.co.uk

Printed and bound in Belgium

ISBN 978-90-5662-734-8

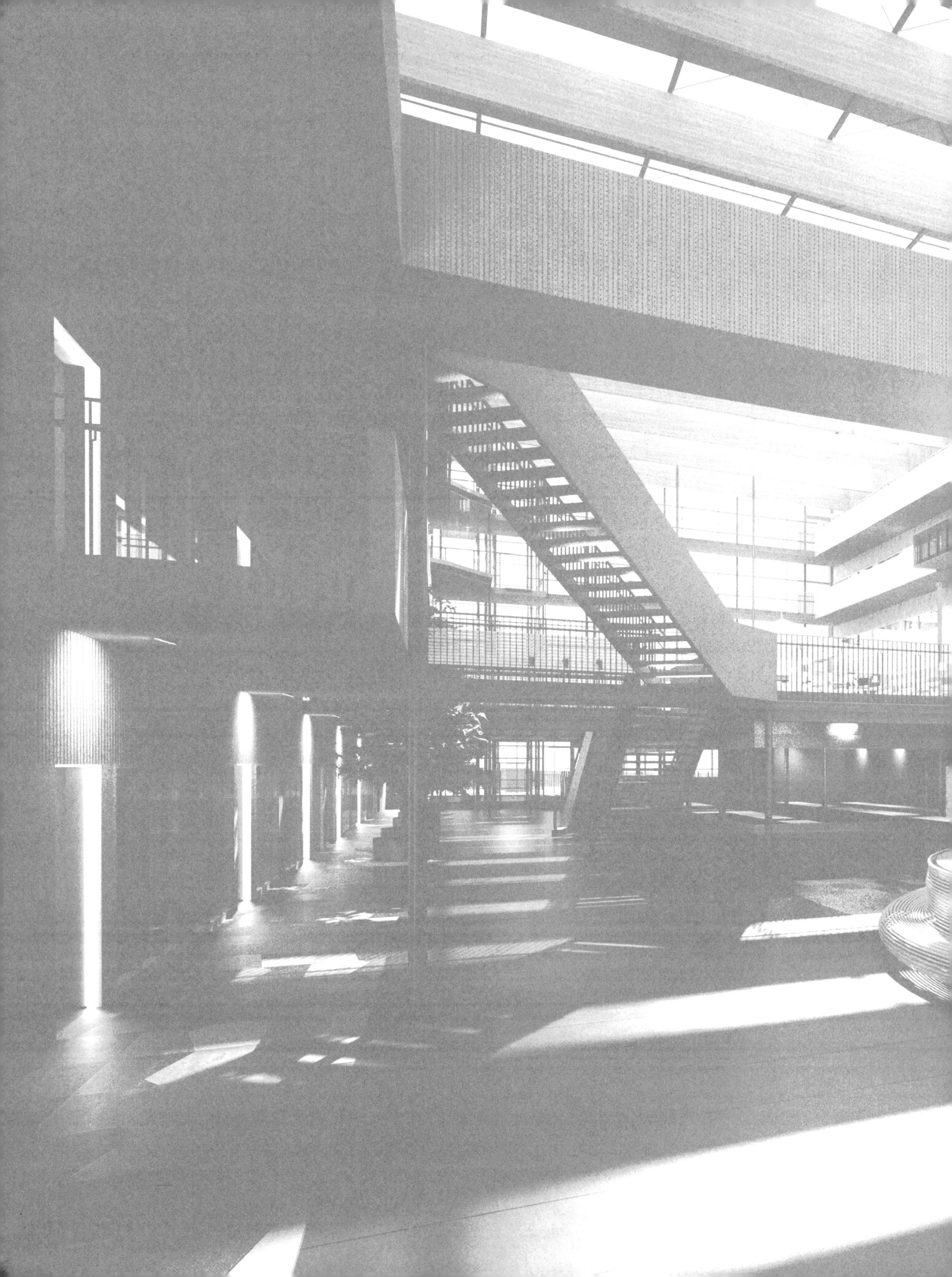